VOLUME 3

MODERN PRACTICE IN ORTHOGNATHIC AND RECONSTRUCTIVE SURGERY

VOLUME 3

MODERN PRACTICE IN ORTHOGNATHIC AND RECONSTRUCTIVE SURGERY

Edited by

WILLIAM H. BELL

Professor, Department of Oral and Maxillofacial Surgery,
Baylor College of Dentistry, Dallas, Texas

Formerly, Professor, Department of Surgery,
Division of Oral and Maxillofacial Surgery,
University of Texas Southwestern Medical Center,
Dallas, Texas

W.B. SAUNDERS COMPANY
Harcourt Brace Jovanovich, Inc.
Philadelphia – London – Toronto – Montreal – Sydney – Tokyo

W. B. SAUNDERS COMPANY
Harcourt Brace Jovanovich, Inc.
The Curtis Center
Independence Square West
Philadelphia, Pennsylvania 19106

Library of Congress Cataloging-in-Publication Data

Modern practice in orthognathic and reconstructive surgery / edited by William H. Bell.
  p.   cm.
  Includes index.
  ISBN 0-7216-3373-0 (set).—ISBN 0-7216-3407-9 (v. 1).—
ISBN 0-7216-3408-7 (v. 2).—ISBN 0-7216-3409-5 (v. 3)
  1. Jaws—Surgery. 2. Face—Surgery. 3. Surgery, Plastic.
4. Temporomandibular joint—Surgery.   I. Bell, William H.,

  [DNLM: 1. Jaw—Surgery. 2. Surgery, Oral. 3. Surgery, Plastic—
methods. 4. Temporomandibular Joint—Surgery.   WU 600 M689]
RD526.M63 1992
617.5′22059—dc20
DNLM/DLC   91-33754

MODERN PRACTICE IN ORTHOGNATHIC
AND RECONSTRUCTIVE SURGERY

Volume 1   ISBN 0-7216-3407-9
Volume 2   ISBN 0-7216-3408-7
Volume 3   ISBN 0-7216-3409-5
Set   ISBN 0-7216-3373-0

Copyright ©1992 by W. B. Saunders Company.

All rights reserved. No part of this publication may be reproduced or transmitted in any form or by any means, electronic or mechanical, including photocopy, recording, or any information storage and retrieval system, without permission in writing from the publisher.

Printed in the United States of America.

Last digit is the print number: 9   8   7   6   5   4   3   2   1

The mission of this book is one of great hope. Our hopes reside in God first and foremost, but also in the young men and women in our specialty — they are an especially talented group who will live lives characterized by excellence, creativity, and service.

For my family: Sherry, Bryan, Adam, Christine, and Elizabeth, to my mother Mrs. Madeleine Bell, and to my brother Harry L. Bell.

CONTRIBUTORS

A. OMAR ABUBAKER, D.M.D., Ph.D.
Assistant Professor, Department of Oral and Maxillofacial Surgery, School of Dentistry, Medical College of Virginia; Medical College of Virginia Hospitals, Richmond, Virginia
Techniques and Applications of Bicoronal and Hemicoronal Flaps

TOMAS ALBREKTSSON, M.D., Ph.D
Professor and Head, Department of Handicap Research, University of Gothenburg, Gothenburg, Sweden
Branemark: Basic and Beyond

EDWARD P. ALLEN, D.D.S., Ph.D
Clinical Professor, Graduate Periodontics Department, Baylor College of Dentistry, Dallas, Texas
Enhancing Facial Esthetics Through Gingival Surgery

JOSE P. AMPIL, D.M.D., M.S.
Associate Professor, Department of Oral and Maxillofacial Surgery, University of Texas Southwestern Medical Center, Dallas, Texas
Case Presentation, Implants in Orthognathics

STEVEN B. ARAGON, D.D.S., M.D.
University of Colorado Health Sciences; University Hospital, Denver General Hospital, Rose Medical Center, Denver, Colorado
A 2-mm Bicortical Screw Technique for Mandibular Osteotomies

G. WILLIAM ARNETT, D.D.S., F.A.C.D.
Lecturer, Orthognathic Surgery, University of California at Los Angeles and Loma Linda; Clinical Instructor, Orthognathic Surgery, University of California at Los Angeles and Valley Medical Center; Attending Staff, Santa Barbara Cottage Hospital and St. Francis Hospital, Santa Barbara, California
Temporomandibular Joint Ramifications of Orthognathic Surgery

UGO BACILIERO, M.D., D.M.D.
Senior Staff Physician, Department of Maxillofacial Surgery and Center for Craniofacial Deformities, San Bortolo Hospital, Vicenza, Italy
Surgical Correction of Posterior Transverse Facial Deformities: Large Face Syndrome with Masseter Muscle Hypertrophy

WILLIAM H. BELL, D.D.S.
Professor, Department of Oral and Maxillofacial Surgery, Baylor College of Dentistry, Dallas, Texas
Analytical Model Surgery; Fabrication of a Composite Splint for Dual-Arch Surgery; Enhancing Facial Esthetics Through Gingival Surgery; Management of Nasal Deformities; Treatment of Temporomandibular Joint Dysfunction by Intraoral Vertical Ramus Osteotomy; Case Presentation, Implants in Orthognathics; Rehabilitation After Orthognathic Surgery; Oblique Modified Le Fort III Osteotomy; Individualizing the Osteotomy Design for the Le Fort I Downfracture; Malar Midfacial Augmentation; Correction of Mandibular Deficiency by Sagittal Split Ramus Osteotomy (SSRO); Alteration of Mandibular Width by Symphyseal Osteotomy; Transverse (Horizontal) Maxillary Deficiency; The Vertical Dimension and the Deep-Bite Deformity; Genioplasty Strategies; Cheiloplasty; Anterior Mandibular Subapical Osteotomy; Combining Sagittal Split Osteotomy with Reduction Genioplasty; Mandibular Advancement in Children: Special Considerations

MILTON D. BERKMAN, D.M.D., M.S.
Assistant Clinical Professor of Dentistry and Orthodontics, Albert Einstein College of Medicine; Orthodontist, Center for Craniofacial Disorders, Montefiore Hospital Medical Center, Bronx, New York
Hemifacial Microsomia: The Use of Microvascular Groin Flaps in Treatment

NORMAN J. BETTS, D.D.S., M.S.
Assistant Professor, Department of Oral and Maxillofacial Surgery, University of Pennsylvania School of Dental Medicine; Staff, Hospital of the University of Pennsylvania, Children's Hospital of Philadelphia, Presbyterian Medical Center, Philadelphia, Pennsylvania
Soft Tissue Changes Associated with Orthognathic Surgery

MICHAEL S. BLOCK, D.M.D.
Associate Professor, Department of Oral and Maxillofacial Surgery, Louisiana State University School of Dentistry, New Orleans, Louisiana
Hydroxylapatite and Hydroxylapatite-Coated Dental Implants for the Treatment of the Partially and Totally Edentulous Patient; Case Presentations, Implants in Orthognathics

DALE S. BLOOMQUIST, D.D.S., M.S.
Associate Professor, Department of Oral and Maxillofacial Surgery, University of Washington, Seattle, Washington
Bone Grafting and Alternative Procedures: I. Bone Grafting in Dentofacial Deformities

HANS BOSKER, D.D.S., Ph.D.
Staff Member, University Hospital Utrecht, Department of Oral and Maxillofacial Surgery; Department of Oral and Maxillofacial Surgery, Martini Hospital, Groningen, The Netherlands
The Transmandibular Implant

SCOTT B. BOYD, D.D.S., Ph.D.
Program Director and Head, Division of Oral and Maxillofacial Surgery, Henry Ford Hospital, Detroit, Michigan
Rehabilitation After Orthognathic Surgery

MICHAEL J. BUCKLEY, D.M.D., M.S.
Associate Professor, Department of Oral and Maxillofacial Surgery, University of Pittsburgh School of Dental Medicine, Pittsburgh, Pennsylvania
Total Mandibular Subapical Osteotomy

PETER H. BUSCHANG, Ph.D
Associate Professor, Department of Orthodontics, Baylor College of Dentistry, Dallas, Texas
The Effect of Orthognathic Surgery on Growth of the Maxilla in Patients with Vertical Maxillary Excess

ANGELO CAPUTO, Ph.D.
Professor and Chairman, Biomaterials Science Section, University of California at Los Angeles School of Dentistry, Los Angeles, California
Biomechanical Considerations in Oral and Maxillofacial Surgery

ALBERT E. CARLOTTI, Jr., D.D.S.
Clinical Associate Professor, Department of Surgery, Brown University School of Medicine; Surgeon-in-Charge, Division of Oral and Maxillofacial Surgery, Department of Surgery, Miriam Hospital, Providence, Rhode Island
Surgical Management of Short Mandibular Ramus Deformities; Nasolabial Esthetics and Maxillary Surgery

DAVID S. CARLSON, Ph.D.
Professor, Department of Orthodontics and Pediatric Dentistry, Department of Anatomy, Research Scientist, Center for Human Growth and Development, University of Michigan Dental School, Ann Arbor, Michigan
The Effects of Mandibular Immobilization on the Masticatory System: A Review

GEORGE J. CISNEROS, D.M.D., M.Med.Sci.
Associate Professor, Orthodontic and Pediatric Dentistry, and Director, Postgraduate Program in Orthodontics, Albert Einstein College of Medicine, Adjunct Attending, Montefiore Medical Center; Director, Center for Craniofacial Disorders, Montefiore Dental Liaison, Bronx, New York
Improved Diagnosis and Treatment Planning of Dentofacial Deformities: An Update on Skeletal Scintigraphy; Sleep Apnea

LUIGI CLAUSER, M.D., D.M.D.
Senior Staff Physician, Department of Maxillofacial Surgery, and Attending Surgeon, Regional Center for Craniofacial Deformities, San Bortolo Hospital, Vicenza, Italy
Surgical Correction of Posterior Transverse Facial Deformities: Large Face Syndrome with Masseter Muscle Hypertrophy; Case Presentation, Implants in Orthognathics

THOMAS A. COLLINS, D.D.S., M.S.
Midamerica Center for Osseointegration; Attending Staff, St. John's Regional Health Center, Cox Medical Center, and Springfield Community Hospital, Springfield, Missouri
Branemark: Basic and Beyond; Implants in Orthognathics: Introduction

GISELA CONTASTI, D.D.S.
Private Practice, Orthodontics; Lecturer, Orthodontics Department, Central University Dental School, Caracas, Venezuela
Transverse (Horizontal) Mandibular Deficiency

DOUGLAS R. CROSBY, D.D.S., M.S.
Assistant Clinical Professor, Department of Orthodontics, Baylor College of Dentistry, Dallas, Texas
Transverse (Horizontal) Maxillary Deficiency

CAMILLO CURIONI, M.D., D.M.D.
Clinical Professor, University of Ferrara; Professor and Chief, Department of Maxillofacial Surgery and Regional Center for Craniofacial Deformities, San Bortolo Hospital, Vicenza, Italy
Surgical Correction of Posterior Transverse Facial Deformities: Large Face Syndrome with Masseter Muscle Hypertrophy; Case Presentation, Implants in Orthognathics

J. J. DANN, III, M.D., D.M.D.
Assistant Clinical Professor, Department of Oral and Maxillofacial Surgery, University of California at San Francisco School of Dentistry; Adjunct Assistant Professor, University of the Pacific School of Dentistry; Chief, Department of Oral and Maxillofacial Surgery, John Muir Medical Center; Associate Staff, Surgeon Craniofacial and Cleft Palate Team, Children's Hospital Medical Center of Northern California, Oakland, California
Delayed Reconstruction of Injuries in the Orbital Region: Diagnostic and Surgical Considerations

DAVID J. DARAB, D.D.S., M.S.
Private Practice, Hickory, North Carolina
Individualizing the Osteotomy Design for the Le Fort I Downfracture; Review of Surgical Techniques; Correction of Mandibular Deficiency by Sagittal Split Ramus Osteotomy (SSRO); Stability of Mandibular Advancement Surgery: A Review

J. T. DAVILA, D.D.S.
Department of Maxillofacial Surgery, Clinic of Craniofacial Deformities, Hospital "Lic. Adolfo Lopez Mateos," Mexico City, Mexico
Oblique Modified Le Fort III Osteotomy

JEAN DELAIRE, M.D., D.D.S.
Professeur de Clinique de Stomatologie et Chirurgie Maxillo-Faciale, University of Nantes, Nantes, France
Surgical Considerations in Patients with Cleft Deformities

MICHAEL G. DONOVAN, D.D.S.
Program Director, Oral and Maxillofacial Surgery Residency, and Chief, Oral and Maxillofacial Surgery Service, William Beaumont Army Medical Center, El Paso, Texas
Augmentation of the Malar Prominence by Sagittal Osteotomy of the Zygoma and Interpositional Bone Grafting

EDWARD ELLIS, III, D.D.S., M.S.
Associate Professor, Division of Oral and Maxillofacial Surgery, University of Texas Southwestern Medical Center; Attending Staff, Parkland Memorial Hospital, University Medical Center, St. Paul Medical Center, Dallas, Texas
The Effects of Mandibular Immobilization on the Masticatory System: A Review

KIM L. ERICKSON, D.D.S.
Attending Surgeon, Center for Craniofacial Disorders, Butterworth Hospital; Attending Surgeon, Blodgett Memorial Medical Center; Attending Surgeon, St. Mary's Hospital, Grand Rapids, Michigan

Analytical Model Surgery; Hemifacial Microsomia: The Use of Microvascular Groin Flaps in Treatment; Model Surgery for Facial Asymmetry Deformities

ANTHONY FAROLE, D.M.D.
Associate Professor, Division of Oral and Maxillofacial Surgery, Thomas Jefferson Medical College; Assistant Director, Oral and Maxillofacial Surgery Residency Program and Postgraduate Oral and Maxillofacial Surgery Residency Training Program; Staff, Thomas Jefferson University Hospital, Philadelphia, Pennsylvania
The Micro System of Rigid Fixation; Contra-Angle Techniques of Rigid Internal Screw Fixation of the Sagittal Ramus Osteotomy

STEPHEN E. FEINBERG, D.D.S., M.S., Ph.D.
Associate Professor and Chairman, Department of Oral Medicine, Oral Pathology, and Oral and Maxillofacial Surgery, University of Michigan School of Dentistry; Attending Staff, University of Michigan Hospitals, Ann Arbor, Michigan
Reconstruction of the Temporomandibular Joint with Pedicled Temporalis Muscle Flaps

RICHARD A. FINN, D.D.S.
Associate Professor, Department of Surgery and Cell Biology, Division of Oral and Maxillofacial Surgery, University of Texas Southwestern Medical Center; Attending Staff, Parkland Memorial Hospital, Zale Lipshy University Hospital, St. Paul Medical Center, and Veterans Administration Medical Center, Dallas, Texas
Case Presentation, Implants in Orthognathics

CAROLYN FLANARY, D.D.S.
Departments of Orthodontics and Oral and Maxillofacial Surgery, University of Texas Health Science Center, San Antonio, Texas
The Psychology of Appearance and the Psychological Impact of Surgical Alteration of the Face

RAYMOND J. FONSECA, D.D.S.
Professor, Department of Oral and Maxillofacial Surgery, and Dean, University of Pennsylvania School of Dental Medicine; Staff, Hospital of the University of Pennsylvania and Children's Hospital of Philadelphia, Philadelphia, Pennsylvania
Soft Tissue Changes Associated with Orthognathic Surgery

CHRISTOPHER R. FORREST, M.D.
Clinical Fellow, Division of Plastic Surgery, Sunnybrook Medical Center, Toronto, Ontario, Canada
Craniofacial Osteotomies and Rigid Fixation in the Correction of Post-Traumatic Craniofacial Deformities

KENNETH S. GAMBRELL, M.F.T., C.D.T.
Head Maxillofacial Technician, Department of Oral Surgery, The University of Texas Southwestern Medical Center; Staff, Zale Lipshy University Hospital, Parkland Memorial Hospital, and Children's Medical Center, Dallas, Texas
Fabrication of a Composite Splint for Dual-Arch Surgery

DAVID A. GARBER, D.M.D., B.D.S.
Clinical Professor of Periodontology, and Clinical Professor of Prosthodontics, Medical College of Georgia School of Dental Medicine, Atlanta, Georgia
Problem of the High Lipline—The Gummy Smile

J. M. GARCIA y SANCHEZ, D.D.S.
Head, Department of Maxillofacial Surgery, and Co-Chairman, Clinic of Craniofacial Deformities, Hospital "Lic. Adolfo Lopez Mateos," Mexico City, Mexico
Oblique Modified Le Fort III Osteotomy

LAWRENCE P. GARETTO, Ph.D.
Assistant Professor, Departments of Orthodontics and Physiology and Biophysics, Indiana University Schools of Dentistry and Medicine, Indianapolis, Indiana
Endosseous Implants for Rigid Orthodontic Anchorage

G. E. GHALI, D.D.S.
Senior Resident, Department of Surgery, Division of Oral and Maxillofacial Surgery, Parkland Memorial Hospital; Resident, John Peter Smith Hospital, Fort Worth; and Veterans Administration Medical Center, Zale Lipshy University Hospital, and Childrens Medical Center, Dallas, Texas
Anesthesia for Orthognathic and Craniofacial Surgery

A. H. GIESECKE, M.D.
Jenkins Professor and Chairman, Department of Anesthesiology, University of Texas Southwestern Medical Center, Dallas, Texas
Anesthesia for Orthognathic and Craniofacial Surgery

DOUGLAS H. GOLDSMITH, D.D.S.
Assistant Clinical Professor, Department of Surgery, Oral and Maxillofacial Surgery Section, Albert Einstein College of Medicine; Attending Oral and Maxillofacial Surgeon, Montefiore Hospital and Medical Center, North Central Bronx Hospital, White Plains Hospital, Scarsdale, New York
Analytical Model Surgery; Hemifacial Microsomia: The Use of Microvascular Groin Flaps in Treatment; Model Surgery for Facial Asymmetry Deformities

CARY E. GOLDSTEIN, D.M.D.
Special Lecturer in Esthetic Dentistry, Emory University, Atlanta, Georgia
Is Your Case Really Finished?

RONALD E. GOLDSTEIN, D.D.S.
Adjunct Clinical Professor of Prosthodontics, Boston University; Clinical Professor of Restorative Dentistry, Medical College of Georgia School of Dentistry, Augusta, Georgia
Is Your Case Really Finished?

THOMAS S. GOLEC, D.D.S., M.S.
Private Practice; Dental Staff, Palomar Medical Center, Escondido, California
Hydroxylapatite and Hydroxylapatite-Coated Dental Implants for the Treatment of the Partially and Totally Edentulous Patient

A. B. GOMEZ PEDROZO, D.D.S.
Department of Maxillofacial Surgery, Clinic of Craniofacial Deformities, Hospital "Lic. Adolfo Lopez Mateos," Mexico City, Mexico
Oblique Modified Le Fort III Osteotomy

JOSEPH S. GRUSS, M.B., F.R.C.S.(C)
Professor of Surgery, University of Washington; Attending

xii / CONTRIBUTORS

Surgery, Faculty of Medicine, Kyoto University, Kyoto, Japan
Arthroscopy of the Temporomandibular Joint

RAVINDRA NANDA, B.D.S., M.D.S., Ph.D.
Professor, Department of Orthodontics, and Director, Orthodontic Clinic, University of Connecticut School of Dental Medicine, Farmington, Connecticut
Biological and Clinical Foundation for Orthognathic Surgery in Growing Patients

GARY J. NISHIOKA, D.M.D., M.D.
Staff, Department of Surgery, Division of Otolaryngology — Head and Neck Surgery, University of Missouri Hospital and Clinics, Columbia, Missouri
The Lip Lift

FELICE O'RYAN, D.D.S.
Director, Oral and Maxillofacial Surgery, Kaiser Permanente Hospital, Oakland, California
Nasolabial Esthetics and Maxillary Surgery; Lipectomy of the Face and Neck

GARY T. PATTERSON, D.M.D.
Assistant Professor of Surgery, Division of Plastic and Maxillofacial Reconstructive Surgery, University of Pittsburgh Health Center Hospitals, Pittsburgh, Pennsylvania
Techniques and Applications of Bicoronal and Hemicoronal Flaps

DAVID POOR, D.D.S.
Associate Clinical Professor, Highland General Hospital, Oakland, California
Lipectomy of the Face and Neck

JEFFREY C. POSNICK, D.M.D., M.D., F.R.C.S.(C), F.A.C.S.
Assistant Professor, Department of Surgery, Faculty of Medicine, University of Toronto; Associate Professor, Faculty of Dentistry, University of Toronto; Medical Director, Craniofacial Program, Division of Plastic Surgery, Department of Surgery, The Hospital for Sick Children, Toronto, Ontario, Canada
Craniosynostosis: Diagnosis and Treatment in Infancy and Early Childhood; Craniofacial Dysostosis: A Surgical Approach to the Midface Deformity

DAVID S. PRECIOUS, D.D.S. M.Sc., F.R.C.D.(C)
Professor and Chair, Oral and Maxillofacial Surgery Dalhousie University; Head, Department of Oral and Maxillofacial Surgery, Victoria General Hospital, Halifax, Nova Scotia, Canada
Surgical Considerations in Patients with Cleft Deformities

JAMES H. QUINN, D.D.S.
Professor, Oral and Maxillofacial Surgery, Louisiana State University Medical Center School of Dentistry; Attending Staff, St. Tammany Parish Hospital, Highland Park Hospital, Covington; East Jefferson General Hospital, Hotel Dieu, and Charity Hospital, New Orleans, Louisiana
Pain Mediators and Chondromalacia in Internally Deranged Temporomandibular Joints

JEFFREY L. RAJCHEL, D.D.S.
Private Practice, Oral and Maxillofacial Surgery, Dallas, Texas
Anatomic Considerations in Mandibular Ramus Osteotomies

JOHN A. RATHBONE, D.D.S.
Orthodontist, Private Practice, Santa Barbara, California
Temporomandibular Joint Ramifications of Orthognathic Surgery

JAMES F. RIPLEY, D.D.S.
Private Practice; Staff, Southwest Texas Methodist Hospital, Humana San Antonio Hospital, and Santa Rosa Northwest Hospital, San Antonio, Texas
Composite Splint for Dual-Arch Surgery

W. EUGENE ROBERTS, D.D.S., Ph.D.
Professor and Chairman of Orthodontics, Indiana University School of Dentistry; Professor, Physiology and Biophysics, Indiana University School of Medicine; Adjunct Professor, Engineering and Technology School, Purdue University at Indianapolis; Adjunct Professor of Implantology and Maxillofacial Reconstructive Surgery, University of Lille; Craniofacial Anomalies Team, Riley Hospital; Indiana University Medical Center, Indianapolis, Indiana
Endosseous Implants for Rigid Orthodontic Anchorage

RICHARD D. ROBLEE, D.D.S., M.S.
Assistant Professor, Department of Operative Dentistry, and Assistant Professor, Department of Orthodontics, Baylor College of Dentistry, Dallas, Texas
A Comprehensive Approach to Dentofacial Treatment

RODNEY J. ROHRICH, M.D., F.A.C.S.
Associate Professor, Department of Surgery, Division of Plastic and Reconstructive Surgery, University of Texas Southwestern Medical Center; Chief of Plastic Surgery, Parkland Memorial Hospital, Dallas, Texas
Management of Nasal Deformities

STEVEN M. ROSER, D.M.D., M.D.
Associate Professor, Clinical Dentistry, School of Dental and Oral Surgery and College of Physicians and Surgeons of Columbia University; Director, Oral and Maxillofacial Surgery, and Associate Attending and Director, Dental Service, Columbia Presbyterian Medical Center, New York, New York
Preoperative, Intraoperative, and Postoperative Care

A. HOWARD SATHER, D.D.S.M.S.
Associate Professor in Dentistry, Mayo Medical School; Staff, Rochester Methodist Hospital and St. Marys Hospital, Rochester, Minnesota
Presurgical and Postsurgical Orthodontics for the Maxillary Deficient Patient

STEPHEN A. SCHENDEL, M.D., D.D.S.
Associate Professor, Division of Plastic and Reconstructive

Surgery, Department of Surgery, Stanford University Medical Center, Stanford, California
Cephalometrics and Orthognathic Surgery; Nasolabial Esthetics and Maxillary Surgery; Lipectomy of the Face and Neck; Surgical Management of Short Mandibular Ramus Deformities

RAINER SCHWESTKA, D.M.D.
Senior Staff Member, Department of Orthodontics, University Hospital, Goettingen, Germany
Intraoperative Control of Condylar Position in Maxillary Osteotomies with Rigid Skeletal Fixation

LEONARD SHARZER, M.D.
Associate Clinical Professor, Plastic Surgery, Albert Einstein College of Medicine; Attending Surgeon, Montefiore Medical Center, Bronx, New York
Hemifacial Microsomia: The Use of Microvascular Groin Flaps in Treatment

VIVEK SHETTY, B.D.S., Dr.Med.Dent.
Adjunct Assistant Professor, Section of Oral and Maxillofacial Surgery, University of California at Los Angeles School of Dentistry, Los Angeles, California
Biomechanical Considerations in Oral and Maxillofacial Surgery

RONA Z. SILKISS, M.D.
Instructor, Pacific Presbyterian Medical Center Department of Ophthalmology, San Francisco; Assistant Clinical Professor, University of California at Berkeley School of Optometry; Active Staff, Merritt Hospital, Oakland, and John Muir Medical Center, Walnut Creek, California
Delayed Reconstruction of Injuries in the Orbital Region: Diagnostic and Surgical Considerations

KIRK E. SIMMONS, D.D.S., Ph.D.
Assistant Professor of Orthodontics and Pharmacology and Toxicology, Indiana University Schools of Dentistry and Medicine; Attending Orthodontist, Riley Hospital, Indianapolis, Indiana
Endosseous Implants for Rigid Orthodontic Anchorage

PETER M. SINCLAIR, D.D.S., M.S.D.
Associate Professor and Graduate Program Director, Orthodontic Department, University of North Carolina School of Dentistry, Chapel Hill, North Carolina
Common Complications in Orthognathic Surgery: Etiology and Management

STEEN SINDET-PEDERSEN, D.D.S.
Associate Professor, Faculty of Medicine, Århus University; Chief, Department of Oral and Maxillofacial Surgery, Kommuhe Hospital, Århus, Denmark
The Transmandibular Implant

DOUGLAS P. SINN, D.D.S.
Professor and Chairman, Department of Oral and Maxillofacial Surgery, University of Texas Southwestern Medical Center, Dallas, Texas
Correction of Mandibular Deficiency by Sagittal Split Ramus Osteotomy (SSRO); Mandibular Deficiency Secondary to Juvenile Rheumatoid Arthritis

BRIAN R. SMITH, D.D.S., M.S.
Assistant Professor of Oral and Maxillofacial Surgery, University of Texas Health Science Center at San Antonio; Active Staff, Medical Center Hospital, San Antonio; Consulting Staff, Audie Murphy Veterans Administration Hospital, San Antonio; Consulting Staff, Ben Taub General Hospital, Houston, Texas
Anatomic Considerations in Mandibular Ramus Osteotomies

CESAR E. SOLANO, D.M.D.
Assistant Clinical Professor, Department of Oral and Maxillofacial Surgery, University of Missouri, Kansas City, School of Dentistry, Kansas City, Missouri
Zygomatic Complex Reduction—System for Accurate Bilateral Symmetric Reduction

GEORGE C. SOTEREANOS, D.M.D., M.S.
Associate Professor, Department of Oral-Maxillofacial Surgery, School of Dental Medicine, and Associate Professor, Department of Surgery, School of Medicine, University of Pittsburgh; Attending Staff, Presbyterian-University Hospital, Montefiore University Hospital, Children's Hospital of Pittsburgh, Veterans Administration Hospital, Pittsburgh, Pennsylvania
Techniques and Applications of Bicoronal and Hemicoronal Flaps

JAMES A. TAMBORELLO, D.D.S., M.S.
Clinical Instructor, University of California at Los Angeles and Valley Medical Center, Attending Staff, Santa Barbara Cottage Hospital, St. Francis Hospital, Santa Barbara, California
Temporomandibular Joint Ramifications of Orthognathic Surgery

CLARK O. TAYLOR, M.D., D.D.S.
Associate Professor, Department of Surgery, Division of Oral and Maxillofacial Surgery, University of Nebraska Medical Center; Director, Fellowship Training in Facial Plastic and Reconstructive Surgery, Medcenter One, Bismarck, North Dakota
Osseointegrated Implants and Total Facial Rehabilitation

TERRY D. TAYLOR, D.D.S., M.S.
Associate Professor, Oral and Maxillofacial Surgery, University of Texas Health Science Center at Houston, Dental Branch; Staff, The Methodist Hospital, Hermann Hospital, Ben Taub General Hospital, M.D. Anderson Hospital, and St. Luke's Hospital, Houston, Texas
Post-Traumatic Maxillomandibular Deformities

PAUL LOUIS TESSIER, M.D.
Private Practice, Paris, France
Surgical Correction of Treacher Collins Syndrome

PAUL M. THOMAS, D.M.D., M.S.
Assistant Clinical Professor, Departments of Orthodontics and Oral and Maxillofacial Surgery, University of North Carolina School of Dentistry; Attending Staff, Durham County General Hospital, Chapel Hill, North Carolina
Common Complications in Orthognathic Surgery: Etiology and Management

NORMAN TRIEGER, D.M.D., M.D.
Professor, Albert Einstein College of Medicine; Chairman, Department of Dentistry, Montefiore Medical Center; Chairman, Staff and Alumni Committee, Montefiore Medical Center, Bronx, New York
Sleep Apnea

MYRON R. TUCKER, D.D.S.
Associate Professor and Director of Graduate Training, Department of Oral and Maxillofacial Surgery, University of North Carolina School of Dentistry, Chapel Hill, North Carolina
Common Complications in Orthognathic Surgery: Etiology and Management

JEAN-FRANÇOIS TULASNE, M.D., D.D.S.
Private Practice, Paris, France
Surgical Correction of Treacher Collins Syndrome

TIMOTHY A. TURVEY, D.D.S.
Professor, Department of Oral and Maxillofacial Surgery, University of North Carolina School of Dentistry; Staff, North Carolina Memorial Hospitals, Chapel Hill, North Carolina
Bone Grafting and Alternative Procedures: I. Bone Grafting in Dentofacial Deformities

LINDA D. VALLINO, Ph.D.
Assistant Professor, Division of Speech Pathology, Faculty of Medicine and Associate Member, School of Graduate Studies, University of Toronto; Speech-Language Pathologist, Department of Speech-Language Pathology and Member of the Craniofacial Treatment and Research Centre, The Hospital for Sick Children, Toronto, Ontario, Canada
Speech Problems in Patients with Dentofacial or Craniofacial Deformities

JOSEPH E. VAN SICKELS, D.D.S.
Professor, Director of Residency Education, Department of Oral and Maxillofacial Surgery, University of Texas, Health Science Center at San Antonio; Medical Center Hospital, San Antonio, Texas
A 2-mm Bicortical Screw Technique for Mandibular Osteotomies; The Lip Lift

D. L. VARGAS, D.D.S.
Department of Maxillofacial Surgery, Clinic of Craniofacial Deformities, Hospital, "Lic. Adolfo Lopez Mateos," Mexico City, Mexico
Oblique Modified Le Fort II Osteotomy

KARIN VARGERVIK, D.D.S.
Professor, Department of Growth and Development; Adjunct Professor, Department of Surgery, and Director, Center for Craniofacial Anomalies, University of California at San Francisco; Medical Staff, University of California at San Francisco Medical Center, San Francisco, California
Hemifacial Microsomia: Diagnosis and Management

PETER D. WAITE, M.P.H., D.D.S., M.D.
Associate Professor, University of Alabama School of Dentistry; Associate Professor of Surgery, University of Alabama Hospital, Birmingham, Alabama
Maxillomandibular Advancement: A Surgical Treatment of Obstructive Sleep Apnea

PER-LENNART WESTESSON, D.D.S., Ph.D.
Associate Professor of Clinical Dentistry and Radiology, University of Rochester School of Medicine and Dentistry; Senior Research Associate of Orthodontics, Eastman Dental Center, Rochester, New York
The Diagnosis of TMJ Disturbances by Imaging Techniques

MARY ANNE WITZEL, Ph.D.
Associate Professor, Faculty of Medicine, Associate Member, School of Graduate Studies, and Associate in Dentistry, Faculty of Dentistry, University of Toronto; Director, Department of Speech-Language Pathology and Member of the Craniofacial Treatment and Research Centre, The Hospital for Sick Children, Toronto, Ontario, Canada
Speech Problems in Patients with Dentofacial or Craniofacial Deformities

LARRY M. WOLFORD, D.D.S.
Clinical Professor of Oral and Maxillofacial Surgery, Baylor College of Dentistry; Full-time Teaching Staff, Baylor University Medical Center; Dallas, Texas
Bone Grafting and Alternative Procedures: II: The Use of Porous Block Hydroxyapatite; The Effect of Orthognathic Surgery on Growth of the Maxilla in Patients with Vertical Maxillary Excess

VIRGIL WOOTEN, M.D.
St. Vincent Infirmary Medical Center, Little Rock, Arkansas; Former Head, Sleep Disorders Center, UAB Hospital, Birmingham, Alabama
Maxillomandibular Advancement: A Surgical Treatment of Obstructive Sleep Apnea

YOSHINURI YAMAGUCHI, D.D.S., Ph.D.
Assistant Professor, Department of Oral and Maxillofacial Surgery, Shiga University of Medical Science; Oral and Maxillofacial Surgeon, Shiga University Hospital, Otsu, Shiga, Japan
Treatment of TMJ Dysfunction by Intraoral Vertical Ramus Osteotomy

ZHIHAO YOU, D.D.S., M.S., Ph.D.
Assistant Professor, Department of Oral and Maxillofacial Surgery, School of Stomatology, Beijing Medical University; Clinical and Research Fellow, The University of Texas Southwestern Medical Center, Department of Surgery, Division of Oral and Maxillofacial Surgery, Dallas, Texas
Treatment of TMJ Dysfunction by Intraoral Vertical Ramus Osteotomy; Individualizing the Osteotomy Design for the Le Fort I Downfracture

JOSEPH ZERNIK, D.M.D., Ph.D.
Assistant Professor, Department of Orthodontics, University of Connecticut School of Dental Medicine; Director of Undergraduate Orthodontics, University of Connecticut Health Center, Farmington, Connecticut
Biological and Clinical Foundation for Orthognathic Surgery in Growing Patients

ACKNOWLEDGMENTS

No man climbs a mountain alone. To be human is to be dependent. *From the cradle to the grave, we depend on the efforts of many other men and women. We build on the past, and we are all the products of our parents, our teachers, our colleagues, and the talents and challenges that God provides us.*

To men like Dr. Sumpter Arnim, Dr. Barnet M. Levy, Dr. Edward C. Hinds, and Dr. Robert V. Walker, I am deeply indebted—these men have provided me the opportunity and environment both to continue animal and clinical investigations and to keep one foot in the clinical arena.

I would like to thank my other surgical and professional colleagues for their teaching, training, and tolerance: Richard A. Finn, Douglas P. Sinn, Stephen C. Hill, Edward P. Ellis, Wayne H. Speer, Joe D. Jacobs, Jose P. Ampil, Kevin L. McBride, Harry L. Legan, George Garcia, and Ronald Hathaway.

For the past 19 years, I have had the privilege of working with 27 young and very talented oral and maxillofacial surgery residents in our research laboratory at the University of Texas Health Science Center at Dallas: Drs. John J. Dann, Raymond J. Fonseca, Stephen A. Schendel, James W. Kennedy, Heidi Opdebeeck, Richard A. Finn, John A. Brammer, Gregory B. Scheideman, Scott B. Boyd, Craig C. Johnston, Michael R. Warner, Kenneth A. Storum, Hideaki Nagura, Jaime G. Quejada, Hiroshi Kawamura, Joseph Schoenaers, Xi-en Zhang, Philip Washko, Silas DeTulio, Waldemar Polido, Aurora Morino, Yoshinoro Yamaguchi, David Darab, Nestor Karas, Chawkett Mannai, and Zhihao You.

I want to extend special thanks to many dental and medical colleagues who have entrusted the surgical care of their patients to me during the developmental phase of orthognathic surgery. By their support and close collaboration, these colleagues have made possible some of the present surgical advances.

I owe an enormous debt to the many contributors to the books. They have waited with unusual patience throughout the gestation of these volumes, and it is in large part to them that I owe the currentness and clinical insight found there.

Special thanks must be extended to many unsung heroes who have helped prepare the manuscript—Mrs. Donna Walker and Ms. Bonnie Boehme, manuscript editors, and Mr. Matt Andrews, illustration specialist, all of the W.B. Saunders Company, and my secretaries, Ms. Judy L. Lewis and Joanne Kresge. Personal thanks are also due the editors and staff of the W.B. Saunders Company—Mr. John Dyson, Mrs. Lorraine Kilmer, Mr. David Kilmer, and Mr. Frank Polizzano—for their support and patient collaboration.

WILLIAM H. BELL

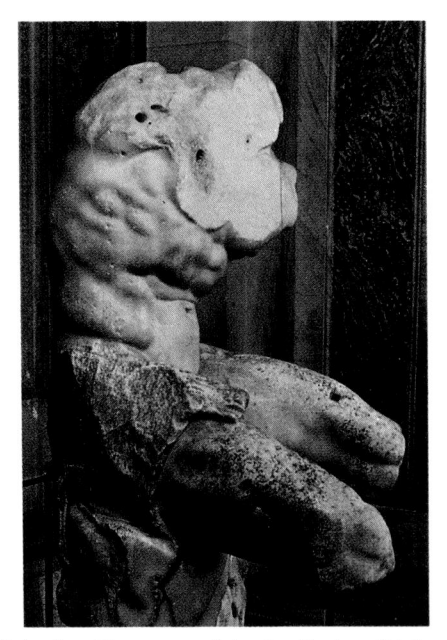

Sala delle Muse: Belvedere Torso, a work by Apollonios of Athens, ca. first century B.C. (Reprinted by permission.)

Looking at this piece of art reminds us that we can learn from one another.

The first century sculptor Apollonios was an inspiration for the great Renaissance sculptors such as Michelangelo. Even the "greatest" use models as they develop their skills and knowledge on the theme; our knowledge is based on multiple sources—many that we have no idea about.

"So many are the links, upon which the true Philosophy depends, of which, if anyone be loose, or weak, the whole chain is in danger of being dissolv'd; it is to begin with the Hands and Eyes, and to proceed on through the Memory, to be continued by the Reason; nor is it to stop there, but to come about to the Hands and Eyes again, and so, by a continual passage round from one Faculty to another, it is to be maintained in life and strength, as much as the body of man is by the circulation of the blood through the several parts of the body, the Arms, the Fat, the Lungs, the Heart, and the Head."

—HOOKE: *Micrographia*, 1567

PREFACE

Orthognathic surgery was in its infancy when *Surgical Correction of Dentofacial Deformities* was published in 1980 (Volumes 1 and 2) and 1985 (Volume 3). Since then, it has evolved into a complex specialty that demands expertise in several surgical disciplines and an understanding of many allied dental and medical specialties. Because orthognathic surgery has been and remains evolutionary, the modern surgeon's training is a continuum. During the past 15 years, quantum leaps have occurred in scientific knowledge, in technology, and in some treatment planning aspects of this dynamic field.

The concept of beauty is central to all human cultures and is deeply rooted in the nature of man. In various ways, human esthetics is woven into the tradition of human civilizations. Physical appearance has always played a significant role in the development of self-concept and self-esteem, in the establishment of interpersonal relationships, in employment opportunities, and even in the quality of life.

A review of our previously treated patients and past publications clearly reveals that many of our orthognathic surgical procedures achieve esthetic facial proportions, improve jaw function, and accomplish occlusal stability. In selected cases, however, the result was compromised because the independent soft tissue components were not systematically analyzed and treated.

Of all the human family, the modern surgeon should be the most vigilant and accurate recorder of facial esthetics. Today's oral and maxillofacial surgeon must be trained in cosmetic facial surgery and must be competent to diagnose and treat both skeletal and soft tissue problems. By virtue of the present level of training, he or she has unique diagnostic and technical skills to address and correct both hard and soft tissue aberrations. During the past decade, great strides have been made to incorporate these two disciplines: An interdisciplinary philosophy has thus evolved.

Sections I and II of *Modern Practice in Orthognathic and Reconstructive Surgery* focus on treatment planning and set forth objective criteria for the appreciation of facial esthetics and beauty. A variety of elements that relate to the structural beauty of the dental, facial, and craniofacial composition are described. Therapeutic means of altering the human morphopsychological features of dentocraniofacial deformities by restorative, gingival, orthognathic, and craniofacial procedures are described in detail.

A large proportion of adults and adolescents with dentocraniofacial deformities manifest a spectrum of functional problems (Sections III and IV). A balanced biomechanical relationship between the masticatory muscles, jaws, temporomandibular joints, and teeth is necessary to achieve normal function after surgical repositioning of the jaws. Proper planning, precise surgical technique, efficient orthodontics used in concert with small bone plate and screw osteosyntheses, and systematic muscular rehabilitation—all increase treatment efficiency and frequently *improve jaw function*. In the treatment of temporomandibular joint pain and dysfunction through balancing the biomechanical relationships between the masticatory muscles, jaws, temporomandibular joints, and teeth, the common denominator of success is that the patient have an appropriate range of motion and be free of pain. Can improved function be explained on the basis of improved occlusion? Is the concept of a pathologic occlusion legitimate? To validate these concepts, the concept of occlusion must be broadened not only to the contact relationships of the teeth and their controlling neuromuscular system but additionally and more importantly to the function and dysfunction of the masticatory system. In this context, malocclusion may be considered pathologic. A new mind set has been developed that considers the relationships between the teeth, temporomandibular joints, muscles, and jaws. In this context, orthognathic surgical procedures not only may improve the interdigitation of the teeth but also may have a positive impact on function by creating a balanced environment for the teeth, temporomandibular joints, muscles, and jaws. It is impossible to master orthognathic surgical techniques without also being a student of the temporomandibular joint. The interrelationship between the teeth, joints, muscles, and jaws as part of a functional unit must be understood. Only when we know how this masticatory system was designed to work can we know what is wrong with it when it is not functioning correctly.

The results to date in patients with TMJ disorders and chronic pain treated with selective orthognathic surgical procedures and additional experience with other patients, with or without malocclusions, provide support for the selective use of maxillary and mandibular osteotomies in treating temporomandibular joint pain and dysfunction. In addition, surgical repositioning of the jaws may have a positive impact on patients who manifest obstructive sleep apnea and speech disorders.

When the limited available procedures in preprosthetic surgery failed to resolve the dilemma of the complete or partially edentulous patient, research on osseointegrated implants, bone grafting techniques, reconstructive tissue techniques, and development of compatible ceramic materials opened new vistas for treatment of the preprosthetic and reconstructive surgery patient. Treatment of the completely or partially edentulous patient was revolutionized with the introduction of the concept of implant osseointegration. This concept came to Branemark serendipitously during microvascular bone marrow studies on live rabbits. He observed that screw-configured titanium vital microscopic chambers were inseparably incorporated within living tissue and were impossible to remove. Thereafter, a series of investigations ultimately led to the clinical application of osseointegration. The functional restoration of the dental occlusion and associated structures with implants is described in Section V. Impressive successes with both maxillary and mandibular implants have been duplicated in multicenter replication studies with various implant systems. Osseointegrated implants have since become a leading edge in the integration of surgery into medical and dental specialties; indeed, it has touched all healing disciplines.

The successful utilization of osseointegration for bone anchorage in the prosthetic management of craniofacial defects has been repeated by various investigators. Today, a seemingly endless variety of prosthetic, craniofacial, and orthopedic combinations can be employed to replace missing parts of the body.

Anatomic model surgery in concert with the use of extraoral vertical referents has made three-dimensional repositioning of the jaws feasible, more precise, and more predictable than had been possible with traditional methods. Individualization of osteotomy designs based upon anatomic, biomechanical, biologic, functional, and esthetic criteria has contributed significantly to the development of new surgical procedures with more predictable, stable, functional, and esthetic results.

Rigid internal fixation has been well accepted by patients and most professionals actively involved in orthognathic surgery. The use of bone plate and screw osteosynthesis has virtually eliminated the need for maxillomandibular fixation and dramatically altered postsurgical neuromuscular and occlusal rehabilitation. Additionally, the concepts of selectively altering the occlusal plane, managing short mandibular ramus deformities, and rotating the mandible counterclockwise have come of age through the modification of rigid internal and skeletal fixation techniques.

Properly planned and precisely positioned osteotomies in concert with orthopedic appliances facilitate an increase of the arch length in both the maxilla and the mandible and permit surgical orthodontic treatment of the majority of dentofacial deformity patients, without extraction of teeth. Such therapy greatly improves treatment efficiency and effectiveness.

CHARLES LINDBERGH: *"What kind of men would live where there is no daring? I don't believe in taking foolish chances, but nothing can be accomplished without taking any chance at all."*

A specialty derives its standards from selected individuals who emerge to take their place in history. I have attempted to select some of these individuals who have made and will continue to make a significant impact on the specialty of oral and maxillofacial surgery. Each contributor is active and dynamic in a particular field of interest.

Volumes 1, 2, and 3 of *Modern Practice in Orthognathic and Reconstructive Surgery* describe the work of visionaries, creative thinkers, and pioneers who dared to take "the first step." Through their efforts, our specialty continues to move forward to new heights.

As a family of oral and maxillofacial surgeons, we possess the powerful force of our specialty spirit. We must spread to people throughout the world the good things we have learned through our parents, our teachers, and our colleagues. The world stands to benefit from all the values we have been so fortunate and privileged to learn as professionally trained people.

Haughty, selfish specialty pride and "turf building" limit progress and the good that can be done. The surgical procedures and methods of treatment (which must be correctly taught) described in these books should be available to all patients and specialists throughout the world. May these books contribute to this end.

Science is a universal language successfully spoken at all international meetings. We live in an age of immediate communications. That the knowledge found in these books will touch people the world over is an exciting thought that prompted me to pursue the writing and editing of these three volumes containing information from contributors all over the world.

In the course of reading these books, it is hoped that you will want to do much experimenting with the bones and soft tissues that make up the human face. After all, it is your participation that will make the adventure most rewarding both for you and for the patients we have the privilege of serving.

WILLIAM H. BELL

CONTENTS

VOLUME 1

I. TREATMENT PLANNING ... 1

1
THE PSYCHOLOGY OF APPEARANCE AND THE PSYCHOLOGICAL IMPACT OF SURGICAL ALTERATION OF THE FACE ... 2
Carolyn Flanary

2
BIOLOGICAL AND CLINICAL FOUNDATION FOR ORTHOGNATHIC SURGERY IN GROWING PATIENTS ... 22
Ravindra Nanda and Joseph Zernik

3
COMMON COMPLICATIONS IN ORTHOGNATHIC SURGERY: ETIOLOGY AND MANAGEMENT ... 48
Peter M. Sinclair, Paul M. Thomas, and Myron R. Tucker

4
CEPHALOMETRICS AND ORTHOGNATHIC SURGERY ... 84
Stephen A. Schendel

5
PREOPERATIVE, INTRAOPERATIVE, AND POSTOPERATIVE CARE ... 100
Steven M. Roser and James R. Hupp

6
ANESTHESIA FOR ORTHOGNATHIC AND CRANIOFACIAL SURGERY ... 128
M. D. Hilley, G. E. Ghali, and A. H. Giesecke

7
ANALYTICAL MODEL SURGERY ... 154
Kim L. Erickson, William H. Bell, and Douglas H. Goldsmith

Composite Splint for Dual-Arch Surgery ... 206
James F. Ripley

Fabrication of a Composite Splint for Dual-Arch Surgery ... 210
William H. Bell and Kenneth S. Gambrell

II. ENHANCING FACIAL ESTHETICS ... 217

8
IS YOUR CASE REALLY FINISHED? ... 218
Ronald E. Goldstein and Cary E. Goldstein

9
ACHIEVING THE ESTHETIC SMILE ... 235

  I. Enhancing Facial Esthetics Through Gingival Surgery 235
  Edward P. Allen and William H. Bell

  II. Problems of the High Lipline — The Gummy Smile 252
  David A. Garber

10
MANAGEMENT OF NASAL DEFORMITIES ... 262
Rodney J. Rohrich and William H. Bell

11
NASOLABIAL ESTHETICS AND MAXILLARY SURGERY ... 285
Felice O'Ryan, Stephen A. Schendel, and Albert E. Carlotti, Jr.

12
RHINOPLASTY TECHNIQUE ... 318
Brent D. Kennedy

13
LIPECTOMY OF THE FACE AND NECK ... 372
Felice O'Ryan, David Poor, and Stephen A. Schendel

14
SURGICAL CONSIDERATIONS IN PATIENTS WITH CLEFT DEFORMITIES ... 390
David S. Precious and Jean Delaire

15
EXCESSIVE TRANSVERSE FACIAL WIDTH: SURGICAL CORRECTION OF MASSETER MUSCLE HYPERTROPHY ... 426
Tadahiko Iizuka

16
SURGICAL CORRECTION OF POSTERIOR TRANSVERSE FACIAL DEFORMITIES: LARGE FACE SYNDROME WITH MASSETER MUSCLE HYPERTROPHY ... 440
Camillo Curioni, Luigi Clauser, and Ugo Baciliero

III. TREATMENT OF TEMPOROMANDIBULAR JOINT DYSFUNCTION AND PAIN ... 455

17
FUNCTIONAL ANALYSIS OF THE TEMPOROMANDIBULAR JOINT IN THE TREATMENT OF DENTOFACIAL DEFORMITY ... 456
Richard P. Harper

18
PAIN MEDIATORS AND CHONDROMALACIA IN INTERNALLY DERANGED TEMPOROMANDIBULAR JOINTS 470
James H. Quinn

19
THE DIAGNOSIS OF TMJ DISTURBANCES BY IMAGING TECHNIQUES .. 482
Per-Lennart Westesson

20
TEMPOROMANDIBULAR JOINT RAMIFICATIONS OF ORTHOGNATHIC SURGERY 522
G. William Arnett, James A. Tamborello, and John A. Rathbone

21
ARTHROSCOPY OF THE TEMPOROMANDIBULAR JOINT 594
Ken-Ichiro Murakami

22
INTRAOPERATIVE CONTROL OF CONDYLAR POSITION IN MAXILLARY OSTEOTOMIES WITH RIGID SKELETAL FIXATION 628
Hans G. Luhr, Rainer Schwestka, and Dietmar Kubein-Meesenburg

23
ARTHROSCOPY AND ARTHROTOMY OF THE TEMPOROMANDIBULAR JOINT 640
Ralph G. Merrill

24
TREATMENT OF TEMPOROMANDIBULAR JOINT DYSFUNCTION BY INTRAORAL VERTICAL RAMUS OSTEOTOMY 676
William H. Bell, Yoshinuri Yamaguchi, and Zhihao You

25
SURGICAL MANAGEMENT OF INTERNAL DERANGEMENTS OF THE TEMPOROMANDIBULAR JOINT 702
Stephen C. Hill

26
RECONSTRUCTION OF THE TEMPOROMANDIBULAR JOINT WITH PEDICLED TEMPORALIS MUSCLE FLAPS 716
Stephen E. Feinberg and Peter E. Larsen

27
TOTAL TEMPOROMANDIBULAR JOINT RECONSTRUCTION 736
Kevin L. McBride

VOLUME 2
IV. RECONSTRUCTIVE SURGERY 829

46
REHABILITATION AFTER ORTHOGNATHIC SURGERY 1652
William H. Bell, Nestor D. Karas, and Scott B. Boyd

47
IMPROVED DIAGNOSIS AND TREATMENT PLANNING OF
DENTOFACIAL DEFORMITIES: AN UPDATE ON SKELETAL
SCINTIGRAPHY 1676
George J. Cisneros

48
SPEECH PROBLEMS IN PATIENTS WTH DENTOFACIAL AND
CRANIOFACIAL DEFORMITIES 1686
Mary Anne Witzel and Linda D. Vallino

49
A COMPREHENSIVE APPROACH TO DENTOFACIAL TREATMENT 1736
Richard D. Roblee

VOLUME 3

50
OBLIQUE MODIFIED LE FORT III OSTEOTOMY 1770
*J. M. Garcia y Sanchez, J. T. Davila, A. B. Gomez Pedrozo, H. S. Mendoza,
D. L. Vargas, and W. H. Bell*

51
QUADRANGULAR LE FORT I AND II OSTEOTOMIES 1790

Presurgical and Postsurgical Orthodontics for the Maxillary-
Deficient Patient 1791
A. Howard Sather

Quadrangular Le Fort I and II Osteotomies 1797
E. E. Keller

52
CRANIOSYNOSTOSIS: DIAGNOSIS AND TREATMENT IN INFANCY AND
EARLY CHILDHOOD 1838
Jeffrey C. Posnick

53
CRANIOFACIAL DYSOSTOSIS: A SURGICAL APPROACH TO THE
MIDFACE DEFORMITY 1888
Jeffrey C. Posnick

54
THE EFFECTS OF ORTHOGNATHIC SURGERY ON GROWTH OF THE
MAXILLA IN PATIENTS WITH VERTICAL MAXILLARY EXCESS 1932
Frank J. Mogavero, Peter H. Buschang, and Larry M. Wolford

55
BIOMECHANICAL CONSIDERATIONS IN ORAL AND MAXILLOFACIAL
SURGERY 1956
Vivek Shetty and Angelo Caputo

VII. ORTHOGNATHIC SURGERY 1979

56
A 2-mm BICORTICAL SCREW TECHNIQUE FOR MANDIBULAR OSTEOTOMIES 1980
Joseph E. Van Sickels, Thomas S. Jeter, and Steven B. Aragon

57
SURGICAL MANAGEMENT OF SHORT MANDIBULAR RAMUS DEFORMITIES 1996
Albert E. Carlotti, Jr., and Stephen A. Schendel

58
SLEEP APNEA 2020
George J. Cisneros and Norman Trieger

59
MAXILLOMANDIBULAR ADVANCEMENT: A SURGICAL TREATMENT OF OBSTRUCTIVE SLEEP APNEA 2042
Peter D. Waite and Virgil Wooten

60
SURGICAL MANAGEMENT OF SKELETAL OPEN BITE BY RAMUS OSTEOTOMIES 2060
Ulrich Joos

61
MANDIBULAR PROGNATHISM 2110
  I. Intraoral Surgery 2111
     H. David Hall

  II. Orthodontic Considerations 2140
     Ronald R. Hathaway

62
SOFT TISSUE CHANGES ASSOCIATED WITH ORTHOGNATHIC SURGERY 2170
Norman J. Betts and Raymond J. Fonseca

63
MAXILLARY AND MIDFACE DEFORMITY 2210
  I. Individualizing the Osteotomy Design for the Le Fort I Downfracture 2211
     William H. Bell, David Darab, and Zhihao You

  II. Case Reports 2272

  III. Special Adjunctive Considerations 2289
     1. Malar Midfacial Augmentation, 2289
        William H. Bell
     2. Augmentation of the Malar Prominence by Sagittal Osteotomy of the Zygoma and Interpositional Bone Grafting, 2298
        Michael G. Donovan
     3. Zygomatic Complex Reduction—System for Accurate Bilateral Symmetric Reduction, 2304
        Cesar E. Solano

4. Model Surgery for Facial Asymmetry Deformities, 2306
   Kim Erickson and Douglas Goldsmith

5. Orthopedic-Assisted Maxillary Advancement in the Cleft Lip and Palate Patient, Using External Headframe Traction, 2315
   Lance L. Lerner and Jeffrey A. Lane

6. Orthopedic Correction of Maxillary Deficiency, 2322
   Ronald R. Hathaway

7. The Lip Lift, 2331
   Thomas S. Jeter, Joseph Van Sickels, and Gary J. Nishioka

64

MANDIBULAR DEFICIENCY 2334
Review of Surgical Techniques 2335
David J. Darab

I. Orthodontic Sequencing, Decisions, and Techniques 2338
   Harry L. Legan

II. Anatomic Considerations in Mandibular Ramus Osteotomies 2347
    Brian R. Smith and Jeffrey L. Rajchel

III. Correction of Mandibular Deficiency by Sagittal Split Ramus Osteotomy (SSRO) 2361
     William H. Bell, David Darab, and Douglas Sinn

IV. Stability of Mandibular Advancement Surgery: A Review .. 2377
    David J. Darab

V. Transverse (Horizontal) Mandibular Deficiency 2383
   Cesar Guerrero and Gisela Contasti

VI. Special Adjunctive Considerations 2403

   1. Transverse (Horizontal) Maxillary Deficiency, 2403
      Douglas R. Crosby, Joe D. Jacobs, and William H. Bell

   2. The Vertical Dimension and the Deep-Bite Deformity, 2431
      William H. Bell

   3. Genioplasty Strategies, 2439
      William H. Bell and Kevin McBride

   4. Cheiloplasty, 2488
      William H. Bell

   5. Mandibular Angle Deficiency, 2488
      Cesar Guerrero

   6. Anterior Mandibular Subapical Osteotomy, 2495
      William H. Bell

   7. Total Mandibular Subapical Osteotomy, 2500
      Michael J. Buckley

   8. Combining Sagittal Split Osteotomy with Reduction Genioplasty, 2503
      William H. Bell

   9. Mandibular Deficiency Secondary to Juvenile Rheumatoid Arthritis, 2506
      Douglas P. Sinn

   10. Lateral Facial Reconstruction, 2511
       Cesar Guerrero

   11. Mandibular Advancement in Children: Special Considerations, 2516
       William H. Bell

INDEX i
Volume 3 contains a cumulative index for all three volumes.

VOLUME 3

MODERN PRACTICE IN ORTHOGNATHIC AND RECONSTRUCTIVE SURGERY

50 OBLIQUE MODIFIED LE FORT III OSTEOTOMY

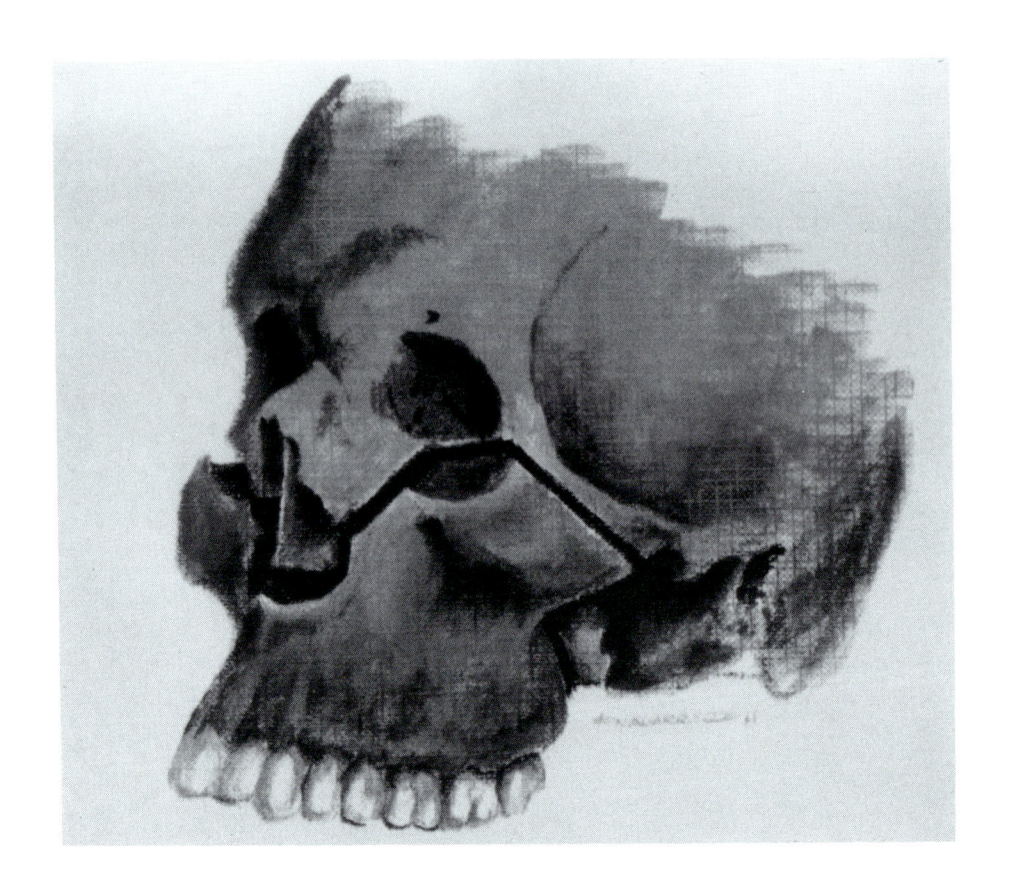

50

ADVANTAGES OF THE OBLIQUE
MODIFIED LE FORT III OSTEOTOMY

SURGICAL TECHNIQUE

CASE STUDIES

J. M. GARCIA Y SANCHEZ
J. T. DAVILA
A. B. GOMEZ PEDROZO
H. S. MENDOZA
D. L. VARGAS

Severe anteroposterior and vertical facial deformities of the middle and inferior third of the face frequently require surgical procedures to achieve optimal functional and esthetic results. The severity of facial disharmony may defy treatment by simultaneous repositioning of the maxilla, mandible, and chin because in the presence of middle-third facial hypoplasia—simple repositioning cannot correct pseudoprognathism—the globes remain unprotected and the esthetic result is unsatisfactory.

Correction of such facial deformities mandates several different methods of treatment because of the variable esthetic manifestations and because of the magnitude of the underjet. The maxillomandibular disharmony, which may be in excess of 12 mm, may require a combination of Le Fort III, Le Fort I, mandibular setback, and genioplasty procedures. It is of prime importance to diagnose and consider the role of each functional and esthetic problem when analyzing the soft and hard tissues. Proper treatment must be individualized and designed to correct each esthetic and functional problem. Numerous different Le Fort III osteotomy designs may be used to advance the midface, including infraorbital rims, supraorbital rims, and the nose depending on the type of deformity. [8,9,19,20,24,26,65]

This chapter focuses on a modified Le Fort III osteotomy design that excludes the nose. The modified LeFort III sagittal osteotomy described by others gives excellent results with advancements of 8 mm or less without bone grafting. Our modified surgical procedure, however, allows advancement up to 15 mm frequently without bone grafting.

Minor vertical discrepancies (4 mm or less) may be corrected simultaneously by the present technique because of the oblique osteotomies that are directed inferosuperiorly. Depending on each individual case, since the present technique involves upward oblique osteotomies, such movements tend to shorten the facial height.

ADVANTAGES OF THE OBLIQUE MODIFIED LE FORT III OSTEOTOMY

The design of the Le Fort III osteotomy for advancement of the middle third of the face has been modified many times to improve the esthetic and functional results. With the original Le Fort III osteotomy,[67,85] bone grafts were always used to stabilize the advanced midface. When, however, oblique cuts are positioned over the zygomatic arch, the root of the zygoma, and the inferior aspect of the lateral orbital walls, the middle third of the face can be advanced with the following advantages:

1. Stabilization of the middle third of the face with bone grafts is frequently unnecessary.
2. Operating time is decreased.
3. Stability from screw and plate osteosynthesis is enhanced.
4. Bony interfacing between the osteotomy sites after large midface advancements usually occurs. Stabilization of repositioned maxillary fragments is facilitated with position screws or bone fixation miniplates placed with minimal contouring and preventing the osteotomized segments from moving when the bone screws are placed.
5. With other techniques large unesthetic defects may occur, since osteotomies of the lateral wall of the orbit require bone grafts to facilitate advancement and stabilization. With the oblique modified Le Fort III osteotomy, the midface is advanced at the expense of the root of the zygoma minimizing unesthetic defects from occurring on the lateral orbital wall.
6. Increased interfacing of the osteotomized segments occurs despite large movements of the zygomatic-maxillary complex; because of the oblique osteotomy design, the zygomatic arch can be "elongated" anteroposteriorly.
7. The superior repositioning combined with anterior advancement (ramping) of the zygomatic maxillary complex favors postoperative protection of the inferior sclera, typically shown in patients with hypoplasia of the middle third of the face resulting in persistent conjunctival dryness. The oblique and sagittal osteotomies over the zygomatic arch and root of the zygoma are designed to compensate for the necessary amount of midface advancement. The direction of movement depends on the inclination of the osteotomy. When the cut is made parallel to the horizontal plane, the result is an even posteroanterior advancement and a slight superior projection of the maxillomalar complex. On the other hand, if the cut is made obliquely toward a more vertical plane, posteroanterior advancement is lessened. Superior movement of the maxillomalar complex, however, may control the posteroanterior and superior movement, depending on the degree of the angle of certain bone cuts. This is important in patients who manifest both hypoplasia of the middle third of the face and vertical maxillary excess. Meticulous cephalometric planning studies, anatomic model surgery (see Chapter 7), and intraoperative measurement of the planned anterior-posterior and vertical movements are essential to achieve these objectives.

SURGICAL TECHNIQUE

Surgical Exposure of Osteotomy Sites

With the patient under general hypotensive nasoendotracheal anesthesia, the nasotracheal tube is positioned laterally to provide accessibility to the oral and midfacial regions. After placement of tarsorrhaphy sutures, the facial part of the procedure is accomplished. A subciliary incision 2.5 to 3.0 cm long is made 2 to 3 mm subjacent and parallel to the lower eyelid margin. The incision extends from an area to 2 to 3 mm lateral to the inferior punctum to the lateral canthus, where it angles inferiorly 0.5 cm. Designing the incision in this manner provides access to both the malar and the lateral orbital regions. An infraorbital rim incision provides access to the orbital rim, floor of the orbit, lateral orbital rim, and malar eminence.

The initial incision is made through the skin and subcutaneous tissue. With the skin margin carefully elevated with skin hooks, the skin and subcutaneous tissue are undermined inferiorly, superficial to the orbicularis oculi muscle, to the level opposite the infraorbital rim. After the bony orbital margin is palpated, a retractor is positioned superiorly to retract the orbital contents back into the orbit. Now a sharp incision is made through the orbicularis oculi and periosteum onto the anterior aspect of the infraorbital rim. Making the incision in this manner avoids cutting through the septum orbitale, which in turn prevents herniation of the periorbital fat.

The lower margin of the periosteum along the periorbital rim is then detached inferiorly down to the infraorbital foramen. This procedure involves detachment of the levator labii superioris alaeque nasi and the lower head of the orbicularis oculi, which, as such, are not recognizable. The infraorbital neurovascular bundle is identified where it exits from the infraorbital foramen and is exposed and dissected free of its enveloping facial soft tissues. The subperiosteal undermining is continued inferiorly medial to the infraorbital nerve toward the lateral piriform rim.

Next, the periorbita is reflected upward over the infraorbital margin and from the orbital floor until the lacrimal fossa is identified medially and the inferior orbital fissure is identified posterolaterally. The periorbita is detached from the lateral orbital rim to the level of the lateral canthal ligament. Next, the reflection is continued from the exposed lateral orbital rim to the posterior aspect of the orbital floor.

The infraorbital rim incision affords excellent access to the malar bone, which must be completely exposed. The lateral aspect of the malar bone, root of the zygoma, and inferolateral aspect of the zygomatic arch are exposed by meticulous subperiosteal tunneling beneath the superior margin of the subciliary incision. The most anterior fibers of the masseter muscle attachment to the inferior aspect of the zygomatic arch are incised and detached to facilitate visualization and dissection.

Osteotomies

The bone cuts, which are made with a tapering fissure bar, are often made easier from a position above the patient. A vertical osteotomy is made through the inferior orbital rim anterior and lateral to the lacrimal apparatus extending posteriorly, approximately 6–7 mm. This bone incision is extended inferiorly to the anterior aspect of the maxilla lateral to the piriform aperture at the level of the anterior insertion of the inferior turbinates without cutting into the lateral piriform rim of the nose. This osteotomy is more precisely completed later intraorally. The osteotomy may also be carried more inferiorly to the inferior-lateral aspect of the piriform rim to facilitate more stable bone plate osteosynthesis.

Through the infraorbital rim incision, the lateral osteotomy is made through the inferolateral orbital margins and orbital floor approximately 8 mm posterior toward, but not to, the inferior orbital fissure. The lateral and medial orbital floor bone cuts are connected with a fine curved osteotome malletted approximately 4 to 6 mm posterior to the infraorbital rim. The orbital floor is sectioned very carefully to prevent transection of the infraorbital neurovascular bundle. The planned oblique osteotomy is inscribed diagonally along a line extending from the inferior edge of the zygomatic arch through the root of the zygoma, terminating at the lateral orbital edge where the lateral orbital wall and orbital floor intersect at an angle. The internal orbital cut is made laterally and anteriorly over the orbital floor to the junction of the medial and inferior orbital rims (inferolateral orbital angle). The magnitude of anterior and superior repositioning of the maxillomalar complex depends on the previously calculated angle of oblique osteotomy based upon careful clinical assessment of the relationship between the infraorbital rim and the anterior aspect of the globe. With the surgical field well illuminated by a fiberoptic light attached to a Langenbeck retractor, the osteotomy is commenced with a reciprocating saw blade with a blunt anterior edge, at the junction of the medial and inferior orbital walls (inferolateral orbital angle), and extended posteroinferiorly through the root of the zygoma to the inferior edge of the zygomatic arch. To complete the osteotomy over the relatively thin zygomatic arch, the saw blade must be inserted into the depth of the retracted wound margins. To transect the entire thickness of the relatively dense more anterior and superior maxillomalar buttress, the saw cut must be made relatively deep. With the same cut, the lowest possible portion of the posterior wall of the maxillary sinus is reached, so that later on when the osteotomy of the posterior wall of the maxillary sinus is made, it will be necessary to extend the cut intraorally toward the ptergyomaxillary buttress. The osteotomy continues superiorly and anteriorly until the orbital rim is reached, where, with the help of an eye retractor, the globe is elevated and protected as the osteotomy is extended to the inferolateral orbital angle. The intraorbital osteotomy is accomplished with a fissure bur in a straight handpiece and osteotome.

The osteotomy is made over the previously marked line on the orbital floor, anterior and lateral to the lacrimal sac. Fine spatula osteotomes are used to check for completeness of the orbital osteotomies, which are made in a similar fashion bilaterally to ensure symmetric advancement of the maxillo-malar complex through the medial orbital rim, lateral orbital rim, and malar bone.

The piriform rims of the nose and anterior nasal spine are exposed through the anterior aspect of a circumvestibular incision extending from the first molar area of one side to the contralateral first molar area. The mucoperiosteum is reflected from the lateral nasal walls to the base of the inferior turbinates and nasal floor. The piriform rims and anterior nasal crest of the maxilla are exposed similarly. An attempt is made to maximize the soft tissue pedicle to the advanced facial bones. The medial vertical orbital rim osteotomies that were previously made inferiorly toward the piriform apertures are identified and completed by extending the bone cuts medially immediately subjacent to the anterior aspect of the inferior turbinate.

A nasoseptal osteotome is malletted posteriorly to separate bony nasal septum from the maxilla. The surgeon's finger is positioned transorally in the region of the posterior nasal spine to feel the end of the nasal septal osteotome. With the nasal mucoperiosteum protected by a malleable retractor, a fine spatula osteotome is used to section the anterior aspect of the lateral nasal walls.

The margins of the posterior aspect of the circumvestibular incisions are undermined subperiosteally to the pterygoid-maxillary junction. After separating the posterior maxilla from the pterygoid plates, the posteotomy is extended from the pterygoid-maxillary suture superiorly and anteriorly toward the inferior orbital fissure (Fig. 50–31).

A thin curved osteotome is malleted superiorly and medially to section the posterolateral aspect of the maxilla. The "blind" cut terminates in the inferior orbital fissure. This osteotomy is accomplished carefully so as to not extend the bone cut into the area of the internal maxillary artery and pterygoid vascular plexus.

Mobilization of the Maxillo-Malar Complex

Carroll Girard bone screws placed in the malar eminences bilaterally through the infraorbital incisions may be used adjunctively to mobilize and reposition the maxillomalar complex. Mobilization of the maxillomalar complex is achieved extraorally from above and behind the patient's head with the aid of disimpaction forceps. The complex is rocked back and forth until passive mobility is achieved. Initially the direction of force is applied with the forceps inferiorly to downfracture the midface complex. As the force is applied, the orbital-malar osteotomy sites are observed bilaterally to determine whether or not the zygomatic-orbital osteotomies are separating symmetrically to avoid inadvertent fracturing of the malar bones. After the initial mobilization of the midface, the maxillo-malar complex must be made freely movable anteriorly. This is accomplished by deliberate continuous movement with adjunctive intraoral traction on the posterior part of the maxilla (similar to mobilization of the Le Fort I osteotomy). Such manipulations must be continued until the complex can be passively repositioned anteriorly with digital pressure. To do so requires careful and patient effort. The complex is advanced into the planned relationship with the mandible and stabilized with bone plates and/or screws. The use of a composite splint in concert with an extraoral vertical referent facilitates achievement of the desired three-dimensional movements of the complex if and when simultaneous movement of the mandible is planned. This can frequently be accomplished with minimal bone grafting.

When the maxillo-malar complex is repositioned anteriorly and *superiorly,* the proximal segment may be purposely telescoped over the labial buccal aspect of the proximal segment and stabilized with long obliquely placed (2 mm in diameter) position screws. Sculpting of the lateral aspect of the proximal segment and medial aspect of the distal segment may be necessary to achieve ideal bony contact between the segments and stability or the maxillomalar complex. Superior repositioning of the complex may also positively affect the relationship between the infraorbital rims and amount of inferior scleral exposure by decreasing the amount of inferior scleral exposure. On the other hand, if there is a lack of tooth exposure with the upper lip in repose, it may be necessary to inferiorly reposition the maxillomalar complex by interpositional bone grafting, alter the design of the modified Le Fort III osteotomy, or employ the more versatile Le Fort I osteotomy. If the maxilla is positioned asymmetrically, a low-level Le Fort I osteotomy may be done simultaneously with the modified oblique Le Fort III osteotomy to achieve the desired three-dimensional changes.

Midfacial osteotomies should be designed to correct the individual's aberrant anatomic form by advancing the maxillomalar complex. Simultaneous advancement of the malar bones and the maxilla as separate units is somewhat more complex than surgical advancement of the intact maxillomalar complex. Facial or dental asymmetry, anterior open bite, a large disparity between the distance the maxilla should be advanced and the distance the malar bones and infraorbital rims should be advanced, and palatal crossbite are some of the clinical indications for simultaneous advancement of the maxilla by low level Le Fort I osteotomy and modified Le Fort III osteotomy as separate units. (Case 1, Figs. 50–1 to 50–6.)

CASE STUDIES

CASE 1 (Figs. 50–1 to 50–6)

ADVANCEMENT OF MAXILLOMALAR COMPLEX BY TRADITIONAL MODIFIED LE FORT III OSTEOTOMY

A 26-year-old female first saw her orthodontist for treatment of her Class III skeletal malocclusion and severe anteroposterior maxillary deficiency.

FIGURE 50–1. Preoperative facial view of infraorbital deficiency, excessive scleral exposure, and increased lower anterior facial height.

FIGURE 50–2. Postoperative view.

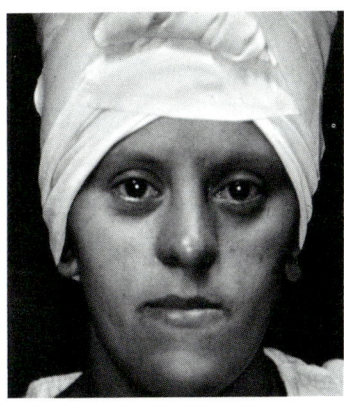

FIGURE 50–1

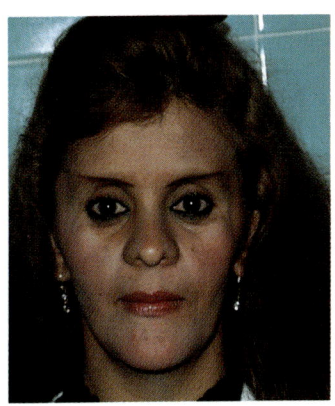

FIGURE 50–2

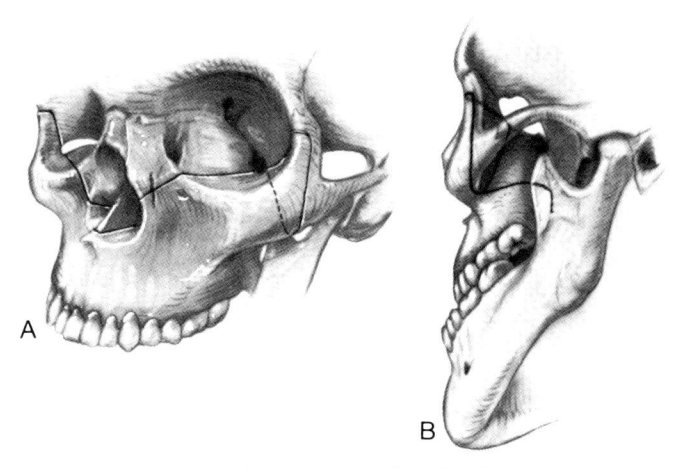

FIGURE 50-3. *A, B,* Intraoperative view showing advancement along lateral orbital wall.

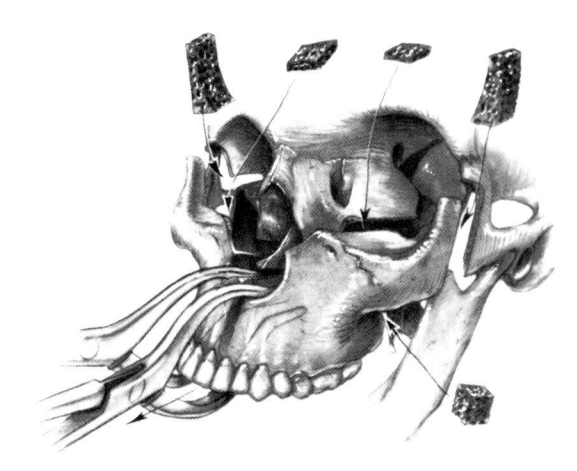

FIGURE 50-4. Mid-face advancement stabilized with interpositional bone graft and transosseous wires.

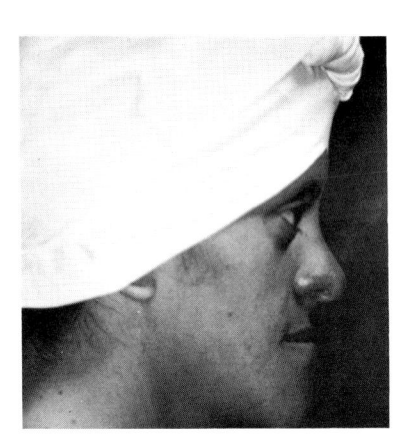

FIGURE 50-5. Lateral preoperative view showing severe maxillary and infraorbital hypoplasia, mandibular prognathism, and concave profile.

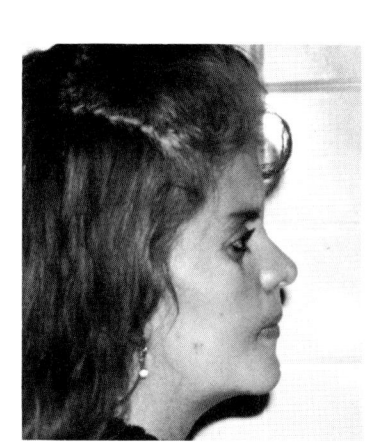

FIGURE 50-6. Lateral postoperative view; the anteroposterior deficiency of the infraorbital rim and malar bone was corrected.

PROBLEMS

Esthetic
Frontal: Infraorbital and paranasal deficiency, vertical maxillary hyperplasia, vertical excess of lower anterior facial third (Fig. 50-1).
Profile: Mandibular prognathism combined with anteroposterior maxillary deficiency; infraorbital, paranasal, and malar hypoplasia; obtuse gonial angle; and acute nasolabial angle (Fig. 50-5).

TREATMENT

1. Modified Le Fort III osteotomy with interpositional bone grafts to advance the middle third of the face (Figs. 50-3 and 50-4).
2. Superior repositioning of maxilla by Le Fort I osteotomy to correct vertical maxillary excess (5 mm).
3. Mandibular setback by intraoral vertical ramus osteotomies (4 mm).
4. Osteotomy of inferior border of mandible to increase chin prominence and decrease chin height (6 mm).

Surgeon — Dr. J. M. Garcia y Sanchez
Orthodontist — Dr. G. G. Lara

CASE 2 (Figs. 50-7 to 50-16)

Champy Technique of Modified Le Fort III Osteotomy

A 20-year-old male was referred by his orthodontist following a year of presurgical orthodontic treatment in preparation for surgery to correct vertical maxillary hyperplasia and middle-third facial hypoplasia.

Problems

Esthetic
Frontal: Vertical maxillary hyperplasia, excessive incisor tooth exposure with lips in repose, and lack of malar prominence (Fig. 50-7).
Profile: Concave, with noticeable deficiency in malar and paranasal regions and acute nasolabial angle. Lip incompetence, obtuse gonial angle, downturned nasal tip, mandibular prognathism, microgenia, and maxillary anteroposterior hypoplasia with a 15-mm underjet.

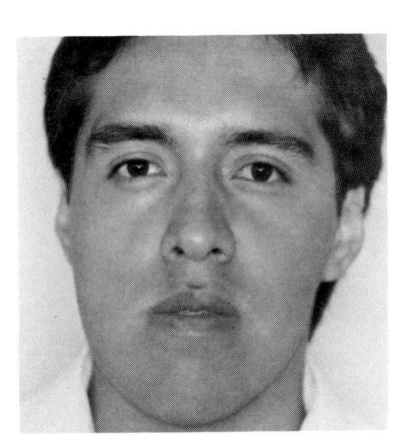

FIGURE 50-7. Preoperative facial view: Note infraorbital, malar, and paranasal deficiency.

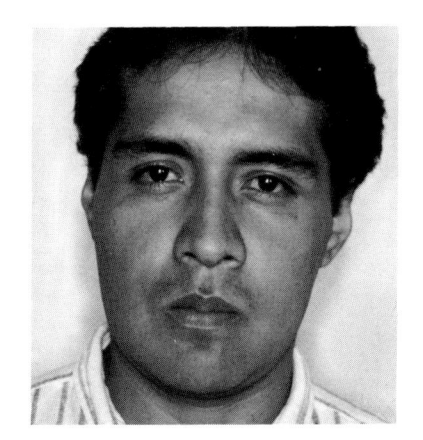

FIGURE 50-8. Postoperative balanced facial proportions.

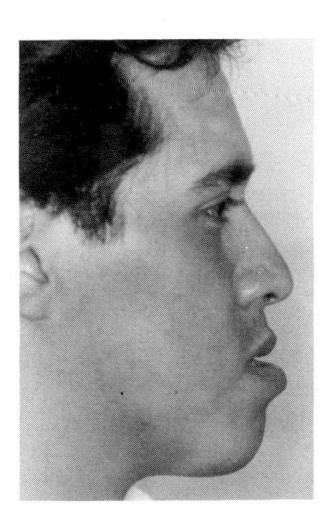

FIGURE 50-9. Preoperative facial appearance: anteroposterior maxillary deficiency and mandibular prognathism.

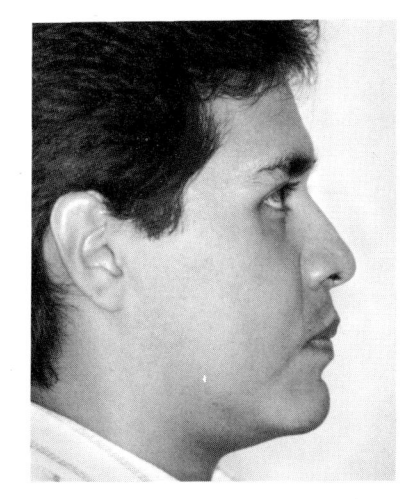

FIGURE 50-10. Postoperative view showing correction of midface deficiency by modified oblique Le Fort III osteotomy technique. A small irregularity of the inferior lateral orbital wall is identifiable.

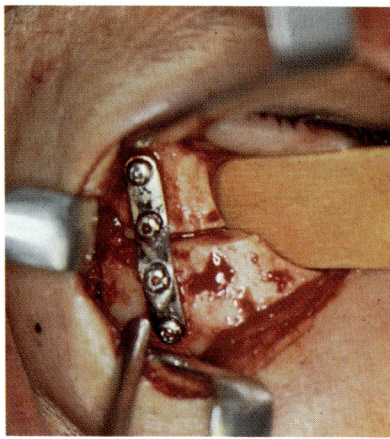

FIGURE 50–11. Intraoperative view showing midface advancement. A miniplate is used on the lateral orbital wall to provide fixation of the maxillomalar complex.

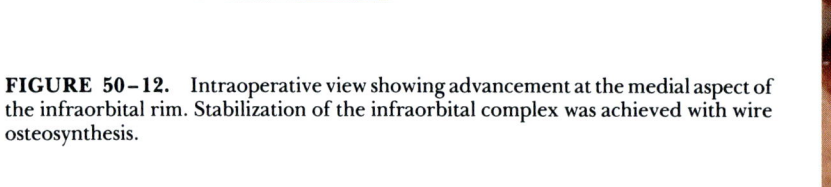

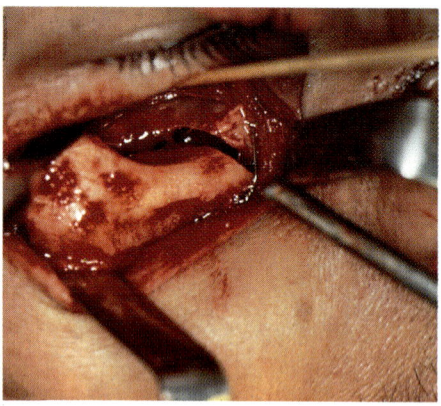

FIGURE 50–12. Intraoperative view showing advancement at the medial aspect of the infraorbital rim. Stabilization of the infraorbital complex was achieved with wire osteosynthesis.

Cephalometric Analysis (Fig. 50–13)

1. Hypoplasia of middle half of face
2. Vertical maxillary excess
3. Mandibular prognathism
4. Microgenia
5. Lip incompetence
6. 15-mm underjet
7. Satisfactory inclination of upper and lower incisors

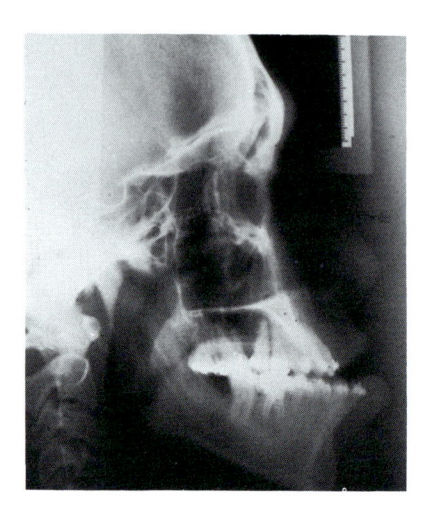

FIGURE 50–13. Preoperative cephalometric radiograph.

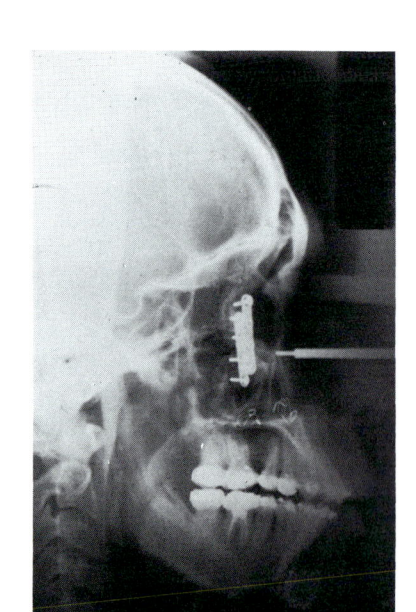

FIGURE 50–14. Postoperative cephalometric radiograph.

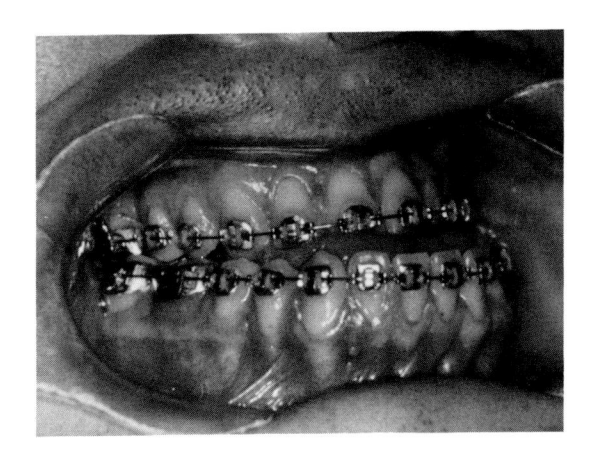

FIGURE 50-15. Preoperative occlusion.

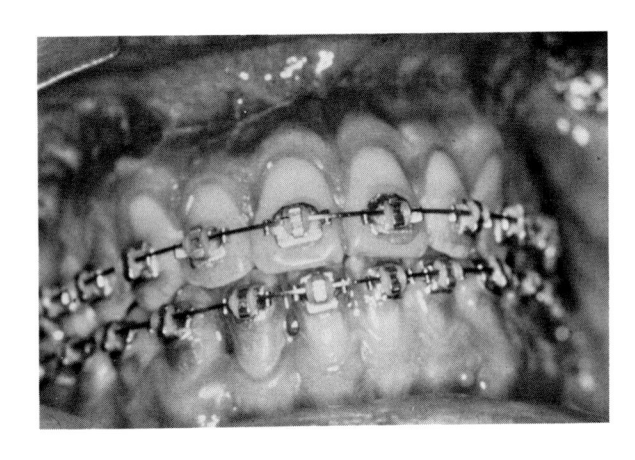

FIGURE 50-16. Postoperative occlusion.

Occlusal Analysis (Fig. 50-15)

The form of the maxillary and mandibular dental arches was symmetric in both the transverse and anteroposterior dimensions with excellent alignment of the teeth in each arch.

Surgical Plan

1. Modified Le Fort III sagittal osteotomy for 5-mm advancement of middle third of the face.
2. Le Fort I osteotomy to superiorly reposition maxilla 4 mm to correct vertical maxillary excess.
3. 7-mm mandibular setback by intraoral vertical ramus osteotomies.
4. Osteotomy of inferior border of mandible to increase chin prominence (5 mm).
5. Positioning of a stainless steel miniplate for stabilizing the Le Fort III osteotomy along the lateral orbital wall. Wire osteosynthesis to stabilize the medial osteotomy as well as the advancement genioplasty (Fig. 50-11).

Surgeon—Dr. J. M. Garcia y Sanchez
Orthodontist—Dr. G. G. Lara

CASE 3 (Figs. 50-17 to 50-42)

Treatment of Maxillomalar Deficiency by Oblique Modified Le Fort III Osteotomy and Simultaneous Le Fort I Osteotomy

A 15-year-old female presented to her orthodontist complaining of upper incisor crowding and severe anterior open bite; additionally, she was unhappy with her protruding lower jaw.

Problems

Esthetic

1. Labial incompetence
2. Excessive upper incisor exposure at rest
3. Excessive gingival exposure (5 mm) when smiling
4. Deficiency of infraorbital, malar, and paranasal regions
5. Excessive inferior scleral exposure

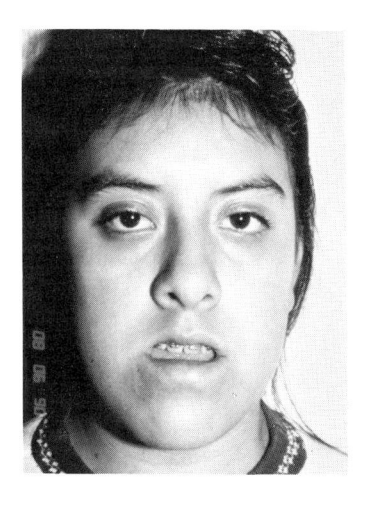

FIGURE 50–17. Preoperative frontal view demonstrating infraorbital, paranasal, and malar deficiency, vertical maxillary excess, and lip incompetence.

Profile

1. Anteroposterior maxillary deficiency
2. Malar, infraorbital, and paranasal deficiency
3. Concave facial profile
4. Nasal tip downturned
5. Obtuse gonial angle
6. Mandibular prognathism
7. Acute nasolabial angle

CEPHALOMETRIC ANALYSIS (FIGS. 50–18 AND 50–20)

1. Vertical maxillary excess
2. Middle-third facial hypoplasia
3. Mandibular prognathism
4. Posterior inclination of palatal plane
5. Proclination of upper incisors
6. Proclination of lower incisors
7. Anterior open bite
8. 15-mm anterior crossbite
9. Lip incompetence

Text continued on page 1785

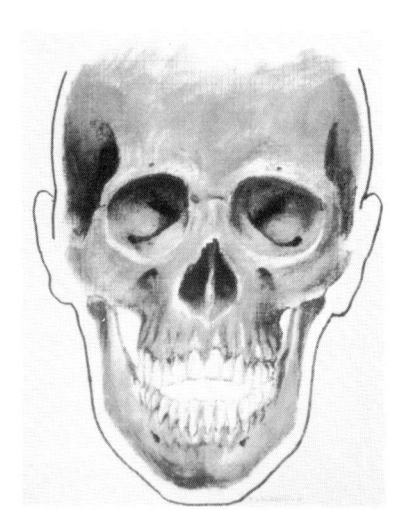

FIGURE 50–18. Schematic view of dentofacial deformity.

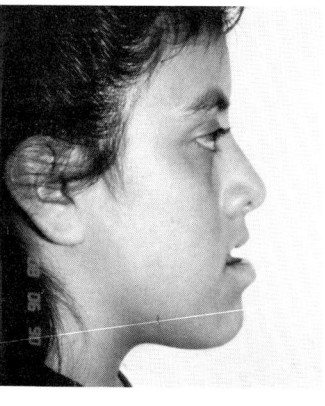

FIGURE 50–19. Preoperative facial profile showing middle-third facial hypoplasia, concave profile, mandibular prognathism, and lip incompetence.

50 — OBLIQUE MODIFIED LE FORT III OSTEOTOMY / **1781**

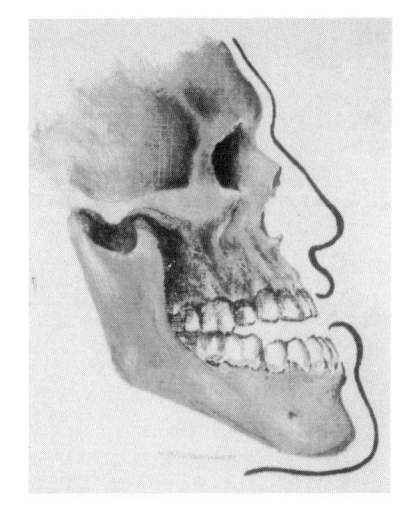

FIGURE 50-20. Preoperative deformity; severe anterior open bite.

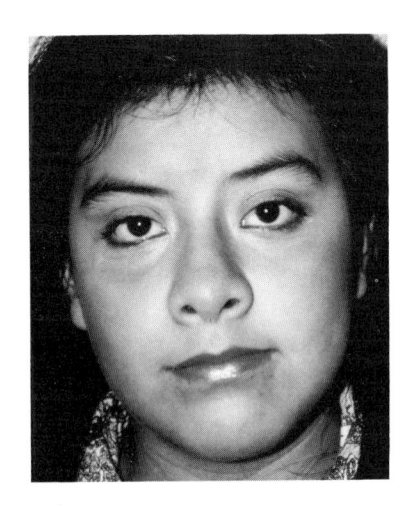

FIGURE 50-21. Postoperative facial appearance.

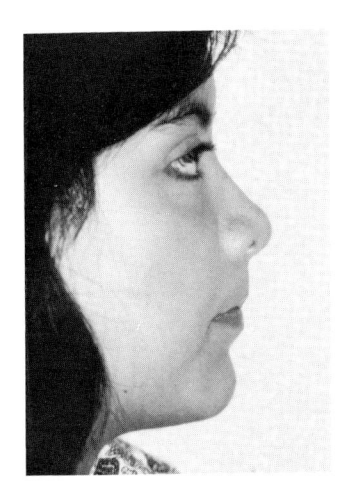

FIGURE 50-22. Postoperative facial appearance.

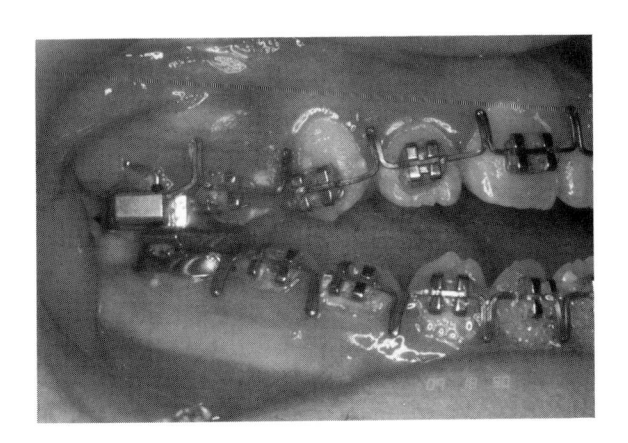

FIGURE 50-23. Preoperative occlusion.

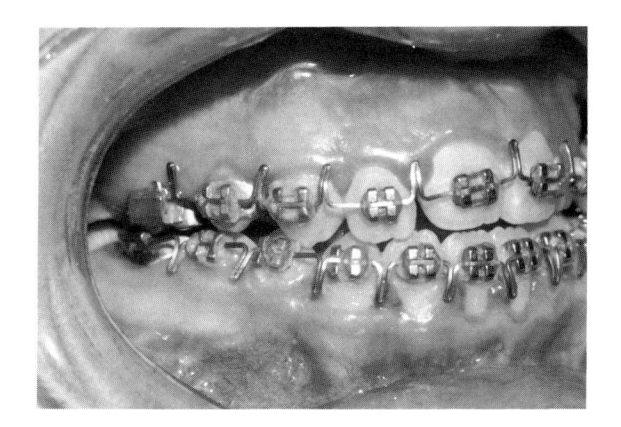

FIGURE 50-24. Postoperative occlusion.

1782 / VI—FUNCTIONAL RESTORATION OF OCCLUSION

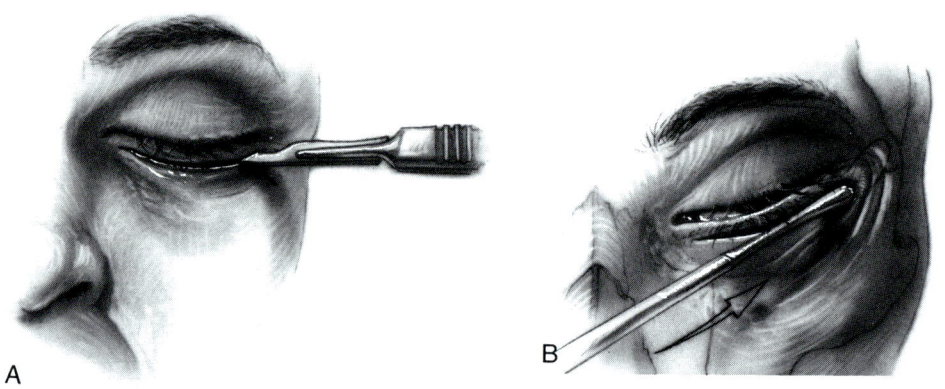

FIGURE 50–25. *A, B,* Infraorbital rim incision. A vertical osteotomy is made through the inferior orbital rim, lateral to the lacrimal apparatus. This bone incision is extended inferiorly to the anterior aspect of the maxilla lateral to the piriform aperture at the level of the anterior insertion of the inferior turbinate. An osteotomy is not made through the piriform rim.

FIGURE 50–26. Surgical approach using oblique cut extending from the inferior lateral aspect of the orbital wall to the posteroinferior portion of the zygomatic arch.

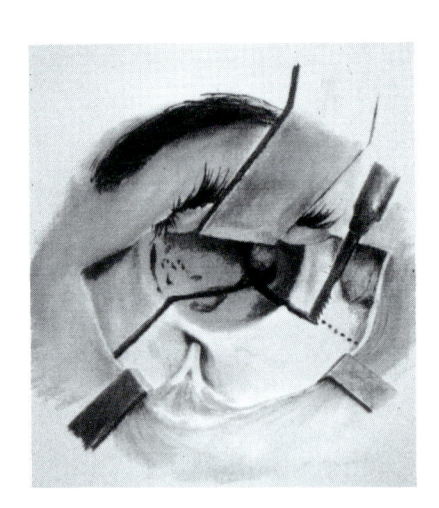

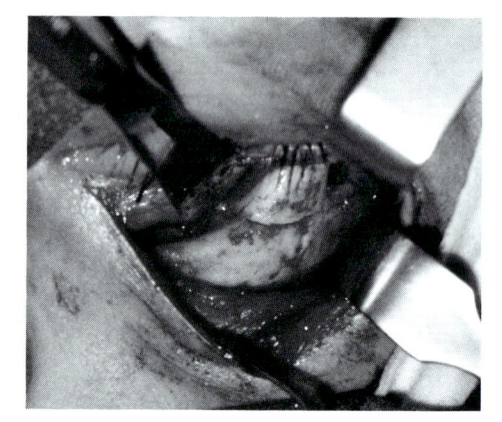

FIGURE 50–27. Through the infraorbital rim incision, the bone cut is extended laterally through the orbital floor 6 to 8 mm posterior to the rim in the direction of the inferior orbital fissure.

FIGURE 50–28. Oblique bone cut extending from the inferolateral aspect of the orbital wall to the posteroinferior portion of the zygomatic arch.

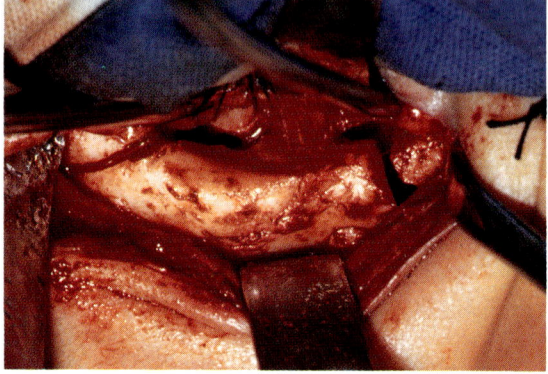

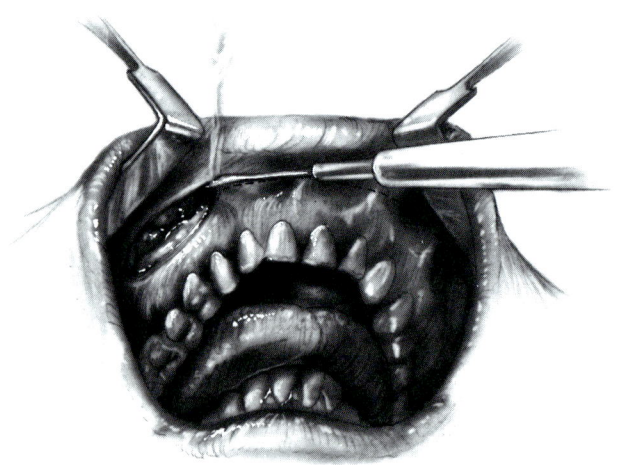

FIGURE 50–29. An electrosurgical cutting blade is used to make a horizontal incision in the maxillary vestibule.

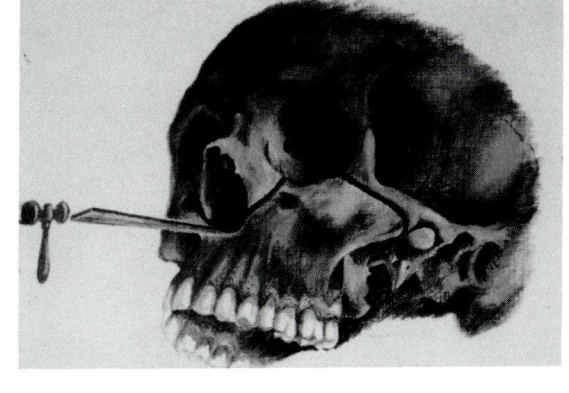

FIGURE 50-30. Nasoseptal osteotome positioned above the anterior nasal spine parallel with the hard palate is malletted to the posterior edge of the nasal septum to separate the nasal septum from the maxilla.

FIGURE 50-31. Osteotomy is made superiorly and medially to section posterior lateral aspect of the maxilla.

FIGURE 50-32. Surgical plan to advance maxillomalar complex as a single unit. Currently, bone plate and/or screw osteosynthesis is used to stabilize the repositioned complex.

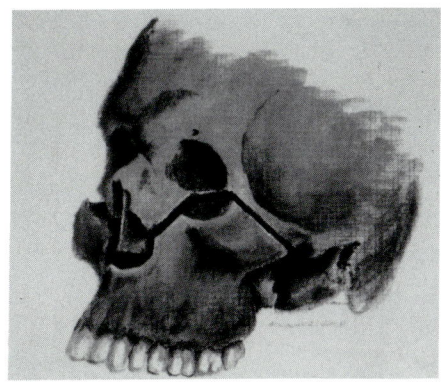

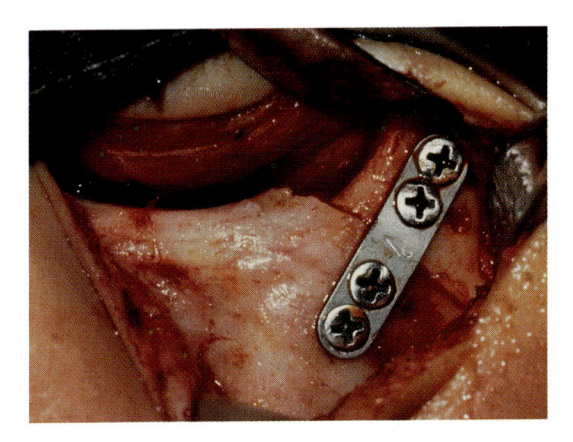

FIGURE 50-33. The lateral wall of infraorbital bone and inferior orbital rim shows an inferolateral osteotomy of the rim made in an oblique direction toward the inferior surface of the zygomatic-malar structure.

FIGURE 50-34. A segment of biocompatible osteoconductive polymer (BOP) is placed in the osseous gap created by advancing the orbital floor.

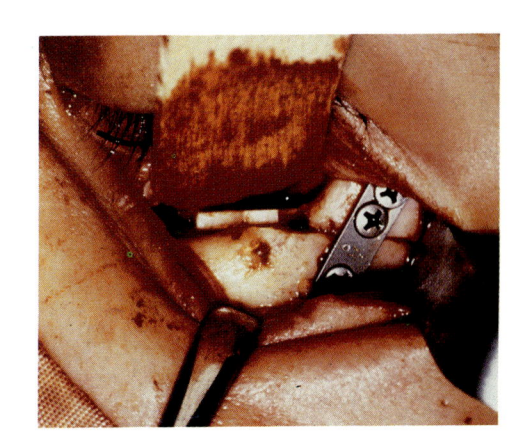

1784 / VI—FUNCTIONAL RESTORATION OF OCCLUSION

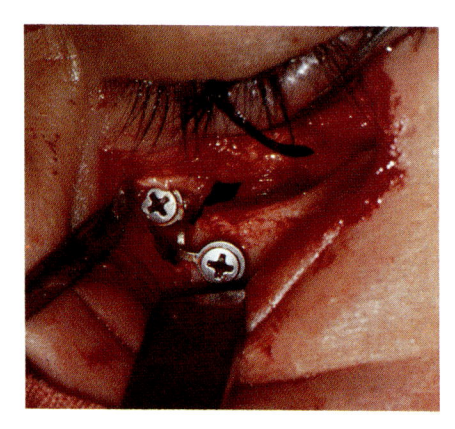

FIGURE 50-35. Miniplate fixation along the medial osteotomy.

FIGURE 50-36. Stabilizing plate used in Le Fort I osteotomy 5 years after repositioning the maxillomalar complex.

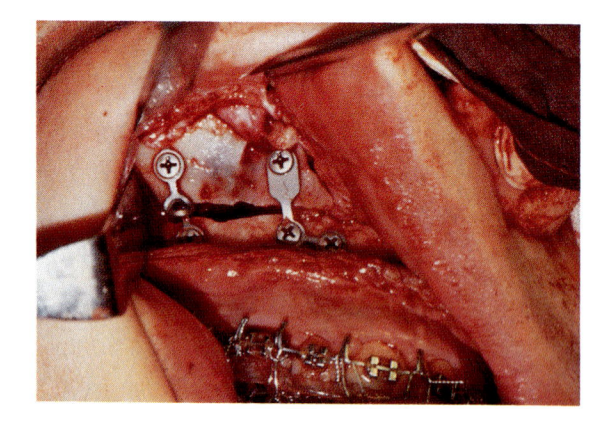

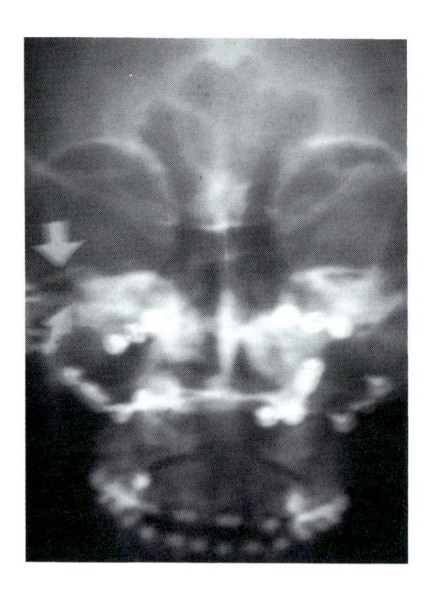

FIGURE 50-37. Postoperative tomographic view.

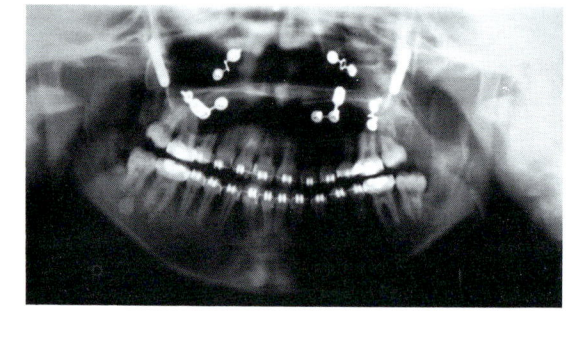

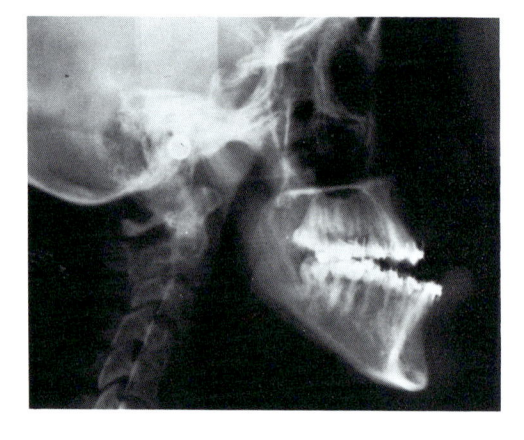

FIGURE 50-38. Panoramic radiograph after surgery.

FIGURE 50-39. Preoperative cephalogram.

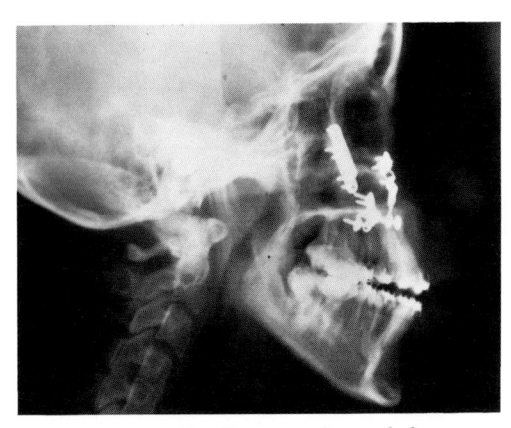

FIGURE 50-40. Postoperative cephalogram.

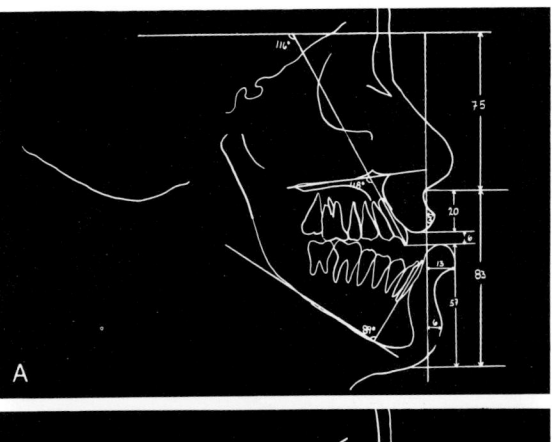

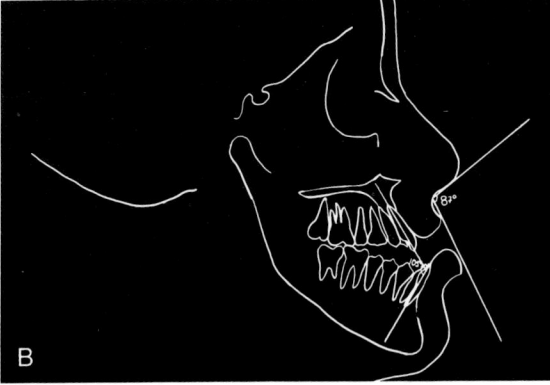

FIGURE 50-41. Preoperative cephalometric tracings showing vertical and anteroposterior disproportionality.

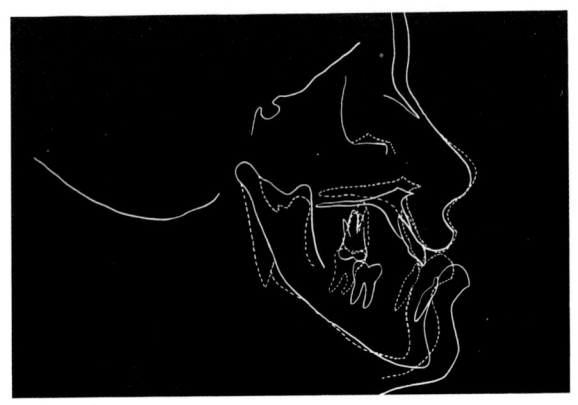

FIGURE 50-42. Superimpositions of preoperative and 3-month postoperative cephalometric tracings.

Vertical Proportions

1. 1-Stms = 6 mm
2. G-Sn = 75 mm/Sn-Me' = 83 mm
3. Sn-Stms = 20 mm/Stmi-me = 57 mm
4. ILG = 6 mm

Anteroposterior Proportions

1. SnV-ULP = 3 mm
2. SnV-LLP = 13 mm
3. Snv-Po' = 6 mm
4. NLA = 105 degrees
5. ULD = 105 degrees

Position of Incisors

1. 1-HP = 116 degrees
2. 1-PP = 118 degrees
3. 1-GoMe = 89 degrees

Occlusal Analysis

Dental arch form: Symmetry of maxillary and mandibular arches in both anteroposterior and transverse dimensions.

Dental alignment: Good dental alignment with small spaces between upper canines and premolars; upper incisors proclined with slightly retroclined mandibular incisors —15-mm underjet, 8-mm open bite.

Treatment Plan

1. Modified oblique Le Fort III osteotomy without bone grafting was performed by 6-mm advancement and 3-mm superior repositioning to correct the middle-third facial hypoplasia and excessive incisor exposure (Figs. 50-27 to 50-34).

2. Superior repositioning of maxilla by Le Fort I osteotomy. Maxilla was raised 7 mm in posterior and 5 mm in anterior for correction of posterior inclination of the palatal plane and vertical maxillary excess.

3. Vitallium miniplates were positioned along the lateral and medial orbital walls to stabilize the repositioned segments of the modified oblique Le Fort III osteotomy.

1786 / VI—FUNCTIONAL RESTORATION OF OCCLUSION

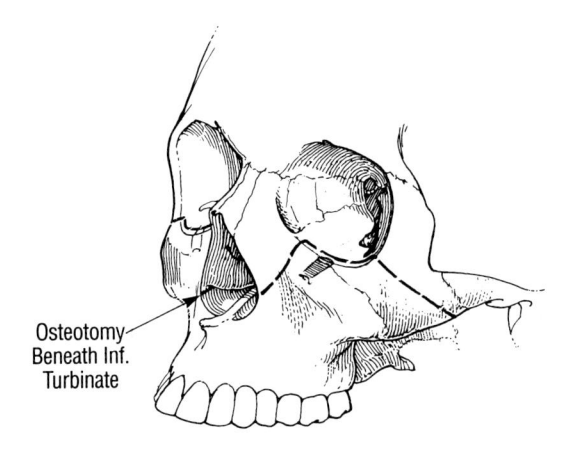

FIGURE 50-43. Surgical plan to advance maxillomalar complex by oblique modified Le Fort III osteotomy.

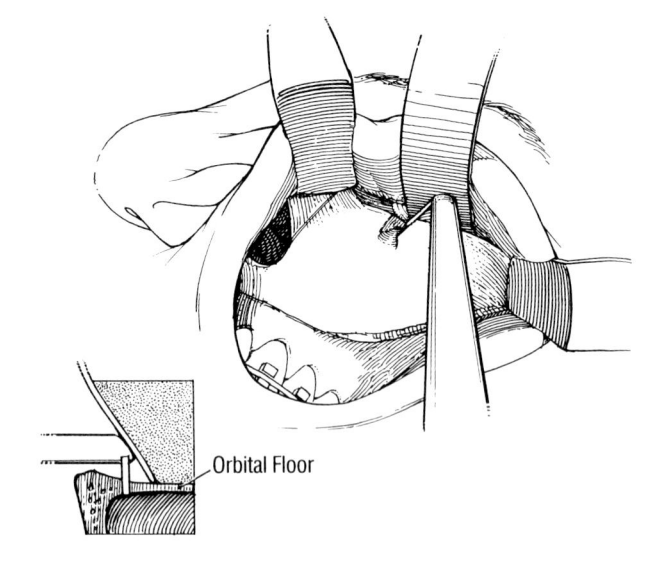

FIGURE 50-44. Oblique modified Le Fort III osteotomy accomplished intraorally—anterior surface of the maxilla, malar bones, infraorbital rims and zygomatic arches exposed by subperiosteal dissection. Osteotomy of the orbital floor is made with a short right-angled oscillating saw blade 4–6 mm posterior to the infraorbital rim.

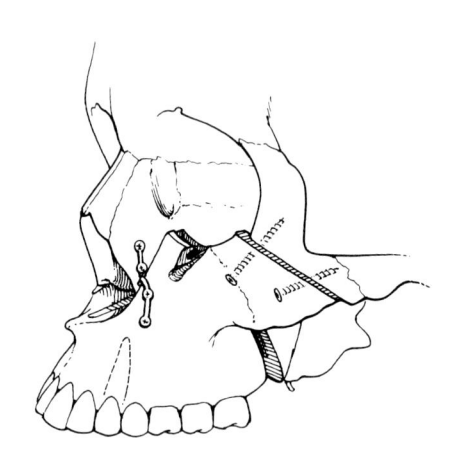

FIGURE 50-45. Stabilization of the repositioned maxillomalar complex with positional screws and mini bone plate.

The Le Fort I level osteotomy was stabilized with miniplates positioned along the zygomatic-maxillary buttress and pyriform aperture (Figs. 50–35 and 50–36).

4. Intraoral vertical ramus osteotomies for 6-mm mandibular setback. Maxillomandibular fixation was utilized for 3 weeks.

Surgeon—Dr. J. M. Garcia y Sanchez
Orthodontist—Dr. Salvador Garcia, Dr. A.R.E. Gutierrez

Recently the soft tissue incisions and osteotomy design for oblique modified Le Fort III osteotomy have been successfully modified so that the entire procedure is done intraorally. Experience with four such cases indicated that accessibility has been adequate. The entire anterior surface of the maxilla, malar bones, and lateral and inferior surfaces of the zygomatic arches are exposed by subperiosteal dissection. The dissection is carried from one pterygopalatine fissure and tuberosity to the contralateral pterygopalatine fissure and tuberosity. Traditionally the osteotomy of the orbital floor has been extended posteriorly to the infraorbital fissure. With the limited accessibility to the orbital floor afforded by the intraoral approach, the osteotomy of the orbital floor is located in the fragile anterior region some 4–6 mm posterior to the infraorbital rim. Stabilization of the maxillomalar complex has been achieved with the use of long position screws (2 mm diameter, 16–26 mm long) through the malar bones. Good stability of the anteriorly repositioned complex has been achieved without maxillomandibular fixation and sometimes without bone grafting.

The oblique modified Le Fort III osteotomy is not as flexible as the various types of Le Fort I osteotomies. Consequently, the technique may not be applicable when (1) there is a significant disparity between the anterior-posterior deficiency of the infraorbital rims and the maxilla, (2) differential vertical movements of the right and left sides are indicated, (3) segmentation of the maxilla with significant expansion is indicated and (4) a large alteration of the occlusal plane is indicated.[50] In such cases it may be prudent to combine Le Fort I osteotomy with augmentation of the malar bones and infraorbital areas. In selected cases Le Fort I osteotomy may be done simultaneously with modified Le Fort III osteotomy. Careful attention must be given to proper soft tissue flap design and osteotomy design.

REFERENCES

1. Bachmayer DI, Ross RB: Stability of Le Fort III advancement surgery in children with Crouzon's, Apert's, and Pfeiffer's syndromes. Cleft Palate J 23(suppl I):69, 1986.
2. Beals SP, Munro IR: The use of mini-plates in cranio-maxillofacial surgery. Plast Reconstr Surg 79:33, 1987.
3. Bell WH, Proffit WR: Maxillary excess. *In* Bell WH, Proffit WR, White RP (eds): Surgical Correction of Dentofacial Deformities. Vol. I. Philadelphia, WB Saunders Company, 1980.
4. Bell WH, Proffit WR, Jacobs JD: Maxillary and midface deformities. (Part A). *In* Bell WH, Proffit WR, White RP (eds): Surgical Correction of Dentofacial Deformities. Philadelphia, WB Saunders Company, 1980.
5. Bell WH, White RP, Hall HD: Mandibular excess (Part A). *In* Bell WH, Proffit WR, White RP (eds): Surgical Correction of Dentofacial Deformities. Vol II. Philadelphia, WB Saunders Company, 1980.
6. Bell WH, Jacobs J, Quejada J: Simultaneous repositioning of the maxilla, mandible, and chin. Am J Orthod 89:28, 1986.
7. Bjork A, Skieller V: Growth in width of the maxilla studied by implant method. Scand J Plast Reconstr Surg 8:26, 1974.
8. Block MS, Zide M: Orbital decompression by midfacial advancement. Oral Surg 57:479, 1984.
9. Brusati R, Sesenna E, Raffaini M: On the feasibility of intraoral maxillo-malar osteotomy. J. Craniomaxillofac Surg 17:110, 1989.
10. Bu B, Kaban LB, Vargervik K: Effect of Le Fort III osteotomy on mandibular growth in patients with Crouzon and Apert syndromes. J Oral Maxillofac Surg 47:666–671, 1989.
11. Bütow KW: A lateral photometric analysis for aesthetic-orthognathic treatment. J Maxillofac Surg 12:201, 1984.
12. Bütow KW: An extension of cephalo-photometric analysis. J Craniomaxillofac Surg 16:266, 1988.
13. Casson PR, Bonnano PC, Converse JM: The midface degloving procedure. Plast Reconstr Surg 53:102, 1974.
14. Conway H, Smith TW, Behrman SJ: Another method of bringing the midface forward. Plast Reconstr Surg 46:325, 1970.
15. Converse JM, Ransohoff J, Mathews ES, et al: Oculo-hypertelorism and pseudohypertelorism: Advances in surgical treatment. Plast Reconstr Surg 45:1, 1970.
16. Converse JM, Horowitz SL, Valauri AJ: The treatment of nasomaxillary hypoplasia: A new pyramidal naso-orbital maxillary osteotomy. Plast Reconstr Surg 45:527, 1970.
17. Converse JM, Wood-Smith D, McCarthy JG: Report on a series of 50 cranio-facial operations. Plast Reconstr Surg 55:283, 1975.
18. Champy M, Lodde JP, Muster D, et al: Osteosynthesis using miniaturized screw-on plate in facial and cranial surgery. Ann Chir Plast Esthet 22:261–264, 1977.
19. Champy M, Lodde JP, Wilk A: A propos de 30 cas d'osteotomies transfacial intermediaires. Ann Chir Plast 24:351, 1979.
20. Champy M, Lodde JP, Wilk A: Surgical treatment of midface deformities. Head Neck Surg 2:451, 1980.
21. Dann John J: Applications of high midface procedures in the management of dentofacial deformities. *In* Current Advances in Oral and Maxillofacial Surgery: Orthognathic Surgery 5:316, 1986.
22. Delaire J, Tessier P, Tulasne JR, Resche F: Aspects cliniques et radiographiques de la dysostose maxillo-nasale: "Syndrome naso-maxillo-vertebral" a propos de 34 nouveaux cas. Rev Stomatol Chir Maxillofac 1979.
23. Delaire J, Tessier P, Tulasne JR, Resche F: Clinical and radiologic aspects of maxillonasal dysostosis (Birden syndrome). Head Neck Surg 3:105, 1980.
24. Epker BN, Wolford M: Middle-third facial osteotomies: Their use in the correction of acquired and developmental dentofacial and craniofacial deformities. J Oral Surg 33:491, 1975.
25. Epker BN, Wolford M: Middle-third facial osteotomies: Their use in the correction of congenital and craniofacial deformities. J Oral Surg 34:324, 1976.
26. Epker BN, Wolford M: Middle-third facial advancement: Treatment considerations in atypical cases. J Oral Surg 37:31–41, 1979.
27. Epker BN, Wolford LM: Dentofacial Deformities: Surgical-Orthodontic Correction. St. Louis, The CV Mosby Company, 1980.
28. Epker BN, Fish LC: Dentofacial Deformities. Chapter 13: True midface dentofacial deformity. St. Louis, The CV Mosby Company, 1986.
29. Fish L, Epker BN: Dentofacial deformities related to midface deficiencies. J Clin Orthod 21:654, 1987.
30. Fish L, Epker BN: Dentofacial deformities related to midface deficiencies: Integrated orthodonthic-surgical correction. J Clin Orthod 21:664, 1987.

31. Freihofer HP: Results of osteotomies of the facial skeleton in adolescence. J Maxillofac Surg 5:276, 1972.
32. Freihofer HP: Latitude and limitation of midface movements. Br J Oral Maxillofac Surg 22:393, 1984.
33. Fornas DW, De Feu DR, Kusske JA: Gabelard osteotomy and orbital craniotomies with microscopic control for correction of hypertelorism: A preliminary report of micro-craniofacial surgery in two patients. Plast Reconstr Surg 70:51, 1982.
34. Frost DE, Krutnick AW: Alternative stabilization of the maxilla during simultaneous jaw-mobilization procedures. Oral Surg 56:125–127, 1983.
35. Garcia y Sanchez JM, Vargas LD, Lara GG: Osteomía. Le Fort III. Sagital en combinación con Osteotomía Le Fort I, Osteotomía Vertical Subsigmoides intraoral y Genioplastía. Rev Lat Am Cirug Taumatol Maxillofac 1:22, 1989.
36. Gillies H, Harrison SH: Operative correction by osteotomy of recessed malar-maxillary compound in a case of oxycephaly. Br J Plast Surg 3:123, 1950.
37. Harsha BC, Terry BC: Stabilization of Le Fort I osteotomies utilizing small bone plates. Int Adult Orthod Orthogn Surg 1:69, 1986.
38. Henderson D, Jackson IT: Naso-maxillary hypoplasia: The Le Fort II osteotomy. Br J Oral Surg 11:77, 1973.
39. Henderson D: The assessment and management of bony deformities of the middle and lower face. Br J Plast Surg 27:287, 1974.
40. Henderson D: Maxillary and midface deformity in correction of dentofacial deformities. In Bell WH, Proffit WR, White RP (eds): Surgical Correction of Dentofacial Deformities. Philadelphia, WB Saunders Company, 1980.
41. Hogeman KE, Willmar K: On Le Fort III osteotomy for Crouzon's disease in children. Scand J Plast Surg 8:169, 1974.
42. Holmstrom H: Surgical correction of the nose and midface in maxillonasal dysplasia (Binder's syndrome). Plast Reconstr Surg 78:568, 1986.
43. Hopkin GB: Hypoplasia of the middle third of the face associated with congenital absence of the anterior nasal spine, depression of the nasal bones and the angle Class III malocclusion. Br Plast Surg 16:147, 1963.
44. Horster W: Experience with functionally stable plate osteosynthesis after forward displacement of the upper jaw. J Maxillofac Surg 8:176, 1980.
45. Jabaley ME, Edgerton ME: Surgical correction of congenital midface retrusion in the presence of mandibular prognathism. Plast Reconst Surg 44:1, 1969.
46. Jackson IT, Khursheed MF, Sharpe DT: Total surgical management of Binder's syndrome. Ann Plast Surg 7:25, 1981.
47. Jackson IT, Munro IR, Salyer, KE, Whitaker LA: Maxillary surgery and repair of facial clefts. In Atlas of Craniomaxillofacial Surgery. St. Louis, The CV Mosby Company, 1982.
48. Jackson IT, Somers PC, Kjar JG: The use of Champy miniplates for osteosynthesis in craniofacial deformities and trauma. Plast Reconstr Surg 77:729–736, 1986.
49. Kaban LB, West B, Conover M, Murray J: Midface position after Le Fort III advancement. Plast Reconstr Surg 73:758, 1984.
50. Keller E, Howard S: Intraoral quadrangular Le Fort II osteotomy. J Oral Maxillofac Surg 45:223–232, 1987.
51. Kellman RM, Schilli W: Fijacion con placa en fracturas de la parte media y superior dela cara. Clin Otorrinolaringol Norte Am 3:591–603, 1987.
52. Kinnebrew MC, Zide MF, Kent JN: Modified Le Fort II procedure for simultaneous correction of maxillary and nasal deformities. J Oral Maxillofac Surg 41:295, 1983.
53. Kinnebrew MC, Dzyak WR: Modification in the Le Fort III osteotomy. J Oral Maxillofac Surg 43:995, 1985.
54. Kufner J: Four year experience of major maxillary osteotomies for retrusion. J Oral Surg 29:549, 1971.
55. Leonard M, Walker GF, Arbor A: A cephalometric guide to the diagnosis of midface hypoplasia at the Le Fort II level. J Oral Surg 35:21, 1977.
56. Luhr HG: Sistemas de Luhr con uso de placas y tornillos de Vitalium para cirugia de recostruccion del esqueleto facial. Clin Otorrinolaringol Norte Am 3:605–639, 1987.
57. Luhr HG: A micro-system for cranio-maxillo-facial skeletal fixation. J Craniomaxillofac Surg 16:312, 1988.
58. Manson PM, Hoops JE: Structural pillar of the facial skeleton: An approach to the management of Le Fort fractures. Plast Reconstr Surg 66:54, 1980.
59. Marchac D, Coohignon J, Vander Meulen J, Bouchta M: A propos des osteotomies d'avancement du crane et de la face. Ann Chir Plast 19:370, 1974.
60. McBride KL, Bell WH: Chin surgery. In Bell WH, Proffit WR, White RP (eds): Surgical Correction of Dentofacial Deformities. Vol. II. Philadelphia, WB Saunders Company, 1980, pp 1211–1279.
61. McCarthy JG, Grayson B, Bookstein F, et al: Le Fort III advancement osteotomy in the growing child. Plast Reconstr Surg 74:343, 1984.
62. Michelet FX, Deymes J, Dessus B: Osteosynthesis with miniaturized screwed plates in maxillofacial surgery. J Maxillofac Surg 1:79–84, 1973.
63. Munro IR, Sinclair WJ, Rudd NL: Maxillonasal dysplasia (Binder's syndromes). Plast Reconstr Surg 63:657, 1979.
64. Murray JE, Lennard T, Swanson T: Midface osteotomy and advancement for craniosynostosis. Plast Reconstr Surg 41:299, 1968.
65. Obwegeser HL: Surgical correction of small or retrodisplaced maxilla. Plast Reconstr Surg 43:351, 1969.

66. Obwegeser HL, Lello GE, Farmand M: Correction of secondary cleft deformities. *In* Bell WH, Proffit WR, White RP (eds): Surgical Correction of Dentofacial Deformities. New Concepts, Vol. III. Philadelphia, WB Saunders Company, 1985.
67. Ortiz Monasterio F, Fuente del Campo A, Carrillo A: Advancement of the orbits and the midface in one piece, combined with frontal repositioning for the correction of Crouzon's deformities. Plast Reconstr Surg 51:507, 1968.
68. Popescu VC: Advancement of the middle third of the face without bone grafting in a case of Crouzon's disease. J Maxillofac Surg 2:219–223, 1974.
69. Pospisil OA: Supra-apical midfacial osteotomies: New surgical techniques and their application. J Craniomaxillofac Surg 16:110, 1988.
70. Precious D, Delaire J: Balanced facial growth: A schematic interpretation. Oral Surg Oral Med Oral Pathol 63:637, 1987.
71. Proffit WR, Epker BN, Hohl T: Treatment planning for dentofacial deformities. *In* Correction of Dentofacial Deformities. Philadelphia, WB Saunders Company, 1982.
72. Psillakis JM, Lapa F, Spina V: Surgical correction of midface retrusion (nasomaxillary hypoplasia) in the presence of normal dental occlusion. Plast Reconstr Surg 51:67, 1973.
73. Raveh J, Vuillemin T: The one-stage surgical management of combined cranio-maxillo-facial and frontobasal fractures: Advantage of the subcranial approach in 374 cases. J Craniomaxillofac Surg 16:160, 1988.
74. Raveh J, Vuillemin T: Advantages of an additional subcranial approach in the correction of craniofacial deformities. J Craniomaxillofac Surg 16:350, 1988.
75. Resche F, Tulasne JF, Tessier P, Delaire J: Malformations de la charniere craniorachidienne. Et du rachis cervical associees ala dysplasie maxillo-nasale de Binder. Rev Stomatol Chir Maxillofac 1979.
76. Rosen HM: Miniplate fixation of Le Fort I osteotomies. Plast Reconstr Surg 78:748–754, 1986.
77. Schilli W, Ewers R, Niederdellman H: Bone fixation with screws and miniplates in the maxillo-facial regions. Int J Oral Surg 10(suppl 1):329–332, 1981.
78. Sifferman RA, Danielson PA, Quatela V, et al: Retrospective analysis of surgically treated Le Fort fractures: Is suspension necessary? Arch Otolaryngol 109:446–448, 1983.
79. Souyris F, Caravel JB, Reynaud JP: Osteotomies "Intermediaires" de l'etage moyen de la face. Ann Chir Plast 18:149–154, 1973.
80. Steidler NE, Cook RM, Read PC: Residual complications in patients with major middle third facial fractures. J Oral Surg 9:259–266, 1980.
81. Steinhauser EW: Variations of Le Fort II osteotomies for correction of midfacial deformities. J Maxillofac Surg 8:258, 1980.
82. Steinhauser EW: Bone screw and plate in orthognathic surgery. Int J Oral Surg 11:209, 1982.
83. Stricker M, et al: Les osteotomies du crane et de la face. Ann Chir Plast 17:233, 1972.
84. Tessier P, Guiot G, Rougerie J, et al: Osteotomies cranio-naso-orbito-facial for hypertelorism. Ann Chir Plast 12:103, 1967.
85. Tessier P: Osteotomies totales de la face; syndrome de Crouzon; syndrome D'Apert; oxycephalies, scaphocephalies, turricephalies. Ann Chir Plast 12:273, 1967.
86. Tessier P: Relationship of craniostenoses to craniofacial dysostoses and to faciostenoses. Plast Reconstr Surg 48:224, 1971.
87. Tessier P: The definitive plastic surgical treatment of the severe facial deformities of cranio-facial dysostosis: Crouzon's and Apert's disease. Plast Reconstr Surg 48:419, 1971.
88. Tessier P: The conjunctival approach to the orbital floor and maxilla in congenital malformation and trauma. J Maxillofac Surg 1:3–8, 1973.
89. Tessier P: Anatomical classification of facial, craniofacial, and laterofacial clefts. J Maxillofac Surg 4:69, 1976.
90. Tessier P, Tulasne JF, Delaires J, Resche F: Aspects therapeutiques de la dysostose maxillo-nasale de Binder. Rev Stomatol Chir Maxillofac 1979.
91. Turvey TA, Hall DJ: Maxillary and midface deformity (Part C). *In* Bell WH, Proffit WR, White RP (eds): Surgical Correction of Dentofacial Deformities. Vol. I. Philadelphia, WB Saunders Company, 1980, pp. 644–683.
92. Van Der Meulen JCH, Vaandragep JM: Surgery related to the correction of hypertelorism. Plast Reconstr Surg 71:6, 1983.
93. Van Sickels JE, Jeter TD, Aragon SB: Rigid fixation of maxillary osteotomies: A preliminary report and technique article. Oral Surg 60:262–265, 1985.
94. Walker RV, Hayward JD, Poulton DR, Bell WH: Mandibular excess. *In* Bell WH, Proffit WR, White RP (eds): Surgical Correction of Dentofacial Deformities. Vol. II. Philadelphia, WB Saunders Company, 1982.
95. Wedgewood D: An Approach to Le Fort II osteotomy. Br J Oral Maxillofac Surg 22:87, 1984.
96. Whitaker LA, Munro IR, Salyer KE: Combined report of problems and complications in 793 craniofacial operations. Plast Reconstr Surg 64:198, 1979.
97. Wolfe SA, Berkowitz S: High maxillary osteotomies requiring an extraoral approach (Le Fort II and Le Fort III osteotomies). *In* Plastic Surgery of the Facial Skeleton. Boston, Little, Brown & Company, 1989.
98. Wolfford LM, Epker BN: The combined anterior and posterior maxillary osteotomy: A new technique. J Oral Surg 33:842, 1975.
99. Worthington P, Champy M: Osteosíntesis monocortical con miniplaca y tornillos. Clín Otorrinolaringol Norte Am 3:641–654, 1987.
100. Zide B, Grayson B, McCarthy JG: Cephalometric analysis for upper and lower midface surgery: Part II. Plast Reconstr Surg 68:961, 1981.

51 QUADRANGULAR LE FORT I AND II OSTEOTOMIES

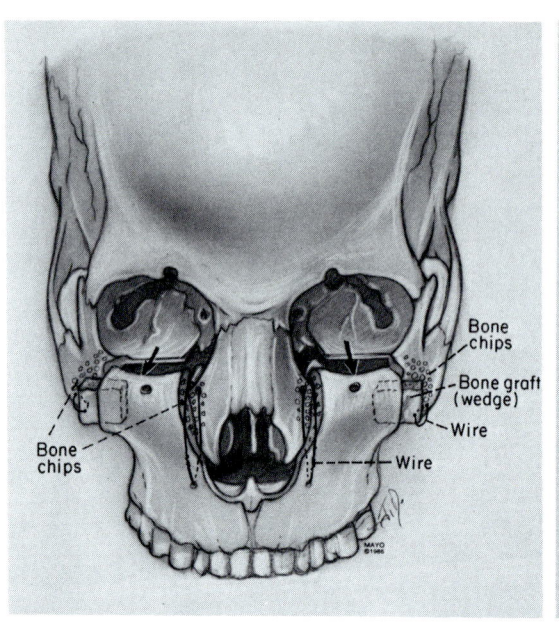

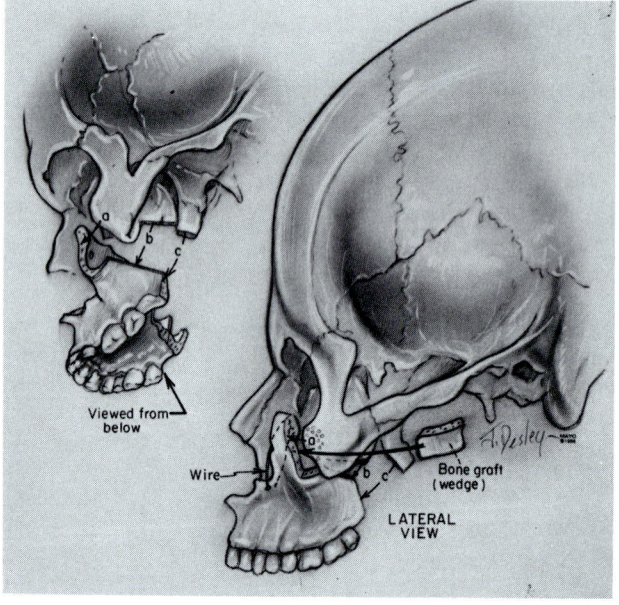

51

PRETREATMENT RECORDS AND EXAMINATION
DIAGNOSTIC CONSIDERATIONS
TREATMENT PLANNING
ORTHODONTIC APPLIANCE CONSTRUCTION CONSIDERATIONS
ORTHODONTIC APPLIANCE CONSIDERATIONS AT SURGERY
POSTSURGICAL ORTHODONTIC APPLIANCE MANIPULATION
RETENTION CONSIDERATIONS FOR THE MAXILLARY-DEFICIENT PATIENT

QUADRANGULAR LE FORT I OSTEOTOMY
   Review of Literature
   Indications
   Surgical Procedure
   Patient Presentations
   Discussion
QUADRANGULAR LE FORT II OSTEOTOMY
   Review of Literature
   Indications
   Surgical Procedure
   Immediate Postsurgical Management
     (Quadrangular Le Fort I and II Osteotomy)
   Patient Presentations
   Discussion

E. E. KELLER

PRESURGICAL AND POSTSURGICAL ORTHODONTICS FOR THE MAXILLARY–DEFICIENT PATIENT
A. HOWARD SATHER

The orthodontic treatment to be rendered to a patient with maxillary deficiency must be viewed as an integral portion of the overall treatment plan. Therefore, the orthodontist must be involved in the initial diagnosis, in conjunction with the surgeon and other health professionals who may be responsible for the patient's care. Ideally, both the surgeon and the orthodontist should see the patient and do a thorough clinical examination. Treatment possibilities and ramifications should be discussed with the patient prior to obtaining elaborate diagnostic records. If, on preliminary review, the patient has no interest in treatment, it is far better to stop at this point than after considerable time and money have been spent on a complete diagnostic workup. In addition, if either the surgeon or the orthodontist does not believe that a combined treatment approach has possible merit for the patient, this divergence of initial opinion should be resolved before making complete records and the formal evaluation.

PRETREATMENT RECORDS AND EXAMINATION

The pretreatment diagnostic records for a patient are extremely important for proper diagnosis, for communication among the team members involved in treatment, and for communication of the treatment plan to the patient. In addition, in view of the prevalence of litigation in our society, the importance of excellent pretreatment records for medicolegal reasons cannot be overemphasized. The American Association of Orthodontists has approved a document entitled *Guidelines for Quality Assessment of Orthodontic Care.*[*] These guidelines contain a list of pretreatment diagnostic records that would be a minimum for the orthognathic surgery patient. They list the following eight records:

1. Patient and/or parent/guardian objectives
2. Medical/dental history
3. Clinical examination findings

---

[*] *Guidelines for Quality Assessment of Orthodontic Care.* St. Louis, MO, American Association of Orthodontists, 1988.

4. Dental casts
5. Full-face and profile photographs
6. Intraoral photographs
7. Lateral cephalometric radiograph
8. Complete intraoral or panoramic radiographic coverage

This list concludes with the following statement: "Other diagnostic material/data may be appropriate." When we consider that maxillary deficiency is frequently combined with other facial skeletal malrelationships, it may be viewed as one of the most complex facial deformities, therefore frequently demanding use of other diagnostic material. In patients with multiple sites of craniofacial skeletal imbalance, such as those with particular syndromes, e.g., Crouzon's and Apert's syndromes, computerized tomographic (CT) scanning of the head in the coronal, frontal, and lateral views should be done to define the extent of the deformity as well as to plan the design of the facial skeletal reconstruction. Techniques are available that allow for computerized three-dimensional analysis and shifting of outlined anatomic parts to define the specific shape and volume of bone grafts that will be needed to achieve optimal correction.

Patients who have significant discrepancies between centric relation and centric occlusion may require the use of mounted dental casts for proper evaluation. The casts should be mounted on a hinge-axis articulator with a carefully obtained centric relationship bite. If a significant vertical component to the discrepancy is present or if significant vertical alteration is planned, then a hinge-axis determination should be made.

If, in obtaining the history or during the clinical examination of the patient, temporomandibular joint (TMJ) pathology or symptoms are discovered, the pathology or symptoms should be thoroughly investigated. Tomograms of the joints are recommended if hard tissue pathology is suspected, and magnetic resonance imaging (MRI) should be ordered if disk dysfunction or soft tissue pathology is the suspected cause of symptoms. Intracranial or infratemporal fossa soft tissue pathology may also be ruled out if an MR scan is obtained.

Patients who are candidates for orthognathic surgery are frequently motivated to seek care because of a desire not only to change their facial appearance but also to improve their jaw dysfunction. In the evaluation of this aspect of the patient's concerns, care must be used to determine if the patient's expectations of treatment are realistic. To learn about the individual patient's personality, it is advisable to do an in-depth interview of the patient and/or to use a personality assessment test, such as the Minnesota Multiphasic Personality Inventory (MMPI) (see Chapter 1). Through this assessment, a greater understanding of the patient's concerns and desires will be obtained, and patients with personality characteristics that would contraindicate surgery may be identified and counseled to forgo surgical intervention. This diagnostic information also assists the surgeon and other health care providers in helping the patient deal with the stress of the perioperative and postoperative periods.

DIAGNOSTIC CONSIDERATIONS

The basic concepts of orthodontic treatment for patients with maxillary deficiency are the same as those for other diagnostic categories requiring orthognathic surgery. Briefly, these concepts include placement of teeth over supporting basal bone and removal of dentoalveolar compensations that have occurred with the development of the malocclusion. When possible, one should use arch-wire mechanics that tend to increase the severity of the vertical and/or horizontal aspects of the malocclusion; for example, in the patient with open bite, intrusive forces should be placed on the anterior teeth. This practice allows relapse forces after the completion of treatment to improve the overbite. The same principle should be used for horizontal movement. This type of presurgical mechanics also allows the maximal surgical correction to be accomplished. In many instances of severe maxillary deficiency, arch length analysis may dictate the removal of teeth in the maxillary arch. In addition, compensatory incisor flaring or procumbency may indicate that extraction is needed to provide space to position the teeth upright over the supporting structures.

In a patient with maxillary deficiency in whom there is borderline maxillary arch length deficiency, or in whom retraction of anterior teeth to close an extraction site would place them upright more than desired, a segmentalized surgical procedure should be considered. This procedure allows anterior movement of the posterior segment or segments to complete the space closure and maintain good inclination of the incisors. In addition, in selected cases the maxilla can be segmented to create a small interdental space, increase the arch length, and correct the arch length deficiency more efficiently than does nonextraction. Transverse segmentalization of the maxilla, however, is limited to the routine Le Fort I osteotomy procedure. If quadrangular Le Fort I or Le Fort II osteotomy procedures are planned, a midline osteotomy may be performed for transverse deficiency correction (up to 10 mm in Le Fort I and up to 6 mm in Le Fort II). Generally, the orthodontics is designed to keep the arch intact either by a nonextraction approach or by completing space closure prior to surgery. If this goal is accomplished, significant reduction in operating time and surgical morbidity is realized. Differential extractions may be utilized to advantage, and space closure anchorage, altering mechanics such as adding lingual root torque to the incisor segment, may be needed to obtain the correct amount of anterior and posterior tooth movement.

TREATMENT PLANNING

To provide maximal correction for the patient, it is essential that the orthodontist understand and observe the previously discussed diagnostic concepts. The decision regarding the need for orthognathic surgery in a patient must be made at the time of the original diagnosis and treatment planning so that the orthodontic treatment is not initiated with the idea of "seeing how far we can get" and then finishing with surgery. This type of treatment approach leads to dental compensations, which, if not sufficient to correct the malocclusion, will lead to relapse postsurgically and to an unstable, partially corrected end result. In addition, the opportunity to gain optimal esthetics from the orthognathic surgical procedure is forfeited. This approach may also lead to excessively long treatment times, as efficient tooth movement toward a predetermined goal is not accomplished. The outline in Table 51–1 is a useful guide to the orthodontist and surgeon in treatment planning.

ORTHODONTIC APPLIANCE– CONSTRUCTION CONSIDERATIONS

Orthodontic appliances used for patients undergoing orthognathic surgery should be well constructed and secure so that intermaxillary fixation wires and wiring into an interdental splint can be accomplished without appliance failure. It is recommended that all molars be banded and teeth anterior to the molars be banded or bonded using stainless steel attachments. The use of plastic or ceramic brackets may create problems during the surgery and/or fixation stage of treat-

TABLE 51-1. TREATMENT PLANNING FOR THE ORTHODONTIST AND SURGEON

CONDITION	SOLUTION		
	Le Fort I and Le Fort I Quadrangular	Le Fort II and Le Fort II Quadrangular	Le Fort III
Satisfactory alignment	Place orthodontic appliances with passive arch wire to maintain arches during surgery.	Same	Same
Crowded maxillary arch	a. Expand to achieve alignment if proper inclination of teeth over basal bone can be maintained. b. Extract maxillary first premolars, align, and close space. c. Extract maxillary second premolars, align, and close space. d. Extract maxillary first premolars and utilize a segmentalized surgical procedure to obtain desired inclinations and space closure.	a. Same b. Same c. Same d. Consider an orthodontic compromise or a separate segmental surgical procedure.	a. Same b. Same c. Same d. Consider an orthodontic compromise or a Le Fort I segmentalized secondary procedure for proper space closure, incisor inclination, and further Class III correction if needed.
Maxillary incisor proclination	a. If arch is spaced, close space and position incisors upright. b. If arch is crowded, extract maxillary first premolars, align, and position incisors upright to close space. c. Extract maxillary first premolars and utilize a segmentalized surgical procedure to obtain desired inclinations and space closure.	a. Same b. Same c. Consider an orthodontic compromise or a separate segmental surgical procedure.	a. Same b. Same c. Same
Asymmetric arch	a. Use differential extractions to produce dental arch symmetry; use surgery to correct skeletal asymmetry. b. Use differential extractions and segmental surgery if asymmetry is large.	a. Use differential extractions to produce dental arch symmetry; surgery is limited to 3-mm rotation or side shift. b. Use differential extractions; surgery is limited to 3 mm of rotation or side shift; plan subsequent segmental Le Fort I surgery to achieve greater movement.	a. Use differential extractions to produce dental arch symmetry; first-stage surgery is very limited; plan a subsequent second-stage Le Fort I procedure. b. Use differential extractions; first-stage surgery is very limited; plan subsequent second-stage Le Fort I procedure.

ment if bracket loss or fracture is encountered. Bracket placement on the teeth is typical for the usual orthodontic patient, except in the area of a planned osteotomy. If the osteotomy is to be done between the roots of two adjacent teeth for which no extraction is planned, then it is advisable to tip the brackets on two adjacent teeth so that a straight wire will cause root divergence during the presurgical orthodontic treatment phase (Fig. 51-1). The alternative to this approach is to use arch-wire bends that produce the desired root movements (Fig. 51-2). The advantage of placing the tip in the bracket is that the root movement bends do not have to be incorporated in each arch wire as the wires are changed. The disadvantage is that

FIGURE 51-1. Brackets of the teeth are tipped toward the osteotomy site so that the placement of a straight arch wire will cause root divergence. By permission of Mayo Foundation.

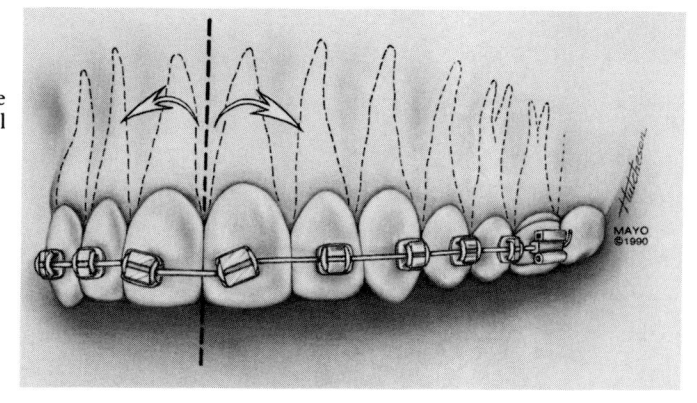

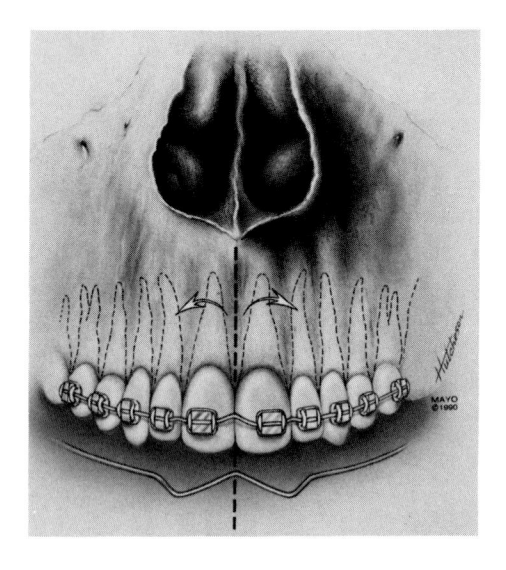

FIGURE 51-2. The arch wire is bent as illustrated to put root-divergence forces on the teeth adjacent to the osteotomy site. By permission of Mayo Foundation.

the brackets must be repositioned or significant reverse arch-wire bends must be placed after surgery during the finishing mechanics. The reverse situation is obviously the case if arch-wire bends are used.

ORTHODONTIC APPLIANCE CONSIDERATIONS AT SURGERY

The use of a maxillary transpalatal arch wire or a mandibular lingual arch wire may be part of the presurgical orthodontic mechanics. These arch wires may be used to control molar rotations, axial inclinations, and arch widths. The lingual arch wires should be removed prior to obtaining the presurgical models so that an accurate impression of the lingual soft tissues is obtained. The interdental or palatal splint serves to maintain arch width corrections during the fixation period.

The labial arch wires that are to be used during the surgical fixation phase of treatment should be passive in contour. The interdental splint, which is carefully constructed and completely seated during surgery, is the appliance used to control arch segments and tooth positions during healing. The arch wires serve as a means of attachment for the interdental wiring. The use of a variety of looped arch wires, soldered spur arch wires, and full-sized rectangular wires has been reported. A round stainless steel arch wire that nearly fills the bracket slot — e.g., 0.016 or 0.018 round wire for 0.018 slotted edgewise brackets or 0.020 or 0.022 for 0.022 edgewise brackets — is usually the arch wire of choice. The round wire is suggested to avoid third-order torque forces that might inadvertently be placed and create unwanted movement during fixation. The intermaxillary wires should be looped around the upper and lower arch wires to distribute the fixation force to the four adjacent brackets rather than directly around the upper and lower brackets (Fig. 51-3). Intermaxillary wire forces placed directly against either bands or bonds will likely dislodge them if these forces are considerable. It is also recommended that 0.010 or 0.012 ligature wires be used for intermaxillary fixation. Very sufficient

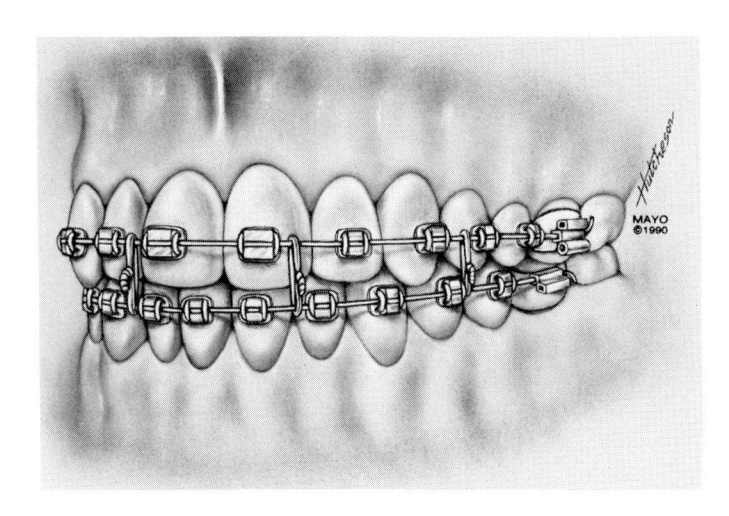

FIGURE 51-3. The intermaxillary wires are placed around the arch wire between the brackets to distribute the force to the four adjacent brackets. By permission of Mayo Foundation.

intermaxillary forces can be developed between the arch wires with this size of wire ligature, and the risk of bracket or bond dislodgment is reduced. Use of intermaxillary wires to force surgical segments into the surgical splint is to be discouraged. Bracket breakage and orthodontic relapse from inadvertent tooth movement are undesirable sequelae.

POSTSURGICAL ORTHODONTIC APPLIANCE MANIPULATION

The use of a carefully constructed, good-fitting interdental splint during the 6-week postsurgical healing phase dictates that passive arch-wire mechanics are indicated, and the only orthodontics needed is for the maintenance of appliance security and comfort of the patient. If rigid fixation devices are used and intermaxillary fixation is maintained for a period of only 7 to 10 days, then light vertical elastic forces on the canines with a Class III component of force should be used in conjunction with the interdental splint as a muscle-training device. The amount and direction of the forces should be carefully considered before application. In the patient with vertical excess in whom maxillary impaction has been accomplished, very minimal vertical forces should be employed, whereas in the patient with deep bite conditions, considerable vertical elastic force in the molar regions may encourage desirable posterior tooth extrusion.

At 6 weeks, the interdental splint should be removed, and the training elastics should be continued for another 1 or 2 weeks. At this time, active finishing orthodontic mechanics may be initiated. If tipped brackets were used presurgically in osteotomy sites, these should be removed and replaced with brackets in the ideal position or slightly tipped in the reverse direction to achieve good root parallelism in the finished occlusion. Intermaxillary elastic traction may be utilized as needed to achieve the final interdigitation of the posterior teeth and the desired midline and overbite-overjet corrections. The patient's occlusal relationship should be completed with as modest an overcorrection as possible in all dimensions.

RETENTION CONSIDERATIONS FOR THE MAXILLARY-DEFICIENT PATIENT

The tooth positioner appliance is used by many orthodontists as the initial finishing retainer. This tooth positioner can be utilized in the maxillary-deficient patient for a short time (2 to 6 weeks) immediately after appliance removal but should not be relied upon on a long-term basis. In cases in which significant transverse corrections have been accomplished, fixed banded or bonded lingual arch retainers are desirable. The lingual arch-wire retainer can be bonded to numerous teeth as needed to maintain space closure rotations, or it can be combined with a removable Hawley-type retainer. It should be recognized that in maxillary advancement procedures significant soft tissue stretch may be present and will require long-term retention. In the higher level Le Fort procedures, use of a face mask for continued anterior traction (from a fixed lingual arch) may be indicated.

QUANDRANGULAR LE FORT I AND II OSTEOTOMIES
E. E. KELLER

Maxillofacial osteotomy procedures approximating anatomically the Guerin-Le Fort fracture classification for correction of midfacial deficiency have been described and modified by surgeons since the late 1920s. The first Le Fort osteotomy was described by Wassmund[1] in 1927 and was performed at the Le Fort I level for correction of a skeletal open-bite deformity. In 1950, Sir Harold Gillies and Harrison[2] performed a Le Fort osteotomy approximating the Le Fort III level for correction of a midfacial deficiency. In 1970, Converse and colleagues[3] described an osteotomy somewhat approximating the classic Le Fort II fracture. Anatomically, this osteotomy included the premaxilla and nasal complex. This osteotomy was biologically and anatomically flawed and has not been reported by subsequent authors. In 1973, Henderson and Jackson[4] presented a landmark paper describing a classic Le Fort II osteotomy that anatomically approximated the Guerin-Le Fort II fracture classification. This procedure was performed through cutaneous and intraoral incisions and included the nasomaxillary complex medial to the infraorbital foramen. As described in their original article,[4] a majority of the infraorbital rim and the total zygomatic complex were left intact. Since a majority of midface-deficient patients require infraorbital and zygomatic advancement, the original Le Fort II procedure described by Henderson and Jackson[4] has been utilized infrequently by oral-maxillofacial surgeons. In contrast, the quadrangular Le Fort II osteotomy, first described by Kufner[5] in 1971, and the high Le Fort I osteotomy, first described by Obwegesser[6] in 1969 and named the quadrangular Le Fort I osteotomy by Keller and Sather[7] in 1989, allowed advancement or augmentation, or both, of the infraorbital rim and a portion of the zygomatic complex. Of major significance is that quadrangular Le Fort I and II osteotomies are performed totally via a transoral approach. This chapter reviews the development, clinical indications, surgical technique, immediate postoperative management, and clinical examples of the quadrangular Le Fort I and quadrangular Le Fort II osteotomies.

QUADRANGULAR LE FORT I OSTEOTOMY

Review of Literature

In 1969, Obwegesser[6] described a Le Fort I osteotomy procedure in which bone cuts were made "as high as possible, from the tuberosity area around the whole maxilla, staying just beneath the infraorbital foramen." Stabilizing bone grafts were placed posteriorly between the pterygoid process of the sphenoid bone and palatine bone and the advanced mobilized maxilla. In addition, bone graft placement was provided anteriorly "from the zygomatic rest to the piriform aperture." Obwegesser[6] acknowledged the large antral communication with the bone graft when it was placed in this manner but indicated healing was uncomplicated, "as shown by Gillies."[8] He also indicated that bone grafts could be extended superiorly to lie as an onlay graft on the infraorbital rim, providing an esthetic benefit as well as skeletal stability (interpositional portion inferiorly) for the advanced maxillary segment.

Keller and Sather[7] performed a high modified Le Fort I osteotomy and reported their experience (1989) in 54 consecutive patients. They utilized the Le Fort I osteotomy as described by Obwegesser. Following complete mobilization and advancement, iliac bone grafts were placed on the infraorbital rim and zygoma superiorly (onlay) and extending into the maxillary antrum posterior to the anterior antral wall (interpositional) inferiorly. This procedure was named the quadrangular Le Fort I osteotomy because its indications, osteotomy shape and level, and projected clinical outcome were quite similar to those of the quadrangular Le Fort II osteotomy described initially by Kufner[5] and later modified by Souyris and associates,[9] Champy,[10] Steinhauser,[11] and Keller and Sather.[12]

Indications

Patients with maxillary-zygomatic horizontal deficiency on clinical and cephalometric examination who have a Class III skeletal malocclusion but exhibit a normal nasal projection are potential candidates for the quadrangular Le Fort I osteotomy. Unless these patients have a coexisting mandibular protrusion, they typically have a normal or shortened throat length. In contrast to patients in whom the quadrangular Le Fort II osteotomy is performed, patients who have undergone a quadrangular Le Fort I procedure may also exhibit significant maxillary midline shift (>5 mm) or significant transverse deficiency (>5 mm). In addition, this procedure (quadrangular Le Fort I osteotomy) offers increased versatility in those patients with significant maxillary vertical excess or deficiency. Since the inferior orbital rims are not mobilized with this osteotomy, its versatility is increased significantly over that of the quadrangular Le Fort II procedure (where the infraorbital rim is attached to the mobilized segment).

Surgical Procedure (Fig. 51-4)

After induction of general anesthesia, nasoendotracheal intubation, and preparation for an intraoral procedure, an incision is made approximately 4 mm above the mucogingival junction from the right to the left first premolar. The entire surface of the anterior maxilla is exposed by subperiosteal dissection extending from the right to the left posterior tuberosity and superiorly to the infraorbital rim (identical to the exposure provided in the quadrangular Le Fort II osteotomy procedure). The infraorbital nerve is completely isolated, and the orbital rim periosteum is completely reflected to allow passive placement of the interpositional-onlay iliac bone graft. Care is taken not to violate the periorbita or infraorbital nerve. The mucosa of the floor of the nose is elevated to expose the maxillary rostrum. It is important to maintain the integrity of the nasal mucosa, especially in patients in whom significant surgical widening (two-piece osteotomy) is accomplished. At this time, the cartilaginous septum and vomer are separated from the palatal midline by curette anteriorly and chisel posteriorly (Fig. 51-4). The maxillary rostrum is then removed by chisel technique. The latter significantly increases access and visibility for exposure of the remainder of the nasal floor and lateral wall. The lateral nasal wall and posterior nasal floor are exposed by subperiosteal dissection up to and frequently above the anterior attachment of the inferior turbinate and posteriorly to expose the posterior nasal spine and area where the palatine artery is identified after downfracture (Fig. 51-4).

An osteotomy cut is placed bilaterally with an oscillating saw through the piri-

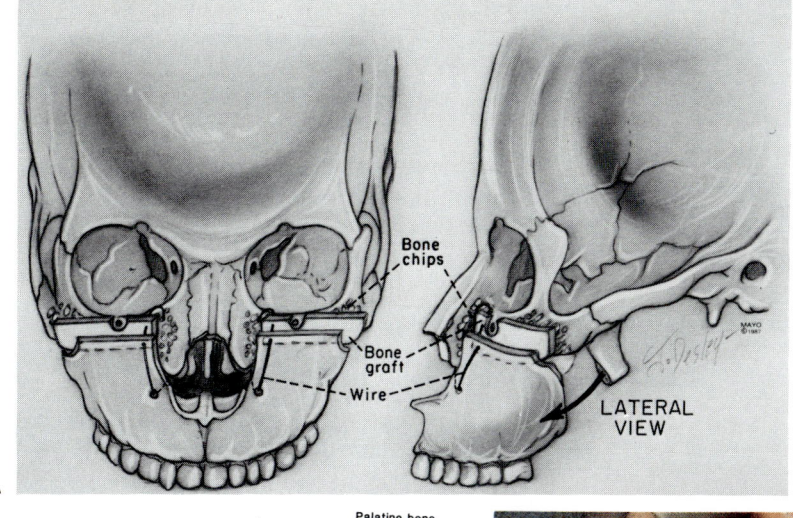

FIGURE 51–4. QUADRANGULAR LE FORT I OSTEOTOMY. *A*, Diagram illustrating quadrangular Le Fort I osteotomy level, bone graft placement, and transosseous wire stabilization. *B*, Diagram illustrating the downfracture exposure and identification of the palatine artery in the posterolateral nasal wall. Paperthin bone (palatine bone) separates the vessel from the antrum (laterally) and nasal cavity (medially). *C*, Diagram illustrating the mobilization of the maxilla with a transpalatal wire traction and retrotuberosity and retronasal finger dissection. *D, E, F,* Intraoperative photographs illustrating lateral osteotomy position, nasal floor exposure, and lateral interpositional bone graft position).

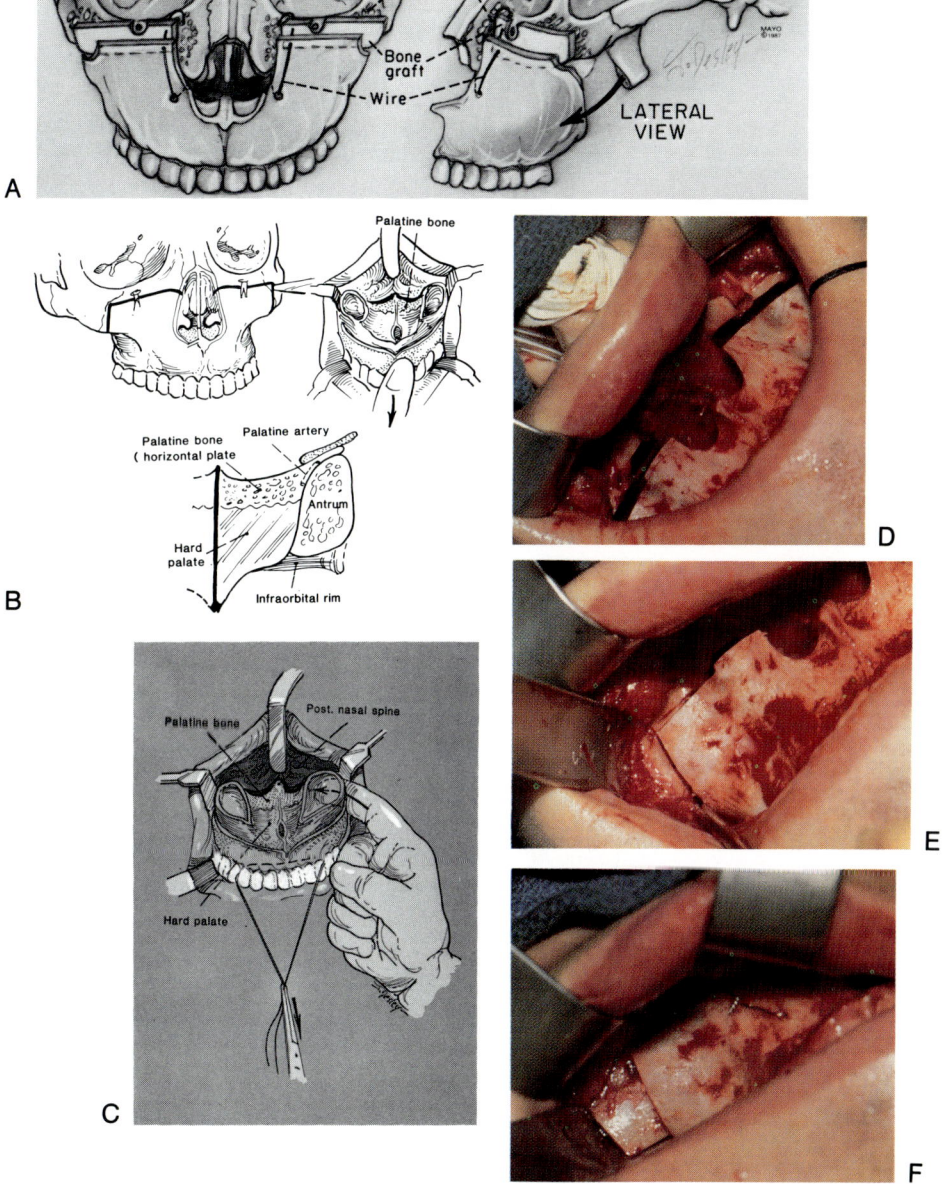

form aperture at the level of the infraorbital nerve and is extended laterally just below the infraorbital foramen to the tuberosity–pterygoid plate region posteriorly (Fig. 51–4). An inferior step in the osteotomy cut is frequently necessary at the anterior margin of the maxillary buttress. Because of the high position of the osteotomy, the posterior osteotomy may need to be accomplished by chisel technique.

The maxilla is then downfractured by finger pressure and completely mobilized (by a disimpaction forceps in selected cases). Pterygoid chisels have not been used to date, as the fracture line consistently follows the maxillary-palatine fissure laterally and fractures (greenstick) occur transversely across the palatine bone medial and posterior to the palatine foramen. The palatine vessels are then identified, isolated, and cauterized (Fig. 51–4). With the maxilla suspended forward with a transpalatal wire, all posterior palatal and tuberosity soft tissue attachments are released by finger dissection (Fig. 51–4). The maxilla is placed passively into a prefabricated splint, and maxillomandibular fixation is applied. The splint is kept as small as possible (interocclusal) to permit oral (versus nasal) air exchange if needed postoperatively. If segmentalization is performed, the splint is extended to cover, but not contact, the palatal tissues.

The cartilaginous septum and vomer are exposed in the midline with a sharp molt curette, and deflections, if present, are corrected by excision-incision techniques. Vertical septal height reductions are also accomplished at this time. Inferior vomer bone spurs are frequently encountered and removed. The nasal midline wound is closed by continuous suture beginning just posterior to the nasopalatine vessels and extending anteriorly to cover the exposed cartilaginous septum completely. Nasal mucosal defects, if present, are closed with interrupted suture (everted nasally). Transosseous suspension wires are placed from the medial orbital rim to the inferior portion of the piriform aperture. Modified channel retractors are utilized above the oribital rim to facilitate transosseous wire placement and protect the globe. These wires are not tightened at this stage. In advancement cases, the proper vertical force is applied when the wire is placed as far posterior as possible on the piriform aperture of the mobilized segment. This position frequently is just mesial or distal to the cuspid root. Segmentalization (two piece) is also done in selected patients in whom transverse deficiency is present. When width increases in the 7- to 10-mm range are required, it is frequently necessary to incise the palatal tissue longitudinally to get passive seating of the segments in the palatal-intraocclusal splint. The osteotomy is also placed in the midline (rather than parapalatal). If the nasal mucosa has not been violated, predictable healing without oronasal fistula will occur. Thin segments of bone from the lateral nasal wall are placed over the midline osseous palatal defect (when present) as autogenous bone grafts prior to final positioning and tightening of the transosseous wires.

Block corticocancellous bone grafts are harvested from the superomedial anterior iliac crest and placed as an onlay-interpositional stabilizing block (Fig. 51–4). The proper bone graft width (amount of maxillary advancement) can, in selected cases, be measured directly in situ, as the maxilla at this stage may be fixed to the stable mandible, which has not been operated on. In bimaxillary osteotomy cases, the mandibular procedure is accomplished either before or after the maxillary procedure, and skeletal fixation is applied (using threaded pins). An interim splint may be used in selected cases in which it is desirable to stabilize the mobilized maxilla prior to performing the mandibular osteotomy. Careful preoperative and intraoperative measurements allow accurate maxillary positioning and osseous anatomic approximation. When an interim splint is not used in bimaxillary procedures, the surgeon is offered the flexibility of positioning the maxilla to maximize bone contacts and bone graft stability without significantly altering the surgical and orthodontic objectives. In this situation, the mandibular procedure is performed after final maxillary positioning. Avoidance of an interim splint also prevents potential errors of incomplete condylar seating during bite registration. The bone graft extends to the superior level of the infraorbital rim and extends laterally to cover the zygomatic prominence to various degrees, depending on the cosmetic requirements in individual cases. Proper and equal bilateral contouring of the blocks is important, as irregular and unequal contours are noticeable in the midface after resolution of edema. The bone graft corticocancellous blocks are also notched to accommodate the infraorbital nerve. After final bone graft contouring, the transosseous suspension wires are placed through the graft for graft stabilization, and the mandible-maxilla is autorotated into the correct vertical position (when only the maxilla is operated on or when the mandible is operated on first). In vertical augmentation cases, the correct vertical height of the mobilized segment and bone graft is determined intraoperatively by direct measurement from bone marks placed before the osteotomy.

After the correct height is determined by observation of lip and tooth position through the use of extraoral vertical referents, bone measurements, and preoperative clinical measurements, the transosseous suspension wires are tightened. At this stage, accuracy is very important; overshortening is quite possible because vertical bone stops may be absent when significant maxillary advancement has been accomplished. Additional transosseous iliac graft stabilizing wires are placed laterally on the zygomatic buttress in most cases. Miniplate or screw skeletal fixation devices may also be utilized in selected cases to stabilize further the lateral graft to the advanced maxilla or underlying zygoma. Cancellous chips are then packed in the lateral nasal and lateral orbital-zygoma areas to achieve a symmetric contour and to eliminate dead space. Two to four long-acting (polyglycolic acid) resorbable sutures are placed to approximate the midline nasal and lip musculature, which in turn helps achieve desirable alar width. Sutures placed previously to close the midline nasal wound also assist in achieving stability of the alar wings. The mucosal incision is closed in a watertight fashion with a continuous horizontal mattress suture and an overlying continuous baseball stitch. Mucosal V-Y closure is not used because the midline lip-nasal muscle closure has already provided the desired lip-nasal width and esthetics.

In recent years, coinciding with the use of skeletal fixation, intermaxillary fixation time has been reduced when mandibular osteotomy procedures are accomplished in the same surgical setting. Skeletal miniplate fixation of both the quadrangular Le Fort I and the quadrangular Le Fort II osteotomies is technically difficult because of the high level of the osseous cut and has not been possible in the author's experience to date; however, the stabilizing interpositional graft has allowed us to reduce the intermaxillary fixation time in most patients to 2 or 3 weeks. Light anterior vertical intermaxillary elastics in concert with the surgical splint are maintained in most cases up to 6 weeks, and the patients are allowed a pureed soft diet during this period of limited function. The splint may be removed during oral intake or brief periods of social or work-related activities to improve esthetics and phonetics. When segmentalization is performed (particularly when significant widening is accomplished), the splint is kept wired to the maxillary teeth 6 to 8 weeks, irrespective of the intermaxillary fixation period. For postsurgical management, refer to Immediate Postsurgical Management under Quadrangular Le Fort II Osteotomy, further on.

Patient Presentations

PATIENT NUMBER 1 (Fig. 51-5)

This 17-year-old boy presented to his orthodontist with a Class III skeletal malocclusion. Facial growth and development were judged to be complete.

CLINICAL EVALUATION
Facial Analysis (Fig. 51-5A)

1. The profile is pseudoprognathic secondary to normal throat length and deficiency of the infraorbital, paranasal, and zygomatic anatomy.
2. The face is long and tapering, with lip incompetence secondary to horizontal jaw growth discrepancy and increased anterior mandibular vertical height.
3. Facial symmetry was satisfactory except for a slight (2 to 3 mm) left deviation of the chin.
4. The nose had normal projection and acceptable form but was narrow inferiorly.

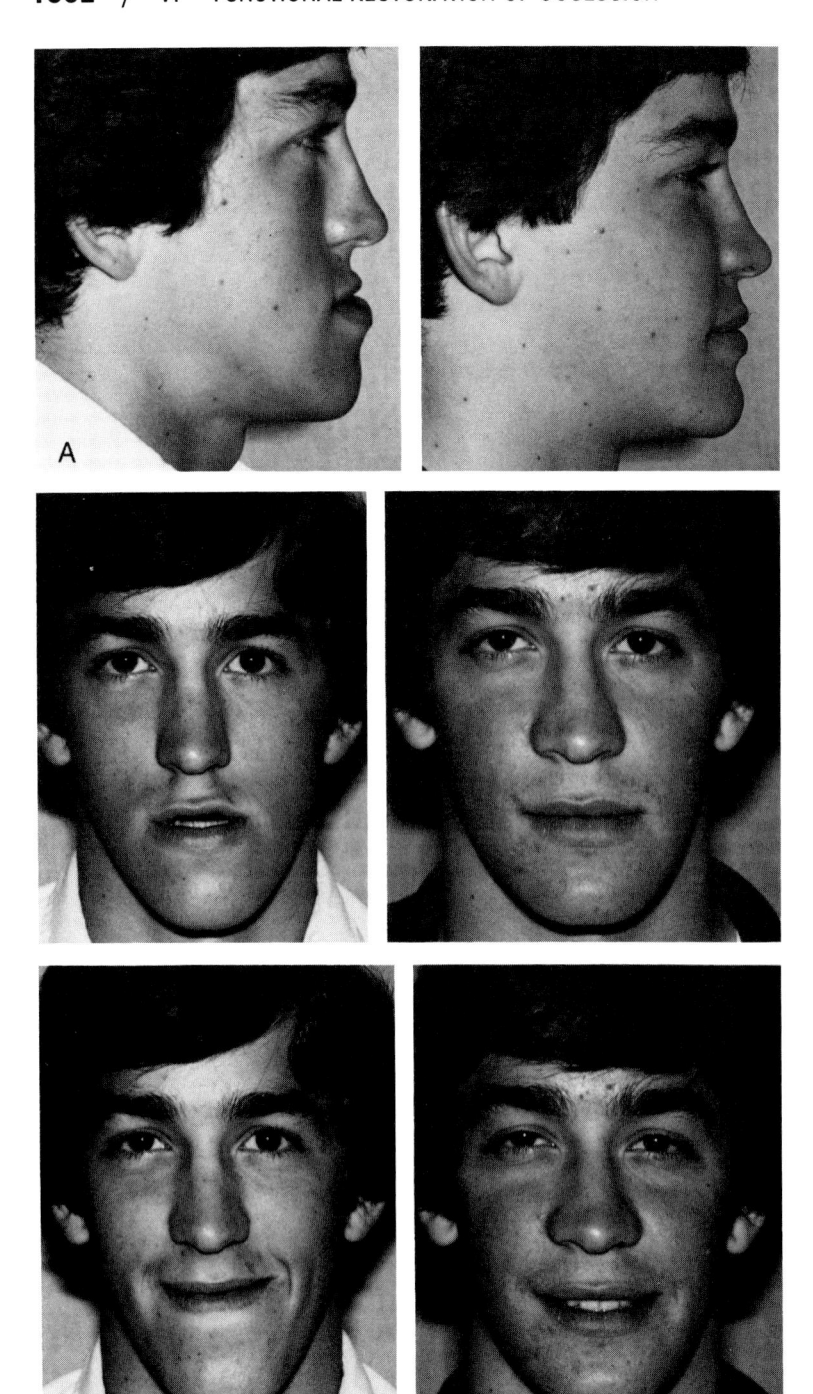

FIGURE 51–5. *A*, Pretreatment *(left)* and 4-year post-treatment *(right)* lateral *(upper)*, anterior *(middle)*, and anterior with smile *(lower)* facial views. Note infraorbital, paranasal, and zygomatic augmentation. Also note improvement in the lower lip-chin relationship secondary to an anterior horizontal osteotomy of the mandible.

5. The lower lip appeared prominent because of the horizontal pogonion deficiency and increased anterior mandibular vertical height.

6. The upper lip had normal length and thickness but was redundant from maxillary horizontal deficiency; the nasolabial angle was acute.

Cephalometric Analysis (Fig. 51–5*B*, left)

1. Class III skeletal open-bite pattern.
2. Maxillary horizontal deficiency (vertical height normal).
3. Mild mandibular horizontal excess.
4. Horizontal deficiency of pogonion.
5. Mandibular anterior vertical excess.

Occlusal Analysis (Fig. 51–5C)

1. Class III cuspid and molar relationship.
2. Crossbite (bilateral posterior and anterior).
3. Missing teeth (maxillary right lateral incisor).
4. Dental midlines normal in relation to face and each other.

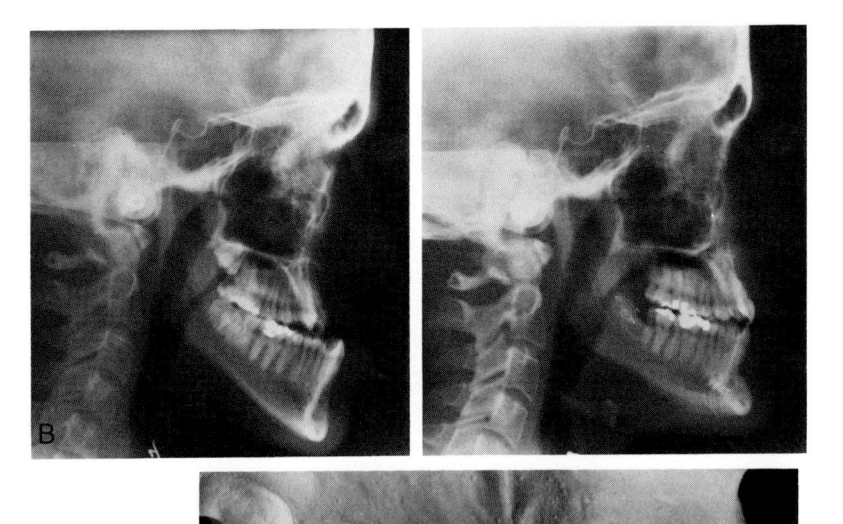

FIGURE 51–5 *Continued. B,* Pretreatment *(left)* and 4-year post-treatment *(right)* lateral cephalograms. Infraorbital transosseous wires were removed in this patient, as they were extended to the orthodontic arch wire (rather than piriform aperture) in the early case (1981). Also note the mandibular transosseous wiring. *C,* Pretreatment dental occlusion (note the missing maxillary right lateral incisor).

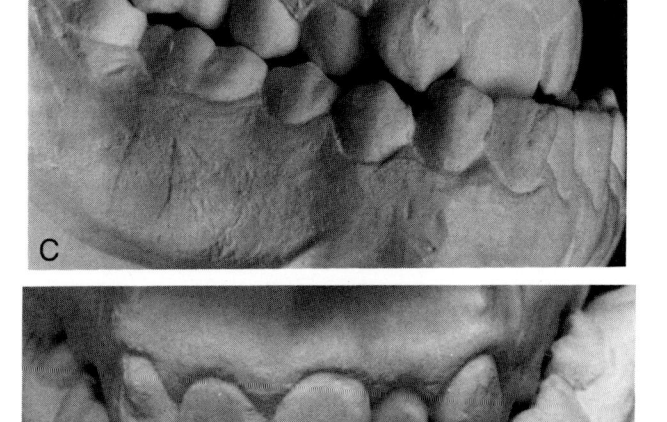

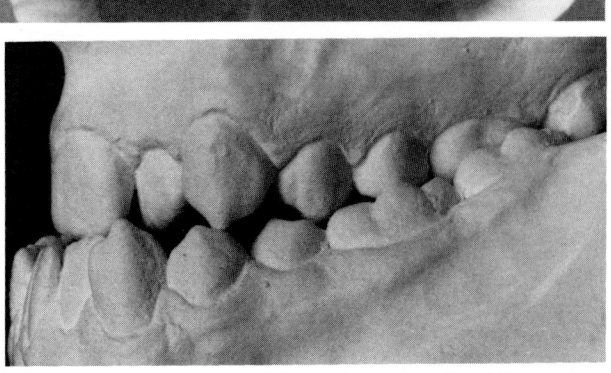

Illustration continued on following page

1804 / VI—FUNCTIONAL RESTORATION OF OCCLUSION

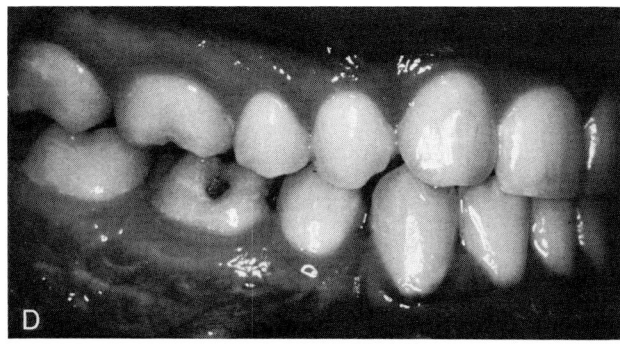

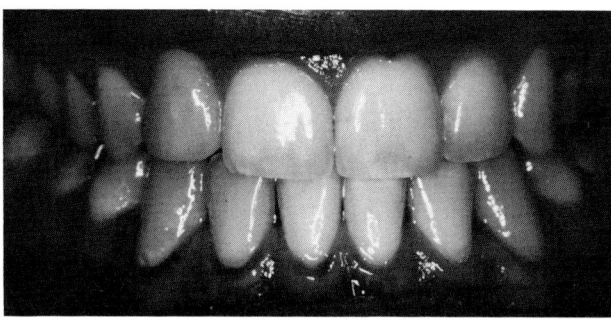

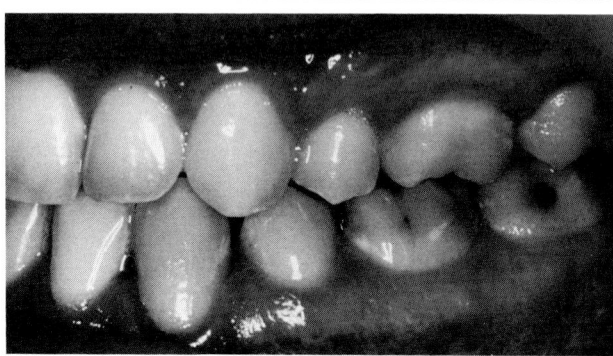

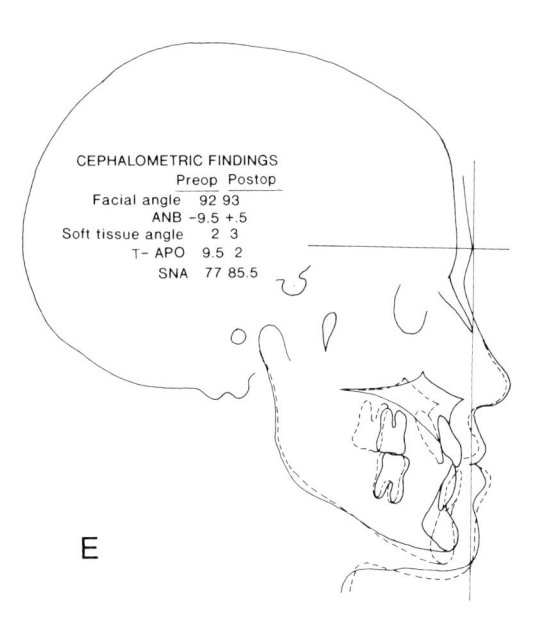

FIGURE 51–5 *Continued.* *D*, Post-treatment dental occlusion (note recontouring and positioning of the maxillary right cuspid to mimic the missing lateral incisor). *E*, Pretreatment *(dashed line)* and 4-year postsurgical *(solid line)* composite tracing of the lateral cephalogram with abbreviated cephalometric analysis and subnasale-vertical reference line. Note the nasal tip and upper lip advancement following maxillary advancement osteotomy. (Orthodontic treatment was provided by Dr. Donald Nelson, Section of Orthodontics, Mayo Clinic, Rochester, MN.)

Presurgical Orthodontic Treatment

1. Tooth removal (maxillary left first bicuspid and mandibular right and left first bicuspids).
2. Maxillary arch: first bicuspid extraction site closed and maxillary right cuspid rotated to simulate lateral incisor.
3. Mandibular arch: segmented alignment of anterior teeth, leaving bilateral osteotomy sites in first premolar area.
4. Eleven months in duration.

Surgical Treatment (Fig. 51–5*B*, right; age 18)

1. Maxillary quadrangular Le Fort I osteotomy with advancement (8 mm).
2. Iliac bone graft (autogenous for infraorbital and zygomatic augmentation onlay) and osteotomy stabilization (interpositional).
3. Mandibular bilateral ramus sagittal osteotomy (3-mm setback).
4. Mandibular bilateral body osteotomy (space closure and posterior segment uprighting).
5. Mandibular anterior horizontal osteotomy for vertical reduction (6 mm) and advancement (8 mm).
6. Intermaxillary fixation maintained five weeks; anterior vertical training elastics maintained an additional 3 weeks.

Postsurgical Orthodontic Treatment

1. Mandibular arch: parallel roots in osteotomy sites and coordination of arch form; establishment of final interdigitation.
2. Maxillary arch: detailing arch form and coordinating with mandibular teeth.
3. Twelve months in duration.

Treatment Results (Fig. 51–5A, D, and E)

1. Excellent skeletal and dental stability was documented at 4-year postsurgical examination.
2. No treatment or post-treatment complications were identified.
3. Esthetic and functional improvements were substantial.
4. Midfacial augmentation in concert with anterior mandibular height reduction produced a straight (rather than concave) lateral facial profile and a more square masculine anterior facial profile.

PATIENT NUMBER 2 (Fig. 51–6)

This 14½-year-old girl presented to her orthodontist with a Class III skeletal malocclusion. Facial growth and development were judged to be near completion, so orthodontic treatment was initiated; growth was complete 18 months later at the surgical date.

CLINICAL EVALUATION

Facial Analysis (Fig. 51–6A)

1. The profile was pseudoprognathic, with a normal throat length and mild to moderate deficiency of the infraorbital, paranasal, and zygomatic anatomy.
2. The face was mildly long and square, with tapering in the lower one third.
3. The nose had normal form and projection.
4. The upper lip had normal form and protrusion; the maxillary incisors were 5 mm below the inferior edge.
5. The lower lip was prominent from lower incisor protrusion.

Cephalometric Analysis (Fig. 51–6B, left, and E)

1. Class III skeletal open-bite pattern.
2. Moderate maxillary horizontal deficiency and mild vertical hyperplasia.
3. Prominent bony pogonion with normal soft tissue covering form.
4. Mild mandibular horizontal excess.

Occlusal Analysis (Fig. 51–6C)

1. Class III molar and cuspid relationship.
2. Crossbite (bilateral posterior and anterior).
3. Impacted right maxillary cuspid.
3. Dental midlines normal in relation to face and each other.

Presurgical Orthodontic Treatment (Fig. 51–6B, right)

1. Impacted maxillary right cuspid and left first bicuspid removal.
2. Maxillary arch: extraction sites closed and normal arch form established; minimal posterior arch expansion.
3. Mandibular arch: leveling of occlusal plane and arch form coordination.
4. Eighteen months in duration.

Surgical Treatment (Fig. 51–6B, right; age 16 years)

1. Maxillary quadrangular Le Fort I osteotomy with advancement (5 mm) and vertical impaction (4 mm anterior and 5 mm posterior).
2. Mandibular bilateral ramus sagittal osteotomy (5-mm setback).
3. Septoplasty (septum reduced 5 mm).
4. Intermaxillary fixation maintained 4 weeks; anterior vertical training elastics maintained an additional 2 weeks.
5. Bone grafting not required because of the high-level osteotomy (infraorbital foramen level) with simultaneous vertical impaction of 5 mm and advancement of 5 mm.

Postsurgical Orthodontic Treatment

1. Establishment of final interdigitation and arch form coordination with fixed appliances.
2. Twelve months in duration.

Treatment Results (Fig. 51–6A, D, and E)

1. Three-year postsurgial examination documented skeletal and dental stability (except for posterior transverse dimensions, where a mild relapse was noted).
2. Facial esthetics were significantly improved in the midface, where augmentation and vertical reduction produced a more convex profile and a more tapering anterior profile.
3. No surgical or orthodontic compromise or complications were encountered, and the patient was very pleased with the cosmetic and functional improvement.

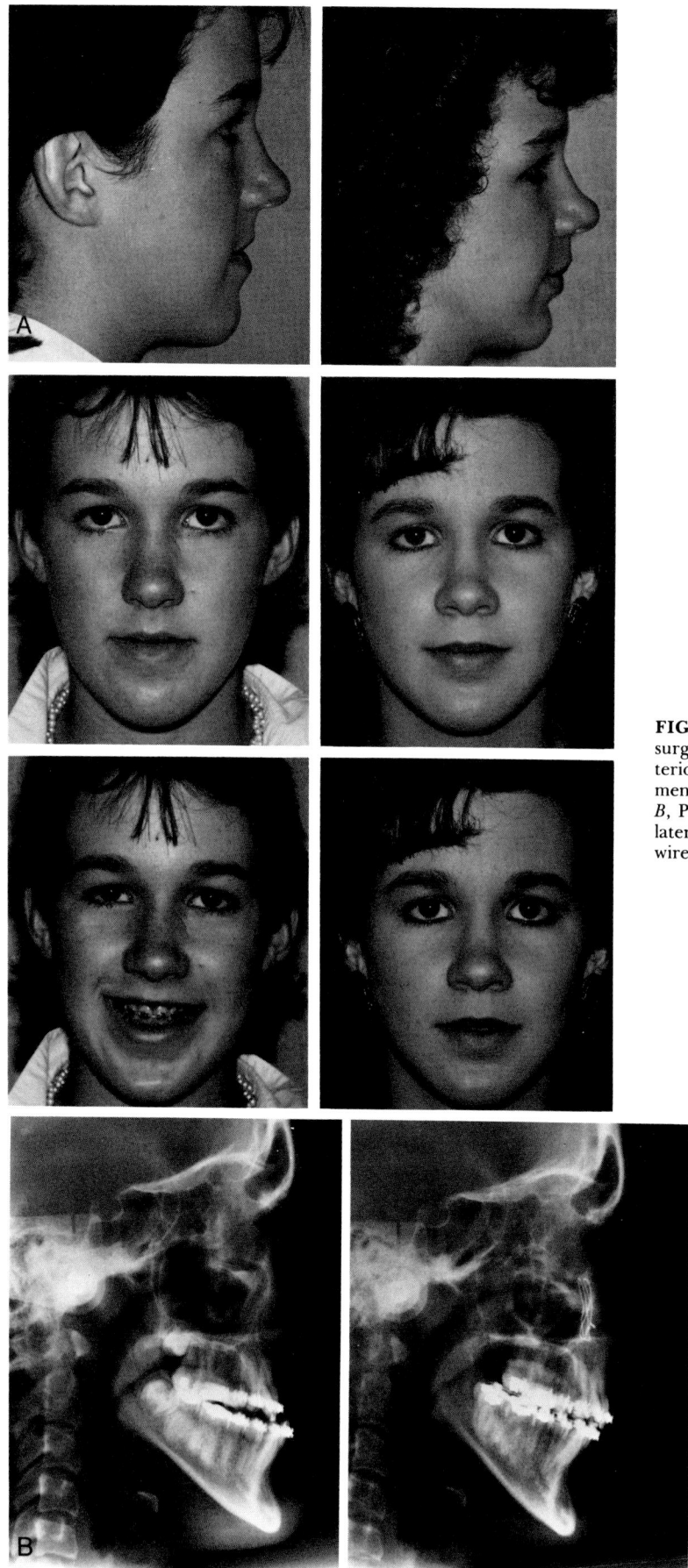

FIGURE 51–6. *A*, Presurgical *(left)* and 3-year postsurgical *(right)* lateral *(upper)*, anterior *(middle)*, and anterior with smile *(lower)* facial views. Note the improvement in midfacial esthetics and change in facial form. *B*, Presurgical *(left)* and 12-month postsurgical *(right)* lateral cephalograms. Note the maxillary transosseous wires.

FIGURE 51–6 *Continued. C,* Presurgical dental occlusion. *D,* Post-treatment (3-year postsurgical) dental occlusion. *E,* Presurgical *(dashed line)* and 3-year postsurgical *(solid line)* composite tracing of the lateral cephalogram with abbreviated cephalometric analysis and subnasale-vertical reference line. (Orthodontic treatment was provided by Gary B. Blodgett, D.D.S., Mason City, IA.)

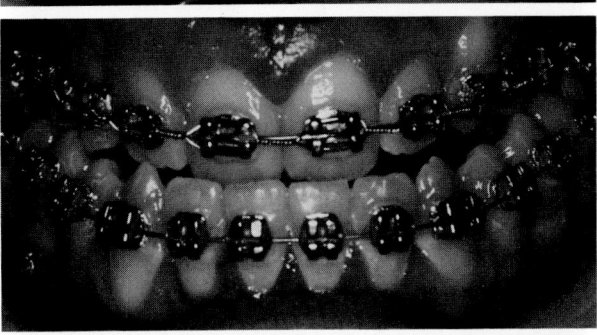

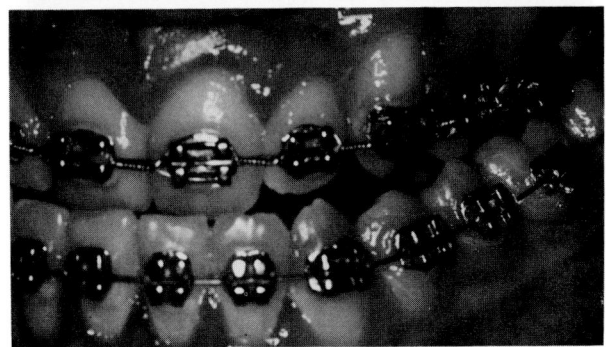

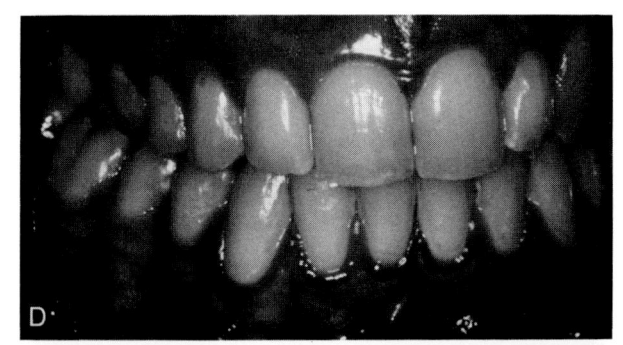

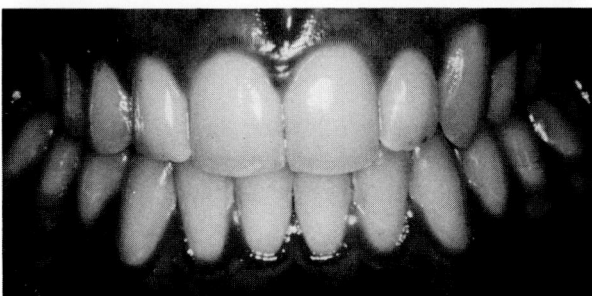

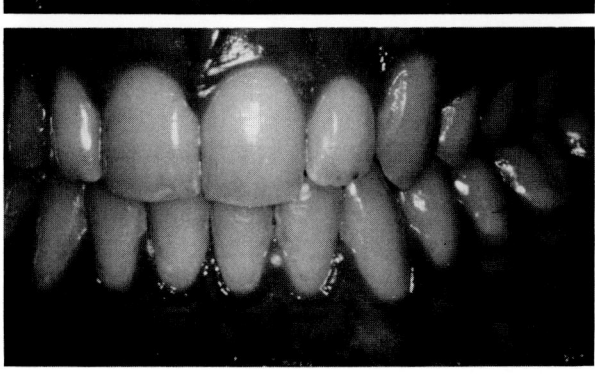

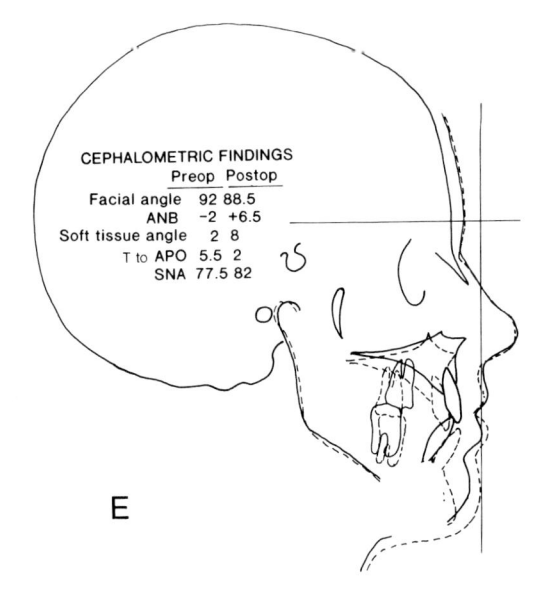

CEPHALOMETRIC FINDINGS
	Preop	Postop
Facial angle	92	88.5
ANB	−2	+6.5
Soft tissue angle	2	8
T to APO	5.5	2
SNA	77.5	82

1808 / VI—FUNCTIONAL RESTORATION OF OCCLUSION

PATIENT NUMBER 3 (Fig. 51–7)

This 15-year-old girl presented to her orthodontist with a Class III skeletal malocclusion. After 1 year of growth observation, orthodontic treatment was initiated. At age 17 (surgical date), facial growth stability was documented by cephalometric analysis.

CLINICAL EVALUATION

Facial Analysis (Fig. 51–7A)

1. The profile was prognathic secondary to moderate midfacial deficiency (infraorbital, paranasal, zygomatic maxillary) and mild mandibular protrusion. Throat length was minimally increased.
2. This patient had a tapering facial form and normal symmetry.
3. Nasal form and projection were acceptable.

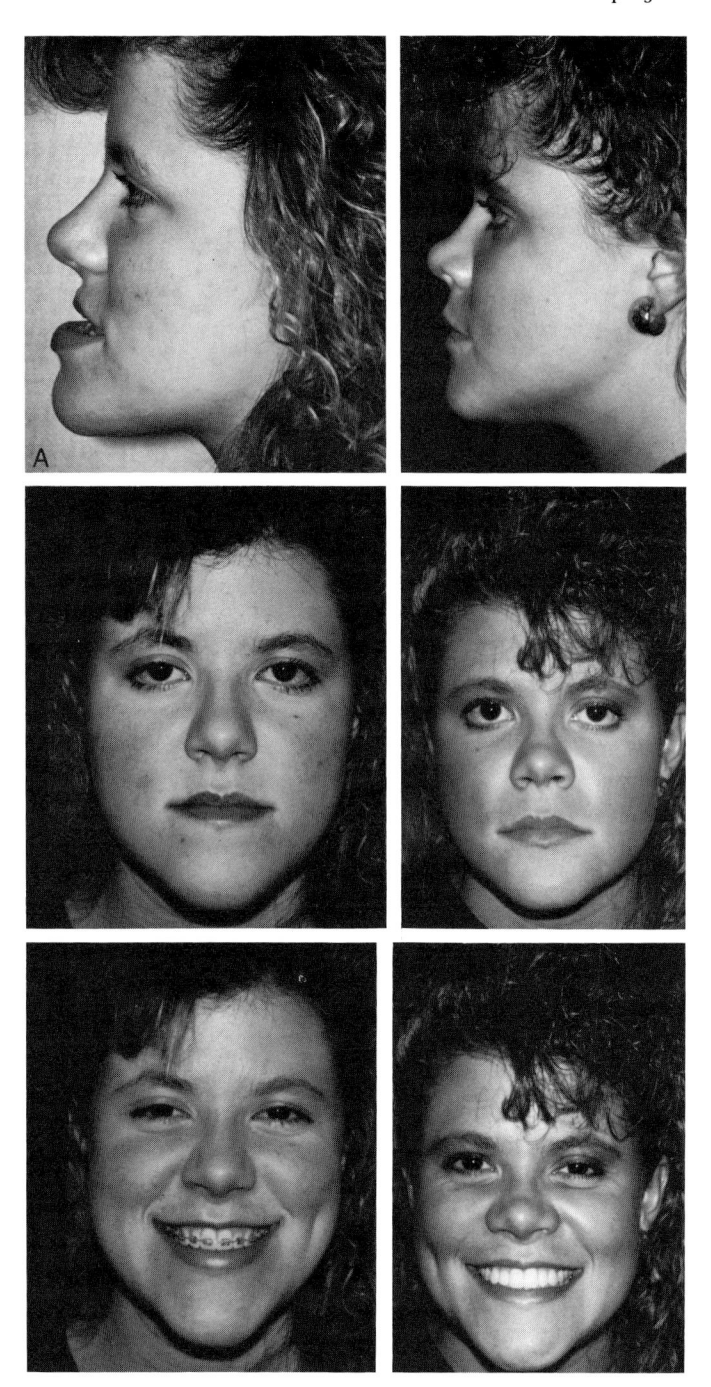

FIGURE 51–7. *A*, Presurgical *(left)* and 18-month postsurgical *(right)* lateral *(upper)*, anterior *(middle)*, and anterior with smile *(lower)* facial views. Note the change in midfacial esthetics; also, alar width was unchanged following maxillary advancement.

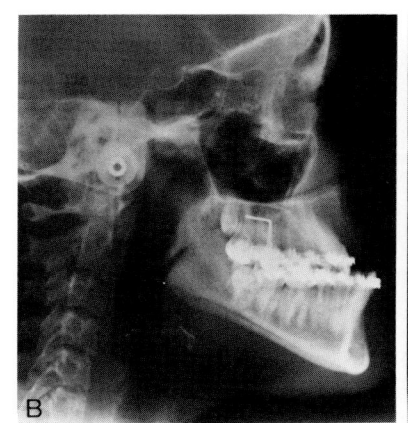

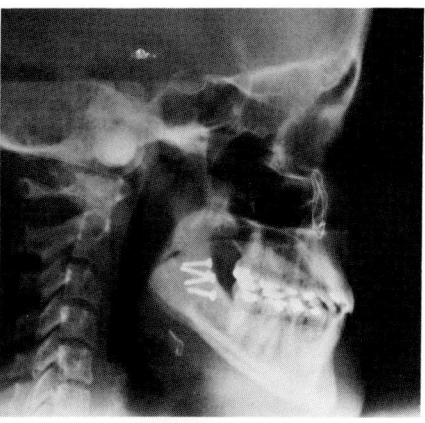

FIGURE 51–7 *Continued. B,* Presurgical *(left)* and 18-month postsurgical *(right)* lateral cephalograms. Note the maxillary transosseous wires and mandibular skeletal fixation screws. *C,* Presurgical dental occlusion.

Illustration continued on following page

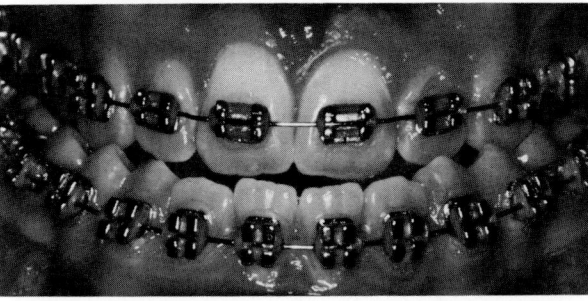

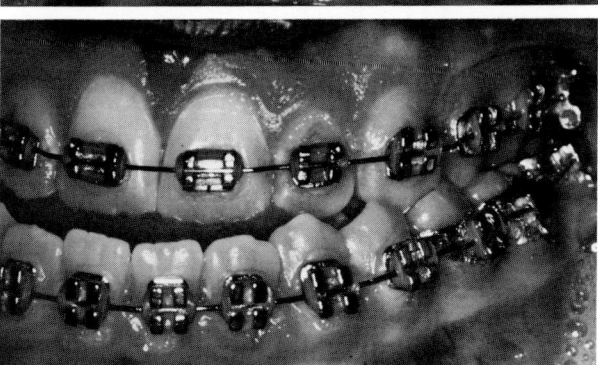

4. Vertical facial height and vertical facial proportions were normal.
5. Lip incompetence (3 mm) was related to horizontal jaw discrepancy. Lip form, size, and position at rest were normal.

Cephalometric Analysis (Fig. 51–7B, left, and E)

1. Class III skeletal pattern.
2. Maxillary horizontal deficiency.
3. Mandibular protrusion.
4. Normal facial height size and proportion.
5. Normal soft and hard tissue pogonion.

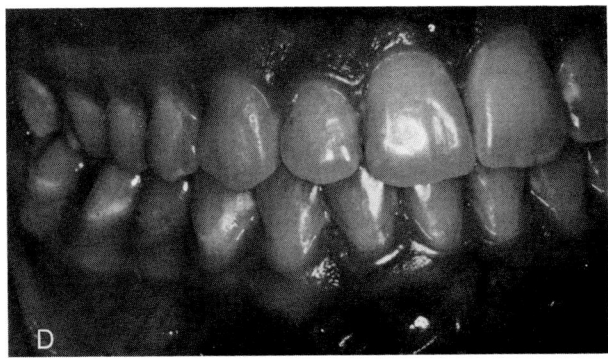

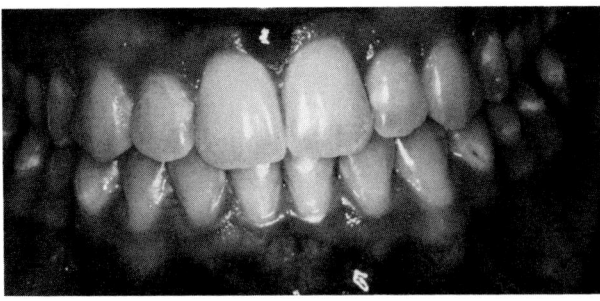

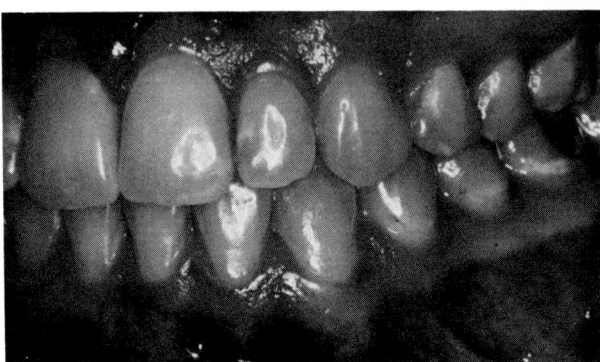

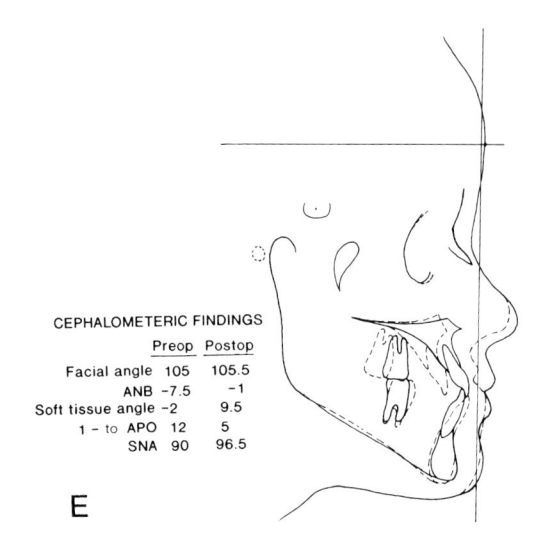

FIGURE 51–7 *Continued.* D, Postsurgical (18 months) dental occlusion. E, Presurgical *(dashed line)* and 18-month postsurgical *(solid line)* composite tracing of the lateral cephalograms with abbreviated cephalometric analysis and subnasale reference line. Note significant nasal tip and upper lip advancement following maxillary Le Fort I advancement; also note that the nasolabial angle remained unchanged. (Orthodontic treatment was provided by Thomas A. Molin, D.D.S., Willmar, MN.)

Occlusal Analysis (Fig. 51–7C, presurgical)

1. Class III cuspid and molar relation.
2. Crossbite (bilateral posterior and anterior).
3. Mild maxillary and mandibular crowding (pretreatment).
4. Maxillary middle 1 mm to right.

Presurgical Orthodontic Treatment

1. Nonextraction approach.
2. Maxillary and mandibular arch form coordination and alignment with fixed appliances.
3. Twelve months duration.

Surgical Treatment (Fig. 51–7B, right, and E; age 17)

1. Maxillary quadrangular Le Fort I osteotomy with advancement (10 mm).
2. Iliac (autogenous) bone graft for infraorbital, paranasal, and zygomatic augmentation (onlay) and osteotomy stabilization (interpositional).
3. Osteotomy stabilization (interpositional).
4. Septoplasty (4 mm vertical reduction) to correct left inferior deflection.
5. Mandibular bilateral ramus sagittal osteotomy (setback of 3 mm and slight counterclockwise rotation).
6. Intermaxillary fixation maintained 3 weeks; anterior vertical training elastics continued an additional 4 weeks.

Postsurgical Orthodontic Treatment

1. Fixed appliance finishing mechanics to establish final interdigitation and complete arch form coordination.
2. Twelve months in duration.

Treatment Results (Fig. 51–7A, D, and E)

1. Dental and skeletal stability was documented at the 18-month postsurgical appointment.
2. Midfacial deficiency was substantially reduced, and lip position was normalized.
3. No surgical or orthodontic compromise or complications were noted during or following treatment.
4. The patient was pleased with the functional and esthetic improvement.

PATIENT NUMBER 4 (Fig. 51–8)

This 18-year-old man presented to his orthodontist with a Class III skeletal malocclusion and a previously repaired maxillary left cleft lip–palate deformity. The patient had received comprehensive orthodontic treatment some years previously and, according to him, "had continued to grow." His facial growth and development were judged to be complete at this time.

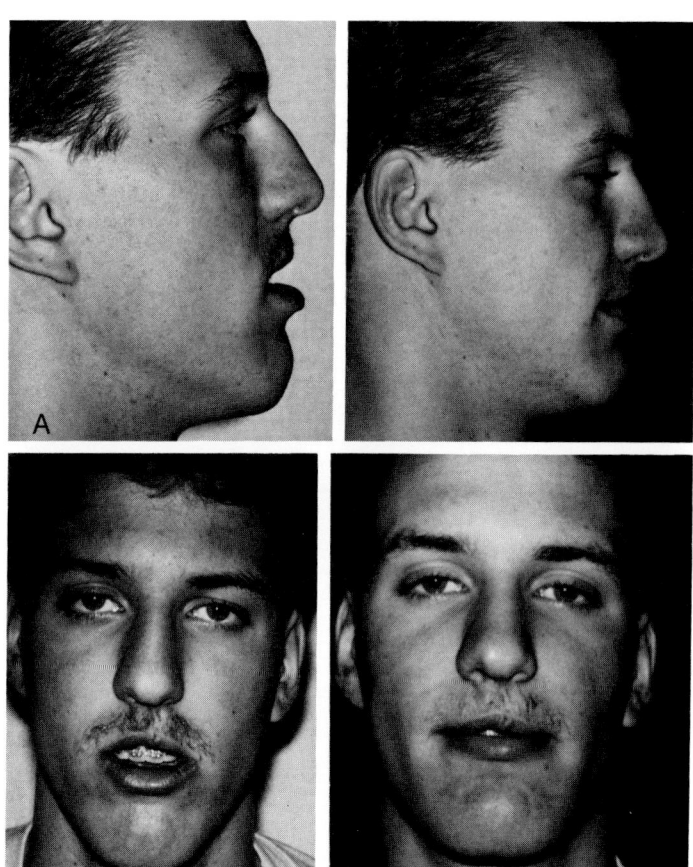

FIGURE 51–8. *A*, Presurgical *(left)* and 12 months postsurgical *(right)* lateral *(upper)*, anterior *(middle)*, and anterior with smile (postsurgical only) *(lower)* facial views. Note the marked improvement in midfacial esthetics and the reduction of lip incompetence. Vertical facial height reduction resulted in a shorter and more square anterior facial form.

Illustration continued on following page

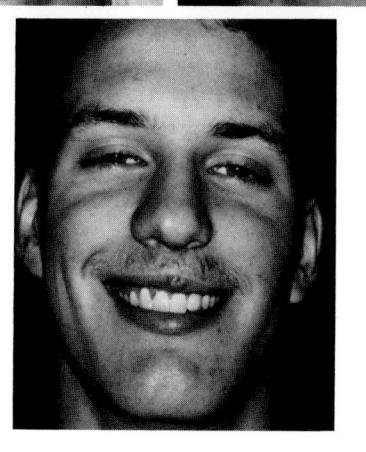

CLINICAL EVALUATION

Facial Analysis

1. The profile was pseudoprognathic secondary to normal throat length and deficiency of the infraorbital, paranasal, and zygomatic anatomy.
2. The face was long and tapering, with lip incompetence of 7 mm; maxillary incisors were positioned 5 mm below the upper lip.
3. Nasal form and projection were normal except for narrowing of the alar area.
4. Mandibular anterior height was increased (also, chin was narrow inferiorly).
5. The upper lip was thin and short secondary to previous cleft deformity and surgical repair.
6. The lower lip was everted from chronic lip incompetence and mentalis muscle hyperactivity.

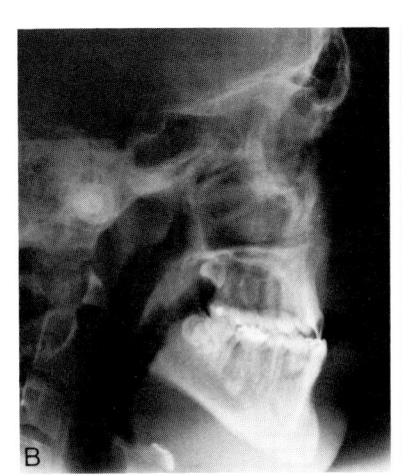

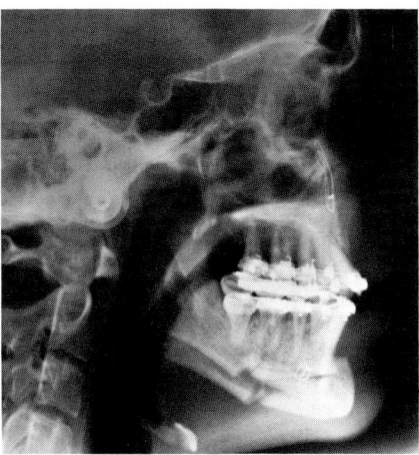

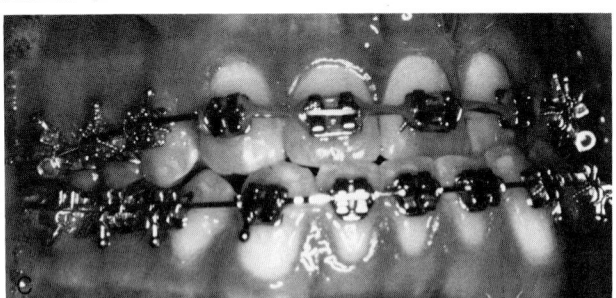

FIGURE 51–8 *Continued.* *B*, Presurgical *(left)* and postsurgical *(right)* lateral cephalograms. Note the maxillary and mandibular transosseous wires. Also note the 3- to 4-mm horizontal overcorrection with maxillary advancement. *C*, Pretreatment dental occlusion (note missing bilateral lateral incisors and one mandibular incisor).

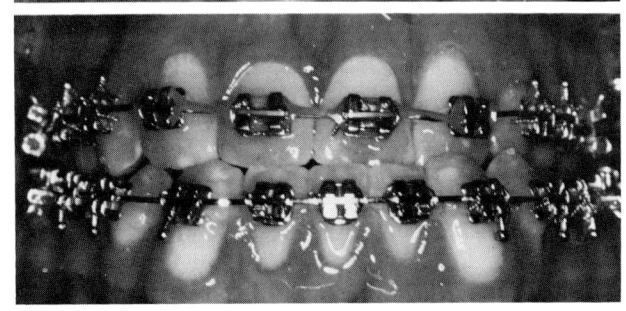

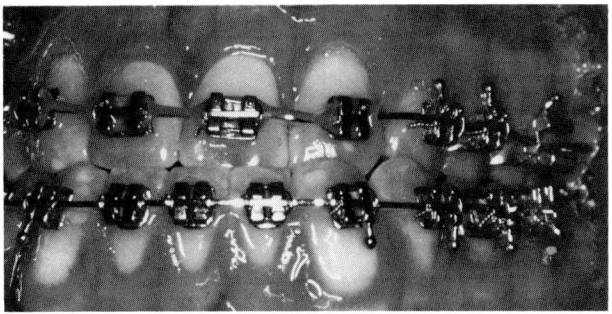

CEPHALOMETRIC FINDINGS

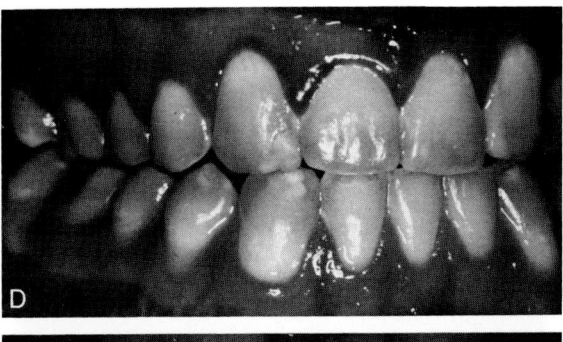

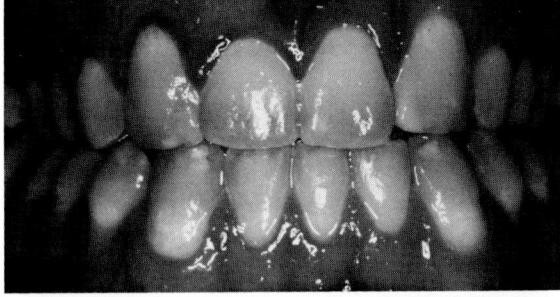

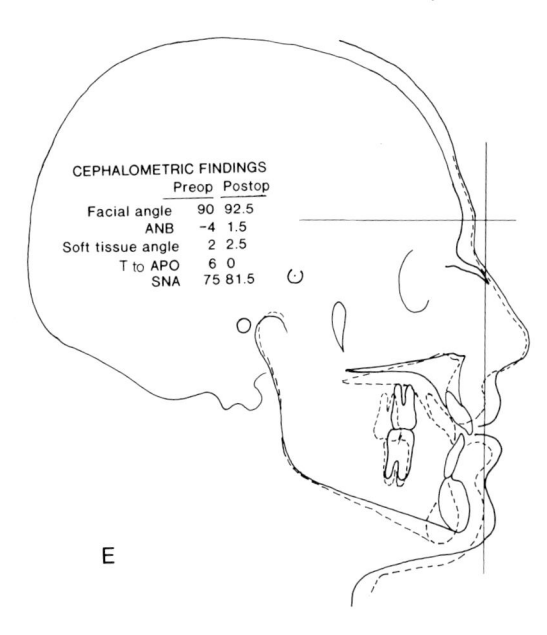

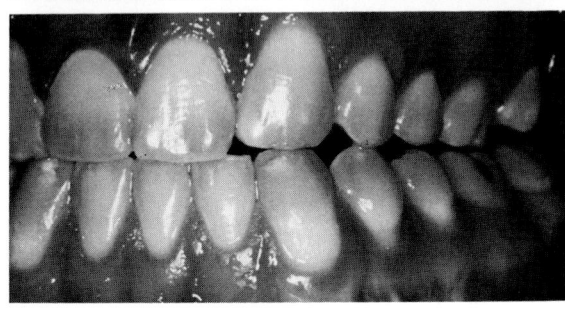

	Preop	Postop
Facial angle	90	92.5
ANB	-4	1.5
Soft tissue angle	2	2.5
T to APO	6	0
SNA	75	81.5

FIGURE 51-8 *Continued.* D, Post-treatment dental occlusion; interdigitation is compromised by missing incisors (three). E, Presurgical *(dashed line)* and postsurgical *(solid line)* composite tracing of the lateral cephalogram with abbreviated cephalometric analysis and subnasale-vertical reference line. (Orthodontic treatment was provided by John Kanyusik, D.D.S., Mankato, MN.)

7. The pogonion was deficient horizontally, and the mandible had excessive vertical height anteriorly.

Cephalometric Analysis (Fig. 51-8B, left)

1. Class III skeletal pattern.
2. Maxillary horizontal deficiency and vertical hyperplasia.
3. Anterior mandibular vertical excess.

Occlusal Analysis (Fig. 51-8C)

1. Class III cuspid and molar relationship.
2. Maxillary right and left lateral incisors missing.
3. Mandibular incisor missing.
4. Anterior crossbite.

Presurgical Orthodontic Treatment

1. Maxillary and mandibular arch form coordination with fixed appliances.
2. Nonextraction treatment (both maxillary lateral incisors and mandibular incisor previously missing).
3. Twelve months in duration.

Surgical Treatment (Fig. 51-8B, right; age 19 years)

1. Maxillary quadrangular Le Fort I osteotomy with advancement (6 mm) and vertical impaction (5 mm posterior and anterior).
2. Mandibular anterior horizontal osteotomy with advancement (6 mm) and vertical reduction (7 mm).
3. Septoplasty (correction of right deviation and 6 mm of vertical reduction).
4. Intermaxillary fixation maintained 2 weeks; anterior vertical training elastics maintained an additional 5 weeks.

Postsurgical Orthodontics

1. Maxillary and mandibular arch form coordination and completion of interdigitation refinement.
2. Nine months in duration.

Treatment Results (12 Months After Surgery; Fig. 51–8A, D, and E)

1. Excellent skeletal and dental stability was documented at the 12-month post-surgical examination.
2. Facial esthetics improved because of midfacial advancement and reduction of vertical facial height.
3. Minimal lip incompetence persists owing to congenital deficiency and surgical scarring.
4. Dental interdigitation is compromised because of missing maxillary lateral incisors and mandibular incisor.
5. No surgical or orthodontic complications or compromised results were noted during the treatment or post-treatment observation. The patient was pleased with the esthetic and functional improvements.

Discussion

Patients who have midfacial deficiency, including the infraorbital rims medially and zygoma laterally, and who have acceptable nasal projection should undergo a maxillary advancement procedure commensurate with their deformity. The procedure of choice for these patients is the quadrangular Le Fort II osteotomy initially described by Kufner[5] and later modified by others.[9-12] With this procedure, both the dentoalveolar and the infraorbital-zygomatic deficiencies are corrected. If the same group of patients also have significant maxillary vertical deficiency, maxillary vertical excess, maxillary transverse excess or deficiency, or maxillary asymmetry, the quadrangular Le Fort I osteotomy described in this section offers an acceptable alternative procedure. Potentially, the final esthetic result can be equal to that of the quadrangular Le Fort II procedure if the onlay-interpositional bone grafting is contoured, properly placed, and stabilized correctly. In the author's experience, the bone graft placement is technically more difficult in the quadrangular Le Fort I procedure than in the quadrangular Le Fort II procedure. One would also expect increased bone resorption of the infraorbital onlay bone graft in the quadrangular Le Fort I procedure. To compensate for this, significant overcontouring of the infraorbital-zygomatic onlay-interpositional graft is provided. Patients are advised preoperatively of this. When the quadrangular Le Fort II osteotomy is performed intraorally, an occasional patient may, upon surgical exposure, be found to have a significant thinning of the lateral nasal-infraorbital bone. The downfracture maneuver in this situation is technically very difficult or impossible. In these patients, the surgeon may decide intraoperatively to perform the quadrangular Le Fort I osteotomy and potentially achieve equal esthetic, dental, and functional results. Preoperative preparation and postoperative management are, for most patients, identical in both procedures, particularly if an intraoperative procedure change is anticipated preoperatively.

Patients with *maxillary alveolar-palatal cleft* frequently have horizontal growth deficiency involving the midportion of the face; in addition, they often have dentoalveolar asymmetry and transverse or vertical maxillary deficiency. In this group of patients (congenital maxillary cleft), the quadrangular Le Fort I osteotomy is an excellent procedure[13]; it is frequently performed in our patient population (17 of 54 patients in a recent report).[7] These patients with maxillary cleft deformity also often require a follow-up nasal-lip reconstructive procedure and may also be candidates for the Le Fort II (pyramidal) or Le Fort III osteotomy procedure (for nasal deficiency correction) in combination with a low-level Le Fort I osteotomy (for sagittal, transverse, and vertical corrections).[13] Two surgical settings are required in these patients (the higher level osteotomy is generally accomplished first).

The surgical technique for the quadrangular Le Fort I osteotomy as described can be accomplished predictably without significant intraoperative complications, as documented in a recent survey of 54 consecutive patients.[7] Strict adherence to an intraoperative and paraoperative anesthesia and surgical protocol is mandatory.

Intraoperative blood replacement was reported in the previously mentioned survey[7] and was done according to an autologous blood replacement protocol.[14]

All patients who are candidates for the quadrangular Le Fort I osteotomy undergo horizontal advancement; however, as documented in a recent survey of 54 consecutive patients, a significant number undergo vertical (39 per cent) and transverse (26 per cent) augmentation.[7] The transverse and vertical corrections for this group of patients can be greater than 5 mm; in contrast, 5 mm is the maximal allowable transverse, vertical, or midline correction acceptable in the quadrangular Le Fort II procedure (described in the next section). Segmentalization is more easily accomplished in the lower level osteotomy, and the quadrangular Le Fort I osteotomy is often used in the patient with maxillary cleft in whom significant width and symmetry problems are common.[13]

Intermaxillary fixation time has varied considerably in our group of patients since this surgical procedure was initiated into our surgical treatment protocol in 1981, in part reflecting a change in fixation hardware and treatment philosophy. We currently provide 2 to 3 weeks of intermaxillary fixation in all patients undergoing the quadrangular Le Fort I osteotomy either alone or in combination with mandibular procedures (in which skeletal fixation is routinely utilized). The onlay-interpositional bone grafting, in combination with the infraorbital–nasal aperture transosseous wiring, provides rigid advancement stability with osseous (skeletal) interlocking. In selected patients with marginal bone contacts who have had significant vertical lengthening in addition to advancement, 3 or 4 weeks of intermaxillary fixation is provided. All patients use anterior vertical training elastics nocturnally in conjunction with the surgical interocclusal splint for varying periods after release of intermaxillary fixation; a soft, pureed diet is permitted during this period. Considerable variation exists in the length of time patients use continuous or nocturnal interarch elastics. In patients with maxillary vertical hyperplasia with lip incompetence and nocturnal oral breathing, nocturnal vertical elastics may be continued 3 to 4 months postsurgically to ensure nasal versus oral breathing during the healing period when function (nasal air flow) can alter internal nasal anatomy.

Postoperative complications that occur in patients undergoing the quadrangular Le Fort I osteotomy[7] were categorized as follows in a recent report of 54 patients: infection, sequestra without infection, neurologic problems, irregular orbital contour, nasolacrimal duct dysfunction, transosseous wire problems, infraorbital air in tissue, iliac crest seroma, and oronasal fistula. The most potentially serious complication involved infection, which was noted in 4 of 54 patients.[7] This infection, occurring 18, 20, 21, and 30 days postoperatively, was associated with infraorbital and buccal swelling. In all four patients, the incision line was opened intraorally for drainage, and antibiotics were given orally for up to 2 weeks. No untoward sequelae occurred, and the graft was not lost in any of these patients. Early dependent surgical drainage (intraoral and antronasal) and aggressive antibiotic therapy are important. To date, we have not had to remove any infraorbital-zygomatic onlay-interpositional iliac bone graft in any patient for any reason in the quadrangular Le Fort I or II procedure. In three patients with congenital maxillary cleft lip–palate deformity, sequestra formation occurred without sepsis in sites of mucosal closure in alveolar (two patients) or palatal (one patient) cleft areas. Meticulous closure of mucosa over bone clefts should prevent this problem; however, closure is frequently difficult when osteotomy and cleft grafting procedures are combined. It is advisable to separate the alveolar-palatal bone grafting and the orthognathic surgical procedure in patients with large clefts or bilateral clefts or those in whom large maxillary advancement is planned.[13] The risk of blood supply compromise or wound dehiscence is greatly reduced. In addition, the surgeon is required to have differing "mind sets" to achieve the surgical objectives in the alveolar-palatal bone grafting versus the orthognathic surgical procedures.

The question of *short-* or *long-term stability* in a group of patients undergoing maxillary advancement via a quadrangular Le Fort I osteotomy has not been scientifically evaluated. Our clinical results suggest that stability has been suitable during the past 7 years because reoperation for any cause (including skeletal relapse) has not been required in a group of 54 patients recently reported on and followed from 1 to 7 years.[7] The relapse most frequently encountered is posterior transverse relapse, especially in patients with cleft deformities (in whom scar tissue is a limiting factor), when orthodontic expansion was attained presurgically, or when complete surgical mobilization was not accomplished (segment not passively seated in splint). We routinely horizontally overcorrect 2 to 3 mm to counteract compression of the postcondylar tissues in patients undergoing maxillary advancement with an intact mandible (or bimaxillary procedures in which internal skeletal fixation is provided in the mandible). If this overcorrection is not lost immediately after release of intermaxillary fixation, it will be utilized by the orthodontist to achieve proper interdigitation and arch form during the postsurgical orthodontic treatment. We have not encountered a patient in whom overcorrection (maxillary horizontal) was a problem and who occasionally could utilize an additional amount of maxillary forward positioning. Long-term stability of the occlusion or the infraorbital bone graft has, to date, been clinically acceptable but not documented scientifically. The overall surgical-orthodontic stability is related to the achievement of proper correction of the total facial deformity in the horizontal, vertical, and transverse dimensions as well as to the provision of proper surgical and orthodontic procedures. Long-term neuromuscular, cutaneous, and skeletal balance should be maintained if achieved completely at the initial treatment.

QUADRANGULAR LE FORT II OSTEOTOMY

Review of Literature

In 1971, Kufner[5] described a maxillary osteotomy procedure that was "in essence a combination of the osteotomy according to the Le Fort I and Le Fort II classifications." He described this "middle" osteotomy and reported its use in 5 of his 61 patients, with the remainder receiving the "low osteotomy" (48 patients) or the "high osteotomy" (8 patients). Kufner gave few written details of the "middle" osteotomy but supplied a clear diagram. He stated that bone grafts were utilized in spaces created by the skeletal advancement and that internal suspension wires were used for segment stabilization. He also mentioned use of a paranasal suspension wire from a frontal "nail" when large advancements were performed.

In 1973, Souyris and colleagues[9] described an "intermediate" osteotomy that was similar to the "middle" osteotomy of Kufner; however, the lateral orbital wall osteotomy was placed at various levels, depending on the cosmetic requirements in individual patients.

In 1980, Champy[10] described an "intermediary" osteotomy that was identical to that described by Kufner, except for the lateral horizontal osteotomy, which was kept level with the orbital floor and extended laterally through the lateral orbital wall and body of the zygoma; this modification made it necessary to perform vertical zygomatic arch osteotomy, as in the classic Le Fort III osteotomy.

In a landmark article in 1980, Steinhauser[11] reviewed the literature on the Le Fort II osteotomy and provided an anatomic classification, which follows:

I. Anterior Le Fort II osteotomy (first described by Converse, 1971[3])

II. Pyramidal Le Fort II osteotomy (first described by Henderson and Jackson, 1973[4])

III. Quadrangular Le Fort II osteotomy (first described by Kufner, 1971[5])

Steinhauser[11] noted that the qudrangular Le Fort II osteotomy was "more often indicated than the two other techniques" in his experience. He mentioned a significant relapse tendency with the Le Fort II osteotomy in general but noted that the self-retaining interpositional bone graft on the malar process in the quadrangular osteotomy provided excellent skeletal stabilization and a decided advantage over the pyramidal Le Fort II procedure. Steinhauser also placed bone grafts in the orbital floor defect after advancement.

Kufner,[5] Souyris,[9] Champy,[10] and Steinhauser[11] performed the quadrangular Le Fort II osteotomy through cutaneous and intraoral incisions and utilized block interpositional bone grafts and suspension wiring to stabilize the advanced segment. Keller and Sather (1987)[12] modified the quadrangular Le Fort II osteotomy: The surgical procedure was performed entirely through intraoral incisions, and the advanced segment was stabilized by interpositional iliac bone grafts and internal transosseous suspension wires.

Brusati and colleagues (1989)[15] reported on an "intra-oral maxillo-malar osteotomy which verified the feasibility of the Kufner osteotomy via an intra-oral route only." They varied the amount of infraorbital rim advancement by placing the medial osteotomy either medial or lateral to the infraorbital nerve. They also attempted to advance more of the body of the zygoma by extending the lateral osteotomy posterior to the anterior attachment of the masseter muscle. They also modified the osteotomy in certain patients by placing the osteotomy just below the infraorbital rim (as in the quadrangular Le Fort I osteotomy described in this section).

Indications

Patients who present with maxillary-zygomatic deficiency on clinical and cephalometric examinations and exhibit a Class III skeletal malocclusion, but who exhibit a normal nasal projection, are potential candidates for this procedure. Because positional change of the infraorbital rim affects orbital contents and volume, this procedure is not indicated when significant lateral or vertical (increase or decrease) shift of the maxilla is required (generally more than 5 mm). In addition, a significant maxillary width increase (greater than 5 mm) via a two-piece osteotomy is not recommended. Segmentalization (other than a two-piece segmentalization via a midline osteotomy) is technically difficult and not recommended. When significant maxillary transverse widening, vertical lengthening, impaction, or midline shift is required in patients who otherwise fulfill the primary indications for a quadrangular Le Fort II osteotomy, a quadrangular Le Fort I osteotomy is performed.[7]

In patients with nasomaxillary deficiency, a pyramidal Le Fort II osteotomy or Le Fort III (or modifications of) osteotomy is selected. Patients with skeletal open-bite deformity of mandibular origin or with mandibular prognathism require additional surgical procedures (in addition to the quadrangular Le Fort II osteotomy) to normalize their facial deformity completely.[16] Patients with maxillary alveolar–palatal cleft deformity and normal nasal projection are candidates for this procedure; however, the alveolar-palatal bone graft should be accomplished well ahead of the osteotomy procedure.[17]

Surgical Procedure (Fig. 51–9)

After induction of nasoendotracheal anesthesia and preparation for an intraoral procedure, an incision is made 4 to 5 mm above the mucogingival junction from the right to the left maxillary buttress. The entire anterior surface of the maxilla and zygoma is exposed, extending superiorly over the infraorbital rim and posteriorly to the pterygopalatine fissure. The periosteum of the infraorbital rim is detached from the lacrimal fossa medially to the vertical portion of the orbital rim laterally. The anterior attachment of the masseter muscle is not disturbed. The

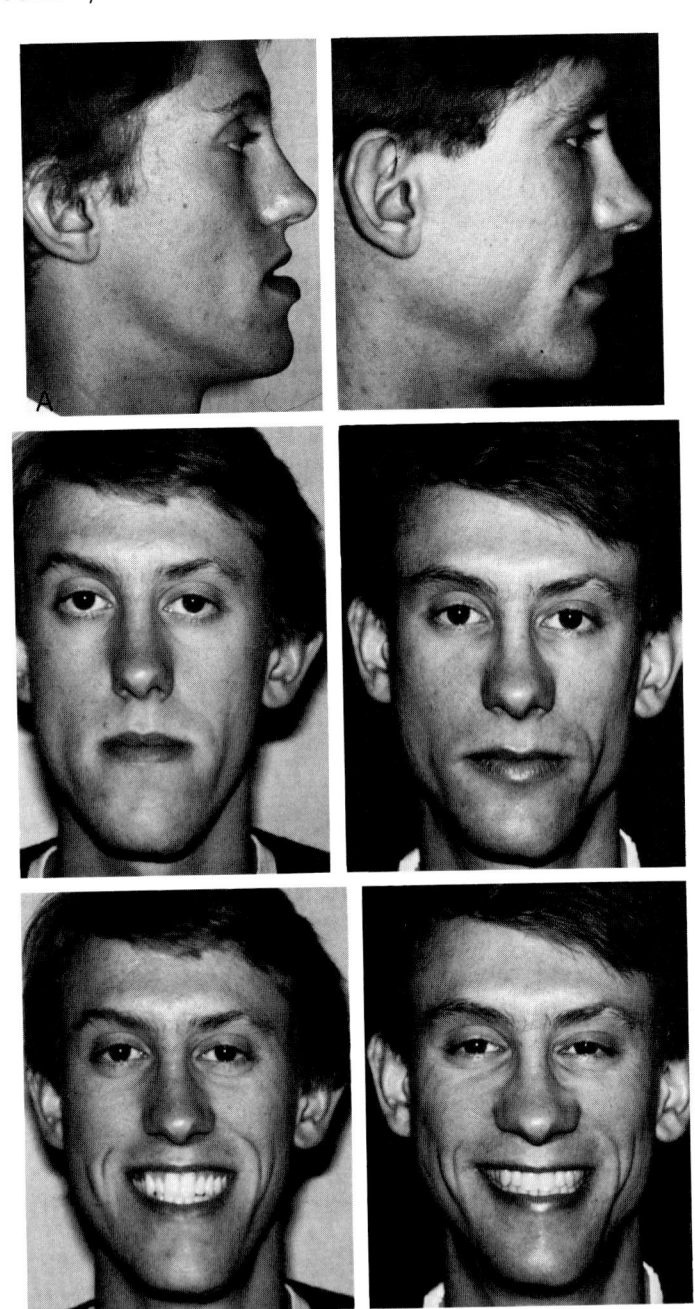

FIGURE 51–10. *A,* Pretreatment *(left)* and 3-year post-treatment *(right)* lateral *(upper),* anterior *(middle),* and anterior with smile *(lower)* facial views. Note the long, tapering face and moderate midfacial deficiency; the latter was seen to improve significantly in post-treatment photographs. Alar width was increased following maxillary advancement. *B,* Pretreatment *(left)* and 3-year post-treatment *(right)* lateral cephalograms. Note the upper lip advancement and overall facial height reduction; also note the maxillary transosseous wires. Wire fixation was not utilized in the mandible (intraoral vertical ramus osteotomy).

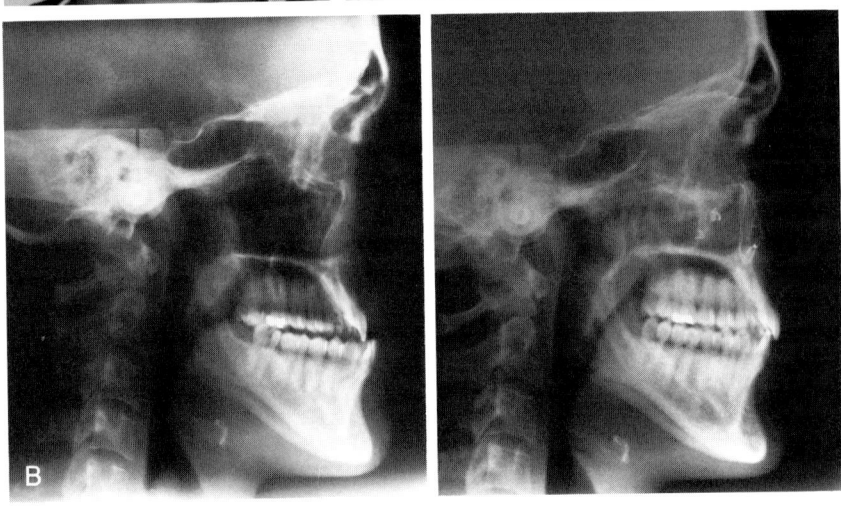

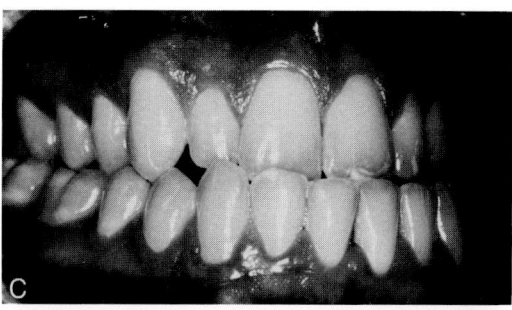

51 — QUADRANGULAR LE FORT I AND II OSTEOTOMIES / **1823**

FIGURE 51–10 *Continued.* *C,* Pretreatment dental occlusion (note midline discrepancy). *D,* Post-treatment (3 years after surgery) dental occlusion (note dental midline correction). *E,* Pretreatment *(dashed line)* and 3-year postsurgical *(solid line)* composite tracing of the lateral cephalogram with abbreviated cephalometric analysis and subnasale-vertical reference line. Note that the nasal tip was advanced slightly after maxillary advancement and impaction. (Orthodontic treatment was provided by Lloyd Truax, D.D.S., Rochester, MN.)

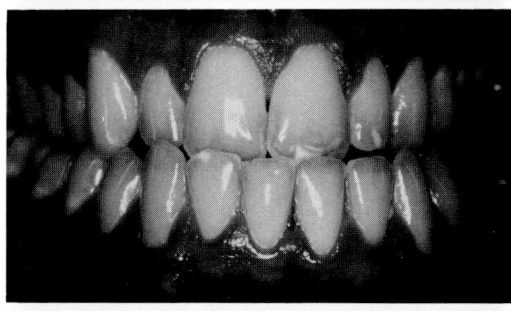

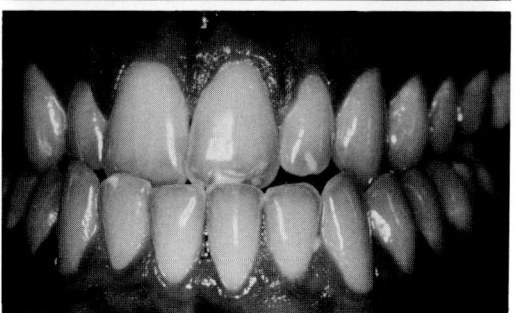

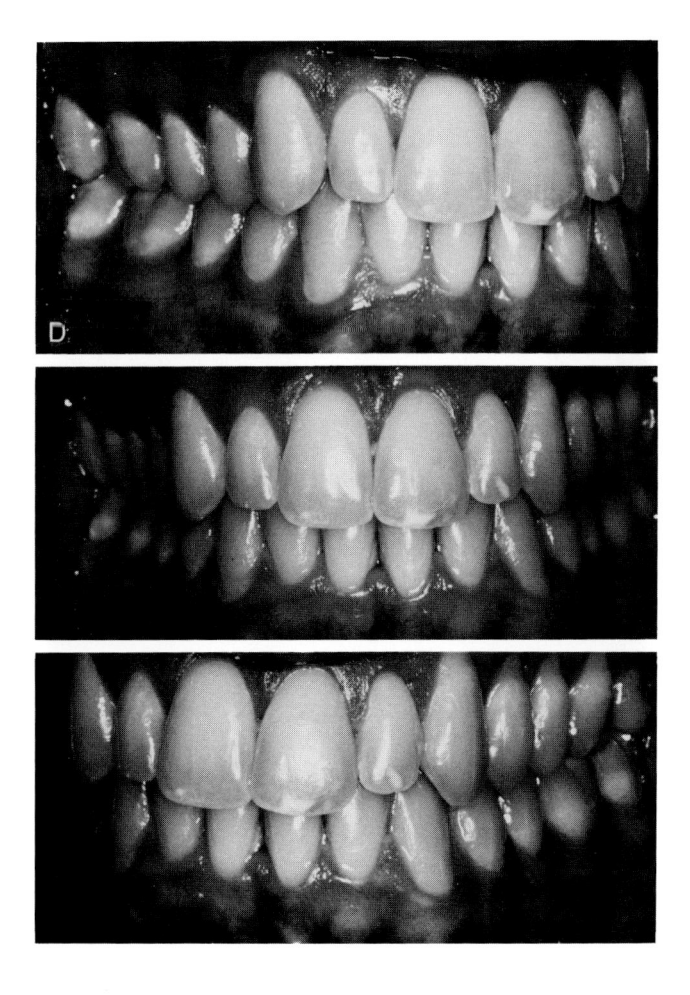

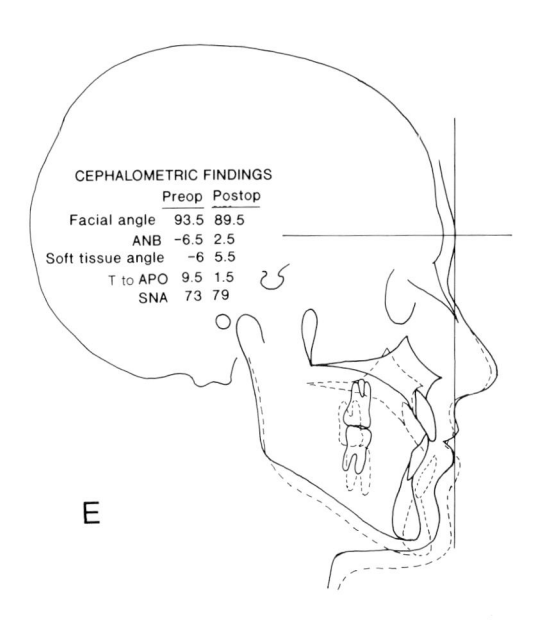

CEPHALOMETRIC FINDINGS

	Preop	Postop
Facial angle	93.5	89.5
ANB	−6.5	2.5
Soft tissue angle	−6	5.5
T to APO	9.5	1.5
SNA	73	79

PATIENT NUMBER 6 (Fig. 51-11)

This 13-year-old girl presented to the orthodontist with a Class III skeletal malocclusion. After 2 years of growth observation and orthodontic treatment, she was referred for surgical evaluation and treatment.

CLINICAL EVALUATION

Facial Analysis (Fig. 51-11A)

1. The profile was pseudoprognathic secondary to maxillary, infraorbital, paranasal, and zygomatic deficiency; throat length was normal.
2. Facial symmetry was normal except for mild left mandibular deviation (3 mm).
3. The patient exhibited a square facial form.
4. Nasal projection and form were acceptable.
5. Lip incompetence of 3 mm was present owing to anteroposterior jaw discrepancy.

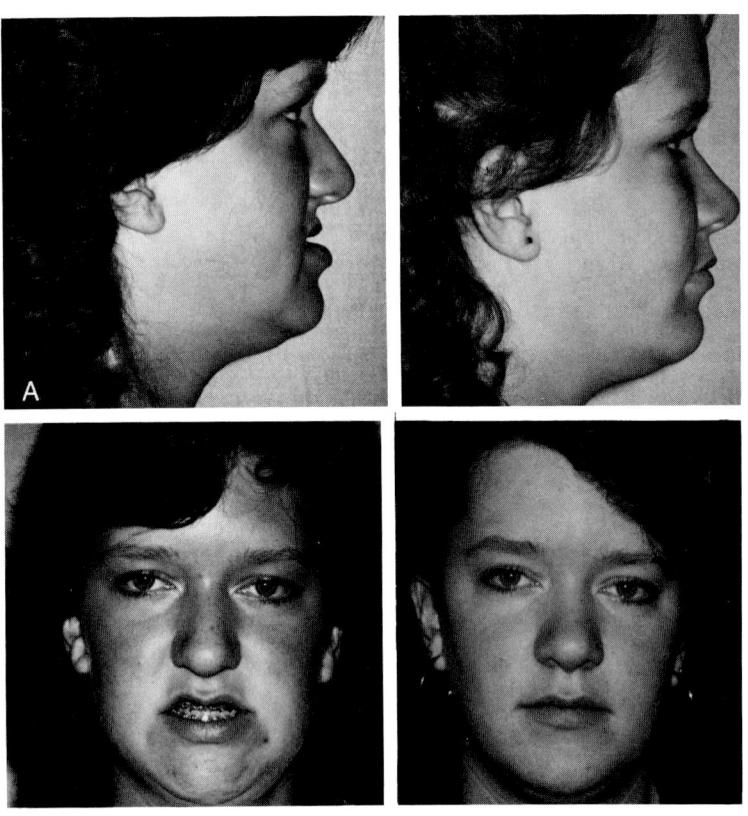

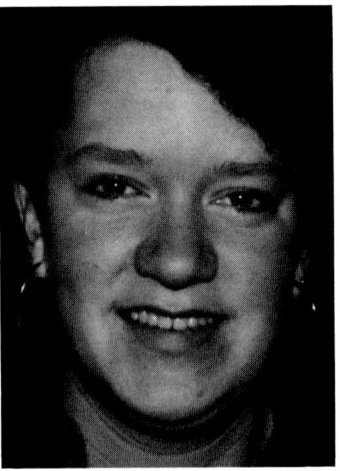

FIGURE 51-11. *A*, Presurgical *(left)* and 18-month postsurgical *(right)* lateral *(upper)*, anterior *(middle)*, and anterior with smile (postsurgical only) *(lower)* facial views. Note the marked improvement in midfacial anatomy and lip posture. Also, alar width was maintained following maxillary advancement.

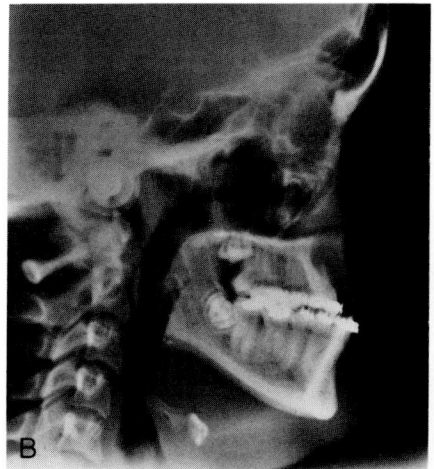

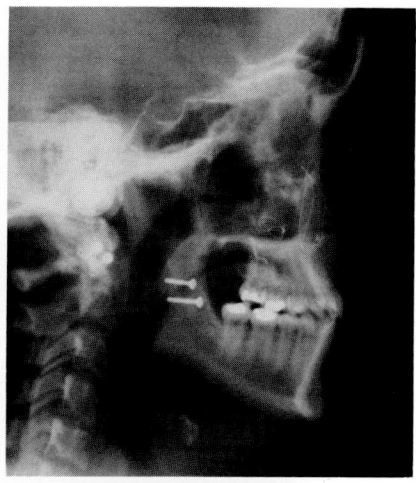

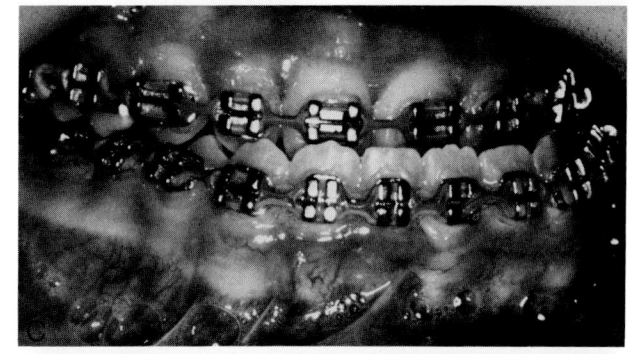

FIGURE 51–11 *Continued.* B, Presurgical *(left)* and postsurgical *(right)* lateral cephalograms. Note the transosseous fixation wires (maxilla) and skeletal fixation screws (mandible). C, Presurgical dental occlusion. Note the midline discrepancy.

Illustration continued on following page

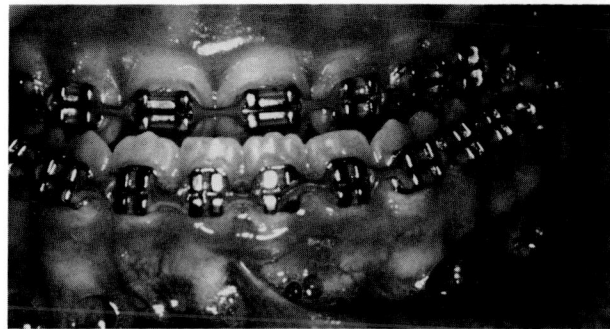

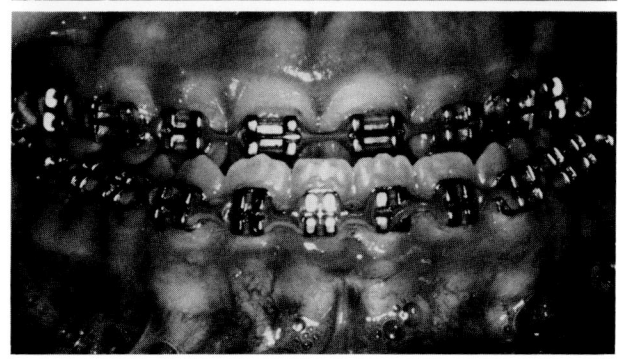

6. The lower lip was prominent and redundant secondary to mentalis hyperactivity.
7. The upper lip was short and redundant secondary to inactivity.

Cephalometric Analysis (Fig. 51–11B, left, and E)

1. Class III skeletal pattern.
2. Maxillary horizontal deficiency.
3. Normal facial vertical proportions.
4. Flat bony pogonion but normal soft tissue pogonion.

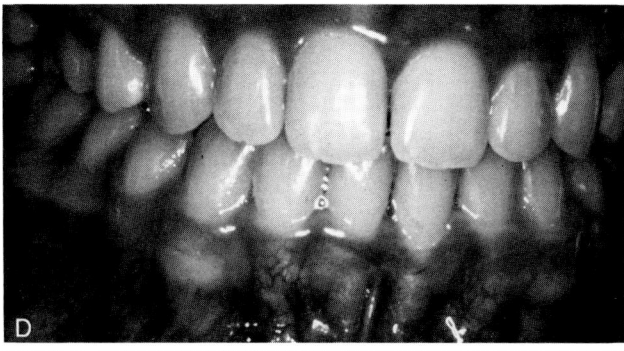

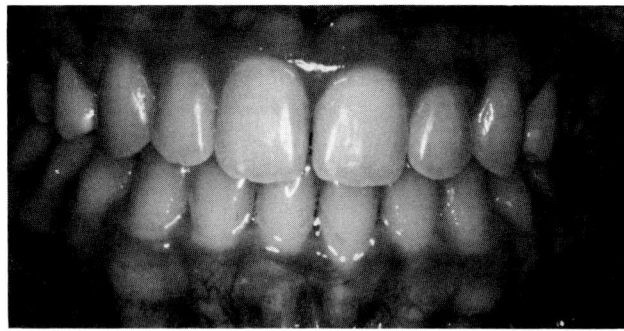

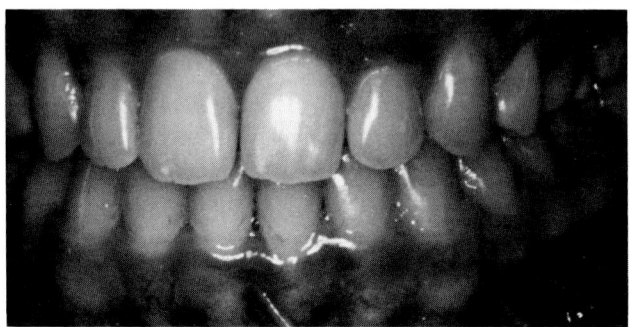

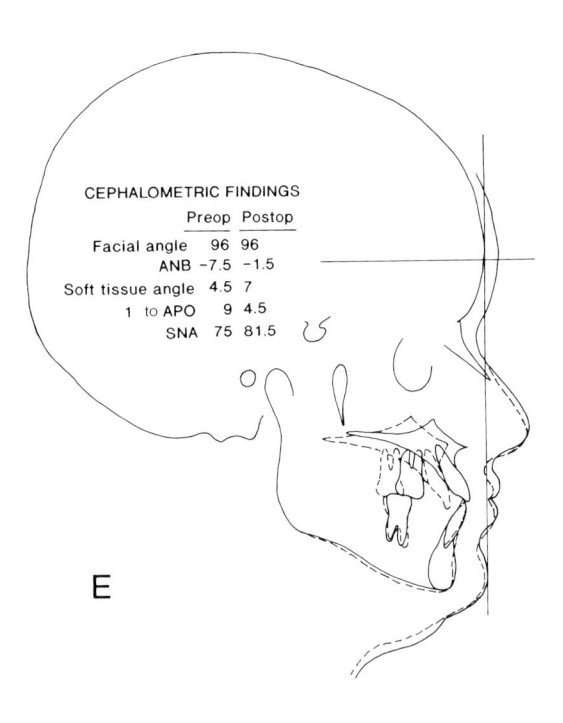

FIGURE 51–11 *Continued.* D, Postsurgical (18 months) dental occlusion. E, Pretreatment *(dashed line)* and 18-month postsurgical *(solid line)* composite tracing of the lateral cephalogram with abbreviated cephalometric analysis and subnasale-vertical reference line. (Note the upper lip and nasal tip advancement.) (Orthodontic treatment was provided by Gary B. Blodgett, D.D.S., Mason City, IA.)

Occlusal Analysis (Fig. 51–11*C*)

1. Class III cuspid and molar relationship.
2. Crossbite (anterior and left posterior).
3. Maxillary right and left first bicuspids removed prior to orthodontic treatment because of upper arch crowding.

Presurgical Treatment

1. Removal of maxillary right and left first bicuspid.
2. Maxillary arch: first bicuspid extraction site closure and arch form coordination.
3. Mandibular arch: (nonextraction) arch form coordination.
4. Two years in duration.

Surgical Treatment (Fig. 51–11*B*, right; age 15)

1. Maxillary quadrangular Le Fort II osteotomy with advancement (9 mm) and vertical impaction (2 mm).
2. Iliac autogenous bone graft for zygomatic augmentation (onlay) and osteotomy stabilization (interpositional).
3. Mandibular right ramus sagittal osteotomy (3-mm right shift).
4. Impacted maxillary and mandibular third molar removal.
5. Intermaxillary fixation of 2 weeks; an additional 4 weeks of anterior vertical training elastics.

Postsurgical Orthodontic Treatment

1. Finishing refinement of interdigitation and arch form coordination.
2. Nine months in duration.

Treatment Results (Fig. 51–11A, D, and E)

1. Excellent skeletal and dental stability was documented at the 18-month postsurgical examination.
2. Midfacial esthetics were much improved, and lip position was normal after skeletal correction.
3. The patient was quite pleased with the esthetic and functional improvement.

PATIENT NUMBER 7 (Fig. 51–12)

This 17-year-old boy presented to his orthodontist with a Class III skeletal malocclusion. After 1 year of observation, growth was documented to be complete, and orthodontic treatment was initiated.

CLINICAL EVALUATION

Facial Analysis (Fig. 51–12A)

1. The profile was pseudoprognathic secondary to maxillary, infraorbital, paranasal, and zygomatic deficiency. Throat length was normal, and the face was symmetric except the mandible, which was deviated slightly (3 mm) to the left.

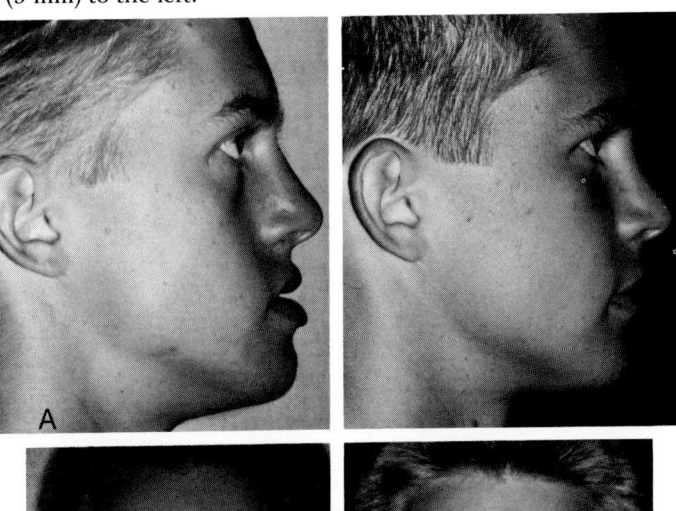

FIGURE 51–12. *A*, Presurgical *(left)* and 13-month postsurgical *(right)* lateral *(upper)*, anterior *(middle)*, and anterior with smile *(lower)* facial views. Note midfacial esthetic improvement and improved lip contour and position. Also, alar width was maintained following maxillary advancement.

Illustration continued on following page

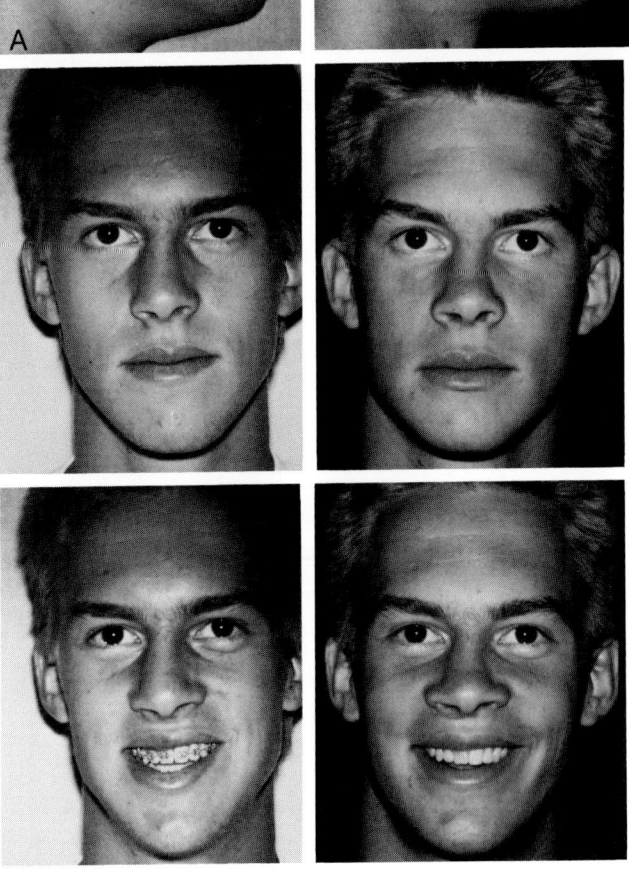

2. Nasal form and projection were acceptable.
3. Minimal lip incompetence (3 mm) was present in the resting position.
4. The upper lip was short and somewhat redundant owing to inactivity.
5. The lower lip was thickened and redundant from mentalis hyperactivity.

Cephalometric Analysis (Fig. 51–12*B*, left, and *E*)

1. Class III skeletal open-bite pattern.
2. Maxillary horizontal deficiency and mild posterior hyperplasia.

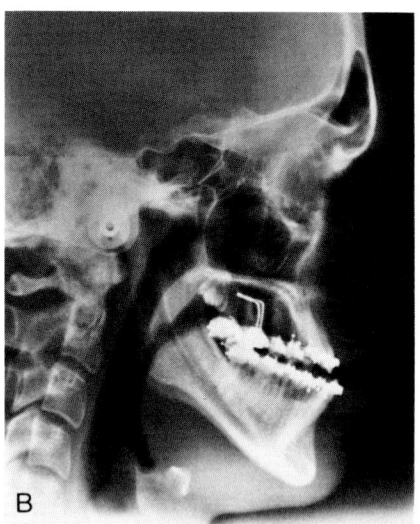

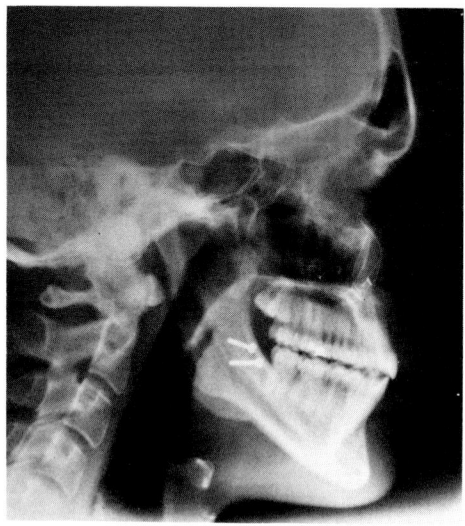

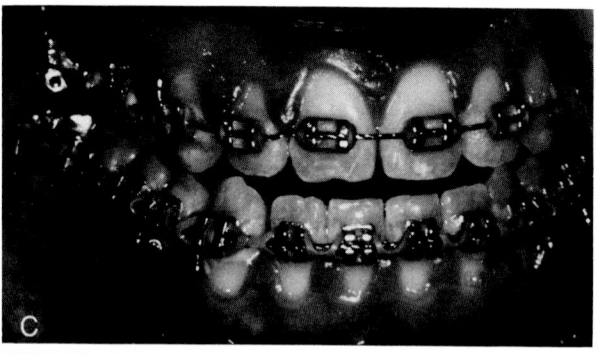

FIGURE 51–12 *Continued. B,* Pretreatment *(left)* and 13-month post-treatment *(right)* lateral cephalograms. Note the maxillary transosseous wires and mandibular right ramus skeletal fixation screws. *C,* Presurgical dental occlusion.

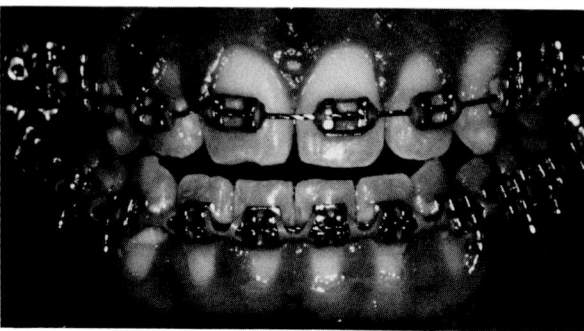

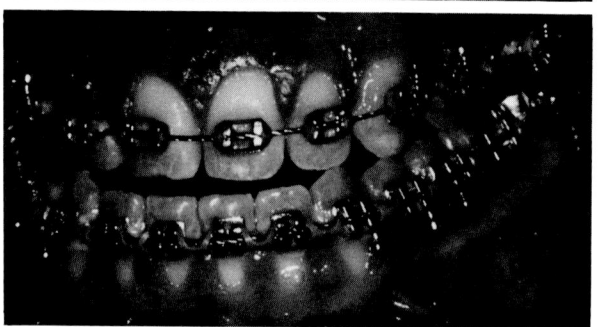

FIGURE 51–12 *Continued. D,* Post-treatment dental occlusion. *E,* Pretreatment *(dashed line)* and 13-month postsurgical *(solid line)* composite tracing of the lateral cephalogram with abbreviated cephalometric analysis and subnasale-vertical reference line. Note the minimal nasal tip advancement.) (Orthodontic treatment was provided by Steven J. Nedrelow, D.D.S., Willmar, MN.)

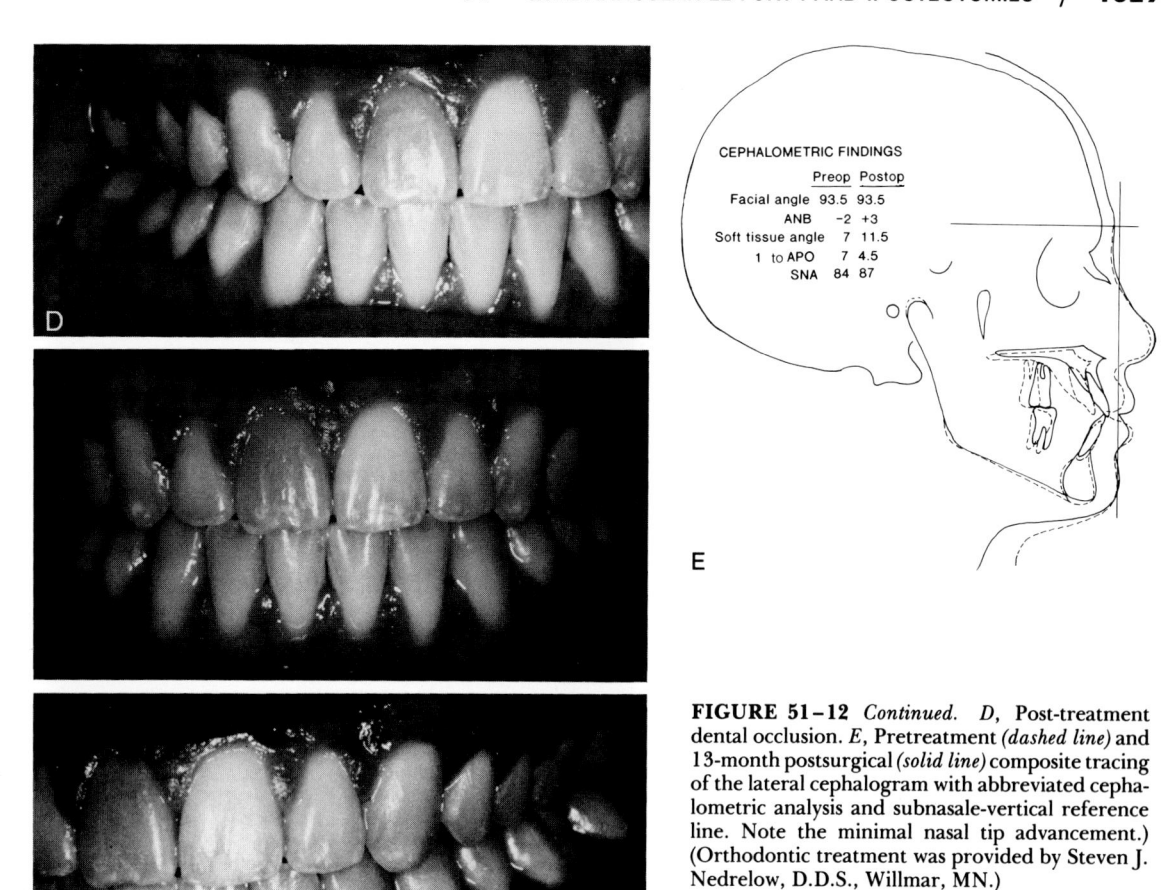

3. Anterior facial height slightly increased (owing to maxillary posterior hyperplasia).

Occlusal Analysis (Fig. 51–12C)

1. Class III cuspid and molar relation.
2. Crossbite (anterior and bilateral posterior).
3. Maxillary and mandibular dental midline shifted to left (3 mm).

Presurgical Orthodontic Treatment

1. Nonextraction treatment.
2. Maxillary and mandibular arch form coordination with fixed appliances.
3. Twelve months in duration.

Surgical Treatment (Fig. 51–12B, right; age 19)

1. Maxillary quadrangular Le Fort II osteotomy with advancement (8 mm), right rotation (3 mm), and posterior impaction (2 mm).
2. Iliac autogenous bone graft for zygomatic augmentation (onlay) and osteotomy stabilization (interpositional).
3. Septoplasty (vertical reduction of 4 mm).
4. Mandibular right ramus sagittal osteotomy (3-mm right rotation).
5. Intermaxillary fixation maintained 2 weeks; anterior vertical training elastics continued an additional 4 weeks.

Postsurgical Orthodontic Treatment

1. Maxillary and mandibular fixed appliances for finishing interdigitation and arch form coordination refinement.
2. Twelve months in duration.

PATIENT NUMBER 8 (Fig. 51-13)

This 17-year-old boy presented to the orthodontist with a Class III skeletal malocclusion. His facial growth and development were complete.

CLINICAL EVALUATION

Facial Analysis (Fig. 51-13A)

1. The profile was pseudoprognathic secondary to maxillary, infraorbital, paranasal, and zygomatic deficiency; mild mandibular protrusion and normal throat length were present.
2. The facial form was long and tapering secondary to maxillary vertical excess.
3. Facial symmetry was normal in all areas.
4. Nasal form and projection were normal, except for a moderately narrow alar width.
5. Mild lip incompetence was present in the resting position.
6. Upper and lower lip position and form were normal in the resting position.

Cephalometric Analysis (Fig. 51-13B, left, and E)

1. Class III skeletal pattern.
2. Maxillary horizontal deficiency and mild vertical excess.
3. Normal soft and hard tissue pogonion.

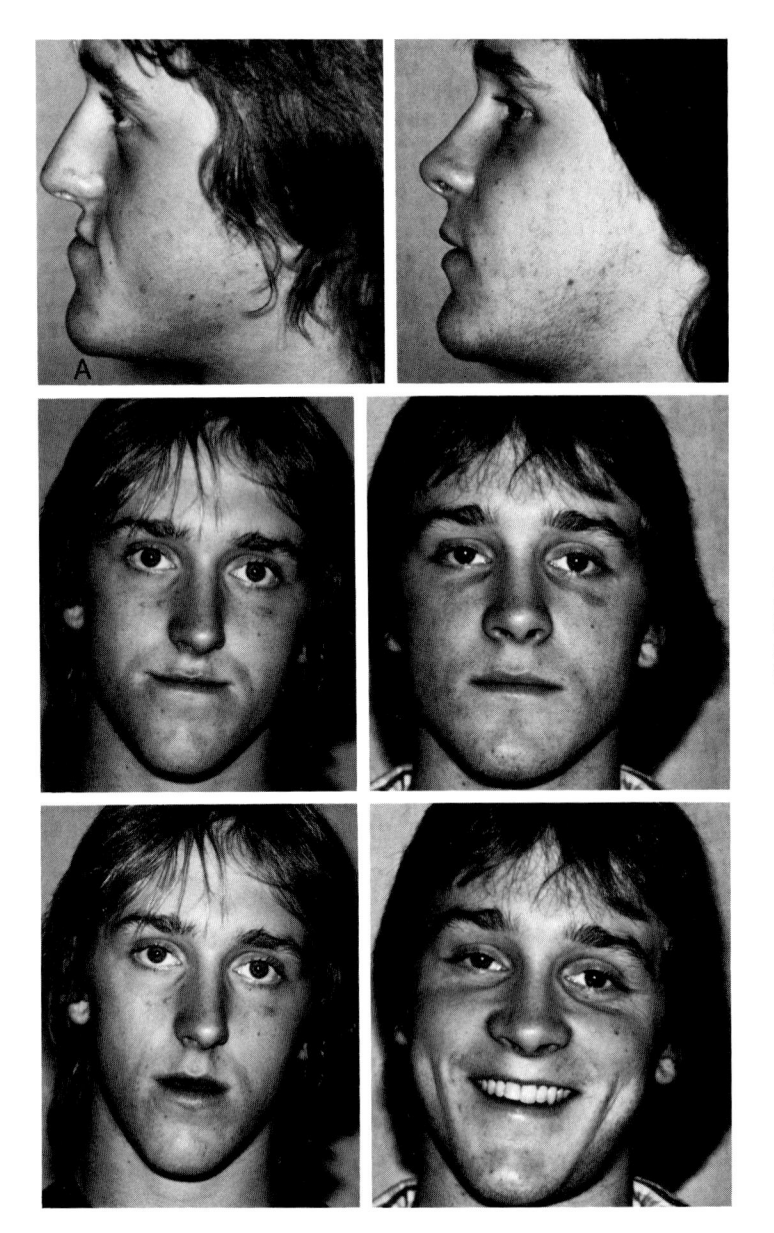

FIGURE 51-13. *A*, Presurgical *(left)* and 14-month postsurgical *(right)* lateral *(upper)*, anterior *(middle)*, and anterior with smile *(lower)* facial views. Note the significant improvement in midfacial esthetics and lip posture.

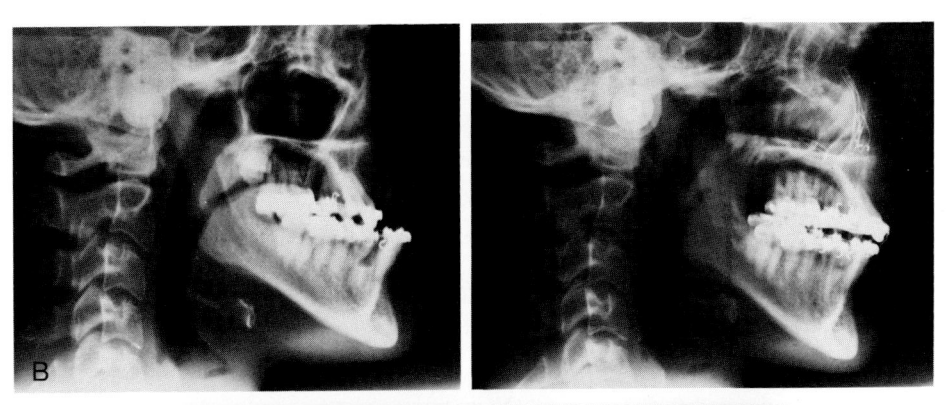

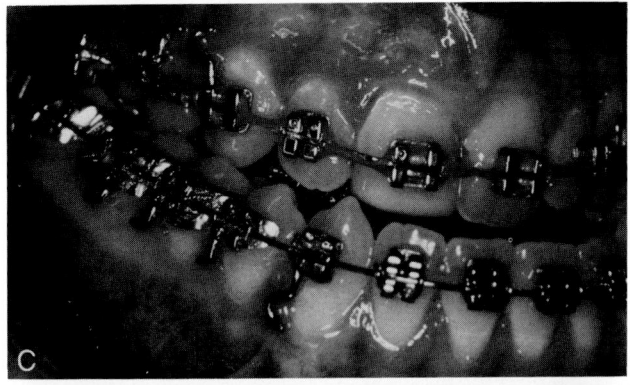

FIGURE 51-13 *Continued. B,* Presurgical *(left)* and 14-month postsurgical *(right)* lateral cephalograms. Note the maxillary transosseous wire fixation. *C,* Presurgical dental occlusion.
Illustration continued on following page.

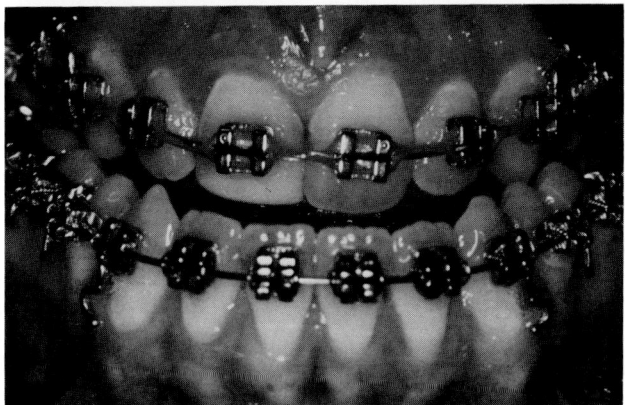

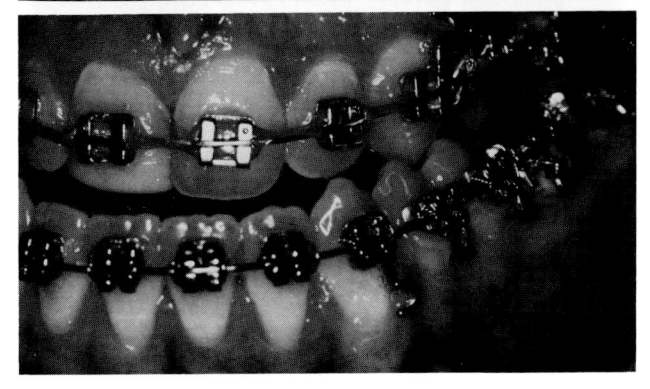

Occlusal Analysis (Fig. 51-13C)
1. Class III cuspid and molar relation (bilateral).
2. Crossbite (bilateral posterior and anterior).
3. Maxillary dental midline shifted to right (3 mm).

Presurgical Orthodontic Treatment
1. Maxillary right and left first bicuspid removal.
2. Maxillary arch: closure of extraction sites and arch coordination with fixed appliances.

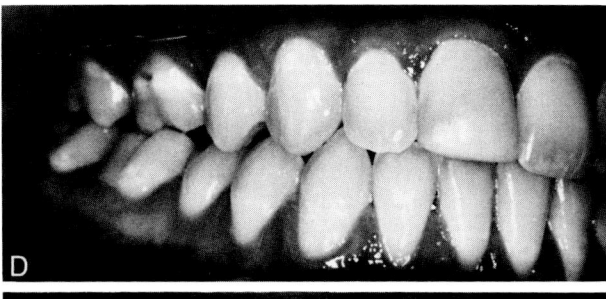

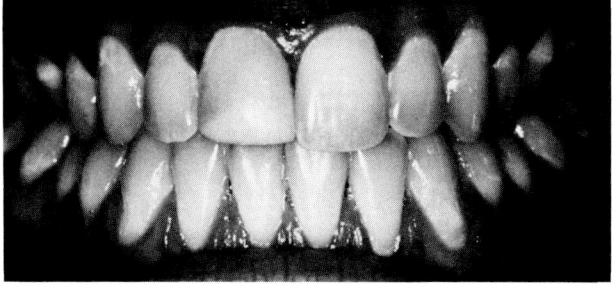

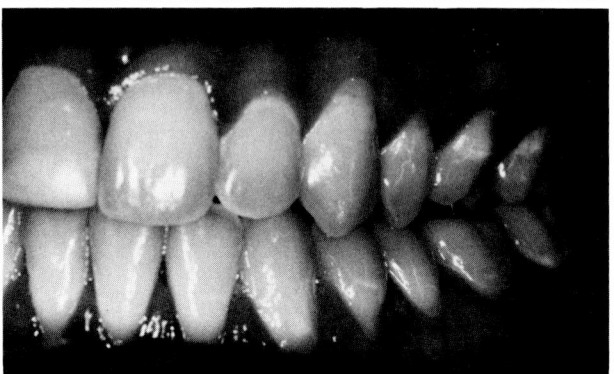

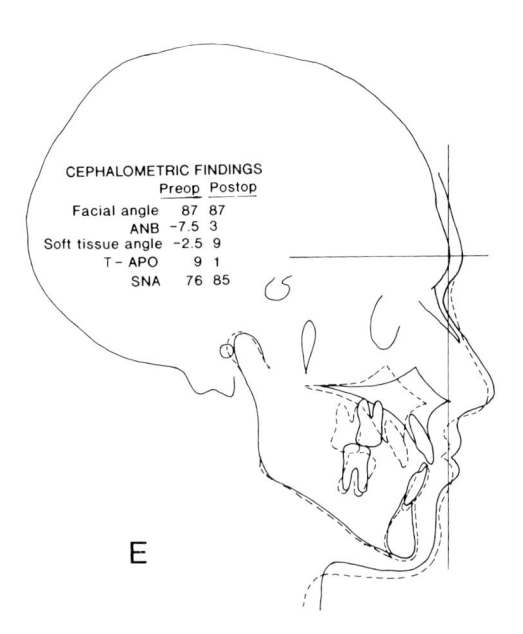

FIGURE 51–13 *Continued.* *D,* Post-treatment (14 months after surgery) dental occlusion. Note the mild maxillary posterior residual transverse deficiency. *E,* Pretreatment *(dashed line)* and 14-month postsurgical *(solid line)* composite tracing of the lateral cephalogram with abbreviated cephalometric analysis and subnasale-vertical reference line. Note the nasal tip elevation and upper lip advancement following maxillary surgical advancement. (Orthodontic treatment was provided by John Kanyusik, D.D.S., Mankato, MN.)

3. Mandibular arch: nonextraction, arch coordination with fixed appliances.
4. Twelve months in duration.

Surgical Treatment (Fig. 51–13*B*, right; and *E*)

1. Maxillary Le Fort II osteotomy with advancement (12 mm) and vertical impaction (5 mm posterior and 3 mm anterior) and left rotation (3 mm).
2. Septoplasty (5-mm vertical reduction).

Postsurgical Orthodontics

1. Maxillary and mandibular fixed appliance midlines to refine interdigitation and arch form coordination.
2. Eight months in duration.

Treatment Result (Fig. 50–13*A*, *D*, and *E*)

1. At the 14-month postsurgical examination, excellent skeletal and dental stability was documented. The posterior occlusion tended toward end to end, indicating some posterior transverse relapse.
2. The midfacial esthetic improvement was substantial, and lip competence and position were normal.
3. The narrow alar width increased to normal width following maxillary advancement and impaction.
4. The patient was quite pleased with the functional and esthetic improvement, which he had not anticipated when he initially presented for treatment.

Discussion

The maxillary osteotomy procedure described by Kufner[5] can be performed through extraoral and intraoral incisions or, as recently described, the intraoral approach alone.[12,15] If the intraoral method is selected, it is necessary to limit the lateral vertical osteotomy (the most lateral position is where the infraorbital and lateral orbital rims join). When this approach is used, the interpositional bone graft extended laterally on the body of the zygoma will provide skeletal stability to the advanced maxilla and at the same time provide malar augmentation (to varying degrees, depending on the cosmetic requirements of each patient). These laterally positioned bone grafts should be initially overcontoured, as significant reduction can be expected during the revascularization and remodeling phase of bone graft healing. Sufficient time must be taken to ensure that symmetric contours are achieved bilaterally. Firm wire, screw, or miniplate fixation of the bone grafts is also required. When the surgeon wishes to advance the lateral orbital rim or body of the zygoma, extraoral incisions in the infraorbital or lateral orbital areas are required in addition to the usual intraoral incisions and exposure (these patients may be better managed with a Le Fort III osteotomy via a coronal approach). Interpositional autogenous bone grafts should be placed with appropriate stabilization in the gaps created by the advancement. Allogeneic graft materials could be considered for minimal advancement procedures,[18] or it may be possible to avoid bone grafts or allogeneic materials completely (especially in patients in whom minimal advancement and anterior vertical impaction are accomplished simultaneously). The latter situation (bone grafting not required) is illustrated in a patient treated with the quadrangular Le Fort I osteotomy (see Fig. 51–6).

The advanced maxilla is stabilized through the intraoral exposure and consists of transosseous wire suspension from the medial orbital rim superiorly (anterior to the nasolacrimal groove) to the piriform aperture and lateral nasal wall inferiorly. Placement of the medial infraorbital wire may be technically difficult; proper positioning of the medial vertical osteotomy (3 to 4 mm lateral to the nasal wall) and protection of the orbital and nasolacrimal apparatus with a small, modified channel retractor assist in acccomplishing proper transosseous wire placement.

Proper mobilization (downfracture) of the quadrangular Le Fort II osteotomy requires adequate strength and thickness of the lateral piriform aperture and infraorbital bone. If this bone is quite thin on surgical exposure, it may be prudent in selected patients to perform the quadrangular Le Fort I procedure (as described in the previous section). With proper bone graft placement, the desired esthetic results are potentially equal (however, in the author's opinion, they are more easily achieved and theoretically more stable with the Le Fort II procedure). If the osteotomized segment is not readily mobilized, it is prudent to re-examine all osteotomy sites, especially the medial and lateral infraorbital area. Use of a fine, curved chisel directed posteriorly and laterally (or medially) in these sites cuts bone in the floor of the orbit, which can be relatively thick in selected patients. The remainder of the orbital floor on either side of the infraorbital nerve is generally thin and fractures during the mobilization maneuver. If the medial and lateral osteotomies are not angled properly to provide unobstructed downfracture, proper mobilization is unlikely and undesirable fractures of the infraorbital area will occur. Pterygoid osteotomies for separation of the maxillary tuberosity from the vertical portion of the palatine bone or osteotomy of the horizontal process of the palatine bone have not been required in the author's experience. A greenstick fracture generally occurs through the horizontal process of the palatine bone posterior to the greater palatine foramen. This fracture is completed following downfracture through the midline nasal approach with a wedging osteotome.

After complete maxillary downfracture, an attempt is made to identify the palatine artery as it lies lateral to the lateral nasal wall in the horizontal process of the palatine bone posterior to the greater palatine foramen. This identification is technically more difficult than in the quadrangular Le Fort I osteotomy, as the anterior antral wall and infraorbital rim restrict visualization of this area. Reducing the lateral nasal wall anteriorly with a pear-shaped bur and curetting the posterior lateral nasal wall with a sharp molt curette generally expose the vessel. The vessel may also be visualized as it traverses the greenstick fracture of the posterolateral palatine bone (Fig. 51-9). If identified, the vessel is electrocoagulated in its canal posteriorly. Osteotomy of the posterior horizontal palatine bone with fine or wedging osteotomes and complete mobilization of the maxilla can then proceed with minimal hemorrhage. Complete separation of soft tissue from the posterior tuberosity and hard palate is critical and is generally accomplished by finger dissection while the maxilla is being held forward with a transpalatal wire secured through an acrylic interocclusal palatal splint (Fig. 51-9). It is imperative that the maxilla be completely mobilized and positioned into maxillary-mandibular fixation with minimal anterior force. If vertical impaction is required, obstructing bone is removed posteriorly and anteromedially by bur technique as the maxilla is autorotated superiorly and hinged on the mandibular condyles. Complete removal of posterior bone contact is necessary to avoid vertical unseating force on the mandibular condyles. To compensate for vertical condylar sag while the patient is under general anesthesia (particularly in patients with skeletal open bite), 1 to 2 mm of overcorrection is frequently provided when posterior maxillary impaction is used.

Patients requiring the quadrangular Le Fort II osteotomy for horizontal maxillary-zygomatic deficiency generally require significant advancement (8 to 15 mm) for complete correction and cosmetic improvement. The author feels that significant relapse potential exists in these patients during the first 12 months after advancement, during which complete bone (including grafted bone) healing and remodeling occur. For this reason, a 2- to 4-mm overcorrection is provided during model surgery and splint construction. If skeletal stabilization is achieved by miniplate application or by interpositional grafts secured by transosseous wires, the initial relapse should be minimal. Long-term relapse forces from the functional soft tissue matrix and morphogenetic pattern are still present after initial bone healing (miniplates and wires become passive) and through an indefinite period (most likely the remainder of the patient's life). If all vertical and horizontal maxillary and mandibular growth discrepancies are completely normalized so that soft tissue, muscular, and skeletal anatomy is properly matched, excellent long-term stability should be achieved. The author has not overadvanced a maxilla to the point where subsequent relapse or orthodontic management could not achieve a correct occlusion; on the other hand, it is not uncommon to be desirous of an additional amount of anterior maxillary positioning to achieve ideal dental intercuspation (especially in patients undergoing Le Fort II and III osteotomies).

As illustrated in the seven cases reported by Keller and Sather,[12] a large amount of posterior and anterior maxillary impaction can also be accomplished along with the maxillary advancement. Anterior impaction or lengthening should be less than 5 mm to avoid significant steps in the infraorbital rims and altered orbital outline and volume. Posterior maxillary impaction can be greater than 5 mm if the patient can tolerate the increased infraorbital rim advancement from the added rotational effect. The amount of potential advancement that can be done esthetically appears to be greater with the quadrangular Le Fort II osteotomy than with the lower classic Le Fort I osteotomy procedure; with large advancement at a low level, cosmetic improvement is compromised in the paranasal and infraorbital area.

The quadrangular Le Fort II procedure is frequently not indicated in a patient with a congenital maxillary cleft because of the common need for nasal advancement. However, if significant vertical or transverse deficiency exists, the quadrangular Le Fort II procedure, followed in 6 months by nasal reconstruction, can give a satisfactory result.[13] In addition, if required, alveolopalatal bone grafting can be accomplished with adequate exposure in the quadrangular Le Fort II osteotomy (rather than the pyramidal Le Fort II osteotomy) because the nasal floor and lateral nasal walls are well exposed, as in the Le Fort I osteotomy. If the alveolar-palatal cleft has not been previously bone grafted (previous cleft bone grafting is preferable in patients undergoing quadrangular Le Fort II osteotomy), a substantial, firmly fixed occlusal-palatal splint must be in place prior to the downfracture maneuver.

Maxillary midline shift must be kept to a minimum to avoid significant asymmetry in the superior portion of the mobilized segment. Similarly, maxillary arch expansion or constriction must be kept symmetric and limited in amount because of its effect on the positioning of the superior portion of the Le Fort II segment. Patients with true nasomaxillary deficiency (Binder's syndrome) who have a skeletal open bite and constricted maxillary arch can be treated by the pyramidal Le Fort II osteotomy followed 6 months later by a Le Fort I osteotomy or, as in one of the patients in a report,[12] by a combination of the intraoral quadrangular Le Fort II osteotomy followed 6 months later by nasal bone graft reconstruction.

The amount of blood lost with the intraoral modified Le Fort II osteotomy alone has been similar to that lost with the Le Fort I procedures. With controlled surgical and hypotensive anesthetic techniques, the need for blood replacement should be minimal. Blood replacement needs are satisfied by having the patient donate blood 48 hours (or longer) preoperatively (autologous donation).[14] Operating time is also similar to that in the Le Fort I procedure, with the added time for bone graft harvesting.

Operative complications have been minimal and center on the mobilization of the osteotomized segment. All osteotomy cuts must be complete. The central portion of the orbital floor must fracture during the downfracture maneuver; at the same time the palatine bone–tuberosity separation occurs, the horizontal process of the palatine bone fracture occurs. An unfavorable fracture may begin just below the infraorbital foramen if the infraorbital medial and lateral cuts are not angled correctly to allow unobstructed movement. These areas are observed closely during mobilization. If an unfavorable infraorbital fracture begins, additional bone cutting should be accomplished before proceeding.

Because of the quantity and quality of bone grafting needed in all of the patients in whom we have performed this procedure, corticocancellous iliac crest blocks are preferred. By keeping the laterosuperior cortex of the iliac crest and associated musculature intact, low morbidity and early ambulation are achieved (documented in a group of 160 consecutive patients[17] undergoing iliac bone harvesting). A 4- to 5-day hospital stay is typical and coincides with our experience with other orthognathic and jaw reconstructive procedures combined with iliac bone grafting.[7,12,13,16,19-24] Homogeneous, heterogeneous, or allogeneic graft material is not used in this group of patients.

Potential postsurgical complications after the quadrangular Le Fort II osteotomy would be similar in type and frequency to those of the quadrangular Le Fort I osteotomy, which were discussed in the previous section and based on a report of 54 consecutive patients. Similar types of complications are discussed: infection, sequestra, neurologic problems, nasolacrimal duct dysfunction, orbital complications, iliac crest problems, and miscellaneous complications.

Postsurgical infection, if present, would be expected to produce recurrent pain and swelling in the infraorbital and upper lip region 3 to 6 weeks after surgery. The patient may also complain of nasal and/or pharyngeal drainage and odor, as the antrum may serve as an area of dependent drainage. Since the lateral wall of the nose and associated mucosa is violated in the Le Fort I and II osteotomies, excellent antral drainage is invariably present. The author routinely passes a large, curved hemostat through the nares bilaterally into the antrum prior to final maxillary positioning and stabilization to confirm an adequate nasoantral communication (also for the Le Fort I procedure). Treatment of postsurgical sepsis, as described previously, would involve establishment of dependent drainage through the previous intraoral incision and maintenance of optimal antibiotic therapy for a minimum of 2 weeks. Prompt resolution should occur unless a problem exists with instability of the bone graft, mobilized maxilla, or foreign bodies used for fixation (e.g., wires and screws), or if antral dependent drainage (via nose) is inadequate. This type of infection has not been encountered in our patient population to date but has been seen in four patients who had undergone quadrangular Le Fort I osteotomy, as described previously. Long-term recurrent antral sepsis could occur if proper dependent drainage is not established intraoperatively or at some time postoperatively (if sepsis occurs).

Sequestra could occur secondary to sepsis or from dehiscence of intraoral wounds. Care is taken not to overcontour bone grafts excessively, and watertight everted incision closure is mandatory to prevent wound breakdown. This complication has not occurred in the patients who have undergone the Le Fort II procedure but was encountered in three patients who had had the Le Fort I osteotomy (all were patients with cleft deformities in whom alveolar-palatal grafting was combined with the orthognathic procedure).

Infraorbital nerve anesthesia and paresthesia are present in all patients undergoing this osteotomy as the infraorbital foramen is advanced and the bony canal is disrupted in the orbital floor. Resolution occurs over a period of months and varies considerably (in time and degree of recovery) from patient to patient, depending on the degree of trauma. Since the nerve injury is quite peripheral, complete resolution is frequently prompt and complete, as judged by follow-up comments by patients (no scientific study has been conducted on neurosensory function in patients who have had Le Fort II or III osteotomy) (see Chapter 34).

Nasolacrimal duct dysfunction of minor degree is frequently seen in patients undergoing Le Fort II osteotomy procedures. If the osteotomy is properly placed and the lacrimal apparatus protected during transosseous wire placement, the dysfunction (increased tearing) will be of short duration and secondary to surgical edema of the duct and surrounding soft tissue. If the duct is lacerated, the lacrimal secretions will generally exit into the nose at a higher level, as the nasal mucosa and lateral nasal wall are also violated with the Le Fort II level osteotomy. Long-term dysfunction requiring surgical intervention has not been encountered.

Orbital complications are grouped as follows: diplopia, endophthalmos, subconjunctival ecchymosis, chemosis, and irregular rim contour. *Diplopia* in all excursions is commonly seen and is secondary to extraocular muscle spasm. This muscle guarding is secondary to trauma to the infraorbital floor and periorbita. Resolution is invariably seen in 48 to 72 hours but has persisted for up to 10 days after surgery. All patients are advised of this potential for diplopia. *Endophthalmos* is a significant potential complication (especially if unilateral) that is secondary to fat herniation occurring when the periorbita is violated. This complication can be prevented by avoiding disruption of the orbital floor periosteum when performing the initial subperiosteal exposure of the maxilla. Repair of this disruption, if it does occur, with sutures and possibly with orbital floor grafts is advisable if endophthalmos is to be avoided. This complication has not occurred in our patient population. *Subconjunctival ecchymosis* and *chemosis* are only temporary cosmetic problems that may be encountered after the Le Fort II osteotomy (they are much more common in patients who have had pyramidal Le Fort II and Le Fort III osteotomies). *Irregular infraorbital contours* (also zygoma) are secondary to unequal and/or overcontoured medial (paranasal) or lateral (zygoma onlay graft) graft margins. Meticulous surgical technique prevents these cosmetic defects, which can be very noticeable and disconcerting to the patient. Secondary surgical procedures will be required if these contour defects are of any great size.

Iliac crest donor site complications are infrequent, as documented in a recent report of 160 consecutive patients.[17] If the lateral iliac crest cortex and associated musculature are left intact, early ambulation is predictable, and long-term gait problems or contour defects are not encountered. To date, all patients require graft thickness in the 6- to 12-mm range, which allows preservation of the lateral iliac crest cortex.

Miscellaneous potential complications include infraorbital emphysema (due to vigorous postsurgical nose blowing), transosseous wire prominence or exposure (after graft recontouring in the medial infraorbital and paranasal area), and oronasal fistula (which occurs if significant maxillary widening is accomplished via a two-piece osteotomy and simultaneous unrepaired nasal mucosa tears exist).

Relapse tendency has been noted by Steinhauser[11] and Freihofer[25] in Le Fort II osteotomy procedures. Freihofer reviewed the results in 20 adolescents with maxillary advancement and attributed most of the relapses to continued mandibular growth, concluding that "osteotomies of the jaws in adolescence should be deferred until growth has ceased." The long-term stability of this procedure awaits further study. The quadrangular Le Fort II osteotomy offers a better chance to place stabilizing interpositional bone grafts, and thus has a decided advantage over the pyramidal Le Fort II osteotomy. For this reason, the quadrangular Le Fort II osteotomy is our choice in patients with moderate-to-severe horizontal maxillary-zygomatic deficiency and acceptable nasal projection.

REFERENCES

1. Wassmund M: Lehrbuch der praktischen Chirurgie des Mundes und der Kiefer. 1st bd. Leipzig, Meusser, 1935.
2. Gillies H, Harrison SH: Operative correction by osteotomy of recessed malar maxillary compound in a case of oxycephaly. Br J Plast Surg 3:123, 1950.
3. Converse JM, Horowitz SL, Valauri AJ, et al: The treatment of nasomaxillary hypoplasia: A new pyramidal naso-orbital maxillary osteotomy. Plast Reconstr Surg 45:527, 1970.
4. Henderson D, Jackson IT: Naso-maxillary hypoplasia—the Le Fort II osteotomy. Br J Oral Surg 2:77, 1973.
5. Kufner J: Four-year experience with major maxillary osteotomy for retrusion. J Oral Surg 29:549, 1971.
6. Obwegesser HL: Surgical correction of small or retrodisplaced maxillae: The "dish-face" deformity. Plast Reconstr Surg 43:351, 1969.
7. Keller EE, Sather AH: Quadrangular Le Fort I osteotomy: Surgical technique and review of 54 consecutive patients. J Oral Maxillofac Surg 48(1):2, 1990.
8. Gillies HG: *In* Row NL, Killie HC: Fractures of the Facial Skeleton. Edinburgh, E & S Livingstone, 1955.
9. Souyris F, Carvel J-B, Reynaud JP: Osteotomies "intermédiaires" de l'étage moyen de la face. Ann Chir Plast 18:149, 1973.
10. Champy M: Surgical treatment of midface deformities. Head Neck Surg 2:451, 1980.
11. Steinhauser EW: Variations of Le Fort II osteotomies for correction of midfacial deformities. J Maxillofac Surg 8:258, 1989.
12. Keller EE, Sather AH: Intraoral quadrangular Le Fort II osteotomy. J Oral Maxillofac Surg 45:223, 1987.
13. Keller EE, Jackson IT: Treatment of skeletal deformities in the cleft patient. *In* Bardach J, Morris H (eds): Multidisciplinary Management of Cleft Lip and Palate. Philadelphia; WB Saunders Company, 1990.
14. Triplett WW, Lund BA, Keller EE, Taswell HF: Preoperative donation of autologous blood: Technique, experience, and community applications. Oral Surg Oral Med Oral Pathol 65:286, 1988.
15. Brusati R, Sesenna E, Raffaini M: On the feasibility of intraoral maxillo-malar osteotomy. J Cranio-Max-Fac Surg 17:110, 1989.
16. Keller EE, Hill AJ, Sather AH: Orthognathic surgery: Review of mandibular body procedures. Mayo Clin Proc 51:117, 1976.
17. Keller EE, Triplett WW: Iliac bone grafting: Review of 160 consecutive cases. J Oral Maxillofac Surg 45:11, 1987.
18. Wardrop RW, Wolford LM: Maxillary stability following downgraft and/or advancement procedures with stabilization using rigid fixation and porous block hydroxyapatite implants. J Oral Maxillofac Surg 47:336, 1989.
19. Brennan MD, Jackson IT, Keller EE, et al: Multidisciplinary management of acromegaly and its deformities. JAMA 253:682, 1985.
20. Jackson IJ, Meland NB, Keller EE, Sather AH: Surgical correction of the acromegalic face. A one stage procedure with team approach. J Cranio-Max-Fac Surg 17:2, 1989.
21. Keller EE, Desjardins RP, Eckert SE, Tolman DE: Composite bone grafts and titanium implants in mandibular discontinuity reconstruction. Int J Oral Maxillofac Implants 3:261, 1988.
22. Keller EE, Van Roekel NB, Desjardins RP, Tolman DE: Prosthetic-surgical reconstruction of the severely resorbed maxilla with iliac bone grafting and tissue-integrated prostheses. Int J Oral Maxillofac Implants 2:155, 1987.
23. Tolman DE, Desjardins RP, Keller EE: Surgical-prosthodontic reconstruction of oronasal defects utilizing the tissue-integrated prosthesis. Int J Oral Maxillofac Implants 3:31, 1988.
24. Tidstrom KD, Keller EE: Reconstruction of mandibular discontinuity with autogenous iliac bone graft: Report of 34 consecutive patients. J Oral Maxillofac Surg 48(4):336, 1990.
25. Freihofer HPM Jr: Results of osteotomies of the facial skeleton in adolescence. J Maxillofac Surg 5:267, 1977.
26. Cutting C, Grayson B, Bookstein F, et al: Computer-aided planning and evaluation of facial and orthognatic surgery. Clin Plast Surg 13:449, 1986.
27. Salyer K, Taylor DP, Billmire DE: Three-dimensional CAT scan reconstruction—pediatric patients. Clin Plast Surg 13:463, 1986.
28. Cutting C, Bookstein FL, Grayson B, et al: Three-dimensional computer-assisted design of craniofacial surgical procedures: Optimization and interaction with cephalometric and CT-based models. Plast Reconstr Surg 77:877, 1986.

52 CRANIOSYNOSTOSIS: DIAGNOSIS AND TREATMENT IN INFANCY AND EARLY CHILDHOOD

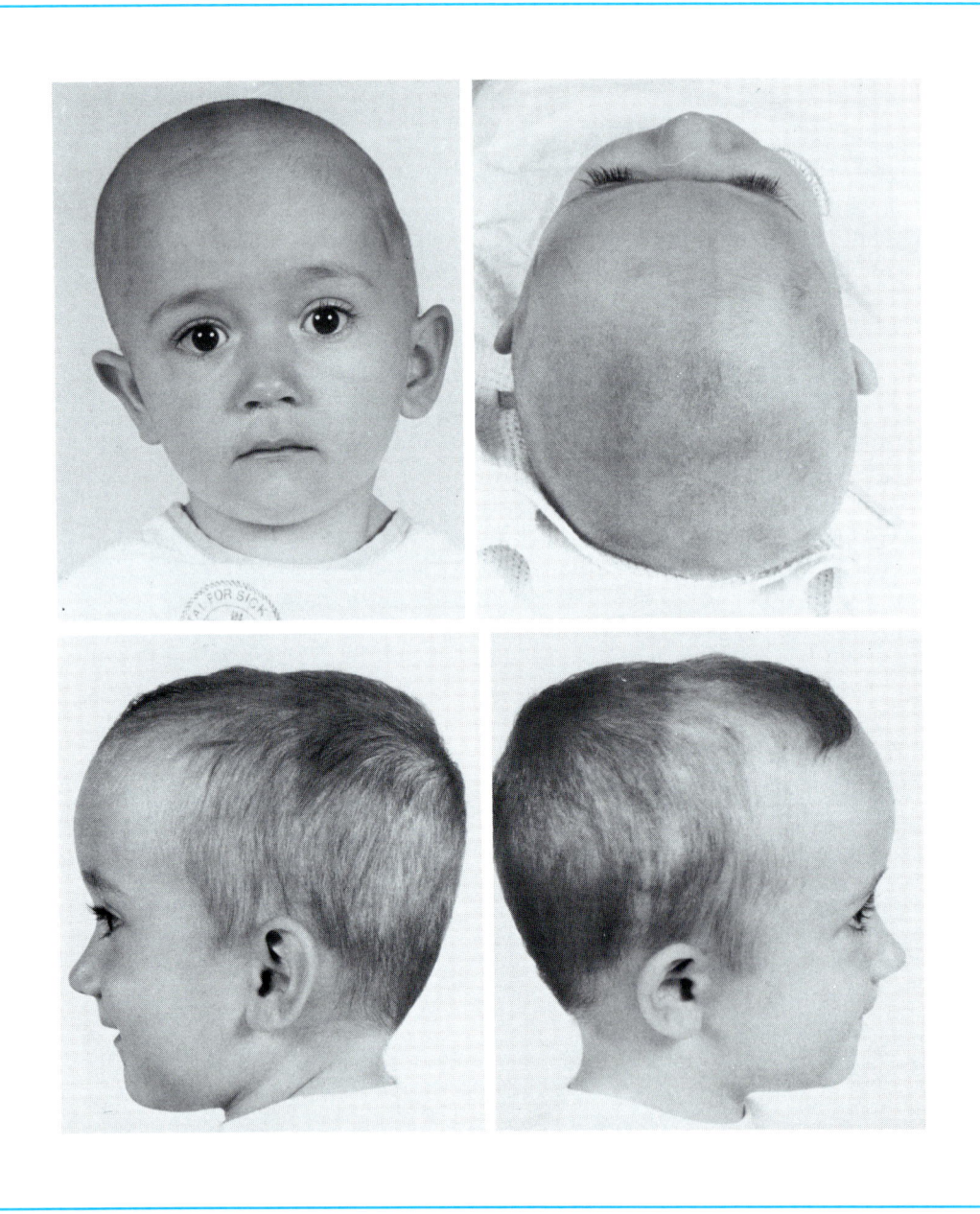

HISTORICAL PERSPECTIVE

FUNCTIONAL PROBLEMS IN CRANIOSYNOSTOSIS

  Brain Growth
  Intracranial Pressure
  Effects on Vision
  Hydrocephalus
  Airway Management
  Dental Effects
  Speech Effects
  Extremity Anomalies

ESTHETIC CONSIDERATIONS

  Fronto-forehead Region

SURGICAL APPROACH

  Historical Perspective
  Current Surgical Approach: Staging of Reconstruction

CLASSIFICATION SYSTEM

  External (Posture) Skull Molding
  Craniosynostosis
  Craniofacial Dysostosis

CASE REPORTS

JEFFREY C. POSNICK

HISTORICAL PERSPECTIVE

Premature fusion of the cranial vault sutures has been recognized since the time of the ancient Greeks. In 1842 Galen introduced the term *oxycephaly* to describe the condition. Later, Virchow coined the term *craniosynostosis* and formulated the classic theory known as Virchow's law, which states that premature fusion (synostosis) of a cranial vault suture inhibits normal skull growth perpendicular to the fused suture and that compensatory growth occurs at the open sutures, with the general direction of growth being parallel to the fused sutures.[158]

Familial types of craniofacial dysostosis were described by Apert in 1906[8] and Crouzon in 1912.[28] The incidence of craniosynostosis is about 0.4 per 1000 in the general population.[4,23] Most cases of simple craniosynostosis are sporadic. However, if both a parent and a child are affected, the risk for each subsequent child approaches 50 per cent. Syndromal craniosynostosis is usually genetic.[46] It may be either autosomal dominant, as in Crouzon syndrome, or less commonly, autosomal recessive, as in Apert syndrome.[24,27,33,57]

The treatment for these conditions has been surgical, but the timing, type, and effectiveness of therapy have not been well studied. This chapter explains a rationale for treatment intervention.

FUNCTIONAL PROBLEMS IN CRANIOSYNOSTOSIS

Brain Growth

Brain volume in the normal child almost triples during the first year of life (Table 52–1). By age 2 years, the cranial capacity is four times that at birth. If this tumor-like brain growth is to proceed unhindered, the open sutures at the level of the cranial vault and base must spread during phases of rapid growth, resulting in marginal ossification.

In craniosynostosis, premature suture fusion is combined with continuing brain growth. The orbital and cranial vault shape is determined by Virchow's law.[158] Depending on the number and location of prematurely fused sutures and the timing of closure, the growth potential of the brain may be limited. If surgical intervention, with suture release and reshaping to restore a more normal intracra-

TABLE 52-1. CRANIAL AND BRAIN GROWTH DURING THE FIRST 20 YEARS OF LIFE*

AGE	VOLUME OF BRAIN (cm³)	CRANIAL CAPACITY (cm³)
Newborn	330	350
3 months	550	600
6 months	575	775
9 months	675	925
1 year	750	1000
2 years	900	1100
3 years	960	1225
4 years	1000	1300
6 years	1060	1350
9 years	1100	1400
12 years	1150	1450
20 years	1200	1500

* From Blinkov SM, Glezer II: The Human Brain in Figures and Tables. A Quantitative Handbook. Translated from the Russian by B. Haigh. Original Russian text published by Meditsina Press, Leningrad, 1964. Copyright © 1968 by Plenum Press and Basic Books, Inc. Reprinted by permission of Basic Books, New York.

nial volume, does not reverse the process, diminished intelligence is often the end result.[120]

Intracranial Pressure

Elevated intracranial pressure is a major functional problem that is frequently associated with premature suture fusion. Its late and devastating effect can be identified on plain radiographs from the fingerprinting or beaten-copper appearance of the inner table of the cranial vault. Early signs of pressure apparent from a CT scan include the loss of cisternae, but this is considered a soft finding. If intracranial hypertension goes untreated, it affects brain function. Funduscopic examination reveals papilledema, and later optic atrophy develops.

Intracranial hypertension can be documented invasively by means of a craniotomy used to place an epidural pressure sensor or by lumbar puncture monitoring.[129] Increased intracranial pressure is most likely to affect those with the greatest disparity between brain growth and intracranial capacity and may occur in as many as 42 per cent of untreated children with more than one suture affected (Fig. 52-1).[129] Work is now underway to verify the efficacy of standard computed tomography (CT) scans as a method of indirect measurement of intracranial vol-

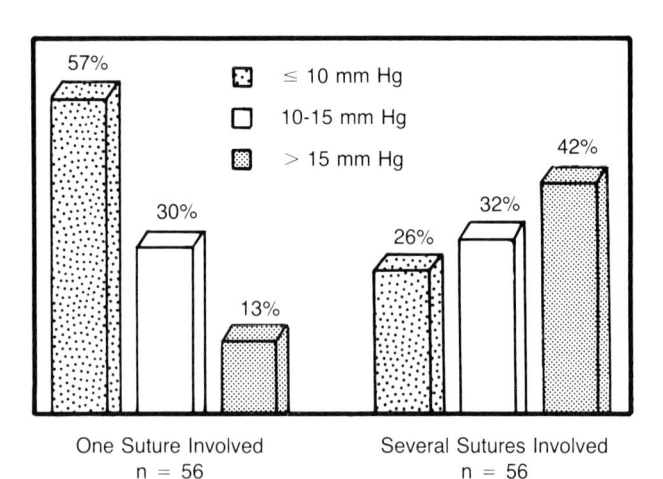

FIGURE 52-1. Craniosynostosis and intracranial pressure. (From Marchac D, Renier D: Craniofacial Surgery For Craniosynostosis. Boston, Little, Brown, 1982.)

ume.[42,125] This noninvasive method can be used to measure intracranial volume in children with craniosynostosis. It might then be possible to select those individuals who are at high risk for developing increased ICP and would benefit the most from early surgery.

Effects on Vision

Increased intracranial pressure, if left untreated, leads to papilledema. Eventually optic atrophy develops, resulting in partial or complete blindness. If the orbits are shallow (exorbitism) and the eyeballs bulge (exophthalmos), the cornea may be exposed and abrasions may occur. An eyeball sitting in a shallow orbit is also at risk for trauma. Some forms of craniosynostosis may involve orbital hypertelorism, which may lead to compromised visual acuity and restricted binocular vision. If the orbit is deformed, an asymmetry (orbital dystopia) may be present. Divergent or convergent nonparalytic strabismus or exotropia occurs frequently and should be looked for.[32,48,100] The incidence of unilateral or bilateral upper eyelid ptosis is also increased.

Hydrocephalus

Hydrocephalus affects 10 to 20 per cent of patients with craniosynostosis. It is particularly common in patients with Crouzon syndrome, Apert syndrome, and kleeblattschädel anomaly.[40,45,54] Although the etiology is not clear, hydrocephalus may be secondary to a generalized cranial base stenosis with constriction of all cranial base foramina. It may be identified from a CT scan or magnetic resonance imaging (MRI) as bilaterally enlarged ventricles. A high index of suspicion should be maintained, with early diagnosis and prompt ventriculoperitoneal shunting when indicated.

Airway Management

All newborn infants are obligate nasal breathers. Breathing is generally satisfactory in craniosynostosis and no special management is required. In some forms of craniofacial dysostosis, a generalized craniofacial atresia exists in which the nasal and nasopharyngeal spaces are markedly diminished.[72] An affected child is forced to breathe through his or her mouth, which may be abnormally filled with a normal tongue that is confined within a small oropharyngeal space.[47] This method of breathing requires a tremendous expenditure of energy and forces the infant into a catabolic state (negative nitrogen balance), in these rare cases, unless treatment is given (i.e., tracheostomy or, occasionally, early monobloc osteotomy with advancement).[72] Sleep apnea of either central or peripheral origin may occur.[47,92] If a peripheral origin of sleep apnea is documented in the sleep laboratory, a tracheostomy may be indicated. Central apnea may result from poorly treated intracranial hypertension.

Dental Effects

Children with Apert syndrome, Crouzon syndrome, and kleeblattschädel anomaly have dental and oral anomalies. The palate is often high-arched and constricted in width. The incidence of cleft palate in patients with Apert syndrome approaches 30 per cent. Dental development is often delayed, and the teeth may be malformed or congenitally absent. The small maxillary arch causes severe crowding of the teeth. In Apert syndrome patients, the soft palate and the uvula are long and hang down into the pharynx, which may further obstruct air passage during sleep.

Speech Effects

In craniofacial dysostosis syndromes, abnormalities of the jaws, teeth, nasal passages, and palate frequently lead to speech and language problems.[164] The diminished intranasal volume often results in hyponasal speech resonance. If a cleft palate is present, hypernasal speech may also occur. Sibilant distortions resulting from anterior malocclusions (e.g., Class III malocclusion, anterior open-bite deformity) are common.[163]

Extremity Anomalies

Apert syndrome results in joint fusion and bony and soft-tissue syndactylism of the digits of all four limbs.[18] Partial or complete fusion of the shoulder or elbow is frequent. Broad thumbs, broad great toes, and partial soft-tissue syndactyly of the hands may be seen in Pfeiffer syndrome, but these are variable features.[68,124] Preaxial polysyndactyly of the feet may be seen in Carpenter syndrome.[20,142]

ESTHETIC CONSIDERATIONS

The surgeon must examine the entire craniofacial region meticulously. Both the skeleton and the soft tissue must be assessed with a standard method to identify all normal and abnormal anatomy. Specific findings tend to occur in particular malformations, but each patient is unique. CT scanning with three-dimensional reconstruction of the abnormal skull helps to confirm clinical impressions.[49,50,89-91,153,154,157] Standard CT scans are becoming increasingly useful for measuring variations from normal in the cranio-orbito-zygomatic regions.[21,160] The standard cephalometric analysis remains a useful tool for assessment of the lower face. When examining the cranium and face, the surgeon must remain aware of normal and abnormal growth patterns common to particular anomalies because these influence the ideal timing and type of reconstruction.

Fronto-forehead Region

The position of the forehead is critically important to overall facial balance. The forehead can be thought of as containing two parts, the supraorbital ridge and the superior forehead.[80,81] The supraorbital ridge includes the supraorbital rim, glabella region, frontozygomatic suture, and temporoparietal bone extension. The morphology and position of the supraorbital ridge are key to upper face esthetics. At the level of the frontonasal suture, an angle, which should range from 90 to 110 degrees, is formed by the supraorbital ridge and the nose as seen in the sagittal plane. The overlying eyebrows should be anterior to the globe when viewed in the sagittal plane. When the supraorbital ridge is viewed from above, the rims should arc posteriorly to achieve a gentle 90-degree angle at the temporal fossa with the center point at the level of the frontozygomatic suture. The superior forehead (about 1.0 to 1.5 cm up from the supraorbital ridge) has a gentle posterior curve when seen in the sagittal plane. This should describe an arc of about 60 degrees, leveling out at the coronal suture region.

SURGICAL APPROACH

Historical Perspective

The first recorded surgical approaches to craniosynostosis were performed by Lannelongue[71] in 1890 and Lane[70] in 1892, who completed strip craniectomies. Their aim was exclusively to control the functional problem of brain compression within a small intracranial volume (increased intracranial pressure).

The classic neurosurgical techniques developed over the ensuing decades have generally been geared toward releasing the synostotic sutures in the hope that the freed-up skull would then reshape itself and continue to grow in a normal and symmetric fashion.[1,2,6,7,15,51,52,98,99,111,137] The strip craniectomy was supposed to allow for the creation of a new suture line at the site of previous synostosis. With the realization that this was inadequate treatment, attempts have been made to fragment the cranial vault surgically with pieces of flat bone used as grafts to refashion the cranial vault shape. These techniques occasionally resulted in adequate cerebral decompression, but they rarely produced an adequate shape[10,127] because of postoperative postural molding that resulted in significant distortions. Furthermore, reossification after craniectomy was unpredictable; often there was excessively rapid reossification and at other times there were significant cranial vault defects.

The application of craniofacial techniques was pioneered by Tessier,[144] who introduced a new way of thinking. He proposed that, when indicated, cranial vault, orbital, and midface reshaping through a combined intracranial and extracranial approach should occur simultaneously with suture release. The coronal incision was often combined with lower eyelid incisions. Autogenous bone grafts were harvested from the hip and rib cage. Stabilization was achieved with well-planned step-cut osteotomies and direct transosseous wires. External pin-fixation devices were used as needed for additional fixation and stabilization. Tracheostomy was generally required for perioperative airway management.

Rougerie et al[132] applied this concept of simultaneous suture release and cranial vault reshaping to infants in 1972 and others have followed their example. Later, in 1976, Hoffman and Mohr[53] advanced the concept of suture release and a degree of cranial vault and orbital reshaping for unilateral coronal synostosis in infancy. They coined the term *lateral canthal advancement* to describe the procedure. In 1977, Whitaker et al[161] proposed a more formal cranial vault and orbital reshaping for unilateral coronal synostosis. In 1979 Marchac and Renier[84] published their experience with the floating forehead technique for simultaneous suture release and cranial vault and orbital reshaping to manage either unilateral or bicoronal synostosis in infancy. They postulated that the growing brain would further push the forehead, orbits, and midface forward and allow for further correction over time.[86,88]

Current Surgical Approach: Staging of Reconstruction

In most cases, once craniosynostosis is recognized, suture release and cranial vault and orbital reshaping are mandatory before the patient reaches 12 months of age.[34,35,53,59,81,84,87,88,93,94,96,121,122,155,161,162] An intracranial approach is used for cranial vault and orbital osteotomies, with reshaping and advancement of bony segments for ideal age-appropriate bony morphology. Close intraoperative cooperation is required between the craniofacial surgeon, neurosurgeon, and pediatric anesthetist.

The child must undergo full craniofacial team assessments preoperatively and at postoperative intervals. Planning the timing and type of surgical intervention must take into account the functions, future growth, and development of the craniofacial skeleton, as well as the maintenance of a normal body image.[9,74,75,118,120]

In recalcitrant or severe forms of craniosynostosis or craniofacial dysostosis, additional intracranial revision of the cranial vault and orbits is necessary during infancy or early childhood to further increase intracranial volume, thereby allowing for continued brain growth and avoiding or relieving intracranial hypertension.[104]

If the cranial base and facial sutures are also involved, as is the case in Apert syndrome, Crouzon syndrome, or kleeblattschädel anomaly,[12,16,19,36-38,41,43,56,61,63,67,69,76,101,102,112,116,126,128,130,131,133-135,138,139,143,146] continuing midface and orbital deficiency requires further reconstruction (i.e., monobloc, monobloc bipartition, or Le Fort III osteotomy) later in childhood or early adolescence.[5,44,58,77-79,83,85,87,103,105,113-115,117,145-152,156] Cranio-orbital and facial esthetics should be reassessed at 5 to 7 years of age, when the brain and eyes and their associated cranial and orbital bones are approximately 85 to 90 per cent of adult size.[160] Any reconstructive surgery undertaken in this region at that time is more or less permanent. Psychosocial considerations weigh heavily in deciding the timing of midface surgery.[9,74,75,118]

Examination of the craniofacial skeleton reveals varied degrees of residual exorbitism (shallow orbits), exophthalmos (bulging eyes), and midface deficiency. If the SOR remains posterior (short anterior cranial base) despite early cranial vault surgery; the orbits are shallow; and the zygomas, nose, and maxilla are deficient, a monobloc advancement is indicated.[5,83,103,114,115,152] If a degree of orbital hypertelorism is also present and requires simultaneous correction, bipartition of the monobloc (facial bipartition) is indicated.[152,156] If, on the other hand, the supraorbital ridge is well positioned, a Le Fort III osteotomy is carried out to correct the flat infraorbital rims (shallow orbits) and generalized midface deficiency.[44,79,85,97,105,113,117,145-152]

For either a monobloc, facial bipartition, or Le Fort III osteotomy, stabilization is provided by bone miniplates and microplates,[103] as well as autogenous cranial bone grafts. Perioperative airway management is accomplished with endotracheal intubation and not tracheostomy. The role of intermaxillary fixation is limited.

Total midface surgery (monobloc, monobloc bipartition, or Le Fort III osteotomy) carried out after the age of 5 years should establish the final position and shape of the orbits.[160] The mandible continues to grow, but the maxilla (at the Le Fort I level) does not keep up. In patients with the moderate to severe forms of Crouzon syndrome and all patients with Apert syndrome and kleeblattschädel anomaly, a Le Fort I osteotomy and genioplasty are needed in conjunction with major orthodontic intervention during mid to late adolescence.[106-109] The Le Fort I osteotomy is stabilized with bone miniplates and screws and iliac corticocancellous bone grafts to limit postoperative skeletal relapse. The need for intermaxillary fixation is diminished when miniplate and screw fixation is used.

CLASSIFICATION SYSTEM

The most commonly used classification of craniosynostosis is based on the shape of the skull, which usually reflects the underlying prematurely closed suture(s). The major cranial vault sutures that may be involved include the left and right coronal, metopic, sagittal, and left and right lambdoid. In the craniofacial dysostosis syndromes, additional cranial base or facial suture or synchondrosis may be involved. These forms of synostosis (cranial base and facial) are more difficult to identify by radiographic techniques, and their resulting deformities are less consistent (i.e., the variation is greater).

External (Posture) Skull Molding

External molding must not be confused with true synostosis because the natural history and the timing and form of intervention differ.[13] Torticollis commonly results in postural molding both of the ipsilateral forehead, which looks similar to unilateral coronal synostosis, and of the contralateral occipitoparietal region, which resembles lambdoid synostosis.[73,165] Klippel-Feil anomaly also results in gross asymmetry and distortion of the craniofacial skeleton but without a true synostosis.[62] Skull molding may result from extraocular muscle dysfunction when the child must angle the head to prevent or limit diplopia.[48] Rotatory subluxations of the cervical spine (C1–C2) may also lead to skull asymmetries resembling true synostosis. Rotatory subluxations of the cervical spine (C1–C2) may also occur in combination with congenital torticollis and skull asymmetry. Skull molding may also result from other forms of repetitive skull positioning, such as that which occurs when a newborn is allowed to lie with the head in one unvaried position. This condition also occurs when partial or complete craniectomy for craniosynostosis has been performed. The skull grows back in a flattened position that reflects the frequent head position during the reossification phase. In some primitive cultures, a ritualistic form of skull molding is achieved by serially banding the forehead to establish flattening of the forehead.[13]

Craniosynostosis

ANTERIOR PLAGIOCEPHALY: UNILATERAL CORONAL SYNOSTOSIS (CASE 1, FIG. 52–2)

The word *plagiocephaly* is derived from the Greek for oblique head. Plagiocephaly from a unilateral coronal synostosis results in flatness or obliquity on the ipsilateral side of the forehead and supraorbital ridge region. This form of suture synostosis must be distinguished from a secondary external skull molding deformity (i.e., torticollis or cervical spine anomalies such as Klippel-Feil) caused by head-positioning patterns without true suture synostosis.

Anterior plagiocephaly, or unilateral coronal synostosis, always results in asymmetric morphology. There are characteristic morphologic features on the affected ipsilateral side. The frontal bone is flat, and the supraorbital ridge and lateral orbital rim are recessed. The affected orbit is shallow and the anterior cranial base is short in the anteroposterior (AP) dimension. The sphenoid wing is elevated, producing a harlequin appearance on the plain radiograph or CT scan. The root of the nose is constricted and deviated to the affected side. The zygoma and infraorbital rim may also be flat and recessed.

Compensatory changes are likely to occur on the opposite (contralateral) side as a result of pushing by the growing brain and distortion of the bones according to Virchow's law.[158] The frontal bone may bulge, leading to anterior and inferior displacement of the supraorbital ridge and lateral orbital rim. In addition, the inferior orbital rim may be displaced inferiorly. The tip of the nose is often deviated to the side opposite the synostosis.

Current Surgical Treatment in Infancy. A variety of surgical approaches for unilateral coronal synostosis have been described.[15,34,35,59,77,80–82,84,93–96,98,99,104,121,123,137,140] Good long-term results are obtained when treatment of unilateral coronal synostosis includes suture release as well as cranial vault and three-quarter orbital osteotomies with reshaping and advancement in infancy. I prefer to perform these procedures at 10 months to 1 year of age. Although the cause is a unilateral synostosis, a bilateral deformity exists morphologically. My belief is that to achieve symmetry, it is necessary to use a bilateral surgical approach. Symmetry of the cranial vault and orbits must be achieved on the operating room table, since results generally do not improve over time. Osteotomy and reshaping of the squamosal portion of the temporal bone are carried out to correct temporal region asymmetries when indicated.[141] Stabilization is achieved with autogenous cranial bone grafts, direct transosseous wires, and the careful and limited use of microplates for selected regions in difficult cases.

instruments to re-establish the normal orbital rim and anterior cranial base morphology appropriate for the child's age. Orbital hypotelorism is corrected by splitting the supraorbital ridge unit vertically in the midline and adding autogenous cranial bone grafts to increase the intraorbital distance. Osteotomy and reshaping of the squamosal portion of the temporal bones deep to the temporalis muscles and down to the cranial base are carried out to achieve a normal bitemporal width. The abnormally shaped forehead bone that has been removed is cut into sections of appropriate shape for the new forehead configuration. The anterior cranial base, anterior cranial vault, and orbits are given a more correct esthetic shape, and the volume of the anterior cranial vault is increased to give the brain more space. Stabilization is achieved with autogenous cranial bone grafts, direct transosseous wires, and the careful and limited use of micro bone plates for selected regions in difficult cases.

SCAPHOCEPHALY: SAGITTAL SUTURE SYNOSTOSIS (CASES 6 AND 7, FIGS. 52–7 AND 52–8)

The term *scaphocephaly* is derived from the Greek word for boat and is used to describe a head shaped like the keel of a boat. This anomaly results from premature fusion of the sagittal suture. It is believed to be the most common form of cranial vault synostosis and is said to be rarely associated with increased intracranial pressure. Usually the midface and anterior cranial vault sutures are not affected.

Scaphocephaly or sagittal suture synostosis results in compensatory growth of the open sutures (i.e., the lambdoid, coronal, and metopic sutures) as the brain continues to grow rapidly in infancy and early childhood. This results in an elongated anteroposterior dimension and a narrowed transverse dimension to the cranial vault. Midface deficiency is rare, but when it is present, the working diagnosis should be Crouzon syndrome.

Current Surgical Approach. When scaphocephaly is recognized early in infancy, most neurosurgeons believe that simple release of the sagittal suture through a strip craniectomy without simultaneous skull reshaping is adequate treatment.[137] Although this may be satisfactory from a functional point of view, a diminished scaphocephalic shape may still be present.[2] This persistent morphology may cause continued psychosocial concern and make wearing head apparel difficult. Unfortunately, studies of efficiency of the classic neurosurgical approach are lacking. If improvements in cranial vault shape are desired after 1 year of age, a formal total cranial vault reshaping is required. The patient is maintained in the supine position for the surgical procedure but is prepared so that total cranial vault reshaping can be carried out. Stabilization is accomplished with autogenous cranial bone grafts, direct transosseous wires, and the use of miniplate and micro bone plate fixation.

Craniofacial Dysostosis

CROUZON SYNDROME (CASES 8 AND 11, FIGS. 52–9 AND 52–12)

Crouzon syndrome, which affects about one person in every 25,000 of the general population, is inherited as an autosomal dominant trait.[136] It is noted for its variable expressivity.[17,28] A significant family pedigree for the trait may be present, but the occurrence of a fresh mutation is just as likely.[22,27,28,33,57,159] At the level of the cranial vault, the skull is generally brachycephalic (see brachycephaly) as a result of bilateral premature fusion of the coronal suture.[65,116] Although less common, other cranial vault sutures may also fuse prematurely and may involve lambdoid, sagittal, or metopic synostosis.[24]

Crouzon[28] described four characteristics of the disease in a family pedigree:

52—CRANIOSYNOSTOSIS: DIAGNOSIS AND TREATMENT IN INFANCY AND EARLY CHILDHOOD / 1849

exorbitism, retromaxillism, inframaxillism, and paradoxic retrogenia. In addition to premature fusion of multiple cranial vault sutures, the coronal sutures (brachycephaly) being most commonly affected, there is a poorly defined effect on the anterior cranial base and facial sutures and on growth centers that results in a variable degree of symmetric hypoplasia of the orbits, zygomas, and maxilla. In general, the soft-tissue envelope is normal. However, upper eyelid ptosis may be present.[63] The overall midface appearance is generally of bulging eyes (exophthalmos) resulting from shallow orbits (exorbitism) and midface flatness with a Class III malocclusion. The mandible has normal growth potential.[11,26]

Current Surgical Approach. A variety of surgical techniques has been described for the management of Crouzon syndrome. Based on a retrospective institutional review carried out at The Hospital for Sick Children (HSC), I recommend a staged approach to reconstruction in patients with Crouzon syndrome.[107,108] In infancy it is necessary to combine suture release with cranial vault and orbital osteotomies with reshaping and advancement to correct the brachycephalic morphology and increase the intracranial volume (see brachycephaly). Repeat craniotomy with further cranial vault and orbital reshaping and advancement is sometimes required later in infancy or early childhood for the management of significantly elevated intracranial pressure as documented from clinical, neurologic, ophthalmologic, or radiographic examination. This repeat cranial vault surgery is geared toward normalizing the intracranial volume but also further corrects orbital depth and skull morphology. Total midface deficiency requires either a Le Fort III or monobloc osteotomy with reshaping and advancement.[30] I prefer to perform these procedures at 5 to 7 years of age in combination with cranial vault reshaping as indicated to further increase the intracranial volume and relieve pressure in the brain and for improvements in cranial vault morphology. The midface procedure selected depends on the position of the supraorbital ridge and the degree of advancement required. When skeletal maturity has been reached (age 14 to 16 years in females, age 16 to 18 years in males), a maxillary Le Fort I osteotomy and genioplasty are generally required and are performed in conjunction with major orthodontic intervention.

APERT SYNDROME (CASE 9, FIG. 52–10)

Apert syndrome (acrocephalosyndactyly) usually occurs sporadically. However, dominant transmission with complete penetrance has been reported. Advanced paternal age is a factor in producing new mutations.[24] The syndrome has been observed in Caucasian, Black, and Oriental populations. Postmortem studies suggest a reduced growth potential of the cranial base, leading to premature fusion of the midline suture from the occiput to the anterior nasal septum.[112] Other studies[135,138,139] suggest that the sphenoid bone may be the main factor in this facial deformity, through synostosis adjacent to the vomer.

Severe bicoronal synostosis is usually seen at the level of the cranial vault. Severe cranial base and facial synostosis and synchondrosis are always present. In most cases, the mandible is not affected.[11,26]

Apert,[8] in 1906, described the syndrome as a severe cranial vault deformity with associated syndactylism, mental retardation, and blindness. Premature bilateral fusion of the coronal suture as well as fusion of the anterior cranial vault and midface suture(s) or growth center(s) is seen. There is severe, symmetric syndactyly of the hands and feet.[14,119] The syndrome has the same general craniofacial bony morphology as Crouzon syndrome but is much more severe.[21] The midface hypoplasia is more marked (both vertically and horizontally), as are the exorbitism, exophthalmos, and orbital hypertelorism. The incidence of cleft palate approaches 30 per cent.

The soft-tissue drape is often abnormal, and acne vulgaris with extensions to the forearms is common (70 per cent). The facial skin, especially in the nasal region, is often thick, with increased sebaceous discharge. Downward slant of the lateral canthi is common and reflects the underlying bony framework.[39] Upper eyelid ptosis is common. Hydrocephalus occurs frequently and requires ventriculoperitoneal shunting.[40,45,54] A conductive hearing loss may be present.[3,25] In 30 to 40 per cent of cases, there is congenital fixation of the middle ear structures, which is often compounded by inadequately treated otitis media.

Current Surgical Approach. Based on a retrospective institutional review carried out at HSC, surgical treatment is sequenced much the same as for patients with Crouzon syndrome.[106-109] The need for repeat cranio-orbital surgery in infancy to increase intracranial volume for the relief of intracranial pressure is greater, and the overall esthetic results are often less gratifying. Mental retardation is common, but its incidence and etiology are not clear.[120] It may be secondary to inadequate treatment of hydrocephalus[40,45,54] or to craniosynostosis with resulting ineffective intracranial brain volume rather than inherent in the etiology itself.

KLEEBLATTSCHÄDEL ANOMALY (CASE 10, FIG. 52-11)

The word *kleeblattschädel*, which is German for cloverleaf, is used to identify the most severe of the craniosynostosis deformities.[55] Although the degree and severity vary and different sutures may be involved in different patients, the most common form is synostosis of multiple cranial vault, cranial base, and facial sutures with only metopic, sagittal, and squamosal sutures remaining open. When this form occurs, the classic cloverleaf shape is present. All known mutations have been spontaneous. However, since most of the affected infants and children have not survived into adolescence, the true inheritance pattern is not clear.

Kleeblattschädel anomaly (cloverleaf skull) consists of a trilobate skull resulting from craniosynostosis. The most common form involves synostosis of the bilateral coronal, bilateral lambdoid, and cranial base sutures with compensatory bulging through the open metopic, sagittal, and squamosal sutures. There may also be a complete cranial vault synostosis (pansynostosis). Severe exorbitism and exophthalmos always occur in association with severe hypertelorism and striking midface deficiency. The nasal passages are only potential spaces (severe craniofacial atresia), resulting in mouth breathing and severe airway difficulties at birth.[72] Early tracheostomy and gastrostomy are required. Hydrocephalus is always present, and early ventriculoperitoneal shunting is necessary.

Current Surgical Approach. Ideally, early and, if necessary, repeated suture release and cranial vault craniectomy are carried out to relieve brain compression and limit irreversible brain damage. Usually craniectomies are performed within the first 1 to 2 months of life, initially of the posterior cranial vault, with the patient in the prone position. After an interval of 2 to 3 months, these are followed by craniectomies of the anterior cranial vault, with the patient in the supine position. This early aggressive craniectomy approach is necessary to restore some degree of normal intracranial volume and prevent the otherwise inevitable clinical deterioration through intracranial hypertension, papilledema, optic atrophy, eyeball herniation, negative nitrogen balance, general body fatigue, wasting, pneumonia, central apnea spells, cardiopulmonary arrest, and death. Later in infancy or early childhood, these procedures are followed by cranial vault and orbital reshaping and advancement.

Early (i.e., before age 2 years) monobloc osteotomy with advancement is indicated occasionally, but this is usually avoided by tracheostomy, gastrostomy, and early repeated craniectomies. Early monobloc advancement is associated with a high mortality and morbidity rate.[5] Later, monobloc advancement at age 5 to 7 years is always indicated. A bipartition of the monobloc osteotomy is preferred for simultaneous correction of orbital hypertelorism.[156] As part of staging the reconstruction, orthognathic surgery in conjunction with major orthodontic treatment is required in adolescence when the skeleton has matured.

OTHER VARIANTS

Pfeiffer Syndrome. Pfeiffer[124] described a disorder which he claimed was autosomal dominant. Bilateral synostosis of the coronal sutures with midface deficiency, exorbitism, and exophthalmos is present. Broad thumbs, broad great toes, and partial soft-tissue syndactyly of the hands are variable features. This disorder should be distinguished from Apert syndrome, Crouzon syndrome, Saethre-Chotzen syndrome, and simple craniosynostosis.[124]

Saethre-Chotzen Syndrome. Saethre-Chotzen syndrome is characterized by a broad and variable pattern of malformations, including asymmetric craniosynostosis (usually coronal or lambdoid), a low-set anterior hairline, eyelid ptosis, brachydactyly, partial simple syndactyly, and various skeletal anomalies. An autosomal dominant inheritance pattern with a high degree of penetrance and variable expressivity should be expected.[66]

Carpenter Syndrome. Carpenter syndrome is an autosomal recessive syndrome characterized by a variable craniosynostosis pattern (usually involving the sagittal and lambdoid sutures), preaxial polysyndactyly of the feet, and other variable associated anomalies.[20,142] It is frequently confused with Apert syndrome.

CASE REPORTS

CASE 1 (FIG. 52-2)

Diagnosis: Anterior plagiocephaly (unilateral coronal synostosis)

Procedure: Anterior cranial vault and three-quarter orbital osteotomies with reshaping and advancement

An 8-month-old infant had a forehead with a flat left side at birth. He was followed conservatively by the local pediatrician but without resolution. Plain radiographs revealed a unilateral coronal synostosis. He was referred to the craniofacial team at HSC for assessment and treatment.

Examination revealed a healthy infant who was normal apart from his craniofacial asymmetry, divergent strabismus, and amblyopia. The left ipsilateral forehead was flat and retruded. The left supraorbital ridge and lateral orbital rim were displaced posteriorly. The root of the nose was constricted to the left side. The left infraorbital rim and anterior zygoma also displayed a degree of flatness. The right contralateral side of the forehead bulged forward with inferior and anterior displacement of the orbital roof and supraorbital ridge. The tip of the nose was shifted to the right of the facial midline.

A CT scan of the craniofacial skeleton was completed in both the axial and coronal planes, with the axial slices reformatted for three-dimensional reconstruction. The left coronal suture was fused. The craniofacial asymmetry described clinically was also appreciated on radiographic examination. In addition, the left sphenoid wing was elevated superiorly, giving a harlequin appearance. The anterior cranial base was short in the anteroposterior dimension on the left side. The ventricles were of normal size. The patient appeared to have premature closure of the left coronal suture with the resultant craniofacial morphology that would be expected.

PROCEDURE

Intraoperative airway management was achieved with orotracheal intubation secured to the mandible to prevent accidental extubation during the surgical procedure. Temporary tarsorrhaphies were done to prevent corneal abrasions during surgery. Intravenous perioperative prophylactic antibiotic coverage with penicillin and cloxacillin was initiated.

A coronal incision was made with the coronal flap elevated anteriorly in the subperiosteal plane, taking the temporalis muscles with the flap. Bilateral 360-degree periorbital dissection followed, with release of the lateral canthi but careful maintenance of the integrity of the medial canthi and the nasolacrimal apparatus. Subperiosteal dissection continued down along the infraorbital rim and anterior aspect of the maxilla and zygoma. The neurosurgeon completed the bifrontal craniotomy with retraction of the frontal and temporal lobes of the brain without detachment of the olfactory bulbs.

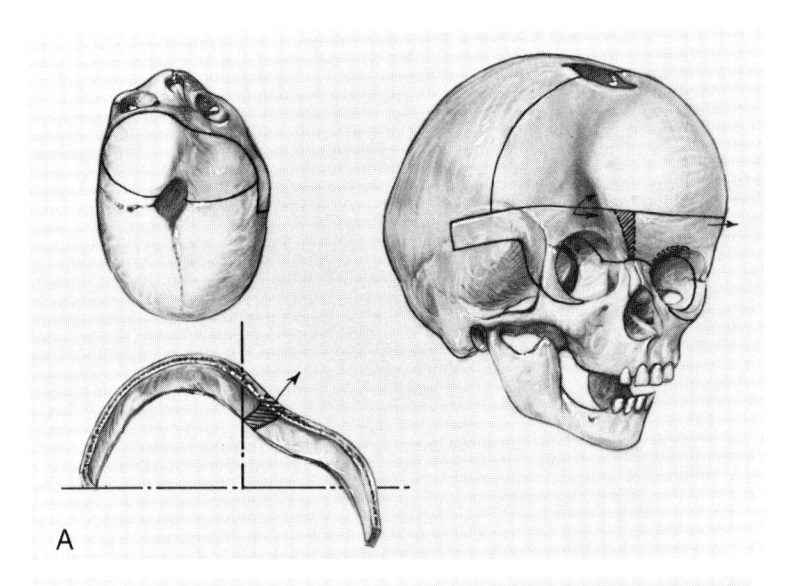

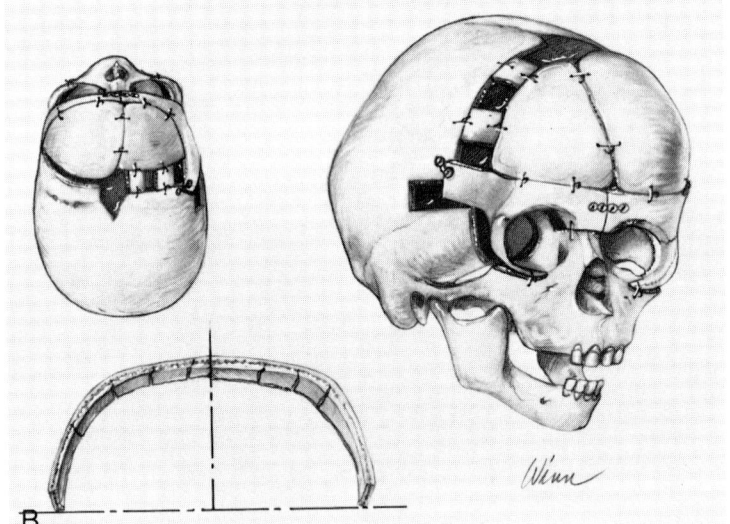

FIGURE 52-2. An 8-month-old infant with unrepaired unilateral coronal synostosis required suture release and anterior cranial vault and three-quarter orbital osteotomies with reshaping and advancement. *A*, Craniofacial morphology resulting from unilateral coronal synostosis. Proposed osteotomies outlined. *B*, Craniofacial morphology after cranial vault and three-quarter orbital osteotomies with reshaping, advancement, and fixation. *C*, Preoperative bird's-eye view. *D*, Bird's-eye view early after reconstruction.

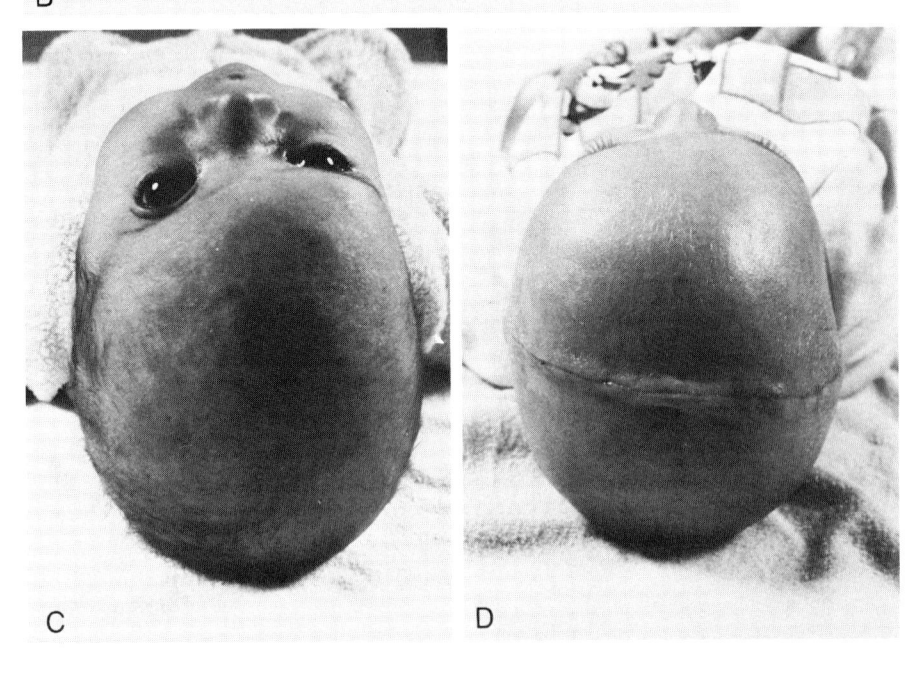

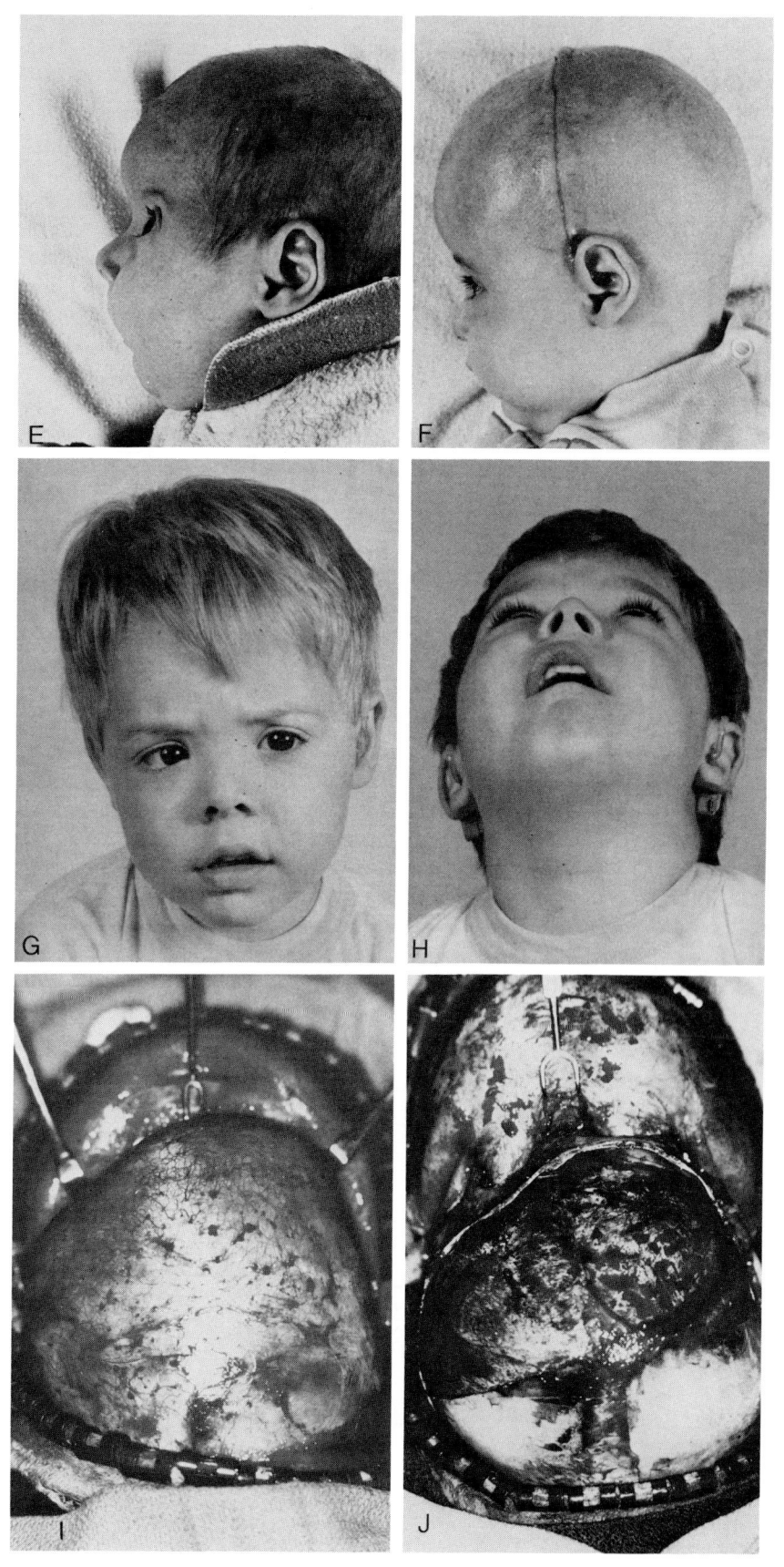

52 — CRANIOSYNOSTOSIS: DIAGNOSIS AND TREATMENT IN INFANCY AND EARLY CHILDHOOD / 1853

FIGURE 52-2 *Continued   E*, Preoperative profile view. *F*, Profile view early after reconstruction. *G*, Frontal view at 3 years of age. *H*, Worm's-eye view at 3 years of age. *I*, Intraoperative bird's-eye view of anterior cranial vault through coronal incision. *J*, Same view after bifrontal craniotomy.

Illustration continued on following page

1854 / VI — FUNCTIONAL RESTORATION OF OCCLUSION

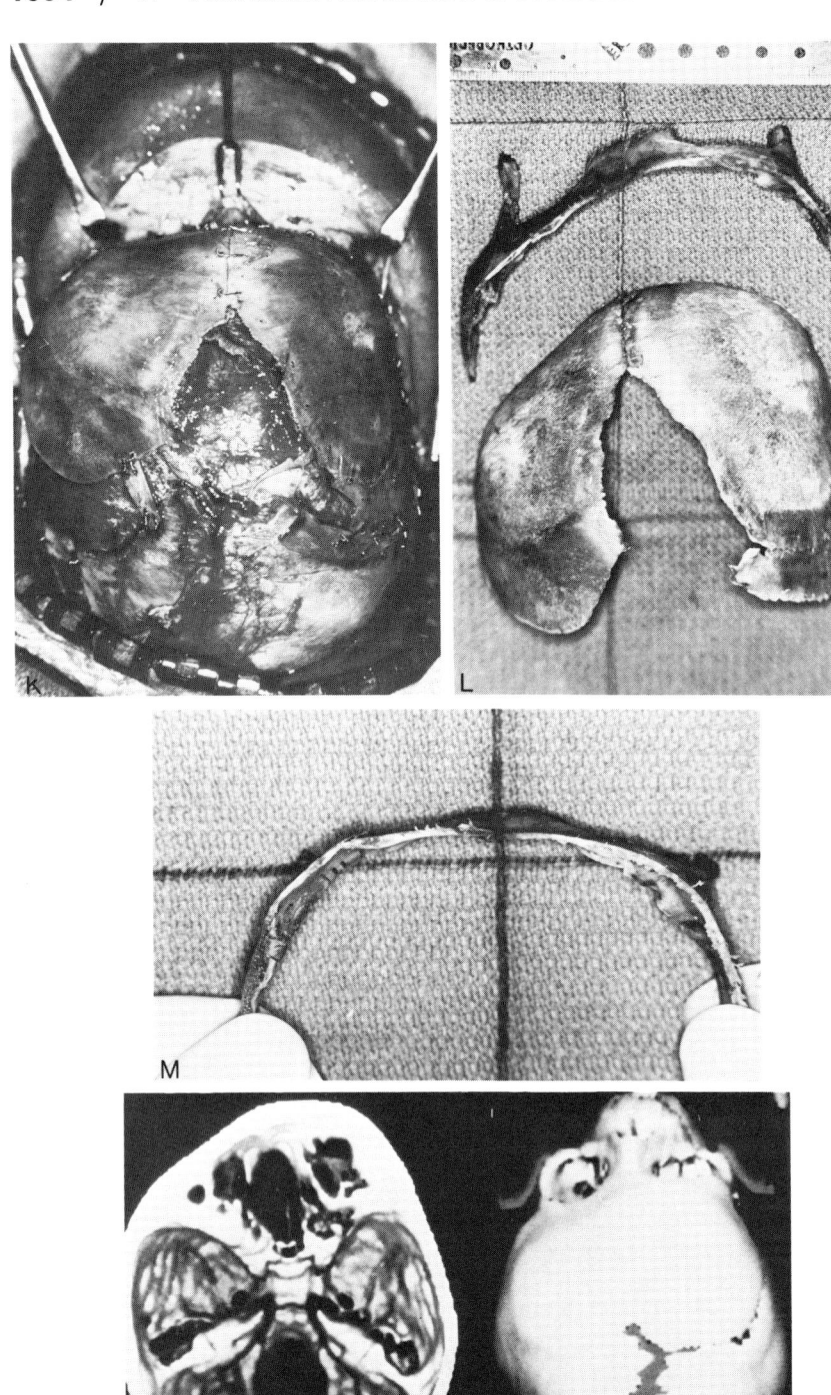

FIGURE 52-2 *Continued* K, Same view after anterior cranial vault and orbital reshaping. L, View of misshapen orbital unit and anterior cranial vault bone before reshaping. M, Same view of orbital unit after reshaping before reinsertion. N, Three-dimensional CT scan reformations. View of the cranial base and craniofacial skeleton in unilateral coronal synostosis.

The three-quarter orbital osteotomies were completed across the orbital roof, lateral orbital wall, orbital floor into the inferior orbital fissure, and down to the mid–infraorbital rim regions with the power and hand-held instruments. The orbital osteotomy units were removed from the field and shaped carefully with a combination of bone-bending instruments, rotary drill, and sagittal saw. It was necessary to stabilize several greenstick fractures with direct transosseous wires. The symmetrically shaped orbital osteotomy units were then re-inset between the ocular globes and the brain. Stabilization was achieved with a direct transosseous wire at the infraorbital rim region on each side, two wires at the nasofrontal region, and direct wires along the tenon extensions of the supraorbital ridges. (Occasionally microplates and screws are preferable for this procedure.) The previously removed anterior cranial vault bone was sectioned and units were selected to reconstruct the new forehead. Additional cranial bone fragments further secured the anterior cranial vault to the posterior cranial vault. Lateral canthopexies were completed and then the coronal incision was closed in layers. Suction drains were placed but no head dressing was required. The temporary tarsorrhaphies and mandibular wire were removed. The patient was extubated and taken to the recovery room in satisfactory condition.

POSTOPERATIVE COURSE

In such cases, no special head protection or postoperative positioning is required. The intravenous line is removed as soon as oral intake is adequate. The day of discharge varies from the fourth to the tenth postoperative day when the scalp sutures are removed. A CT scan is obtained before discharge.

Standard follow-up visits to the craniofacial surgeon, ophthalmologist, and neurosurgeon occur at 6 weeks, 6 months, and 1 year. At the 1-year postoperative visit, and yearly until 5 years of age, a CT scan is obtained.

CASE 2 (FIG. 52-3)

Diagnosis: Posterior plagiocephaly (unilateral lambdoid synostosis)

Procedure: Posterior cranial vault osteotomies with reshaping

One side of the back of a patient's head was noted to be flat when he was born, but there was no evidence of birth trauma. Range of motion of the neck was good. There was no evidence of torticollis. The flatness did not diminish over the ensuing months despite meticulous head positioning to prevent preferential positioning while he lay prone. Plain radiographs showed lambdoid suture synostosis. The patient was referred to the craniofacial team at HSC for evaluation and treatment.

A CT scan of the craniofacial skeleton was obtained in both the axial and coronal planes. A left lambdoid suture synostosis was noted with ridging along the internal table of the skull. Both the anterior and posterior cranial vault regions were markedly asymmetric, and fingerprinting was seen on the inner table of the left parieto-occipital skull region.

There was flatness and obliquity to the left parieto-occipital region. In addition, there was some bulging of the forehead and supraorbital ridge region on the same side. The ear canal and external ear were more anterior on the left side than on the right.

PROCEDURE

Airway management was achieved through nasotracheal intubation secured by suturing it to the septum of the nose. The infant was turned over so that he lay prone with his head resting in a Mayfield head ring. Great care was taken to ensure that the cervical spine was even, without excessive extension or flexion, that there was no pressure on the eyeballs, and that airway control through the nasotracheal tube was satisfactory.

The usual coronal incision was made and then, with subperiosteal dissection, the posterior scalp flap was taken down to the level of the foramen magnum and the mastoid air cell regions. The neurosurgeon completed a posterior craniotomy with care taken to avoid injury to the transverse sinus. When the posterior cranial vault bone had been removed, the posterior cranium was reshaped for improved symmetry and appropriate morphology for his age. Stabilization was achieved with carefully selected micro and mini bone plates and screws.

POSTOPERATIVE COURSE

The postoperative course was similar to that described in Case 1. There was no need for head protection or positioning postoperatively. The follow-up appointments and consultations followed our protocol as described in the previous case report.

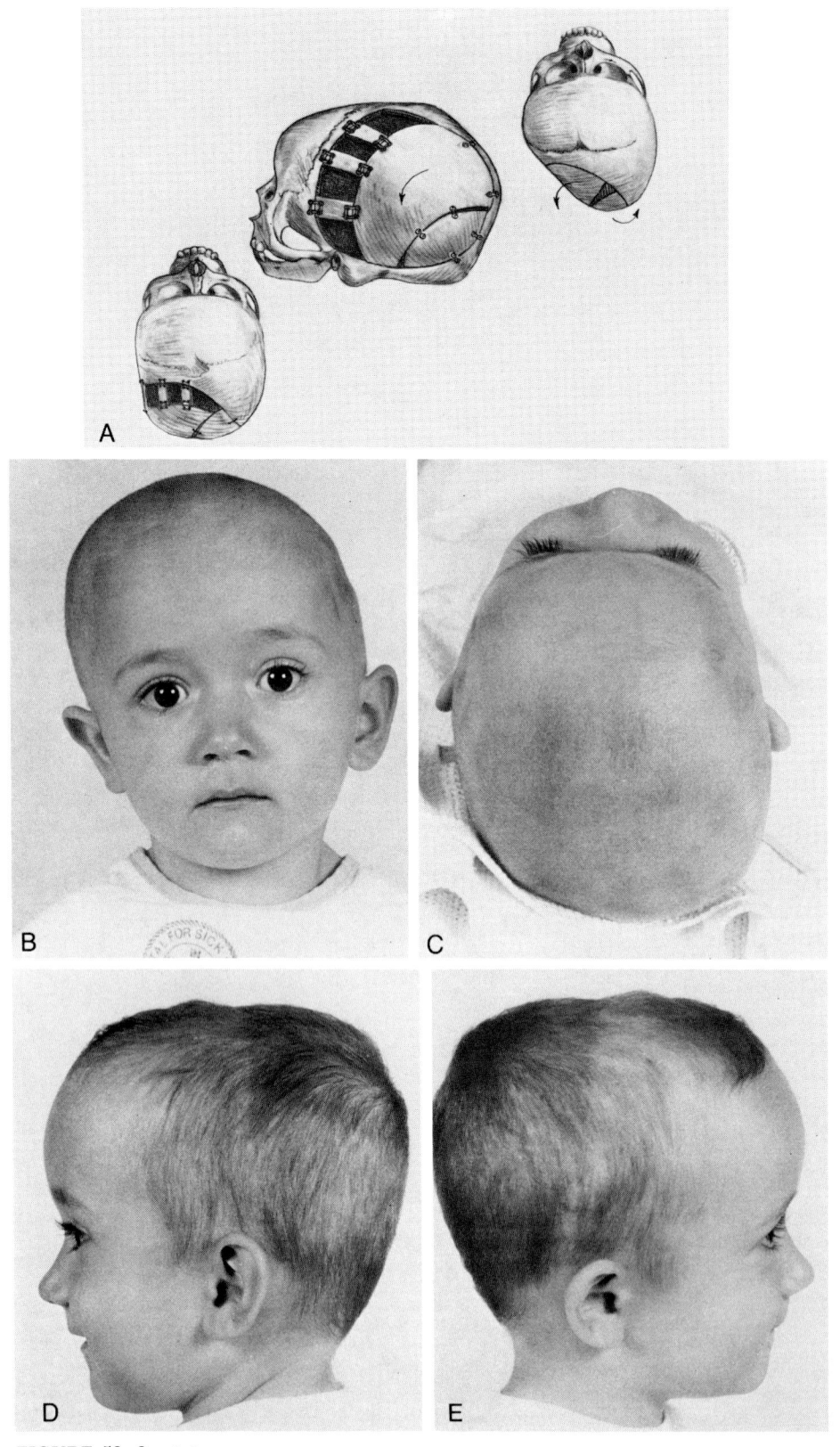

FIGURE 52-3. A 2-YEAR-OLD CHILD WITH UNREPAIRED UNILATERAL LAMBDOID SYNOSTOSIS REQUIRING SUTURE RELEASE AND POSTERIOR CRANIAL VAULT RESHAPING WITH EXPANSION OF THE INTRACRANIAL VOLUME. A, Craniofacial morphology resulting from unilateral lambdoid synostosis. Proposed osteotomies, reshaping, and fixation of the posterior cranial vault. B, Preoperative frontal view. C, Preoperative bird's-eye view. D, Left profile view early after reconstruction. E, Right profile view early after reconstruction.

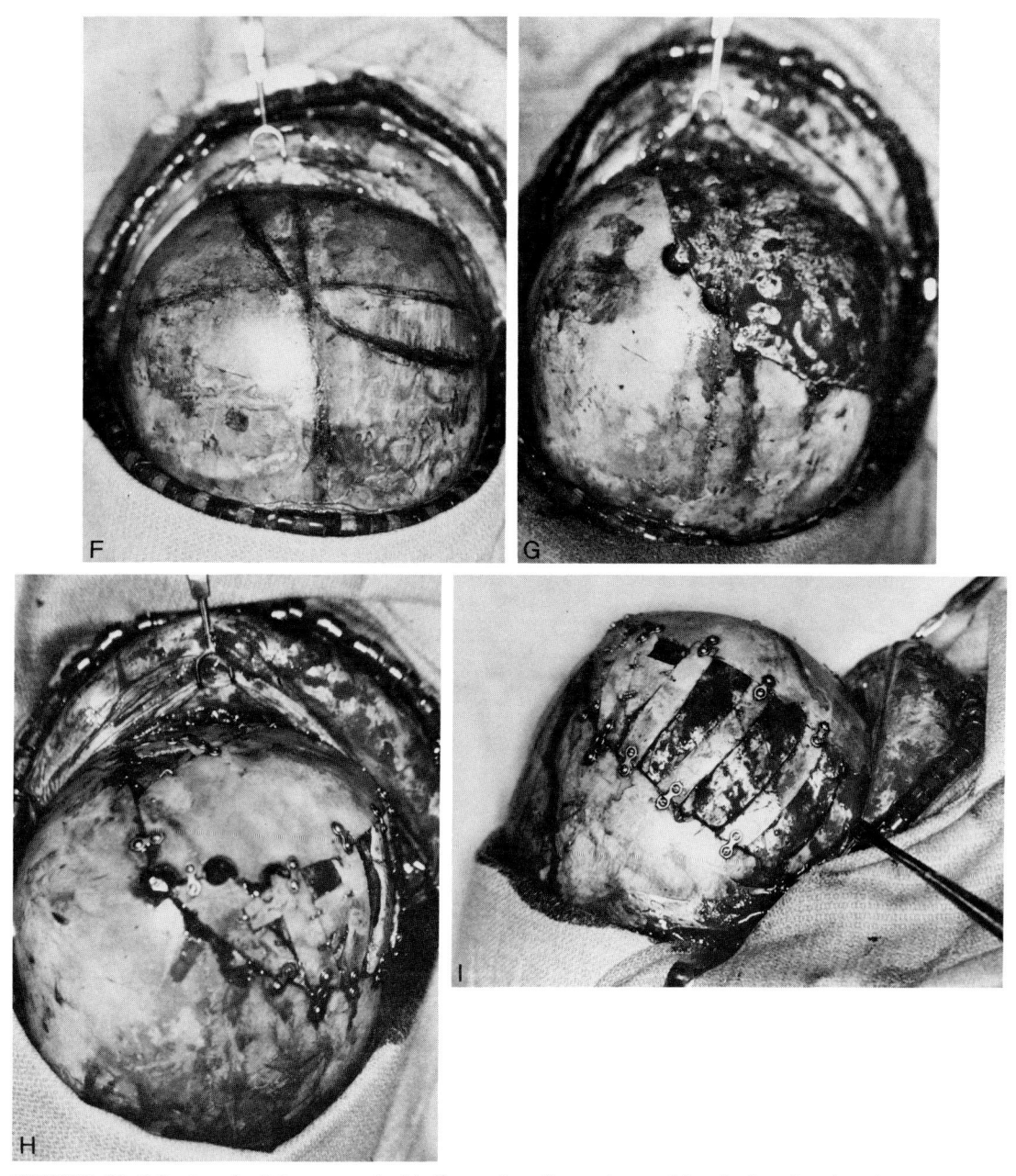

FIGURE 52-3 *Continued* *F*, Intraoperative bird's-eye view of posterior cranial vault after elevation of posterior skull flap (patient in supine position). *G*, Same view after craniotomy. *H*, Same view after reshaping and stabilization with titanium miniplates. *I*, Lateral view after reshaping with expansion of intracranial volume.

Illustration continued on following page

1858 / VI—FUNCTIONAL RESTORATION OF OCCLUSION

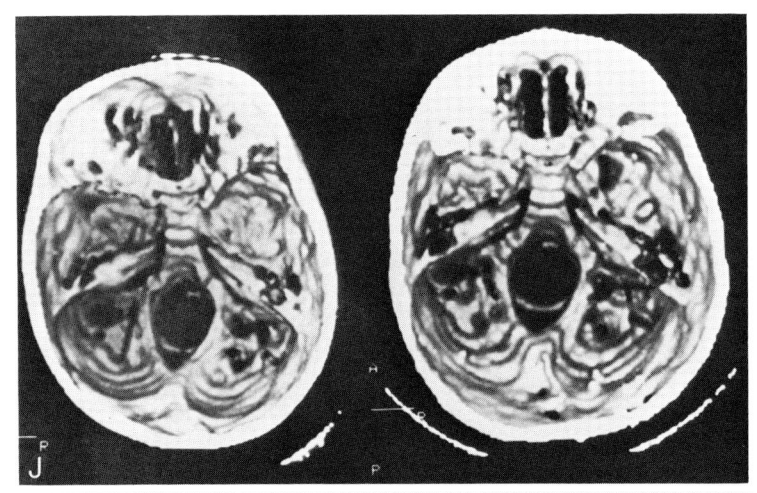

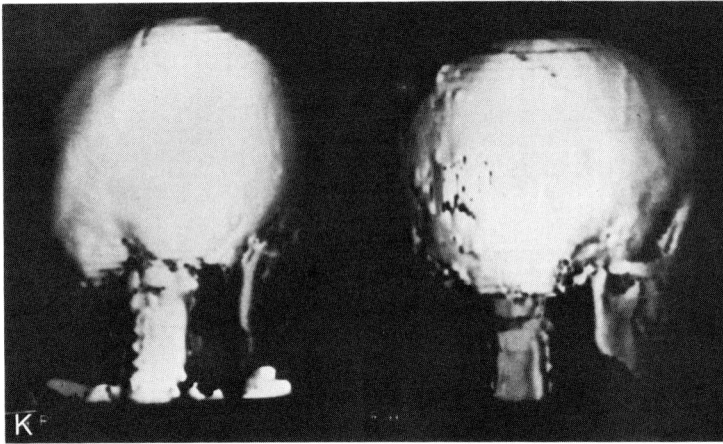

FIGURE 52-3 *Continued* *J*, Three-dimensional CT scan reformations. View of the cranial base before and after reconstruction. *K*, Three-dimensional CT scan reformations. Oblique view of posterior cranial vault before and after reconstruction.

CASE 3 (FIG. 52-4)

Diagnosis: Brachycephaly (bilateral coronal synostosis)

Procedure: Anterior cranial vault and three-quarter orbital osteotomies with reshaping and advancement

The flatness noted in a patient from birth became more noticeable over the ensuing months. There was some bulging of the eyes, and then the anterior fontanelle sealed off prematurely. She was referred by her pediatrician to the craniofacial team at HSC for evaluation and treatment.

Examination revealed a symmetric but peculiar shape to the forehead and upper face. The supraorbital ridges were markedly recessed and, when viewed in the sagittal plane, the eyebrows were posterior to the corneas. The forehead was wide and tall and bulged superiorly. Bony ridges were palpable over the coronal suture regions.

A CT scan of the craniofacial skeleton was obtained in both the axial and coronal planes. The axial CT scan was reformatted for three-dimensional reconstruction. The anterior cranial base was short in the anteroposterior dimension and extremely wide transversely. The orbits were shallow and the eyes bulged. Ridging was evident over the left and right coronal sutures, indicating premature closure. The ventricles were of normal size and the midface appeared normal. The patient appeared to have premature closure of the left and right coronal sutures in conjunction with the expected abnormal craniofacial morphology.

PROCEDURE

The intraoperative management of the airway, incision placement, surgical dissection, osteotomy location, and craniotomy were similar to those described for the patient in Case 1.

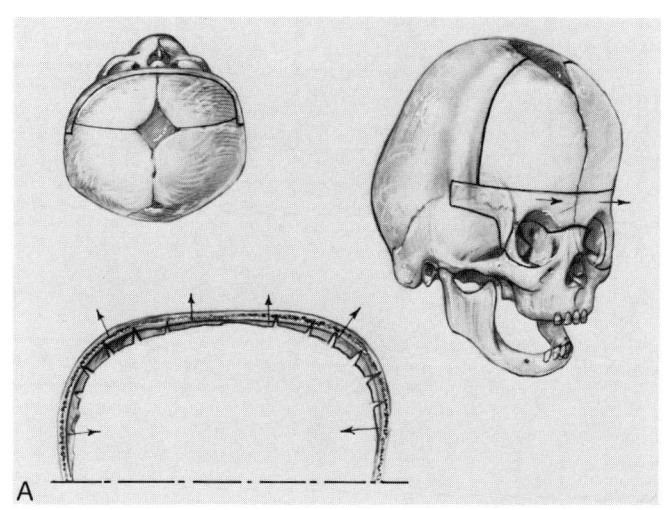

FIGURE 52-4. A 1-YEAR-OLD INFANT WITH UNREPAIRED BICORONAL SYNOSTOSIS REQUIRING SUTURE RELEASE AND CRANIAL VAULT AND THREE-QUARTER ORBITAL OSTEOTOMIES WITH RESHAPING AND ADVANCEMENT. *A*, Craniofacial morphology resulting from bicoronal synostosis. Proposed osteotomies outlined. *B*, Craniofacial morphology after cranial vault and three-quarter orbital osteotomies with reshaping, advancement, and fixation. *C*, Preoperative oblique view. *D*, Oblique view after reconstruction.

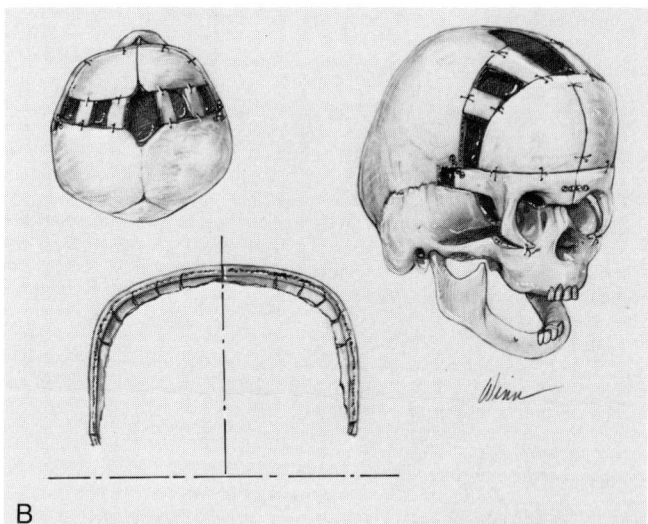

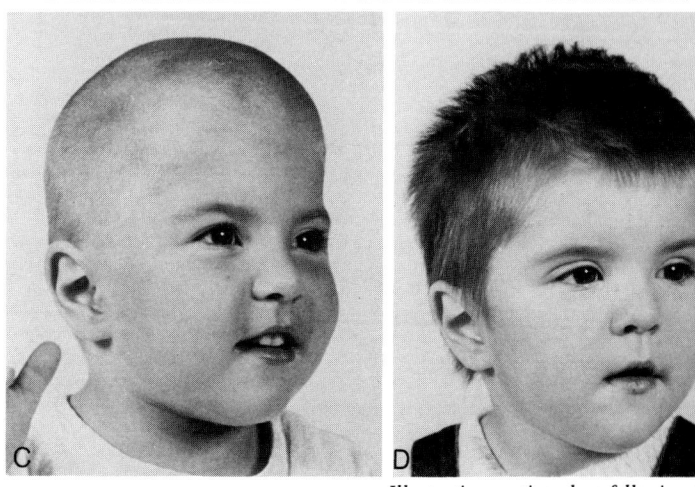

Illustration continued on following page

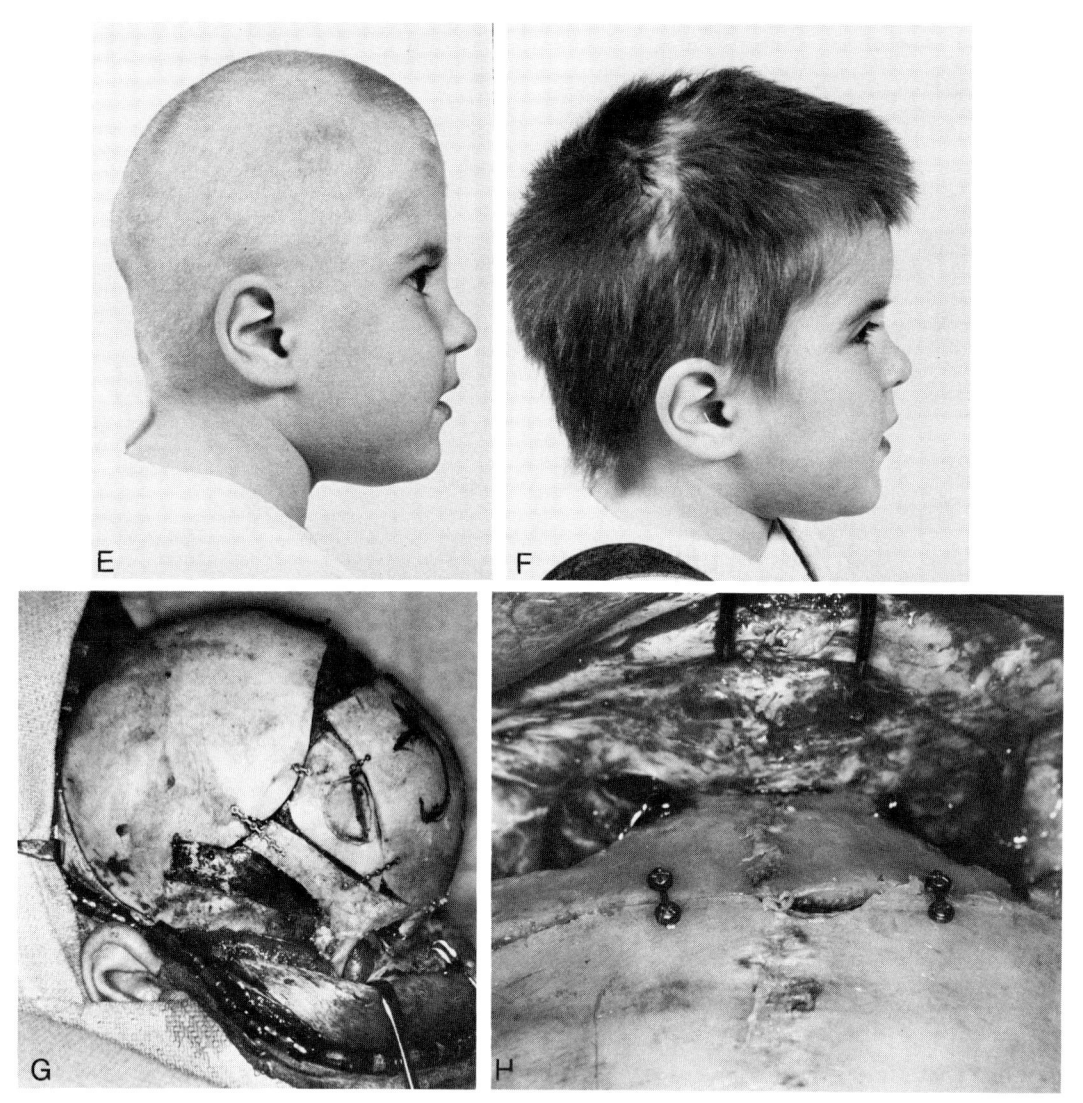

FIGURE 52-4 *Continued* *E*, Preoperative profile view. *F*, Profile view after reconstruction. *G*, Intraoperative lateral view of cranial vault and orbits through coronal incision after reshaping and micro bone plate fixation. *H*, Close-up of anterior cranial vault at supraorbital ridge level demonstrating micro bone plate fixation.

The main objective in reshaping the orbital osteotomies with their tenon extensions was to change the center point of the arc of rotation from its lateral location to one more directly over the frontozygomatic suture region. This had the effect of decreasing the bitemporal (anterior cranial vault) width. The anterior aspect of the supraorbital ridge was also given a more normal arc. The orbital osteotomy unit was reinserted in an advanced position, which gave increased depth to both the orbital cavities and the anterior cranial base. The previously removed anterior cranial vault bone was sectioned appropriately to reconstruct a normal upper forehead configuration.

POSTOPERATIVE COURSE

The postoperative recovery and follow-up were very similar to those described in Case 1.

CASE 4 (FIG. 52-5)

Diagnosis: Oxycephaly (late, bilateral coronal suture synostosis)

Procedure: Total cranial vault and upper orbital osteotomies with reshaping and advancement

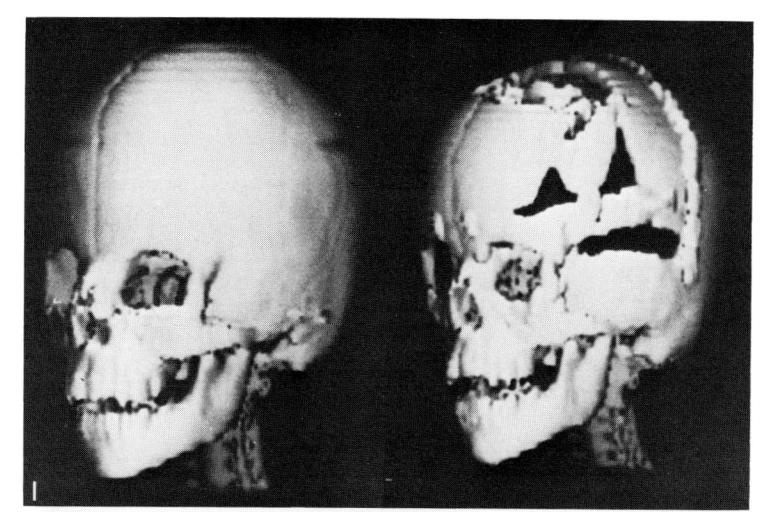

FIGURE 52–4 *Continued* *I*, Three-dimensional CT scan reformations of craniofacial skeleton. Oblique view before and early after reconstruction. *J*, Three-dimensional CT scan reformations. View of the cranial base before and early after reconstruction demonstrating increased depth achieved at the anterior cranial base.

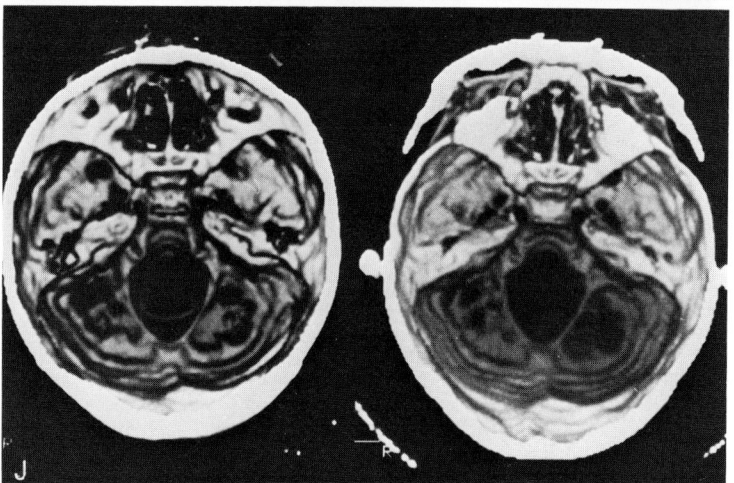

A 9-year-old girl from Indonesia had frequent headaches and a degree of optic atrophy. Fingerprinting was seen on plain radiographic examination. She was 2 years behind in school. She was thought to have a form of craniosynostosis and was referred to the craniofacial team at HSC for evaluation and treatment.

Examination showed a small cranium with decreased head circumference and flat frontonasal angle, as well as recession to the supraorbital ridges. Psychological testing demonstrated the cognitive skills of a 7 year old (a 2-year delay). Funduscopic examination showed mild bilateral optic atrophy.

A CT scan of the craniofacial skeleton was performed in both the axial and coronal planes. The axial scan was reformatted into a three-dimensional image for review. The ventricles were a normal size, and gross brain development appeared normal. The indirect intracranial volume, as measured from the CT scan, was believed to be small, and there was evidence of bilateral coronal synostosis. The orbits were shallow, and the supraorbital ridges were recessed. There was a decreased anteroposterior dimension to the anterior cranial base. The patient appeared to have late, bilateral coronal suture synostosis in conjunction with the expected craniofacial morphology.

PROCEDURE

The intraoperative airway management, incision placement, surgical dissection, and craniotomy were similar to those described in Case 1. Orbital osteotomies were carried down to the mid-lateral orbital rims rather than the infraorbital rim regions because the lower aspect of the orbits was thought to be in a normal location. The total cranial vault, including the squamosal portion of the temporal bone, was removed through craniotomies and osteotomies so that total cranial vault reshaping could be completed. Once the upper orbits were re-inset in the advanced position to give

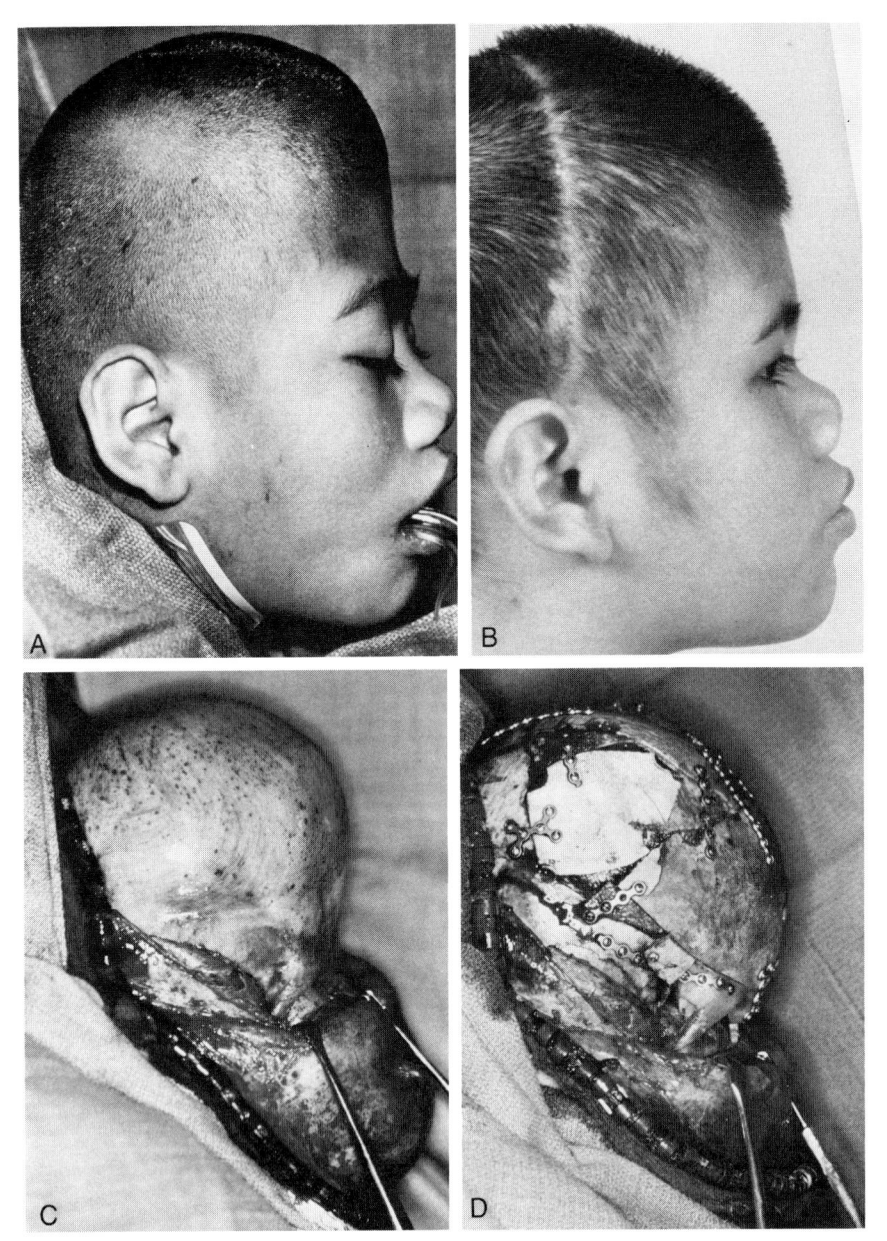

FIGURE 52–5. A 9-YEAR-GIRL WITH UNREPAIRED LATE, BICORONAL SYNOSTOSIS REQUIRING SUTURE RELEASE AND CRANIAL VAULT AND UPPER ORBITAL OSTEOTOMIES WITH RESHAPING AND ADVANCEMENT. *A*, Preoperative profile view. *B*, Profile view after reconstruction. *C*, Intraoperative lateral view of cranial vault and upper orbits after elevation of coronal flap. *D*, Same view after reconstruction. Stabilization with titanium miniplates and screws.

increased depth to the anterior cranial base and orbital cavities, sections of the cranial vault bone were selected to reconstruct the new forehead. The total cranial vault was reshaped, working from anterior to posterior. A full-thickness cranial bone graft was selected for augmentation of the nasal dorsum. Stabilization of all osteotomy units was achieved with multiple titanium miniplates and screws.

Postoperative Course

The postoperative course was similar to that described in Case 1. The patient returned to Indonesia 6 weeks after surgery. She has been followed through written correspondence and is doing well.

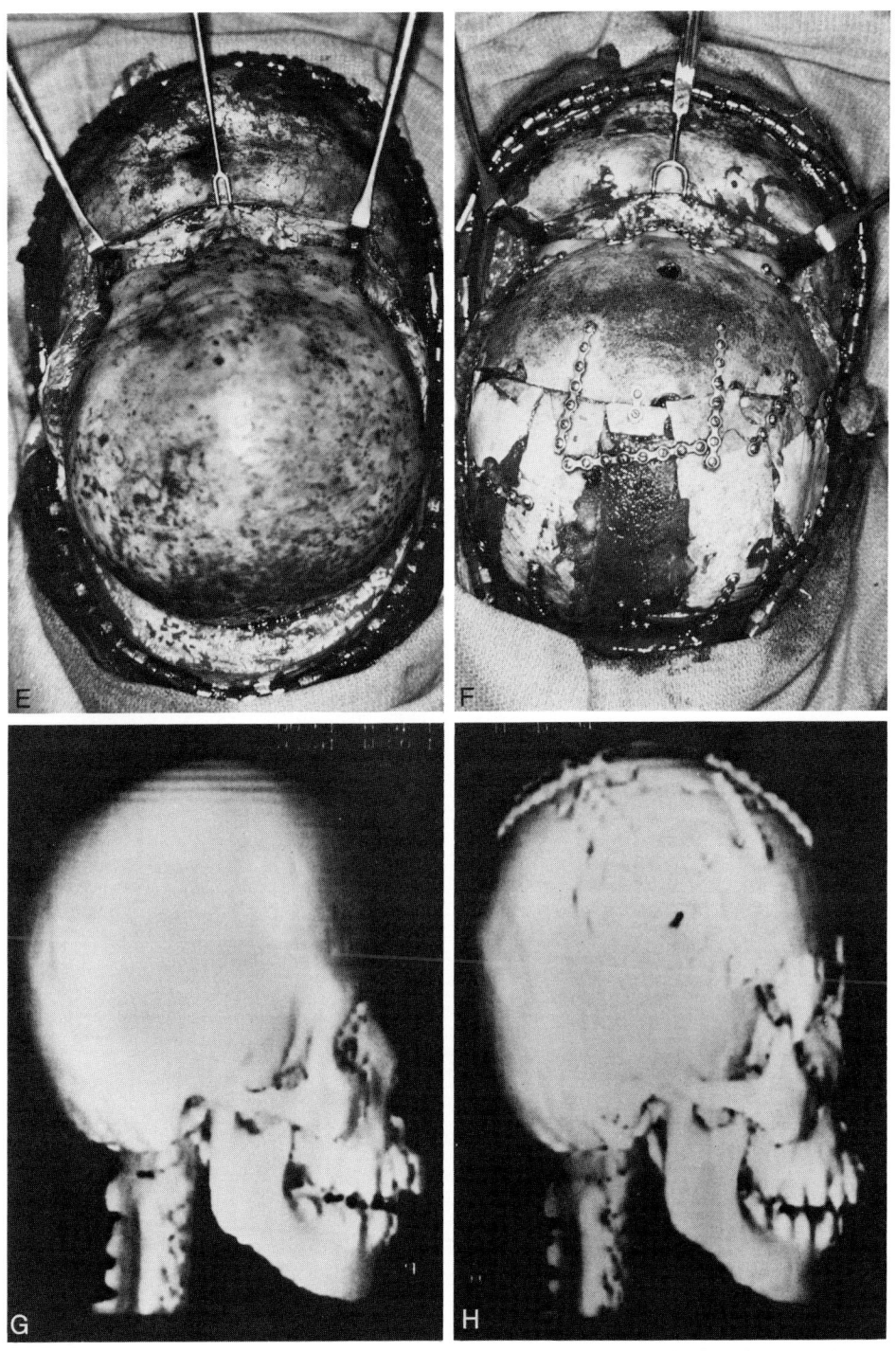

FIGURE 52–5 *Continued* E, Intraoperative bird's-eye view of cranial vault after elevation of anterior and posterior scalp flaps. F, Same view after cranial vault and upper orbital osteotomies with reshaping. Stabilization with titanium bone plates and screws. G, Three-dimensional CT scan reformation of craniofacial skeleton. Lateral view before reconstruction. H, Lateral view after reconstruction. (From Posnick JC et al: Indirect intracranial volume measurements using CT scans: Clinical applications for craniosynostosis. J Plast Reconstr Surg Jan 1992, in press. Copyright 1992. The Williams & Wilkins Co., Baltimore.)

1864 / VI—FUNCTIONAL RESTORATION OF OCCLUSION

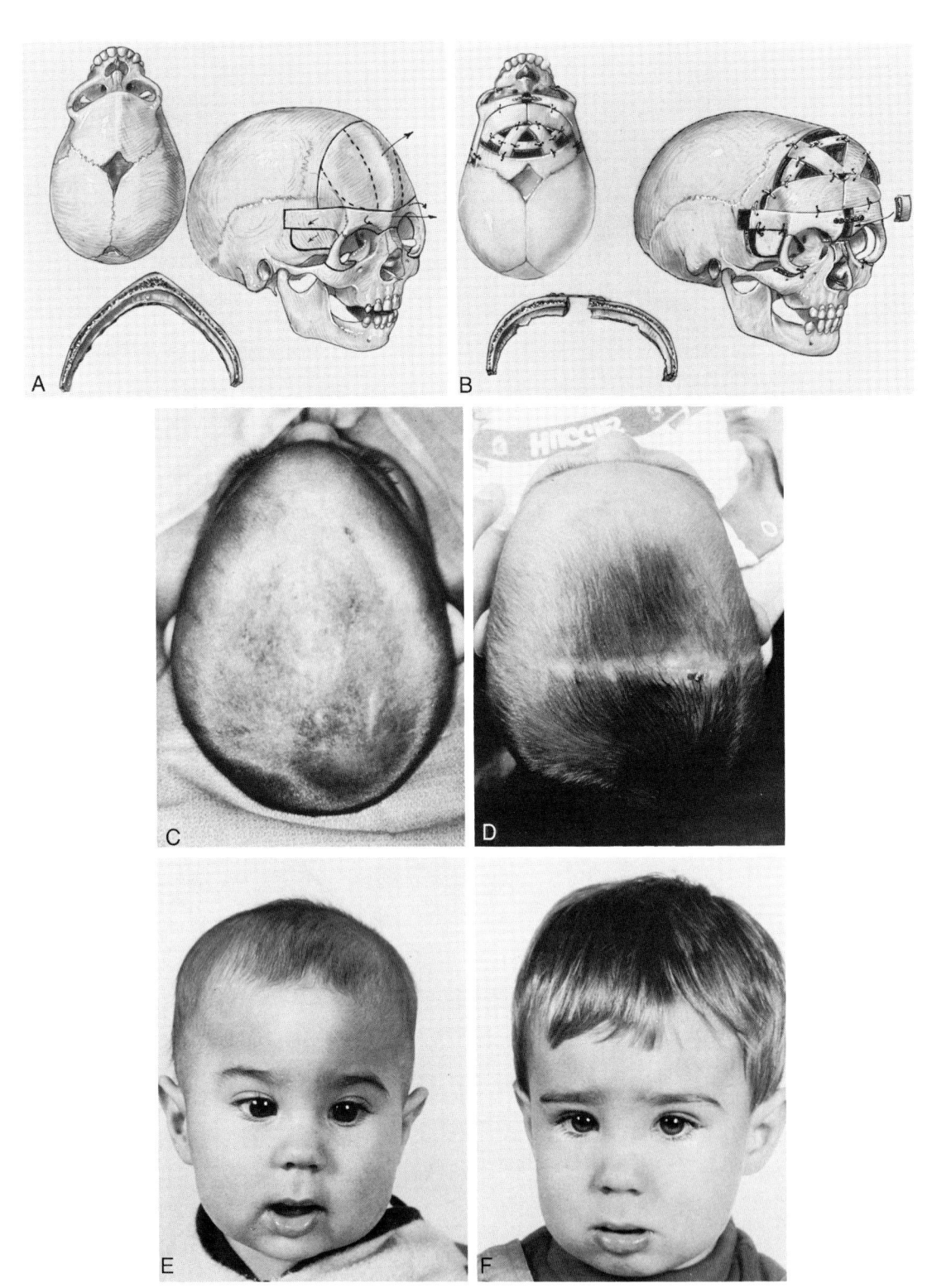

FIGURE 52-6. A 1.5-YEAR-OLD BOY WITH UNREPAIRED METOPIC SYNOSTOSIS REQUIRING CRANIAL VAULT AND THREE-QUARTER ORBITAL OSTEOTOMIES WITH RESHAPING. *A*, Craniofacial morphology resulting from metopic suture synostosis. Proposed osteotomies outlined. *B*, Craniofacial morphology after cranial vault and three-quarter orbital osteotomies with reshaping. *C*, Preoperative bird's-eye view demonstrating trigonocephaly. *D*, Bird's-eye view early after reconstruction. *E*, Preoperative frontal view. *F*, Postoperative frontal view at 1 year.

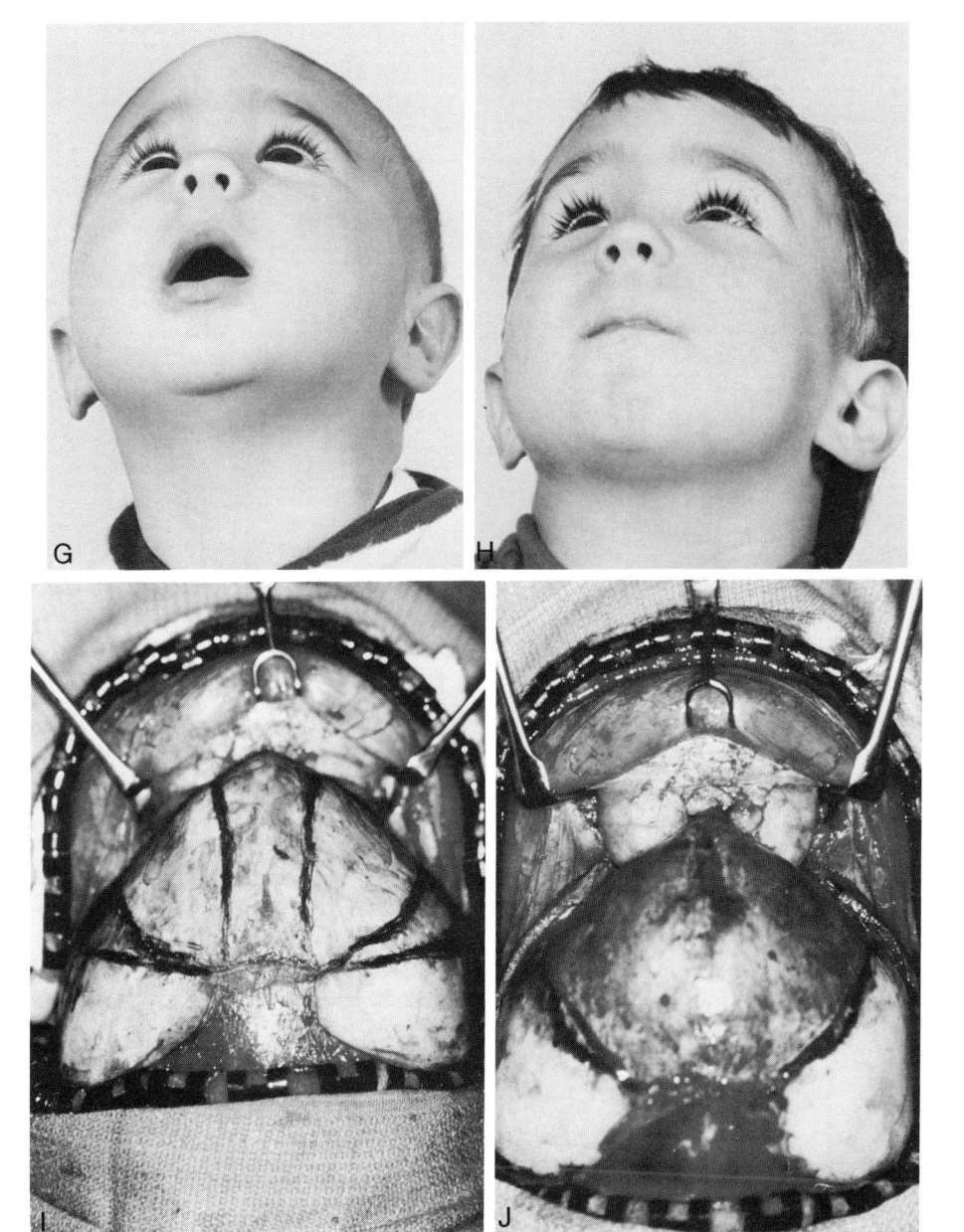

FIGURE 52-6 *Continued G,* Preoperative worm's-eye view. *H,* Postoperative worm's-eye view at 1 year. *I,* Intraoperative bird's-eye view of cranial vault through coronal incision. *J,* Same view after craniotomy and orbital osteotomy units are removed.

Illustration continued on following page

CASE 5 (FIG. 52-6)

Diagnosis: Trigonocephaly (metopic suture synostosis)

Procedure: Anterior cranial vault and three-quarter orbital osteotomies with reshaping and advancement

A newborn was noted to have a vertical ridge over the forehead with flatness to the sides of the skull. Plain-skull radiographs were suggestive of metopic suture synostosis. He was referred to the craniofacial team at HSC for evaluation and treatment.

During examination, the infant appeared normal except for his craniofacial morphology. Vertical ridging of the forehead extending from the nasofrontal region back to the coronal suture area was immediately apparent. A degree of orbital hypotelorism was appreciated. The supraorbital ridges were bilaterally and symmetrically flat and recessed. When looked at from the bird's-eye view, the anterior cranial vault had a triangular shape, with decreased bitemporal width.

A CT scan of the craniofacial skeleton was completed through the axial and coronal planes. Three-dimensional reformation of the axial plane CT scan was completed. Premature closure of the metopic suture was evident. The anterior cranial vault was

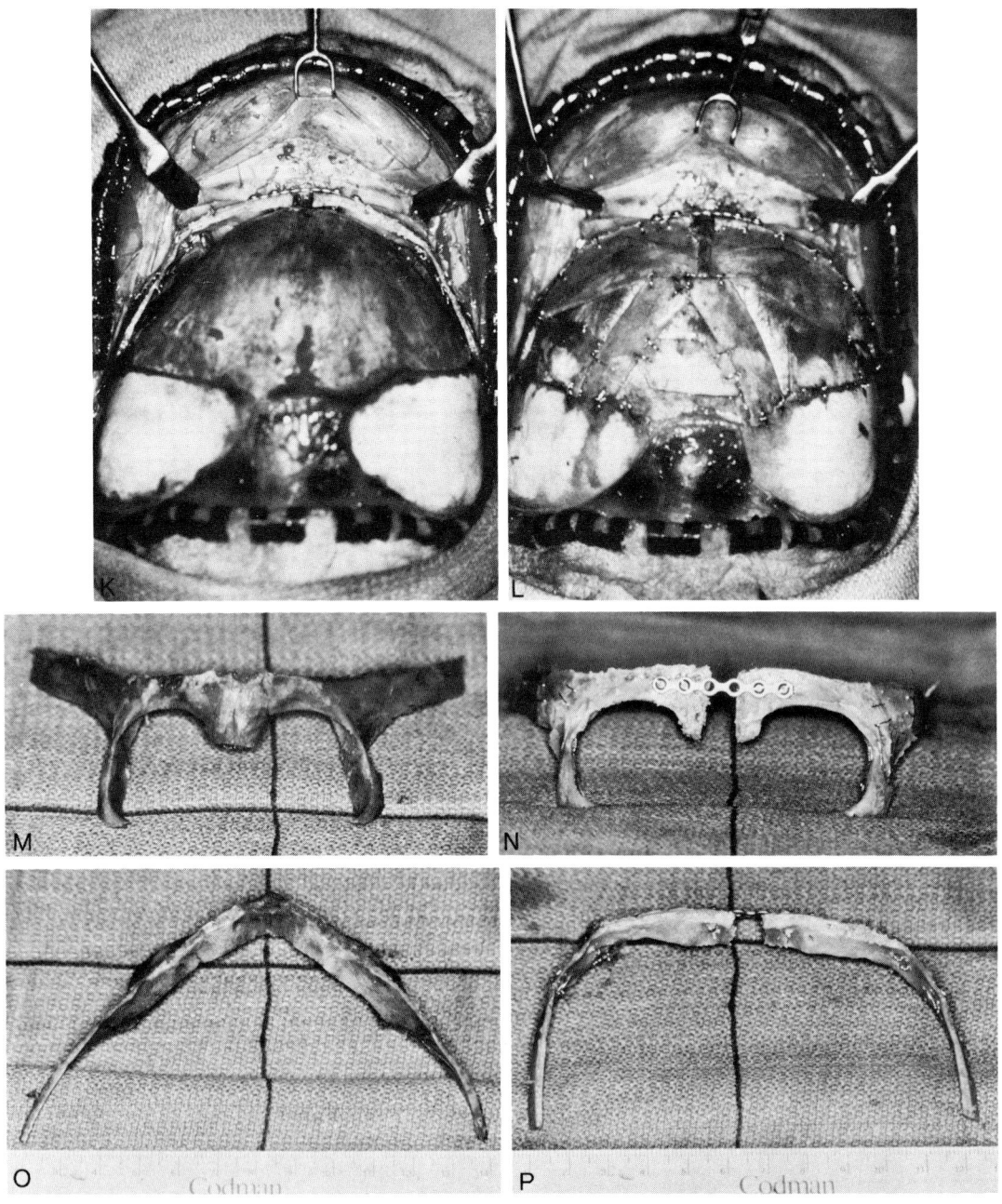

FIGURE 52-6 *Continued* *K*, Same view after three-quarter orbital osteotomy units are reshaped and then re-inset. *L*, After completion of cranial vault and orbital reshaping. *M*, Frontal view of three-quarter orbital osteotomy units with tenon extensions before reshaping. *N*, Same view after orbital unit reshaping with correction of orbital hypotelorism. Stabilization of central orbits with bone plate and screws. *O*, Bird's-eye view of orbital osteotomy units before reshaping. *P*, Bird's-eye view of orbital osteotomy units after reshaping.

diminished in volume and had a triangular shape, with a degree of orbital hypotelorism. The orbits were shallow in their lateral aspects, as was the lateral aspect of the anterior cranial base.

Overall the patient appeared to have premature closure of the metopic suture with the expected resulting craniofacial morphology.

Procedure

Intraoperative management of the airway, incision placement, flap dissection, craniotomy, and osteotomy locations were completed as described for the patient in Case 1. Once the three-quarter orbital osteotomies were completed, reshaping was carried out as described in Case 1. Although the bone requiring reconstruction varies in

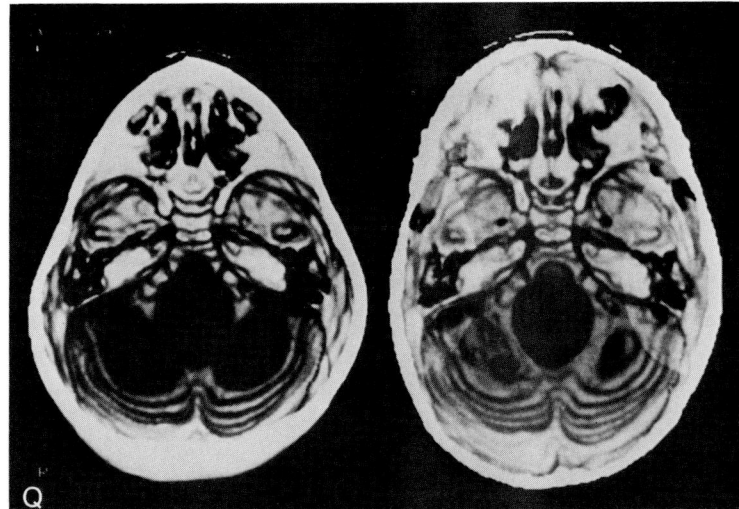

FIGURE 52-6 *Continued* Q, Three-dimensional CT scan reformations. Cranial base views before and 1 year after reconstruction. R, Three-dimensional CT scan reformations. Bird's-eye view before and 1 year after reconstruction. (From Posnick JC, et al: Indirect intracranial volume measurements using CT scans: Clinical application for craniosynostosis. Plast Reconstr Surg. In press.)

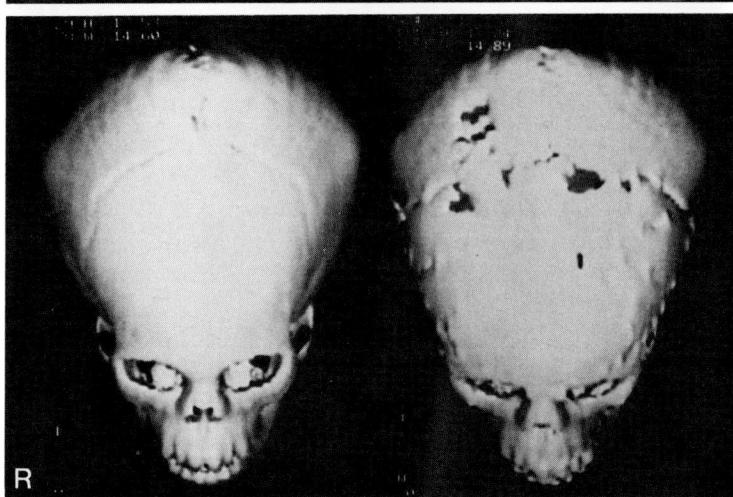

shape (e.g., anterior plagiocephaly, tragiocephaly, brachycephaly), the principles remain the same. In addition, the orbital units were split vertically in the midline, and a gap was created to correct the degree of hypotelorism present. An autogenous cranial bone graft was inset to the defect, and a miniplate and screws were used to stabilize the orbital units in their new relationship to each other. The reshaped orbital osteotomy units were re-inset, and direct transosseous wire stabilization was carried out in the same locations as described in Case 1. Craniotomies of the squamosal portion of the temporal bones were completed. The temporal bones were reshaped to increase the bitemporal width. The previously removed anterior cranial vault bone was further sectioned for reconstruction to create an appropriate anterior cranial vault volume and forehead shape. Stabilization was with additional direct transosseous wire.

POSTOPERATIVE COURSE

Recovery in hospital and standard follow-up assessments at 6 weeks, 6 months, and yearly intervals were similar to those described for the patient in Case 1.

CASE 6 (FIG. 52-7)

Diagnosis: Scaphocephaly (sagittal suture synostosis)

Procedure: Total cranial vault and upper orbital osteotomies with reshaping

Shortly after birth, a patient born and raised in India was noted to have an elongated skull that was constricted in width. Since facilities for his management were not available in his home region, he was referred to the craniofacial team at HSC for evaluation and treatment at age 3.5 years.

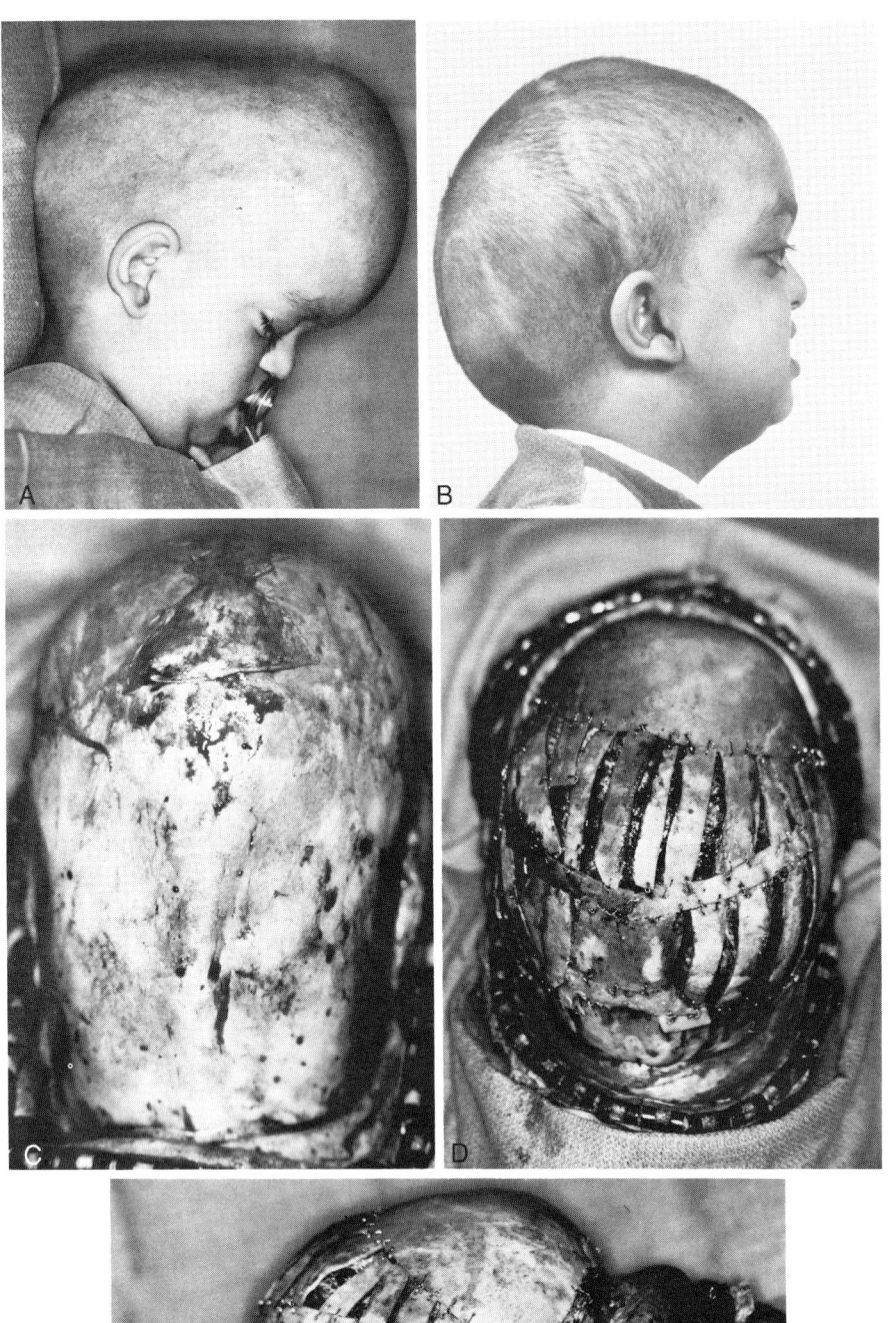

FIGURE 52-7. A 3.5-YEAR-OLD BOY WITH SAGITTAL SUTURE SYNOSTOSIS RESULTING IN SEVERE SCAPHOCEPHALY REQUIRING CRANIAL VAULT AND UPPER ORBITAL OSTEOTOMIES WITH RESHAPING. *A*, Preoperative profile view. *B*, Profile view early after reconstruction. *C*, Intraoperative bird's-eye view of cranial vault through coronal incision. Sagittal suture ridging can be seen. *D*, Same view of cranial vault after reconstruction. *E*, Lateral view of cranial vault after reconstruction. Note that a solid unit of skull is selected to reconstruct the forehead esthetic unit.

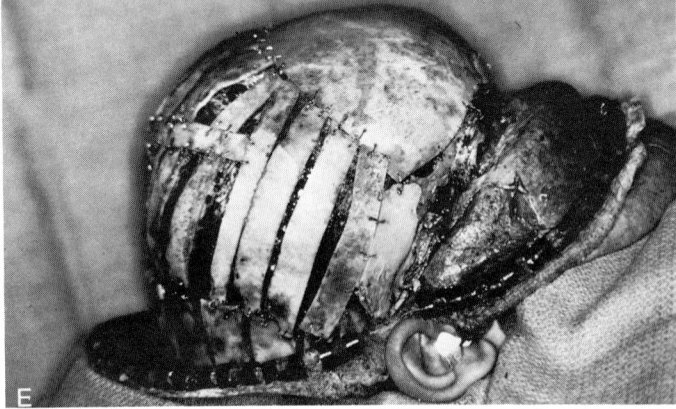

During examination, the boy displayed a good sense of humor and a normal psychological profile. He had tremendous anteroposterior elongation of his skull with diminished bitemporal width. His orbits were shallow and his midface was deficient. There was no family history of craniosynostosis. Ophthalmologic examination revealed strabismus and amblyopia, but funduscopic examination was normal.

CT scan of the axial and coronal planes showed ridging over the sagittal suture and a symmetric midface deficiency with shallow orbits. The shape of the cranial vault was consistent with a neglected severe sagittal suture synostosis. The ventricles were moderately enlarged, indicating a degree of hydrocephalus.

The patient appeared to have a sagittal suture synostosis associated with midface hypoplasia. His father had shallow orbits and slightly bulging eyes; a presumed diagnosis of Crouzon syndrome was made.

Procedure

Intraoperative management of the airway and incision placement were basically as described in Case 1. Dissection of the anterior scalp flap was also similar. The posterior scalp flap was taken back in the subperiosteal plane as far as the occiput, almost to the foramen magnum. Craniotomy involved the total cranial vault with osteotomies of the upper half of the orbits down to the midlevel of the lateral orbital rims. After reshaping, the upper orbital osteotomy unit was inset in a more posterior position. A section of cranial vault bone was selected from the posterior skull and used to construct a new forehead. The reconstructed forehead was also significantly posterior in position. Osteotomies of the squamous portion of the temporal bones down to the level of the cranial base were completed with reshaping and positioning to increase the bitemporal width. The remainder of the cranial vault bone was cut into strips, which were placed individually to achieve a more normally configured cranial vault. Stabilization was achieved with multiple direct transosseous wires. This was a time-consuming process. I now prefer micro and minibone plates and screws.

Postoperative Course

Postoperatively the patient did well. He returned to India 6 weeks after the operation. He will likely require a midface osteotomy with advancement to correct his midface deficiency.

CASE 7 (Fig. 52–8)

Diagnosis: Scaphocephaly (sagittal suture synostosis)

Procedure: Total cranial vault and upper orbital osteotomies with reshaping

Shortly after birth, a patient was noted to have an elongated and constricted cranial vault. Surgery had been suggested to the family early on, but their concern about operative morbidity prevented their following through. By the age of 9 years, the child was being teased at school and in the neighborhood to such an extent that he was referred to the craniofacial team at HSC for evaluation and treatment.

The boy had a normal psychological profile but had tremendous anteroposterior elongation of his skull and diminished bitemporal width. The midface seemed normal with a Class I occlusion. Ophthalmologic examination revealed a strabismus and amblyopia and upper eyelid ptosis, but funduscopic examination was normal.

CT scan of the axial and coronal planes showed ridging over the sagittal suture and a symmetric well-developed midface. The shape of the cranial vault was consistent with a neglected severe sagittal suture synostosis. The ventricles were normal in size and shape and were symmetric.

Procedure

Intraoperative management of the airway and incision placement were similar to those described in Case 1. Dissection of the scalp flaps with exposure to the total cranial vault, location of craniotomies, and orbital osteotomies were similar to those described in Case 6. After reshaping, the upper orbital osteotomy unit was re-inset in a more posterior position. The total cranial vault was reshaped to decrease the anteroposterior dimension and increase the bitemporal width. The importance of the craniotomies of the squamous temporal bone cannot be overstated in order to achieve the desired increased bitemporal width. It was necessary to section the cranial vault bone into units and then reunite it with multiple titanium miniplates and screws for stabilization of the bony units.

Postoperative Course

Recovery in the hospital and then standard follow-up assessments at 6 weeks, 6 months, and yearly intervals were similar to those described in Case 1. Surgical repair for strabismus and upper eyelid ptosis is planned.

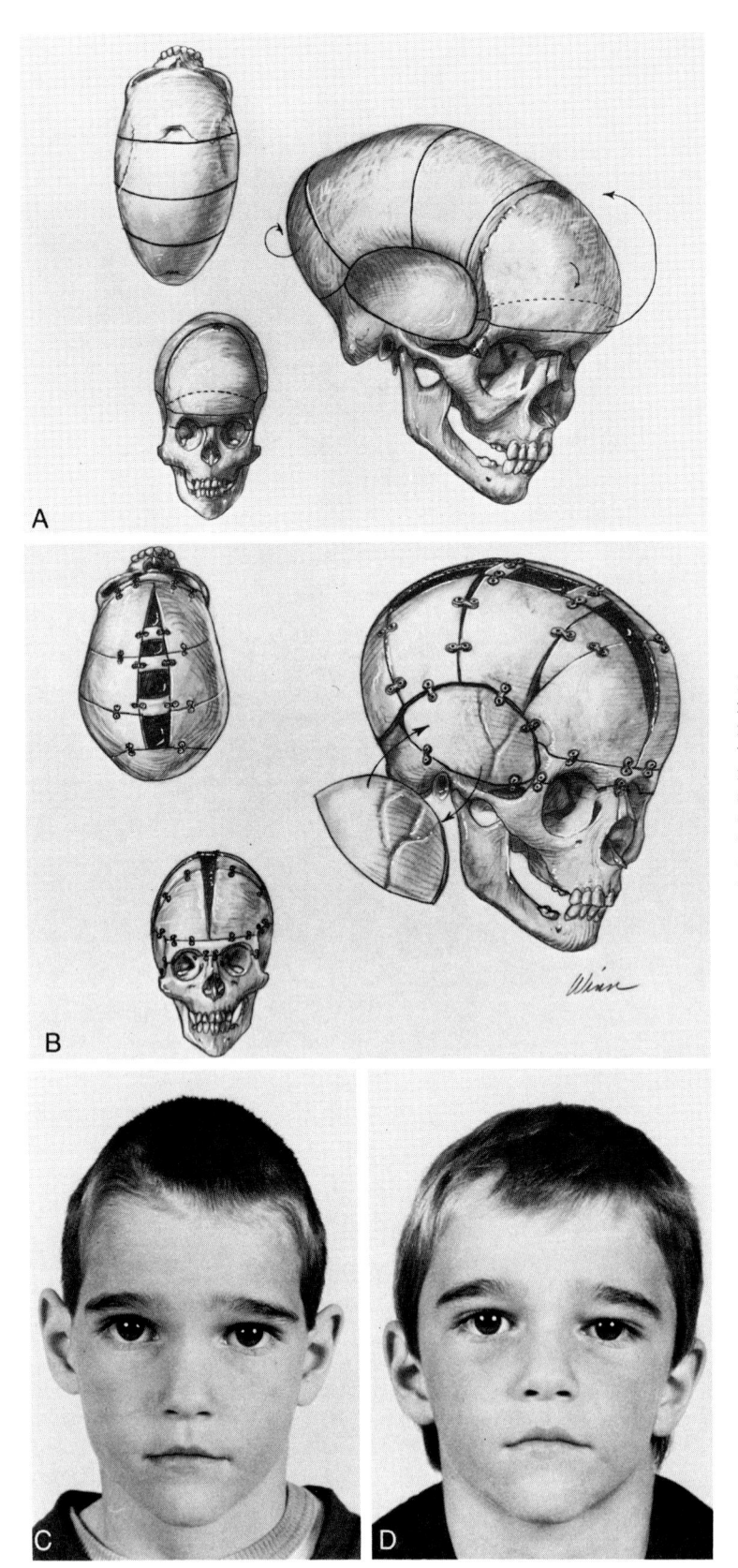

FIGURE 52-8. A 9-YEAR-OLD BOY WITH UNREPAIRED SAGITTAL SUTURE SYNOSTOSIS RESULTING IN MARKED SCAPHOCEPHALY REQUIRING TOTAL CRANIAL VAULT AND UPPER ORBITAL OSTEOTOMIES WITH RESHAPING. *A*, Craniofacial morphology resulting from sagittal suture synostosis. Proposed osteotomies outlined. *B*, Craniofacial morphology after cranial vault and upper orbital osteotomies with reshaping. *C*, Preoperative frontal view. *D*, Frontal view at 1 year after reconstruction.

FIGURE 52-8 *Continued E*, Preoperative oblique view. *F*, Oblique view at 1 year after reconstruction. *G*, Preoperative profile view. *H*, Profile view at 1 year after reconstruction. *I*, Intraoperative bird's-eye view after cranial vault reshaping. Stabilization with titanium mini plates and screws.

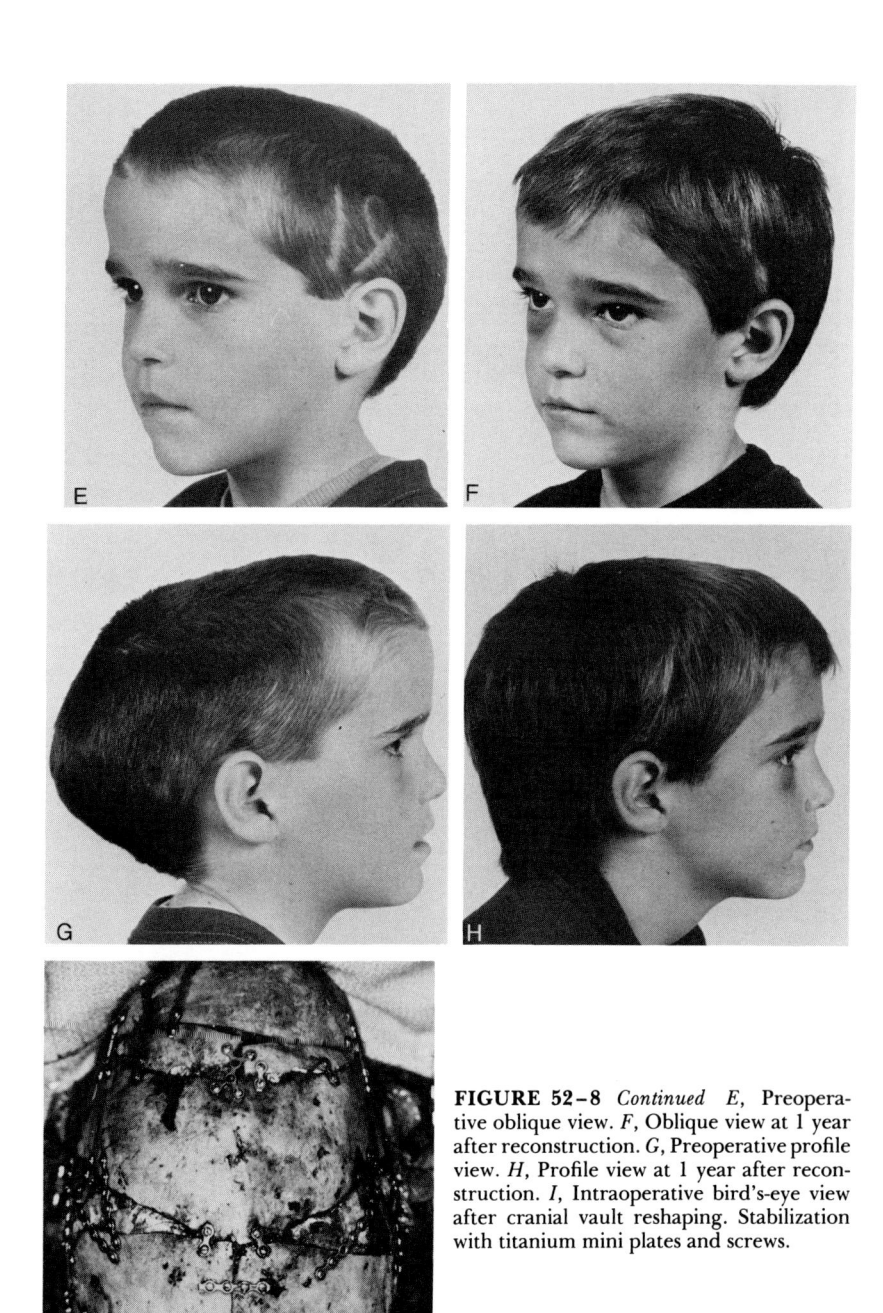

Illustration continued on following page

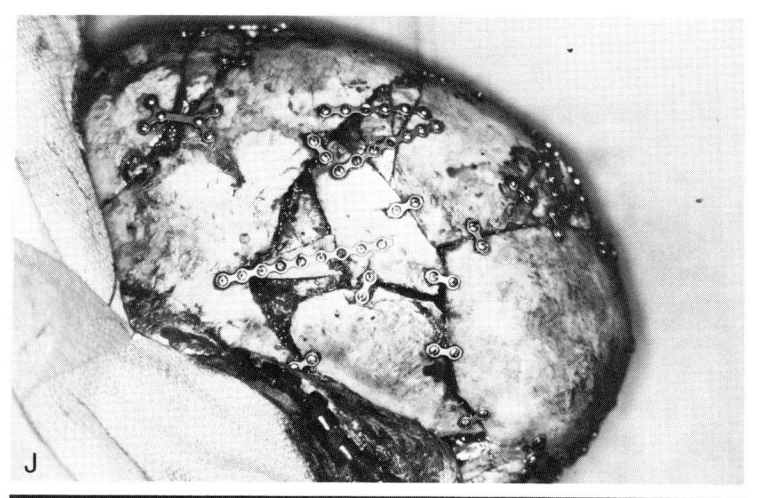

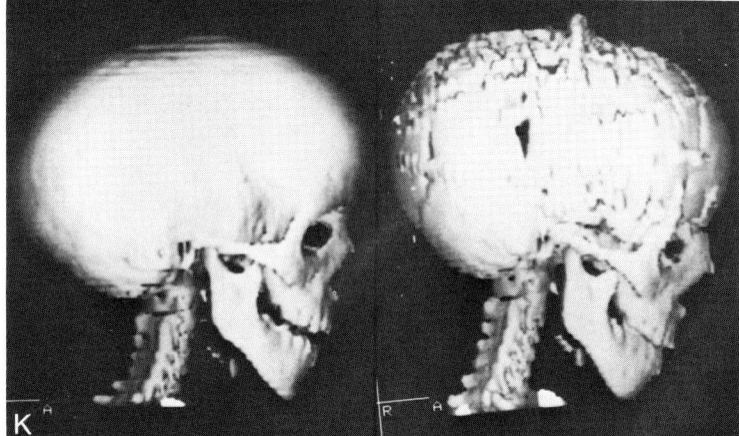

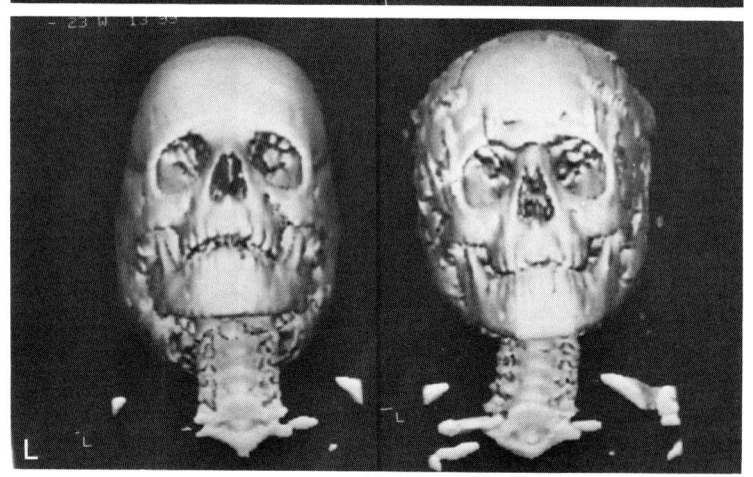

FIGURE 52-8 *Continued* *J*, Intraoperative lateral view of cranial vault after reshaping. *K*, Three-dimensional CT scan reformations. Lateral view before and after reconstruction. *L*, Three-dimensional CT scan reformations. Worm's-eye view before and after reconstruction.

CASE 8 (FIG. 52-9)

Diagnosis: Crouzon syndrome (bilateral coronal synostosis)

Procedure: Anterior cranial vault and three-quarter orbital osteotomies with reshaping and advancement

A patient who had abnormal craniofacial morphology at birth also had a positive family history for Crouzon syndrome: Father had a degree of midface hypoplasia, shallow orbits, and bulging eyes; one sibling had a congenital midline dermoid cyst over the sagittal suture; another had bicoronal suture synostosis and midface hypoplasia. Examination of this patient revealed symmetric bony recession at the level of

FIGURE 52-9. A 10-month-old girl with unrepaired bilateral coronal synostosis as part of Crouzon syndrome requiring suture release and anterior cranial vault and three-quarter orbital osteotomies with reshaping and advancement. *A*, Preoperative frontal view. *B*, Frontal view early after reconstruction. *C*, Preoperative profile view. *D*, Profile view early after reconstruction.

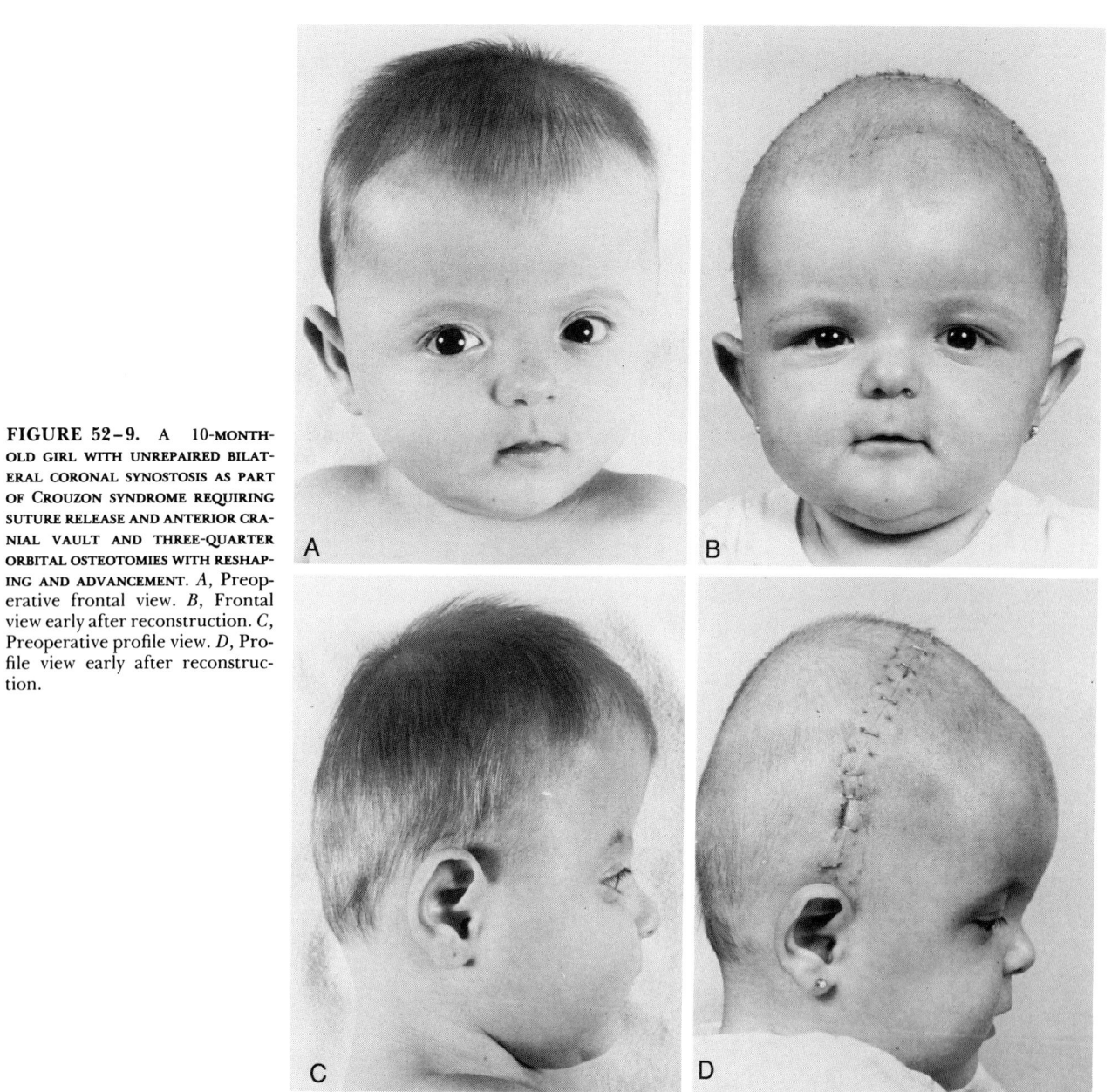

Illustration continued on following page

the supraorbital ridges with resulting shallow orbits and bulging eyes. The forehead was wide and there was compensatory bulging superiorly. Bony ridges were palpable over the coronal suture regions. Midface hypoplasia was minimal.

A CT scan of the craniofacial skeleton was obtained in both the axial and coronal planes. The axial CT scan was reformatted for three-dimensional reconstruction. The anterior cranial base was short and wide, indicative of brachycephaly. The orbits were shallow with globe protrusion and without evidence of orbital hypertelorism. Review of the midface suggested the presence of hypoplasia.

Procedure

The procedure carried out was similar to that described in Case 3.

Postoperative Course

The early postoperative course varied little from that described for Case 1. A staged reconstruction is required for Crouzon syndrome; therefore, further surgery is planned.

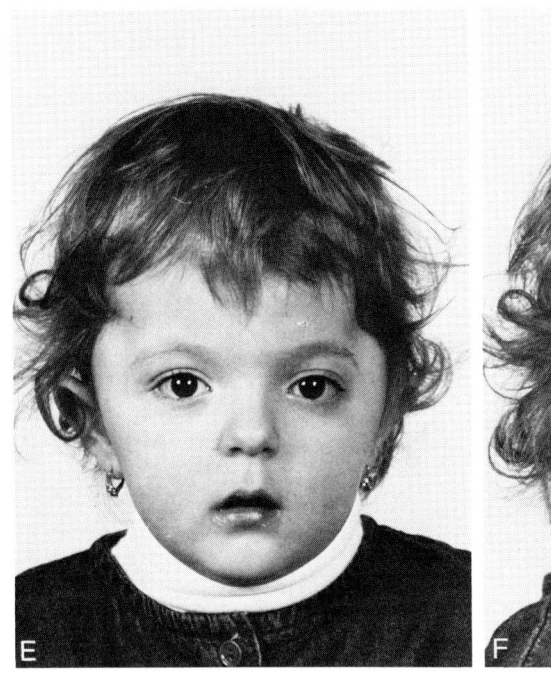

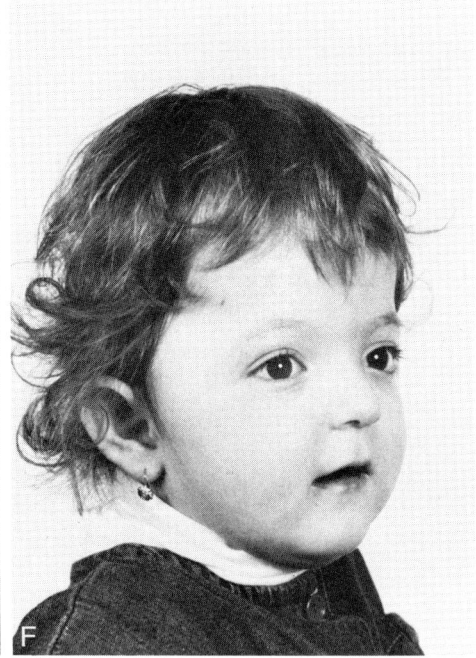

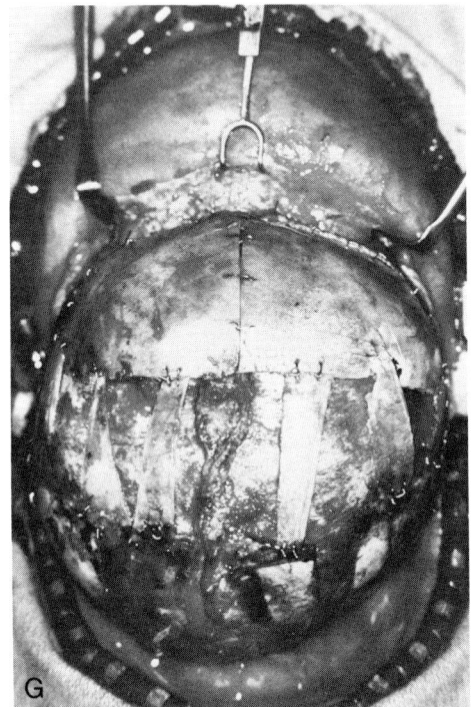

FIGURE 52-9 *Continued* *E*, Frontal view at 3 years of age. *F*, Oblique view at 3 years of age. *G*, Intraoperative bird's-eye view of cranial vault through coronal incision after reconstruction.

CASE 9 (FIG. 52-10)

Diagnosis: Apert syndrome (bilateral coronal synostosis)

Procedure: Anterior cranial vault and three-quarter orbital osteotomies with reshaping and advancement

When abnormal craniofacial morphology and four-limb complex syndactylies were appreciated at birth, a female infant was referred by her pediatrician to the craniofacial team at HSC for evaluation and treatment.

Examination revealed ridging over the bicoronal suture, a short and wide anterior cranial base, shallow orbits, bulging eyes, and a degree of orbital hypertelorism in

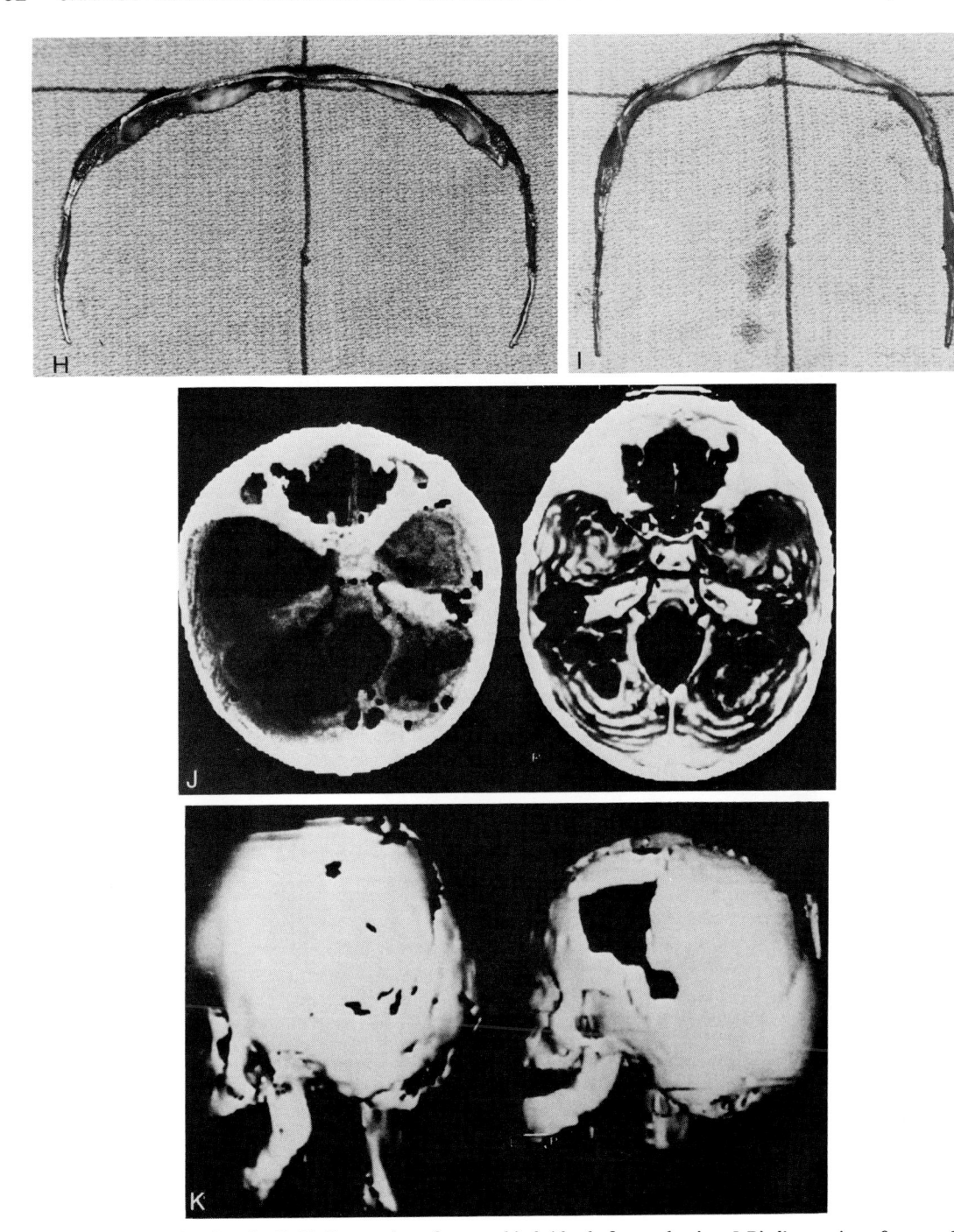

FIGURE 52–9 *Continued* H, Bird's-eye view of supraorbital ridge before reshaping. I, Bird's-eye view of supraorbital ridge after reshaping. J, Three-dimensional CT scan reformations. View of cranial base before and 1 year after reconstruction demonstrating improvement in brachycephalic shape. K, Three-dimensional CT scan reformations. Profile view before and early after reconstruction.

combination with midface hypoplasia. There was a large soft spot over the region where the metopic suture might normally be expected.

A CT scan of the craniofacial skeleton was obtained in both the axial and coronal planes. The axial CT scan was reformatted for three-dimensional reconstruction. The anterior cranial base was short in the AP dimension and extremely wide transversely. The orbits were shallow, the eyes were bulging, and a degree of orbital hypertelorism was present. Ridging was evident over the left and right coronal sutures, and a bony defect was noted over the metopic suture region. The ventricles were a normal size and the midface was hypoplastic. The patient appeared to have

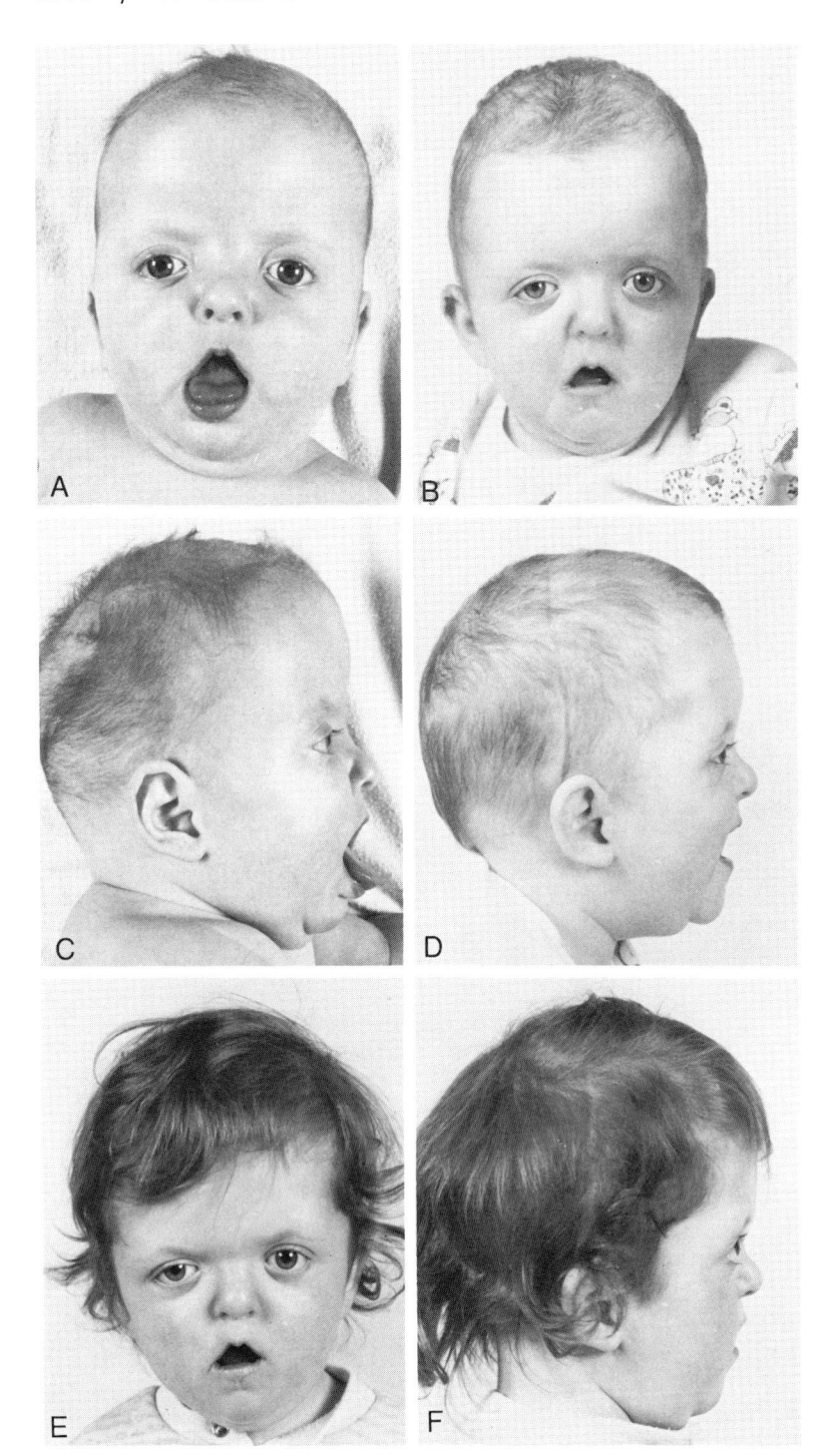

FIGURE 52–10. A 10-month-old infant with unrepaired bicoronal synostosis as part of Apert syndrome requiring suture release and cranial vault and three-quarter orbital osteotomies with reshaping and advancement. *A,* Preoperative frontal view. *B,* Frontal view early after reconstruction. *C,* Preoperative profile view. *D,* Profile view early after reconstruction. *E,* Frontal view at 2.5 years of age. *F,* Profile view at 2.5 years of age.

premature closure of the left and right coronal suture with additional orbital and midface findings suggestive of Apert syndrome.

Procedure

The intraoperative management was very similar to that described in Case 3.

Postoperative Course

The early postoperative recovery and follow-up appointments were very similar to those described in Case 1. A staged reconstruction is required for Apert syndrome; therefore, further surgery is planned.

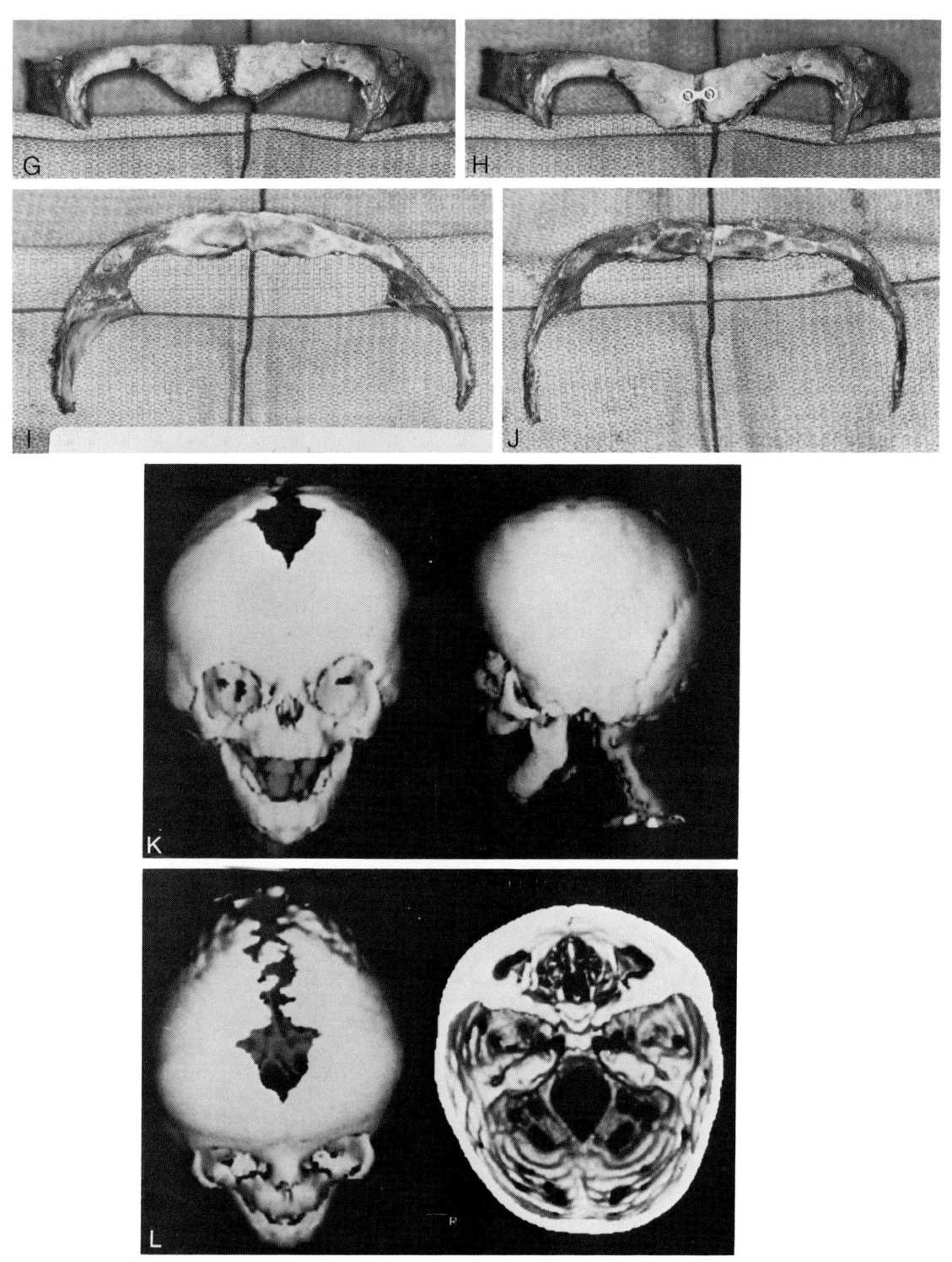

FIGURE 52–10 *Continued* G, Frontal view of orbital osteotomy unit before reshaping. H, Same view after reshaping. Stabilization with titanium mini plate and screws. I, Bird's-eye view of orbital osteotomy unit before reshaping. J, Same view after reshaping. K, Three-dimensional CT scan reformations. Views before surgery. L, Additional three-dimensional CT scan reformations before surgery showing marked brachycephaly.

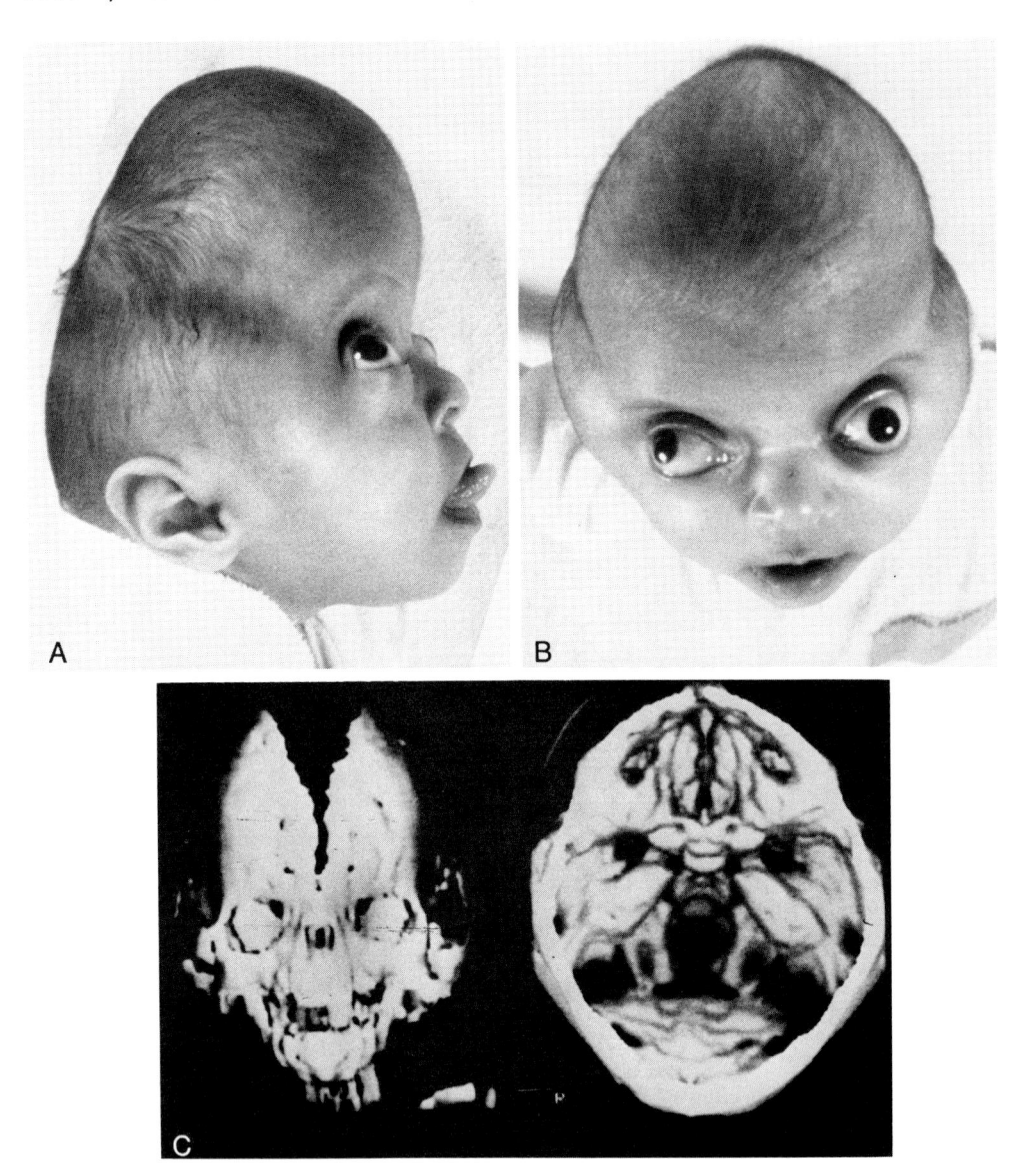

FIGURE 52–11. A 3.1-YEAR-OLD GIRL WITH KLEEBLATTSCHÄDEL ANOMALY. SHE INITIALLY UNDERWENT UPPER ORBITAL AND CRANIAL VAULT RESHAPING TO RELIEVE INTRACRANIAL PRESSURE. SHE LATER UNDERWENT POSTERIOR CRANIAL VAULT RESHAPING IN ORDER TO FURTHER INCREASE THE INTRACRANIAL VOLUME. SHE WILL BE UNDERGOING MONOBLOC OSTEOTOMY WITH ADVANCEMENT AT THE AGE OF 4 YEARS. *A*, Preoperative profile view. *B*, Preoperative bird's-eye view. *C*, CT scan reformations of craniofacial skeleton before surgery.

CASE 10 (FIG. 52–11)

Diagnosis: Kleeblattschädel anomaly

Procedure: Total cranial vault and three-quarter orbital osteotomies with reshaping and advancement, and posterior cranial vault craniotomies and reshaping

A patient noted at birth to have a cloverleaf shape to the craniofacial skeleton had difficulty with air management as a neonate and required early tracheostomy for breathing and gastrostomy for feeding. She was referred to the craniofacial team at HSC for further evaluation and treatment.

Examination at approximately 10 months of age revealed a symmetric and peculiar shape to the cranial vault with bulges laterally and one superiorly. The orbits were extremely shallow with marked globe protrusion. Past globe herniation had required emergency reduction. There was severe midface hypoplasia with limited nasal air flow.

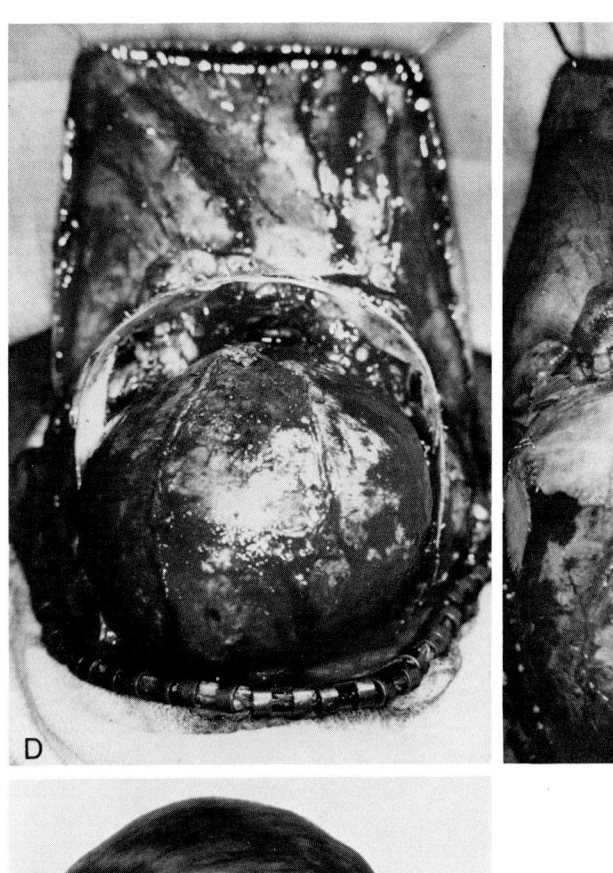

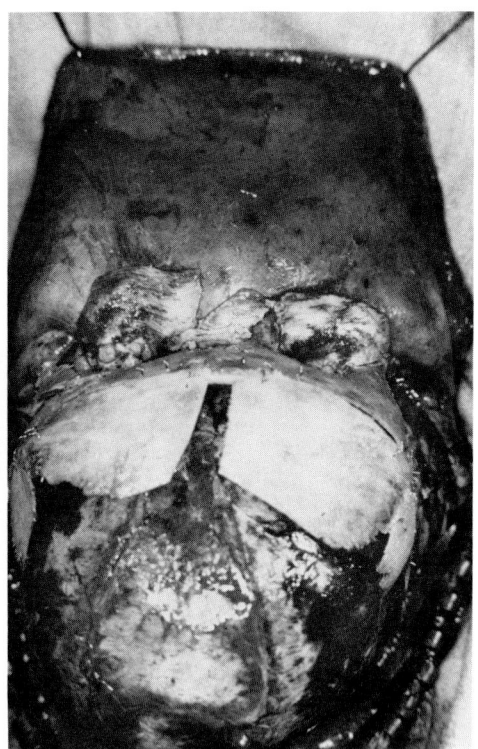

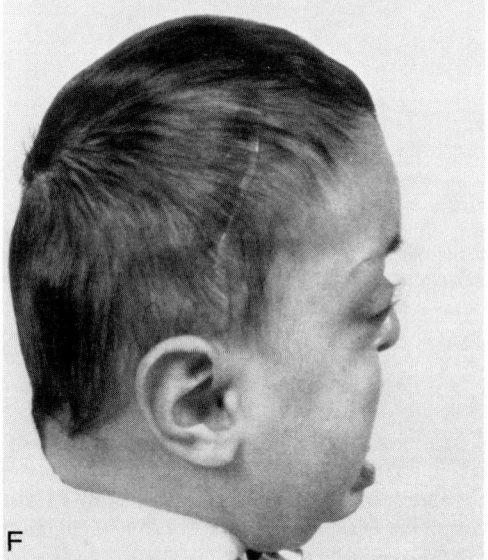

FIGURE 52-11 Continued D, Intraoperative bird's-eye view through coronal incision after orbital osteotomies with reshaping and extensive advancement. E, Same view after initial cranial vault bone reconstruction. F, Profile view early after reconstruction.
Illustration continued on following page

A CT scan of the craniofacial skeleton was obtained in both the axial and coronal planes. The axial CT scan was reformatted for three-quarter dimensional reconstruction. The scan confirmed the diagnosis of kleeblattschädel anomaly. There were cranial vault openings in the region of the metopic and sagittal sutures as well the squamosal sutures of the temporal bone regions bilaterally. The ventricles were slightly dilated, indicating mild to moderate hydrocephalus. The patient appeared to have kleeblattschädel anomaly with fusion of all sutures except the squamosal, metopic, and anterior sagittal sutures.

Procedure

The intraoperative management of the airway was through the previous tracheostomy. The incision was bicoronal with dissection in the subperiosteal plane until the total cranial vault, orbits, squamous portion of temporal bones, anterior maxilla, and zygomas bilaterally were exposed.

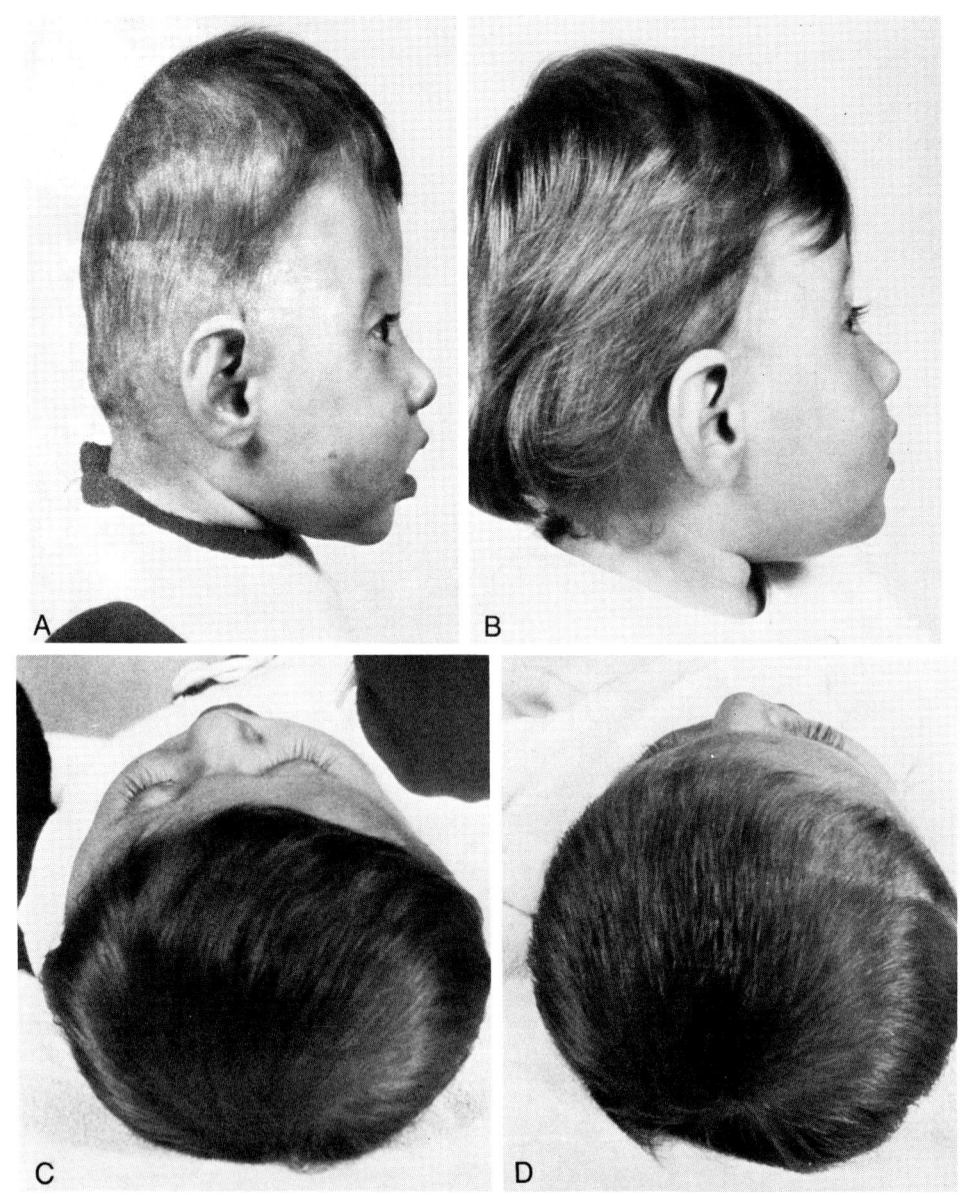

FIGURE 52–12. A 2.5-YEAR-OLD FEMALE INFANT BORN WITH CROUZON SYNDROME. SHE PREVIOUSLY UNDERWENT BILATERAL LATERAL CANTHAL ADVANCEMENT FOR CORONAL SUTURE RELEASE AND RESHAPING. SIGNS OF INCREASED INTRACRANIAL PRESSURE DEVELOPED AND SHE THEREFORE UNDERWENT REPEAT CRANIOTOMY WITH CRANIAL VAULT AND THREE-QUARTER ORBITAL OSTEOTOMIES WITH RESHAPING AND ADVANCEMENT TO FURTHER INCREASE THE INTRACRANIAL VOLUME AND RELIEVE PRESSURE. *A*, Preoperative profile view before repeat craniotomy. *B*, Profile view after second-stage cranio-orbital reconstruction to increase intracranial volume. *C*, Preoperative bird's-eye view before repeat craniotomy. *D*, Bird's eye view after second-stage reconstruction.

During examination, the infant was found to have an extremely short anteroposterior dimension to the cranial vault with shallow orbits and bulging eyes. The bitemporal width was enlarged.

A CT scan of the craniofacial skeleton was completed through the axial and coronal planes. Three-dimensional reformation of the axial CT scan was completed. A ventriculoperitoneal shunt was well positioned, and the ventricles were normal in size and symmetric. The anterior cranial base was short and extremely wide. The cephalic height was increased, resulting in an oxycephalic shape to the cranial vault.

Overall, the patient appeared to have oxycephaly resulting from refusion of the bicoronal sutures with an overall diminished anteroposterior skull dimension and increased bitemporal width.

PROCEDURE

Intraoperative management of the airway, incision placement, flap dissection, initial craniotomy, and orbital osteotomies were similar to those described in Case 1. Increased intraoperative blood loss and dural tears associated with repeat craniotomy occurred as expected. The cranial vault bone was thin and brittle.

Once the three-quarter orbital osteotomies were completed, reshaping was carried out with the methods similar to those described in Case 3. Further craniectomy of the posterior cranial vault was required to carry out total cranial vault reshaping. Once the orbital units were reshaped and inset, the cranial vault bone was pieced together, beginning with the forehead and then working posteriorly. Stabilization in this patient was achieved with multiple direct intraosseous wires.

POSTOPERATIVE COURSE

The postoperative recovery and follow-up were very similar to those described in Case 8.

REFERENCES

1. Acquaviva R, Tamic PM, Lebascle J, et al: Les craniostenoses en milieu marocain, a propos de 140 observations. Neuro-chirurgie 12:561, 1966.
2. Alberius P, Brandt L, Selvik G: Calvarial growth after linear craniectomy in scaphocephaly as evaluated by X-ray stereophotogrammetry. J Craniomaxillofac Surg 15:2, 1987.
3. Alberti PW, Ruben RJ (eds): Otologic Medicine and Surgery. New York, Churchill Livingstone, 1988.
4. Alderman BW, Lammer EJ, Joshua SC, et al: An epidemiologic study of craniosynostoses: Risk indicators for the occurrence of craniosynostosis in Colorado. Am J Epidemiol 128:431, 1988.
5. Anderl H, Muhlbauer W, Twerdy K, Marchac D: Frontofacial advancement with bony separation in craniofacial dysostosis. Plast Reconstr Surg 71:303, 1983.
6. Anderson FM, Geiger L: Craniostenosis: A survey of 204 cases. J Neurosurg 22:229, 1965.
7. Andersson H, Gomes SP: Craniosynostosis: Review of the literature and indications for surgery. Acta Paediatr Scand 57:47, 1968.
8. Apert E: De l'acrocephalosyndactylie. Bull Mem Soc Med Hop Paris 23:1310, 1906.
9. Barden RC, Ford ME, Jensen AG, et al: Effects of craniofacial deformity in infancy on the quality of mother-infant interactions. Child Dev 60:819, 1989.
10. Benattar A: La craniectomie extensive dans le traitement des craniostenoses: Etude de 37 cas. Th med Paris 5, Necker-Enfants Malades, 1977.
11. Binghong BU, Kaban LB, Vargervik K: Effect of Le Fort III osteotomy on mandibular growth in patients with Crouzon and Apert syndromes. J Oral Maxillofac Surg 47:666, 1989.
12. Bjork A: Cranial base development. Am J Orthod 41:198, 1955.
13. Bjork A, Bjork L: Artificial deformation and cranio-facial asymmetry in ancient Peruvians. J Dent Res 43:353, 1964.
14. Blank CE: Apert's syndrome (a type of acrocephalosyndactyly)—observations on a British series of thirty-nine cases. Ann Hum Genet 24:151, 1960.
15. Blundell JE: Early craniectomies for craniofacial dysostosis. In Converse JN, McCarthy JG, Wood-Smith D (eds): Symposium on Diagnosis and Treatment of Craniofacial Anomalies. St Louis, CV Mosby, 1979, p 311.
16. Bookstein FC: Describing a craniofacial anomaly: Finite elements and the biometrics of landmark locations. Am J Phys Anthropol 74:495, 1987.
17. Breitbart AS, Eaton C, McCarthy JG: Crouzon's syndrome associated with acanthosis nigricans: Ramifications of the craniofacial surgeon. Ann Plast Surg 22:310, 1989.
18. Buchanan RC: Acrocephalosyndactyly or Apert's syndrome. Br J Plast Surg 21:406, 1968.
19. Burdi AR, Kusnetz AB, Venes JL, Gebarski SS: The natural history and pathogenesis of the cranial coronal ring articulations: Implications in understanding the pathogenesis of the Crouzon craniostenotic defects. Cleft Palate J 23:28, 1986.
20. Carpenter G: Two sisters showing malformations of the skull and other congenital abnormalities. Rep Soc Study Dis Child (London) 1:110, 1901.
21. Carr M, Posnick JC, Armstrong D: Cranio-orbital-zygomatic measurements from standard CT scans in unoperated Crouzon and Apert patients: Comparison to normal controls. Proceedings of the 47th Annual Meeting, American Cleft Palate/Craniofacial Association, St. Louis, Missouri, May 1990, p 59.
22. Chana HS, Klauss V: Crouzon's craniofacial dysostosis in Kenya. Br J Ophthalmol 72:196, 1988.
23. Cohen MM Jr (ed): Craniosynostosis—Diagnosis, Evaluation and Management. New York, Raven Press, 1986.
24. Cohen MM Jr: An etiologic and nosologic overview of craniosynostosis syndromes. Birth Defects 11:137, 1975.
25. Corey JP, Caldarelli DD, Gould HJ: Otopathology in cranial facial dysostosis. Am J Otol 8:14, 1987.
26. Costaras-Volarich M, Pruzansky S: Is the mandible intrinsically different in Apert and Crouzon syndrome? Am J Orthod 85:475, 1984.

27. Cross HE, Opitz JM: Craniosynostosis in the Amish. J Pediatr 75:1037, 1969.
28. Crouzon O: Dysostose cranio-faciale herediataire. Bull Soc Med Hop Paris 33:545, 1912.
29. Cutting CB, McCarthy JG, Berenstein A: Blood supply of the upper craniofacial skeleton: The search for composite calvarial bone flaps. Plast Reconstr Surg 74:603, 1984.
30. Cutting CB, McCarthy JG, et al: Three-dimensional shape of the midface in Crouzon's disease in relation to the methods for correction. Proceedings of the 46th Annual Meeting, The Cleft Craniofacial Association, April 1989, p 29.
31. De Myer W, Zeman W, Palmer CG: The face predicts the brain: Diagnostic significance of median facial anomalies for holoprosencephaly (arhinencephaly). Pediatrics 34:256, 1964.
32. Diamond GR, Whitaker L: Ocular motility in craniofacial reconstruction. Plast Reconstr Surg 73:31, 1984.
33. Dodge HW, Wood MW, Kennedy RLJ: Craniofacial dysostosis: Crouzon's disease. Pediatrics 23:98, 1959.
34. Edgerton MT, Jane JA, Berry FA, Fisher JC: The feasibility of craniofacial osteotomies in infants and young children. Scand J Plast Reconstr Surg 8:164, 1974.
35. Edgerton MT, Jane JA, Berry FA: Craniofacial osteotomies and reconstruction in infants and young children. Plast Reconstr Surg 54:13, 1974.
36. Enlow DH, Azuma M: Functional growth boundaries in the human and mammalian face. Birth Defects 11(7):217, 1975.
37. Enlow DH, McNamara JA Jr: The neurocranial basis for facial form and pattern. Angle Orthod 43:256, 1973.
38. Enlow DH: Handbook of Facial Growth, 2nd ed. Philadelphia, WB Saunders, 1982.
39. Farkas LG, Kolar JC, Munro IR: Craniofacial disproportions in Apert's syndrome: An anthropometric study. Cleft Palate J 22:253, 1985.
40. Fishman MA, Hogan GR, Dodge PR: The concurrence of hydrocephalus and craniosynostosis. J Neurosurg 34:621, 1971.
41. Ford EHR: Growth of the human cranial base. Am J Orthod 44:498, 1958.
42. Gault D, Brunelle F, Renier D, Marchac D: The calculation of intracranial volume using CT scans. Child's Nerv Syst 4:271, 1988.
43. Giblin N, Alley A: Studies in skull growth. Coronal suture fixation. Anat Rec 88:143, 1944.
44. Gillies H, Harrison SH: Operative correction by osteotomy of recessed malar maxillary compound in case of oxycephaly. Br J Plast Surg 3:123, 1950.
45. Golabi M, Edwards MSB, Ousterhout DK: Craniosynostosis and hydrocephalus. Neurosurgery 21:63, 1987.
46. Cohen MM, Levin LS: Syndromes of the Head and Neck, 3rd ed. New York, Oxford University Press, 1990.
47. Guilleminault C: Obstructive sleep apnea syndrome and its treatment in children: Areas of agreement and controversy. Pediatr Pulmonol 3:429, 1987.
48. Helveston EM: Symposium: Head posture and strabismus. Am Orthoptic J 33:1, 1983.
49. Hemmy DC, David DJ, Herman GT: Three-dimensional reconstruction of craniofacial deformity using computed tomography. Neurosurgery 13:534, 1983.
50. Hemmy DC, Tessier PL: CT of dry skulls with craniofacial deformities: Accuracy of three-dimensional reconstruction. Radiology 157:113, 1985.
51. Hoffman HJ: Early craniectomy and stripping in craniofacial synostosis. In Converse JM, McCarthy JG, Wood-Smith D (eds): Symposium on Diagnosis and Treatment of Craniofacial Anomalies. St Louis, CV Mosby, 1979, p 287.
52. Hoffman HJ, Hendrick EB: Early neurosurgical repair in craniofacial dysmorphism. J Neurosurg 51:796, 1979.
53. Hoffman HJ, Mohr G: Lateral canthal advancement of the supraorbital margin: A new corrective technique in the treatment of coronal synostosis. J Neurosurg 45:376, 1976.
54. Hogan GR, Bauman ML: Hydrocephalus in Apert's syndrome. J Pediatr 79:782, 1971.
55. Holtermuller K, Wiedemann HR: Kleeblattschadel-syndrome. Med Monatsschr 14:439, 1960.
56. Hoyte DA: A critical analysis of the growth in length of the cranial base. Birth Defects 11:255, 1975.
57. Hunter AGW, Rudd NL: Craniosynostosis. Coronal synostosis: Its familial characteristics and associated clinical findings in 109 patients lacking bilateral polysyndactyly or syndactyly. Teratology 15:301, 1977.
58. Israele V, Siegel JD: Infectious complications of craniofacial surgery in children. Rev Infect Dis 2(1):9, 1989.
59. Jane JA, Park TS, Zide BM, et al: Alternative techniques in the treatment of unilateral coronal synostosis. J Neurosurg 61:550, 1984.
60. Kaban LB, West B, Conover M, et al: Midface position after Le Fort III advancement. Plast Reconstr Surg 73:758, 1984.
61. Kaye CI, Matalon R, Pruzansky S: The natural history of Apert syndrome, with speculations on pathogenesis. Teratology 17:28A, 1978.
62. Klippel M, Feil A: Un ceas d'absence des vertebres cervicales. Nouv Iconogr Salpet 25:223, 1912.
63. Kolar JC, Munro IR, Farkas LG: Patterns of dysmorphology in Crouzon syndrome: An anthropometric study. Cleft Palate J 25:235, 1988.
64. Kreiborg S, Aduss H: Pre- and postsurgical facial growth in patients with Crouzon's and Apert's syndromes. Cleft Palate J (Suppl) 23:78, 1986.
65. Kreiborg S, Bjork A: Description of a dry skull with Crouzon syndrome. Scand J Plast Reconstr Surg 16:245, 1982.
66. Kreiborg S, Pruzansky S, Pashayan H: The Saethre-Chotzen syndrome. Teratology 6:287, 1972.

67. Kreiborg S: Crouzon syndrome. A clinical and roentgencephalometric study. Scand J Plast Reconstr Surg 18:1 (Suppl), 1981.
68. Kroczek RA, Muhlbauer W, Zimmermann I: Cloverleaf skull associated with Pfeiffer syndrome: Pathology and management. Eur J Pediatr 145:442, 1986.
69. Kushner J, Alexander E Jr, Davis CH Jr, et al: Crouzon's disease (craniofacial dysostosis) modern diagnosis and treatment. J Neurosurg 37:434, 1972.
70. Lane LC: Pioneer craniectomy for relief of mental imbecility due to premature sutural closure and microcephalus. JAMA 18:49, 1892.
71. Lannelongue M: De la cranectomie dans la microcephalie. Compte-Rendu Acad Sci 110:1382, 1890.
72. Lauritzen C, Lilja J, Jarlstedt J: Airway obstruction and sleep apnea in children with craniofacial anomalies. Plast Reconstr Surg 77:1, 1986.
73. Lawrence WT, Azizkhan RG: Congenital muscular torticollis: A spectrum of pathology. Ann Plast Surg 23(6):523, 1989.
74. Lefebvre A, Barclay S: Psychosocial impact of craniofacial deformities before and after reconstructive surgery. Can J Psychiatry 27:579, 1982.
75. Lefebvre A, Travis F, Arndt EM, Munro IR: A psychiatric profile before and after reconstructive surgery in children with Apert's syndrome. Br J Plast Surg 39:510, 1986.
76. Lewin ML: Facial deformity in acrocephaly and its surgical correction. Arch Ophthalmol 47:321, 1952.
77. Longacre JJ, Destefano GA, Holmstrand K: The early versus the late reconstruction of congenital hypoplasia of the facial skeleton and skull. Plast Reconstr Surg 27:489, 1961.
78. Losken HW, Morris WMM, Uys PB, et al: Crouzon's disease. Part I. One-stage correction by combined face and forehead advancement. S Afr Med J 75:274, 1989.
79. Marchac D: Problemes poses par la contention apres osteotomies de type Le Fort III. Rev Stomatol Chir Maxillofac 78:193, 1977.
80. Marchac D: Radical forehead remodeling for craniostenosis. Plast Reconstr Surg 61:823, 1978.
81. Marchac D: Forehead remodeling for craniostenosis. *In* Converse JM, McCarthy JG, Wood-Smith D (eds): Symposium on Diagnosis and Treatment of Craniofacial Anomalies. St. Louis, CV Mosby, 1979, p 323.
82. Marchac D, Cophignon J, Clay C, et al: Reparation des fraces fronto-orbitaires par reposition ou osteotomie et greffes osseuses. Ann Chir Plast 19:41, 1974.
83. Marchac D, Cophignon J, Van der Meulen J, et al: A propos des osteotomies d'advancement du crane et de la face. Ann Chir Plast 19:311, 1974.
84. Marchac D, Renier D: "Le front flottant." Traitement precoce des faciocraniostenoses. Ann Chir Plast 24:121, 1979.
85. Marchac D, Renier D: Cranio-facial surgery for craniosynostosis. Scand J Plast Reconstr Surg 15:235, 1981.
86. Marchac D, Renier D: Craniofacial surgery for craniosynostosis improves facial growth: A personal case review. Ann Plast Surg 14:43, 1985.
87. Marchac D, Renier D: Treatment of craniosynostosis in infancy. Clin Plast Surg 14:61, 1987.
88. Marchac D, Renier D, Jones BM: Experience with the "floating forehead." Br J Plast Surg 41:1, 1988.
89. Marsh JL, Gado MH, Vannier MW, Stevens WG: Osseous anatomy of unilateral coronal synostosis. Cleft Palate J 23:87, 1986.
90. Marsh JL, Vannier MW: The anatomy of the cranio-orbital deformities of craniosynostosis: Insights from 3-D images of CT scans. Clin Plast Surg 14:49, 1987.
91. Marsh JL, Vannier MW: The "third" dimension in craniofacial surgery. Plast Reconstr Surg 71:759, 1983.
92. Martin PR, Lefebvre AM: Surgical treatment of sleep-apnea-associated psychosis. Can Med Assoc J 124:978, 1981.
93. McCarthy JG: New concepts in the surgical treatment of the craniofacial synostosis syndromes in the infant. Clin Plast Surg 6:201, 1979.
94. McCarthy JG, Coccaro PJ, Epstein F, Converse JM: Early skeletal release in the infant with craniofacial dysostosis: The role of the sphenozygomatic suture. Plast Reconstr Surg 62:335, 1978.
95. McCarthy JG, Coccaro PJ, Epstein FJ: Early skeletal release in the patient with craniofacial dysostosis. *In* Converse JM, McCarthy J, Wood-Smith D (eds): Symposium on Diagnosis and Treatment of Craniofacial Anomalies. St Louis, CV Mosby, 1979, p 295.
96. McCarthy JG, Epstein F, Sadove M, et al: Early surgery for craniofacial synostosis: An 8-year experience. Plast Reconstr Surg 73:521, 1984.
97. McCarthy JG, Grayson B, Bookstein F, et al: Le Fort III advancement osteotomy in the growing child. Plast Reconstr Surg 74:343, 1984.
98. McLaurin RL, Matson DD: Importance of early surgical treatment of craniosynostosis. Pediatrics 10:637, 1952.
99. Mohr G, Hoffman HJ, Munro IR, et al: Surgical management of unilateral and bilateral coronal craniosynostosis: 21 years of experience. Neurosurgery 2:83, 1978.
100. Morax S: Oculomotor disorders in craniofacial malformations. *In* Caronni EP (ed): Craniofacial Surgery. Boston, Little, Brown, 1985, p 97.
101. Moss ML: The pathogenesis of premature cranial synostosis in man. Acta Anat 37:351, 1959.
102. Moss ML, Bromberg BE, Song IC, Eisenman G: The passive role of nasal septal cartilage in mid-facial growth. Plast Reconstr Surg 41:536, 1968.
103. Muhlbauer W, Anderl H: Use of miniplates in craniofacial surgery. Proceedings of the 1st International Congress of the International Society of Craniomaxillofacial Surgeons. Berlin, Springer-Verlag, 1987, p 334.

104. Muhling J, Reuther J, Sorenson N: Problems with lateral canthal advancement. Childs Nerv Syst 2:287, 1986.
105. Murray JE, Swanson LT: Mid-face osteotomy and advancement for craniosynostosis. Plast Reconstr Surg 41:200, 1968.
106. Nakano P, Posnick JC: Early morbidity and long term reconstructive results in Apert syndrome. Proceedings of the 71st Annual Meeting of The American Association of Oral and Maxillofacial Surgeons 47(8): 83 (Suppl 1), 1989.
107. Nakano PH, Posnick JC: Long-term results of reconstructive craniofacial surgery in patients with Crouzon and Apert syndrome. Proceedings of the 46th Annual Meeting of The Cleft Palate-Craniofacial Association, April 1989.
108. Nakano PH, Posnick JC: Long-term results of reconstruction in craniofacial dysostosis. Proceedings of the 6th International Congress of Cleft Palate and Related Anomalies, June, 1989.
109. Nakano PH, Posnick JC: Morbidity and long term reconstructive results in Apert syndrome. Proceedings of the 43rd Annual Meeting of The Canadian Society of Plastic Surgeons, June, 1989.
110. Nathan V: Craniofacial dysostosis: Crouzon's disease. West Indian Med J 32:237, 1983.
111. Neill CL: Influence of early cranioplasty for craniostenosis upon cranial and facial configuration. In Smith B, Converse JC (eds): Proceedings of 2nd International Symposium of Plastic and Reconstructive Surgery of the Eye and Adnexa. St. Louis, CV Mosby, 1967, p 302.
112. Norgaard JO, Kvinnsland S: Influence of submucous septal resection on facial growth in the rat. Plast Reconstr Surg 64:84, 1979.
113. Obwegeser HL: Surgical correction of small or retrodisplaced maxillae: The "dish-face" deformity. Plast Reconstr Surg 43:351, 1969.
114. Ortiz-Monasterio F, Fuente del Campo A, Carillo A: Advancement of the orbits and the midface in one piece, combined with frontal repositioning, for the correction of Crouzon's deformities. Plast Reconstr Surg 61:507, 1978.
115. Ortiz-Monasterio F, Fuente del Campo A: Refinements on the bloc orbitofacial advancement. In Caronni EP (ed): Craniofacial Surgery. Boston, Little, Brown, 1985, p 263.
116. Ousterhout DK, Melsen B: Cranial base deformity in Apert's syndrome. Plast Reconstr Surg 69:254, 1982.
117. Ousterhout DK, Vargervik K: Aesthetic improvement resulting from craniofacial surgery in craniosynostosis syndromes. J Craniomaxillofac Surg 15:189, 1987.
118. Palkes HS, Marsh JL, Talent BK: Pediatric craniofacial surgery and parental attitudes. Cleft Palate J 23:137, 1986.
119. Parekh BK, Jakhi SA: Acrocephalosyndactyly. Apert's syndrome—case report of a rarity. Ann Dent 46:31, 1987.
120. Patton MA, Goodship J, Hayward R, Lansdown R: Intellectual development in Apert's syndrome: A long term follow up of 29 patients. J Med Genet 25:164, 1988.
121. Persing JA, Babler WJ, Jane JA, Duckworth PF: Experimental unilateral coronal synostosis in rabbits. Plast Reconstr Surg 77:369, 1986.
122. Persing JA, Babler WJ, Nagorsky MJ, et al: Skull expansion in experimental craniosynostosis. Plast Reconstr Surg 78:594, 1986.
123. Persing JA, Cronin AJ, Delshaw JB, et al: Late surgical treatment of unilateral coronal synostosis using methyl methacrylate. J Neurosurg 66:793, 1987.
124. Pfeiffer RA: Dominant erbliche Akrocephalosyndaktylie. Z Kinderheilkd 90:301, 1964.
125. Posnick JC, Bite U, Nakano P, Davis J: Comparison of direct and indirect intracranial volume measurements. Proceedings of the 6th International Congress on Cleft Palate and Related Craniofacial Anomalies, June 1989.
126. Poswillo D: Mechanisms and pathogenesis of malformation. Br Med Bull 32:59, 1976.
127. Powiertowski H, Matlosz Z: The treatment of craniostenosis by a method of extensive resection of the vault of the skull. In Proceedings of the 3rd International Congress on Neurosurgery. Surg Excerpta Med Internat Cong Series 110:834, 1965.
128. Pruzansky S: Time: The fourth dimension in syndrome analysis applied to craniofacial malformations. Birth Defects 13(3c):3, 1977.
129. Renier D, Sainte-Rose C, Marchac D, Hirsch JF: Intracranial pressure in craniostenosis. J Neurosurg 57:370, 1982.
130. Richtsmeirer JT: Comparative study of normal, Crouzon and Apert craniofacial morphology using finite element scaling analysis. Am J Phys Anthropol 74:473, 1987.
131. Rosen HM, Whitaker LA: Cranial base dynamics in craniofacial dysostosis. J Maxillofac Surg 12:56, 1984.
132. Rougerie J, Derome P, Anquez L: Craniostenosis et dysmorphies cranio-faciales. Principes d'une nouvelle technique de traitement et ses resultats. Neurochirurgie 18:429, 1972.
133. Sarnat BG: Differential craniofacial skeletal changes after postnatal experimental surgery in young and adult animals. Ann Plast Surg 1:131, 1978.
134. Sarnat BG: The postnatal maxillary-nasal-orbital complex: Some considerations in experimental surgery. In McNamara JA (ed): Factors Affecting the Growth of the Midface. Ann Arbor, University of Michigan Press, 1976.
135. Seeger JF, Gabrielsen TO: Premature closure of the frontosphenoidal suture in synostosis of the coronal suture. Radiology 101:631, 1971.
136. Shiller JG: Craniofacial dysostosis of Crouzon: A case report and pedigree with emphasis on heredity. Pediatrics 23:107, 1959.
137. Shillito J Jr, Matson DD: Craniosynostosis: A review of 519 surgical patients. Pediatrics 41:829, 1968.
138. Stewart RE, Dixon G, Cohen A: The pathogenesis of premature craniosynostosis in acrocephalosyndactyly (Apert's syndrome): A reconsideration. Plast Reconstr Surg 59:699, 1977.

139. Stewart RE, Kawamoto HK Jr: Acrocephalosyndactyly (Apert's syndrome): A cause for reconsideration of its pathogenesis. *In* Converse JM, McCarthy JG, Wood-Smith D (eds): Symposium on Diagnosis and Treatment of Craniofacial Anomalies. St. Louis, CV Mosby, 1979, p 258.
140. Stricker M, Montaut J, Hepner H, et al: Les osteotomies du crane et de la face. Ann Chir Plast 17:233, 1972.
141. Tajima S, Nakajima H, Maruyama Y, et al: Temporal double inversion method in reshaping the temporal bulging in a case of Apert's syndrome. J Maxillofac Surg 8:125, 1980.
142. Temtamy SA: Carpenter's syndrome: Acrocephalopolysyndactyly. An autosomal recessive syndrome. J Pediatr 69:11, 1966.
143. Ten Cate AR, Freeman E, Dickinson JB: Sutural development: Structure and its response to rapid expansion. Am J Orthod 71:622, 1977.
144. Tessier P: Osteotomies totales de la face. Syndrome de Crouzon, syndrome d'Apert: Oxycephalies, scaphocephalies, turricephalies. Ann Chir Plast 12:273, 1967.
145. Tessier P: Dysostoses cranio-faciales (syndromes de Crouzon et d'Apert). Osteotomies totales de la face. *In* Transactions of the Fourth International Congress of Plastic and Reconstructive Surgery. Amsterdam, Excerpta Medica, 1969, p 774.
146. Tessier P: Relationship of craniostenoses to craniofacial dysostoses and to faciostenoses: A study with therapeutic implications. Plast Reconstr Surg 48:224, 1971.
147. Tessier P: The definitive plastic surgical treatment of the severe facial deformities of craniofacial dysostosis: Crouzon's and Apert's diseases. Plast Reconstr Surg 48:419, 1971.
148. Tessier P: Total osteotomy of the middle third of the face for faciostenosis or for sequelae of Le Fort III fractures. Plast Reconstr Surg 48:533, 1971.
149. Tessier P: Traitement des dysmorphies faciales propres aux dysostoses cranio-faciales (DCF). Maladies de Crouzon et d'Apert. Osteotomie totale du massif facial. Deplacement sagittal du massif facial. Neurochirurgie 17:295, 1971.
150. Tessier P: Recent improvement in the treatment of facial and cranial deformities in Crouzon's disease and Apert's syndrome. *In* Symposium on Plastic Surgery of the Orbital Region. St Louis, CV Mosby, 1976, p 271.
151. Tessier P: The craniofaciostenoses (CFS): The Crouzon and Apert diseases, the plagiocephalies. *In* Tessier P, Rougier J, Hervouet F, et al (eds): Plastic Surgery of the Orbit and Eyelids. New York, Masson, 1977, p 200.
152. Tessier PL: Apert's syndrome: Acrocephalosyndactyly type I. *In* Caronni EP (ed): Craniofacial Surgery. Boston, Little, Brown, 1985, p 280.
153. Tessier P, Hemmy D: Three dimensional imaging in medicine. A critique by surgeons. Scand J Plast Surg 20:3, 1986.
154. Thaller SR, Powers R, Daniller A: Three-dimensional imaging: A role in acute facial trauma? Med Rev 28:1, 1988.
155. Tressera L, Fuenmayor P: Early treatment of craniofacial deformities. J Maxillofac Surg 9:1, 1981.
156. van der Meulen JCH, Vaandrager JM: Surgery related to the correction of hypertelorism. Plast Reconstr Surg 71:6, 1983.
157. Vannier MW, Marsh JL, Knapp RH: Three-dimensional reconstruction from CT scans. Disorders of the head. Appl Radiol 16:114, 1987.
158. Virchow R: Uber den Cretinismus, nametlich in Franken und uber pathologische Schadelforamen. Ver Phys Med Cesselsch Wurzburg 2:230, 1881.
159. Vulliamy DG, Normandale PA: Cranio-facial dysostosis in a Dorset family. Arch Dis Child 41:375, 1966.
160. Waitzman A, Posnick JC, Armstrong D, Pron G: Normal values and growth trends in paediatric cranio-orbito-zygomatic measurements. Proceedings of the 47th Annual Meeting of the American Cleft Palate/Craniofacial Association, St. Louis, Missouri, May 1990, p 28.
161. Whitaker LA, Schut L, Kerr LP: Early surgery for isolated craniofacial dysostosis. Plast Reconstr Surg 60:575, 1977.
162. Whitaker LA, Bartlett SP, Schut L, Bruce D: Craniosynostosis: An analysis of the timing, treatment, and complications in 164 patients. Plast Reconstr Surg 80:195, 1987.
163. Witzel MA: Articulation before and after facial osteotomy. J Maxillofac Surg 8:195, 1980.
164. Witzel MA: Speech problems in craniofacial anomalies. Commun Disord 8:45, 1983.
165. Wolfort FG, Kanter MA, Miller LB: Torticollis. Plast Reconstr Surg 84(4):682, 1988.

53 CRANIOFACIAL DYSOSTOSIS: A SURGICAL APPROACH TO THE MIDFACE DEFORMITY

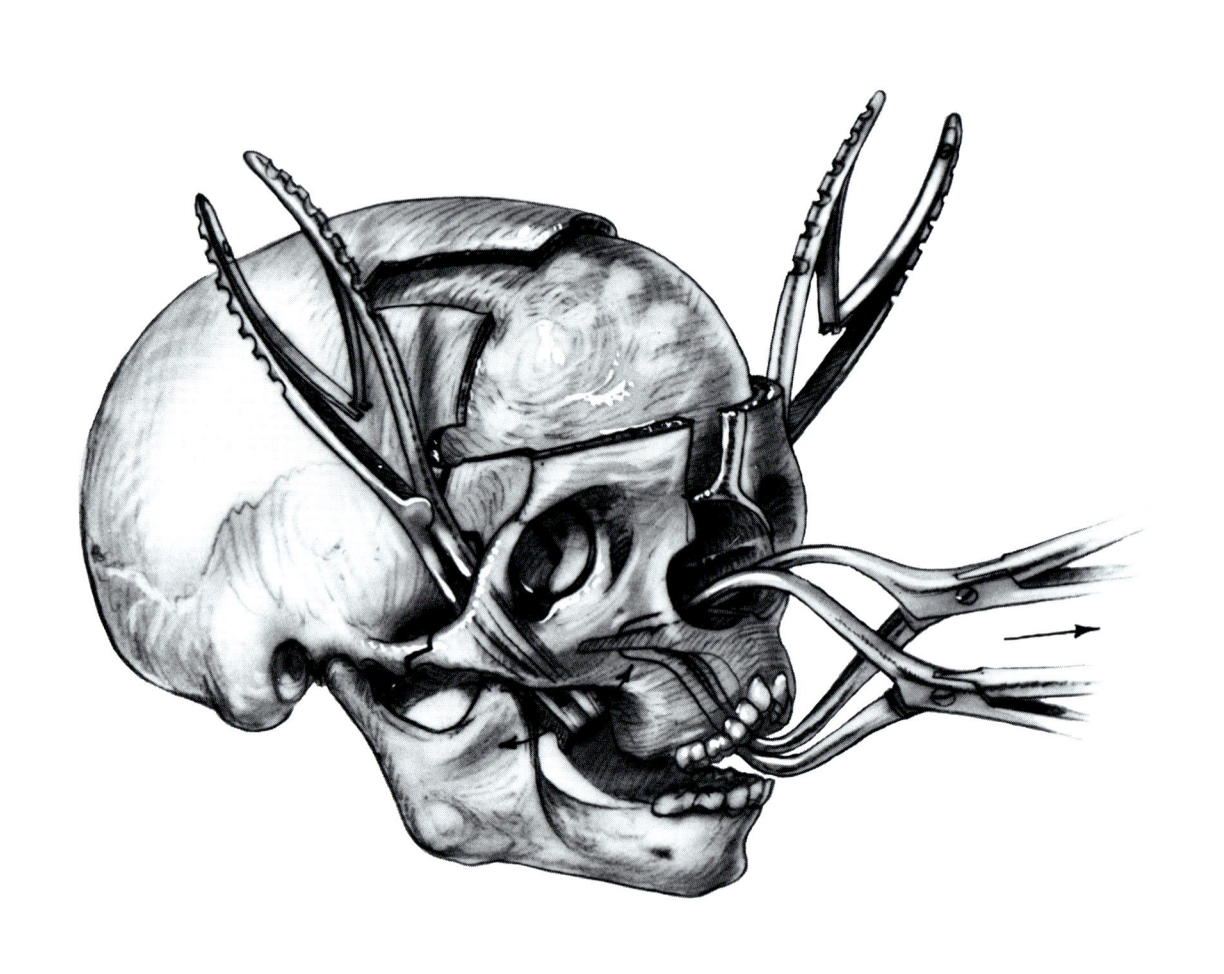

53

HISTORICAL PERSPECTIVE
   The Pioneers
   Bone Grafting and Fixation Techniques
   Craniofacial CT Scanning
   Airway Management

CROUZON SYNDROME
   Morbidity and Long-Term Reconstructive Results
   Current Staged Reconstructive Approach

APERT SYNDROME
   Morbidity and Long-term Reconstructive Results
   Current Staged Reconstructive Approach

SUMMARY

CASE REPORTS

JEFFREY C. POSNICK

HISTORICAL PERSPECTIVE

The Pioneers

The trench warfare of World War I resulted in thousands of combined soft and hard tissue facial injuries that required urgent treatment. During and after World War I and again during World War II, Dr. Varaztad Kazanjian[22] and Sir Herald Gillies[42] laid the foundation for what we now know as craniomaxillofacial surgery. After World War II, Sir Herald Gillies saw increasing numbers of patients with previously untreated congenital craniofacial malformations. He applied the knowledge he had gained in treating war injuries to their problems and in 1950 reported his experience with total midface osteotomy and advancement for Crouzon syndrome.[41] During the postoperative period, however, the patient's midface advancement relapsed to its preoperative position and the patient experienced a return of eye proptosis and Class III malocclusion.

The year 1967 marked the beginning of modern craniofacial surgery. After many years of work in the field, Dr. Paul Tessier described a new approach to the management of Crouzon syndrome and Apert syndrome.[151] To overcome the problems encountered by Gillies, Tessier developed a new basic surgical approach that included new osteotomy locations and the use of autogenous bone grafts. He also applied an external fixation device to maintain bony stability. The following year Dr. Joe Murray from Boston Children's Hospital published his experience with the Tessier midface advancement for Crouzon syndrome.[110] During this same period, Hans Luhr, a young maxillofacial surgeon who was still training in Hamburg, Germany, learned of the benefits of internal fixation (bone plates) for extremity fracture healing. In 1968, he constructed a miniature bone plate and screw system with eccentric holes for compression to use for mandibular fracture fixation.[78] However, despite Dr. Luhr's enthusiasm, his concepts of internal fixation for the craniofacial skeleton did not take hold.

Bone Grafting and Fixation Techniques

Various innovative craniofacial osteotomies were developed by Tessier, Ortiz-Monasterio, and others,[5,119,120,158–161,163,168] but many (e.g., monobloc osteotomy) lost favor because they were associated with major infections (including brain abscess, meningitis, and osteomyelitis).[56,155] It was not until Luhr's concepts of improved osteotomy and bone graft fixation in craniomaxillofacial surgery were further developed through the use of rigid fixation that the next giant leap in craniofacial surgery could occur.[31,53,107,131]

Today, with the use of plate and screw internal fixation techniques, several of the early osteotomies (e.g., monobloc and monobloc bipartition) have resurfaced. When well designed, executed, and stabilized, these osteotomies can often simultaneously solve the problems of diminished intracranial volume, deficient midface, obstructed nasal passages, and shallow, hyperteloric orbits. I have found that the combination of bone plate and screw fixation with autogenous cranial bone grafting reduces the associated morbidity rate to an acceptably low level. However, important questions arise. Should bone plates be used in the growing child? Will the placement of a bone plate inhibit or distort further bone growth? Since definitive answers are not yet available, children in whom bone plates have been used must be followed so that their growth and development can be monitored.

A further advance in craniofacial surgery has occurred with the widespread use of autogenous cranial bone grafts, which have now virtually replaced rib or hip grafts when bone replacement or augmentation is required in cranio-orbital surgery.[27,45,48,57–60,98,131,136,178] This transition can be understood by reviewing experimental studies that used cranial bone grafts.[28,69,106,126,127,130,146,166,175,179,180] From an embryologic point of view, bone is now believed to be either membranous or endochondral in origin.[102] Membranous bone results from the direct differentiation of mesenchymal cells, whereas endochondral bone results from the ossification of a cartilaginous strut. In general, the craniofacial skeleton is membranous in origin, whereas the rib cage and extremities are endochondral.

Peer[126] has shown that human membranous autogenous bone grafts placed in a subcutaneous pocket resorb less over time than do endochondral grafts. Similarly, in studies in New Zealand rabbits in which membranous and endochondral autogenous onlay bone grafts were placed subcutaneously and subperiosteally, Smith[146] found that the membranous grafts resorbed less. He demonstrated histologically that the microarchitecture of the membranous grafts was maintained over time. Working with both New Zealand rabbits and rhesus monkeys, Zins[180] also harvested and placed membranous and endochondral autogenous onlay bone grafts in a subperiosteal pocket but without any form of fixation. Over time he demonstrated less resorption of the membranous bone grafts. Wilkes[175] studied different variables relating to onlay bone grafts in immature and mature New Zealand rabbits, including the influence of periosteum left on the graft, autogenous grafts versus homografts, and membranous versus endochondral grafts. Overall he concluded that membranous grafts resorbed less and that the maintenance of periosteum on the graft was an unimportant variable. Kusiak[69] examined the variables influencing membranous versus endochondral autogenous onlay bone grafts in mature New Zealand rabbits. All of the grafts were placed subperiosteally but without fixation. He demonstrated that the membranous onlay grafts revascularized earlier and resorbed less over time.

Phillips[130] studied onlay autogenous bone grafts in mature sheep from a slightly different perspective. He examined the differences between membranous and endochondral onlay autogenous bone grafts and considered fixation technique to be an additional variable. He concluded that the stable fixation of grafts (lag-screw technique) results in less graft resorption. The nonfixed membranous grafts resorbed less than nonfixed endochondral grafts, but the differences in graft resorption patterns were much less when a stable form of fixation (e.g., lag-screw technique) was used.

My review of these experimental studies indicates that all onlay bone grafts tend to resorb, but resorption occurs to a lesser degree when grafts are stably (i.e., rigidly) fixed, that membranous bone resorbs less in most circumstances than endochondral bone, and that bone graft resorption patterns may vary according to the region grafted. This experimental work coupled with clinical studies has resulted in almost universal use of autogenous cranial bone grafts as a first choice when either onlay or interpositional grafts are required in the cranial vault, orbit, zygoma, or nasal regions.[154]

Craniofacial CT Scanning

Current techniques in craniofacial surgery demand both subjective (qualitative) and objective (quantitative) assessment. Various methods have been used in the past to indirectly analyze the craniofacial region. The morphology, patterns of growth and development, and normative standards involving the craniofacial skeleton have been studied extensively. Cephalometric radiography has traditionally been used for these purposes. Large collections of normative data have been compiled, allowing clinicians to monitor the individual patient's development.

Other methods of quantitative craniofacial analysis have been used to a much more limited extent. Examples of these are anthropometry and multiplane and finite element scaling analysis. Each of these techniques is limited in its ability to develop accurate normative standards for the craniofacial complex, as well as for overall qualitative analysis.

Computed tomography (CT) has now been established as an important modality in the diagnosis, surgical planning, and longitudinal study of craniofacial anomalies. CT is not subject to most of the limitations of either anthropometric or cephalometric analysis. Anthropometry can be influenced to a great extent by the overlying soft tissue, which prevents the clinician from obtaining reliable information about the underlying bone. In the case of cephalometric radiography, enlargement or distortion of the image can occur. The number of anatomic landmarks that can be accurately identified is also limited, and the overlap of structures on the radiographs makes the location of these landmarks difficult. Often landmarks that have been selected as standard points of reference are not true biologic loci and may be of limited use to the clinician. The normative data available are generally derived from lateral projections only. These are strictly two-dimensional and consequently greatly oversimplify the craniofacial form.

With the CT scan, there is no significant enlargement or distortion of the image, structural overlap, or tracing error, and the number of anatomic landmarks is vast. Moreover, three-dimensional representation is possible, which is particularly useful in surgical reconstruction of the upper facial skeleton where standard cephalometric films are of limited use.

At this institution, The Hospital for Sick Children in Toronto, Ontario (HSC), a retrospective study was recently undertaken to define normal values for a series of craniofacial measurements and to evaluate the growth patterns of the craniofacial complex through axial CT. Fourteen measurements were taken from the CT scans of 453 skeletally normal subjects. These variables were then divided into age categories of 1 year each, from ages 1 to 17 years, and into four age groups for those under 1 year of age.[171] The normal range and growth pattern of measurement values for the cranial vault, orbital region, and upper midface were established.

Knowledge of these differential growth patterns and normal measurement values in the craniofacial region will help craniofacial surgeons to make accurate diagnoses, perform reconstructive surgery more precisely, and follow up patients more effectively. With the combination of two- and three-dimensional CT scans of the craniofacial skeleton, we can now gain qualitative impressions as well as make quantitative measurements to assist in surgical reconstruction.

Airway Management

A close working relationship between the skilled and dedicated anesthetist and the craniofacial surgeon has virtually eliminated the need for tracheostomy as a means of perioperative airway management for craniomaxillofacial procedures. For routine cranio-orbital surgery in infancy, childhood, and adolescence, orotracheal intubation is preferred. For routine maxillofacial osteotomy, nasotracheal intubation is a safe and effective means of perioperative airway management. For airway protection during a total midface osteotomy (Le Fort III, monobloc, monobloc bipartition) carried out through an intracranial approach, my preference is to begin surgery with orotracheal intubation, once all osteotomies are complete and the midface complex is disimpacted, then convert to nasotracheal intubation, which allows direct establishment of the occlusion and preferred orbital positioning. The nasotracheal tube remains in place for several days postoperatively. This allows time for the bony passage created by the midface advancement at the level of the anterior cranial vault and nasal cavity to stabilize. Another way of managing the problem of airway control without tracheostomy is to construct a specially designed splint: An orotracheal intubation is completed and the tube is stabilized at the anterior mandibular incisor region with a circomandibular wire. The specially constructed prefabricated acrylic splint has an increased freeway space. This allows a gap anteriorly through which the orotracheal tube can be positioned. With this technique the osteotomies are completed, the occlusion is made ideal, and the osteotomies are stabilized without the need to change the intubation.

CROUZON SYNDROME

The incidence of Crouzon syndrome is 1 in 25,000 in the general population.[4,21] The inheritance pattern is autosomal dominant, and the trait is noted for its variable expression.[16,25,170]

Crouzon described an affected family pedigree in 1912.[26] He listed four major characteristics of their disease: exorbitism, retromaxillism, inframaxillism, and paradoxic retrogenia. Premature fusion of multiple cranial vault sutures may occur at the level of the cranial vault, with bilateral coronal premature fusion being the most common and resulting in a brachycephalic appearance.[19,30,55,66–68,115,138,144] Other forms of premature suture stenosis (i.e., sagittal, lambdoid, or metopic) may also occur in Crouzon syndrome. In addition to cranial vault suture synostosis, there is a poorly defined effect on the anterior cranial base, facial sutures, and facial growth centers which results in a variable degree of symmetric hypoplasia of the orbits, zygomas, and maxilla.[11,12,15,18,34–36,39,40,54,65–67,94,104,105,117,128,129,133,135,139,142,143,150] Usually the mandible grows normally but often with increased vertical height to the chin.[10,24] In general, the soft tissue envelope is normal both quantitatively and qualitatively, except that there may be a variable degree of upper eyelid ptosis and inferiorly positioned lateral canthi (antimongoloid slant).[64] In the typical full-blown case, the cranial vault is either brachycephalic or oxycephalic, the orbits are shallow with bulging eyes, and the midface is flat with a Class III malocclusion. The nasal airway is diminished with partial obstruction and a mouth-breathing habit.

Morbidity and Long-Term Reconstructive Results

Seventy-four patients with Crouzon syndrome who had undergone reconstructive surgery at HSC between 1972 and 1986 were studied retrospectively.[112,113] Details of their surgical procedures, complications associated with each, surgical variables (i.e., length of operation, percentage of blood volume transfused, bone graft donor sites, type of fixation, age at operation, perioperative airway management, number of previous craniotomies, and whether or not the intracranial procedure required osteotomy through the cranial bone), skeletal results, and additional procedures required for the completion of the skeletal reconstruction were reviewed. Patients who were under 6 years old at the time of the study and those whose medical, photographic, and orthodontic records were not complete were excluded. It was thought that children under age 6 years and those with incomplete data could not be adequately judged in terms of residual deformities requiring reconstruction. This left a final study group of 40 patients (21 patients under age 6 years and 13 for whom the data were incomplete).

Analysis of the data revealed many similarities between the Crouzon group and another group of 37 patients with Apert syndrome who were also reviewed.[111,114] The Crouzon deformity required a staged reconstruction consisting of three to four major craniomaxillofacial procedures. These usually included cranial vault reconstruction (cranial vault and supraorbital ridge osteotomy with reshaping and advancement) in infancy. Frequently further revision cranio-orbital reshaping was required in early childhood to expand the intracranial volume and relieve intracranial pressure and papilledema. A total midface osteotomy and advancement (Le Fort III osteotomy) was commonly used in this study group in childhood, and then maxillary repositioning (Le Fort I osteotomy) was often combined with a genioplasty in the teenage years. However, patients with the Crouzon deformity required total midface advancement less frequently than those with Apert syndrome.

In both groups, major complications were a significant factor only in those procedures that involved total midface advancement (Le Fort III). Risk factors for the Crouzon group seemed to be the number of previous craniotomies carried out, the number of additional bone graft donor sites harvested (i.e., rib and hip), and the use of wire rather than plate and screw fixation. The major complication rate for the Le Fort III procedure was 37 per cent in the Crouzon group.

During the years studied, the surgical techniques used were somewhat different from those I would recommend today. For example, perioperative airway management usually depended on a tracheostomy, osteotomy fixation was achieved with direct wires rather than bone plates and screws, the autogenous bone grafts used were generally taken from the hip or rib rather than the cranial bone, and the most common midface procedure selected was the Le Fort III rather than a monobloc osteotomy.

The study indicated that the Crouzon deformity requires a staged reconstruction but that the midface involvement is often less severe than that seen in patients with Apert syndrome.

Current Staged Reconstructive Approach

My current approach to the surgical treatment of Crouzon syndrome is based on both the retrospective study discussed above and personal clinical experience.

Primary Cranio-orbital Surgery in Infants

Primary cranio-orbital surgery in infants is geared toward re-establishing a more normal intracranial volume and morphology, attempting to limit the potential effects of increased intracranial pressure from a rapidly growing brain within a confined skull box.[1,2,6,7,10,14,32,33,49-51,61,70,71,75,76,80-88,93,95,96,100,101,116,129,134,137,140,141,145,149,167,172,174] In the typical brachycephalic skull resulting from bicoronal synostosis, signs of increased intracranial pressure (i.e., papilledema) rarely occur before 6 months to 1 year of age. I prefer to postpone first-stage reconstruction until the patient is close to 1 year of age, if possible. It is my impression that when surgery is carried out very early in infancy (less than 6 months of age) the need for repeat cranial vault reshaping later in childhood is increased.

The surgical procedures required are performed through a coronal incision, which allows access and exposure for the bifrontal craniotomy, orbital osteotomies, and reconstruction. I routinely extend the orbital osteotomies down to the level of the mid-infraorbital rims. The orbital osteotomies with their tenon extensions are removed as free bone grafts. The units are totally reshaped to gain the configuration and morphology appropriate for the child's age and then repositioned with advancement at the level of the anterior cranial base, usually with decreased bitemporal width. The infraorbital rim osteotomy junction serves as the pivot point for the orbital advancement and is stabilized with a direct transosseous wire on each side (i.e., infraorbital rim to stable maxilla). The tenon extensions are fixed to the stable temporal bone with either a direct transosseous wire or a micro bone plate and screws. When the orbital osteotomies are completed as I have described, continuity of the supraorbital and lateral orbital rim is maintained down to and including the lateral aspect of the infraorbital rims. In this way, disruption of the frontozygomatic suture and a resulting step-off at the lateral orbital rim are prevented. When revision orbital osteotomies are carried out later as part of the staged reconstruction, they are easily accomplished without concern about fibrous or malunion of the orbital rims being a limiting factor. Sections of cranial vault bone are selected to reconstruct the new forehead for a more normal shape and configuration but also for a resulting overall increased anterior cranial vault volume.[132] I do not use the Marchac floating forehead technique[84,88] during the procedure because I believe that the incidence of significant bitemporal hollowing or depression is very high, as is the occurrence of a superior forehead depression or bulge in the region where a large bony defect would be left behind.

Repeat Craniotomy in Young Children

Repeat craniotomy with cranial vault and orbital osteotomies, reshaping, and further advancement is sometimes required later in infancy or early childhood for the management of increased intracranial pressure secondary to inadequate intracranial volume. Despite primary suture release and reshaping in infancy, a percentage of children develop signs and symptoms of increased intracranial pressure, including vomiting, headaches, lethargy, papilledema, and, if they are left untreated, optic and brain atrophy. To protect further brain development and vision, revision craniotomy with cranial vault and orbital reshaping geared toward the further expansion of the intracranial volume must be carried out.[132] Thorough preoperative planning is necessary and must include complete craniofacial CT scanning with three-dimensional reformation followed by discussion with the neuroradiologist, ophthalmologist, neurosurgeon, craniofacial surgeon, and family. Special intraoperative problems encountered with repeat craniotomies and reshaping include increased blood loss, an increased number of dural tears, and a generally fragmented and brittle cranial vault. Not uncommonly, a ventriculoperitoneal shunt may have been placed previously for the management of hydrocephalus[38,43,52] and must be carefully protected. Stable fixation with micro bone plates and screws, although used sparingly, can make the difference between success and failure in these repeat reshaping procedures. I use bone plates and screws very cautiously in the infant skull because they may increase growth distortion. Furthermore, if additional repeat craniotomy is required later, osteotomies may be difficult because of metal hardware scattered throughout the cranial vault.

Total Midface Deficiency and Surgical Management

As documented from the HSC retrospective institutional study of patients with Crouzon syndrome, some form of total midface osteotomy with advancement is required in 75 per cent of cases. In general, osteotomy alternatives for the total midface include the Le Fort III osteotomy, monobloc osteotomy, or monobloc bipartition osteotomy.[5,62,76,77,79,83,97,107,110,118,122,151,153,156-159,162,168] The decision whether to use a monobloc or a Le Fort III osteotomy for management of the horizontal midface deficiency depends on the current position of the supraorbital ridge. If the supraorbital ridge with its overlying eyebrows sits in a good position when viewed from the sagittal plane, with adequate depth to the anterior cranial base, then there is no need to reposition this region. In this case, the total midface deficiency is usually managed by a Le Fort III osteotomy. On the other hand, if the supraorbital ridge and anterior cranial base are deficient in the sagittal plane along with the zygomas, nose, lower orbits, and maxilla, then a monobloc osteotomy with differential anterior repositioning may be indicated. If some degree of orbital hypertelorism is also present, the monobloc is split vertically in the midline (monobloc bipartition), a wedge of intraorbital bone is removed, and the orbits are repositioned more immediately while the arch width of the maxilla is increased.

In the past, the Le Fort III osteotomy was used too frequently to overcome total midface deficiency in patients with craniofacial dysostosis. As a result, many patients had unesthetic step-offs in the lateral orbital rim that are difficult to modify later. Excessive lengthening of the nose with flattening of the nasofrontal angle may also occur if a Le Fort III osteotomy is incorrectly selected. With the Le Fort III it is difficult to judge the ideal intraorbital rim advancement, and therefore problems arise from either residual proptosis from undercorrection or enophthalmos from overcorrection. In addition, simultaneous correction of orbital hypertelorism is not possible.

My preference is to manage the total midface deficiency between age 5 and 7 years. By this stage the cranial vault and orbits are approximately 85 to 90 per cent of their adult size,[171] and any reconstructive surgery performed in these regions is more or less permanent once healing has occurred. Psychosocial considerations weigh heavily in selecting the timing of midface advancement after 5 years of age.[9,73,74,123] Occasionally the presence of peripheral sleep apnea is a consideration.[44,72,90] The total midface surgery is carried out solely through a coronal incision without the need for lower eyelid or intraoral incisions. Airway management is achieved through endotracheal intubation without tracheostomy. Autogenous cranial bone grafts are used exclusively, and there is no need for either rib or hip grafts. Fixation is accomplished with a combination of miniplates and microplates without the use of direct wires.

Class III Malocclusion and Surgical Management

The mandible, which has normal growth potential,[10,24] continues to develop throughout childhood and adolescence, but the upper jaw at the Le Fort I level does not keep up, and as a result, a Class III malocclusion usually results.[65,76,86,97,112,113] This residual dentofacial deformity is managed in a routine fashion with a Le Fort I osteotomy (horizontal advancement and vertical lengthening), often combined with a genioplasty (vertical reduction and advancement). Planning for this procedure is done in conjunction with major orthodontic intervention. Stabilization is achieved with bone miniplates and screws and autogenous bone grafts, thereby limiting the importance of intermaxillary fixation.[31,53]

APERT SYNDROME

Most cases of Apert syndrome have occurred sporadically.[20,21,124] Documented pedigrees of dominant transmission with complete penetrance have been reported. However, the numbers of adults with Apert syndrome who have been followed in the past have not been sufficient to ascertain a genetic pattern. Advanced paternal age is thought to be a factor in producing new mutants. This syndrome has been observed in Caucasian, black, and Oriental populations. The incidence of occurrence is thought to be 1 in 100,000 in the general population.[13] Postmortem studies suggest that skeletal deficiencies of the face result from a reduced growth potential of the cranial base, leading to premature fusion of the midline suture from the occiput to the anterior nasal septum.[121,147,148] Some studies suggest that the sphenoid bone may be a factor in this facial deformity, with synostosis of the sphenoid bone to the adjacent vomer.[63]

Apert[8] first described the syndrome as a combination of multiple physical findings, including severe cranial vault deformity, syndactylism, and mental retardation, often associated with blindness. We now know that the craniofacial skeletal abnormality of Apert syndrome is complex and includes bilateral premature coronal suture fusion and fusion of the anterior cranial base and midface suture(s) or growth centers.[11,104,105,139] In addition, the syndrome is characterized by four-limb symmetric complex syndactylies of the hands and feet.[21] Fusion of other joints, including the elbows and shoulders, often occurs. Although the syndrome has the same general craniofacial bony morphology as Crouzon syndrome, expressivity of the trait in Apert syndrome is more consistent and severe, with little variation.[17,138] Shallow orbits (exorbitism) and bulging eyes (exophthalmos) are more severe and a moderate orbital hypertelorism is generally present. Hydrocephalus requiring ventriculoperitoneal shunting is also seen in Apert syndrome.[38,43,52] Apert syndrome is more frequently associated with a degree of developmental delay than is Crouzon syndrome, but the reasons for this remain unclear.[125] Midface hypoplasia is more marked both vertically and horizontally. The incidence of cleft palate approximates 30 per cent, and the uvula is excessively long. The anterior open-bite deformity is usually more severe than in Crouzon syndrome and causes sibilant distortions in speech.[176,177] Apert syndrome is characterized by a marked acne vulgaris, often with extensions to the forearms. The facial skin (especially in the nasal region) is often thick, with increased sebaceous discharge. The soft tissue drape also varies from that of Crouzon syndrome, with a greater downward slant to the lateral canthi and a distinctive upper eyelid ptosis.[37] A conductive hearing loss may be present and is characterized by a 30 to 40 per cent incidence of congenital fixation of the middle ear structures and a high incidence of poorly treated otitis media.[3,23]

Morbidity and Long-Term Reconstructive Results

A retrospective institutional review was carried out to evaluate the long-term reconstructive results and morbidity of craniofacial surgery in 65 children with Apert syndrome deformity who underwent treatment by the craniofacial team at HSC from 1974 to 1986 inclusive.[111,114] Patients with an incomplete data base and those under the age of 6 years were excluded because their reconstructive outcomes and residual deformities could not be judged. Only 37 of the total 65 patients were therefore included in the study group (19 patients under age 6 and 9 with incomplete data).

Data were collected from medical records, serial full-face photographs, and orthodontic records. Details of surgical procedures, complications associated with each surgical variable (i.e., length of operation, per cent blood volume transfused, number of previous craniotomies, bone graft donor sites, type of fixation, age at operation, perioperative airway management, and simultaneous cranial bone osteotomy), skeletal results, and additional procedures required for the completion of the skeletal reconstruction were reviewed.

The procedures carried out in the study group fell into one of four major categories: simple craniotomy, anterior cranial vault and supraorbital ridge osteotomy with reshaping, Le Fort III osteotomy and advancement, and Le Fort I osteotomies and genioplasty.

Within the study group the Le Fort III osteotomy was preferred for total midface surgery, and stabilization was most commonly achieved with a combination of autogenous bone graft (rib or hip) and direct transosseous wiring. A tracheostomy was performed in all cases for perioperative airway management and in many cases a coronal incision was combined with lower eyelid incisions as part of the surgical technique.

Of the 37 patients in the study group, only 34 were available and required a final reconstructive assessment. There were three perioperative deaths and eight other major complications in this group.

Overall, 94 per cent of the patients underwent or required at least one cranial vault procedure in infancy, a total midface advancement, and a Le Fort I osteotomy in adolescence to complete their skeletal reconstruction. Only two patients did not follow this sequence.

The initial cranial vault procedure carried out in infancy was either a strip craniectomy or a more formal cranial vault and supraorbital ridge osteotomy with reshaping and advancement. When a strip craniectomy was the first procedure carried out, a second cranio-orbital revision in infancy was frequently required. These procedures generally had a low perioperative complication rate.

The Le Fort III osteotomy procedure had a major complication rate of 42 per cent. It was our impression that a satisfactory esthetic reconstruction was rare when bony infection occurred after a Le Fort III osteotomy. Of the operative variables reviewed, several risk factors were identified which were thought to be associated with major morbidity. They included the number of previous craniotomies, the use of a tracheostomy for perioperative airway management, the use of multiple distant bone graft donor sources, and the combined intracranial-extracranial approach with simultaneous sectioning of the cranial base. The Le Fort I osteotomy was associated with only minor complications.

This retrospective review documents the need for a staged reconstruction to correct the Apert deformity. Generally one or two cranial vault and supraorbital ridge decompressions/reconstructions was required in infancy. A total midface osteotomy with advancement was carried out later in childhood followed by more routine orthognathic surgery (Le Fort I and genioplasty) performed in conjunction with major orthodontic treatment, which was undertaken when skeletal maturation was reached.

As in the retrospective study on patients with Crouzon syndrome, the surgical techniques used in patients with Apert syndrome differed from those I recommend today. For example, the method of airway management for total midface procedures, and in some cases for cranio-orbital surgery, was a tracheostomy. Today this is no longer required, and perioperative airway management is done with orotracheal or nasotracheal intubation. The method of fixation was direct transosseous wires and step-cut osteotomies. Now, miniplate and microplate fixation is preferred. The use of autogenous cranial bone grafts has greatly reduced the need to harvest rib or hip grafts. Total midface deficiency in Apert syndrome is usually managed with a monobloc bipartition osteotomy rather than the Le Fort III osteotomy. Lower eyelid incisions are not required, since the coronal incision alone gives adequate exposure for all midface osteotomies above the Le Fort I level.

Current Staged Reconstructive Approach

My current approach to the staging of reconstruction for Apert syndrome is similar to that described for Crouzon syndrome. This is based on both the retrospective study discussed above and personal clinical experience.

Primary Cranio-orbital Procedure in Infancy

The primary procedure carried out in infancy is a combination of anterior cranial vault and three-quarter orbital osteotomies with reshaping and advancement carried out between 6 months and 1 year of age. The main goal of the procedure is to increase intracranial volume[132] and decrease the incidence of intracranial hypertension resulting from a normally growing brain within a confined skull box. The orbital depth is also increased, which tends to improve but not correct the proptosis (see "Current Staged Reconstruction Approach" for Crouzon syndrome).

Repeat Craniotomy in Young Children

Repeat craniotomy and further cranial vault and orbital osteotomies with reshaping and advancement are frequently necessary later in infancy or early childhood. This second procedure is carried out if signs of increased intracranial pressure develop that are not secondary to hydrocephalus. Regular monitoring for hydrocephalus is needed and whenever it occurs, treatment with ventriculoperitoneal shunting must be instituted (see "Current Staged Reconstructive Approach" for Crouzon syndrome).[38,43,52]

Total Midface Deficiency and Surgical Management

If possible, a second cranial vault procedure is delayed until the patient reaches age 5 to 7 years. At this point, it can be carried out in conjunction with the monobloc or monobloc bipartition osteotomy. A Le Fort III osteotomy is rarely sufficient to manage the total midface deficiency, since the supraorbital ridge and anterior cranial base are generally posteriorly positioned and require repositioning as well. Usually the degree of hypertelorism is severe enough that bipartition of the monobloc osteotomy is needed to reduce the intraorbital distance and at the same time increase the maxillary arch width. This total midface procedure carried out in childhood not only relieves the eyeball proptosis and concave profile but further improves both the nasal air flow and the Class III malocclusion. It does not totally correct the anterior open bite deformity, which will await orthognathic surgery in adolescence (see "Current Staged Reconstructive Approach" for Crouzon syndrome).

Class III Malocclusion and Surgical Management

The mandible, which has normal growth potential,[10,24] continues to develop throughout childhood and adolescence, but the upper jaw at the Le Fort I level does not keep up; as a result, a Class III malocclusion with an anterior open bite results. A maxillary Le Fort I osteotomy (horizontal advancement and vertical lengthening) is required in combination with a genioplasty (vertical reduction and horizontal advancement) to further correct the lower face deformity. This is carried out in conjunction with major orthodontic intervention planned for completion at skeletal maturation (age 14 to 16 years in females and 16 to 18 years in males). Stabilization is achieved with bone miniplates and screws and autogenous bone graft, thereby limiting the importance of intermaxillary fixation.[31,53]

SUMMARY

The treatment of craniofacial dysostosis, of which Crouzon syndrome and Apert syndrome are the most common forms, requires a concerted team effort.[91,92,99,108,109,173] The team evaluation begins shortly after birth and follows the patient through infancy, childhood, adolescence, and early adulthood. The importance of particular team members in the patient's analysis and treatment varies during different growth phases. For example, in infancy and early childhood, constant combined reassessment by the pediatrician, neurosurgeon, ophthalmologist, neuroradiologist, and craniofacial surgeon, along with the psychosocial team, is essential. Later, in adolescence and early adulthood, the ophthalmologist, neuroradiologist, and neurosurgeon become less important and the orthodontist, speech pathologist, maxillofacial surgeon, and psychosocial team play a much more dominant role.

Major craniofacial centers should develop protocols for patient management and then proceed with a prospective data base collection. Meeting this objective allows us to learn from the past and move ahead.

The modern era of craniofacial surgery began with Tessier in 1967.[151] During the past decade, craniomaxillofacial surgery has advanced in a number of major ways. The first advance is the use of autogenous bone grafting for onlay or interpositional use. Cranial bone has supplanted the need to harvest rib or hip grafts for use in the upper face regions. The second is the refinement of stable bone-fixation techniques. In the past, stainless steel wires were combined with step-cut osteotomies, often leaving gross mobility to the osteotomy units and resulting in a relatively high rate of relapse and infection when total midface osteotomies were performed. The modern use of plate and screw internal fixation has greatly freed the surgeon's approach in craniofacial skeletal reconstruction. In general, compression plates are not required or preferred. Advances in the design and technology have improved so that miniplates or microplates, when they are selected, are not visible through the skin and do not jeopardize the results of the reconstruction. The concern about infection and relapse, while ever present, has diminished. The need for intermaxillary fixation has also been reduced. The third advance is the reintroduction of creative osteotomies such as the monobloc and monobloc bipartition, especially when they are combined with plate and screw fixation and cranial bone grafting for management of the midface deformity. The fourth is the development of CT scanning techniques applied to the craniofacial skeleton. Three-dimensional reformations of axial-sliced CT scans give an improved global (qualitative) view of the bony deformity. More recently, quantitative measurements have been made which influence the timing of surgery (i.e., intracranial volume measurements) and the directional moves carried out (i.e., normalization of orbital depth and separation).[46,47,89,164,165,169,171] Finally, the use of innovative endotracheal tube management by dedicated craniofacial anesthetists has virtually eliminated the need for tracheostomy in perioperative airway management. These refinements have led to truly successful functional and esthetic results.

The recognition of the need for a staged surgical approach in the correction of deformities caused by Apert and Crouzon syndromes has led to a clearer understanding of reconstructive goals. Surgeons can now take advantage of differential craniofacial skeletal growth rates, as they do for cleft lip and palate patients. We must continue to define our reasons for intervention at different time intervals: for example, cranial vault surgery in infancy (i.e., to relieve increased intracranial pressure and papilledema), total midface advancement in childhood (to increase intracranial and intraorbital volume and improve nasal airflow, occlusion, and body image), nasal or cheekbone augmentation later in the growth phase (to restore esthetics), and orthognathic surgery in adolescence (to improve occlusion, speech, and esthetics). By selecting the best time for intervention, we may maximize long-term functional and esthetic improvements.

1908 / VI—FUNCTIONAL RESTORATION OF OCCLUSION

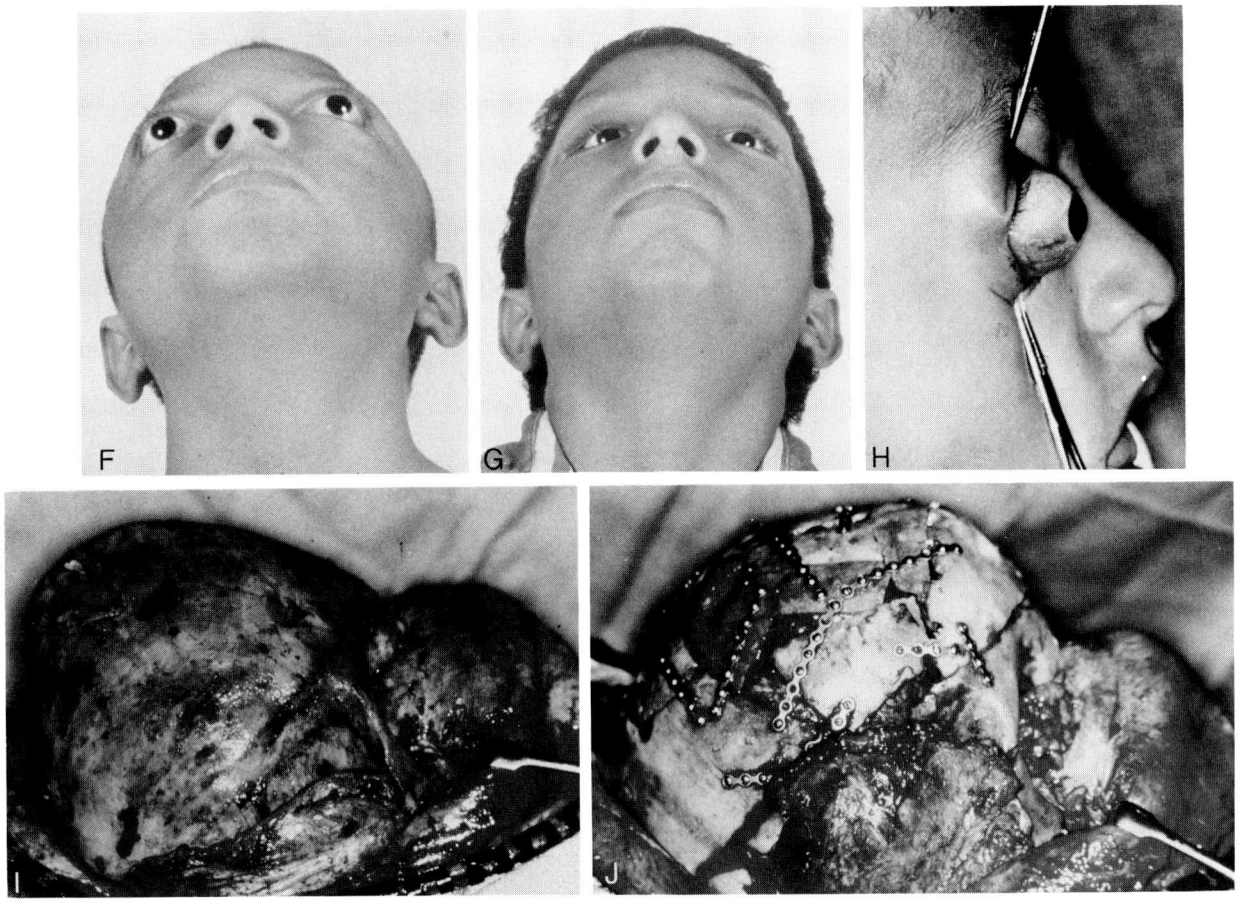

FIGURE 53-3 *Continued.* *F*, Preoperative worm's eye view. *G*, Postoperative worm's eye view. *H*, Extent of preoperative eyeball proptosis demonstrated with hemostats touching orbital rims (positive Tessier sign). *I*, Intraoperative lateral view of cranial vault and orbits through coronal incision before osteotomies. *J*, Same view after osteotomies, cranial bone grafting, and titanium bone plate and screw fixation.

CT scan radiographic examination revealed the oxycephalic appearance of the cranial vault and fingerprinting along the inner table of the skull and cranial base. The ventricles were of normal size. The orbits were shallow and the midface was deficient.

The patient's clinical impression was characteristic of Crouzon syndrome with bicoronal synostosis and total midface deficiency that was greater at the supraorbital ridge level than at the occlusal level.

Surgical Approach

The airway was managed initially with orotracheal intubation, but after the monobloc osteotomy was completed this was converted to nasotracheal intubation so that the correct occlusal relationship could be obtained. Temporary tarsorrhaphies were completed to prevent corneal abrasions during surgery. The surgical procedure was undertaken through a coronal incision only; no lower eyelid incisions were needed. The bifrontal craniotomy was completed first, followed by a monobloc osteotomy. Then the posterior cranial vault bone was removed through further craniotomy. The monobloc unit was brought forward 18 mm at the level of the supraorbital ridge and 2 mm at the maxillary incisor edge. The jaws were wired together. Stabilization was then achieved at the supraorbital ridge level of the monobloc, with bone miniplates placed back to the stable temporal bone region bilaterally. Titanium miniplates were also placed across the zygomatic arches extending from the anterior maxilla back to the squamous portion of the temporal bone on each side. A section of the cranial vault was selected for the new forehead and stabilized with multiple miniplates and screws. The residual cranial vault bone was sectioned and pieced together working from anterior to posterior until the total cranial vault was reconstructed. Fixation of each unit was with multiple miniplates and screws. Lateral canthopexies were completed as described in Case 2. The coronal incision was closed in layers. The intermaxillary fixation was released, and the temporary tarsorrhaphies were removed.

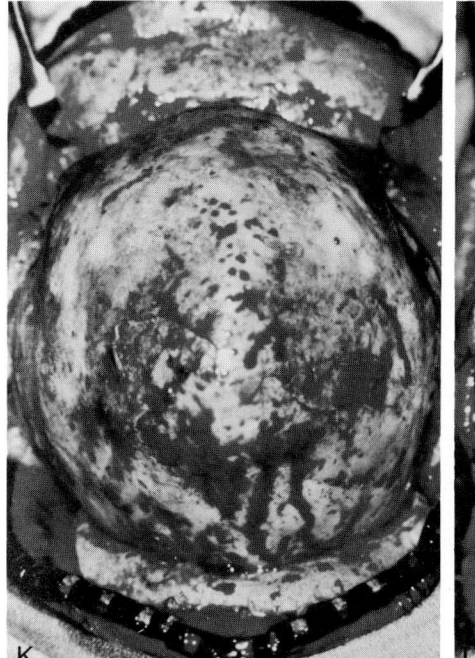

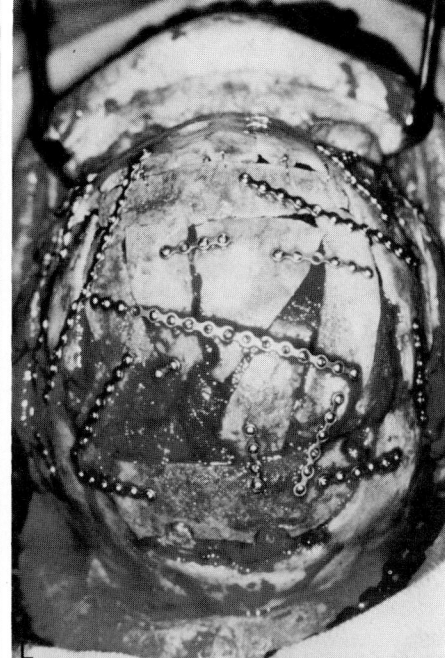

FIGURE 53-3 *Continued. K,* Intraoperative bird's eye view of cranial vault through coronal incision before osteotomies. *L,* Same view after cranial vault reshaping with cranial bone grafting and titanium bone plate and screw fixation. *M,* Three-dimensional CT scan reformations. Lateral views before and after reconstruction. (From Posnick JC, Nakano P: Craniofacial dysostosis: Staging of reconstruction and management of the midface deformity. Neurosurg Clin North Am 2(3):683–702, 1991.)

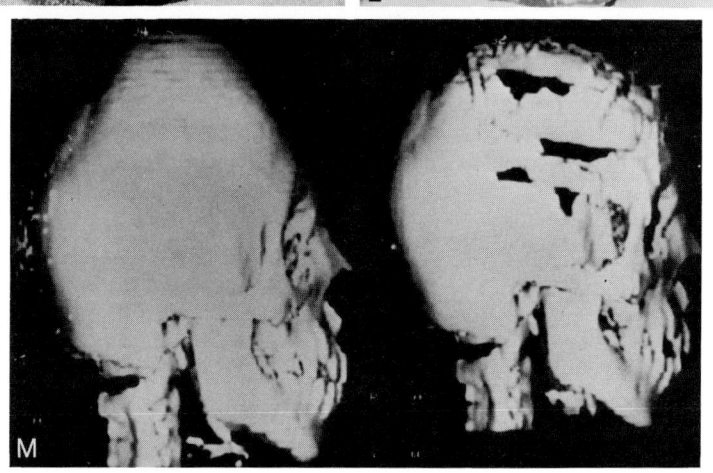

POSTOPERATIVE COURSE

The patient remained electively intubated for 3 days in the intensive care unit. This allowed time for the bony passage created by the midface advancement at the level of the anterior cranial vault and nasal cavity to stabilize. Intravenous antibiotics consisting of penicillin and cloxacillin, which were initiated just before surgery, were discontinued on the tenth postoperative day and the patient was discharged from hospital. After an additional 6-week stay in the Toronto area, he returned to his home town in Nicaragua.

CASE 4 (FIG. 53-4)

Diagnosis: Crouzon syndrome
Previous surgery: Suture release and forehead reshaping at 3 months
  Redo cranial vault reshaping at 9 months
  Le Fort III osteotomy and cranial vault reshaping at 2 years
Procedure: Cranial vault, monobloc, Le Fort I, and genioplasty osteotomies with reshaping and advancement

A 14-year-old girl who was born with Crouzon syndrome underwent bicoronal suture release and cranial vault reshaping at 3 months of age. Additional craniectomy and

1910 / VI—FUNCTIONAL RESTORATION OF OCCLUSION

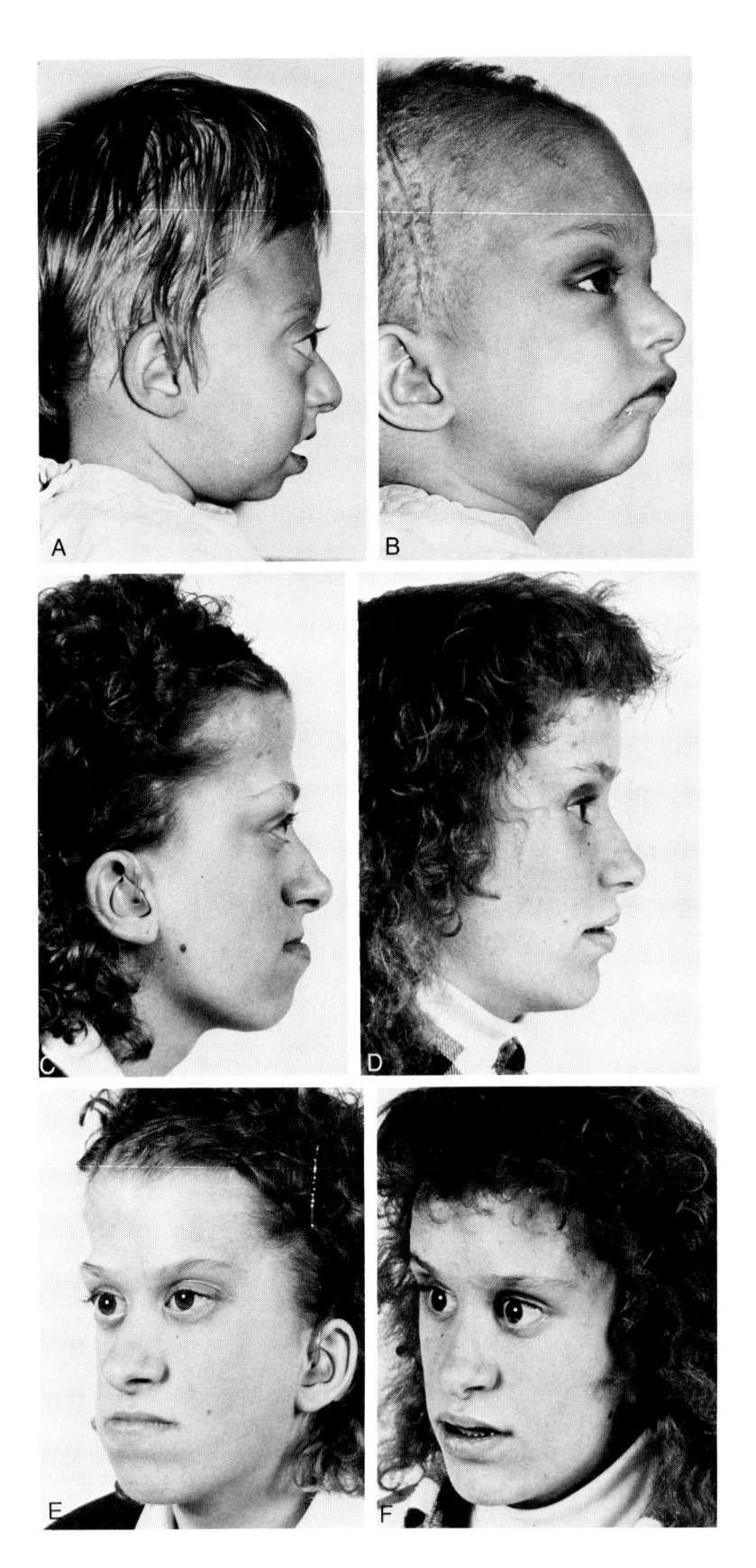

FIGURE 53-4. A 14-YEAR-OLD GIRL BORN WITH CROUZON SYNDROME. SHE UNDERWENT BICORONAL SUTURE RELEASE AND CRANIAL VAULT RESHAPING AT 3 MONTHS OF AGE. ADDITIONAL CRANIECTOMY AND CRANIAL VAULT RESHAPING WERE COMPLETED WHEN SHE WAS 9 MONTHS OLD. AT 2 YEARS OF AGE, SHE UNDERWENT A LE FORT III TOTAL MIDFACE ADVANCEMENT COMBINED WITH CRANIAL VAULT RESHAPING THROUGH AN INTRACRANIAL APPROACH. SHE PRESENTS NOW FOR REPEAT MIDFACE OSTEOTOMY TO INCLUDE SIMULTANEOUS CRANIAL VAULT, MONOBLOC, LE FORT I, AND CHIN OSTEOTOMIES WITH RESHAPING AND THREE-DIMENSIONAL REPOSITIONING. *A*, Profile view at 1 year of age after two intracranial cranial vault and orbital procedures. *B*, Profile view at 2 years of age shown early after additional cranial vault and Le Fort III osteotomies with advancement. *C*, Profile view at 14 years of age demonstrating residual cranial vault, orbital, and midface deformities. *D*, Profile view at 1 year after combined cranial vault, monobloc, Le Fort I, and chin osteotomies with reshaping. *E*, Oblique view before reconstruction. *F*, Oblique view at 1 year after cranial vault, monobloc, Le Fort I, and chin osteotomies.

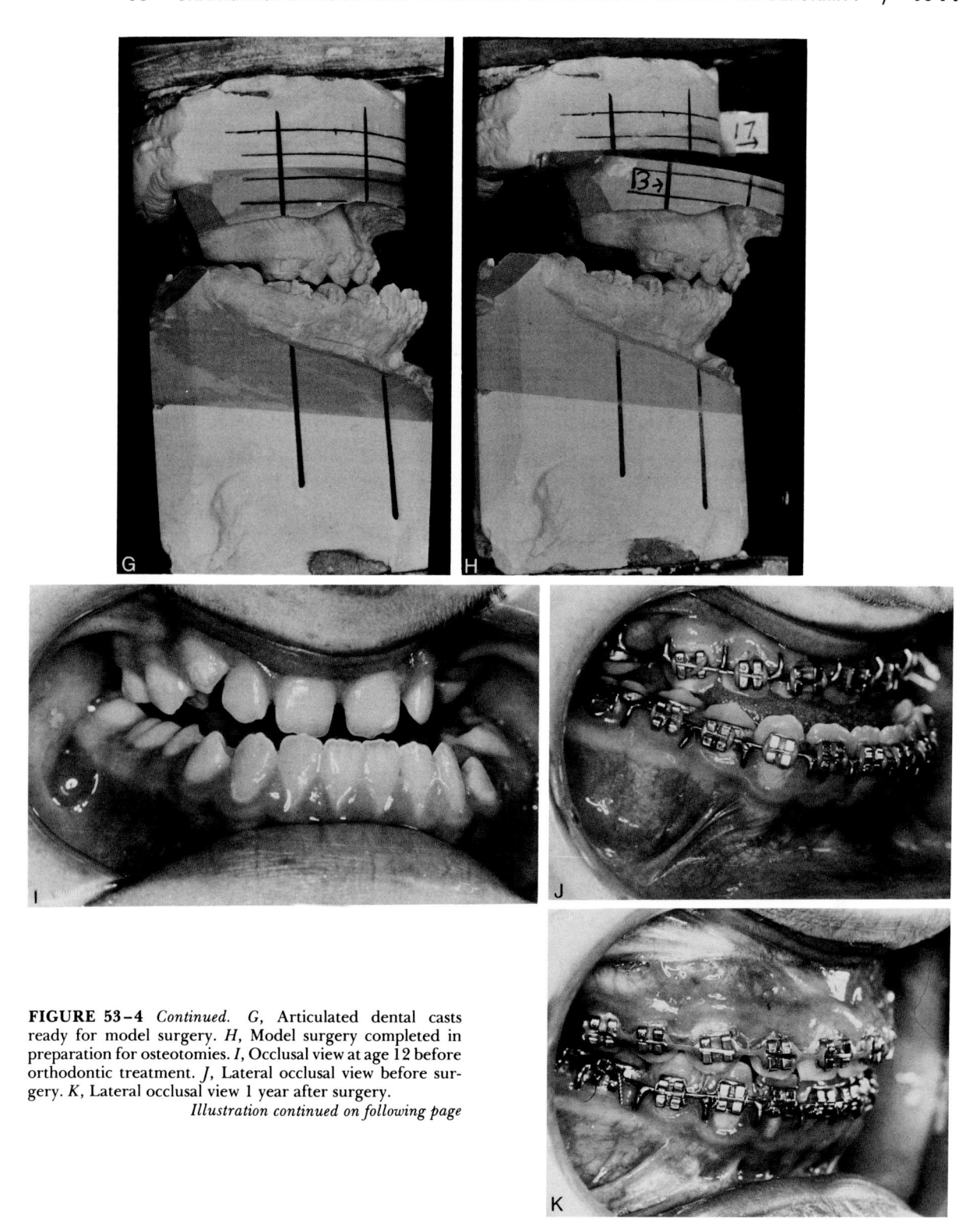

FIGURE 53-4 *Continued.* *G,* Articulated dental casts ready for model surgery. *H,* Model surgery completed in preparation for osteotomies. *I,* Occlusal view at age 12 before orthodontic treatment. *J,* Lateral occlusal view before surgery. *K,* Lateral occlusal view 1 year after surgery.

Illustration continued on following page

cranial vault reshaping were completed when she was 9 months old. At 2 years of age she underwent a Le Fort III total midface advancement combined with cranial vault reshaping through an intracranial approach.

Physical examination revealed marked cranial vault dysplasia with a constrictive band across the forehead just above the supraorbital ridges and bilateral temporal bone depressions. Multiple cranial vault bony defects were present, the orbits were shallow with bulging eyes, and the orbital dystopia was asymmetric. There were palpable step-offs at the lateral orbital rim region where the previous Le Fort III osteotomy

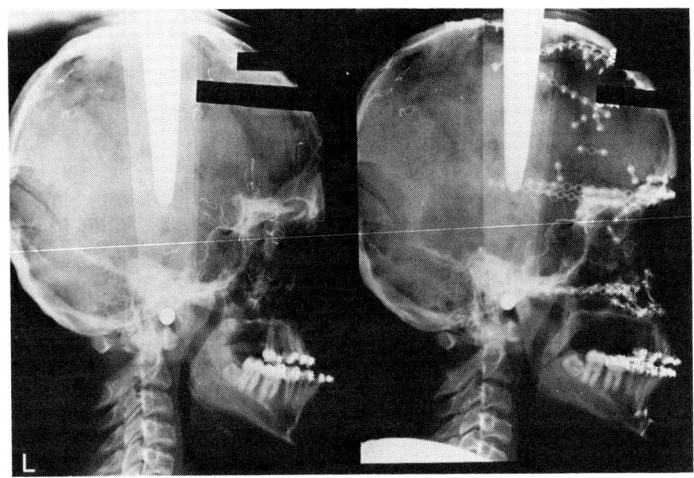

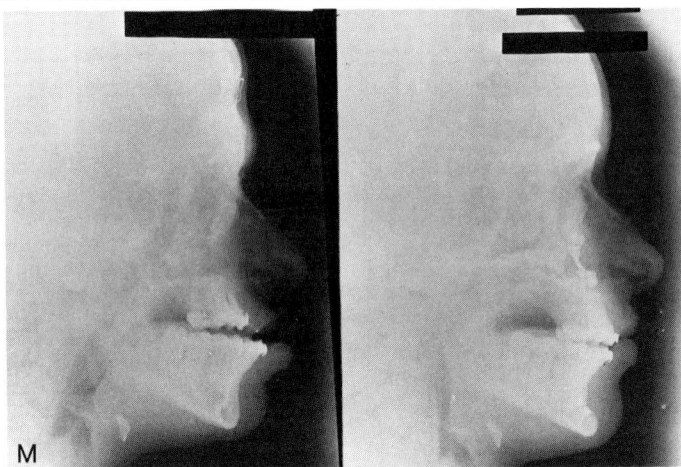

FIGURE 53-4 *Continued.* L, Lateral cephalometric radiographs before and after cranial vault, monobloc, Le Fort I, and chin osteotomies. M, Soft tissue lateral cephalometric radiographs before and after cranial vault, monobloc, Le Fort I, and chin osteotomies.

had been carried out. The total midface was deficient and the maxilla was extremely hypoplastic both vertically and horizontally. There was a severe full Class III malocclusion and an anterior open bite deformity. The six maxillary permanent molar teeth were not present. The chin appeared retrognathic.

Funduscopic examination revealed mild optic atrophy bilaterally. There was severe strabismus and amblyopia, as well as astigmatism that improved somewhat with eyeglasses. The left cornea showed signs of previous ulceration from exposure keratitis. The patient suffered from a marked bilateral conductive hearing loss and required placement of bone-conducted hearing aids. She had previously undergone surgery for upper eyelid ptosis and for blockage of her nasolacrimal apparatus after her previous midface surgery. Unfortunately, the upper eyelid ptosis remained. She was developmentally delayed as a result of longstanding intracranial hypertension. She was mildly depressed, had a poor self-image, and demonstrated behavior problems that probably resulted from the constant ridicule she experienced both at school and in her neighborhood.

Surgical Procedure

Airway management was achieved initially through orotracheal intubation. This was later converted to nasotracheal intubation after the monobloc osteotomy was completed. Temporary tarsorrhaphies were completed to prevent corneal abrasions during the surgical procedure. Perioperative intravenous antibiotics included penicillin and cloxacillin.

The previously placed coronal incision was opened and the anterior scalp flap was developed in the subperiosteal plane. A 360-degree periorbital dissection followed. Great care was taken to avoid injury to or detachment of the medial canthi and the nasolacrimal apparatus. With the dissection complete, there was bony exposure of the total cranial vault, orbits, and squamous portion of the temporal bones, zygomas, dorsum of the nose, and anterior maxilla. A bifrontal craniotomy was performed, the frontal and temporal lobes of the brain were retracted, and the monobloc osteotomy was completed. The monobloc was further disimpacted with a combination of Tessier disimpaction forceps placed in the nose and mouth and pterygomaxillary suture spreaders inserted through the coronal incision deep to the zygomas and through the infratemporal fossa. With the monobloc disimpacted, the orotracheal intubation was converted to nasotracheal intubation and the prefabricated intermediate acrylic splint was wired between the maxillary and mandibular teeth with the maxilla in both a horizontally and vertically advanced position.

Through the coronal incision, titanium bone plates and screws were placed across the tenon extensions of the supraorbital ridges back into the stable temporal bone, and the orbits were carefully advanced to increase and idealize the orbital depth. Additional titanium bone plates and screws were placed across each zygomatic arch extending from the anterior maxilla back to the stable squamous temporal bone regions. A segment of cranial vault bone was selected for the new forehead, and this was stabilized with multiple titanium bone plates and screws. Additional cranial vault segments were selected and pieced together for total reconstruction of the skull. Interpositional cranial bone grafts were placed along bone gaps at the zygomatic arches and tenon extensions of the supraorbital ridges. Bilateral canthopexies were completed as previously described. The coronal incision was closed in layers.

The patient was reprepared and draped for intraoral maxillofacial surgery. The previously placed intermediate splint was removed. A Le Fort I osteotomy was performed. The prefabricated final acrylic splint was wired between the maxillary and mandibular teeth with the maxilla further advanced both horizontally and vertically to its desired final position. Four titanium bone plates were placed, one at each zygomatic buttress and one at each piriform aperture. Attention was turned to the chin, and a vestibular incision was made with exposure of the bony chin. A vertical reduction and advancement genioplasty were completed. Stabilization was with titanium miniplates and screws. The wounds were irrigated and closed. The jaws were unwired, and the occlusion was checked and found to be satisfactory. The patient was taken to the intensive care unit in satisfactory condition.

POSTOPERATIVE COURSE

The patient remained electively intubated for 3 days, after which the nasotracheal tube was removed. This allowed time for the bony passage created by the midface advancement at the level of the anterior cranial vault and nasal cavity to stabilize. The intravenous antibiotics were continued for 10 days. The scalp sutures were removed and the patient was discharged from the hospital. She remained on a wired-jaw diet for 8 weeks, after which the interocclusal splint was removed and postoperative orthodontic detailing of the occlusion continued.

CASE 5 (FIG. 53–5)

Diagnosis: Apert syndrome
Previous surgery: Suture release and forehead reshaping at 6 months
Staged syndactyly reconstruction
Procedure: Total cranial vault and monobloc bipartition osteotomies with reshaping and advancement

This 5-year-old girl was born with Apert syndrome. She underwent suture release and forehead reshaping at 6 months of age. She was in the process of staged reconstruction of her four-limb syndactyly. She had strabismus and amblyopia for which she wore eyeglasses and was undergoing eye patching.

She presented with a retruded and wide anterior cranial base (residual bradycephaly). The forehead was flat at the supraorbital ridge level with bitemporal constrictions and bulged superiorly. The orbits were shallow with bulging eyes and a moderate degree of orbital hypertelorism. The midface lacked a normal convexity when viewed from above. The total midface was deficient, with a marked anterior open bite and full Class III malocclusion. Nasal airflow was poor, and the patient habitually breathed through her mouth.

A craniofacial CT scan was completed in both the axial and coronal planes. The axial CT scan was reformatted for three-dimensional reconstruction. The ventricles were of normal size and shape. There was evidence of fingerprinting along the inner table

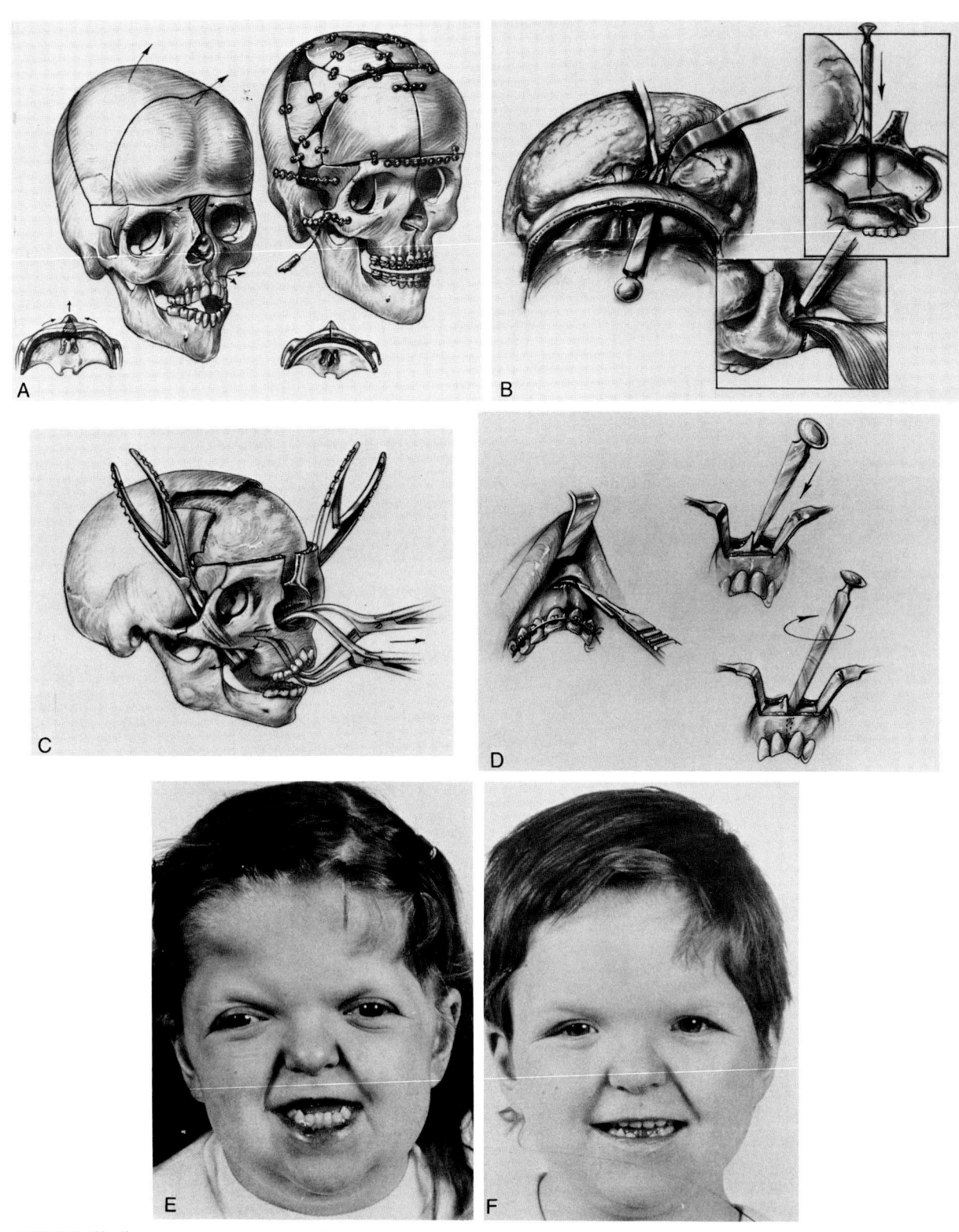

FIGURE 53-5. A 5-YEAR-OLD GIRL WITH APERT SYNDROME WHO UNDERWENT SUTURE RELEASE AND FOREHEAD RESHAPING AT 6 MONTHS OF AGE. SHE PRESENTS NOW FOR CRANIAL VAULT AND MONOBLOC BIPARTITION OSTEOTOMIES WITH RESHAPING AND ANTERIOR REPOSITIONING. *A,* Preoperative craniofacial morphology, planned and completed osteotomies with reshaping. Stabilization is with cranial bone grafts and miniplate fixation. *B,* Osteotomies requiring completion with a chisel. Osteotomy of medial orbital wall completed remaining posterior to medial canthi and nasolacrimal apparatus, with chisel placement through anterior cranial base; osteotomy through anterior cranial base down through bony septum of nose; osteotomy through coronal incision and infratemporal fossa to pterygomaxillary suture, which is then fractured. *C,* Completed monobloc bipartition osteotomies. Tessier disimpaction forceps placed through nose and mouth with pterygomaxillary spreader forceps placed through coronal incision and infratemporal fossa to pterygomaxillary suture regions for disimpaction of midface. *D,* Illustration of intraoral buccal vestibular incision, dissection down to anterior nasal spine region with osteotomy down midline of hard palate as part of monobloc bipartition osteotomy. *E,* Preoperative frontal view. *F,* Postoperative frontal view at 1 year after reconstruction.

FIGURE 53–5 *Continued. G*, Preoperative lateral view. *H*, Postoperative lateral view at 1 year after reconstruction. *I*, Intraoperative lateral view of cranial vault, orbits, and zygomatic arch through coronal incision after osteotomies. Stabilization with cranial bone grafts and miniplate fixation. *J*, Pre- and postoperative axial-sliced CT scans through mid-orbits, demonstrating improvement in orbital hypertelorism and orbital depth with diminished eyeball proptosis. *K*, Three-dimensional CT scan reformations. Oblique views before and after reconstruction. (From Posnick JC, Nakano P: Craniofacial dysostosis: Staging of reconstruction and management of the midface deformity. Neurosurg Clin North Am 2(3):683–702, 1991.)

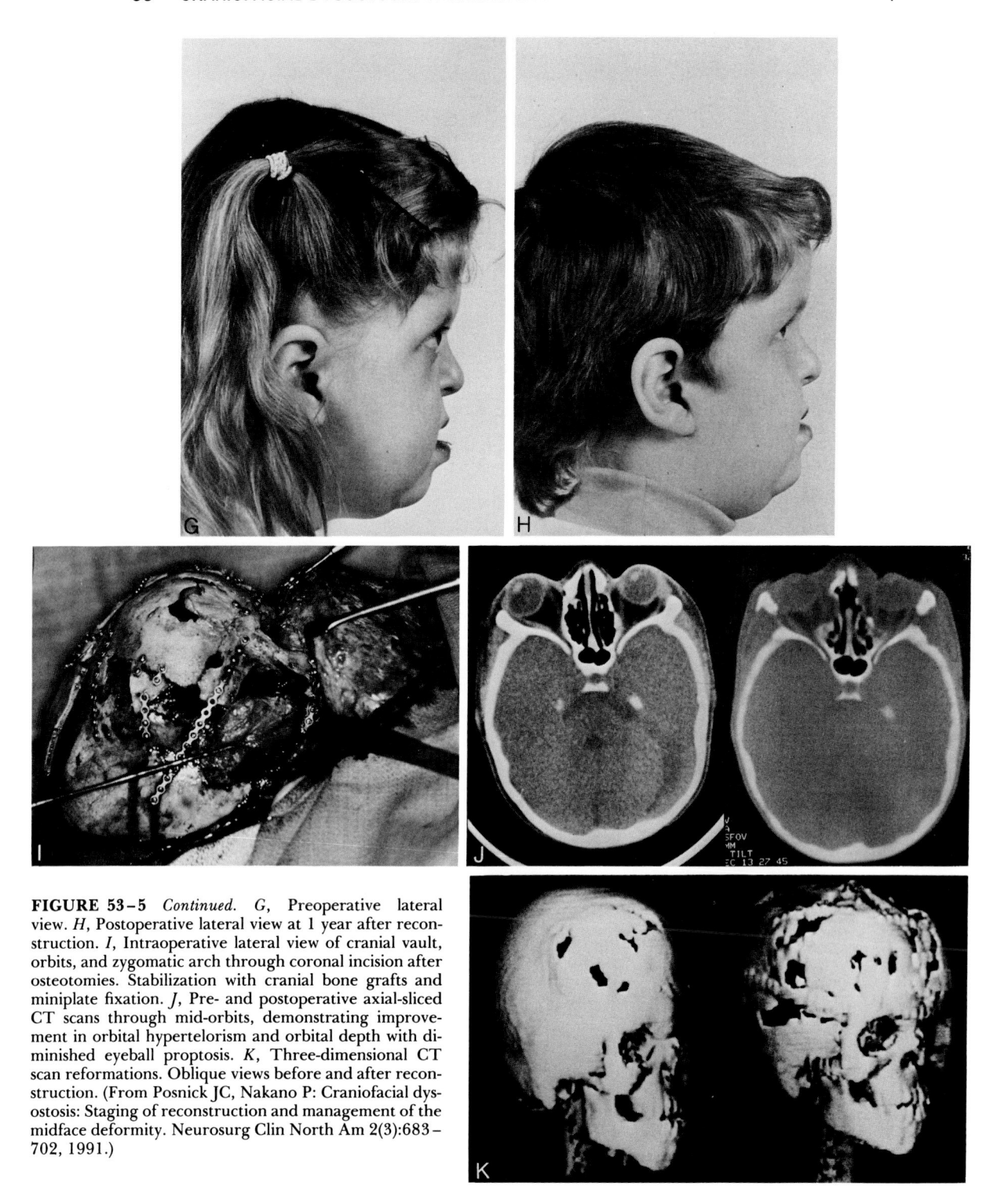

of the cranial vault and anterior cranial base. The CT scan confirmed that the anterior cranial base was short, with bitemporal constrictions and a recessed supraorbital ridge. The superior forehead bulged anteriorly. The orbits were shallow and moderate orbital hypertelorism was present. The total midface was deficient and the nasal air passages were diminished.

The patient appeared to have Apert syndrome with residual cranial vault dysplasia, exorbitism, exophthalmos, orbital hypertelorism, and total midface deficiency.

Surgical Procedure

General anesthesia was administered through orotracheal intubation. Temporary tarsorrhaphies were completed, and perioperative prophylactic intravenous penicillin and cloxacillin were given. The previous coronal incision was incised and carried down to bone, and the anterior scalp flap was developed as previously described. With the craniofacial skeleton exposed through the coronal incision, the bifrontal craniotomy was completed, the frontal and temporal lobes of the brain were retracted, and the monobloc osteotomy was completed. The monobloc was further disimpacted with a combination of the Tessier disimpaction forceps and the pterygomaxillary spreaders as described previously. Bipartition of the monobloc was completed next, first by resection of a wedge of bone in the midline between the orbits. This included nasal bone, supraorbital ridge, and nasal septum. Great care was taken to avoid injury or detachment of the medial canthi or nasolacrimal apparatus.

A small intraoral midline maxillary vestibular incision was then carried down to bone with subperiosteal dissection and exposure of the anterior nasal spine and the floor of the nose. With an osteotome and mallet the maxilla was split in the midline between the two central incisor teeth, completing the monobloc bipartition and separating the facial skeleton into two halves. Working through the coronal incision, additional bone was removed from the posterior floor of the nose and maxilla. Care was taken to avoid perforation of the palatal mucosa during the surgical procedure. Next a titanium bone plate and screws were placed across the supraorbital ridge, bringing the two halves of the face toward the midline and correcting the orbital hypertelorism. In the transverse plane, the monobloc was arched to take on a more normal convex appearance to the facial halves when viewed from above.

At this point attention was turned to the oral cavity. Erich arch bars were placed on the maxillary and mandibular teeth and the jaws were wired together to correct the Class III malocclusion, posterior crossbites, and anterior open bite deformities.

Attention was returned to the orbits through the coronal incision, and titanium bone plates and screws were placed along the supraorbital ridge tenon extension back to stable temporal bone with the orbits in the advanced position. Additional bone plates and screws were placed across the zygomatic arches extending from the anterior maxilla back to the squamous portion of the temporal bones. Additional posterior cranial vault bone was removed for reshaping of the cranial vault. Sections of skull bone were selected for the new forehead and were secured in place with titanium bone plates and screws. The cranial vault was reconstructed from anterior to posterior until its reshaping was complete. Interpositional cranial bone grafts were placed along the gaps of the zygomatic arches. Bilateral lateral canthopexies were completed, and the scalp was closed in layers. The patient remained intubated and was taken to the intensive care unit in satisfactory condition.

Postoperative Course

The patient was electively extubated on the third postoperative day and transferred from the intensive care unit to the ward. Intravenous antibiotics were continued for 10 days, after which the coronal sutures were removed. She was discharged from hospital on the sixteenth postoperative day and returned to British Columbia on a wired-jaw diet. When she returned at the 6-week postoperative interval her jaws were unwired and the Erich arch bars were removed under intravenous sedation.

At 1 year after surgery, she has maintained good function and esthetics. It is anticipated that a Le Fort I osteotomy and genioplasty will be required in combination with orthodontic treatment when the skeleton reaches maturity.

CASE 6 (Fig. 53-6)

Diagnosis: Apert syndrome
Previous surgery: Bilateral lateral canthal advancement and morcelization of the cranial vault at 2 months
Ventriculoperitoneal shunting at 8 months
Staged syndactyly reconstruction
Procedure: Total cranial vault and monobloc osteotomies with reshaping and advancement

A 2.5-year-old child born with Apert syndrome had undergone bilateral lateral canthal advancement procedures (Hoffman procedure)[51] and cranial vault morcelization to release the prematurely closed coronal sutures and reshape her skull. By 8 months of age, she had severe hydrocephalus which necessitated ventriculoperitoneal shunting. She was in the process of undergoing staged reconstruction for her four-limb congenital syndactyly when she presented to our team.

On presentation at 2.5 years of age, the patient had severe oxycephaly with multiple cranial vault bony defects. Her orbits were shallow (exorbitism) and her eyes bulged (exophthalmos). There was total midface deficiency with a severe anterior open bite deformity. The palate was high-arched but without bony clefting. A sleep apnea study showed evidence of obstruction, with the majority of obstructive episodes associated with moderate oxygen desaturation. Ophthalmologic examination showed strabismus, amblyopia, and mild optic atrophy.

A craniofacial CT scan was completed in both the axial and coronal planes. The axial CT scan was reformatted for three-dimensional reconstruction. The ventricles were mildly dilated and the ventriculoperitoneal shunt was in place. Fingerprinting could be seen along the inner table of the anterior cranial base and skull, suggesting intracranial hypertension. The orbits were extremely shallow and the eyes bulged. There was no true bony stenosis of the nasal passages, but they were extremely constricted because of severe midface hypoplasia. Multiple full-thickness cranial bone defects were present as a result of previous surgery.

The patient appeared to have Apert syndrome with residual severe cranial vault dysplasia, exorbitism, exophthalmos, orbital hypertelorism, and total midface deficiency.

Surgical Procedure

General anesthesia was administered initially through orotracheal intubation. This was later converted to nasotracheal intubation after a monobloc bipartition osteotomy was completed. Temporary tarsorrhaphies were completed, and perioperative prophylactic intravenous penicillin and cloxacillin were given. Despite its anterior location, the previous coronal incision was used. The incision was carried down to bone and the anterior scalp flap was developed as previously described. The posterior scalp flap was taken back to the occiput with care to avoid exposing the previously placed ventriculoperitoneal shunt. With the craniofacial skeleton exposed, a bifrontal craniotomy was completed, the frontal and temporal lobes of the brain were retracted, and a monobloc osteotomy was completed as previously described. With the monobloc osteotomy completed and further disimpacted for release of scar tissue, the orotracheal intubation was converted to nasotracheal intubation as previously described. Attention was turned to the oral cavity, and Erich arch bars were placed on the maxilla and mandible. The jaws were wired together through a prefabricated acrylic splint, giving a 15-mm advancement at the incisal edge. The orbits were then reconstructed through the coronal incision, and titanium bone plates and screws were placed along the supraorbital ridge tenon extensions back to the stable temporal bone. This allowed a 20-mm advancement at the level of the supraorbital ridges. Additional bone plates and screws were placed across the zygomatic arches extending from the anterior maxilla and then back to the squamous portion of the temporal bones. The posterior cranial vault bone was removed next through a further craniotomy. A section of skull bone was selected for the new forehead, and this was secured with additional titanium bone plates and screws. The cranial vault was further reconstructed from anterior to posterior until the reshaping was complete. Interpositional cranial bone grafts were placed along the gaps of the zygomatic arches. Bilateral lateral canthopexies were completed and the scalp was closed in layers. The patient was taken to the intensive care unit with the nasotracheal tube in place.

Postoperative Course

The patient remained electively intubated until the third postoperative day when she was extubated and transferred from the intensive care unit to the ward. Intravenous antibiotics were continued for 10 days, after which the scalp sutures were also removed. She remained on a wired-jaw diet for 8 weeks. The intermaxillary fixation was then released and the arch bars were removed.

At age 5 (i.e., 2.5 years after monobloc and cranial vault osteotomy), she has maintained good cranial vault shape, depth of orbits, and midface projection. Since her total midface osteotomy was carried out at a young age (2.5 years), the expected additional growth of the cranial vault and orbits may result in residual orbital dystopia. Repeat total midface surgery may be required. In any case, a Le Fort I osteotomy and genioplasty in combination with orthodontics will be required when the skeleton matures.

1918 / VI — FUNCTIONAL RESTORATION OF OCCLUSION

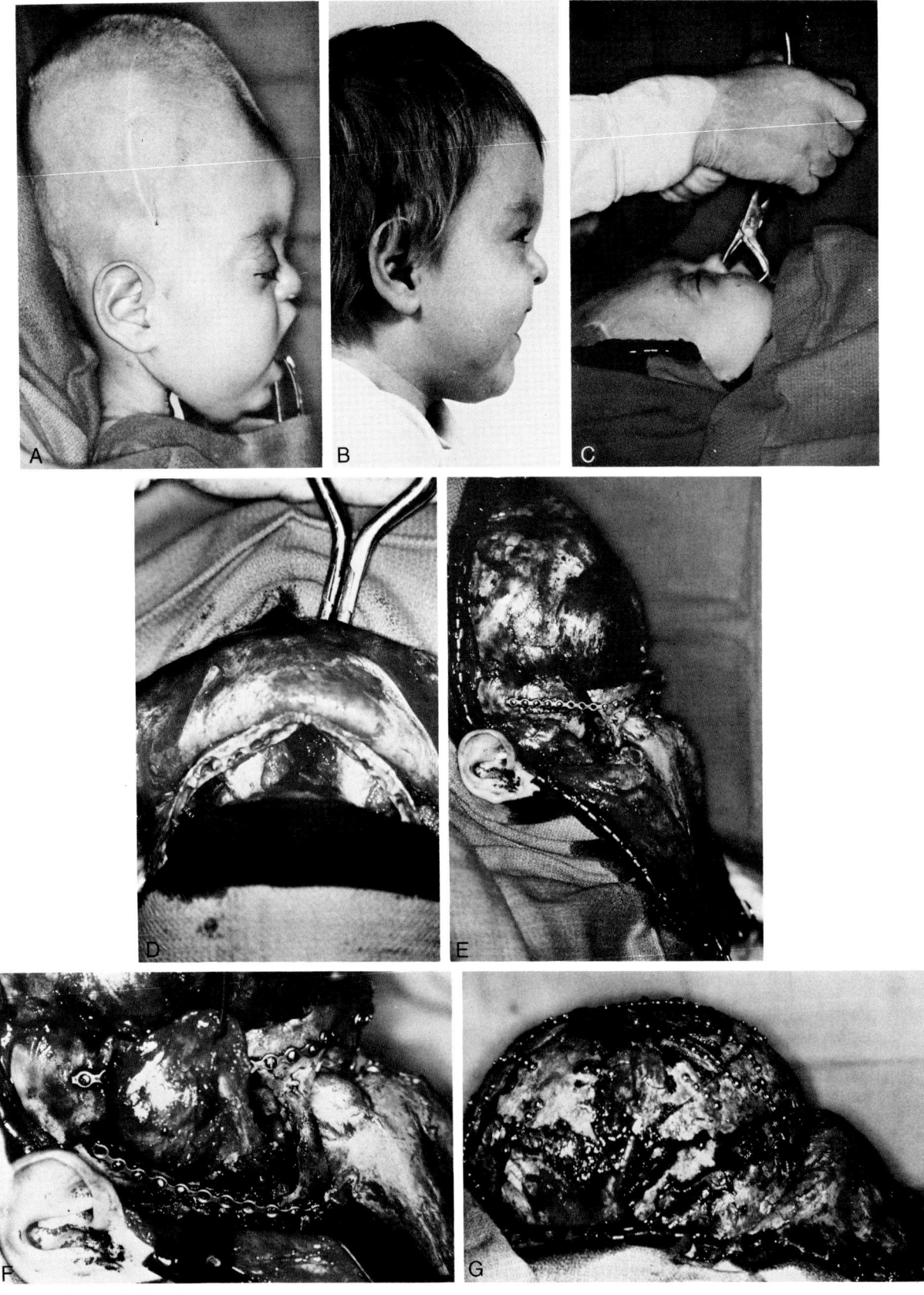

See opposite page for legend

CASE 7 (FIG. 53-7)

Diagnosis: Pfeiffer's syndrome
Previous surgery: Bilateral lateral canthal advancement
Ventriculoperitoneal shunt placement
Procedure: Total cranial vault and monobloc osteotomies with reshaping and advancement

A 7-year-old boy who was born with Pfeiffer's syndrome underwent bilateral lateral canthal advancement through an intracranial approach at approximately 3 months of age. Later, he required placement of a ventriculoperitoneal shunt for management of hydrocephalus. He was referred to our unit because of poor nasal airflow, obstructive sleep apnea, developmental delay, corneal exposure, and herniation of his globe, which had required emergency reduction in the past.

Physical examination revealed multiple cranial vault bony defects, a decreased head circumference, bulging eyes, and vertical orbital dystopia. The total midface was hypoplastic with severe Class III malocclusion and anterior open bite deformity. The nasal air flow was poor and a sleep study revealed obstructive sleep apnea. Papilledema with mild optic atrophy combined with severe strabismus, amblyopia, corneal exposure, and upper eyelid ptosis was present.

A CT scan was completed in both axial and coronal planes. The axial CT scan was reformatted for three-dimensional reconstruction. The ventricles were mildly enlarged and a ventriculoperitoneal shunt was in place. Multiple cranial vault bony defects were present, and fingerprinting was observed along the inner table of the skull and the anterior cranial base, caused by longstanding increased intracranial pressure. The orbits were extremely shallow with asymmetric globe proptosis. There was severe hypoplasia of the midface, which was also documented through cephalometric analysis. The mandible showed a normal anteroposterior growth pattern as documented by the SNB angle.

SURGICAL PROCEDURE

Details of the procedure carried out were very similar to those described for Cases 1 and 3. After the monobloc osteotomy was complete and disimpaction satisfactory, the supraorbital ridge level was advanced approximately 25 mm. Horizontal advancement at the occlusal level was 14 mm.

POSTOPERATIVE COURSE

The patient remained electively intubated for 5 days, after which the nasotracheal tube was removed. He was discharged from the hospital approximately 2.5 weeks after surgery. He returned after 8 weeks for removal of arch bars and the interocclusal acrylic splint.

A 1-year postoperative sleep study revealed resolution of the previous significant oxygen desaturation. Corneal exposure and globe herniation were no longer problems. Papilledema was resolved, but mild optic atrophy remained. Occlusion and chewing were improved, but the Class III malocclusion remained. A Le Fort I osteotomy and genioplasty in combination with orthodontic treatment will be required when the skeleton matures.

FIGURE 53-6. A 2.5-YEAR-OLD CHILD BORN WITH APERT SYNDROME. SHE HAD UNDERGONE BILATERAL LATERAL CANTHAL ADVANCEMENT PROCEDURES AND CRANIAL VAULT MORCELIZATION IN EARLY INFANCY. SHE LATER REQUIRED VENTRICULOPERITONEAL SHUNTING. SHE PRESENTS NOW FOR TOTAL CRANIAL VAULT AND MONOBLOC OSTEOTOMIES WITH RESHAPING AND ADVANCEMENT. *A*, Preoperative lateral view. *B*, Postoperative lateral view at 4.5 years of age. *C*, Intraoperative view after monobloc osteotomies with Tessier disimpaction forceps in place. *D*, With disimpaction forceps in place and the coronal incision down, the degree of advancement achieved at the level of the anterior cranial base is demonstrated. *E*, Intraoperative lateral view of anterior cranial vault and orbits through coronal incision demonstrating miniplate fixation of orbital ridge to temporal bone. *F*, Intraoperative close-up lateral view after osteotomies demonstrating stabilization with miniplate fixation across zygomatic arch–anterior maxilla and supraorbital ridge–temporal bone with temporalis muscle sandwiched in between. *G*, Intraoperative lateral view demonstrating cranial vault after reshaping. Stabilization with cranial bone grafts and miniplate fixation.

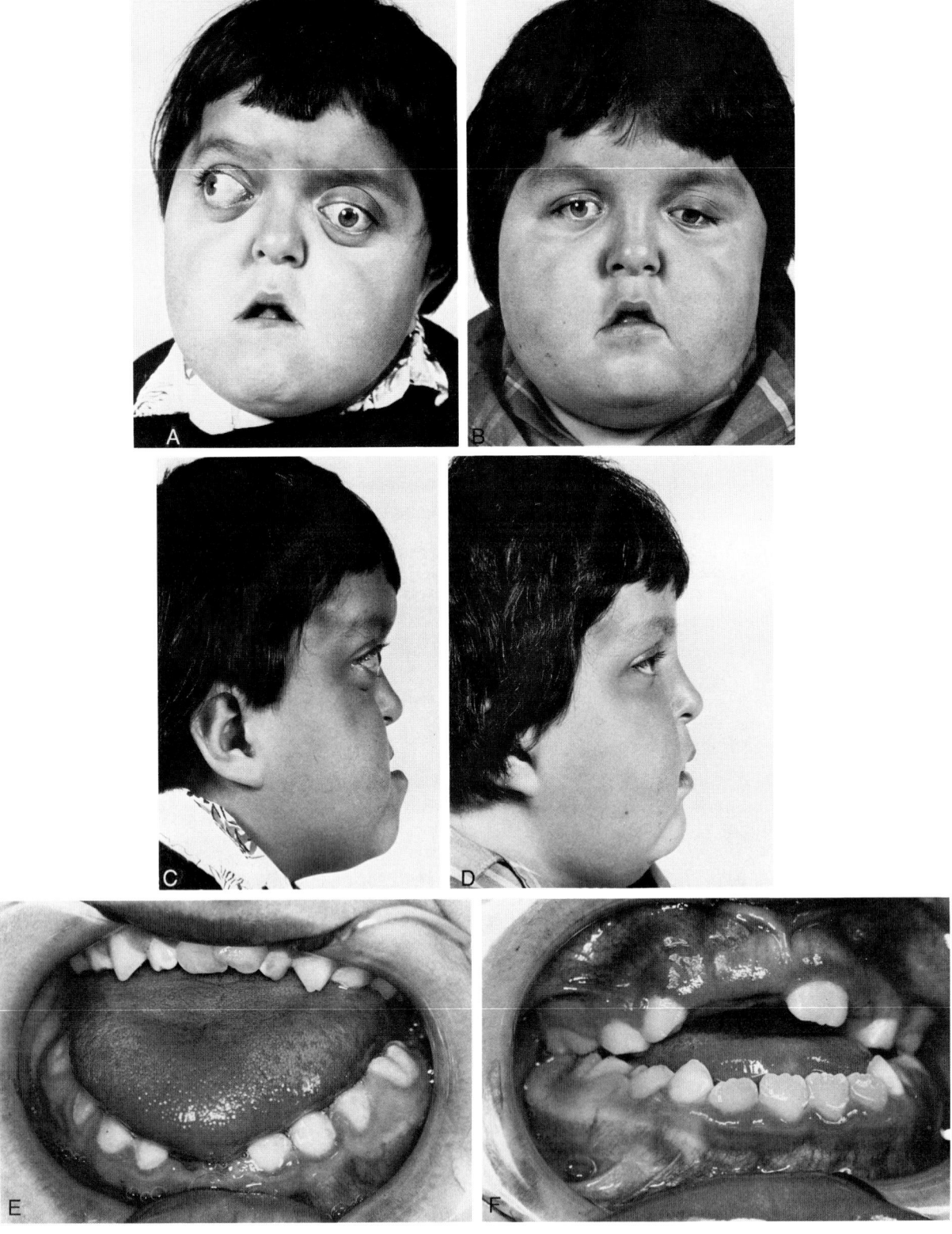

FIGURE 53–7. A 7-YEAR-OLD BOY BORN WITH PFEIFFER'S SYNDROME UNDERWENT BILATERAL LATERAL CANTHAL ADVANCEMENTS THROUGH AN INTRACRANIAL APPROACH AT 3 MONTHS OF AGE. HE LATER REQUIRED PLACEMENT OF A VENTRICULOPERITONEAL SHUNT. HE PRESENTS NOW FOR TOTAL CRANIAL VAULT AND MONOBLOC OSTEOTOMIES WITH RESHAPING AND ADVANCEMENT. *A*, Preoperative frontal view. *B*, Postoperative frontal view at 1 year after reconstruction. *C*, Preoperative lateral view. *D*, Postoperative lateral view at 1 year after reconstruction. *E*, Preoperative occlusion. *F*, Postoperative occlusion at 1 year after reconstruction. (From Posnick JC, Nakano P: Craniofacial dysostosis: Staging of reconstruction and management of the midface deformity. Neurosurg Clin North Am 2(3):683–702, 1991.)

CASE 8 (FIG. 53-8)

Diagnosis: Apert syndrome
Previous surgery: Strip craniectomy (coronal sutures)
    Anterior cranial vault and upper orbital osteotomies with advancement
    Attempted cranioplasty
    Attempted Le Fort III osteotomy
    Ventriculoperitoneal shunt placement three times
Procedure: Total cranial vault and monobloc bipartition osteotomies with reshaping and advancement
    Repair of encephalocele and orbital defects

An 8-year-old girl who was born with Apert syndrome underwent strip craniectomy of the stenotic coronal sutures in infancy while living in Saudi Arabia. When signs of increased intracranial pressure occurred, she was taken to Lebanon, where upper orbital and cranial vault osteotomies were performed. Her surgery was complicated by infection and loss of bone in the right fronto-orbital region. A cranioplasty was later attempted, but further infection occurred. Herniation of the brain through the resulting defect in the orbital roof and medial orbital wall resulted in further orbital dystopia and proptosis. She was taken to England where a Le Fort III osteotomy was attempted. Ventriculoperitoneal shunting was carried out on three occasions.

She presented to the craniofacial team at HSC as a cheerful, good-natured child whose intelligence was just below normal. Strabismus, amblyopia, and astigmatism with mild optic atrophy were present. She had four-limb complex syndactylies that had not been previously surgically reconstructed. Previous infections and fistula tracts had resulted in multiple well-healed scars over her forehead. A large encephalocele was evident through the bony defect in the right medial supraorbital ridge, orbital roof, and medial orbital wall region. The orbits were shallow and the eyes were bulging; a degree of orbital hypertelorism was present. A Class III malocclusion with an anterior open bite was also present. The patient experienced poor nasal air flow and habitually breathed through her mouth. Her forehead was flat and wide, indicative of unresolved brachycephaly.

SURGICAL PROCEDURE

The surgical procedure carried out was similar to that described in Case 5. The dissection and reconstruction were complicated by the presence of a right fronto-orbital encephalocele that required neurosurgical repair and duroplasty. Additional bony reconstruction required at the level of the supraorbital ridge, orbital roof, and medial orbital wall was completed with a cranial bone graft. The previous aborted Le Fort III osteotomy also complicated the reconstruction. Only fibrous unions were present at the lateral orbital rim regions. These required stabilization with cranial grafts and bone miniplates before monobloc osteotomy disimpaction.

POSTOPERATIVE COURSE

This patient's postoperative course was also similar to that described for the patient in Case 5. Three months postoperatively, the staged four-limb syndactyly release and reconstruction got under way. A Le Fort I osteotomy and genioplasty in combination with orthodontic treatment will be required when the skeleton reaches maturity. Residual deformity and hypoplasia over the bridge of the nose may also require further skeletal augmentation later in adolescence.

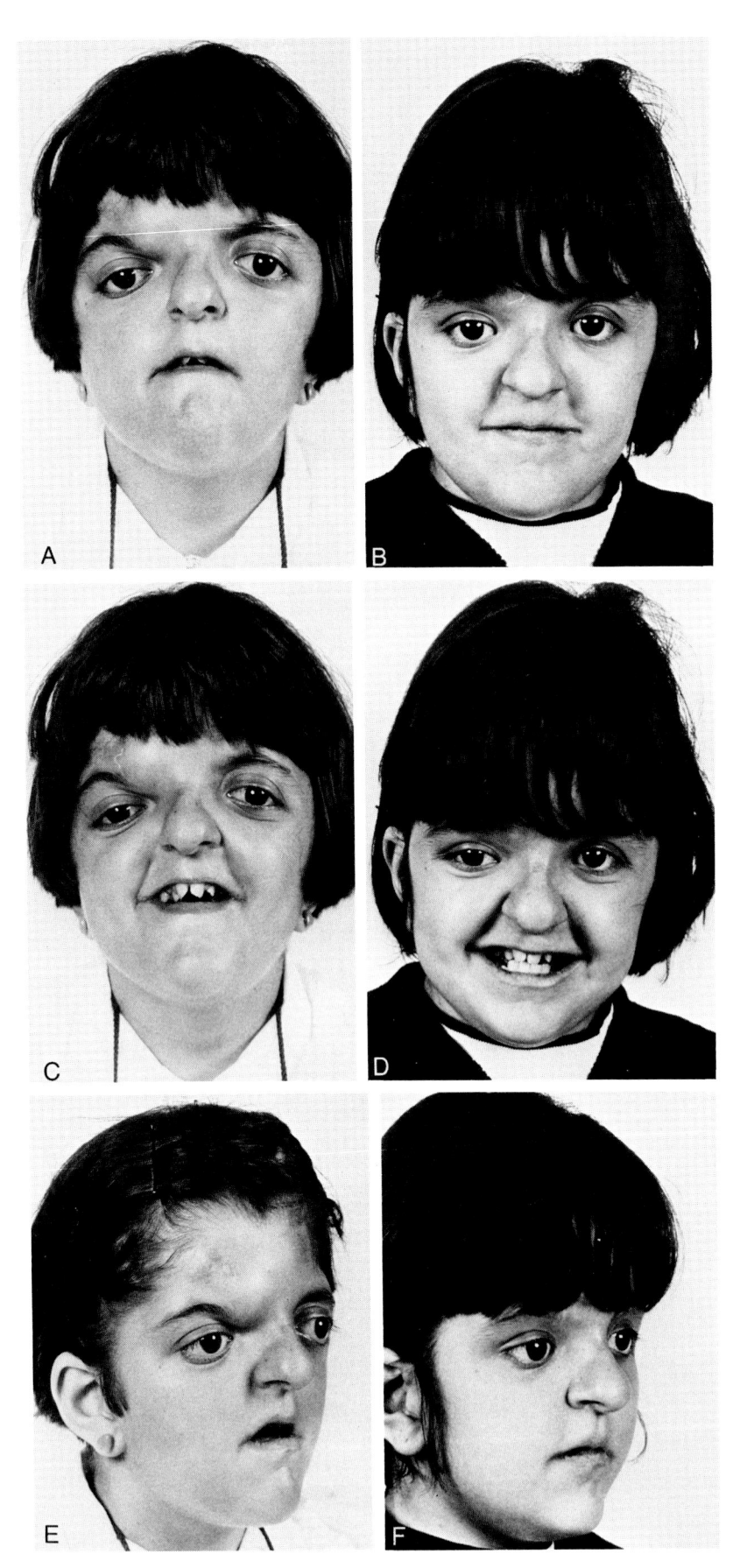

FIGURE 53-8. An 8-year-old girl who was born with Apert syndrome had undergone multiple intracranial surgical procedures in the past, including an attempted Le Fort III osteotomy. She was referred for management of her residual problems and underwent repair of fronto-orbital encephalocele, reconstruction of orbital wall defects combined with total cranial vault and monobloc bipartition osteotomies with reshaping and advancement. *A*, Preoperative frontal view. *B*, Postoperative frontal view at 1 year after reconstruction. *C*, Preoperative frontal view with smile. *D*, Postoperative frontal view with smile at 1 year after reconstruction. *E*, Preoperative oblique view. *F*, Postoperative oblique view at 1 year after reconstruction.

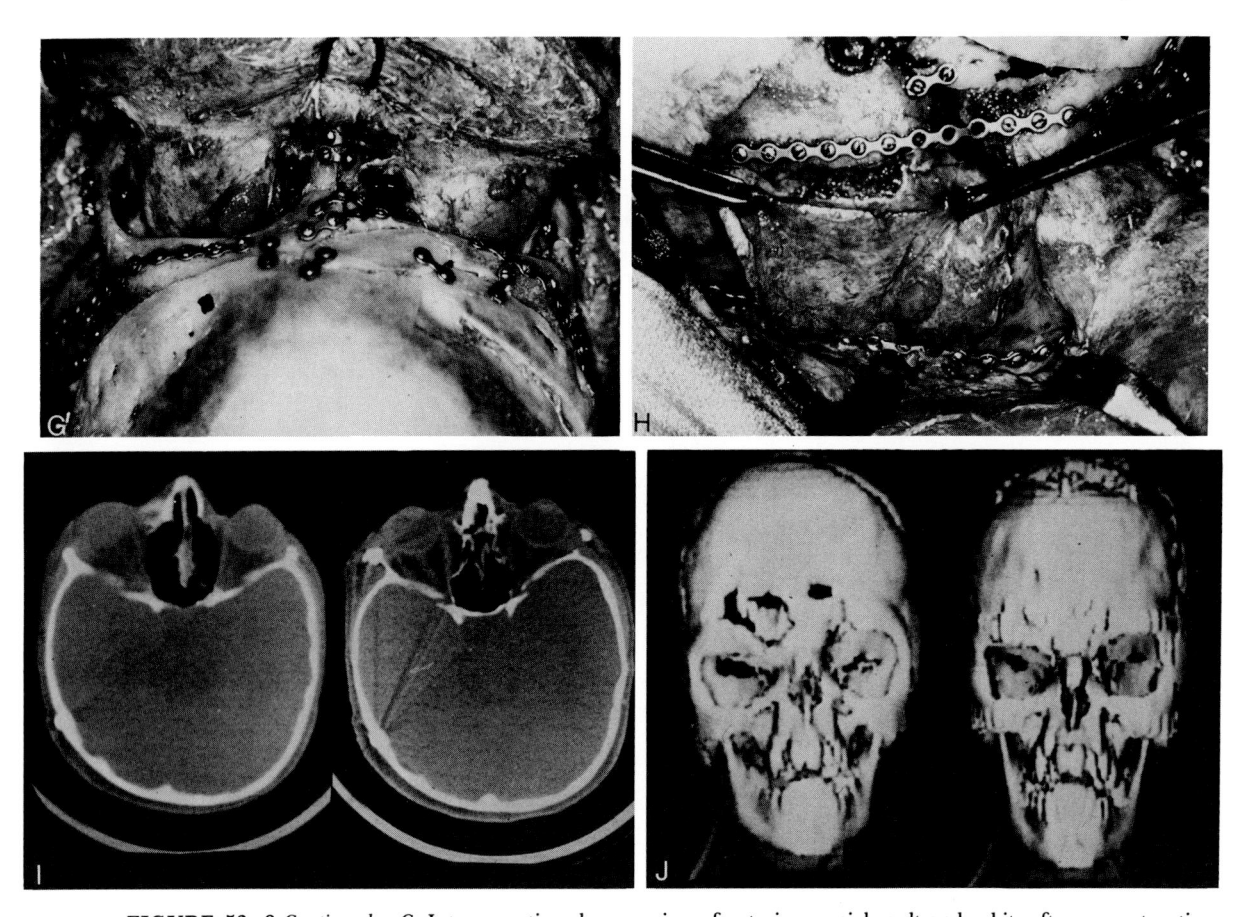

FIGURE 53–8 *Continued.* *G*, Intraoperative close-up view of anterior cranial vault and orbits after reconstruction. Stabilization with cranial bone grafts and miniplate fixation. *H*, Intraoperative close-up lateral view through coronal incision of fixation across zygomatic arch–anterior maxilla and supraorbital ridge–temporal bone region. *I*, Axial sliced CT scans through mid-orbits before and after reconstruction, demonstrating diminished orbital proptosis and correction of orbital dystopia and hypertelorism. *J*, Three-dimensional CT scan reformations of craniofacial skeleton. Frontal views before and after reconstruction.

CASE 9 (FIG. 53–9)

Diagnosis: Crouzon syndrome
Previous surgery: None
Procedure: Anterior cranial vault and monobloc osteotomies with reshaping and advancement

A 6-year-old girl who was born with Crouzon syndrome had a positive family history: Her mother had bicoronal synostosis, proptosis, and midface deficiency. The child was developing constant headaches and difficulty with her vision when her mother brought her for medical examination.

Physical examination revealed a flat, wide forehead with recessed supraorbital ridges, shallow orbits, and bulging eyes. The total midface was flat with a Class III malocclusion. There was evidence of poor nasal airflow and a mouth-breathing habit. Funduscopic examination revealed papilledema with mild optic atrophy, strabismus, and amblyopia.

A CT scan was completed in both the axial and coronal planes. The axial CT scan was reformatted for three-dimensional reconstruction. The ventricles were mildly enlarged. Fingerprinting was obvious along the inner table of the skull and the anterior cranial base, resulting from longstanding increased intracranial pressure. The orbits were shallow with ocular proptosis. The midface deficiency was also confirmed through cephalometric analysis, which revealed an SNA angle greater than 2 standard deviations below the norm. The SNB angle was within normal limits.

1924 / VI — FUNCTIONAL RESTORATION OF OCCLUSION

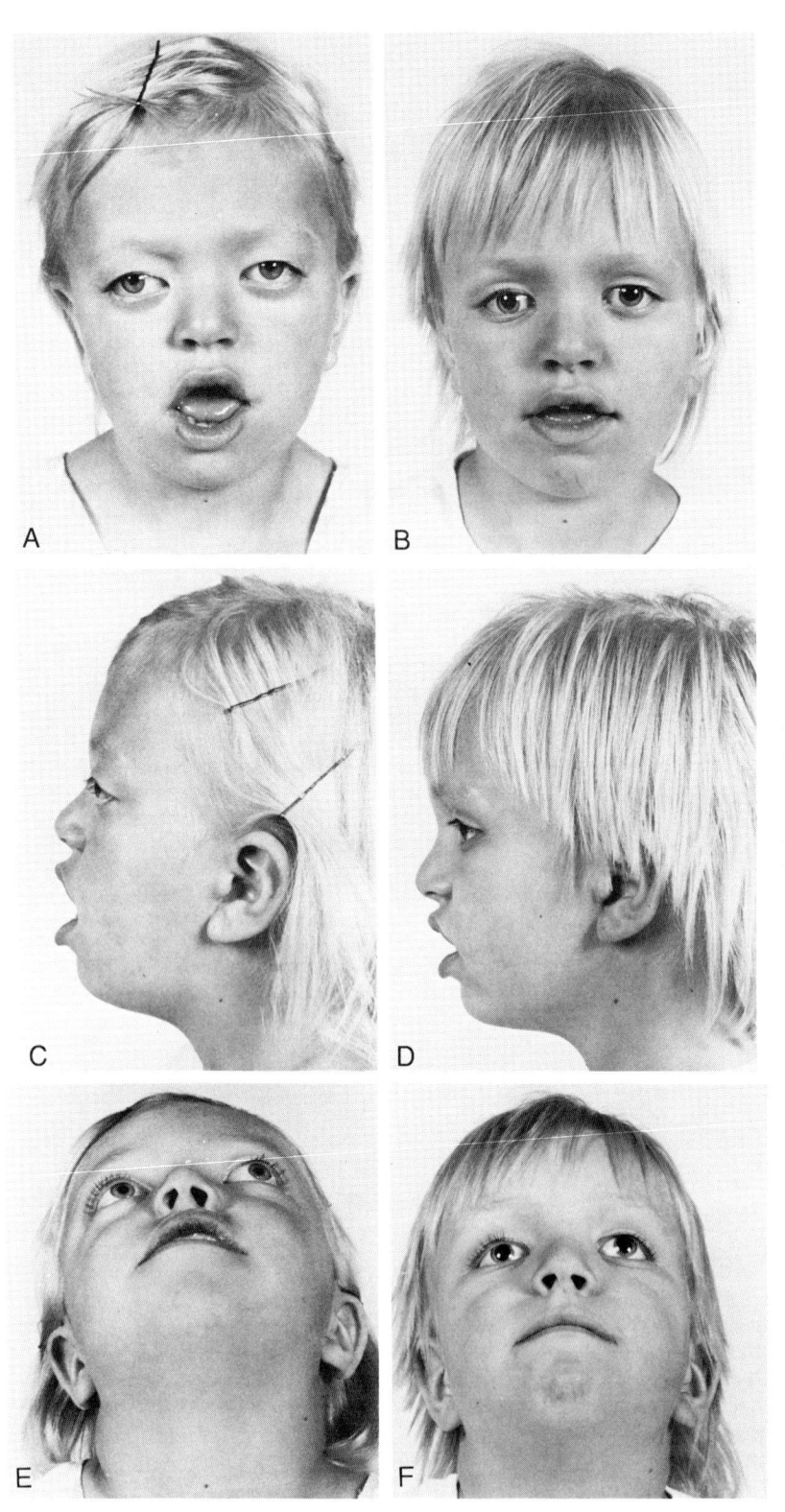

FIGURE 53–9. A 6-YEAR-OLD GIRL WHO WAS BORN WITH CROUZON SYNDROME UNDERWENT ANTERIOR CRANIAL VAULT AND MONOBLOC OSTEOTOMIES WITH RESHAPING AND ADVANCEMENT. *A*, Preoperative frontal view. *B*, Postoperative frontal view at 1 year after reconstruction. *C*, Preoperative lateral view. *D*, Postoperative lateral view at 1 year after reconstruction. *E*, Preoperative worm's eye view. *F*, Postoperative worm's eye view at 1 year after reconstruction.

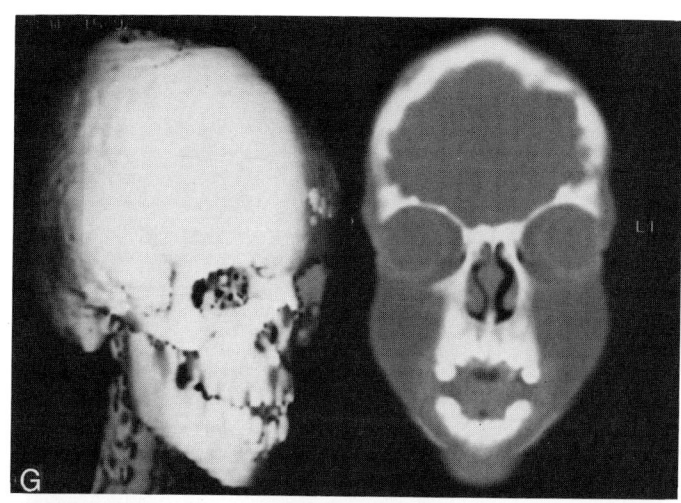

FIGURE 53-9 *Continued.* G, Three-dimensional CT scan reformations before operation. H, Three-dimensional CT scan reformations after reconstruction. I, Additional three-dimensional CT scan reformations after reconstruction including cranial base view demonstrating increased anteroposterior dimension achieved. (From Posnick JC, Nakano P: Craniofacial dysostosis: Staging of reconstruction and management of the midface deformity. Neurosurg Clin North Am 2(3):683–702, 1991.)

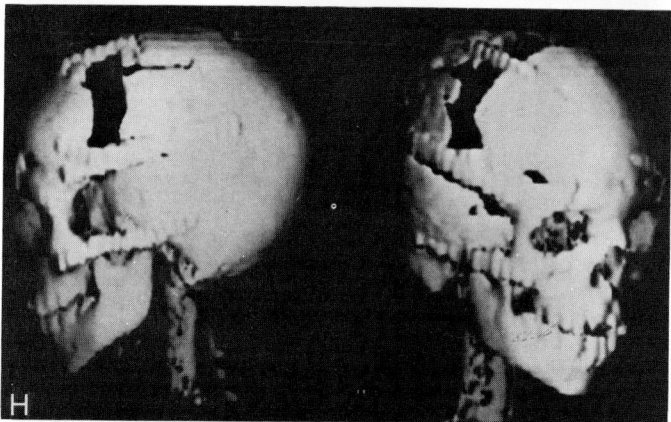

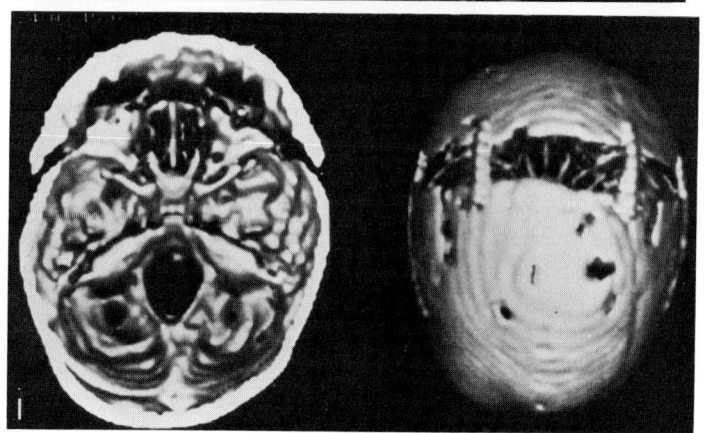

Surgical Procedure

The procedure carried out was almost identical to that described for the patient in Case 1. The intraoperative airway management varied. A prefabricated acrylic splint had been constructed from the dental models after the maxilla was horizontally advanced 14 mm. The models were articulated on a Hanau articulator with a facebow transfer. The freeway space was opened up approximately 8 mm, and the acrylic splint was increased in thickness by the same amount. The anterior central portion of the splint adjacent to the mandibular incisor teeth was left hollowed out, providing enough clearance for the orotracheal tube.

During surgery, the patient was intubated orotracheally. The orotracheal tube was secured to the anterior mandible after the passage of a 26-gauge circomandibular wire. After completion of the monobloc osteotomy, the prefabricated acrylic splint was applied and secured to the mandible with two additional circomandibular wires.

An Erich arch bar was applied to the maxillary teeth, the midface was horizontally advanced, the maxillary teeth were secured to the splint, and the jaws were wired together.

POSTOPERATIVE COURSE

The patient remained electively intubated for 3 days, after which the orotracheal tube was removed. This allowed time for a degree of healing to occur at the level of the anterior cranial base without concern for positive pressure penetration of nasal cavity fluid into this region. The postoperative course was similar to that described for patients in previous cases.

This patient will require a Le Fort I osteotomy and genioplasty in combination with orthodontic treatment when the skeleton matures.

REFERENCES

1. Acquaviva R, Tamic PM, Lebascle J, et al: Les craniosténoses en milieu marocain, a propos de 140 observations. Neurochirurgie 12:561, 1966.
2. Alberius P, Brandt L, Selvik G: Calvarial growth after linear craniectomy in scaphocephaly as evaluated by x-ray stereophotogrammetry. J Craniomaxillofac Surg 15:2, 1987.
3. Alberti PW, Ruben RJ: Otologic Medicine and Surgery. Vol 2. New York, Churchill Livingstone, 1988, p 1096.
4. Alderman BW, Lammer EJ, Joshua SC, et al: An epidemiologic study of craniosynostoses: Risk indicators for the occurrence of craniosynostosis in Colorado. Am J Epidemiol 128:431, 1988.
5. Anderl H, Mühlbauer W, Twerdy K, Marchac D: Frontofacial advancement with bony separation in craniofacial dysostosis. Plast Reconstr Surg 71:303, 1983.
6. Anderson FM, Geiger L: Craniostenosis: A survey of 204 cases. J Neurosurg 22:229, 1965.
7. Andersson H, Gomes SP: Craniosynostosis: Review of the literature and indications for surgery. Acta Paediatr Scand 57:47, 1968.
8. Apert E: De l'acrocéphalosyndactylie. Bull Mem Soc Méd d'Hôp de Paris 23:1310, 1906.
9. Barden RC, Ford ME, Jensen AG, et al: Effects of craniofacial deformity in infancy on the quality of mother-infant interactions. Child Dev 60:819, 1989.
10. Bu BH, Kaban LB, Vargervik K: Effect of Le Fort III osteotomy on mandibular growth in patients with Crouzon and Apert syndromes. J Oral Maxillofac Surg 47:666, 1989.
11. Björk A: Cranial base development. Am J Orthod 41:198, 1955.
12. Björk A, Björk L: Artificial deformation and cranio-facial asymmetry in ancient Peruvians. J Dent Res 43:353, 1964.
13. Blank CE: Apert's syndrome (a type of acrocephalosyndactyly) — observations on a British series of thirty-nine cases. Ann Hum Gen 24:151, 1960.
14. Blundell JE: Early craniectomies for craniofacial dysostosis. In Converse JN, McCarthy JG, Wood-Smith D (eds): Symposium on Diagnosis and Treatment of Craniofacial Anomalies. St Louis, CV Mosby, 1979, p 311.
15. Bookstein FC: Describing a craniofacial anomaly: Finite elements and the biometrics of landmark locations. Am J Phys Anthropol 74:495, 1987.
16. Breitbart AS, Eaton C, McCarthy JG: Crouzon's syndrome associated with acanthosis nigricans: Ramifications of the craniofacial surgeon. Ann Plast Surg 22:310, 1989.
17. Buchanan RC: Acrocephalosyndactyly or Apert's syndrome. Br J Plast Surg 21:406, 1968.
18. Burdi AR, Kusnetz AB, Venes JL, Gebarski SS: The natural history and pathogenesis of the cranial coronal ring articulations: Implications in understanding the pathogenesis of the Crouzon craniostenotic defects. Cleft Palate J 23:28, 1986.
19. Chana HS, Klauss V: Crouzon's craniofacial dysostosis in Kenya. Br J Ophthalmol 72:196, 1988.
20. Cohen MM Jr (ed): Craniosynostosis: Diagnosis, Evaluation and Management. New York, Raven Press, 1986.
21. Cohen MM Jr: An etiologic and nosologic overview of craniosynostosis syndromes. Birth Defects 11:137, 1975.
22. Converse JM, Kazanjian VH (eds): Surgical Treatment of Facial Injuries, 2nd ed. Baltimore, Williams & Wilkins, 1982.
23. Corey JP, Caldarelli DD, Gould HJ: Otopathology in craniofacial dysostosis. Am J Otol 8(1):14, 1987.
24. Costaras-Volarich M, Pruzansky S: Is the mandible intrinsically different in Apert and Crouzon syndrome? Am J Orthod 85:475, 1984.
25. Cross HE, Opitz JM: Craniosynostosis in the Amish. J Pediatr 75:1037, 1969.
26. Crouzon O: Dysostose cranio-faciale héréditaire. Bull Soc Méd Hôp Paris 33:545, 1912.
27. Cutting CB, McCarthy JG, Berenstein A: Blood supply of the upper craniofacial skeleton: The search for composite calvarial bone flaps. Plast Reconstr Surg 74:603, 1984.
28. Dado DV, Izquierdo R: Absorption of onlay bone grafts in immature rabbits: Membranous versus enchondral bone and bone struts versus paste. Ann Plast Surg 23:39, 1989.
29. Diamond GR, Whitaker L: Ocular motility in craniofacial reconstruction. Plast Reconstr Surg 73:31, 1984.
30. Dodge HW, Wood MW, Kennedy RLJ: Craniofacial dysostosis: Crouzon's disease. Pediatrics 23:98, 1959.

31. Drommer P, Luhr HG: The stabilization of osteotomized maxillary segments with Luhr miniplates in secondary cleft surgery. J Maxillofac Surg 9:166, 1981.
32. Edgerton MT, Jane JA, Berry FA, Fisher JC: The feasibility of craniofacial osteotomies in infants and young children. Scand J Plast Reconstr Surg 8:164, 1974.
33. Edgerton MT, Jane JA, Berry FA: Craniofacial osteotomies and reconstruction in infants and young children. Plast Reconstr Surg 54:13, 1974.
34. Enlow DH, Azuma M: Functional growth boundaries in the human and mammalian face. Birth Defects 11(7):217, 1975.
35. Enlow DH, McNamara JA Jr: The neurocranial basis for facial form and pattern. Angle Orthod 43:256, 1973.
36. Enlow DH: Handbook of Facial Growth, 2nd ed. Philadelphia, WB Saunders, 1982.
37. Farkas LG, Kolar JC, Munro IR: Craniofacial disproportions in Apert's syndrome: An anthropometric study. Cleft Palate J 22:253, 1985.
38. Fishman MA, Hogan GR, Dodge PR: The concurrence of hydrocephalus and craniosynostosis. J Neurosurg 34:621, 1971.
39. Ford EHR: Growth of the human cranial base. Am J Orthod 44:498, 1958.
40. Giblin N, Alley A: Studies in skull growth. Coronal suture fixation. Anat Rec 88:143, 1944.
41. Gillies H, Harrison SH: Operative correction by osteotomy of recessed malar maxillary compound in case of oxycephaly. Br J Plast Surg 3:123, 1950.
42. Gillies H, Millard DR: The Principles and Art of Plastic Surgery. Boston, Little, Brown & Company, 1957.
43. Golabi M, Edwards MSB, Ousterhout DK: Craniosynostosis and hydrocephalus. Neurosurgery 21:63, 1987.
44. Guilleminault C: Obstructive sleep apnea syndrome and its treatment in children: Areas of agreement and controversy. Pediatr Pulmonol 3:429, 1987.
45. Harsha BC, Turvey TA, Powers SK: Use of autogenous cranial bone grafts in maxillofacial surgery: A preliminary report. J Oral Maxillofac Surg 44:11, 1986.
46. Hemmy DC, David DJ, Herman GT: Three-dimensional reconstruction of craniofacial deformity using computed tomography. Neurosurgery 13:534, 1983.
47. Hemmy DC, Tessier PL: CT of dry skulls with craniofacial deformities: Accuracy of three-dimensional reconstruction. Radiology 157:113, 1985.
48. Hendel PM: The harvesting of cranial bone grafts: A guided osteotome. Plast Reconstr Surg 76:642, 1985.
49. Hoffman HJ: Early craniectomy and stripping in craniofacial synostosis. In Converse JM, McCarthy JG, Wood-Smith D (eds): Symposium on Diagnosis and Treatment of Craniofacial Anomalies. St Louis, CV Mosby, 287, 1979.
50. Hoffman HJ, Hendrick EB: Early neurosurgical repair in craniofacial dysmorphism. J Neurosurg 51:796, 1979.
51. Hoffman HJ, Mohr G: Lateral canthal advancement of the supraorbital margin: A new corrective technique in the treatment of coronal synostosis. J Neurosurg 45:376, 1976.
52. Hogan GR, Bauman ML: Hydrocephalus in Apert's syndrome. J Pediatr 79:782, 1971.
53. Horster W: Experience with functionally stable palate osteosynthesis after forward displacement of the upper jaw. J Maxillofac Surg 8:176, 1980.
54. Hoyte DA: A critical analysis of the growth in length of the cranial base. Birth Defects 11:255, 1975.
55. Hunter AGW, Rudd NL: Craniosynostosis. Coronal synostosis: Its familial characteristics and associated clinical findings in 109 patients lacking bilateral polysyndactyly or syndactyly. Teratology 15:301, 1977.
56. Israele V, Siegel JD: Infectious complications of craniofacial surgery in children. Rev Infect Dis 11:9, 1989.
57. Jackson IT, Adham M, Bite U, Marx R: Update on cranial bone grafts in craniofacial surgery. Ann Plast Surg 18:37, 1987.
58. Jackson IT, Hide TAH, Barker DT: Transposition cranioplasty to restore forehead contour in craniofacial deformities. Br J Plast Surg 31:127, 1978.
59. Jackson IT, Pellett C, Smith JM: The skull as a bone graft donor site. Ann Plast Surg 11:527, 1983.
60. Jackson IT, Smith J, Mixter RC: Nasal bone grafting using split skull grafts. Ann Plast Surg 11:533, 1983.
61. Jane JA, Park TS, Zide BM, et al: Alternative techniques in the treatment of unilateral coronal synostosis. J Neurosurg 61:550, 1984.
62. Kaban LB, West B, Conover M, et al: Midface position after Le Fort III advancement. Plast Reconstr Surg 73:758, 1984.
63. Kaye CI, Matalon R, Pruzansky S: The natural history of Apert syndrome, with speculations on pathogenesis. Terotology 17:28A, 1978.
64. Kolar JC, Munro IR, Farkas LG: Patterns of dysmorphology in Crouzon syndrome: An anthropometric study. Cleft Palate J 25:235, 1988.
65. Kreiborg S, Aduss H: Pre- and postsurgical facial growth in patients with Crouzon's and Apert's syndromes. Cleft Palate J (Suppl) 23:78, 1986.
66. Kreiborg S, Björk A: Description of a dry skull with Crouzon syndrome. Scand J Plast Reconstr Surg 16:245, 1982.
67. Kreiborg S: Crouzon syndrome. A clinical and roentgen cephalometric study. Scand J Plast Reconstr Surg (Suppl) 18:1, 1981.
68. Kushner J, Alexander E Jr, Davis CH Jr, et al: Crouzon's disease (craniofacial dysostosis) modern diagnosis and treatment. J Neurosurg 37:434, 1972.

69. Kusiak JF, Zin JE, Whitaker LA: The early revascularization of membranous bone. Plast Reconstr Surg 76:510, 1985.
70. Lane LC: Pioneer craniectomy for relief of mental imbecility due to premature sutural closure and microcephalus. JAMA 18:49, 1892.
71. Lannelongue M: De la cranectomie dans la microcephalie. Compte Rendu Acad Sci 110:1382, 1890.
72. Lauritzen C, Lilja J, Jarlstedt J: Airway obstruction and sleep apnea in children with craniofacial anomalies. Plast Reconstr Surg 77:1, 1986.
73. Lefebvre A, Barclay S: Psychosocial impact of craniofacial deformities before and after reconstructive surgery. Can J Psychiatry 27:579, 1982.
74. Lefebvre A, Travis F, Arndt EM, Munro IR: A psychiatric profile before and after reconstructive surgery in children with Apert's syndrome. Br J Plast Surg 39:510, 1986.
75. Lewin ML: Facial deformity in acrocephaly and its surgical correction. Arch Ophthalmol 47:321, 1952.
76. Longacre JJ, Destefano GA, Holmstrand K: The early versus the late reconstruction of congenital hypoplasia of the facial skeleton and skull. Plast Reconstr Surg 27:489, 1961.
77. Losken HW, Morris WMM, Uys PB, et al: Crouzon's disease. Part I. One-stage correction by combined face and forehead advancement. S Afr Med J 75:274, 1989.
78. Luhr HG: Zur stabilen Osteosynthese bei Unterkieferfrakturen. Deutsch Zahnaerztl Z 23:754, 1968.
79. Marchac D: Problèmes posés par la contention après ostéotomies de type Le Fort III. Rev Stomatol Chir Maxillofac 78:193, 1977.
80. Marchac D: Radical forehead remodeling for craniostenosis. Plast Reconstr Surg 61:823, 1978.
81. Marchac D: Forehead remodeling for craniostenosis. *In* Converse JM, McCarthy JG, Wood-Smith D (eds): Symposium on Diagnosis and Treatment of Craniofacial Anomalies. St. Louis, CV Mosby, 1979, p 323.
82. Marchac D, Cophignon J, Clay C, et al: Réparation des fraces fronto-orbitaires par reposition ou ostéotomie et greffes osseuses. Ann Chir Plast 19:41, 1974.
83. Marchac D, Cophignon J, Van der Meulen J, et al: A propos des ostéotomies d'advancement du crâne et de la face. Ann Chir Plast 19:311, 1974.
84. Marchac D, Renier D: "Le front flottant" traitement précoce des facio-craniosténoses. Ann Chir Plast 24:121, 1979.
85. Marchac D, Renier D: Cranio-facial surgery for craniosynostosis. Scand J Plast Reconstr Surg 15:235, 1981.
86. Marchac D, Renier D: Craniofacial surgery for craniosynostosis improves facial growth: A personal case review. Ann Plast Surg 14:43, 1985.
87. Marchac D, Renier D: Treatment of craniosynostosis in infancy. Clin Plast Surg 14:61, 1987.
88. Marchac D, Renier D, Jones BM: Experience with the "floating forehead." Br J Plast Surg 41:1, 1988.
89. Marsh JL, Vannier MW: The "third" dimension in craniofacial surgery. Plast Reconstr Surg 71:759, 1983.
90. Martin PR, Lefebvre AM: Surgical treatment of sleep-apnea-associated psychosis. Can Med Assoc J 124:978, 1981.
91. Matthews D: Craniofacial surgery—indications, assessment and complications. Br J Plast Surg 32:96, 1979.
92. Matthews DN: Experiences in major craniofacial surgery. Plast Reconstr Surg 59:163, 1977.
93. McCarthy JG: New concepts in the surgical treatment of the craniofacial synostosis syndromes in the infant. Clin Plast Surg 6:201, 1979.
94. McCarthy JG, Coccaro PJ, Epstein F, Converse JM: Early skeletal release in the infant with craniofacial dysostosis: The role of the sphenozygomatic suture. Plast Reconstr Surg 62:335, 1978.
95. McCarthy JG, Coccaro PJ, Epstein FJ: Early skeletal release in the patient with craniofacial dysostosis. *In* Converse JM, McCarthy J, Wood-Smith D (eds): Symposium on Diagnosis and Treatment of Craniofacial Anomalies. St Louis, CV Mosby, 1979, p 295.
96. McCarthy JG, Epstein F, Sadove M, et al: Early surgery for craniofacial synostosis: An 8-year experience. Plast Reconstr Surg 73:521, 1984.
97. McCarthy JG, Grayson B, Bookstein F, et al: Le Fort III advancement osteotomy in the growing child. Plast Reconstr Surg 74:343, 1984.
98. McCarthy JG, Zide BM: The spectrum of calvarial bone grafting: Introduction of the vascularized calvarial bone flap. Plast Reconstr Surg 74:10, 1984.
99. McCarthy JG: The concept of a craniofacial anomalies center. Clin Plast Surg 3(4):611, 1976.
100. McLaurin RL, Matson DD: Importance of early surgical treatment of craniosynostosis. Pediatrics 10:637, 1952.
101. Mohr G, Hoffman HJ, Munro IR, et al: Surgical management of unilateral and bilateral coronal craniosynostosis: 21 years of experience. Neurosurgery 2:83, 1978.
102. Moore KL: The Developing Human: Clinically Oriented Embryology, 3rd ed. Philadelphia, WB Saunders, 1982.
103. Morax S: Oculomotor disorders in craniofacial malformations. *In* Caronni EP (ed): Craniofacial Surgery. Boston, Little, Brown & Company, 1985, p 97.
104. Moss ML: The pathogenesis of premature cranial synostosis in man. Acta Anat 37:351, 1959.
105. Moss ML, Bromberg BE, Song IC, Eisenman G: The passive role of nasal septal cartilage in mid-facial growth. Plast Reconstr Surg 41:536, 1968.
106. Mowlem R: Editorial. Br J Plast Surg 4:231, 1952.
107. Muhlbauer W, Anderl H: Use of miniplates in craniofacial surgery. Proceedings of the 1st

International Congress of the International Society of Craniomaxillofacial Surgeons. Berlin: Springer-Verlag, 1987, p 334.
108. Munro IR: Orbito-cranio-facial surgery: The team approach. Plast Reconstr Surg 55:170, 1975.
109. Munro IR, Sabatier RE: An analysis of 12 years of craniomaxillofacial surgery in Toronto. Plast Reconstr Surg 76:29, 1985.
110. Murray JE, Swanson LT: Mid-face osteotomy and advancement for craniosynostosis. Plast Reconstr Surg 41:299, 1968.
111. Nakano P, Posnick JC: Early morbidity and long term reconstructive results in Apert's syndrome. Proceedings of the 71st Annual Meeting of the American Association of Oral and Maxillofacial Surgeons 47(8):83 (Suppl 1), 1989.
112. Nakano PH, Posnick JC: Long-term results of reconstructive craniofacial surgery in patients with Crouzon syndrome and Apert syndrome. Proceedings of the 46th Annual Meeting of the Cleft Palate-Craniofacial Association, April, 1989, p 26.
113. Nakano PH, Posnick JC: Long-term results of reconstruction in craniofacial dysostosis. Proceedings of the 6th International Congress of Cleft Palate and Related Anomalies, June, 1989, p 56.
114. Nakano PH, Posnick JC: Morbidity and long term reconstruction results in Apert's syndrome. Proceedings of the 43rd Annual Meeting of the Canadian Society of Plastic Surgeons, June, 1989, p 1.
115. Nathan V: Craniofacial dysostosis: Crouzon's disease. West Indian Med J 32:237, 1983.
116. Neill CL: Influence of early cranioplasty for craniostenosis upon cranial and facial configuration. In Smith B, Converse JC (eds): Proceedings of 2nd International Symposium of Plastic and Reconstructive Surgery of the Eye and Adnexa. St. Louis, CV Mosby, 1967, p 302.
117. Norgaard JO, Kvinnsland S: Influence of submucous septal resection on facial growth in the rat. Plast Reconstr Surg 64:84, 1979.
118. Obwegeser HL: Surgical correction of small or retrodisplaced maxillae: The "dish-face" deformity. Plast Reconstr Surg 43:351, 1969.
119. Ortiz-Monasterio F, Fuente del Campo A, Carillo A: Advancement of the orbits and the midface in one piece, combined with frontal repositioning, for the correction of Crouzon's deformities. Plast Reconstr Surg 61:507, 1978.
120. Ortiz-Monasterio F, Fuente del Campo A: Refinements on the bloc orbitofacial advancement. In Caronni EP (ed): Craniofacial Surgery. Boston, Little, Brown & Company, 1985, p 263.
121. Ousterhout DK, Melsen B: Cranial base deformity in Apert's syndrome. Plast Reconstr Surg 69:254, 1982.
122. Ousterhout DK, Vargervik K: Aesthetic improvement resulting from craniofacial surgery in craniosynostosis syndromes. J Craniomaxillofac Surg 15:189, 1987.
123. Palkes HS, Marsh JL, Talent BK: Pediatric craniofacial surgery and parental attitudes. Cleft Palate J 23:137, 1986.
124. Parekh BK, Jakhi SA: Acrocephalosyndactyly. Apert's syndrome — case report of a rarity. Ann Dent 46:31, 1987.
125. Patton MA, Goodship J, Hayward R, Lansdown R: Intellectual development in Apert's syndrome: A long term follow up of 29 patients. J Med Genet 25:164, 1988.
126. Peer LA: Transplantation of Tissues. Vol 1. Baltimore, Williams & Wilkins, 1955.
127. Perren SM: Physical and biological aspects of fracture healing with special reference to internal fixation. Clin Orthop 138:175, 1979.
128. Persing JA, Babler WJ, Jane JA, Duckworth PF: Experimental unilateral coronal synostosis in rabbits. Plast Reconstr Surg 77:369, 1986.
129. Persing JA, Babler WJ, Nagorsky MJ, et al: Skull expansion in experimental craniosynostosis. Plast Reconstr Surg 78:594, 1986.
130. Phillips JH, Rahn BA: Fixation effects on membranous and endochondral onlay bone-graft resorption. Plast Reconstr Surg 82:872, 1988.
131. Posnick JC, Seagle MB, Armstrong D: Nasal reconstruction with full-thickness cranial bone grafts and rigid internal fixation. Plast Reconstr Surg 1990 (in press).
132. Posnick JC, Bite U, Nakano P, et al: Indirect Intracranial Volume Measurements Using CT Scans: Clinical Applications for Craniosynostosis. Plast Reconstr Surg (in press).
133. Poswillo D: Mechanisms and pathogenesis of malformation. Br Med Bull 32:59, 1976.
134. Powiertowski H, Matlosz Z: The treatment of craniostenosis by a method of extensive resection of the vault of the skull. In Proceedings of the 3rd International Congress on Neurosurgery. Surg Excerpta Med Internat Cong Series 110:834, 1965.
135. Pruzansky S: Time: The fourth dimension in syndrome analysis applied to craniofacial malformations. Birth Defects 13(3c):3, 1977.
136. Psillakis JM, Grotting JC, Casanova R, et al: Vascularized outer-table calvarial bone flaps. Plast Reconstr Surg 78:309, 1986.
137. Renier D, Sainte-Rose C, Marchac D, Hirsch J-F: Intracranial pressure in craniostenosis. J Neurosurg 57:370, 1982.
138. Richtsmeirer JT: Comparative study of normal, Crouzon and Apert craniofacial morphology using finite element scaling analysis. Am J Phys Anthropol 74:473, 1987.
139. Rosen HM, Whitaker LA: Cranial base dynamics in craniofacial dysostosis. J Maxillofac Surg 12:56, 1984.
140. Rougerie J, Derome P, Anquez L: Craniosténosis et dysmorphies craniofaciales. Principes d'une nouvelle technique de traitement et ses résultats. Neurochirurgie 18:429, 1972.
141. Sarnat BG: Differential craniofacial skeletal changes after postnatal experimental surgery in young and adult animals. Ann Plast Surg 1:131, 1978.
142. Sarnat BG: The postnatal maxillary-nasal-orbital complex: Some considerations in experimental

surgery. *In* McNamara JA (ed): Factors Affecting the Growth of the Midface. Ann Arbor, University of Michigan Press, 1976.
143. Seeger JF, Gabrielsen TO: Premature closure of the frontosphenoidal suture in synostosis of the coronal suture. Radiology 101:631, 1971.
144. Shiller JG: Craniofacial dysostosis of Crouzon: A case report and pedigree with emphasis on heredity. Pediatrics 23:107, 1959.
145. Shillito J Jr, Matson DD: Craniosynostosis: A review of 519 surgical patients. Pediatrics 41:829, 1968.
146. Smith JD, Abramson M: Membranous vs endochondral bone autografts. Arch Otolaryngol 99:203, 1974.
147. Stewart RE, Dixon G, Cohen A: The pathogenesis of premature craniosynostosis in acrocephalosyndactyly (Apert's syndrome): A reconsideration. Plast Reconstr Surg 59:699, 1977.
148. Stewart RE, Kawamoto HK Jr: Acrocephalosyndactyly (Apert's syndrome): A cause for reconsideration of its pathogenesis. *In* Converse JM, McCarthy JG, Wood-Smith D (eds): Symposium on Diagnosis and Treatment of Craniofacial Anomalies. St. Louis, CV Mosby, 1979, pp 258–262.
149. Stricker M, Montaut J, Hepner H, et al: Les ostéotomies du crâne et de la face. Ann Chir Plast 17:233, 1972.
150. Ten Cate AR, Freeman E, Dickinson JB: Sutural development: Structure and its response to rapid expansion. Am J Orthod 71:622, 1977.
151. Tessier P: Ostéotomies totales de la face. Syndrome de Crouzon, syndrome d'Apert: Oxycéphalies, scaphocéphalies, turricéphalies. Ann Chir Plast 12:273, 1967.
152. Tessier P: Dysostoses cranio-faciales (syndromes de Crouzon et d'Apert). Ostéotomies totales de la face. *In* Transactions of the Fourth International Congress of Plastic and Reconstructive Surgery. Amsterdam, Excerpta Medica, 1969, pp 774–783.
153. Tessier P: Relationship of craniostenoses to craniofacial dysostoses and to faciostenoses: A study with therapeutic implications. Plast Reconstr Surg 48:224, 1971.
154. Tessier P: Autogenous bone grafts taken from the calvarium for facial and cranial applications. Clin Plast Surg 9:531, 1982.
155. Tessier P: The scope and principles—dangers and limitations—and the need for special training—in orbitocranial surgery. *In* Hueston JT (ed): Transactions of the Fifth International Congress of Plastic Surgeons. Australia, Butterworth, 1971, p 903.
156. Tessier P: Total osteotomy of the middle third of the face for faciostenosis or for sequelae of Le Fort III fractures. Plast Reconstr Surg 48:533, 1971.
157. Tessier P: Traitement des dysmorphies faciales propres aux dysostoses cranio-faciales (DCF). Maladies de Crouzon et d'Apert. Ostéotomie totale du massif facial. Déplacement sagittal du massif facial. Neurochirurgie 17:295, 1971.
158. Tessier P: Recent improvement in the treatment of facial and cranial deformities in Crouzon's disease and Apert's syndrome. *In* Symposium on Plastic Surgery of the Orbital Region. St Louis, CV Mosby, 1976, p 271.
159. Tessier P: The craniofaciostenoses (CFS): The Crouzon and Apert diseases, the plagiocephalies. *In* Tessier P, Rougier J, Hervouet F, et al (eds): Plastic Surgery of the Orbit and Eyelids. New York, Masson, 1977, p 200.
160. Tessier PL: Apert's syndrome: acrocephalosyndactyly type I. *In* Caronni EP (ed): Craniofacial Surgery. Boston, Little, Brown & Company, 1985, p 280.
161. Tessier P: Orbital hypertelorism: I. Successive surgical attempts. Materials and methods. Causes and mechanisms. Scand J Plast Reconstr Surg 6:135, 1972.
162. Tessier P: The definitive plastic surgical treatment of the severe facial deformities of craniofacial dysostosis: Crouzon's and Apert's diseases. Plast Reconstr Surg 48:419, 1971.
163. Tessier P, Guiot G, Derome P: Orbital hypertelorism: II. Definite treatment of orbital hypertelorism (OR.H.) by craniofacial or by extracranial osteotomies. Scand J Plast Reconstr 7:39, 1973.
164. Tessier P, Hemmy D: Three dimensional imaging in medicine. A critique by surgeons. Scand J Plast Surg 20:3, 1986.
165. Thaller SR, Powers R, Daniller A: Three-dimensional imaging: A role in acute facial trauma? Med Rev 28:1, 1988.
166. Thompson N, Casson JA: Experimental onlay bone grafts to the jaws. A preliminary study in dogs. Plast Reconstr Surg 46:341, 1970.
167. Tressera L, Fuenmayor P: Early treatment of craniofacial deformities. J Maxillofac Surg 9:1, 1981.
168. van der Meulen JCH, Vaandrager JM: Surgery related to the correction of hypertelorism. Plast Reconstr Surg 71:6, 1983.
169. Vannier MW, Marsh JL, Knapp RH: Three-dimensional reconstruction from CT scans. Disorders of the head. Appl Radiol 16:114, 1987.
170. Vulliamy DG, Normandale PA: Cranio-facial dysostosis in a Dorset family. Arch Dis Child 41:375, 1966.
171. Waitzman A, Posnick J, Armstrong D, Pron G: Normal values and growth trends in pediatric cranio-orbito-zygomatic measurements. Proceedings of the 47th Annual Meeting of the American Cleft Palate Craniofacial Association. St. Louis, May 1990, p 28.
172. Whitaker LA, Bartlett SP, Schut L, Bruce D: Craniosynostosis: An analysis of the timing, treatment, and complications in 164 consecutive patients. Plast Reconstr Surg 80:195, 1987.
173. Whitaker LA, Broennle AM, Kerr LP, Herlich A: Improvements in craniofacial reconstruction: Methods evolved in 235 consecutive patients. Plast Reconstr Surg 65:561, 1980.
174. Whitaker LA, Schut L, Kerr LP: Early surgery for isolated craniofacial dysostosis. Improvement and possible prevention of increasing deformity. Plast Reconstr Surg 60:575, 1977.

175. Wilkes GH, Kernahan DA, Christenson M: The long-term survival of onlay bone grafts—a comparative study in mature and immature animals. Ann Plast Surg 15:374, 1985.
176. Witzel MA, Ross RB, Munro IR: Articulation before and after facial osteotomy. J Maxillofac Surg 8:195, 1980.
177. Witzel MA: Speech problems in craniofacial anomalies. Commun Disord 8:45, 1983.
178. Wolfe SA, Berkowitz S: The use of cranial bone grafts in the closure of alveolar and anterior palatal clefts. Plast Reconstr Surg 72:659, 1983.
179. Zins JE, Kusiak JF, Whitaker LA, Enlow DH: The influence of the recipient site on bone grafts to the face. Plast Reconstr Surg 73:371, 1984.
180. Zins JE, Whitaker LA: Membranous versus endochondral bone: Implications for craniofacial reconstruction. Plast Reconstr Surg 72:778, 1983.

Acknowledgments: I am grateful to Dr. I. R. Munro for the work he did in organizing and developing craniofacial surgery at The Hospital for Sick Children, Toronto, Ontario. He served as the craniofacial surgeon from 1971 until June of 1986. In July of 1986, I became the craniofacial surgeon and the Medical Director of the Craniofacial Program, a position I continue to hold. I also wish to acknowledge the work of Drs. H. J. Hoffman, R. B. Hendrick, J. Drake, J. K. Rutka, and R. P. Humphreys in neurosurgical care and surgical collaboration provided at HSC, and Drs. R. B. Ross and A. P. Dagys for orthodontic care. The consistent dedication by the members of the Departments of Anaesthesia, Neuroradiology, Nursing, Ophthalmology, Otolaryngology, Speech Pathology, Plastic Surgery, Psychiatry, and Social Work, along with others in the planning and ongoing care of these patients, is appreciated. This book chapter was prepared with the assistance of Medical Publications, The Hospital for Sick Children, Toronto, Ontario.

54

THE EFFECTS OF ORTHOGNATHIC SURGERY ON GROWTH OF THE MAXILLA IN PATIENTS WITH VERTICAL MAXILLARY EXCESS

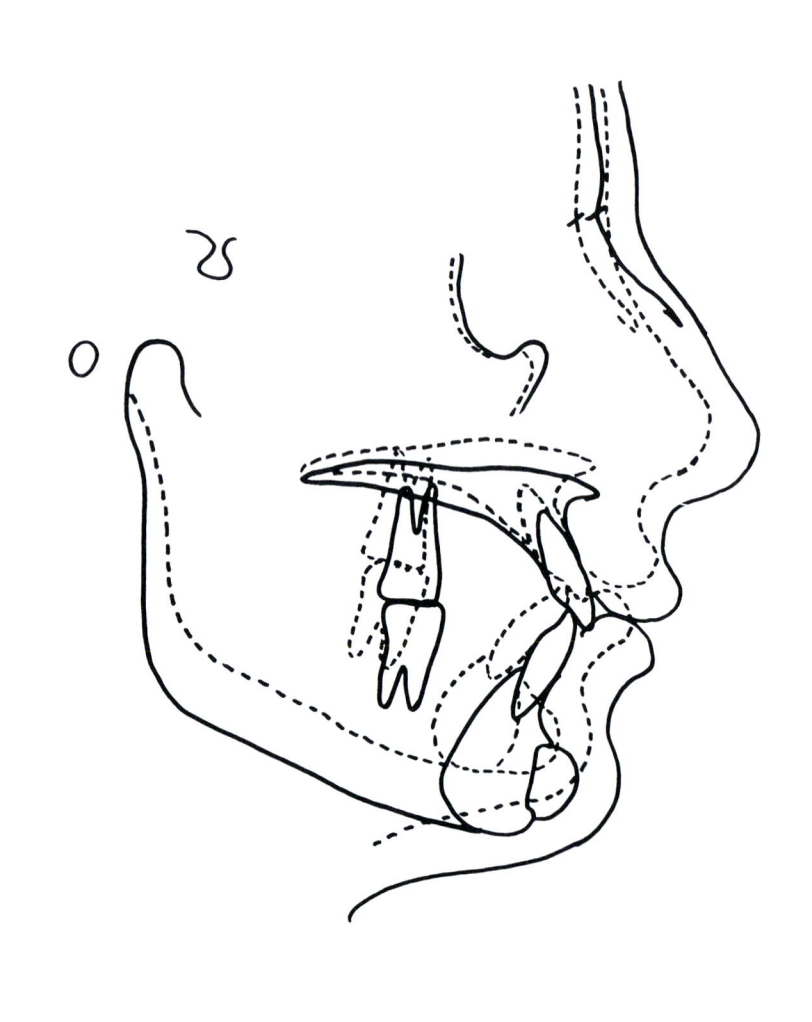

54

CONTROL OF MAXILLARY GROWTH
THE DIRECTION OF MAXILLARY GROWTH
ABNORMAL MAXILLARY GROWTH
ANIMAL STUDIES
POSTSURGICAL STABILITY OF THE MAXILLA
SURGERY IN VERTICALLY EXCESSIVE INDIVIDUALS

COMPARISON OF SURGICAL PATIENTS TO MATCHED CONTROLS
   Surgical Technique
   Data Collection
   Untreated Control
   Results
   Clinical Significance of Results
USE OF THE SURGICAL-ORTHODONTIC APPROACH IN THE VERTICALLY GROWING ADOLESCENT
CASE PRESENTATIONS

FRANK J. MOGAVERO
PETER H. BUSCHANG
LARRY M. WOLFORD

Orthognathic surgery has become a useful and acceptable treatment modality for many patients with skeletal discrepancies in addition to orthodontic problems. In the nongrowing patient, postsurgical changes can usually be attributed to instability at the osteotomy site or to temporomandibular joint (TMJ) problems, such as joint edema, hemarthrosis, condylar malposition, or condylar resorption. Postsurgical change is of greater concern in the growing patient, for whom further growth—or lack of growth—could adversely affect the treatment result. The functional, esthetic, and psychological benefits to the patient when surgery is done during growth must be weighed against the patient's sometimes unpredictable growth potential and the unknown effects of surgery on the growing craniofacial skeleton. The inability to predict growth subsequent to surgery is especially significant for the maxillary complex. Because surgical trauma could affect growth and the long-term surgical-orthodontic outcome for these young patients, practitioners may select a nonsurgical treatment plan with a compromised result.

If most of the anteroposterior maxillary growth is complete by puberty,[44,53] then only minimal effects of maxillary surgery on growth of the maxilla during adolescence should be expected, especially if the cartilage of the nasal septum is considered inactive at this time.[50]

Conversely, it is possible that maxillary growth in normal, untreated patients continues well into adulthood. Behrents,[6] surveying data from 113 young adults followed 25 to 35 years into adulthood, found significant increases in many craniofacial dimensions. Lewis and Roche,[29] in an attempt to estimate ages at which growth ceased, recently found that growth of the cranial base and mandible continues into the second and third decades, albeit at a much reduced rate. Nevertheless, the majority of facial growth is complete following puberty. Approximately 98 to 100 per cent of maxillary growth of 22-year-old males and females is complete by 15.5 years of age.[12]

One important reason for performing early orthognathic surgery relates to the psychological well-being of the patient. Facial appearance is fundamental in determining interpersonal relationships.[30,31] Patients with severe skeletal deformities are likely to be less attractive than their peers when they are entering the teen dating years, and differences in behavior toward attractive versus unattractive individuals are well documented.[1,2] Waiting to do orthognathic surgery until growth is complete or choosing a nonsurgical treatment plan merely to provide teeth that mesh while compromising overall facial esthetics could be detrimental to the patient's self-image during the impressionable teen years. Graber[23] noted that treatment regimens that improve facial appearance appear to produce concomitant improvements in esthetic self-satisfaction and body image. While much work is still required in the evaluation of post-treatment patients, it can be stated that, for the most part, treatment-induced improvements in facial functional and esthetics result in associated improvements in self-esteem.

A dentofacial skeletal discrepancy recognized in adolescence and left untreated until adulthood can also cause or aggravate problems in occlusion, masticatory function, TMJ function and morphology, speech, airway, and esthetics.[37] A major concern when operating on young patients is the presence of unerupted permanent teeth, including the cuspids, bicuspids, and molars, that could be damaged during surgery. These teeth usually are erupted and can be aligned orthodontically by the ages of 12 to 13 years.

CONTROL OF MAXILLARY GROWTH

Normal growth of the maxilla must be carefully considered when attempting to evaluate the effects of maxillary surgery. Unfortunately, the mechanisms of normal growth are not well understood. Beginning with Fick in the 19th century,[20] many researchers have studied the role of the nasal cartilage in attempting to define the mechanism of normal growth.[52]

Scott's theories on the role of the nasal septum as a pacemaker for midfacial growth are perhaps the best known. Scott[47] defined two distinct phases of midfacial growth. During the first 7 years of life, growth of the brain and the eye increases the size of the cranial base and orbits; nasal cartilage forces the maxillary complex away from the sphenoid bone. After 7 years of age, corresponding to closure of the sphenoethmoidal suture, growth of the cranial base and orbits is minimal, and the nasal cartilage ceases to grow. Subsequent maxillary growth is attributed primarily to apposition of bone, with vertical growth predominating and with limited horizontal growth and width changes. Scott[48] concluded that the horizontal component in the growth of the cartilage of the nasal septum can be estimated by the length of the hard palate.

Sarnat and Wexler[41] found that extensive resection of nasal cartilage in young growing rabbits resulted in a marked lack of midfacial growth. Kvinnsland[26] and Gange and Johnston[22] showed similar growth changes in studies involving partial resection of the nasal cartilage in rats.

By contrast, Moss et al subordinated the role of the nasal septum to that of a passive or compensatory response associated with orofacial function.[36] According to the "functional matrix" theory, the nasal cartilage had no direct "morphogenetic" role in the growth of the maxilla. Proponents of the theory believe that it is simply the collapse of the roof of the nasal cavity which leads to growth retardation in surgical patients.

Babula's group[3] concluded that while the cartilaginous nasal septum was significantly shorter in mice fetuses with bilateral clefts of the lip and palate, this finding alone did *not* support the view that the nasal septum acts as a growth center. In a study involving young guinea pigs, Stenstrom and Thilander[55] concluded that the nasal septal cartilage is not a primary growth center for the midfacial skeleton; rather, its main function is related to mechanical support.

Searching for an alternative mechanism, Latham and Scott[28] suggested that the septo-premaxillary ligament pulls the maxilla downward and forward. Latham[27] subsequently proposed that osteogenesis at the posterior and superior maxillary surfaces exerts forces against the circummaxillary pad of fatty tissue to induce sutural adjustment of the maxilla. The roles of sutures and periosteum in maxillary growth have also been examined.[16,34] In general, growth of the maxilla has been attributed to numerous factors, including growth at synchondroses such as the nasal septum, growth at the sutures, remodeling, and the influence of the soft tissue and environmental factors.

THE DIRECTION OF MAXILLARY GROWTH

Björk[9,10] concluded that the increase in height of the maxilla takes place by "growth at its processes; suturally toward the frontal and zygomatic bones and appositionally on the lower aspect of the alveolar process in association with the eruption of teeth." The maxilla tends to rotate forward during growth, but differential remodeling maintains the relationship of the nasal floor to the anterior cranial base. Growth in the length of the maxilla occurs "suturally towards the palatine bones and by apposition on the maxillary tuberosities."

Scott[49] and Enlow[15] note that maxillary growth in both higher primates and humans tends to be oriented more vertically than horizontally. Melsen,[33] evaluating 132 human skulls from India, found that during development, the maxillary complex as a whole moves downward and forward from the time of fully erupted deciduous teeth until the permanent canines and premolars are fully erupted. The direction of growth changes to become mainly downward during the last part of the growth period.

Singh and Savara[44,53] studied the size and rates of maxillary growth for boys and girls 3 to 16 years of age. They found that in girls, height and length of the maxilla grow at approximately the same rates from 3 to 6 years. After a slight lag period, maxillary height grows faster than length from 8 to 16 years of age. An adolescent spurt in maxillary growth was found between 10 and 12 years of age in girls. Growth of the maxilla was similar for boys, who experienced their adolescent spurt 1 to 3 years later than girls.

ABNORMAL MAXILLARY GROWTH

An understanding of the mechanisms and direction of normal growth is important when variations in normal maxillary growth are considered. Sassouni and Nanda[42] analyzed longitudinal cephalograms taken from birth to adulthood of eight individuals with Class II skeletal open bite and eight with Class II skeletal deep bite. The open-bite patients were found to have a greater maxillary dental height at both the incisor and molar levels, as well as unfavorable (clockwise) rotation of the mandible. Schendel and coworkers[45] characterized the open-bite morphology as the "long face syndrome," characterized by excessive lower facial height, extreme clockwise rotation of the mandible, adenoid facies, idiopathic long face, total maxillary alveolar hyperplasia, and vertical maxillary excess (VME). Excessive vertical maxillary growth is described as the "common denominator" for these patients. They generally show an inordinate amount of the maxillary teeth and gingiva upon smiling. Anterior open bites may or may not be present.

When patients with maxillary hyperplasia present for orthodontic treatment as adolescents, the treatment plan of choice for the best functional and esthetic result often calls for orthognathic surgery in conjunction with orthodontics. Surgery commonly involves a Le Fort I osteotomy with superior repositioning of the maxilla.[17,59]

The effects of maxillary surgery on growth of the maxillary complex are poorly understood. Epker and Wolford[17] described the use of Le Fort I osteotomy with complete mobilization of the osteotomized segments and their overcorrection due to relapse. Fixation at that time involved only the use of suspension wires and intermaxillary fixation. They reported some success in treating patients 8 to 12 years old but did not have data regarding their subsequent growth.

While noting that the faces of baboons grow in a much more horizontal direction than those of humans, Siegel[52] found that nasal septal cartilage resection in baboons had an effect on growth of the maxilla; however, if the surgery was done at a later age, more growth had been attained and the effect was less noticeable. They conclude that "what [growth] is lost as a result of surgery is lost forever."

Freihofer,[21] in examining the effects of various surgical procedures on growth in adolescents, found that maxillary advancements performed "too early" would experience "pseudorelapse" because of continued growth of the mandible without apparent maxillary growth. However, 19 of the 20 cases were cleft palate patients, for whom maxillary retrusion is well established. Freihofer was not able to determine whether further growth of the maxilla occurred following surgery.

The problems of maxillary surgery during growth may be compounded when maxillary growth is already deficient, as in patients requiring Le Fort I anterior and inferior repositioning of the maxilla[51] or in craniofacial syndrome patients requiring Le Fort III advancement surgery.[4,32] In patients exhibiting maxillary hypoplasia, a second surgery after completion of facial growth may be indicated.[4]

ANIMAL STUDIES

Conclusions drawn from animal studies assessing the effects of maxillary surgery on growth have also been variable. Kokich and Shapiro,[25] studying six juvenile (27 to 33 months) *Macaca nemestrina* monkeys, found that maxillary Le Fort I advancement osteotomies adversely affected anteroposterior maxillary growth. They suggest that anteriorly directed postsurgical extraoral forces be applied when Le Fort I advancement osteotomy is performed in patients who already have severe hypoplasia due to lack of growth prior to surgery. Nanda and Topazian[37] studied seven experimental and eight control *Macaca fascicularis* monkeys, 30 to 40 months of age. It was found that in the experimental monkeys, who had Le Fort I osteotomies with impaction, the vertical component of growth was "most aberrant" following surgery. The vertical displacement was primarily in a superior direction in four monkeys and in an inferior direction in three monkeys. However, anteroposteriorly the maxilla and mandible were found to grow in a "harmonious fashion" after total maxillary osteotomy; the mandible of each experimental animal showed significantly less growth than did those of the controls, although it was subjected to no surgical intervention. Growth during the first 6 months after surgery was relatively less than in controls, but long-term follow-up showed a "significant increase in growth."

Nanda et al.[38] studied 14 *Macaca fascicularis* monkeys 30 to 41 months old; three received Le Fort I osteotomies with a 4-mm advancement only (Group I), three received Le Fort I osteotomies with a 5-mm advancement and a 2.5-mm impaction (Group II), and eight monkeys served as controls. Transosseous wires without maxillomandibular fixation were used to fix the maxilla into its final position. The mean anterior (horizontal) displacement of the premaxilla in Groups I and II was reduced 37 per cent and 67 per cent, respectively, in relation to the control group 12 months after surgery. With respect to the vertical dimension, the overall incremental change in anterior facial height of the control group, especially of the lower facial height, was significantly greater than that of the experimental groups. The Group II animals, in which the maxilla had been superiorly repositioned as well as advanced, demonstrated the greatest decrease in overall maxillary growth. The authors conclude that injury to the nasal septal complex may have inhibited maxillary growth and displacement. Excision of the nasal septal cartilage *retarded* but *did not stop* the anterior growth of the maxilla. The mandible followed the maxillary growth pattern in both experimental groups.

POSTSURGICAL STABILITY OF THE MAXILLA

Postsurgical stability must be considered if the surgical effects on growth are to be addressed. Previous studies of nongrowing patients having undergone Le Fort I osteotomy *without* rigid fixation have demonstrated that immediately after surgery and during the fixation period (generally 6 weeks), the maxilla was somewhat unstable and continued to move upward, as well as slightly posteriorly at A-point; after the fixation period the results were stable.[8,11,39,46] Interestingly, Denison et al[14] reported greater stability of superiorly repositioned maxillae in nongrowing patients without open bite than in those with open bite malocclusions.

By contrast, Hennes et al[24] studied the stability of maxillary osteotomies with superior repositioning and concomitant mandibular advancement using rigid fixation in nongrowing patients. Postoperatively, the maxilla showed no significant superior vertical movement, although there was a slight tendency for posterior movement at A-point during the 9-month postsurgical period. Similarly Turvey et al[56] found a tendency toward posterior and inferior rotation of the entire maxillomandibular complex following superior repositioning of the maxilla and mandibular advancement using wire fixation. They concluded that double-jaw surgery is more stable than mandibular advancement alone when vertical maxillary excess or open bite is associated with mandibular deficiency. Skoczylas and coworkers[54] examined the short-term (4 to 8 weeks) stability of rigid versus skeletal wire fixation in 30 patients who had undergone superior maxillary repositioning and mandibular advancement. They found no significant difference in stability between the two techniques with regard to nondental maxillary landmarks, although they did note a significantly greater amount of vertical molar movement postsurgically in the skeletal wire fixation group.

Finally, Satrom[43] recently examined the long-term (15 months) stability of rigid internal fixation versus skeletal wire fixation in 33 nongrowing patients who had also undergone superior repositioning of the maxilla with simultaneous mandibular advancement. He found that the maxilla was very stable both horizontally and vertically for both fixation methods. While the rigid fixation sample was moved forward 1.6 mm more at A-point, it showed no tendency for posterior movement at A-point. The wire sample showed a "nonsignificant" tendency for posterior movement postsurgically and a slightly greater tendency for inferior movement of the maxilla after surgery.

SURGERY IN VERTICALLY EXCESSIVE INDIVIDUALS

Few studies examining maxillary postsurgical growth in VME patients have been reported. Epker et al[19] and Washburn et al[58] reported on the effects of superior maxillary positioning in 12 individuals 10 to 16 years of age, treated between 1973 and 1977 with intermaxillary fixation and suspension wiring for stabilization. The average superior movement of the maxilla was 5.3 mm; neither the duration of postsurgical fixation nor the type of surgical splint worn was indicated. The authors found that "slightly less than normal" vertical growth occurred following surgery, and there was no significant change in the anteroposterior dimension of the maxilla with growth. It was concluded that in view of the damage to nasal septal cartilage during maxillary surgery, the surgeon should consider the use of complete maxillary alveolar osteotomy,[18] which requires virtually no septal resection. Some decrease in vertical maxillary growth in these patients was attributed to increased masticatory efficiency following surgery. Later animal studies by Nanda et al[38] supported the view that total alveolar osteotomy may be the treatment of choice for younger individuals.

Recently, Vig and Turvey[57] examined the presurgical and postsurgical lateral cephalograms of 17 females and 3 males between 13.7 and 16.5 years at the time of maxillary superior repositioning. The mean age at surgery was 14.9 years. The "longest follow-up records" ranged from 2 to 7 years, with a mean of 3.3 years.

Results

Presurgically, both plate fixation and wire fixation groups demonstrated significant inferior vertical growth, which was similar in magnitude and not statistically different from that of their matched controls. Vertical growth was excessive compared to published norms for both experimental and control subjects. Both experimental groups and their controls demonstrated modest presurgical horizontal growth, although somewhat reduced in comparison to normally growing children.

There were no differences between the plate fixation and wire fixation groups with respect to median surgical moves. This was important for the comparison of postsurgical effects between the two groups.

Postsurgical vertical growth for both the plate fixation and the wire fixation samples was again excessive compared to published norms, but not significantly different from that of the matched controls. Postsurgical vertical changes for both rigid and wire fixation groups, while not different from those of controls, were somewhat less than presurgical changes. This decrease in vertical growth is expected because most of the patients were past their peak growth following surgery. Vertical growth and treatment changes for ANS and PNS are illustrated in Figures 54–3 and 54–4.

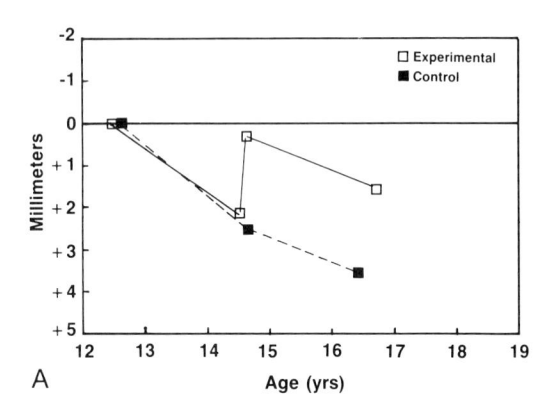

FIGURE 54–3. Vertical changes at ANS (mm) from the initial position show that the growth rates between the experimental subjects and their controls were essentially parallel both presurgically and postsurgically. The sharp step in the experimental curves indicates surgical change between the T2 and T3 occasions. *A*, Plate fixation group. *B*, Wire fixation group.

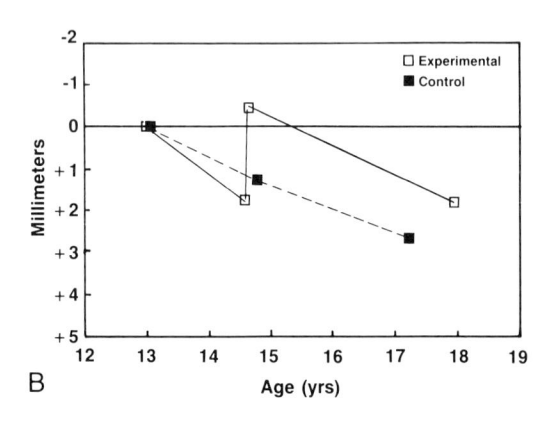

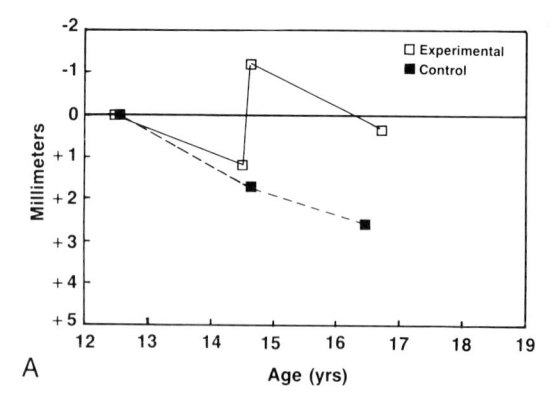

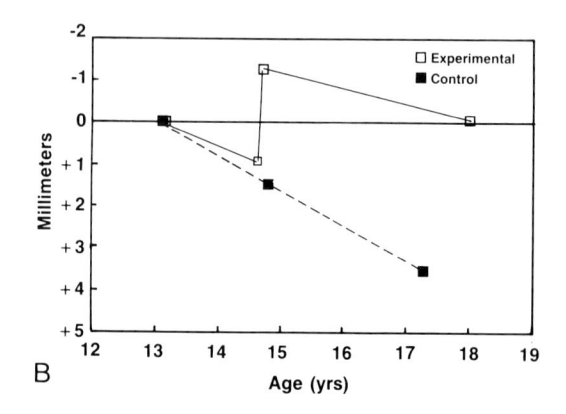

FIGURE 54–4. Vertical changes at PNS (mm) from the initial position show that the growth rates between the experimental subjects and their controls were essentially parallel both presurgically and postsurgically. The sharp step in the experimental curves indicates surgical change between the T2 and T3 occasions. *A*, Plate fixation group. *B*, Wire fixation group.

TABLE 54-1. POSTSURGICAL GROWTH DIFFERENCES BETWEEN EXPERIMENTAL AND CONTROL GROUPS (WILCOXON MATCHED-PAIRS SIGNED-RANKS TEST)

MEASURES	PLATES	WIRES
Horizontal		
A-point	0.010	<0.001
ANS	NS	<0.001
PNS	NS	NS
U1	0.038	0.006
U6	NS	0.007
PNS-A	0.013	<0.001
Angular		
SNA	NS	<0.001

Greater postsurgical variability existed in the horizontal dimensions. The posterior maxilla and palate of the plate fixation group did not show evidence of relapse or decreased growth compared to that of controls except for differences at A-point, reflected in the palatal length PNS-A, and at the upper incisor. Because ANS and the upper molar were not affected, these changes were attributed to postsurgical orthodontics (Table 54-1). Conversely, subjects in the wire fixation group experienced a general horizontal posterior relapse of the entire maxilla. They showed highly significant differences from controls in a posterior direction at every maxillary point except PNS. Horizontal changes with age are illustrated in Figures 54-5 to 54-7.

The larger posterior changes seen postsurgically in the wire fixation sample versus the plate fixation sample are comparable to those seen in previous studies on nongrowing patients, whereas inferior vertical changes demonstrated were much greater than those seen in the literature pertaining to Le Fort I osteotomies performed on nongrowing patients. The observed vertical growth and lack of horizontal growth were not surprising, because according to Enlow[15] and others, the human maxilla is expected to grow vertically, with little anterior component, during adolescence.

Clinical Significance of Results

Several conclusions were drawn from Mogavero's study:

1. Le Fort I osteotomy has little or no effect on postsurgical vertical growth.

FIGURE 54-5. Horizontal changes at A-point (mm) from the initial position. Differences between experimental subjects and their controls were seen in both groups both presurgically and postsurgically, presumably a result of presurgical and postsurgical orthodontic changes involving the maxillary incisor. The sharp step in the experimental curves indicates surgical change between the T2 and T3 occasions. *A*, Plate fixation group. *B*, Wire fixation group.

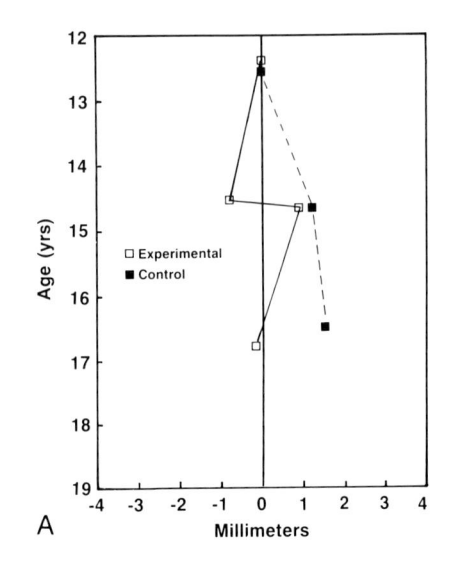

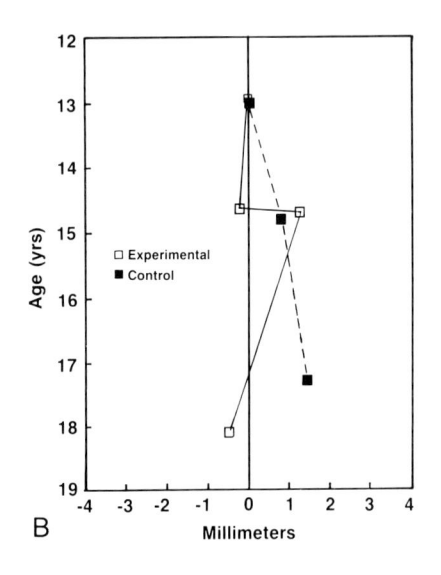

pected outcome of nonsurgical versus surgical treatment, even though the individual may require orthognathic surgery at a later time. Conversely, other adolescents present with severe posterior vertical maxillary excess and a disfiguring "gummy smile" with or without open bite, constricted maxilla, and/or retrusive mandible. It is not reasonable to expect orthodontic treatment alone to provide an acceptable result in these severe cases. Growth modification, which can possibly halt vertical growth, has never been shown to reverse that which has already been expressed.

Rather than wait until growth has been completed, it seems prudent to carry out the correct treatment plan from the beginning and operate on these severe cases early in order to provide the optimal dental, skeletal, functional, and esthetic results. Importantly, earlier treatment might also allow the patient to avoid going through his or her adolescent years with a poor self-image due to an uncorrected skeletal deformity. Proffit and coworkers,[39] in a study of 61 patients who had undergone Le Fort I osteotomy with superior repositioning of the maxilla, separately examined the postsurgical stability of the patients who were less than 18 years old at the time of surgery. One third of the patients were 18 or younger, but the youngest were 14 and mature females. All patients were stabilized using wire fixation. No difference in stability emerged between the younger and older groups, and it was concluded that "after the completion of the adolescent growth spurt, surgical repositioning of the maxilla is as stable as it will be later."

The study by Mogavero[35] is especially relevant because it examined growth compared to matched controls using both rigid and wire fixation. By comparing changes in the experimental groups to those in their matched controls, the presence of vertical growth without horizontal growth could be positively identified in these subjects, just as observed in the untreated controls. Despite this continued vertical growth, the surgeon (LMW) could identify no more generalized long-term postsurgical problems of stability, function, or esthetics in the operated growing patients than he has observed in the nongrowing adult patients in his practice. Even with the continued vertical growth occurring postsurgically, these patients apparently grow in proportion and do not appear to "grow back into a long face syndrome." Nevertheless, a few patients did demonstrate an increase in their tooth-to-lip relationships from the immediate to the long-term postsurgical period.

Mogavero further reported that following superior repositioning of the maxilla in adolescents, rigid fixation appears to provide superior long-term anteroposterior and vertical stability compared to skeletal wire fixation in growing patients. This result is supported by the literature.

It is our conclusion that superior repositioning of the maxilla to correct vertical maxillary excess may be safely undertaken in the adolescent without increased potential for the patient to "grow out" of the surgery, as is known to occur in true mandibular prognathism. This conclusion is supported by Vig and Turvey.[57]

Orthognathic surgery may not be indicated for every patient with vertical maxillary excess, and, like orthodontics, it is not without its own set of inherent problems and failures. Nevertheless, early surgical correction of severe vertical maxillary excess can provide excellent functional and esthetic results in the adolescent, providing the patient with both a beautiful smile and a better self-image.

CASE PRESENTATIONS

CASE 1

This 12-year, 6-month-old female was seen for surgical evaluation to correct her "gummy smile" (see Chapter 9). She had been under orthodontic treatment for approximately 1 year with a good orthodontic result. She had difficulty getting her lips together when chewing and for speech. In addition, she had significant inflammation and hypertrophy of her maxillary gingiva, particularly around the anterior teeth. There was a periodontal concern as well as an esthetic concern (Fig. 54–8).

54 — EFFECTS OF SURGERY ON MAXILLARY GROWTH IN PATIENTS WITH VERTICAL MAXILLARY EXCESS / 1945

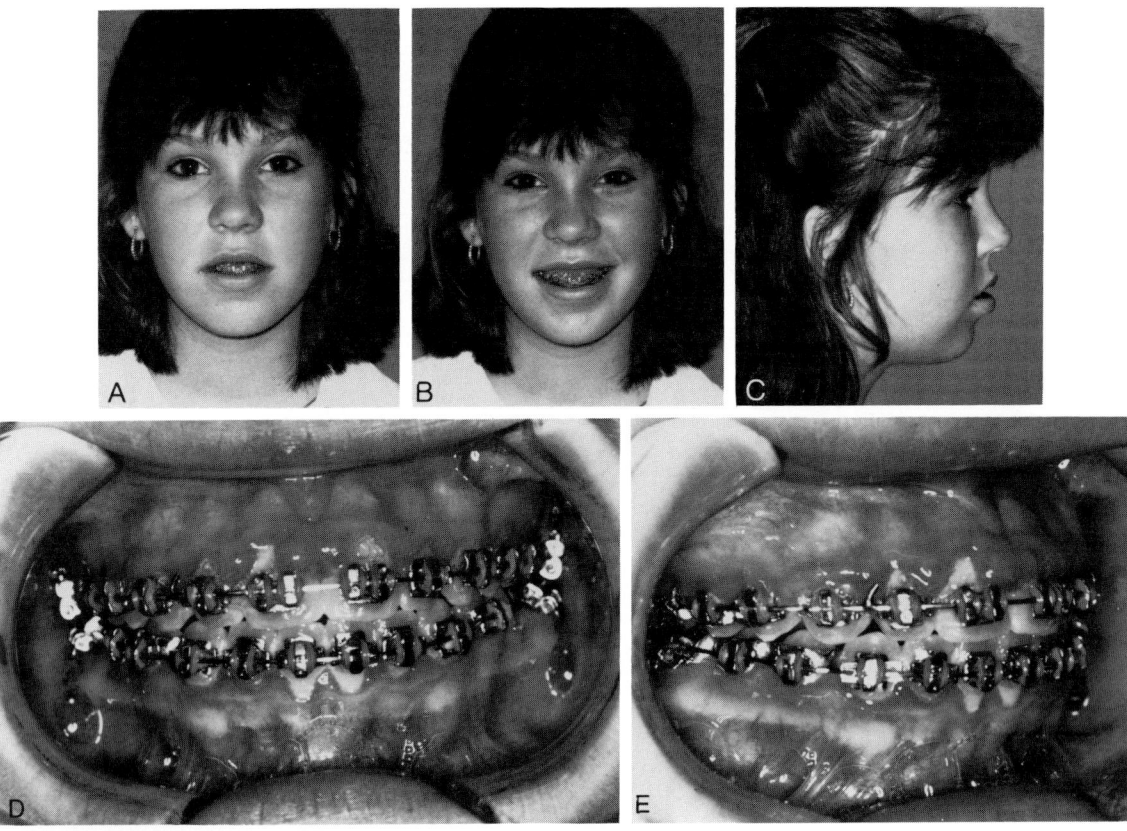

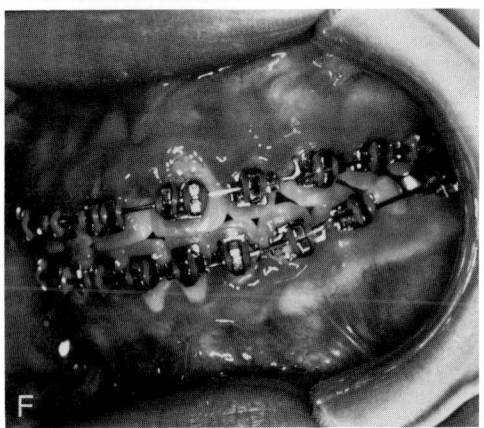

FIGURE 54-8. *A*, This 12-year, 6-month-old female presented for correction of vertical maxillary excess. The lip incompetence is evident. *B*, When smiling, she shows a significant amount of hyperplastic inflamed gingiva. *C*, The profile view demonstrates an increased vertical height of the lower third of the face and AP microgenia. *D* to *F*, The patient has been under orthodontic treatment for 1 year and has a good Class I cuspid-molar relationship.

PROBLEM LIST

Esthetics. In the frontal view, with her lips relaxed, she had significant lip incompetence (Fig. 54–8*A*). In smiling, she showed a significant amount of teeth (6 mm) and gingiva with gingival inflammation and hypertrophy (Fig. 54–8*B*). In profile view, she had a long lower third of the face and significant lip incompetence in a relaxed position. With her lips together, she had hyperfunction of the mentalis muscle. Also, she demonstrated AP deficiency of the chin (Fig. 54–8*C*).

Cephalometric Analysis. Cephalometric analysis demonstrated vertical maxillary excess and AP maxillary deficiency. Also, there was AP microgenia present. The lower third of the face was excessively long secondary to the VME (Fig. 54–9*A*).

Occlusion. The patient had been under orthodontic treatment for approximately 1 year prior to surgical evaluation. The occlusion was essentially a Class I cuspid-molar relationship (Fig. 54–8*D* to *F*).

TREATMENT PLAN

Orthodontic Treatment. The orthodontics had been completed to align and level the teeth and establish a Class I cuspid-molar relationship. No additional orthodontic recommendations were made.

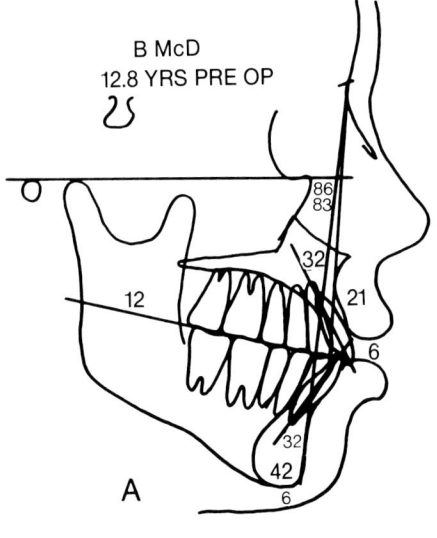

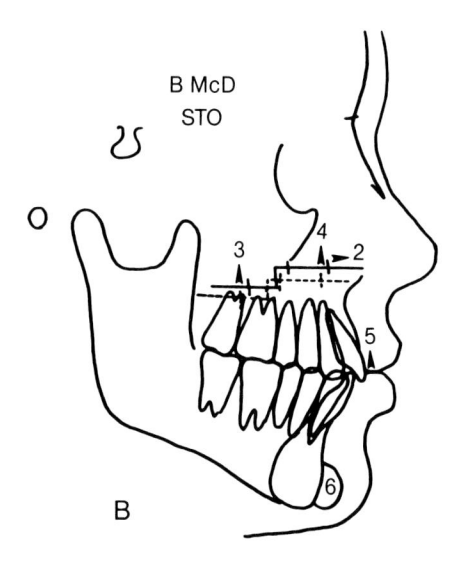

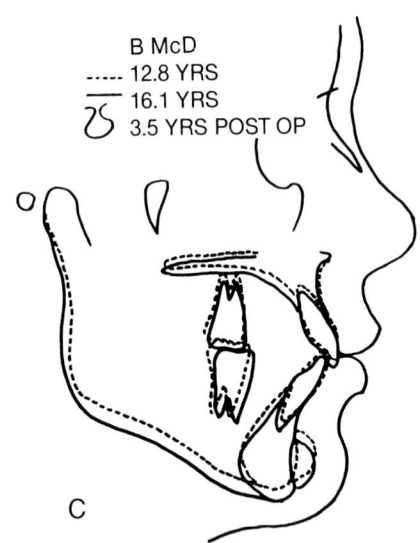

FIGURE 54-9. *A*, Cephalometric analysis demonstrates vertical maxillary excess and slight AP maxillary deficiency. AP microgenia is present, and the lower third of the face is excessively long. *B*, The surgical treatment objective demonstrates superior movement of the maxillary incisors 5 mm and a maxillary advancement of 2 mm. A 6-mm alloplastic chin augmentation was also planned. *C*, Superimposition of the immediate postoperative and 3-year, 5-month follow-up radiographs demonstrates predominantly vertical growth of the maxilla and mandible. The jaws appear to have grown harmoniously.

Surgical Treatment

1. Multiple maxillary osteotomies were performed using the maxillary step osteotomy designed to move the maxilla superiorly and slightly forward. Stabilization was achieved with bone plates. The maxilla was moved superiorly 5 mm at the incisor tip (Fig. 54-9*B*).
2. Augmentation genioplasty of 6 mm to improve chin projection.

Active Treatment. The patient was operated on at the age of 12 years, 8 months. The Class I cuspid-molar relationship was maintained with the surgical procedure, and the maxilla was placed into proper vertical position. Bone plates were used to stabilize the maxilla. No intermaxillary fixation was used, but light anterior vertical elastics were used for approximately 2 or 3 weeks to help control the occlusion. The orthodontic appliances were removed 3 months after surgery.

Long-Term Follow-up. The patient was followed periodically with long-term follow-up at 3 years, 5 months after surgery (Fig. 54-10*A* to *C*). She has continued to have harmonious growth between the maxilla and mandible. The growth vector, however, has been predominantly vertical (see Fig. 54-9*C*). A good Class I cuspid-molar relationship has been maintained, and she has excellent jaw function with no TMJ and/or myofacial pain problems (Fig. 54-10*D* to *F*).

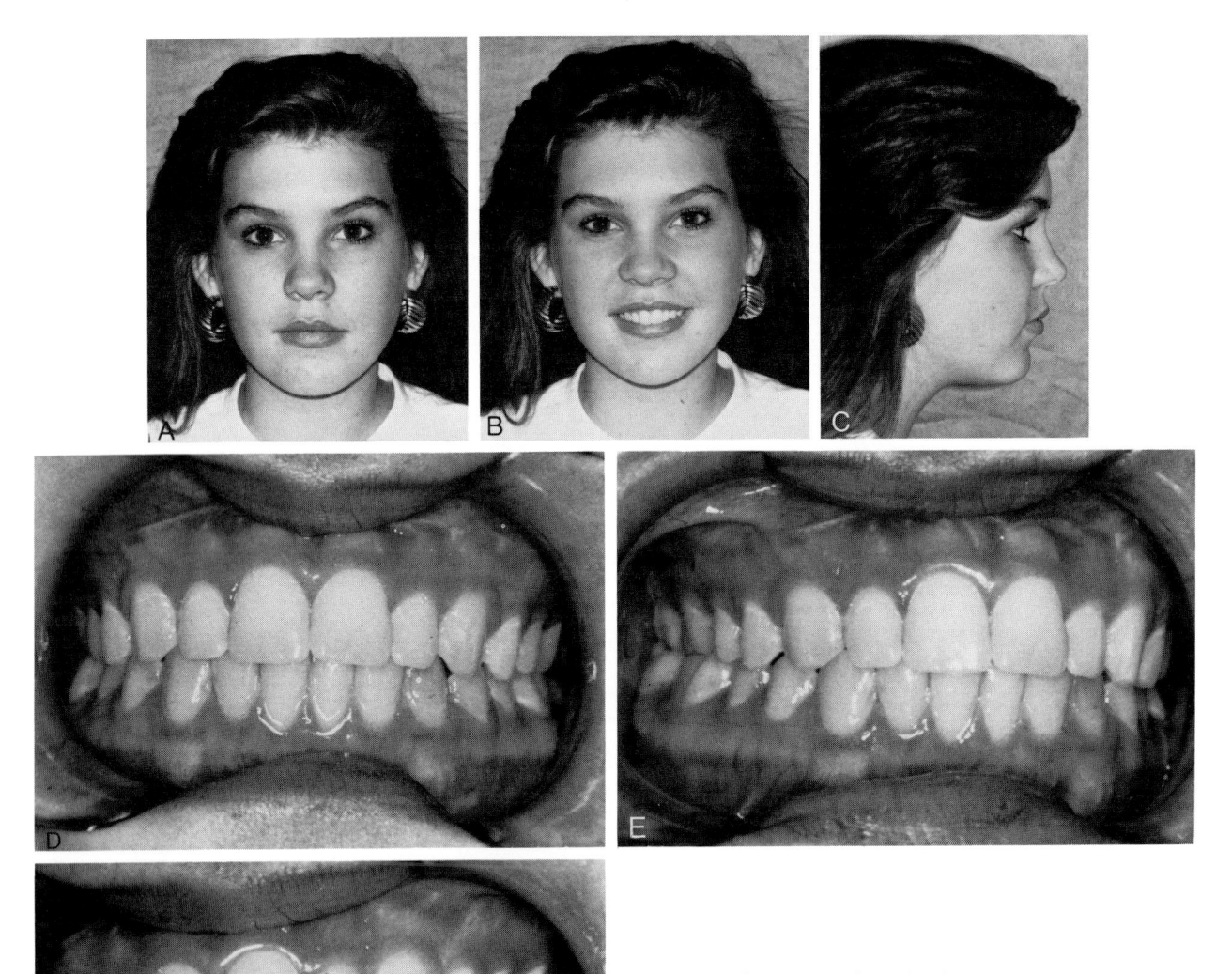

FIGURE 54–10. *A,* The patient is seen 3 years, 5 months after surgery, demonstrating good lip competence. *B,* Upon smiling, she shows a normal amount of tooth and gingiva. The inflammatory and hyperplastic gingival condition has cleared following the corrective surgery and the completion of orthodontics. *C,* Profile view demonstrates establishment of good facial balance. *D* to *F,* A Class I cuspid-molar relationship has been retained with the elimination of the hypertrophied inflammatory gingival condition.

CASE 2

This 13-year, 1-month-old male was evaluated for surgical correction of his facial deformity. The patient's primary concerns were his upper teeth and the peer pressure he was under because of the deformity (Fig. 54–11A and B). He was 13 years, 8 months of age at surgery. The patient actually began orthodontic treatment approximately 5 years earlier and wore a headgear for about 1 year, as well as some appliances and a retainer to try to correct the vertical growth problem of the maxilla, all without success.

Problems List

Esthetics. Frontal view demonstrated significant lip incompetence, an excessive tooth-to-lip relationship (7 mm), and an excessive amount of gingiva when smiling (Fig. 54–11A). In profile view, he had a protrusive upper lip and the nasal tip is upturned. The chin appeared deficient anteroposteriorly (Fig. 54–11B).

Cephalometric Analysis. A cephalometric analysis showed AP maxillary protrusion, VME, AP mandibular deficiency, and AP microgenia. The maxillary and mandibular incisors were overangulated. Tooth-to-lip relationship prior to surgery was 9 mm (Fig. 54–12A).

Occlusion. The patient had a Class II end-on occlusion with an anterior deep-bite relationship of about 4 to 5 mm. There was an overjet of 7 mm. He had a bilateral posterior crossbite tendency when placed in a Class I cuspid-molar relationship (Fig. 54–11C to E). A tooth size discrepancy of approximately 3 mm existed. There was also some gingival inflammation in the maxillary anterior arch. Panographically, there were bony impacted maxillary and mandibular third molars.

Treatment Plan

Presurgical Orthodontics

1. Align the maxilla in three segments:
   Segment 1 — left cuspid through second molar

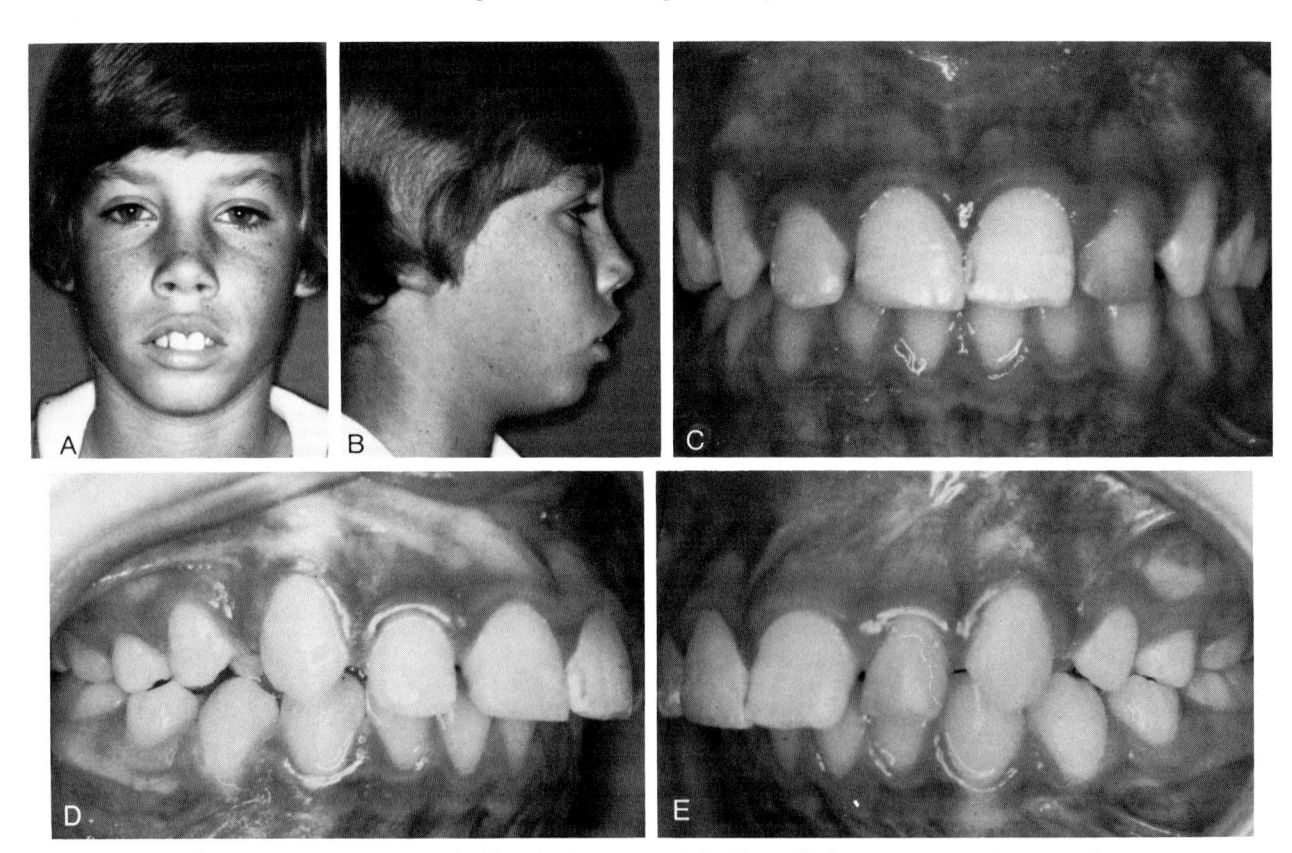

FIGURE 54–11. *A*, This 13-year, 1-month-old male demonstrated significant lip incompetence and an excessive tooth-to-lip relationship. *B*, Profile view demonstrates significant prominence of the maxilla and anterior teeth, and the chin appears retruded anteroposteriorly. *C* to *E*, The patient has a Class II end-on occlusion with an anterior deep bite. There is an overjet of approximately 7 mm.

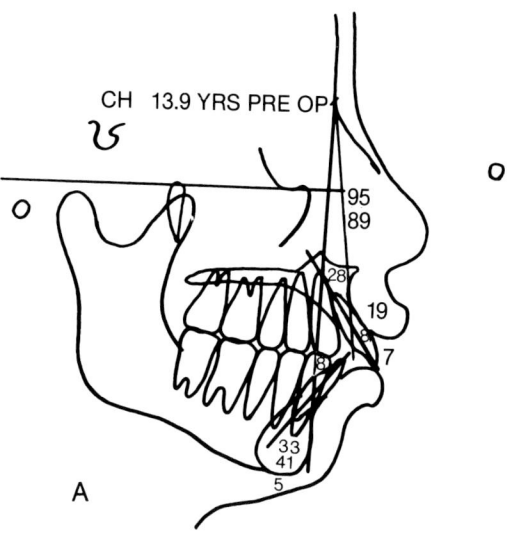

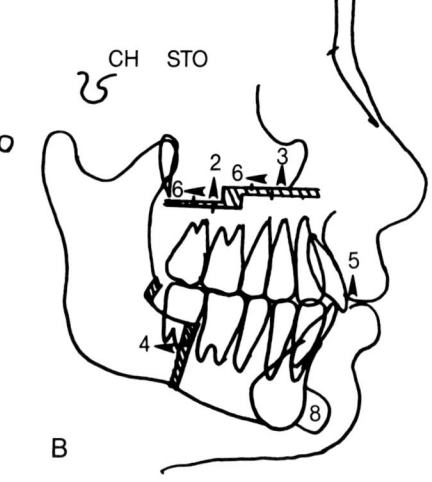

FIGURE 54–12. *A*, Cephalometrically, the patient demonstrated maxillary protrusion and relatively good AP position of the mandible except for the AP microgenia. The maxillary incisors were overangulated and an excessive tooth-to-lip relationship was present. *B*, The STO demonstrates the basic movements made. Maxillary incisors were moved superiorly 5 mm, and the cuspid and posterior aspects of the maxilla were moved superiorly 3 mm. The maxilla was repositioned posteriorly 6 mm, and the mandible was repositioned posteriorly 5 mm, since it would be too strong because of the autorotation of the mandible with the maxillary surgery. An augmentation genioplasty of 6 mm was also planned. *C*, An 8-year, 7-month follow-up radiograph is superimposed on the presurgical radiograph. The subsequent facial growth is seen with virtually no AP growth of the maxilla, although a significant vertical component of growth has occurred.

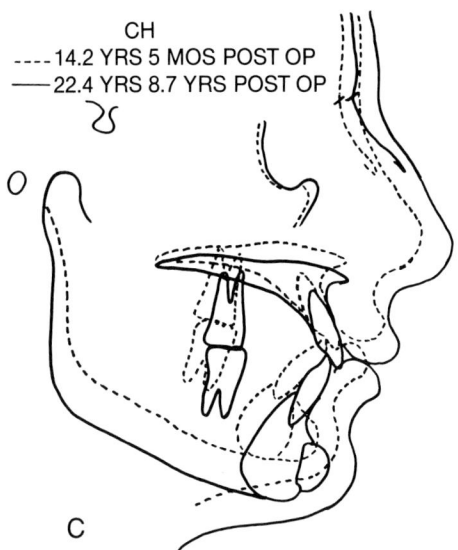

Segment 2—left lateral incisor through right lateral incisor
Segment 3—right cuspid through right second molar
  2. Maintain spacing of 1.5 mm around each maxillary lateral incisor to compensate for the significant tooth size discrepancy.
  3. Align and level the lower arch.

Surgical Treatment

  1. Multiple maxillary osteotomy to move the maxilla superiorly and posteriorly. Upright anterior four teeth to decrease this axial inclination (Fig. 54–12*B*).
  2. Bilateral mandibular ramus osteotomies to rotate the mandible in a counterclockwise direction and to establish a Class I cuspid-molar relationship.
  3. Augmentation genioplasty.
  4. Surgical removal of the four bony impacted third molars.

Active Treatment. The patient was 13 years, 8 months of age at the time of surgery and was treated prior to the use of rigid fixation. The desired occlusion was obtained with the surgical procedure, establishing the proper vertical and AP dimensions of the maxilla and mandible. Intraorbital suspension wires were used to stabilize the maxilla along with an occlusal splint and interosseous wiring. The mandible was stabilized with interosseous wires and circummandibular skeletal stabilization wires. Intermaxillary fixation was maintained for 6 weeks and then released. Orthodontic treatment was resumed at approximately 8 weeks after surgery, and the oral suspension wires and occlusal splint were also removed at that time. Orthodontic appliances were removed 8 months after surgery.

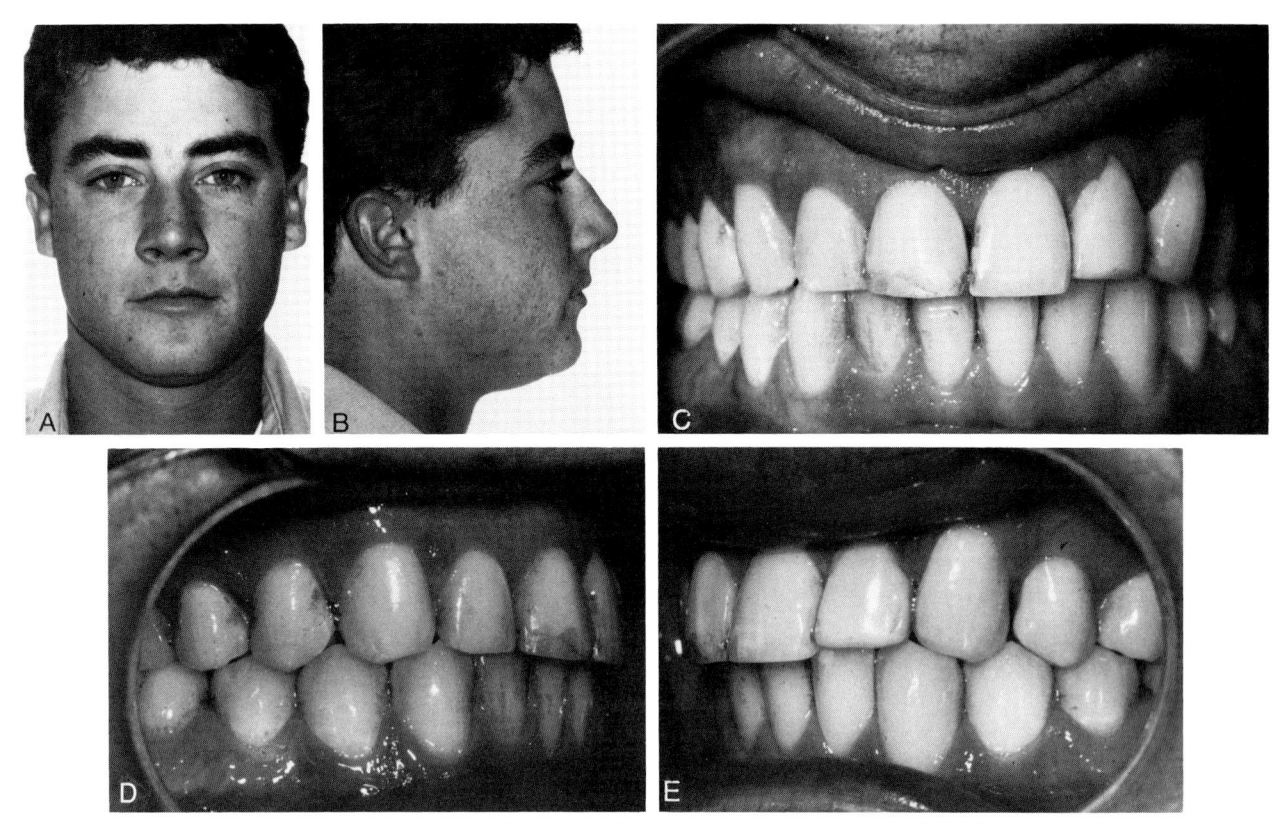

FIGURE 54-13. *A,* The patient is seen 8 years, 7 months after surgery, demonstrating good facial growth and harmony between the jaw structures. *B,* Profile view demonstrates good vertical facial dimension and balance. There appears to be good harmonious growth since surgery. *C* to *E,* The patient's occlusion has remained stable over the 8-year, 7-month postoperative time period.

Long-Term Follow-up. The patient was evaluated periodically, and the longest follow-up records were taken at 8 years, 7 months after surgery. He demonstrated good harmonious growth between the maxilla and mandible and showed maintenance of good, stable Class I occlusion (Fig. 54–13). There was virtually no AP growth of the maxilla, but significant vertical growth occurred (see Fig. 54–12C).

CASE 3

This 12-year, 5-month-old boy presented, on referral from his orthodontist, for surgical treatment considerations (Fig. 54–14). Clinical, radiographic, and dental model analysis revealed the following problem list.

PROBLEM LIST

Esthetics. Frontal view demonstrated lip incompetence, excessive tooth-to-lip relationship (6 mm), and an excessive amount of gingiva when smiling (Fig. 54–14A and B). Profile view demonstrated lip incompetence in the long lower third of the face. The chin appeared slightly retruded (Fig. 54–14C).

Cephalometric Analysis. This revealed a relatively normal maxillary depth but AP mandibular deficiency. The maxilla was vertically excessive, and the lower incisors were slightly overangulated. Occlusal plane angulation was 15 degrees (Fig. 54–15A).

Occlusion. The patient had a Class I cuspid-molar relationship on the right side and a Class II end-on cuspid-molar relationship on the left side. There was a tendency toward crossbite posteriorly, particularly on the left side. There was significant crowding in the lower anterior arch (Fig. 54–14D to F). The patient also had impacted maxillary and mandibular third molars.

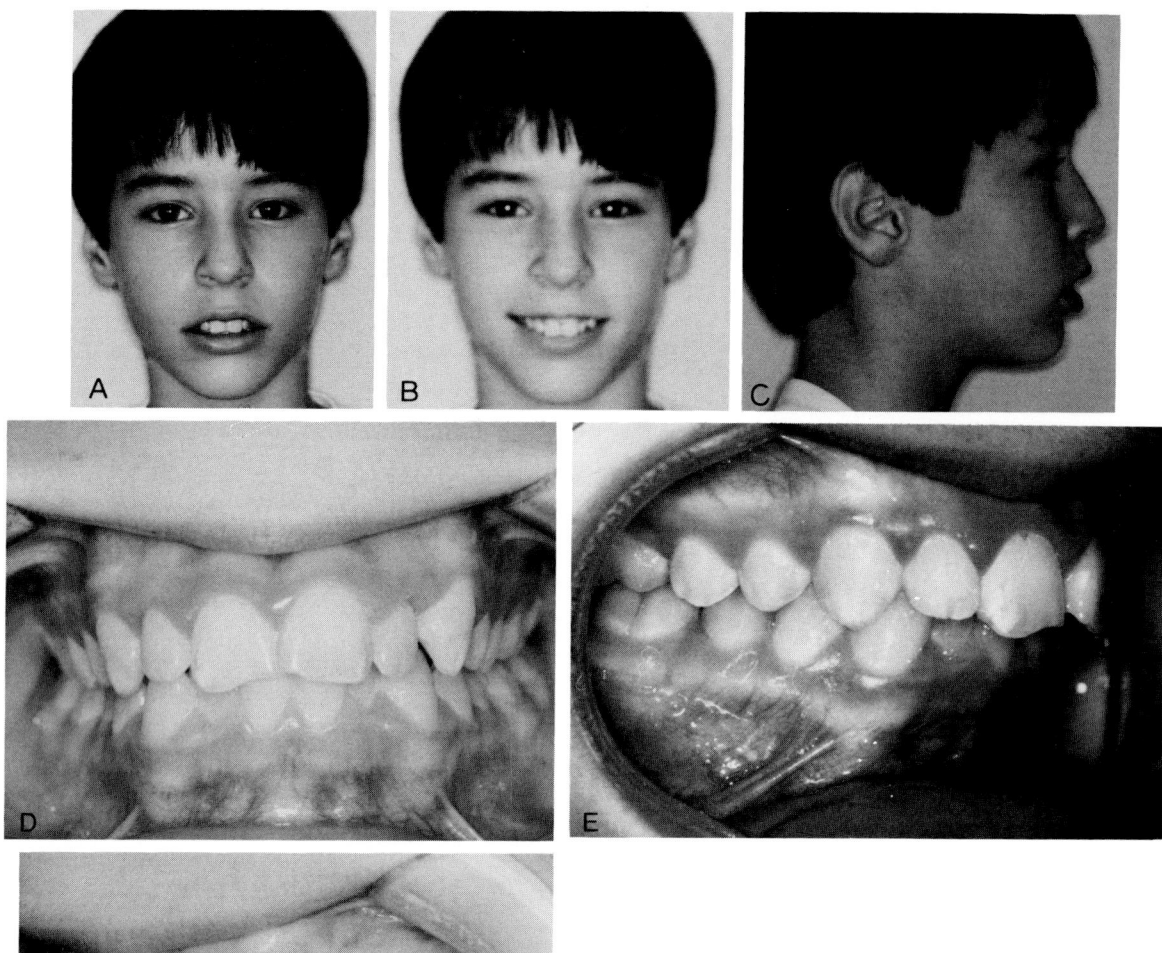

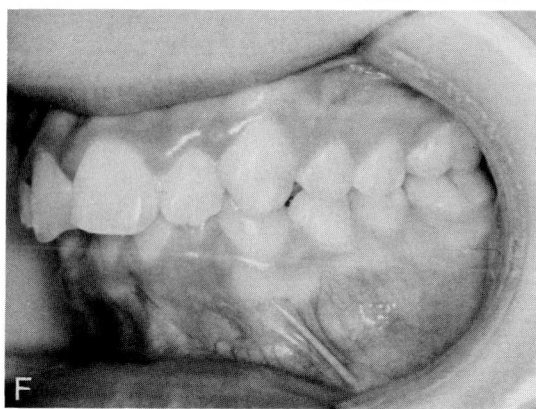

FIGURE 54-14. *A*, This 12-year, 5-month-old boy presented with lip incompetence and an increased lower third facial height. *B*, Upon smiling, he showed an excessive amount of gingiva. *C*, Profile view demonstrated increased lower third facial height and AP deficiency in the chin. *D* to *F*, He had a Class I cuspid-molar relationship on the right side and a Class II end-on cuspid-molar relationship on the left side. Significant crowding existed in the lower arch.

TREATMENT PLAN

Preorthodontic Treatment

1. Remove maxillary left and right second bicuspids.
2. Remove mandibular left and right first bicuspids.
3. Remove mandibular impacted third molars.

Orthodontic Treatment

1. Align and level maxillary arch, closing the extraction space. Lose posterior anchorage so that the anterior teeth are not retracted significantly.
2. Align and level mandibular arch, closing the extraction space and uprighting the teeth over basal bone (Fig. 54-15*B*).

Surgical Treatment

1. Superior repositioning of the anterior maxilla 4 mm and posterior maxilla 2 mm, with expansion of the posterior aspect (Fig. 54-15*C*).
2. Mandibular advancement in a counterclockwise rotation.
3. Augmentation genioplasty with Proplast.

1952 / VII — MANDIBULAR DEFICIENCY

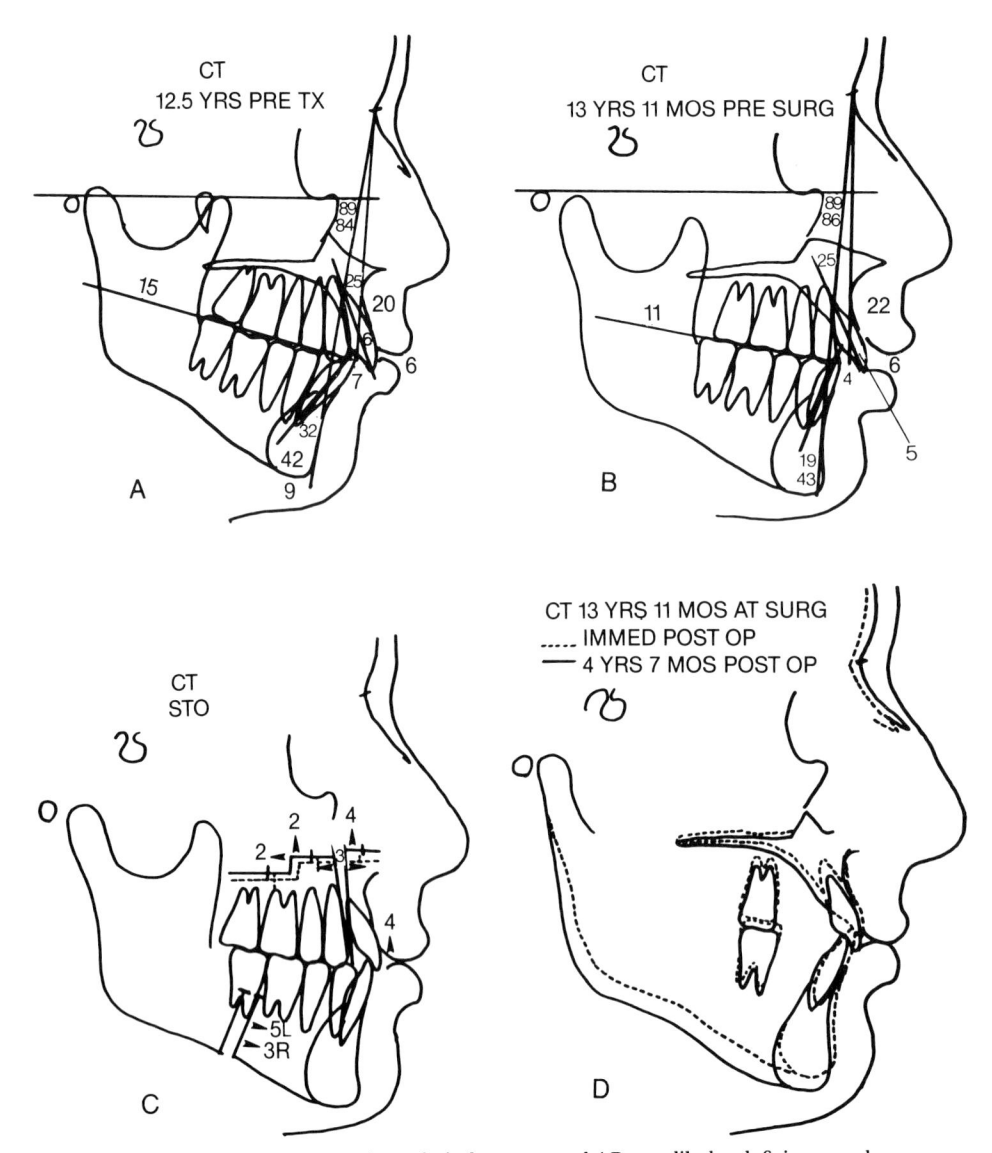

FIGURE 54-15. *A,* Cephalometric analysis demonstrated AP mandibular deficiency and overangulation of the lower incisors. The occlusal plane was overangulated by 15 degrees. Excessive tooth-to-lip relationship of 6 mm was noted. *B,* The patient was re-evaluated cephalometrically following extraction of four bicuspids and presurgical orthodontics. A 6-mm tooth-to-lip relationship existed, but the incisors were better positioned. *C,* The surgical treatment objective demonstrated superior movement of the maxillary central incisors of 4 mm and a posterior movement in the posterior aspect of the maxilla of 2 mm. Bilateral osteotomy cuts were performed between the lateral incisors and cuspids. The mandible was advanced asymmetrically, with the left side advancing 5 mm and the right side 3 mm. *D,* Superimposition of the immediate postsurgical cephalometric radiograph and a 4-year, 7-month postoperative radiograph demonstrates virtually no AP growth of the maxilla and mandible. There is a downward and posterior rotation of the maxilla and mandible as a result of subsequent growth.

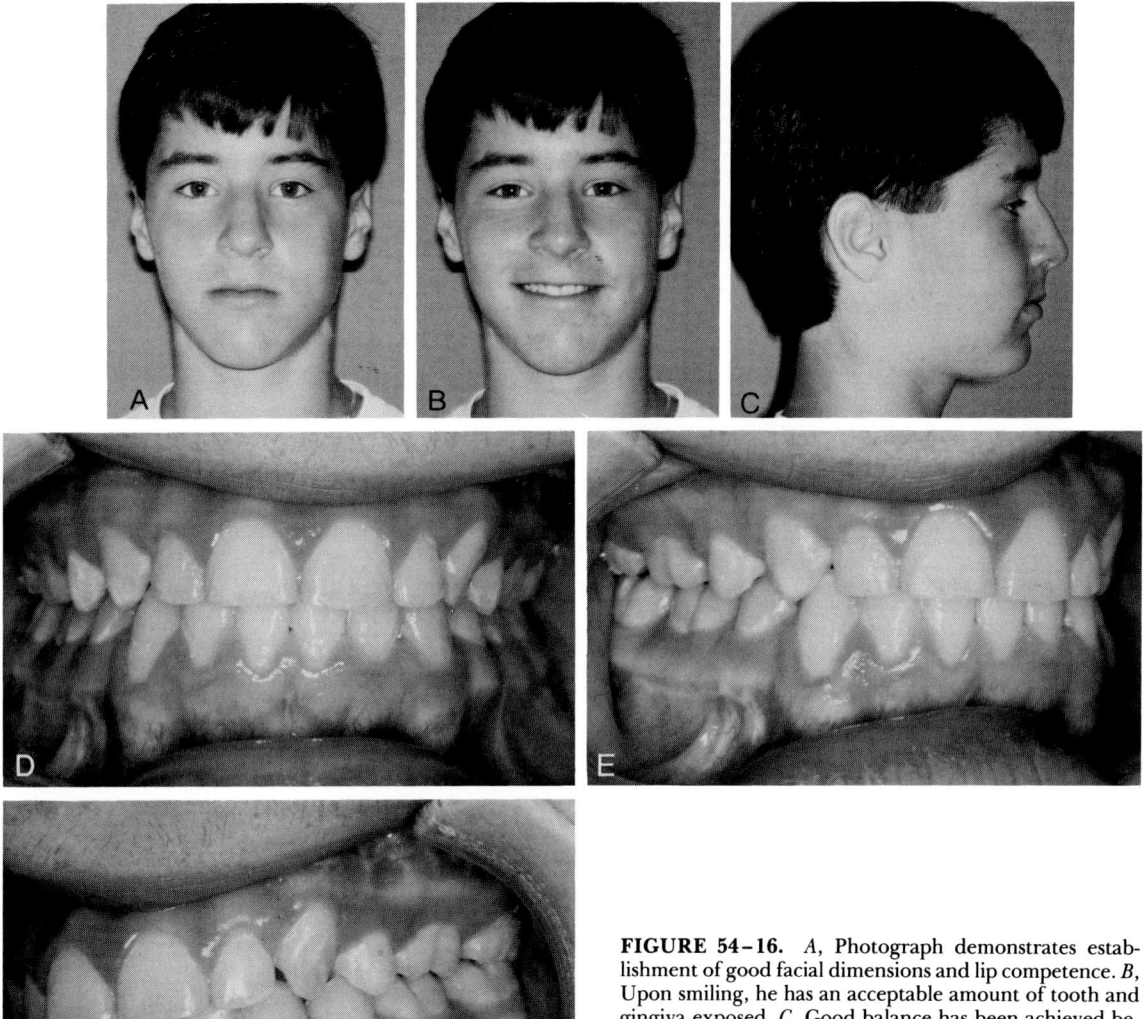

FIGURE 54-16. *A,* Photograph demonstrates establishment of good facial dimensions and lip competence. *B,* Upon smiling, he has an acceptable amount of tooth and gingiva exposed. *C,* Good balance has been achieved between the lips, nose, cheeks, and chin. *D* to *F,* A solid Class I cuspid-molar relationship has been established.

Postsurgical Orthodontics. Refine occlusion.

Active Treatment. The surgery was performed when the patient was 13 years, 11 months of age. A maxillary step osteotomy was performed with superior movement and expansion of the maxilla. Stabilization was achieved using four bone plates with two screws above and two screws below the osteotomy site with each bone plate. Bone screws were used to stabilize the mandible in its new position. An alar base cinch suture was used to control the width of the nose, together with a V-Y closure of the maxillary vestibular incision. No intermaxillary fixation was used following surgery. Light interarch elastics were used after surgery to guide his occlusion. The surgical stabilizing splint was used and removed 1 week after surgery. He progressed extremely well.

Long-Term Follow-Up. The patient was last evaluated 4 years, 7 months after surgery at the age of 18 years, 6 months. Good facial esthetics and balance have been achieved (Fig. 54-16A to C). Occlusion is good and stable (Fig. 54-16D to F), and facial growth appears to be harmonious and relatively complete. A significant component of vertical growth has occurred with no AP growth (see Fig. 54-15D).

REFERENCES

1. Adams GR: Physical attractiveness. *In* Miller A (ed): In the Eye of the Beholder: Contemporary Issues in Stereotyping. New York, Praeger, 1982, pp 253–304.
2. Alley TR: Physiognomy and social perception. *In* Alley TR (ed): Social and Applied Aspects of Perceiving Faces. Hillsdale, NJ, Lawrence Erlbaum Associates, 1988, pp 167–186.
3. Babula WJ Jr, Smiley GR, Dixon AD: The role of the cartilaginous nasal septum in midfacial growth. Am J Orthod 58:250–263, 1970.
4. Bachmayer DI, Ross RB, Munro IR: Maxillary growth following Le Fort III advancement surgery in Crouzon, Apert, and Pfeiffer syndromes. Am J Orthod Dentofac Orthop 90:420–430, 1986.
5. Baughan B, Demirjian A, Levesque GY, Laplame-Chaput L: The pattern of facial growth before and during puberty, as shown by French-Canadian girls. Ann Hum Biol 6:59–76, 1979.
6. Behrents RG: Growth in the aging craniofacial skeleton. Monograph No. 17, Craniofacial Growth Series, Center For Human Growth and Development. Ann Arbor, University of Michigan, 1985.
7. Bennett MA, Wolford LM: The maxillary step osteotomy and Steinmann pin stabilization. J Oral Maxillofac Surg 43:307–311, 1985.
8. Bishara SE, Chu GW, Jakobsen JR: Stability of the Le Fort I one-piece maxillary osteotomy. Am J Orthod Dentofac Orthop 94:184–200, 1988.
9. Björk A: Facial growth in man, studied with the aid of metallic implants. Acta Odont Scand 13:9–34, 1955.
10. Björk A, Skieller V: Growth of the maxilla in three dimensions as revealed radiographically by the implant method. Br J Orthod 4:53–64, 1977.
11. Bundgaard M, Melsen B, Terp S: Changes during and following total maxillary osteotomy (Le Fort I procedure): A cephalometric study. Euro J Orthod 8:21–29, 1986.
12. Buschang PH, Baume RM, Nass GG: A craniofacial growth maturity gradient for males and females between 4 and 16 years of age. Am J Phys Anthrop 61:373–381, 1983.
13. Demirjian A, Brault Dubuc M, Jenicek M: Etude comparative de la croissance de l'enfant canadien d'origine francais à Montreal. Can J Public Health 62:111–119, 1971.
14. Denison TF, Kokich VG, Shapire PA: Stability of maxillary surgery in open bite vs. non-open bite malocclusions. Angle Orthod 59:5–10, 1989.
15. Enlow DH: A comparative study of facial growth in *Homo* and *Macaca*. Am J Phys Anthropol 24:293, 1966.
16. Enlow DH, Harvold EP, Latham RA, et al: Research on control of craniofacial morphogenesis: An NIDR state-of-the-art workshop. Am J Orthod 71:509–530, 1977.
17. Epker BN, Wolford LM: Middle-third facial osteotomies: Their use in the correction of acquired and developmental dentofacial and craniofacial deformities. J Oral Surg 33:491–514, 1975.
18. Epker BN, Wolford LM: Dentofacial Deformities: Surgical-Orthodontic Correction. St. Louis, C.V. Mosby Company, 1980.
19. Epker BN, Schendel SA, Washburn M: Effects of early superior repositioning of the maxilla on subsequent growth: III. Biomechanical considerations. *In* McNamara JA Jr, Carlson DS, Ribbens KA (eds): The Effect of Surgical Intervention on Craniofacial Growth. Ann Arbor, University of Michigan, 1982, pp 231–250.
20. Fish L: Uber die Ursacken der Knockenformen: Experimental Unterrsuchung. Gottingen, G.H. Wigard, 1857.
21. Freihofer HPM Jr: Results of osteotomies of the facial skeleton in adolescence. J Maxillofac Surg 5:267–297, 1977.
22. Gange RJ, Johnston LE: The septopremaxillary attachment and midfacial growth. Am J Orthod 66:71–81, 1974.
23. Graber LW: Psychological considerations of orthodontic treatment. *In* Lucker GW, Ribbens KA, McNamara JA Jr (eds): Psychological Aspects of Facial Form. Ann Arbor, University of Michigan, 1980, pp 81–117.
24. Hennes JA, Wallen TR, Bloomquist DS, Crouch DL: Stability of simultaneous mobilization of the maxilla and mandible utilizing internal rigid fixation. Int J Adult Orthod Orthogn Surg 3:127–141, 1988.
25. Kokich VG, Shapiro PA: The effects of Le Fort I osteotomies on the craniofacial growth of juvenile *Macaca nemestrina*. *In* McNamara JA, Jr, Carlson DS, Ribbens KA (eds): The Effect of Surgical Intervention on Craniofacial Growth. Ann Arbor, University of Michigan, 1982, pp 131–141.
26. Kvinnsland S: Partial resection of the cartilaginous nasal septum in rats: Its influence on growth. Angle Orthod 44:135–140, 1974.
27. Latham RA: An appraisal of the early maxillary growth mechanism. *In* McNamara JA Jr (ed): Factors Affecting the Growth of the Midface. Monograph No. 6, Craniofacial Growth Series, Center for Human Growth and Development. Ann Arbor, University of Michigan, 1976, pp 43–59.
28. Latham RA, Scott JH: A newly postulated factor in the early growth of the human middle face and the theory of multiple assurance. Arch Oral Biol 15:1097–1100, 1970.
29. Lewis AB, Roche AF: Late growth changes in the craniofacial skeleton. Angle Orthod 58:127–135, 1988.
30. Liggett J: *The Human Face*. London, Constable, 1974.
31. Macgregor FC: *Transformation and Identity*. New York, Quadrangle, 1974.
32. McCarthy JG, Grayson B, Bookstein F, et al: Le Fort III advancement osteotomy in the growing child. Plast Reconstr Surg 74:343–354, 1984.
33. Melsen B: A radiographic craniometric study of dimensional changes in the nasal septum from infancy to maturity. Acta Odont Scand 25:541–561, 1967.

34. Mills JRE: A clinician looks at facial growth. Br J Orthod 10:58–72, 1983.
35. Mogavero FJ: An analysis of growth changes and treatment effects following superior repositioning of the maxilla using rigid and non-rigid fixation. Unpublished M.S. Thesis, Baylor College of Dentistry, Dallas, Texas, 1990.
36. Moss ML, Bromberg BE, Song IC, Eisenman G: The passive role of nasal septal cartilage in mid-facial growth. Plast Reconstr Surg 41:536–542, 1968.
37. Nanda R, Topazian RG: Craniofacial growth following Le Fort I osteotomy in adolescent monkeys. In McNamara JA Jr, Carlson DS, Ribbens KA (eds): *The Effect of Surgical Intervention on Craniofacial Growth*. Ann Arbor, University of Michigan, 1982, pp 99–129.
38. Nanda R, Bouayad O, Topazian RG: Facial growth subsequent to Le Fort I osteotomies in adolescent monkeys. J Oral Maxillofac Surg 45:123–136, 1987.
39. Proffit WR, Phillips C, Turvey TA: Stability following superior repositioning of the maxilla by Le Fort I osteotomy. Am J Orthod Dentofac Orthop 92:151–161, 1987.
40. Proffit WR, White RP Jr: Long-face problems. In Proffit WR, White RP Jr (eds): *Surgical-Orthodontic Treatment*. St. Louis, C.V. Mosby Company, 1990, pp 381–427.
41. Sarnat BG, Wexler MR: Postnatal growth of the nose and face after resection of septal cartilage in the rabbit. Oral Surg Oral Med Oral Pathol 26:712–727, 1968.
42. Sassouni V, Nanda S: Analysis of dentofacial vertical proportions. Am J Orthod 50:801–823, 1964.
43. Satrom KD: The stability of double jaw surgery: A comparison of rigid fixation versus skeletal wire fixation. Unpublished M.S. Thesis, Dept. of Orthodontics. Baylor University, Dallas, Texas, 1988.
44. Savara BS, Singh IJ: Norms of size and annual increments of seven anatomical measures of maxillae in boys from three to sixteen years of age. Angle Orthod 38:104–120, 1968.
45. Schendel SA, Eisenfeld J, Bell WH, et al: The long face syndrome: Vertical maxillary excess. Am J Orthod 70:398–408, 1976.
46. Schendel SA, Eisenfeld JH, Bell WH, Epker BN: Superior repositioning of the maxilla: Stability and soft tissue osseous reactions. Am J Orthod 70:663–674, 1976.
47. Scott JH: The growth of the human face. Proc R Soc Med 47:91–100, 1953.
48. Scott JH: Analysis of facial growth. The anteroposterior and vertical dimensions. Am J Orthod 44:507–512, 1958.
49. Scott JH: Analysis of facial growth from fetal life to adulthood. Angle Orthod 33:110–113, 1963.
50. Scott JH: Dentofacial Development and Growth. London, Pergamon Press, 1967, pp 65–137.
51. Shapiro PA, Kokich VG: Treatment alternatives for children with severe maxillary hypoplasia. Euro J Orthod 6:141–147, 1984.
52. Siegel MI: Mechanisms of early maxillary growth—Implications for surgery. J Oral Surg 34:106–112, 1976.
53. Singh IJ, Savara BS: Norms of size and annual increments of seven anatomical measures of maxillae in girls from three to sixteen years of age. Angle Orthod 36:312–324, 1966.
54. Skoczylas LJ, Ellis E, Fonseca RJ, Gallo WJ: Stability of simultaneous maxillary intrusion and mandibular advancement: A comparison of rigid and nonrigid fixation techniques. J Oral Maxillofac Surg 46:1056–1064, 1988.
55. Stenstrom SJ, Thilander BL: Effects of nasal septal cartilage resections on young guinea pigs. Plast Reconstr Surg 45:160–170, 1970.
56. Turvey TA, Phillips C, Zaytoun HS, Proffit WR: Simultaneous superior repositioning of the maxilla and mandibular advancement: A report on stability. Am J Orthod 94:372–382, 1988.
57. Vig KWL, Turvey TA: Surgical correction of vertical maxillary excess during adolescence. Int J Adult Orthod Orthogn Surg 4:119–128, 1989.
58. Washburn MC, Schendel SA, Epker BN: Superior repositioning of the maxilla during growth. J Oral Maxillofac Surg 40:142–149, 1982.
59. Wolford LM, Hilliard FW: Surgical-orthodontic correction of vertical facial deformities. J Oral Surg 39:883–897, 1981.

55 BIOMECHANICAL CONSIDERATIONS IN ORAL AND MAXILLOFACIAL SURGERY

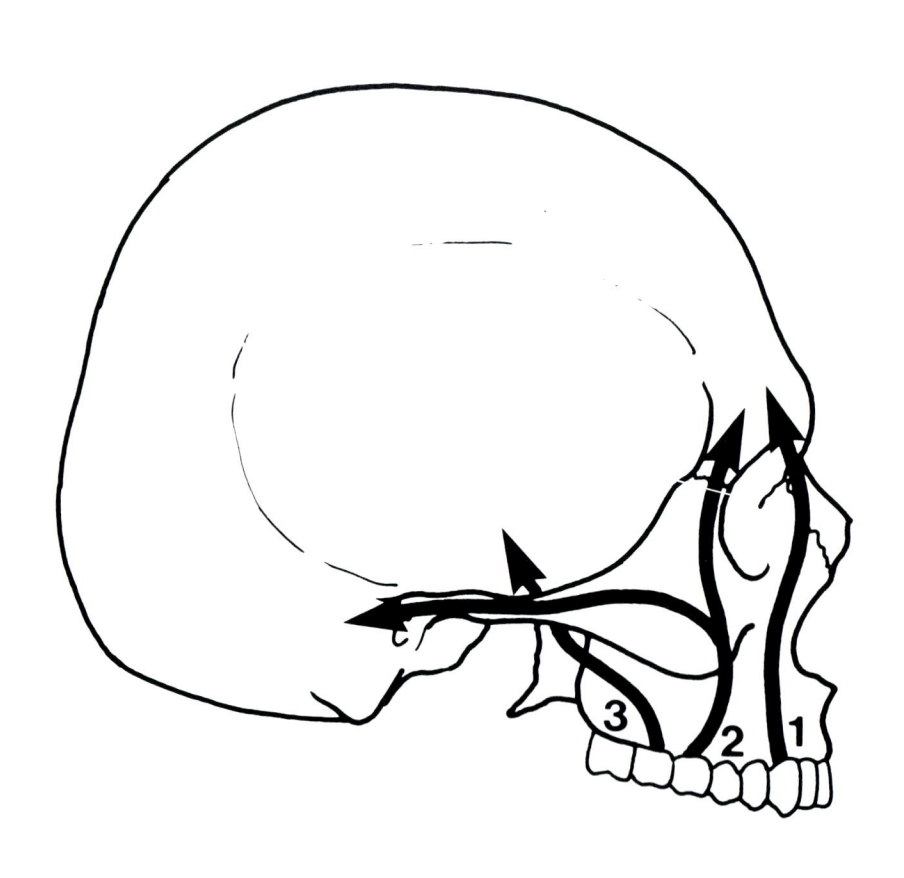

55

HISTOLOGIC RESPONSE TO
MECHANICAL DEMANDS

MUSCLE FORCES
  Mandible
  Midface

STRESS TRAJECTORIES OF THE FACIAL
SKELETON

EXPERIMENTAL ANALYSIS OF STRESS
AND STRAIN
  Stress Patterns in the Mandible
  Stresses Within the Condyle
  Midface

COMPARATIVE EVALUATION OF
INTERNAL FIXATION TECHNIQUES
  Internal Fixation of Mandibular Angle
  Fractures

VIVEK SHETTY
ANGELO CAPUTO

SUMMARY

The human skeleton in general and the facial skeleton in particular are corollaries of a complex evolutionary process that has endowed skeletal structures with the ability to adapt to and withstand the complicated structural demands imposed on them during function and rest. Alterations in the balance of functional forces by surgical correction of facial deformities or trauma elicit complex structural responses. These responses include compensatory bone remodeling and ensure that the skeleton remains suitable for its customary mechanical function. However, latitude for these offsetting osseous changes may be restricted by regional anatomic factors like dental occlusion—the building block of orofacial reconstruction. Alterations that exceed the adaptive capacity of biologic tissues result in damage and deterioration under loads that normally would be withstood without adverse effects. Clinical manifestations of a mismatch between structure and function include relapse of orthognathic surgical procedures, fracture nonunion, and temporomandibular joint disorders.

Increasing sophistication in oral and maxillofacial treatment modalities has led to heightened expectations in terms of the clinical result. Healing alone no longer suffices; it has to be rapid and complete, permitting early return of form and function. Accordingly, the biomechanical consequences of surgical restitution or alteration of orofacial skeletal structure have greater significance than ever before. Knowledge of the mechanical stresses to which the living tissues are subject and the corresponding biologic response provides the surgeon with the option of surgically changing these stresses to promote the desired therapeutic effect. Conversely, procedures performed without regard to the biomechanical consequences increase the chances of complications and treatment failure. An appreciation of biomechanical principles helps predict clinical performance of surgical techniques and provides guidelines for their use. In addition to facilitating improved results, an understanding of biomechanics also forms the groundwork for judicious and effective use of materials and techniques yet to come.

HISTOLOGIC RESPONSE TO MECHANICAL DEMANDS

From a mechanical viewpoint, every break in bone continuity represents a structural interruption that results in impaired transmission of forces. Consequently, all fracture healing is directed toward restoration of the load-bearing ability and abrogation of interfragmentary motion. Spontaneous fracture healing is composed of a histologic cascade involving the sequential formation of granulation tissue, fibrous tissue, fibrocartilage, and ultimately bone. A putative explanation of the interrelationship between the mechanical properties of reparative tissues and existing interfragmentary strain levels was provided by Perren.[1] He hypothesized that the increasing modulus of elasticity of each succeeding tissue is an expression of mechanical adaptation of reparative tissue to the changing strain levels. Accordingly, the complex interplay of mechanical and biologic processes at the fracture site results in a gradual transition from an elastic tissue of high energy-absorbing capacity (granulation tissue) to stiff tissue (bone). The granulation tissue that forms initially helps splint the bone segments and dampens interfragmentary movement. Decreased interfragmentary movement in turn permits the subsequent replacement of the granulation tissue by fibrous tissue. Through an enhanced stabilization of the bone segments, fibrous tissue facilitates successive formation of fibrocartilage. Once the strain levels are within viable tissue limits, mineralization of fibrocartilage occurs, leading to eventual bone formation. Stated simply, each succeeding tissue type gently and progressively limits interfragmentary motion, permitting replacement by tissue with decreasing tolerance to deformation and increasing strength.[2] Relative motion during the healing period of bone interferes with the normal histologic cascade.[2-4] By adversely affecting osseous healing, instability predisposes the fracture site to complications such as postoperative osteitis, osteomyelitis, and nonunion. Conversely, bony union can be achieved even in the presence of infection, provided that the fracture fixation is stable.[5,6]

Healing following rigid fixation is unlike spontaneous fracture healing, in which fluctuating mechanical conditions dictate that osseous healing progress through all stages of tissue differentiation. Under relative stability the healing process is very abbreviated, as the interfragmentary strains are reduced to an extremely low level. Intermediate connective tissue, callus, and cartilage stages are thus absent, with lamellar bone being laid down right from the beginning. Knowledge of the influence of the mechanical situation on the pattern of fracture healing provides an insight into the genesis of common clinical problems. For example, a fibrous nonunion may result from excessive motion across the fracture line during the healing process, thereby preventing formation of the ensuing tissue type. Decreasing strain in interfragmentary tissue by firmly fixing the bone fragments may well suffice to reactivate tissue differentiation and promote healing. This assumption is corroborated by clinical observation; stabilizing a well-vascularized nonunion with a bone plate is often enough to enable the ossification process to continue as in normal fracture healing.[7,8] The histologic response at osteotomy sites to mechanical demands is similar to that in fracture healing. Fixing the bone segments in a constant and stable relationship to one another protects the developing osteotomy sites from displacing muscle forces. By assisting bone in actualizing its healing potential, the surgeon helps minimize the possibility of complications such as relapse that may occur following orthognathic procedures.

MUSCLE FORCES

As primary stress generators of the orofacial complex, muscles elicit characteristic deformations of skeletal structure. The interplay of agonistic muscles generates a complex mix of tensile, compressive, and shear stresses within the bone. Disturbance of natural structural integrity by trauma or elective orthognathic surgery perturbs the equilibrium between muscle pull and bone. Consequently, uncompensated tensile stresses develop at certain sites, causing distraction of the fragments. At other sites, the stresses are essentially compressive in nature. From a biomechanical viewpoint, the distracting tensile forces elicited by attached muscles are deleterious and must be eliminated. Recognition of this phenomenon led Pauwels to apply the tension-band principle to the internal fixation of bone fractures.[9] Tension banding entails judicious placement of a device for force transfer at the site of distraction in order to convert the tensile forces into compressive forces.

There is a concomitant reduction in the compressive forces on the opposite side, thereby distributing forces more equitably over the entire fracture surface. Most of the rigid internal fixation systems currently used in maxillofacial surgery are based on the tension-banding principle. However, effective use of these systems is predicated on a sound knowledge of the muscle forces and their consequences on structure and function of the stomatognathic system.

Mandible

The forces exerted by the muscles of mastication (masseter, temporalis, and pterygoids) and the opposing depressor muscles cause characteristic deformations of the mandible. Functional loading of the mandible results in tension acting predominantly on the alveolar side and compression at the inferior border. In the intercanine region, these forces fluctuate under function, producing a torsional component.[10,11] Following a fracture or osteotomy, the physiologic balance between applied forces and bone resistance is altered, resulting in abnormal muscle pulls. Ensuing distraction forces are compensated by placing the force transfer device at the site of tension. This can be in the form of a dental splint in the dentulous region or a small bone plate in the retromolar region.[12] However, anatomic constraints such as the position of the inferior alveolar nerve or tooth roots often preclude placement of the bone plate in a biomechanically optimal site. This led to the development of force/transfer devices, such as the eccentric dynamic compression plate, which take the biomechanical situation into consideration.[13,14] Aligning the outer compression holes obliquely results in the development of compressive forces at the alveolar border while the axially oriented inner compression holes produce interfragmentary compression. Any torsional component, as is found in the intercanine region, is compensated by the flexural rigidity of the bone plate or by applying an additional miniplate.[15]

By creating a fracture-like situation, surgical correction of dentofacial anomalies effects a modification of muscle function. Altered muscle function results from stretching or shortening the muscle, altering the direction of muscle action, or even changing the mechanical advantage of the muscle by surgically repositioning the jaws.[16] Accompanying changes in masticatory efficiency can be appreciated by considering the mandible as a Class III lever (Fig. 55–1). The condyle acts as fulcrum, the food bolus as resistance, and the combined pull of the elevating muscles as the applied force.[17] Mandibular advancement or setback increases or decreases the distance between the fulcrum and the resistance, i.e., the moment arm. This mobilization induces a corresponding change in the muscle forces needed to maintain equilibrium (Fig. 55–2). One possible outcome of surgically

FIGURE 55–1. Two-dimensional representation of the human mandible. C = Condyle, which acts as a fulcrum; F = resultant masseter force; R_1 = bite force at molars; R_2 = bite force at incisors.

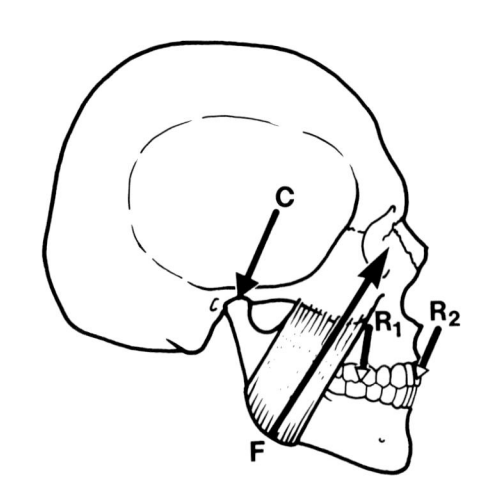

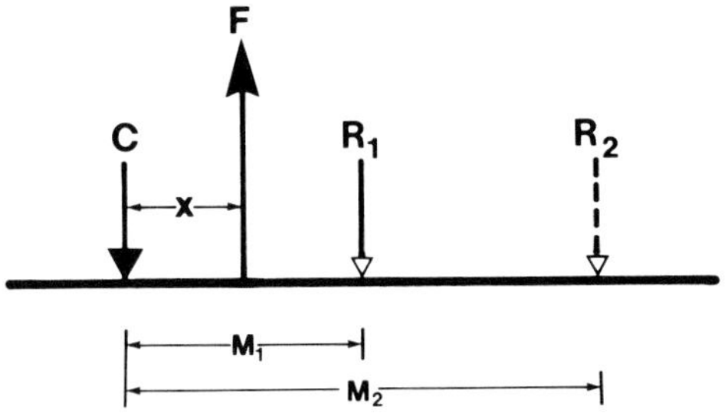

FIGURE 55-2. Schematic representation of the mandible as a Class III lever. Movement of the biting force from molars (R_1) to incisors (R_2) increases the moment arm from M_1 to M_2. This results in a corresponding increase in the muscle force needed to maintain equilibrium or to do work according to the relationship

$$F = \frac{[R_2(M_2 - M_1)]}{x}$$

actuated modifications of mechanical advantage is a more efficient muscle function at any given bite force. In other words, it takes less muscle force to produce an equivalent molar bite force.[18] The potential of orthognathic surgery to enhance the masticatory efficiency of the stomatognathic system was demonstrated by Finn et al.[19] In a group of patients with high-angle mandibular deficiency, superior repositioning of the maxilla with mandibular advancement resulted in a 13 per cent increase in the mechanical advantage of the temporalis muscle and a 21 per cent increase for masseter muscle when compared with mandibular advancement alone. Conversely, jaw repositioning surgery may result in reduced mechanical advantage or inefficient muscle function as manifested by the diminished occlusal forces measured following some orthognathic procedures.[20-22]

Owing to their ability to influence jaw biomechanics, postoperative variations in muscle behavior also affect the stability of orthognathic procedures. Focal areas of immature bone and osteoid are observed between the osteotomized bone segments even at 8 weeks after surgery.[23] During the interim, while the mechanical properties of the reparative tissue are developing, the osteotomy site is vulnerable to the deforming action of muscle forces. Large mandibular mobilizations that produce significant interfragmentary diastemata are particularly damaging. The anomalous force vectors induced by mandibular mobilization tend to accentuate the impaired ability of newly formed woven bone to resist functional forces. Current knowledge is limited in its understanding about the compensatory neuromuscular changes secondary to the abrupt repositioning of skeletal structures. However, in the absence of any significant neuromuscular rehabilitation, the chances of precipitating a relapse are greater.

Because the osteotomy sites initially constitute the weakest part of the masticatory system, surgical management must anticipate the effects of altered muscle mechanics on these sites. The surgical technique employed, choice of internal fixation technique, and duration of maxillomandibular fixation are all contingent on the clinical situation. For example, certain mandibular mobilizations require the use of a sagittal split ramus osteotomy to provide adequate osseous overlap and abet healing. The efficiency of the osteotomy design is augmented by employing a fixation technique that provides a degree of interfragmentary stability capable of withstanding the functional forces at all times through the course of healing. One way of diminishing the relapse potential is to protect the osteotomy sites by "lag" or "position" screw fixation.[24,25] The segments are held in a stable relationship to one another until healing is complete and the newly formed bone can withstand the effects of the condyle-ramus-masticatory muscle complex.[26] By securing functional stabilization of the osteotomized segments in a chosen position, biomechanically competent fixation techniques greatly reduce the period of maxillomandibular fixation as well as the risk of delayed bone union and postoperative relapse. The early return to function contributes to lowering the incidence of temporomandibular dysfunction subsequent to orthognathic surgery.[27] Enhanced stability also translates as an increased predictability of surgical procedures formerly associated with a high relapse rate, such as reduction of anterior open bites by counterclockwise rotation of the mandible.[28]

Midface

Alterations in masticatory muscle forces are not exclusive to mandibular mobilizations. Lengthening or shortening of the maxilla induces corresponding alterations in muscle activity and mechanical efficiency of the masticatory system. As in the mandible, increases in muscular activity aggravate the tendency to produce movement in the maxillary osteotomy sites and potentiate relapse. Deterioration of the surgical result caused by increased biomechanical forces is of particular concern following procedures that involve large advancements or inferior repositioning of the maxilla.[29,30] By effecting a distraction of the mandibular elevator muscles, surgery increases the stresses on the mobilized maxilla and any grafted tissue. Additionally, the constant pumping action of the masticatory muscles contributes to the altered stresses.[30] Subsequent resorption of the osteotomy margins and remodeling of interposed bone grafts precipitates a high incidence of relapse.[20] These indirect effects of stretched masticatory muscles on the stability of orthognathic surgery have also been observed in primate studies. Increasing mandibular elevator muscle length and altering function with bite-opening appliances results in a marked anterior and superior displacement of the maxilla and severe dental intrusion in adult monkeys, even when no surgery of the maxilla has been performed.[31,32]

Minimizing or countering the altered muscular forces that act on the repositioned maxilla has been an underlying theme of the various technical refinements devised to optimize the results of maxillary mobilizations. Methods advocated include the presurgical use of bite-opening splints, myotomies of the masseter and medial pterygoid muscles, and rigid skeletal fixation.[33-35] One option is to design the osteotomy so that mobilization is less likely to stretch the pterygomasseteric muscle sling.[36] During the interval that neuromuscular adaptation is taking place to accommodate an increase in maxillary height, the osteotomy sites and bone grafts must be protected from the occlusal forces. Of the various methods used, bone plate fixation has been found to be particularly useful in countering the adverse effects of muscle-pumping action on graft resorption and postoperative stability.[37-40] Bone plates effect skeletal stabilization principally by reconstructing the stress-dissipating pathways of the midfacial skeleton. Although rigid enough to withstand functional forces, plate fixation needs to be augmented with interpositional bone grafting if maxillary repositioning results in large defects between the bony walls.[29,41] Lack of osseous contact predisposes to delayed or fibrous union, malunion, or even superior telescoping of the maxilla under function.

As with the mandible, occlusion is a major determinant of the success of midfacial procedures. Immediate postoperative stability of the mobilized maxillary complex, for example, is contingent on the occlusion achieved. An equitable distribution of the occlusal forces ensures even dissipation of the forces of mastication. Occlusal prematurities tend to concentrate the masticatory forces in one region and provoke regressive changes, particularly during the early healing stages following maxillary repositioning.[41] The destabilizing effects of an unbalanced occlusion may manifest in the early postoperative period as excessive maxillary mobility. In such instances, the occlusal abnormalities should be treated by occlusal modifications or splint alteration. Redistributing the occlusal forces would permit a gradual stabilization of the mobile maxilla and preclude delayed union or nonunion.[41]

With the exception of the masseter, most of the midfacial muscles attach to the walls of the maxilla and insert into soft tissues. Consequently, their displacing forces are negligible and do not contribute to postsurgical deformity and relapse. In the case of the zygoma, the inserting masseter muscle and the temporalis fascia counteract one another. Disruption of this equilibrium following fracture can lead to relatively large movements of the zygoma by the masseter muscle. An inferior and medial displacement of the zygoma by the masseter muscle is often seen in unstable zygomatic complex fractures. Biomechanical analysis of fixation techniques for zygoma fractures in fresh cadaver skulls has established that even low masseteric forces are capable of displacing an unstable zygomatic complex fracture.[42] The tensile stresses generated within the zygoma by the inserting masseter muscle are seen primarily at the frontozygomatic suture. This stress configuration renders the frontozygomatic suture an ideal site for applying a tension band. It should be noted that a single point of wire fixation applied to this site may not suffice to prevent rotation around a longitudinal or vertical axis, especially in an unstable malar complex. Such clinical situations necessitate supplementary fixation at the inferior orbital rim in order to overcome muscle pulls. However, additional fixation against destabilizing muscle pulls often may be dispensed with by applying a bone plate at the frontozygomatic fracture site. The three-dimensional stability afforded by a single bone plate placed in the tension zone is often sufficient to avoid additional bone grafting.[43-46]

STRESS TRAJECTORIES OF THE FACIAL SKELETON

To appreciate force transmission within the orofacial complex, one must consider the facial skeleton as a stress-receiving and distributing structure. The mandible, for example, is essentially a curved, movable beam that bears against the fixed neurocranium. Although genetically programmed, the structure of the mandible has been modified by function to resist oral forces. As with other stress-bearing bones, much of the adaptation to functional forces is manifested internally. This adaptation is evidenced by the arrangement of the medullary trabeculae, which form stress-distributing arches and struts between alveolar bone and the cortical plates. Bony trabeculae are aligned in a manner that converts the complex forces of mastication into pure tension and compression. In keeping with the trajectorial theory propounded by von Meyer and Wolf, osseous reinforcement in the mandible occurs along the lines of maximum internal stress or trajectories.[47,48] These include the principal tension trajectory along the alveolar portion and the corresponding pressure trajectory along the inferior border of the mandible. Osseous reinforcement along these trajectories is manifest externally as a selective thickening of the shell of cortical bone, as is seen along the lower border of the mandible. Similar trajectories are found in the region of the mandibular angle as well as on the inner surface of the ramus. The rather thick cortical plate of the mental protuberance appears to be an analogous adaptive response to the torsional forces prevalent in the intercanine region.

Using a modified Benninghoff split-line technique, Seipel provided a mechanical interpretation of the mandibular architecture.[49] He obtained the split-line patterns of the mandibles by making a series of punctures in the partially decalcified surface of cadaveric mandibles and subsequently rubbing India ink into them. Based on his trajectorial interpretation of mandibular architecture, Seipel described the inferior basal trajectories of the mandible as compressive and the oblique ridge and alveolar trajectories as tensile in nature. These trajectories were perceived as effects of the muscle forces acting upon the mandible. Incorporation of these trajectorial concepts in fracture management has led to the development of special osteosynthesis systems and their application in biomechanically optimal areas. By restoring the structural effects of stress trajectories and helping effective dissipation of functional forces, these fixation systems provide a milieu for osseous healing to proceed to completion.

Masticatory loads do not dissipate entirely into the mandibular geometry. Some proportion of these loads are transmitted to the craniofacial complex through the temporomandibular articulation. Transmitted stresses are dispersed into the midface and neurocranium via trajectories in the zygomatic arch, canine eminence, orbital rims, nasal bones, and pterygoid plates. Corresponding reinforcement of bone occurs along these trajectories in order to protect the maxilla against the mainly vertically directed forces of mastication. Pneumatization of the remainder of the midfacial skeleton results in a structure with minimal osseous material, yet capable of bearing maximal forces. Masticatory force vectors dissipated along these structural pillars are essentially compressive and unidirectional in nature. This is possibly one of the reasons that fracture nonunion is uncommon in the maxilla. Although bony union in the midface occurs later than in mandibular fractures, functional stability is restored earlier because the fragments are not subject to distracting muscular forces.[50]

The vertical orientation of the structural pillars primarily cushions against vertically directed forces, but renders the maxilla at risk of fracture from transversely oriented impact. An inability to block force vectors that tend to displace the fractured maxillary segment superiorly and posteriorly interferes with the healing process. Owing to its potential to adversely influence the treatment outcome, reconstruction or stabilization of the critical buttresses of the midface should be an integral part of therapy. This is especially true in the case of comminuted midfacial fractures that are characterized by an extensive loss of these stress-dissipating structural pillars. Malunion of midfacial fractures invariably results from inadequate reconstruction of the buttresses of strength of the midface. Restoration of preinjury facial bony architecture may necessitate the use of bone plates and autogenous bone grafts to augment these buttresses. Additionally, early and accurate reconstruction of the midfacial buttresses provides the proper structural framework over which the injured soft tissue may develop scar contracture.[50] Similar considerations influence the use of interpositional bone grafts and miniplates in orthognathic procedures, including inferior repositioning of the maxilla to correct vertical maxillary deficiency.

EXPERIMENTAL ANALYSIS OF STRESS AND STRAIN

The biomechanical consequences of altering facial morphology are better appreciated by first elucidating the normal biomechanics of the facial skeleton. Stresses that develop in the facial skeleton under static conditions have been studied using various experimental techniques. Such approaches include the use of anatomic specimens incorporating strain gauges, photoelastic models of these specimens, or a combination of both. These specimens or their models are loaded under well-defined conditions in the laboratory and the mechanical response is measured. Of these techniques, photoelastic stress analysis is particularly useful as a predictor of biologic response, especially since the structure to be studied is irregularly shaped. In contrast to strain gauges that measure strains only at discrete points, the photoelastic technique permits visualization of the global state of stress within a structure rather than at a selection of isolated points.

Photoelastic stress analysis is based on the property of some transparent materials to exhibit colored patterns when loaded and viewed in polarized light. These patterns occur as the result of alteration of the polarized light by the internal stresses into two waves that travel at different velocities.[51] Developing patterns reflect the distribution of internal stresses and comprise the photoelastic effect. The array of colored patterns (isochromatic fringes) indicates the relative magnitude of the stresses. Black lines (isoclinics) are also observed and are related to the stress direction. The isochromatics and isoclinics can be used in conjunction with appropriate equations of elasticity to calculate individual stresses within the model. Often, the main information of interest is the location and magnitude of stress

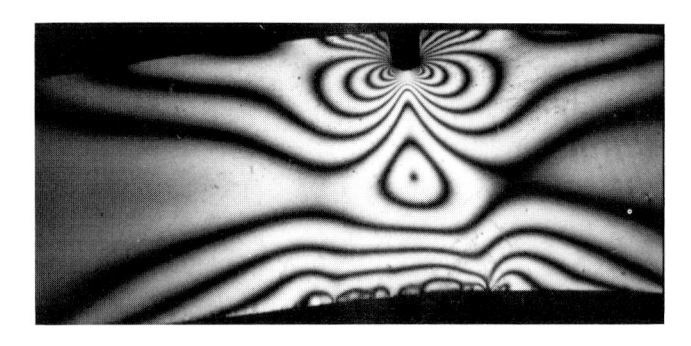

FIGURE 55-3. A birefringent plastic beam under three-point loading in the field of a circular polariscope. Proximity of fringes indicates stress concentration; number of fringes denotes stress intensity.

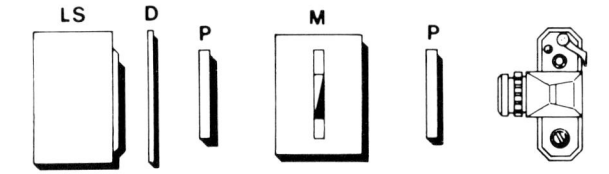

FIGURE 55-4. Plane polariscope arrangement. LS = Light source; D = diffuser; P = polarizing filters; M = model.

concentrations. This information has important clinical implications because these areas of stress concentration are indicative of regions of potential weakness or regions where major biologic responses may be expected. Examination of the isochromatic fringe patterns permits localization and quantification of the magnitude of stress concentration. Interpretation of these fringe patterns is quite straightforward with the use of the following principles: (a) the larger the number of fringes, the higher the stress intensity, and (b) the closer the isochromatic fringes are to each other, the higher the stress concentration (Fig. 55-3).

Using various birefringent plastics to simulate the modulus of teeth, bone, and periodontal ligament, it is possible to fabricate three-dimensional photoelastic models of the human skull and mandible. Skeletal structures including the maxilla, zygoma, vomer, and palatine bones are molded individually and affixed at their sutures with adhesives. Good geometric fidelity is thereby achieved, permitting evaluation of the effects of multiplex force systems. Under loading in a special rig, the models are examined in polarized light and photographed to record the photoelastic patterns (Fig. 55-4). Additionally, some of the birefringent plastics used are capable of "stress freezing," facilitating three-dimensional visualization of induced stresses. For stress freezing, models made from these special plastics are subjected to loads at specific elevated temperatures, and the loads are maintained while the temperature is slowly reduced to room temperature. As a result, the induced stress patterns remain after the loads are removed. Thin slices of the model are obtained and analyzed, from which a composite three-dimensional stress picture is constructed.

Stress Patterns in the Mandible

All applied occlusal forces elicit an internal stress response within the mandible. The nature of these stresses was visualized using the techniques of three-dimensional photoelastic stress analysis.[52] Bilaterally loaded mandible analogues were found to exhibit symmetric isochromatic fringe patterns (Fig. 55-5). The fringe patterns discerned tended to aggregate along the following major stress trajectories:

1. From the angle of the mandible up to the posterior border of the ascending ramus and running into the condyle
2. Obliquely from below the molars through the body of the mandible and ramus to the condyle

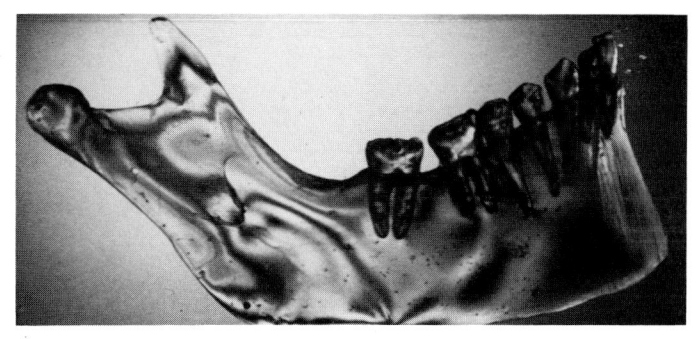

FIGURE 55-5. Photoelastic model of a bilaterally loaded mandible illustrating the four major stress trajectories.

3. From the molar alveolar crests up the anterior border of the ascending ramus and toward the coronoid process
4. Along the margin of the sigmoid notch

Loading the mandibles unilaterally resulted in stress trajectories similar to those observed under bilateral loading. However, variations in intensity and areas of stress concentration were apparent on both the working and balancing sides of the mandibles. Loaded sides demonstrated increased stress intensity in the condyles and their necks, whereas contralateral unloaded sides showed a corresponding decrease in stress levels. The high stress concentrations generated within individual teeth appeared to be modified as they crossed through the periodontal ligament space into the supporting alveolus (Fig. 55–6). By acting as a stress-absorbing cushion, the periodontal ligament seemed to effect a more equitable stress distribution within the trabecular lattice and ultimately into the cortex.

Analysis of horizontal sections obtained at different levels through the body of the mandible following stress freezing showed that the stresses tend to concentrate in areas that correspond to cortical and trabecular thickening in actual human mandibles (Fig. 55–6). Although the photoelastic models were homogenous and did not actually contain trabeculae, their behavior under experimental conditions suggests that a bone shaped like the mandible would require reinforcement exactly where osseous reinforcement exists. Within the body and ramus of the mandible, the distribution of stress concentrations corresponds to the split-line trajectories described by Benninghoff and Seipel.[49,53] Likewise, the isochromatic fringes correlate well with the distribution of trabeculae determined on the basis of radiographic studies of various mandibles by Dovitch and Herzberg.[54] By corroborating the trajectorial nature of stress distribution in the mandible determined by other anatomic studies, photoelastic analysis is able to substantiate the biomechanical basis of current rigid internal fixation techniques, including the compression bone plates. This knowledge is also compatible with the principles of tension banding which permit restoration of the load-bearing capacity of the mandible while using a minimum of implant material.

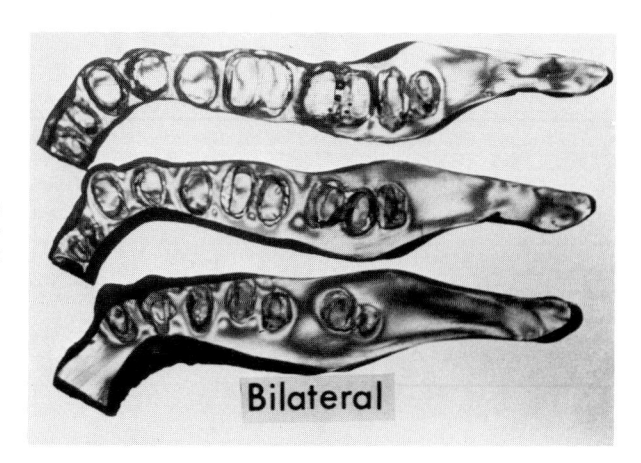

FIGURE 55-6. Horizontal sections taken through the body of a bilaterally loaded mandible following stress freezing. Isoclinics intersect at sites of nonpreferential stress distribution called isotropic points.

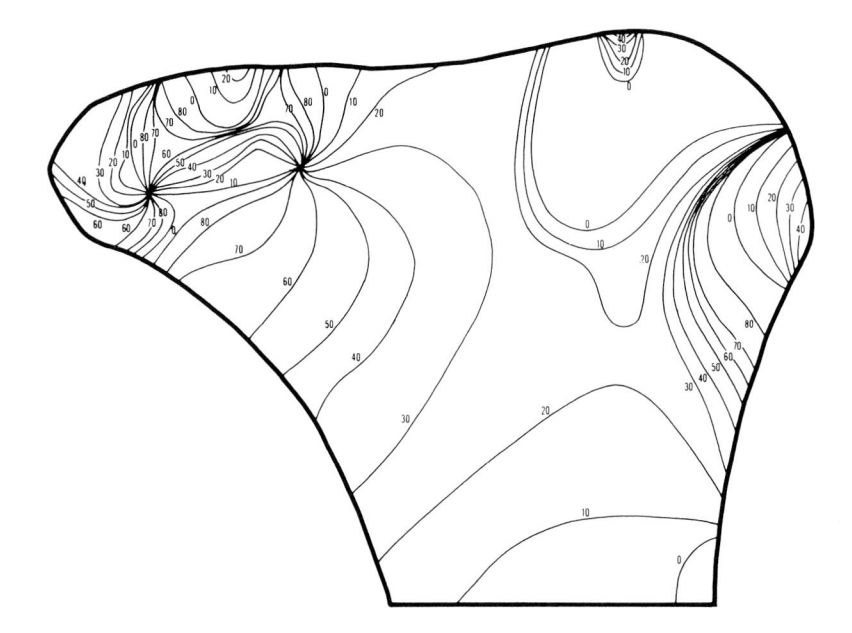

FIGURE 55-7. Composite of isoclinic patterns observed in a frontal section of the condyle during bilateral loading of the mandible.

Stresses Within the Condyle

On analyzing the stress trajectories in the photoelastic mandible analogues, it became apparent that the condyle is the ultimate destination of most of the major stress trajectories. In this way, a major component of the applied masticatory forces is transmitted to the base of the skull. Following stress freezing of mandible analogues loaded under clinically relevant conditions, the condyles were sectioned either in frontal, sagittal, or horizontal planes. Observing the sections in both plane and circularly polarized light permitted three-dimensional visualization of stress intensity and direction within the condyles. Viewed in plane polarized light, the condyle sections revealed isoclinic arrays related to stress direction. By overlaying the isoclinic patterns from the different sections to form a single composite, a more complete picture of stress direction was visible (Fig. 55-7). At those locations where all isoclinic lines intersected (isotropic points), no preferential stress directions existed, implying lack of stimulus for preferential orientation of bony reinforcement.

Horizontal sections through condyles stress-frozen during incisal loading demonstrated isoclinics converging into isotropic points (Fig. 55-8). In the case of

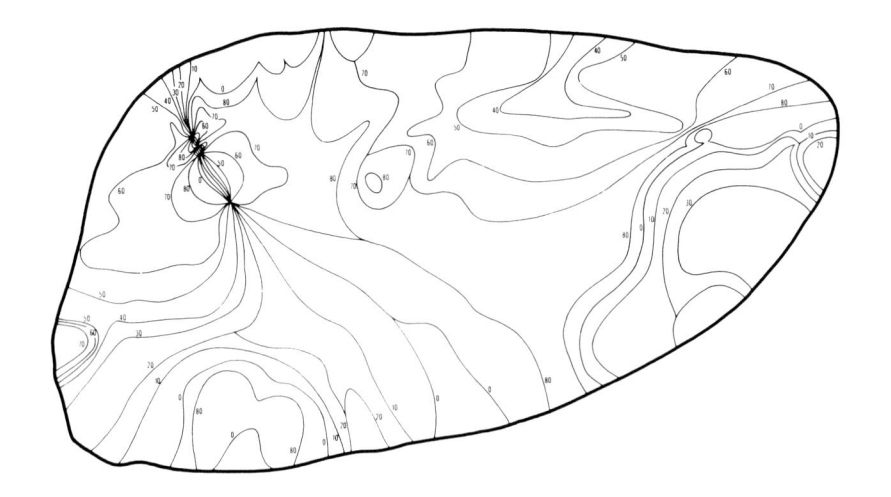

FIGURE 55-8. Composite of isoclinic patterns observed in a horizontal section of the condyle during incisal loading of the mandible.

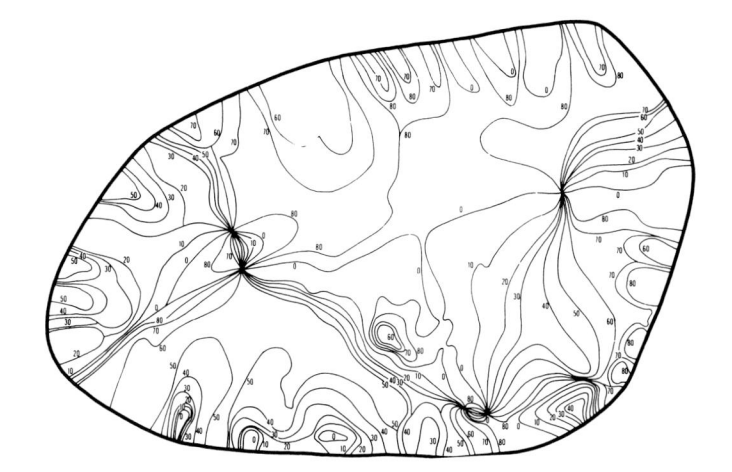

FIGURE 55-9. Composite of isoclinic patterns observed in a horizontal section of the condyle during bilateral loading.

mandibles bilaterally loaded in the posterior region (Fig. 55-9), nonpreferential stress zones in different locations were observed in the horizontal condylar sections. Sagittal sections of the same loading evidenced yet another perspective on these isotropic bands. In contrast, the sagittal views of an anteriorly loaded condyle showed two isotropic points in completely different areas of the condyle. When all the isotropic points were superimposed within a condylar head, they were found to be scattered in a more or less random pattern. In other words, each variation in loading caused different zones of nonpreferential stress distribution to develop within the condyle.

Sectioning the corresponding anatomic specimens disclosed that the condyles were not heavily reinforced by cortical thickness (Fig. 55-10). The uniform distribution of trabecular bone and the extremely thin cortical bone seemed to indicate condylar adaptation to nonpreferential stress distribution as well as low stress levels. These observations are probably related to the fact that the translating nature of the human temporomandibular joint (TMJ) requires the condyle to act as a fulcrum in many different positions. Although the elliptic shape of the condyle helps reduce stress intensity and concentration, the constantly shifting isotropic zones create an environment of nonpreferential stress distribution that may preclude heavy bony reinforcement under functional loading. The condyle appears to be adapted to varied light forces rather than unidirectional, severe, repeated forces. These findings reinforce those theories that assign function a major role in bone remodeling. In this context it is understandable that the condyle degenerates rather than reinforcing when heavy cyclic forces are applied. On the other hand, the condylar neck of the anatomic specimen was highly reinforced in the region where photoelastic study revealed the stresses to be intense, concentrated, and nearly unidirectional.

FIGURE 55-10. Corresponding anatomic specimen sectioned at the level demonstrated in Figure 54-8. Uniform distribution of trabeculae and thin cortical plate evidences adaptation to nonpreferential stress distribution and low stress levels.

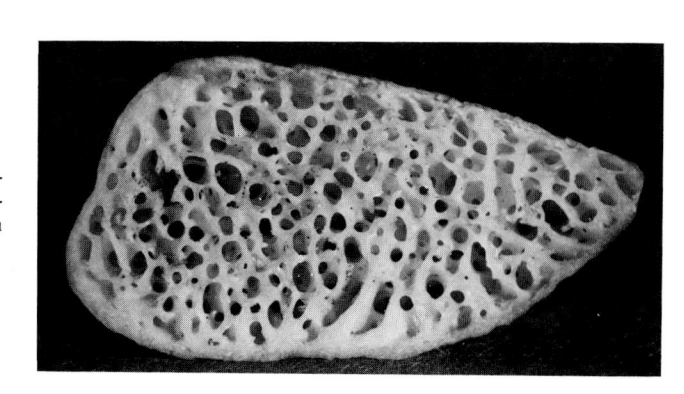

Correlating the photoelastic studies to the anatomic specimens suggests that TMJ disorders, like degenerative disease, may be essentially clinical manifestations of an adverse alteration in TMJ biomechanics. Faulty stress distribution transforms the functional stresses of mastication into unacceptable levels within the tissues of the joint and elicits a pathologic response. Functional forces have been implicated as the most important factors of remodeling and osteoarthrosis in the adult TMJ.[55] When these forces are light and cyclic, progressive remodeling can occur in the articulating surfaces to better accommodate the changes in function. Once masticatory forces become heavy and repeated, regressive remodeling results in the degenerative changes of osteoarthrosis. Hence, adaptive remodeling as well as destructive processes of the TMJ are essentially end products of forces that differ primarily in magnitude or direction. The body initially tries to adapt to increased stresses by forming tissue with corresponding load-bearing abilities. This adaptive response is evidenced by the conversion of fibrous connective tissue to fibrocartilage only in the pressure-bearing areas of the joint.[56] However, exceeding the remodeling capabilities of the body or the presence of existing modeling errors ultimately leads to degeneration of articular bone and cartilage, impeding mechanical function of the joint.

The unforgiving nature of some of the rigid fixation techniques emphasizes the need to be aware of their long-term effects on TMJ function. An example is the sagittal split-ramus osteotomy, in which mandibular mobilization invariably results in diastemas of varying degrees between the segments. The magnitude of these diastemas depends upon the inter-ramus angle, the ramus curvature, and the amount of mandibular advancement and setback. At best, the fragments may be joined only at certain points of contact. In such instances, lag screw fixation would cause compression of the buccal and lingual cortical plates. If the interfragmentary diastemas are large, the resulting closure displaces the condyles and effects torquing about the vertical condylar axis. Condylar displacement, which may be up to 12 mm in the intercondylar distance, results in a chronic compressive loading of the joints.[57,58] Whereas small distractions of the condyle from the glenoid fossa may be accommodated by the adaptive ability of the TMJs, larger displacements manifest as TMJ pain and dysfunction with decreased functional ability.[59,60] These clinical observations have been substantiated by experimental studies demonstrating that extensive condylar displacements result in remodeling, adaptation, and substantial degenerative changes of the joint structures.[61,62] The immutable alteration of presurgical condyle-fossa relationship caused by lag screws has been used as an argument for semirigid wire fixation. However, the trade-off is a low degree of stabilization of the osteotomy site. A viable alternative is to use a technique that rigidly stabilizes the ramal cortices while maintaining the diastemata between them.[25,63-67]

Based on current knowledge, the one common treatment goal of TMJ therapy should be to redistribute functional forces more evenly within the stomatognathic system.[68] Restoration of a structural balance is conducive to early return of pain-free motion and also helps avoid cartilage erosion and long-term traumatic arthrosis. This axiom is especially pertinent to reconstructive or orthognathic procedures that involve the TMJ, either directly or indirectly. Persistently high stress levels within the joint eventually induce degenerative TMJ osteoarthrosis, especially in the absence of the disk as a stress-distributing buffer. Hence, great prudence must be exercised in carrying out radical procedures like meniscectomies. It should be noted that a modulus mismatch between bone and the alloplastic TMJ implants predisposes to the build-up of intolerable stress concentrations. This manifests clinically as failure of the artificial meniscal implants following joint loading.

Improved joint biomechanics is also the rationale for using procedures like intraoral vertical ramus osteotomies for the treatment of TMJ pain and dysfunction with associated anterior disk displacements.[69] The neuromuscular control system provided by the pterygomasseteric sling and lateral pterygoid muscles is used to help realign the proximal fragment to a more functional position. Resolution of symptoms is believed to occur by a repositioning of the condyle anteriorly and inferiorly, thereby unloading the TMJ region.[69] Concomitant control of occlusion is accomplished by maxillomandibular fixation. In essence, this treatment philosophy seeks to alleviate TMJ dysfunction by balancing the biomechanical relationships among masticatory muscles, jaws, TMJs, and teeth.[69]

Midface

Photoelastic analysis of the routes of force transfer to the cranium discloses three major stress trajectories in the upper jaw and midface — the maxillonasal, maxillozygomatic, and the maxillopterygoid (Fig. 55–11). These trajectories arise from the basal part of the alveolar processes and are contiguous with the neurocranium. After originating at the apex of the maxillary canine, the maxillonasal trajectory follows the lateral border of the piriform aperture to join the medial end of the supraorbital rim. The maxillozygomatic stress trajectory arises from the apex of the first maxillary molar and continues into the zygoma through the zygomatic process of the maxilla, where it divides into two components. One component, the zygomaticofrontal, continues upward to reach the frontal bone after crossing the frontozygomatic suture. The other component, the zygomaticotemporal, continues along the zygomatic arch and crosses the zygomaticotemporal suture to dissipate into the temporal bone. Finally, the maxillopterygoid stress trajectory starts from the apices of the second and third molars and reaches the base of the skull through the lateral pterygoid plate.

Based on intensity, the predominant trajectory in the midface passes through the zygoma and the zygomatic arch. Consequently, masticatory forces may be transferred to the neurocranium primarily by the zygomaticotemporal trajectorial component followed by the zygomaticofrontal trajectorial component. Variations in stress intensity are observed on analysis of the fringe patterns across the sutural articulation of the zygoma with the maxilla, frontal, and temporal bone. At the zygomatocomaxillary suture the transmitted stresses are uniformly distributed across the suture (Fig. 55–12). Superiorly, relatively uniform stresses cross the frontozygomatic suture to concentrate along the lateral surface and posterior

FIGURE 55–11. The three major stress trajectories of the upper jaw and midface as determined by the photoelastic technique of stress analysis.

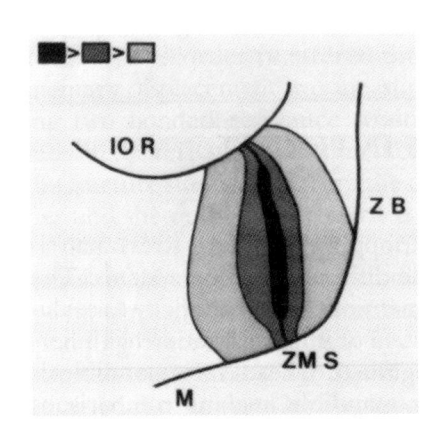

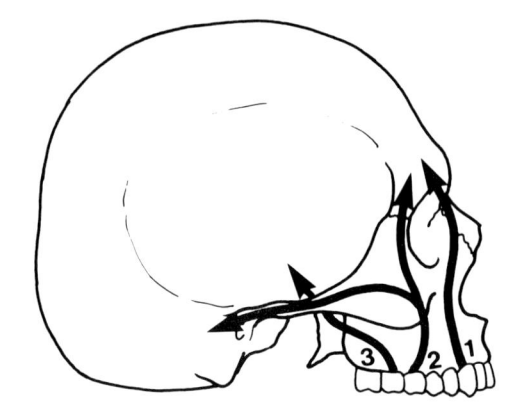

FIGURE 55–12. Schematic representation of the stress intensities observed at the left zygomaticomaxillary suture during occlusal loading. Stresses are evenly distributed across the suture. IOR = Infraorbital rim; ZB = zygomatic bone; ZMS = zygomaticomaxillary suture; M = maxilla.

7. Luhr H-G: Zur stabilen Osteosynthese bei Unterkieferfrakturen. Dtsch Zahnärztl Z 23:754, 1968.
8. Luhr H-G: Infections of the fracture line, pseudarthroses, and defect fractures. *In* Krueger E, Schilli W (eds): Oral and Maxillofacial Traumatology. Chicago, Quintessence Publishing Company, 1982, vol 2, p 423.
9. Pauwels F: Grundriss einer Biomechanik der Frakturheilung. Verh Dtsch Orthop Ges 34:62, 1950.
10. Niederdellmann H, Uhlig G, Joos U: Das elastische Formverhalten der Mandibula unter funktioneller Belastung. Die Quintessenz 32:1113, 1981.
11. Champy M, Lodde JP, Jaeger JH, Wilk A: Ostéosynthéses mandibulaires selon la technique de Michelet. I - Bases biomécaniques. Rev Stomat 77:569, 1976.
12. Spiessl B, Schargus G: Das Okklusionsproblem bei der funktionsstabilen Osteosynthese des bezahnten Unterkiefers. Dtsch Zahn Mund Keiferheilk 57:293, 1971.
13. Niederdellmann H, Schilli W: Zur Plattenosteosynthese bei Unterkieferfrakturen. Dtsch Zahnärztl Z 28:638, 1973.
14. Schmoker R, Spiessl B: Exzentrisch-dynamische Kompressionsplatte. Schweiz Mschr Zahnheilkd 83:1496, 1973.
15. Champy M, Lodde JP: Synthéses mandibularis. Localisation des synthéses en fonction des contraintes mandibularis. Rev Stomat 77:971, 1976.
16. Finn RA, Throckmorton GS, Gonyea WJ, et al: Neuromuscular aspects of vertical maxillary dysplasias. In Bell WH, Proffit WR, White RP (eds): Surgical Correction of Dentofacial Deformities. Philadelphia, WB Saunders Company, 1980, vol 2, p 1712.
17. Hylander WL: The human mandible: Lever or link. Am J Phys Anthropol 43:227, 1975.
18. Throckmorton GS, Finn RA, Bell WH: Biomechanics of differences in lower facial height. Am J Orthod 77:410, 1980.
19. Finn RA, Throckmorton GS, Bell WH, Legan HL: Biomechanical considerations in the surgical correction of mandibular deficiency. J Oral Surg 38:257, 1980.
20. Persson G, Hellem S, Nord PG: Bone-plates for stabilizing Le Fort I osteotomies. J Maxillofac Surg 14:69, 1986.
21. Throckmorton GS, Johnston CP, Gonyea WJ, Bell WH: A preliminary study of biomechanical changes produced by orthognathic surgery. J Prosthet Dent 51:252, 1984.
22. Proffit WR, Turvey TA, Fields HW, Phillips C: The effect of orthognathic surgery on occlusal force. J Oral Maxillofac Surg 47:457, 1989.
23. Bell WH, Schendel SA: Biologic basis for modification of the sagittal split ramus osteotomy. J Oral Surg 35:362, 1977.
24. Spiessl B: Osteosynthese bei sagittaler Osteotomie nach Obwegeser/Dal Pont. Fortschr Kiefer Gesichtschir 18:145, 1974.
25. Niederdellmann H, Shetty V, Collins FJV: Controlled osteosynthesis utilizing the position screw. Int J Adult Orthod Orthognath Surg 2:159, 1987.
26. Reitzik M, Schoorl W: Bone repair in the mandible: A histologic and biometric comparison between rigid and semi-rigid fixation. J Oral Maxillofac Surg 41:215, 1983.
27. Güdel M: Nachuntersuchung bei 29 Progenie-Patienten. Doctoral thesis. Basel University, 1986.
28. Bell W: Personal communication, 1990.
29. Araujo A, Schendel SA, Wolford IM, et al: Total maxillary advancement with and without bone grafting. J Oral Surg 36:849, 1978.
30. Wolford LM, Hillard FW: The surgical orthodontic correction of vertical dentofacial deformities. J Oral Surg 39:883, 1981.
31. Carlson DS, Schneiderman ED: Cephalometric analysis of adaptations after lengthening of the masseter muscle in adult rhesus monkeys. Arch Oral Biol 28:627, 1983.
32. Schneiderman ED, Carlson DS: Growth and remodeling of the mandible following alteration of function in adult rhesus monkeys. Am J Phys Anthropol 54:275, 1981.
33. Bell WH, Scheideman GB: Correction of vertical maxillary deficiency: Stability and soft tissue changes. J Oral Surg 39:666, 1981.
34. Wessberg GA, Epker BN: Intraoral skeletal fixation appliance. J Oral Maxillofac Surg 40:827, 1982.
35. Piecuch J, Tideman H, DeKoomen H: Short-face syndrome: Treatment of myofascial pain dysfunction by maxillary disimpaction. Oral Surg Oral Med Oral Pathol 49:112, 1979.
36. Quejada JG, Bell WB, Kawamura H, Zhang X: Skeletal stability after inferior maxillary repositioning. Int J Adult Orthod Orthognath Surg 2:67, 1987.
37. Hörster W: Experience with functionally stable plate osteosynthesis after forward displacement of the upper jaw. J Maxillofac Surg 8:176, 1980.
38. Drommer R, Luhr H-G: The stabilization of osteotomized maxillary segments with Luhr miniplates in secondary cleft surgery. J Maxillofac Surg 9:166, 1981.
39. Paulus GW, Hardt N, Steinhäuser EW: Miniplattenosteosynthesen bei Mehrfachosteotomien der Maxilla. Dtsch Z Mund Kiefer Gesichtschir 8:245, 1984.
40. Van Sickels JE, Jeter TS, Aragon SB: Rigid fixation of maxillary osteotomies: A preliminary report and technique article. Oral Surg Oral Med Oral Pathol 60:262, 1985.
41. Van Sickels JE, Tucker MR: Management of delayed union and nonunion of maxillary osteotomies. J Oral Maxillofac Surg 48:1039, 1990.
42. Karlan MS, Cassisi NJ: Fractures of the zygoma—a geometric, biomechanical, and surgical analysis. Arch Otolaryngol 105:320, 1979.
43. Champy M, Gerlach K, Kahn J, Pape H: Treatment of zygomatic bone fractures. *In* Oral and Maxillofacial Surgery. Proceedings of the 8th International Conference on Oral and Maxillofacial Surgery. Chicago, Quintessence Publishing Company, 1985, p 226.
44. Düker J, Härle F, Olivier D: Drahtnaht oder miniplatte—Nachuntersuchungen dislozierter Jochbeinfrakturen. Fortschr Kiefer Geisichtschir 22:49, 1977.

45. Härle F, Düker J: Miniplattenosteosynthese am Jochbein. Dtsch Zahärztl Z 31:97, 1976.
46. Stoll P, Schilli W: Primary reconstruction with AO-miniplates after severe cranio-maxillofacial trauma. J Craniomaxillofac Surg 16:18, 1988.
47. von Meyer H: Die Architektur des Spongiosa. Arch Anat Physiol 34:615, 1867.
48. Wolff J: Ueber die innere Architectur der Knochen und ihre Bedeutung für die Frage vom Knochenwachstum. Virchow's Arch Path Anat 50:389, 1870.
49. Seipel CM: Trajectories of the jaws. Acta Odont Scand 8:81, 1948.
50. Manson PN, Hoopes JE, Su CT: Structural pillars of the facial skeleton. An approach to the management of Le Fort fractures. Plast Reconstr Surg 66:54, 1980.
51. Durelli AJ, Riley WF: Introduction to Photomechanics. Englewood Cliffs, NJ, Prentice-Hall, 1965.
52. Ralph JP, Caputo AA: Analysis of stress patterns in the human mandible. J Dent Res 54:814, 1975.
53. Benninghoff A: Ueber die Anpassung der Knochenkompakta an geänderte Beanspruchung. Anat Anz 63:289, 1927.
54. Dovitch V, Herzberg F: A radiographic study of the bony trabecular pattern in the mandibular rami of herbivores, carnivores and omnivores. Angle Orthod 38:205, 1968.
55. Zarb GA, Carlsson GE: TMJ Function and Dysfunction. St. Louis, C.V. Mosby Company, 1979, p 172.
56. Moffett BC, Johnson LC, McCabe JB, Askew HC: Articular remodeling in the adult human temporomandibular joint. Am J Anat 115:119, 1964.
57. Freihofer HP: Modellversuch zur Lageveränderung des Kiefer-köpfchens nach sagittaler Spaltung des Unterkiefers. Schwiez Mschr Zahnheilk 87:12, 1977.
58. Tuinzing DB, Swart IGN: Lageveränderungen des caput mandibulae bei Verwendung von schrauben nach sagittaler Osteotomie des Unterkiefers. Dtsch Z Mund Kiefer Gesichtschir 2:94, 1978.
59. Kundert M, Hadjianghelou O: Condylar displacement after sagittal splitting of the mandibular rami. J Maxillofac Surg 8:278, 1980.
60. Hadjianghelou O: Züricher Erfahrungen mit der Zugschraubenosteosynthese bei der sagittaler Spaltung des Ramus. Fortschr Kiefer Gesichtschir 8:62, 1984.
61. Ewers R: Die temporomandibulären Strukturen Erwachsener und die Reaktion auf operative Verlagerungen. Eine tierexperimentelle Studie an ausgewachsenen Cercopithecus-aethiops Affen. Z Stomatol 81:73, 1984.
62. Sitzmann F: Klinische und tierexperimentelle Untersuchungen über Kiefergelenkveränderungen nach korrektiven Osteotomien bei Dysgnathien. Fortschr Kiefer Gesichtschir 26:75, 1981.
63. Niederdellmann H, Bührmann K, Collins FJV: Stellschraube—Adjuvans in der kieferorthopädischen Chirurgie. Dtsch Z Mund Kiefer Gesichtschir 8:62, 1984.
64. Lindorf HH: Funktionsstabile Tandem-Verschraubung der sagittalen Ramusosteotomie. Dtsch Z Mund Kiefer Gesichtschir 8:367, 1984.
65. Niededellmann H, Shetty V: Technical improvements in the sagittal split ramus osteotomy. Oral Surg Oral Med Oral Pathol 67:25, 1989.
66. Turvey TA, Hall DJ: Intraoral self-threading screw fixation for sagittal osteotomies. Early experiences. Int J Adult Orthod Orthognath Surg 4:243, 1986.
67. Jeter TS, Van Sickels JE, Dolwick MF: Rigid internal fixation of ramus osteotomies. A technique article. J Oral Maxillofac Surg 42:220, 1984.
68. Lerman MD: A unifying concept of the TMJ pain-dysfunction syndrome. J Am Dent Assoc 86:833, 1973.
69. Bell WH, Yamaguchi Y, Poor MR: Treatment of temporomandibular joint dysfunction by intraoral vertical ramus osteotomy. Int J Adult Orthod Orthognath Surg 5:9, 1990.
70. Yanagisawa E: Symposium on maxillofacial trauma. III. Pitfalls in the management of zygomatic fractures. Laryngoscope 88:527, 1973.
71. Hosaka N, Shetty V, Caputo A, Bertolami C: Biomechanical validation of solitary lag screw fixation of mandibular angle fractures. IADR/AADR General Session. Cincinnati, Ohio, March, 1990.
72. Shetty V, Caputo A, Baker S, Bertolami C: Evaluation of internal fixation techniques for mandibular angle fractures. IADR/AADR General Session. Cincinnati, Ohio, March, 1990.
73. Niederdellmann H, Akuamoa-Boateng E: Internal fixation of fractures. Int J Oral Surg 7:252, 1978.
74. Niederdellmann H, Shetty V: Solitary lag screw osteosynthesis in the treatment of fractures of the angle of the mandible. Plast Reconstr Surg 80:688, 1987.
75. Rahn BA, Cordey J, Prein J, Russenberger M: Zur Biomechanik der Osteosynthese der Mandibula. Fortschr Kiefer Gesichtschir 19:37, 1975.
76. Kroon F: *In* Spiessl B: Internal Fixation of the Mandible. Berlin, Springer, 1989, p 26.

VII

ORTHOGNATHIC SURGERY

56 A 2-mm BICORTICAL SCREW TECHNIQUE FOR MANDIBULAR OSTEOTOMIES

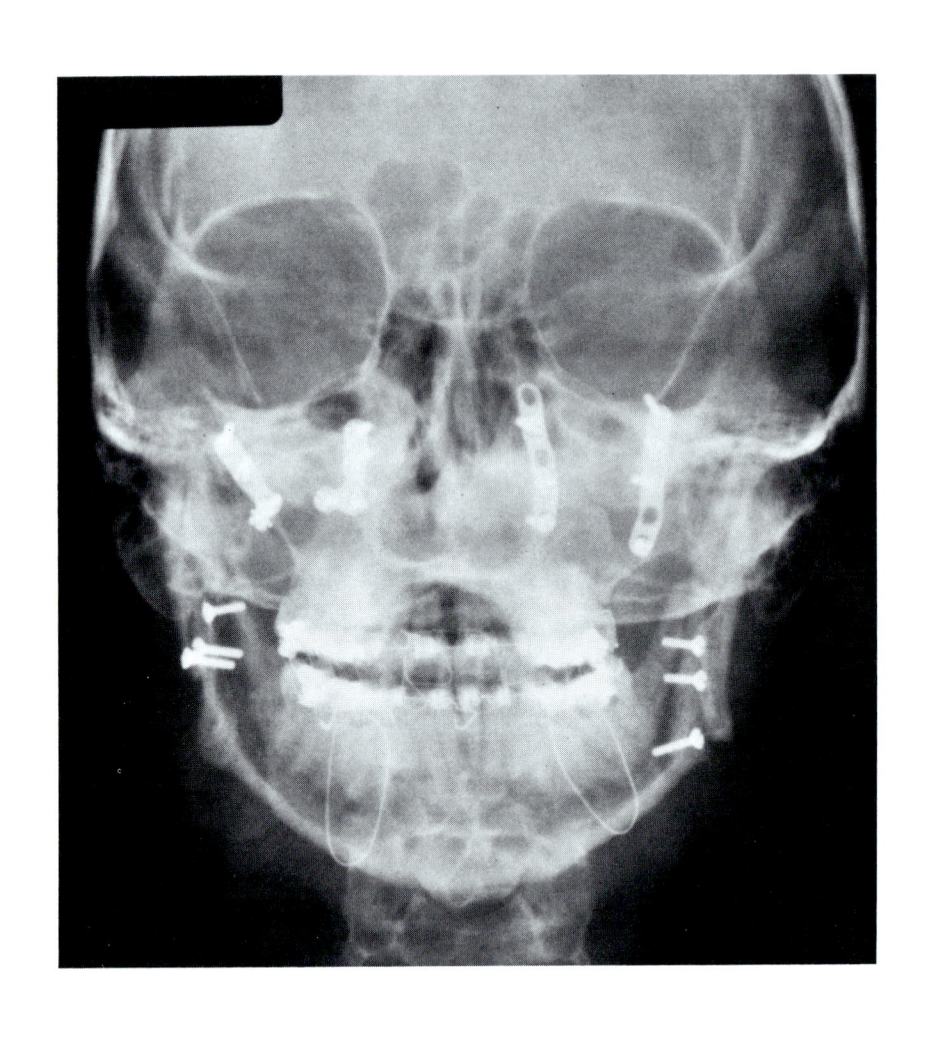

MODIFIED TECHNIQUE FOR 2-mm
BICORTICAL SCREW PLACEMENT

STABILITY OF MANDIBULAR
ADVANCEMENTS
   Relapse
   Occlusal Shifts
   Condylar Position
   TMJ Symptoms

STABILITY OF MANDIBULAR SETBACKS
   Relapse
   Modified Technique

MANAGEMENT OF UNUSUAL BUCCAL
FRAGMENTS

STABILITY OF TWO-JAW PROCEDURES

56

JOSEPH E. VAN SICKELS
THOMAS S. JETER
STEVEN B. ARAGON

While concepts of rigid fixation with fractures have been well established, the necessity of absolutely immobile systems in osteotomies has not been shown. Certainly a degree of rigidity is necessary in order to allow the bony segments to heal properly and to allow patients to function either immediately or shortly after surgery. The size of the screw or the amount of rigidity required to achieve a satisfactory postoperative occlusion is unknown. Several techniques have been employed and are believed to have been successful in the treatment of mandibular deformities. This chapter reviews the 2-mm bicortical screw technique used to stabilize sagittal split osteotomies for both advancements and setbacks. Studies involving patients treated with this method are reported.

MODIFIED TECHNIQUE FOR 2-mm BICORTICAL SCREW PLACEMENT

The following description is a review of our previous work, highlighting some of the technical aspects of the procedure.[11,31] We routinely use a "rigid" technique on all sagittal split osteotomies. When asymmetry cases are treated, one needs to pay particular attention to the preoperative radiographs and planned mandibular movement. Contouring of the fragments is often necessary, and screw placement may need to be modified in order to use this system (Fig. 56–1). Soft tissue dissection is accomplished as described by Bell and associates.[3] We utilize a reciprocating saw for all bony cuts. Although it is not an absolute necessity, we believe that a saw achieves a finer cut than a bur, thereby maximizing the bony surfaces for screw placement. Additionally, we believe that a saw is less likely to cause soft tissue injury. The medial cut is carried distal to the lingula with a bevel of at least 30 degrees and often vertically to the bone if the regional anatomy permits. This is particularly helpful in preventing bony interferences with mandibular setbacks or rotational movements. The saw should penetrate the cortical bone and be 4 to 5 mm superior to the neurovascular bundle (Fig. 56–2). A bony cut in excess of 5 mm above the neurovascular bundle may result in a split that continues up to the condylar process. A bony cut that does not extend posterior to the region of the neurovascular bundle may result in a medial fracture anterior to the neurovascular

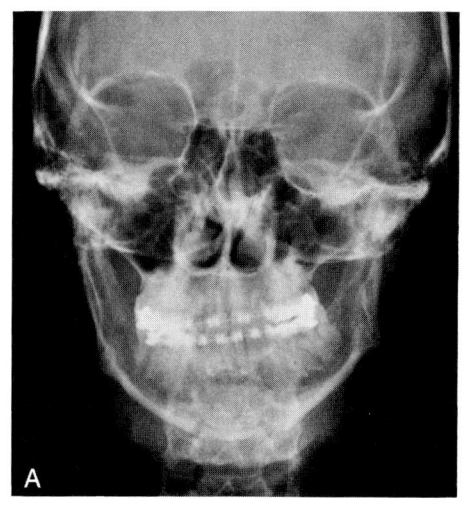

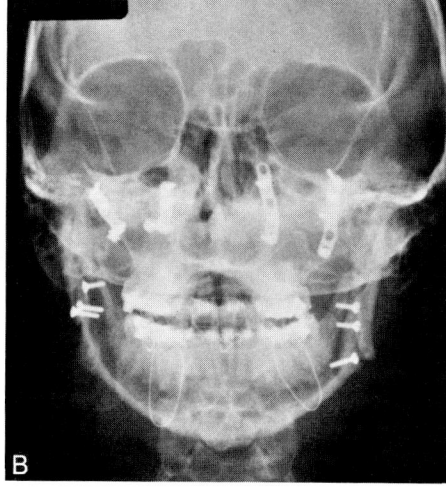

FIGURE 56-1. Preoperative (A) and postoperative (B) anteroposterior cephalometric radiograph of patient with maxillomandibular asymmetry. The proximal and distal fragments often require contouring in order to passively fit together, and screw placement may vary from side to side.

FIGURE 56-2. The medial saw cut must be 4 to 5 mm superior to the neurovascular bundle. A bevel of at least 30 degrees (and preferably a vertical cut) is helpful in preventing irregularities between the proximal and distal segments, thereby requiring less fragment modification prior to stabilization.

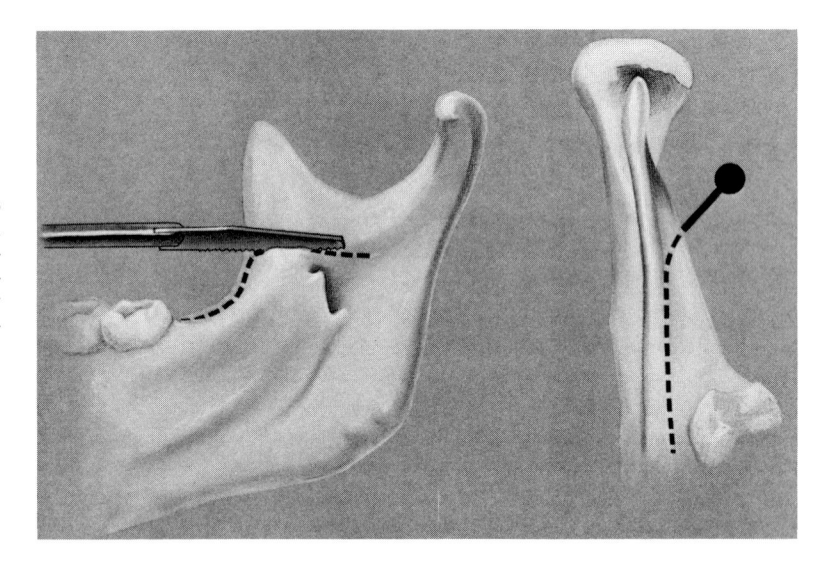

bundle. Care should be taken when retracting on the medial aspect, as a recent study has shown possible injury to the nerve when excessive retraction is used.[12] The medial osteotomy should be carried down the ascending ramus just medial to the external oblique ridge. Approaching the second molar, the saw blade is directed in a more vertical orientation. The lateral vertical osteotomy cut is also beveled posteriorly with respect to the buccal surface of the bone and is generally made in the first and second molar region (Fig. 56-3). The cut should be brought under the inferior border to the lingual aspect of the mandible. Failure to do so may result in the shearing of a buccal fragment. Beveling the buccal vertical cut allows placement of the chisel at the inferior border in the osteotomy in order to direct the split posteriorly. Splitting of the mandible is done by gently prying the fragments apart while using fine osteotomes to complete the bony cuts. Once the splits are complete, the mandible is placed in its preplanned occlusion and stabilized with maxillomandibular fixation (MMF). It is important to make the splint so that the buccal flange is removed between the most posterior occluding molars. This enables one to inspect the occlusion when the fragments are stabilized with a clamp, thereby preventing a posterior open bite. Gross interferences between the proximal and distal segments should be removed. While the segments should ideally lie in perfect apposition along their entire lengths, areas of poor contact are often present. Positioning of the proximal segment is technically a very sensitive component of the procedure. One might produce temporomandibular symptoms

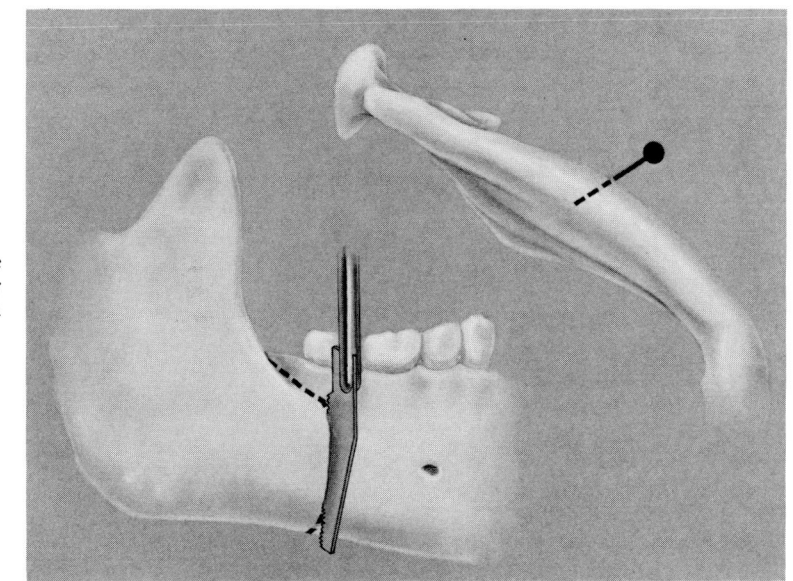

FIGURE 56-3. The lateral osteotomy is made with a posterior bevel in the first and second molar region. This enables one to place the osteotome in a posterior direction for a more controlled split.

by aggressively placing the condyle in its most posterosuperior position within the glenoid fossa.

The following pages describe the general techniques we have been using since 1982. Modifications of this technique are discussed in the section on condylar position. The proximal fragment should be manipulated superiorly and distally with mild pressure. One should not use excessive force when seating the condyles posteriorly, as this may result in postoperative disk dysfunction. Frequently the proximal segment is manipulated several times to make sure the segment is firmly but not forcibly seated. Extraoral palpation helps assure that the inferior borders are aligned as dictated by the cephalometric predictions. A small V wire pusher is used on the inferior aspect of the proximal segment to determine correct position. A modified clamp is then used to stabilize the proximal and distal fragments for screw insertion (Fig. 56-4). The authors recommend the removal of third molars at least 6 months and preferably 1 year in advance of surgery in order to allow mature bone to fill the socket sites. This allows good bone contact, leaves a larger area for screw placement, and decreases the incidence of adverse splits.[31,32] It is important to place the clamp in a region of good bone contact. Once the clamp is

FIGURE 56-4. The bony segments are positioned and stabilized with a modified clamp prior to screw insertion. The clamp is modified in order to avoid excessive compression between the two segments.

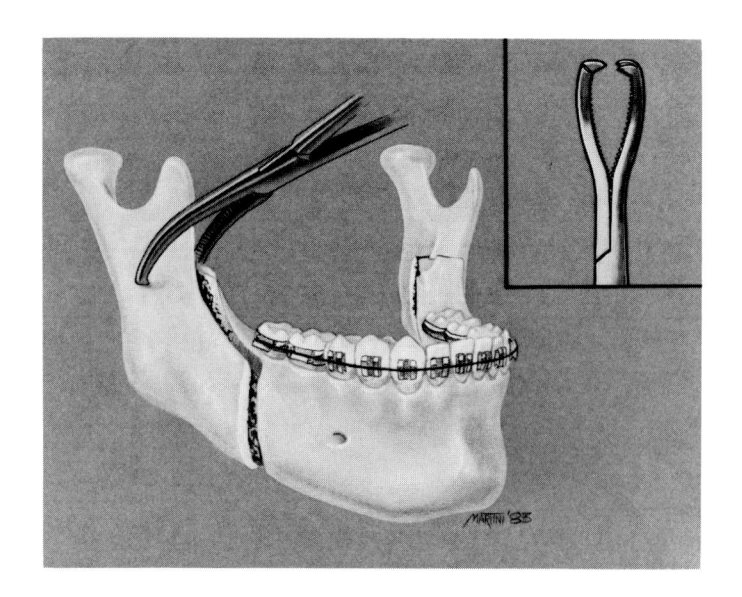

placed, the occlusion must be inspected. If a posterior open bite is created, the clamp should be released and repositioned as established by the predetermined occlusion. This usually requires superior repositioning of the distal fragment prior to replacing the clamp. The proximal segment should be observed for any medial or lateral movement. Such movement suggests that the condyle is being torqued. Placement of the clamp in an area of good bone contact minimizes torquing forces placed upon the fragments. The modified clamp, as shown in the illustration, does not come together at the tips in order to avoid undue pressure and possible fracture. In certain instances when the segments are extremely thin, a Kocher or other instrument is necessary to prevent slippage of the segments prior to screw placement.

Once stabilized, the fragments are inspected for position, orientation, and their effects upon the occlusion. If they lie together in good apposition and the cheek can be easily retracted, it may be desirable to drill and place screws intraorally. The authors, however, usually use a transcutaneous approach. We find the percutaneous approach to be technically easier than an intraoral approach. Furthermore, we believe that when segments tend to splay apart, a perpendicular screw placed in the area of best bone contact may minimize segment displacement. A stab incision is made in the cheek approximately 1.5 to 2.5 cm above the antegonial notch and a small trocar is placed. A 1.5-mm drill or a 0.062-inch threaded Kirschner (K) wire on a mini-pin driver is placed through the trocar, and at least three holes are driven through both the proximal and distal fragments. All three holes are placed distal to the second molar and frequently anterior and superior to the neurovascular bundle. In some cases it may be possible and/or desirable to place two screws above and one below the canal. A recent study showed this configuration to be biomechanically superior to three screws placed at the tension zone.[5] The depth of the hole is measured with a measuring device. If the measurement indicates a size that is not available, one should choose a screw 1 mm longer rather than shorter, since bicortical engagement of the screws is desired. When large-headed screws are used, the hole is countersunk prior to placing the screws in order to place the head more flush with the cortex. When screws with low-profile heads are used, this step is unnecessary. A 2-mm diameter screw of the proper length is brought into the mouth on screw-holding forceps and seated in a previously drilled hole. If the hole is stripped, a larger diameter screw is used. While larger screws may provide greater holding power, we have found the 2-mm diameter screw system adequate for both mandibular advancements and setbacks. The screwdriver is inserted through the trocar and the screw is firmly seated. The other two screws are seated in a similar fashion. Following placement of three screws on the opposite side, the maxillomandibular fixation is removed and the occlusion is checked. While seating the condyles both vertically and distally, the mandible is rotated along its rotational arc and the occlusion is verified. Palpation of the medial aspect of the mandible ensures that no screws protrude through the medial cortex. The surgical site is then closed in the routine manner. Following the release of MMF, the nasoendotracheal tube may be converted to an oral endotracheal tube, enabling one to proceed with concomitant nasal procedures if applicable. The authors differ with regard to postoperative splint usage. The splint is removed and the patient is allowed to function when the postoperative occlusion is stable. When the occlussion is not stable, two of the authors (JVS, SBA) leave the splint in for at least 2 weeks in order to provide a more stable occlusion and possibly prevent minor shifts and potentially altering bone healing.

Two or three box elastics are placed at the end of the procedure, one on either side posteriorly and one in the anterior region. In cases of large advancements, skeletal wires and a period of fixation may be necessary.[33] As the patient adapts to his new occlusion, the number of elastics and the time that they are worn are decreased. Diet is restricted to soft foods for the first 8 weeks, advancing from liquids the first 2 weeks to a regular diet by the eighth week (see previous guidelines).[31] Ideally, with active and passive physiotherapy, the patient can open to 40 mm by 8 weeks. While occasional patients obtain this amount of opening by 8 weeks, most fall short of this arbitrary goal.[1] More vigorous therapy is instituted when hypomobility is noted. Generally within 6 months the preoperative range of motion is achieved.

STABILITY OF MANDIBULAR ADVANCEMENTS

Relapse

Stability of an osteotomy must be evaluated with respect to its effects on occlusion and the bony segments. In this first section, relapse of bilateral sagittal split osteotomies is reviewed.[13,24,28,29] Overall the results seen with this procedure are very stable.[13,24,29] Minimal or no relapse has been seen both horizontally and vertically 6 to 12 months postoperatively in several studies.[13,29] For the average case, when the mandible was brought forward, there was a further long-term advancement secondary to occlusal settling and splint removal.[24,28,29] Although the results are generally very stable, relapse can occur when 2-mm screw fixation is employed, especially with large anterior advancements.

Relapse may be due to a number of factors: (1) failure to seat condyles in the fossa at the time of surgery, (2) soft tissue tension (muscles and paramandibular connective tissue), (3) magnitude of advancement, (4) proximal segment control, (5) condylar resorption, (6) postoperative management, and (7) unknown causes. Failure to seat condyles should be found at the time of surgery, following the release of MMF to confirm condylar position. As discussed earlier, while in surgery, one should seat condyles both vertically and posteriorly and manipulate the mandible into occlusion. Any interference or slide that is posterior to the desired position in the splint must be carefully evaluated. When the deviation is significant, one should replace the maxillomandibular fixation, remove the screws, and reposition the proximal fragments. If an unacceptable occlusion is still present, one should consider wire fixation coupled with skeletal wires.

In a study of 51 patients who underwent mandibular advancements with a bilateral sagittal split osteotomy fixated with 2-mm bicortical screws, the magnitude of advancement had the highest correlation with relapse.[33] The farther the mandible was advanced, the greater the chance for relapse. While the amount of advancement was highly significant it did not account for all the relapse seen in the sample.

Early studies with a 2-mm system have shown excellent maintenance of the proximal segment position both intraoperatively and long-term postoperatively.[29] However, extreme rotation of the proximal fragment in a clockwise fashion may predispose one to relapse as the sling attempts to return to its previous position.

Condylar resorption has been shown to occur following orthognathic surgery.[19] It has been suggested that rigid fixation may increase the load on the condyle and cause late resorption. If this were to happen on a regular basis, one would expect to see relapse occurring late (after 6 weeks to 6 months). This is a controversial area, as studies have shown that in animals the most damaging scenario may be one in which the condyle is placed in the fossa forcibly (compression forces) and followed by immobilization.[9,17] Few clinical studies have addressed this question with respect to rigid fixation. One paper evaluated 29 patients treated with 2-mm screws to assess when relapse occurred.[33] A nonsignificant 0.06-mm relapse was noted during the first 6 weeks, followed by further advancement of the mandible. This suggests that relapse occurred early and was probably at the osteotomy site and not at the condyle.

Postoperative management may play a role in patient outcome. Box elastics in the immediate postoperative period are suggested. The use of "long" Class II elastics (extending from the lower molars to the upper cuspid region) may accentuate the pull of the muscles of mastication and result in relapse. One author (JVS) has observed relapse of the distal fragment with upward movement of proximal fragment in several cases in which the use of long Class II elastics in the immediate postoperative period were used. Studies accomplished with wire osteosynthesis have noted many factors to play a role in relapse. Some of these factors probably play a role in the relapse of sagittal split osteotomies secured by rigid fixation.

Occlusal Shifts

One of the peculiarities that has been noted with rigid fixation is lateral shifts of the occlusion. These are seen in the early postoperative period and may be due to several factors — swelling in the joints and muscles, failure to seat both condyles evenly, and condylar torque. Swelling resolves quickly, and the occlusion is easily managed by training elastics. However, an anteroposterior shift to one side is more problematic. This is most likely due to failure to recognize that a condyle is not seated fully in the fossa at the time of surgery. If a severe shift is present, reoperation is necessary. Mild mandibular shifts of 1 to 2 mm may be managed orthodontically. Most sources believe that this may be due to a slight discrepancy in the condylar positioning during the placement of rigid fixation of the two segments. This discrepancy is typically recognized within the first 6 weeks after surgery.

Once the surgical splints have been removed, the orthodontic management of such a mandibular shift can be handled relatively easily. During the first several weeks after surgery, the orthodontist can begin correction by an exaggerated skewing (bowing) of upper and lower rectangular arch wires opposite the direction of the midline shift (Fig. 56–5). Short Class II and Class III elastics can be worn on opposite sides to further enhance the correction of the midlines. For example, if the mandible shifts 1.5 mm to the right, the mandibular heavy arch wire is skewed to the left while the maxillary arch wire is skewed to the right. Short-span Class II elastics are then worn on the left and short Class III elastics on the right. Small discrepancies of a couple of millimeters are usually corrected within 1 to 2 months using this regimen. Once the correction has been achieved, it is important to remember to recoordinate the upper and lower arch wires to a symmetric shape so that the midlines and arch forms are not allowed to overcorrect in opposite directions.

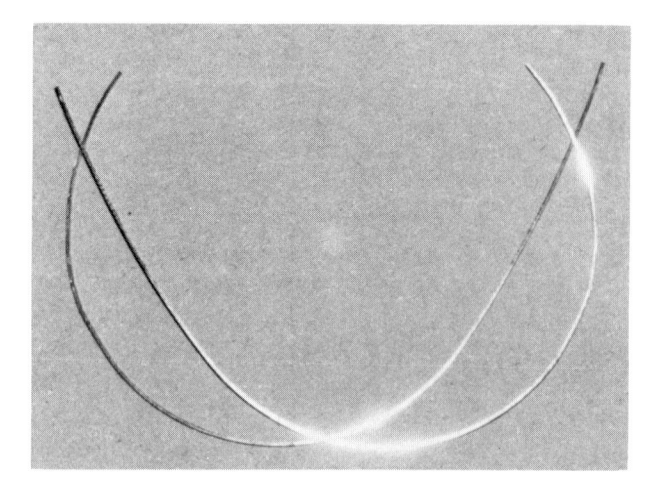

FIGURE 56–5. Right and left skewed arch wires are useful in correcting minor discrepancies soon after splint removal. (Courtesy of Dr. Carolyn Flanary.)

Condylar Position

There is concern that the condyle may become torqued within the fossa with the application of rigid fixation. This may result in anteroposterior or mediolateral changes within the fossa. Investigators have studied anteroposterior changes with lateral tomograms. Kundert and Hadjianghelou[14] compared a group of patients who had undergone bilateral sagittal splits stabilized with circumferential wires versus those with three 2.7-mm bicortical screws. They noted that with advancements of the mandible, the condyle tended to shift posteriorly within the fossa, while the reverse was true with setbacks. They also noted a greater incidence of condylar shifts when screws were employed than with wires. Timmis et al,[26] in a preliminary report, looked at lateral tomograms of advancements and setbacks treated by bilateral sagittal split osteotomies fixated with 2-mm bicortical screws. Similar to the findings of Kundert and Hadjianghelou,[14] they noted that there was a trend for the condyle to be pushed posteriorly in the fossa with advancements while the reverse was true with setbacks. They also noted a normalization of condylar position from the initial postoperative position to that seen at 6 months. Mediolateral shifts have also been of concern when screws were employed. Studies with dried mandibles have noted significant movement of the condyles and condylar torque when the screws were applied.[7,27] A simple geometric model of the mandible suggests that as the mandible is set back the condyles constrict and that they would expand as the mandible is advanced (Figs. 56–6 and 56–7). Spitzer et al[23] examined 10 patients who had undergone mandibular setbacks treated with 2.7-mm bicortical screws and noted no gross displacement of the condylar fragments. Hackney et al[10] examined submental vertex films obtained preoperatively and 6 months after surgery on 15 patients who had undergone bilateral sagittal split osteotomies fixated with 2-mm bicortical screws. Intercondylar width and angle were documented before and 6 months after surgery (Fig. 56–8). There was no significant change in intercondylar angle nor intercondylar width for the group as a whole. However, there was a wide range of variability within the group. The intercondylar angle increased in nine patients, decreased in four, and remained unchanged in two. Intercondylar width increased in five patients, decreased in eight, and remained unchanged in two.

FIGURE 56–6. In order to exactly approximate segments, a simple geometric model suggests that the condyles would rotate medially as the mandible is set back.

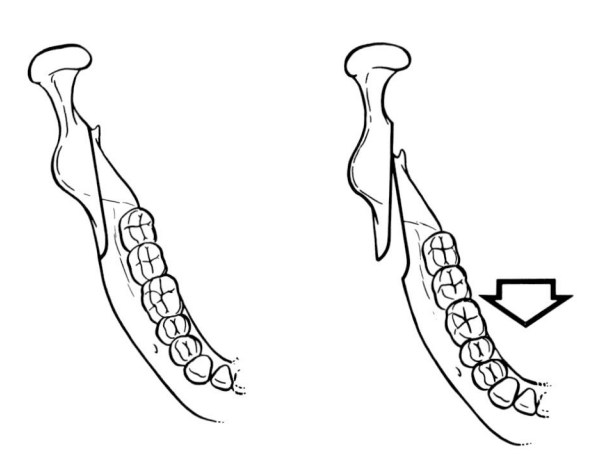

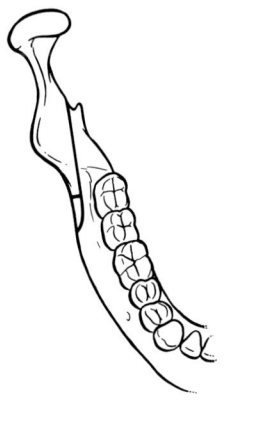

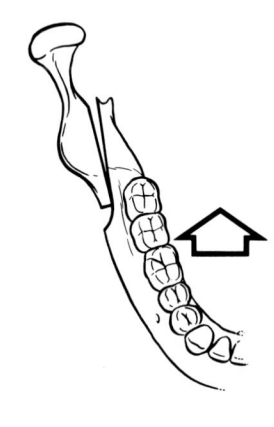

FIGURE 56–7. As the distal segment is advanced, a simple geometric model conversely predicts that the condylar segment rotates laterally.

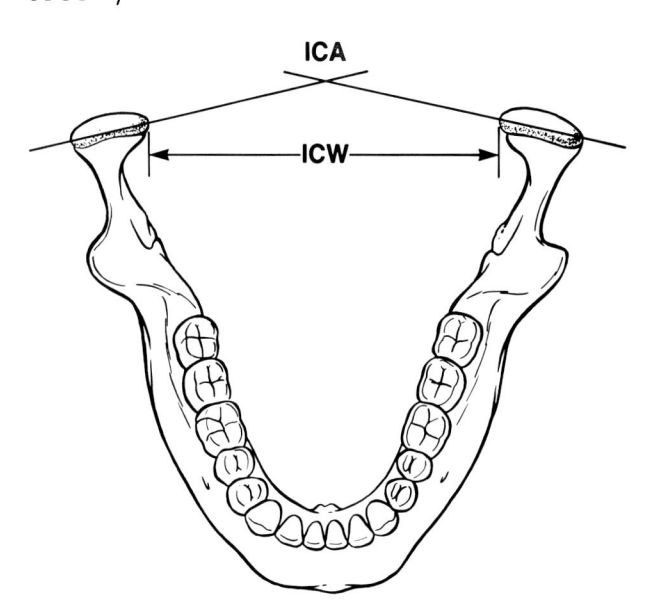

FIGURE 56-8. Intercondylar width and intercondylar angle measurements of the mandible.

These studies suggest that changes in condylar position, both anteroposterior and mediolateral, do occur with screw osteosynthesis. However, those changes do not correspond to a simple geometric model. Anteroposterior changes may be minimized by the technique described earlier. Several techniques have been advocated in order to reproduce condylar position during fixation of the fragments. The benefit of this technique, although based on sound clinical judgment, remains to be proven. One author (JT) uses a measuring device to place the proximal segment near its preoperative position. Prior to splitting the ramus, a hole is placed in the external oblique ridge just distal to the vertical buccal osteotomy. With the mandible in centric relation, a measurement with calipers is made from the hole in the external oblique ridge to a convenient maxillary landmark (usually the buccal tube of the maxillary first molar orthodontic bracket). When a two-jaw procedure is planned, the measurement is taken after fixation of the maxilla. This measurement is then duplicated at the time of fragment stabilization with the bone clamp and screw fixation. Mediolateral changes are related to how the fragments lie together. Clamp placement probably has more influence on this aspect than the geometry of the surgical move. It is unknown how much condylar adaptation can take place with respect to a change in condylar position. It may actually be more important to note the effect on temporomandibular signs and symptoms following the surgical procedure.

Temporomandibular Joint (TMJ) Symptoms

TMJ symptoms are present in the population at large and certainly in a number of individuals who elect to undergo orthognathic surgery.[16] Whether symptoms improve or worsen with orthognathic surgery is certainly of concern. Several investigators have examined this subject with wire osteosynthesis. Freihoffer and Petrosvic[8] noted that 16 of 38 patients experienced TMJ clicking after sagittal split advancement stabilized with wire osteosynthesis. Schendel and Epker,[20] in a multi-institutional study, documented TMJ noise in 12 of 71 patients and TMJ pain in one after advancement. They concluded that there was no increased incidence of pathologic conditions of the TMJ after advancement. Will et al[34] noted a similar incidence of TMJ pain, clicking, and locking in both pre- and postsurgical populations in 41 patients at least 6 weeks after mandibular advancements and maxillomandibular fixation. Kyiak et al[2,15] noted that popping and clicking of the TMJ were reduced in 73 per cent and increased in about 25 per cent of the patients following surgery.

There is less information with rigid fixation. While concern has been raised that rigid fixation causes TMJ symptoms, several studies have not shown this to be a problem. Paulus and Steinhauser[18] noted no difference in TMJ symptoms from the pre- to postoperative periods whether 2.7-mm screws or wires were used to fix sagittal split osteotomies for correction of mandibular prognathism. Timmis et al[25] studied signs and symptoms of TMJ dysfunction in two groups of patients undergoing bilateral sagittal split osteotomies. Fourteen subjects had wire osteosynthesis and 14 had 2-mm screw osteosynthesis. When subjective symptoms and clicking were examined, the wire group had no significant increase in postoperative TMJ dysfunction. The screw group had significant improvement in both subjective complaints and clicks. While these findings suggest that screw osteosynthesis may be superior to wire osteosynthesis, one must be careful in interpreting these results owing to the small sample size and multiple variables between the groups. In the study previously reported by Hackney et al[10] there was no correlation between changes in condylar position and clicking seen prior to or after surgery. These results are encouraging and suggest that there is a certain amount of adaptability in the joint complex.

STABILITY OF MANDIBULAR SETBACKS

Relapse

Mandibular setbacks stabilized by 2.7-mm screws have been studied by several authors. Schmoker et al[21] found a decreased relapse tendency with mandibular setbacks when three screws rather than two were used for bone fixation. Paulus and Steinhauser[18] observed similar results when patients with two screws in vertical ramal setbacks experienced greater relapse than those with three screws in sagittal split setbacks. They noted greater vertical and horizontal stability with the sagittal split group than with the vertical subcondylar group. Spiessel noted only a 4 per cent recurrence following sagittal split osteotomies with three lag screws, compared to 22 per cent recurrence when fixation was achieved with maxillomandibular fixation, Kirschner wires, or one or two lag screws.[22] Franco et al[6] studied 25 patients who had undergone bilateral sagittal split osteotomies for setbacks. One- and two-jaw procedures were included. Even with excellent occlusal results, the chin point tended to rotate forward postoperatively. The pattern of forward rotation at the chin point with loss of anterior facial height was similar to that seen with stable mandibular advancements. There was minimal influence of the maxilla on the mandibular result. The cause of relapse in the two groups differed. With isolated mandibular setbacks, the magnitude of setback was the single factor most responsible for relapse, while with two-jaw surgeries alteration of the proximal fragment was chiefly responsible for relapse. The authors postulated that the two factors were related and could both cause relapse. The farther one moves the distal fragment back, the greater the amount of stretch is placed on the medial attachments of the mandible. Likewise, when one rotates the proximal fragment posteriorly, the lateral attachments are placed under tension. Following this study, minor alterations in technique were suggested to prevent these problems.

Modified Technique

The amount of the setback is determined from models and cephalometric predictions. The bony cuts are made as described above. For a routine case a second cut is made obliquely toward the inferior border of the mandible (Fig. 56–9). This strip, which is wider at the inferior portion of the mandible, is removed, and the

Two weeks after surgery, the patient's occlusion markedly changed. Inspection of the radiographs suggested that there was a horizontal fracture of the left ramus. The patient was taken to surgery, where this finding was confirmed. The mandible was placed in MMF and the proximal fragment was manipulated posteriorly and superiorly. A four-hole plate was placed via a percutaneous incision and an additional bicortical anterior screw was used to stabilize the segments (Fig. 56-12). The patient was also functional immediately without any further sequelae.

STABILITY OF TWO-JAW PROCEDURES

Single-jaw maxillary and mandibular surgeries treated with rigid fixation have been shown to be more stable than those treated with wire osteosynthesis. While one would assume that two-jaw procedures would also be more stable, this is not necessarily so. In this section, two cases are reviewed. In one the results were extremely stable, whereas in the second the results were poor. Factors contributing to the poor result are reviewed.

CASE 1

A 23-year-old man with vertical maxillary excess and horizontal mandibular deficiency was scheduled for a maxillary impaction and advancement, mandibular advancement, and a genial advancement (Fig. 56-13). Total advancement of the chin point was 20 mm. Four plates were placed to stabilize the maxillary osteotomy, and three screws were used per side. Skeletal wires were used and the patient was kept in fixation for 5 days. His 6-week and 6-month radiographs revealed an extremely stable result (Fig. 56-14).

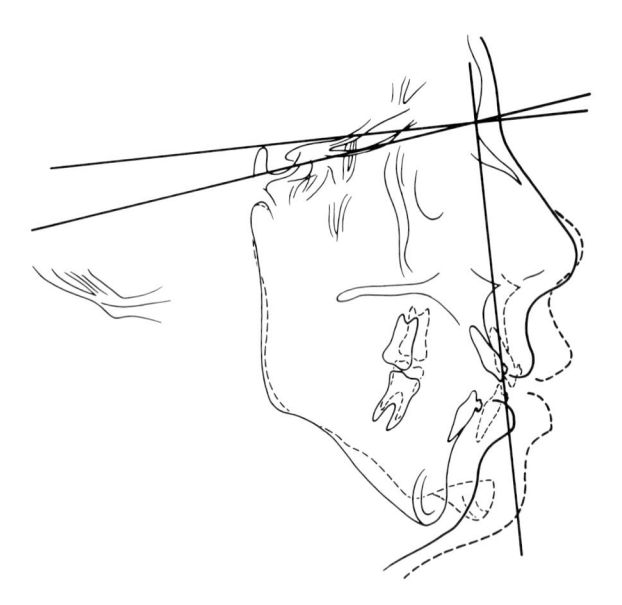

FIGURE 56-13. Preoperative and immediate postoperative cephalometric tracings of a patient following maxillary impaction and advancement with mandibular and genial advancement. The total advancement at the chin measures about 20 mm.

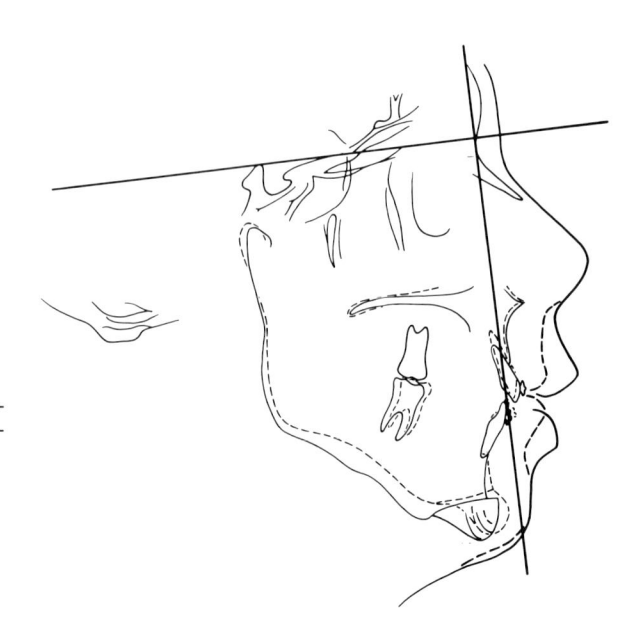

FIGURE 56-14. Immediate postoperative and 6-month postoperative cephalometric tracings showing an extremely stable dental and skeletal result.

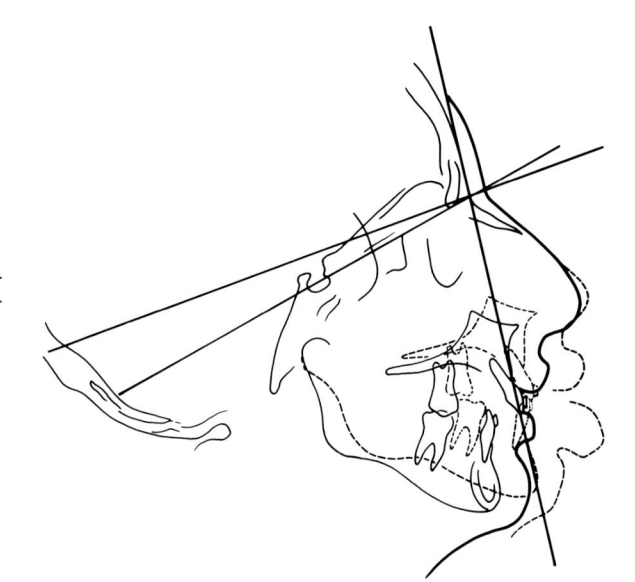

FIGURE 56-15. Preoperative and immediate postoperative cephalometric tracings of a patient following a maxillary impaction with mandibular and genial advancement.

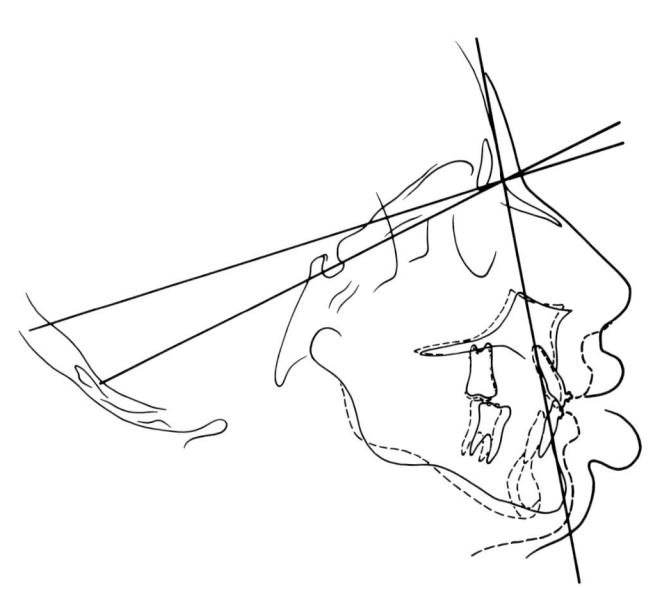

FIGURE 56-16. Comparison of immediate and 2-year postoperative cephalometric tracings showing marked relapse of 8 mm at the chin point and 3 mm relapse at the central incisor.

CASE 2

A 20-year-old woman was planned to have a maxillary impaction, mandibular advancement, and genial advancement. Total movement at the chin point was 15 mm (Fig. 56-15). She had four plates used in the maxilla, three screws per side in the mandible. Her 2-year radiograph showed relapse of 8 mm at the chin point (Fig. 56-16). Her central incisor was 3 mm posterior and 1 mm inferior to the planned position. Analysis of the 6-week radiographs reveal that the majority of the relapse occurred during this time period.

While it is speculative, two factors may have contributed to this result. The initial postoperative film shows that the proximal segments were rotated with the surgery. In the first 6 weeks, the surgeons recognized that the patient did not have a Class I occlusion. Long Class II elastics were placed in an effort to maintain the occlusion. This therapy resulted in the extrusion and retrusion of the maxillary centrals as well as augmentation of the mandibular relapse.

The results of the first case stand in sharp contrast to those of the second. A minimal period of fixation combined with skeletal wires resulted in an extremely stable result. It is tempting to speculate which of these factors is more important in the end result. Skeletal wires and maxillomandibular fixation have been shown to decrease the amount of relapse seen when conventional wire osteosynthesis was used.[4] By tying the skeletal bases to one another, one can prevent movement through the teeth and their periodontal ligaments. On large advancements, the pull of the paramandibular adnexial tissue appears to overcome the holding power of the screws. Therefore, some

57

SURGICAL MANAGEMENT OF SHORT MANDIBULAR RAMUS DEFORMITIES

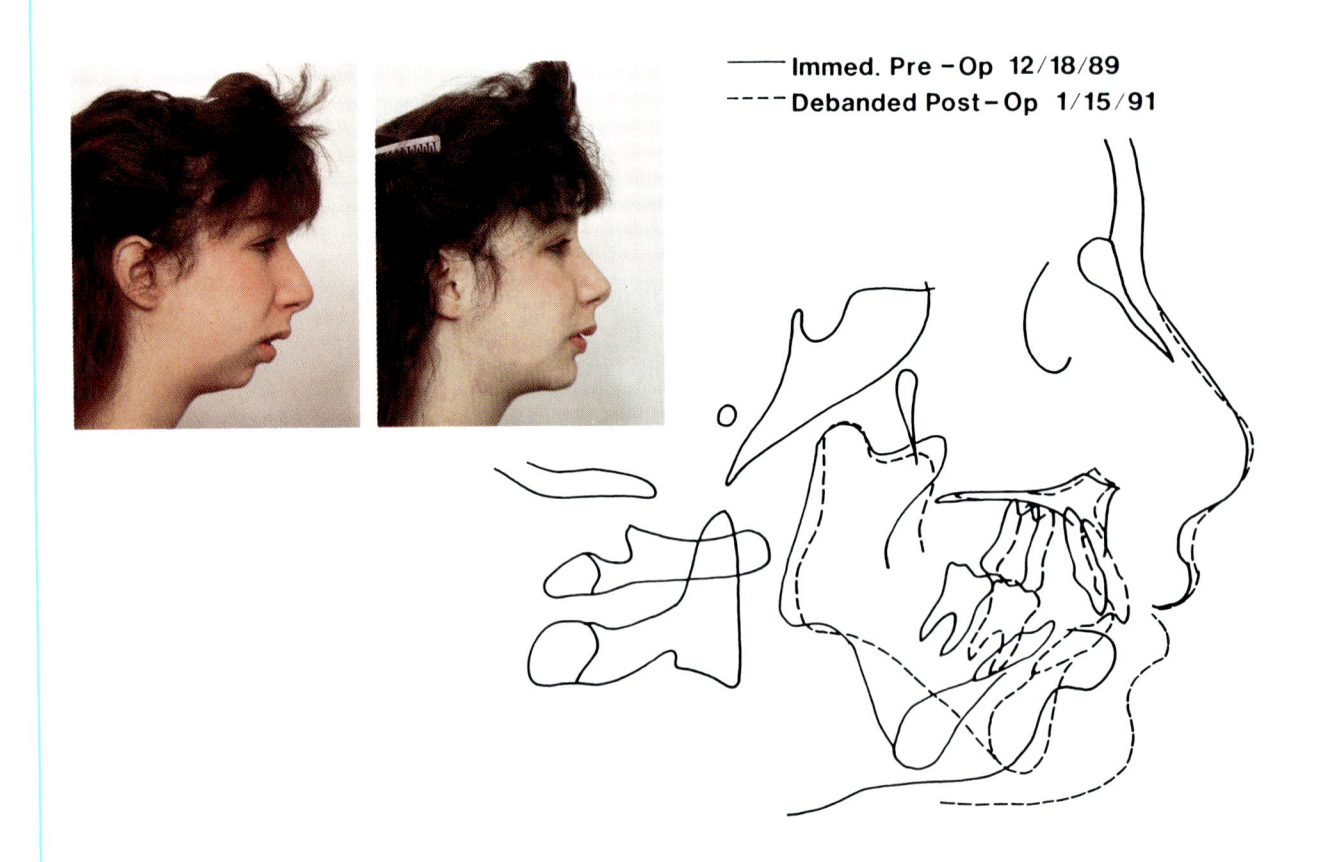

CLINICAL DEFORMITY
SURGICAL TREATMENT
CLINICAL CASES

57

ALBERT E. CARLOTTI, Jr.
STEPHEN A. SCHENDEL

Short mandibular ramus deformities are characterized by a lack of posterior facial height. This is frequently associated with anterior maxillary hyperplasia and always with posterior maxillary hypoplasia.[1-12] Different conditions, either congenital or acquired, may cause this skeletal pattern, including temporomandibular ankylosis, rheumatoid arthritis, bilateral otomandibular dysplasia, and Treacher Collins syndrome. Frequently, however, the deformity appears following growth and development without any obvious cause.

Surgical correction of this deformity is directed to the location of the principal anatomic abnormalities.[6-8,12] The central malformation is the short mandibular ramus resulting in a lack of chin projection and a Class II malocclusion. Failure of development of the mandible also alters the maxilla. Underdevelopment of the posterior maxilla and alteration of the occlusal plane are common. Frequently, this is associated with overdevelopment of the anterior maxilla. Both maxillary and mandibular corrective procedures should be considered in the treatment plan. In this chapter, we discuss the diagnosis and surgical treatment of the short mandibular ramus patient. Surgical treatment deals with the mandibular body and ramus deformities and associated maxillary deformities but does not review temporomandibular joint reconstruction.

CLINICAL DEFORMITY

The clinical appearance of the patient with a short mandibular ramus is characteristic.[12] The mandible is small and retrusive, with microgenia representative of the overall hypoplasia. While the chin lacks anterior projection, it is usually increased in vertical direction. The face tapers rapidly and has been called the "bird-face deformity" by Obwegeser.[7,8] The maxilla can be of normal height anteriorly or may be elongated as in vertical maxillary excess. The occlusal plane is always greatly canted obliquely upward posteriorly.

The nose is quite prominent and often narrow. The upper lip is variable, but it can appear short secondary to the anterior vertical maxillary excess. However, there is almost always lip incompetence because of the maxillary problem and lack of chin projection. This results in a short suprahyoid area and lack of the definite cervicomandibular angle. The lower lip may be either curled outward or tight with perioral muscular hyperfunction.

The radiographic pattern is also characteristic, and the cephalometric analysis has been especially relevant. Subjectively, the mandibular ramus appears short, and the retrogenia with Class II malocclusion is evident. Classic analysis shows a large mandibular plane angle associated with a smaller than normal SNB angle. The lower anterior face height may also be increased. The architectural and structural analysis of Delaire has been especially useful in demonstrating the spectrum of malformations seen here[3,4] (see clinical cases). This analysis compares the jaws to the cranial base and is based upon individual proportions, thereby avoiding statistical averages. A complete description of this analysis is beyond the scope of this paper; only the relevant findings are discussed.

The mandibular ramus is short vertically and is frequently narrow whereas the chin is long vertically. The mandibular body is variable but frequently hypoplastic. The chin lacks anterior projection. The condyles may be small; however, the glenoid fossa is usually low and anterior in position relative to the cranial base. The maxilla is tipped upward and the occlusal plane is accentuated. The posterior palate is superiorly displaced in many cases. The maxillary alveolar height is always short posteriorly. The anterior nasal spine is usually normal in position, but the maxillary anterior alveolar portion may be increased. The anterior facial height is thus generally increased. The maxillary incisors are usually normally inclined. However, secondary to the tipped maxillary occlusal plane, the angle between the upper and lower incisors is closer to 110 degrees. The occlusion is Class II with an open bite tendency with dental crowding, as the arches are frequently narrow.

In a large series of patients operated for an excessive display of maxillary gingiva, we found that a certain percentage of this group actually fell into the short ramus category using the Delaire analysis.[11] It is important to identify these patients and not to confuse them with those with vertical maxillary excess, classically known as the long face syndrome, since the surgical correction for optimal functional and esthetic results is different.

SURGICAL TREATMENT

The main treatment objectives include elongation of posterior facial height and increased projection of the lower face. Leveling the occlusal plane by lowering the posterior maxilla is an integral part of the increase in posterior facial height. Reduction of the anterior facial height is usually needed and consists of two components. Anterior maxillary height may be increased and should be reduced by maxillary ostectomy. Since the chin is usually increased vertically, it also should be reduced in height as it is advanced either by total mandibular rotation or vertical reduction genioplasty. Of course, the plan may consist of any combination of the above depending upon the individual deformity.

Logic dictates that the mandibular deformity be corrected at the site of its anatomic origin, which is the ramus.[1,7,8,12] Maximum elongation/advancement of the mandible can be achieved only by surgically lengthening the ramus with chin surgery. However, surgical procedures to increase the posterior facial height are associated with counterclockwise rotation of the mandible, and they have been shown to result in extensive relapse. Suprahyoid myotomies, overcorrection using splints, cervical collars, and external fixation devices have all been advocated to minimize the relapse.

Sagittal splitting of the ramus, as described by Obwegeser for correction of the bird-face deformity, is applicable in cases of minimal ramus lengthening with modifications.[6-8] The correction of larger deformities is accomplished according to the principles of Delaire as described by Tulasne and Tessier. In both cases, correction of the maxillary and chin deformities should be done concomitantly.

Up to 10 mm of posterior ramus height can be obtained without significant relapse by the sagittal ramus-splitting technique under certain conditions. First, the ramus must be sufficiently broad, thick, and well-developed even though it is short. A small, abnormally shaped ramus as seen in hemifacial microsomia is not a candidate for this procedure. Secondly, the masseteric sling should be completely stripped from both the proximal and distal segments and not reattached during closure. Third, rigid fixation must be utilized.

Large ramus deformities need to be corrected by lengthening the ramus through an extraoral approach. A V or inverted L osteotomy is performed and the defective bone grafted. The masseter and medial pterygoid muscles are again completely detached and are not repositioned at the end of surgery. The graft should be mortised into position and rigid plate fixation utilized. Reduction of the anterior lower facial height improves the stability.

Maxillary surgical correction is accomplished at the same time by a Le Fort I osteotomy using the downfracture technique. The posterior facial height is lengthened by bone grafting the maxillary defect created when the occlusal plane is leveled. At the same time, the anterior maxillary excess is resected and the anterior facial height shortened. Rigid fixation is utilized for increased stability and ease of segment repositioning.

The chin deformity is corrected by a combined advancement/vertical reduction genioplasty. Either the functional genioplasty technique as described by Schendel or the "jumping" bone flap technique of Tessier is utilized.[12] Fixation with these techniques is easily obtained with screws. Multiple horizontal osteotomies of the chin to increase the advancement are not recommended, nor are alloplastic materials in this instance.

The timing of these procedures after puberty is not critical. In young children with this deformity, ramus lengthening can safely be done starting at around 8 years of age.[12] If the joint is abnormal, reconstruction should be completed as early as possible. When the ramus is lengthened in the growing individual, the maxillary deformity can be precluded or minimized in many cases. In those cases with a maxillary component, the maxillary surgery frequently can be avoided, and this aspect of the deformity can be corrected orthopedically according to the principles of Delaire.

Sagittal splitting of the mandible is performed in the usual manner up to the time for detachment of the masseter and medial pterygoid muscles. These muscles are completely detached, and care is taken to detach the sphenomandibular ligament. The osteotomies and splits are accomplished in the usual manner. The segments are mobilized into their new positions and fixed using screws or plates. The technique of Tulasne and Schendel for intraoral rigid plate application following sagittal splitting is recommended.[13] The maxilla is fixed into position prior to the mandibular segments when concomitant maxillary repositioning is performed. The pterygomasseteric sling is not reconstructed at the time of wound closure.

A 3-cm incision is made below the angle of the mandible in the Risdon fashion for the extraoral osteotomy technique. The ramus is then exposed by a wide subperiosteal dissection of the masseter and medial pterygoid muscles. An inverted L or V osteotomy is then performed. It is important at this time to completely free the sphenomandibular ligament, after which the ramus should be easily lengthened and advanced. The maxillary osteotomy is completed and the maxilla repositioned and stabilized. The mandible is repositioned with intermaxillary fixation. Bone grafts are onlayed and inlayed into the ramus defects and fixed to the proximal and distal fragments with rigid plate fixation. The condyles should be carefully repositioned into the glenoid fossa during this part of the procedure. The periosteal layer and the pterygomasseteric muscles are not closed primarily. However, the platysma layer is closed primarily. Postoperative care and rehabilitation are similar to those employed in the management of other high-angle bimaxillary deformities. Maxillomandibular fixation is usually maintained for 6 weeks even with the use of rigid internal fixation. In cases in which the maxilla is not operated simultaneously, but a large posterior open bite is created to allow the maxillary dentoalveolar segments to elongate slowly, the postoperative treatment is somewhat different. The maxillomandibular fixation is removed at 6 weeks, but the splint is left in place for a number of months. The area of the splint anterior to the last molar is gradually removed, allowing the teeth to erupt. After these teeth are completely erupted, the molar area is reduced accordingly and the splint is finally removed. This procedure is usually indicated in growing individuals.

CLINICAL CASES

CASE 1, J.D.

This 50-year-old woman was initially seen with a chief complaint of difficulty chewing, slurred speech, and intermittent jaw joint pain. Facially she appeared to have a retruded chin (Fig. 57–1). The examination at this time revealed the following:

1. Short mandibular ramus syndrome
2. Vertical and transverse maxillary deficiency
3. High-angle mandibular deficiency
4. Class II, Division 1 molar and cuspid malocclusion (Fig. 57–2)
5. Chronic left temporomandibular joint internal derangement with advanced degenerative joint changes

The preoperative radiographs confirm these skeletal findings (Fig. 57–3). The modified Delaire analysis shows a short ramus and mandibular body (Fig. 57–4). The anterior facial height is excessive secondary to the mandibular posteroinferior rotation. There is also slight maxillary vertical excess contributing to the deformity.

Edgewise orthodontic treatment was instituted in August, 1985. A moderate amount of horizontal and vertical bone loss was noted in both arches. The mandibular right third molar was horizontally impacted, and the left third molar was supererupted. The maxillary third molars were missing. The mandibular third molars were removed in September, 1986. A nonextraction orthodontic approach was then instituted (Fig. 57–5).

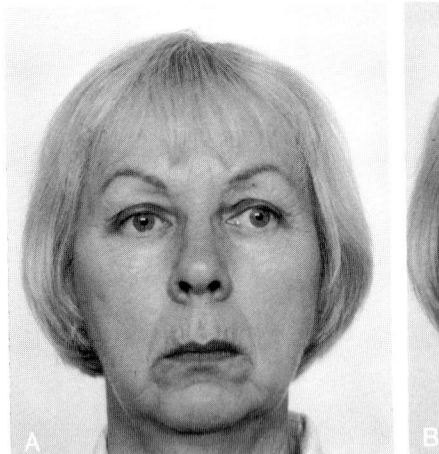

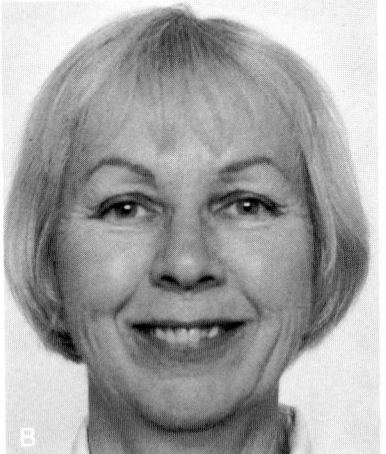

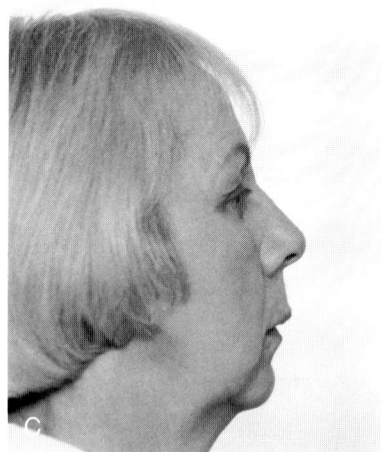

FIGURE 57–1. PREOPERATIVE PHOTOGRAPHS OF CASE 1. *A*, Full face. *B*, Smiling. *C*, Profile. A long lower facial third and microgenia or mandibular retrusion are apparent.

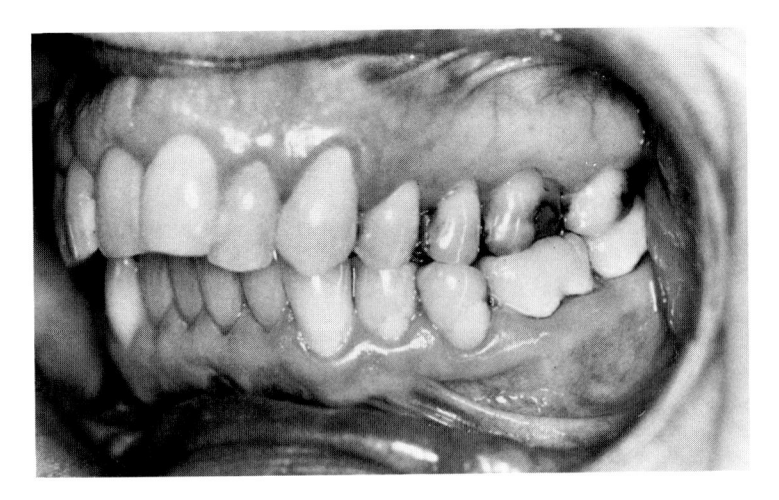

FIGURE 57–2. Preoperative occlusion of Case 1. Class II malocclusion with crowding prior to orthodontic treatment.

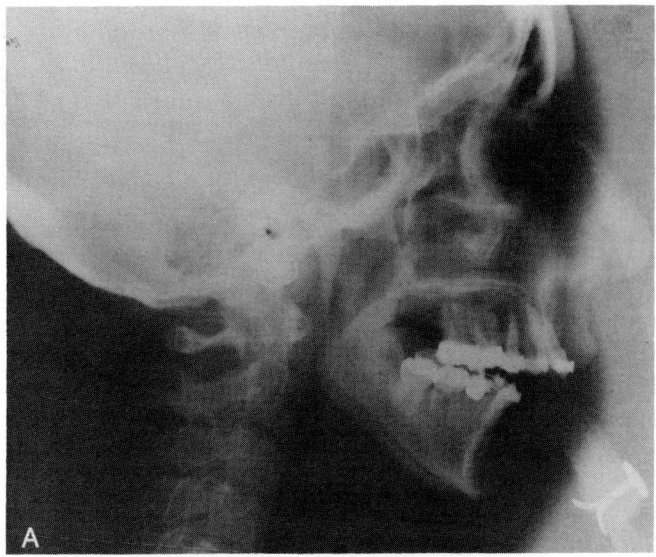

57 — SURGICAL MANAGEMENT OF SHORT MANDIBULAR RAMUS DEFORMITIES / **2001**

FIGURE 57-3. PREOPERATIVE RADIOGRAPHS OF CASE 1. *A*, Lateral cephalometric radiograph. *B*, Panoramic radiograph.

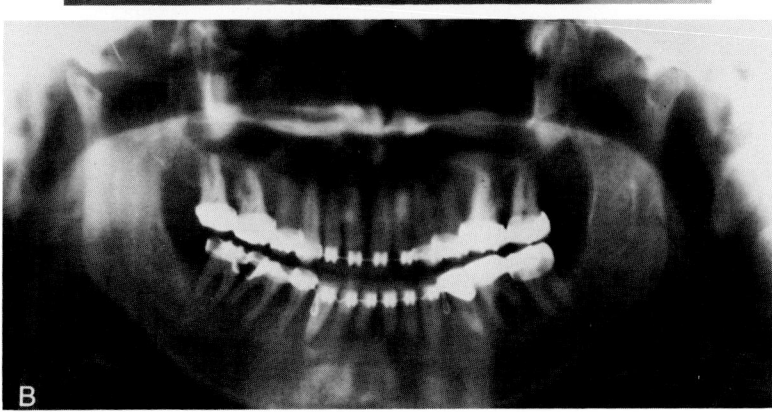

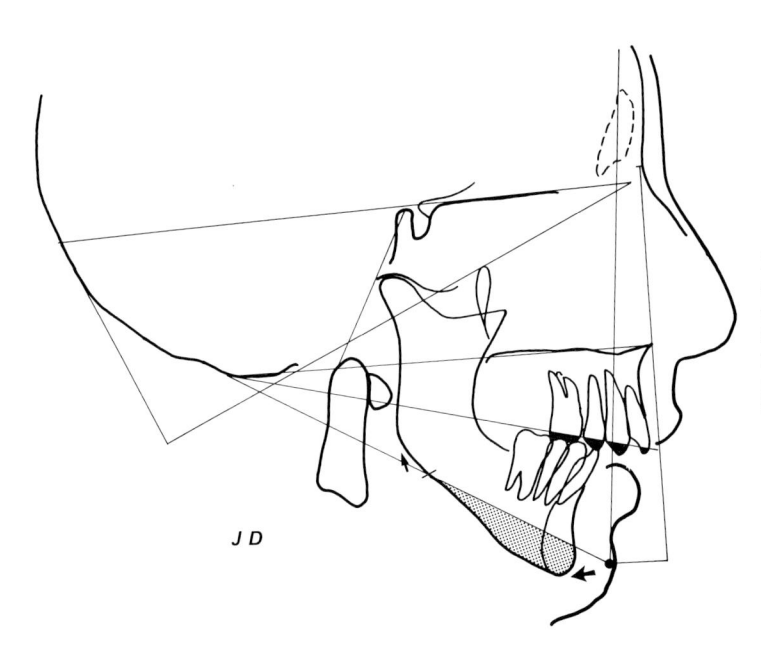

FIGURE 57-4. DELAIRE ANALYSIS OF CASE 1. Maxillary excess is demonstrated by the solid color and mandibular excess by the stippled areas. Maxillary anteroposterior position is normal. The mandibular body and chin are retruded, as seen by the large arrow from the ideal menton point. The small arrow indicates the shortness of the ramus from its ideal point in this analysis.

2002 / VI—ORTHOGNATHIC SURGERY

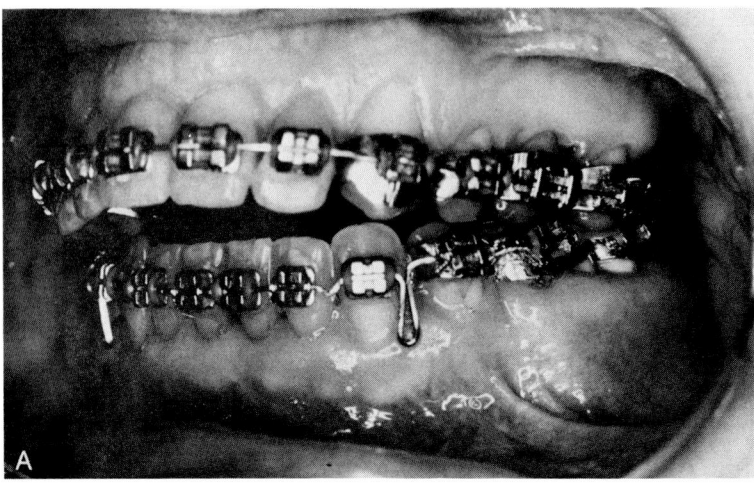

FIGURE 57-5. Preoperative occlusion after orthodontic therapy in Case 1.

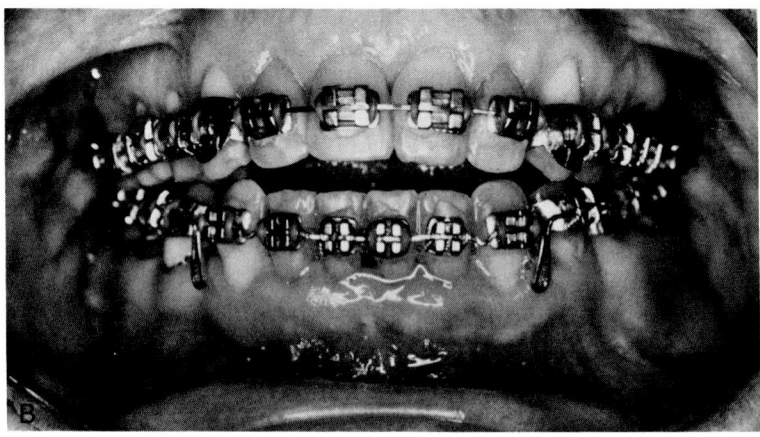

FIGURE 57-6. SURGICAL DRAWINGS OF CASE 1. *A,* The planned osteotomies are marked and include a Le Fort I osteotomy for reduction of slight maxillary vertical excess and bilateral inverted L osteotomies to both lengthen the ramus and advance the mandibular body. *B,* The completed maxillary and mandibular osteotomies. The mandible has been lengthened and a bone graft inserted. Rigid fixation is assured by a Ti-Mesh Plate on either side.

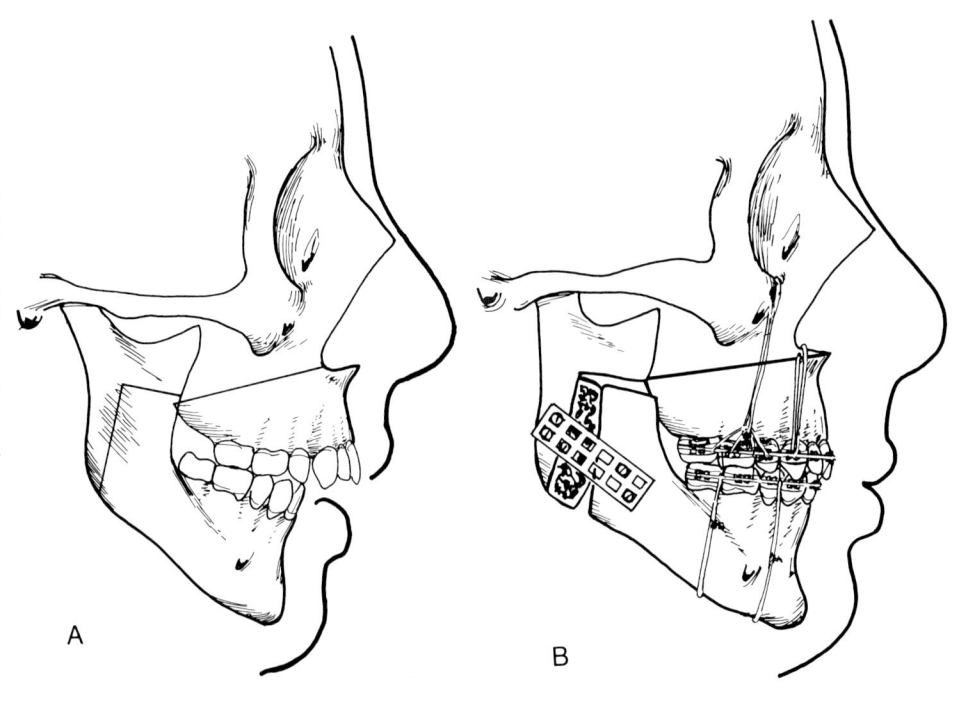

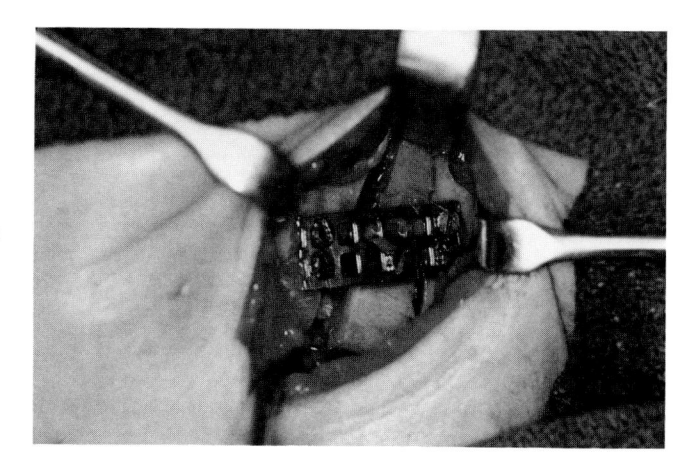

FIGURE 57-7. Bone plate. The mesh bone plate has been fixed into position.

Surgery consisted of the following:

1. A Le Fort I osteotomy in two segments with midline split and expansion utilizing autogenous iliac crest bone graft
2. Bilateral extraoral mandibular inverted L ramus osteotomies with advancement utilizing interpositional cortical cancellous bone grafts and TiMesh bone plates (Figs. 57-6 and 57-7)
3. Skeletal suspension consisting of four circumandibular wires and infraorbital and piriform rim wires
4. Intermaxillary fixation with a surgical stabilizing splint

Six weeks postoperatively, the intermaxillary fixation was released, and the skeletal fixation appliances were removed 1 week later. Six months postoperatively, all active orthodontic appliances were removed. She has since demonstrated a stable Class I occlusion with a normal overbite/overjet relationship and no evidence of transverse disharmonies (Figs. 57-8 and 57-9). The maximum interincisal opening is 35 mm, with slight deviation to the left upon opening. Cephalometric radiographs obtained 1 year postoperatively revealed excellent stability (Fig. 57-10).

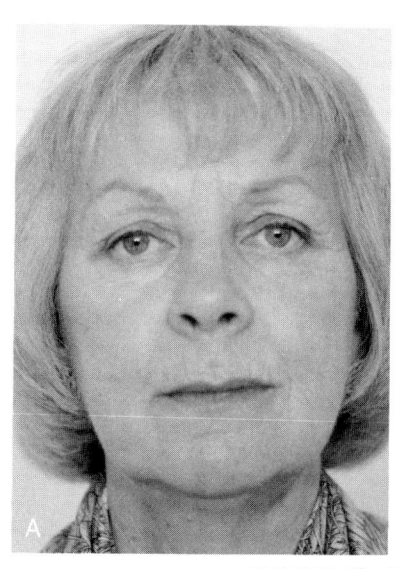

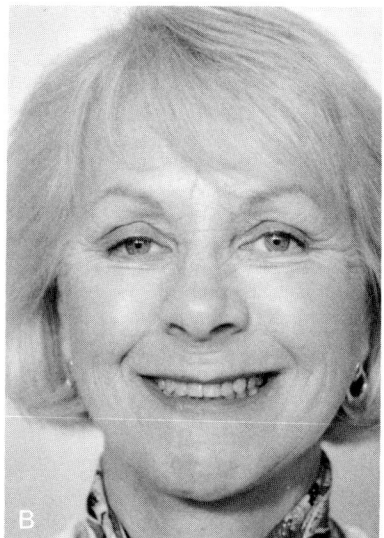

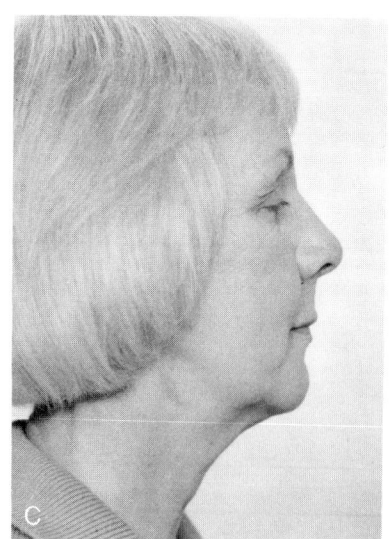

FIGURE 57-8. POSTOPERATIVE FACIAL PHOTOGRAPHS OF CASE 1. *A*, Full face. *B*, Smiling. *C*, Profile.

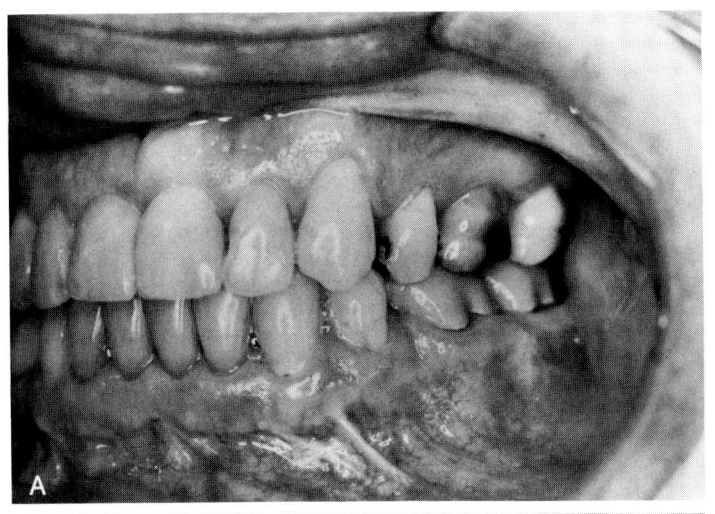

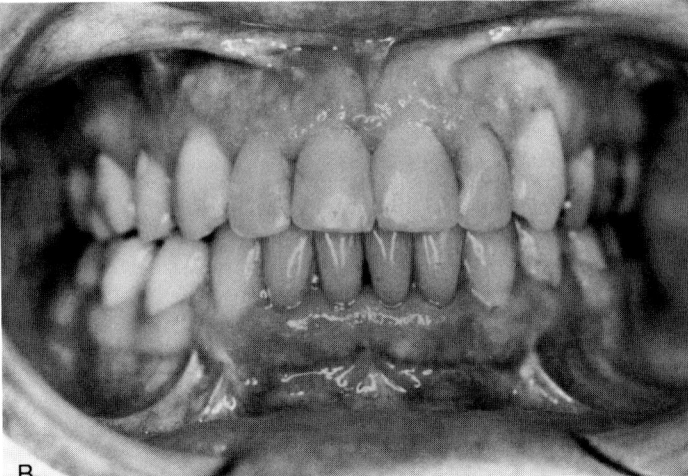

FIGURE 57-9. Postoperative occlusion of Case 1.

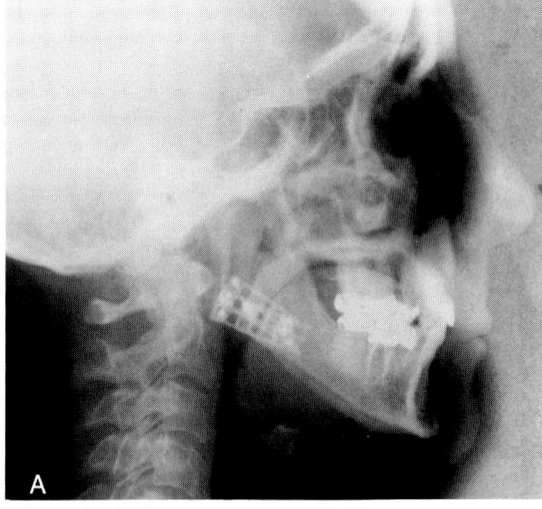

FIGURE 57-10. Long-term postoperative cephalometric and panoramic radiographs of Case 1. Excellent bony healing and stability are seen.

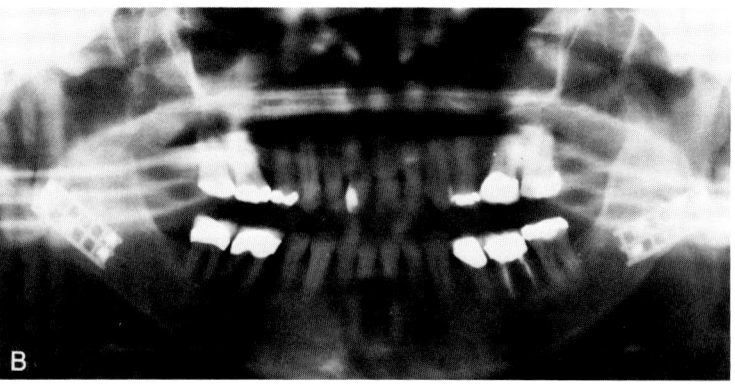

CASE 2, K.G.

The patient was initially evaluated at age 5. Clinical examination at that time was consistent with left hemifacial microsomia. At that time, she demonstrated a Class II malocclusion with deviation to the left upon opening and limited exursive movements of the mandible to the right (Fig. 57–11). The patient was lost to follow-up until age 13. At that time, the asymmetry had increased in severity and the malocclusion was unchanged (Fig. 57–12). In May, 1984, at age 19, she returned for re-evaluation. At that time, she complained of difficulty chewing, slurred speech, and concern about the facial asymmetry as it related to normal socialization. The maximum interincisal opening was 44 mm, with deviation to the left upon opening. The maxillary arch was narrow and tapered with a high palatal vault. The maxillary occlusal plane was canted inferiorly on the right side. The maxillary third molars were missing. The mandibular arch demonstrated an excessive curve of Spee. The mandibular left second molar was horizontally impacted with the root apices almost perforating the inferior border of the mandible. The mandibular left third molar, first molar, and right third molar were missing (Fig. 57–13). She demonstrated a Class II, Division 1 malocclusion with an overjet of 8 mm and an overbite of 5 mm.

FIGURE 57–11. Facial view at age 5 of Case 2. Note the facial asymmetry.

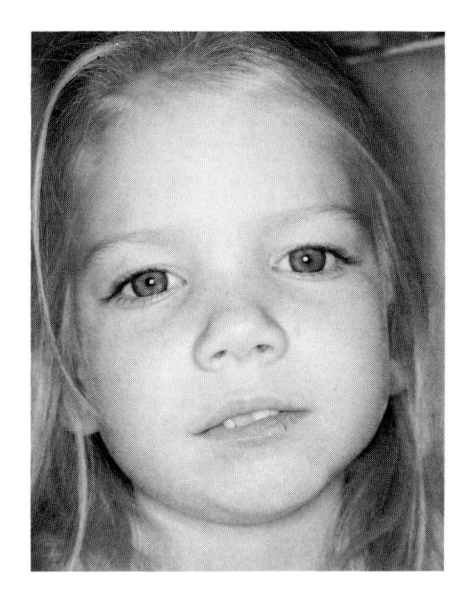

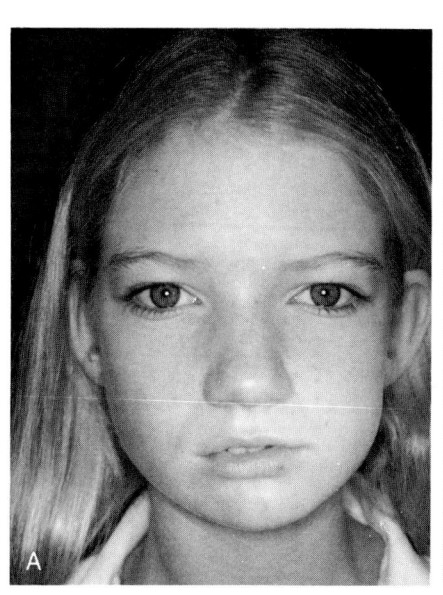

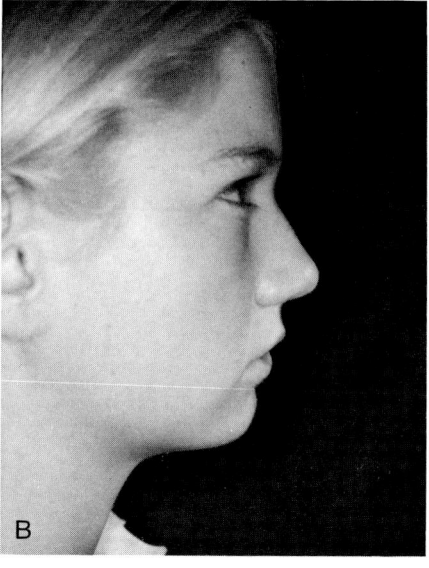

FIGURE 57–12. Full face (*A*) and profile (*B*) views of Case 2. Patient at age 13 with increased facial asymmetry and mandibular retrusion.

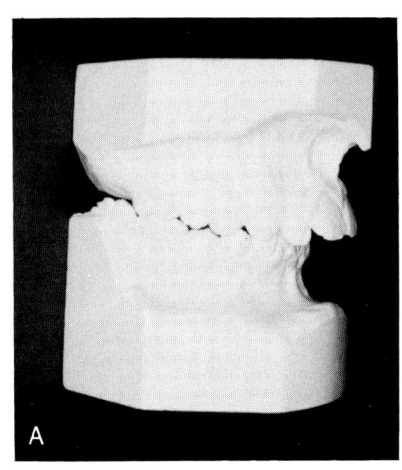

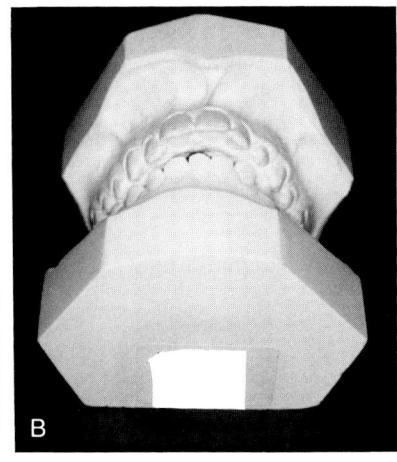

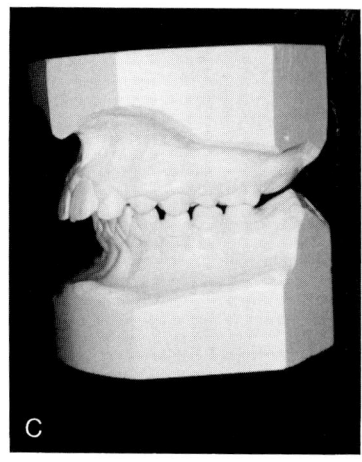

FIGURE 57-13. Dental models of Case 2. Class II malocclusion and a tilted occlusal plane are evident.

Active edgewise orthodontic therapy was started in September of 1985. Examination of the patient at this time revealed the following (Figs. 57-14 and 57-15):

1. Left hemifacial microsomia with agenesis of the left mandibular condyle, short mandibular ramus, and pseudoarthrosis
2. Compensatory left vertical maxillary hypoplasia
3. Severe mandibular deficiency
4. Class II, Division 1 molar and cuspid malocclusion
5. Left ear deformity without associated hearing loss

These changes can be seen in the initial radiographs (Figs. 57-16 and 57-17). The cephalometric analysis clarifies these abnormalities (Fig. 57-18). The facial asymmetry is apparent in both lateral and anteroposterior analyses. A short ramus is identified on one side by the arrow and a long ramus on the other. The anteroposterior analysis shows the left facial shortness with midline rotation to the same side.

Surgery was performed on July 21, 1986. The following procedures were done (Figs. 57-19 and 57-20):

1. Right mandibular sagittal ramus osteotomy
2. A left transoral mandibular inverted L osteotomy with an interpositional iliac crest bone graft and rigid plate fixation
3. A Le Fort I osteotomy with midline split and downgrafting of the left maxilla utilizing an interpositional iliac crest bone graft

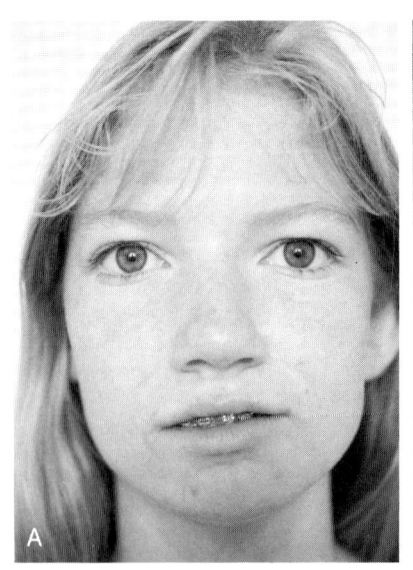

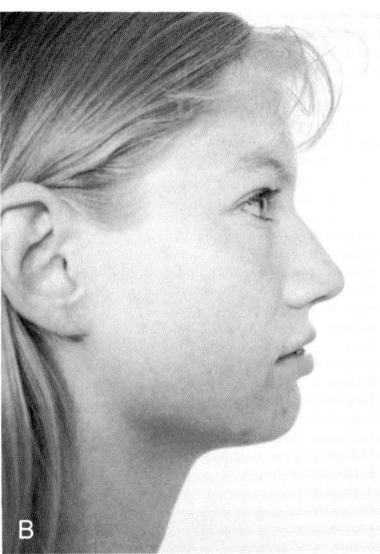

FIGURE 57-14. Pretreatment full face (A) and profile (B) views of Case 2. Facial asymmetry and mandibular retrusion are present. There is also slight lower face shortness.

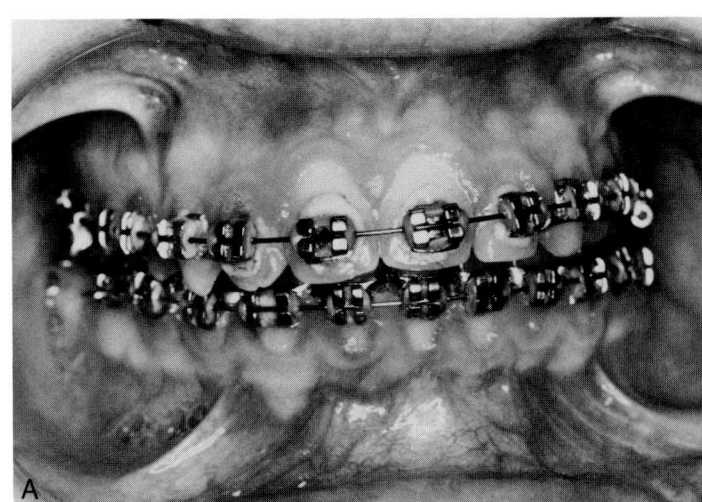

FIGURE 57-15. Presurgical occlusion of Case 2. Occlusion ready for surgery following preliminary orthodontic treatment.

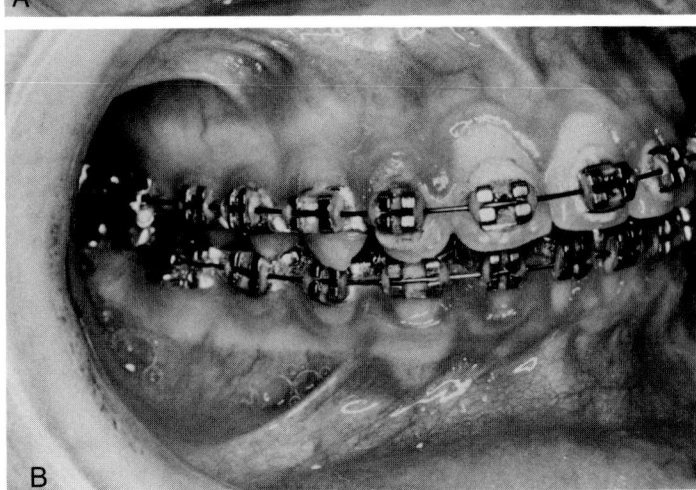

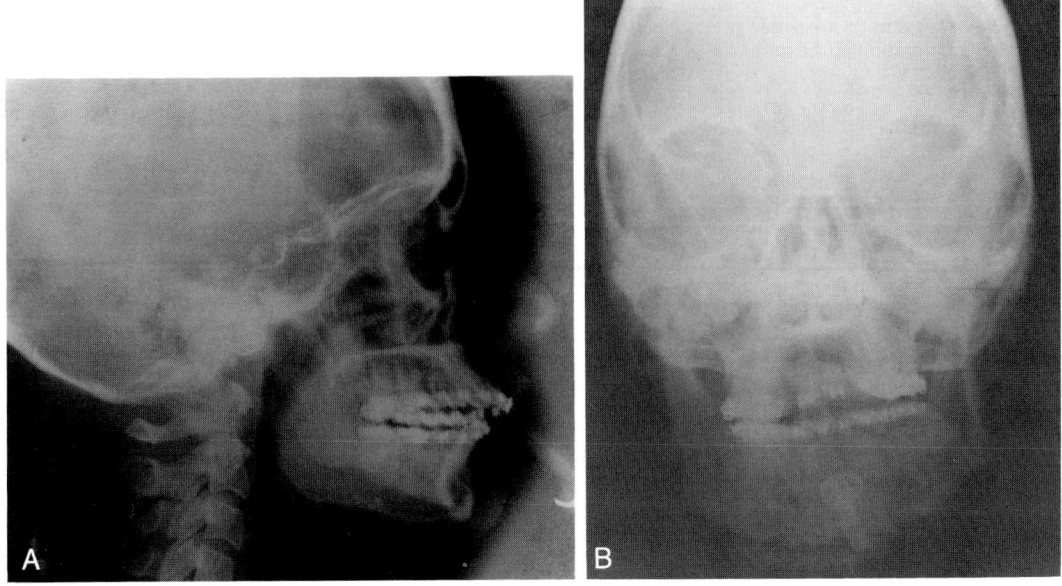

FIGURE 57-16. CEPHALOMETRIC RADIOGRAPHS OF CASE 2. *A*, Lateral. *B*, Posteroanterior.

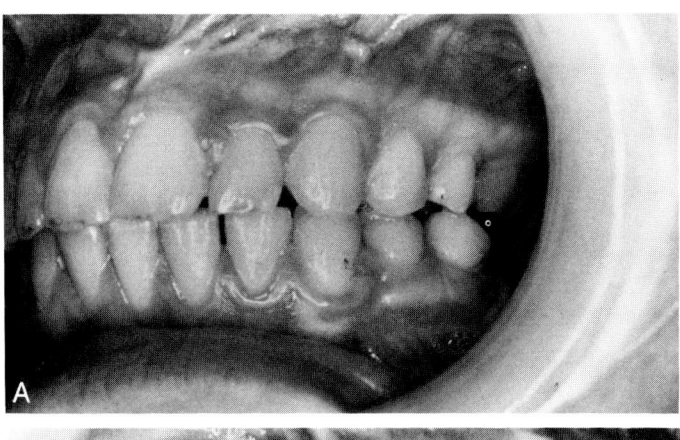

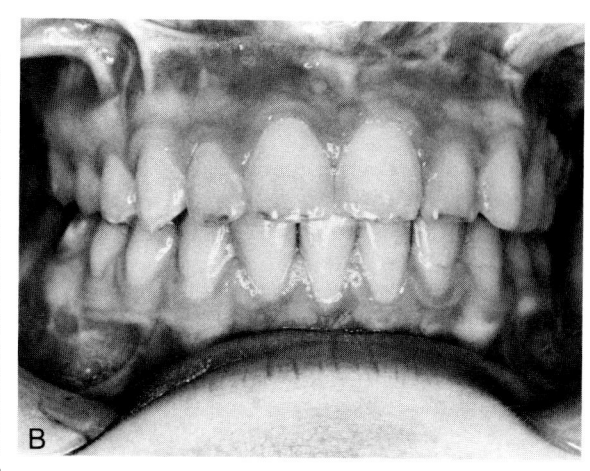

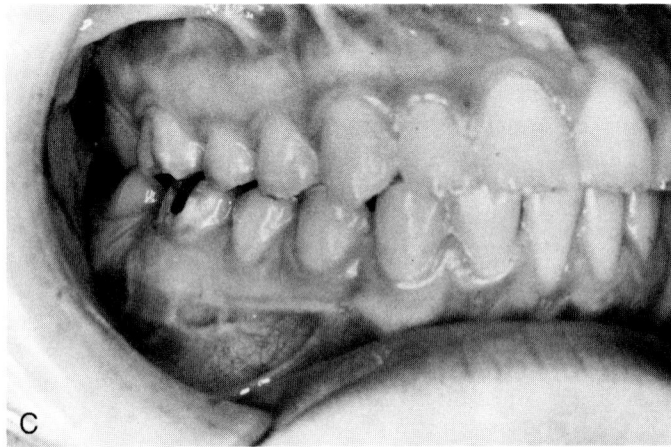

FIGURE 57-22. Postoperative occlusion of Case 2.

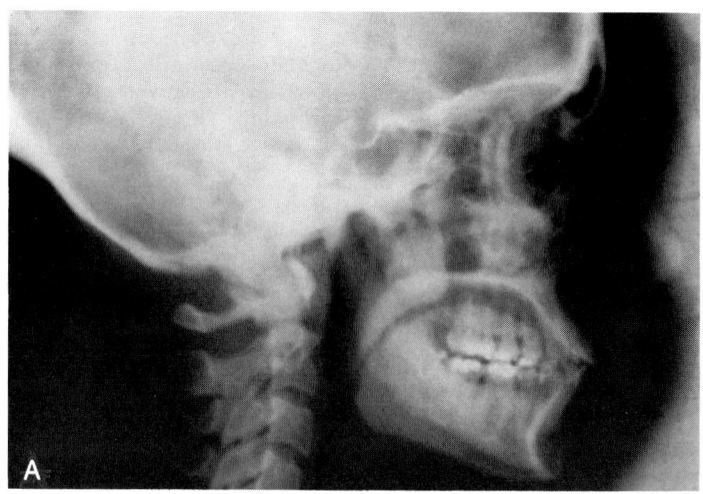

FIGURE 57-23. POSTOPERATIVE RADIOGRAPHS OF CASE 2. *A*, Cephalometric radiograph. *B*, Panoramic radiograph. Both radiographs were taken at 1 year postoperatively.

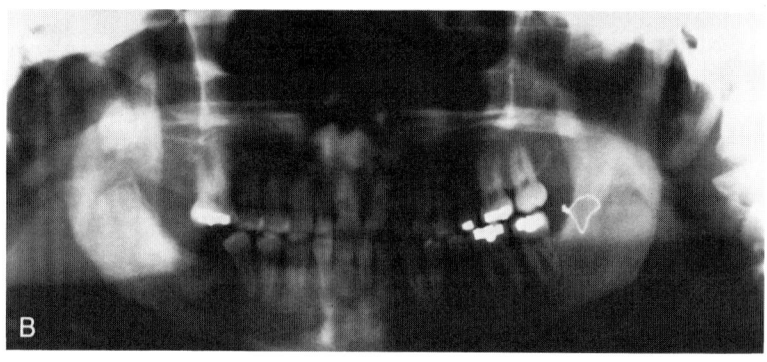

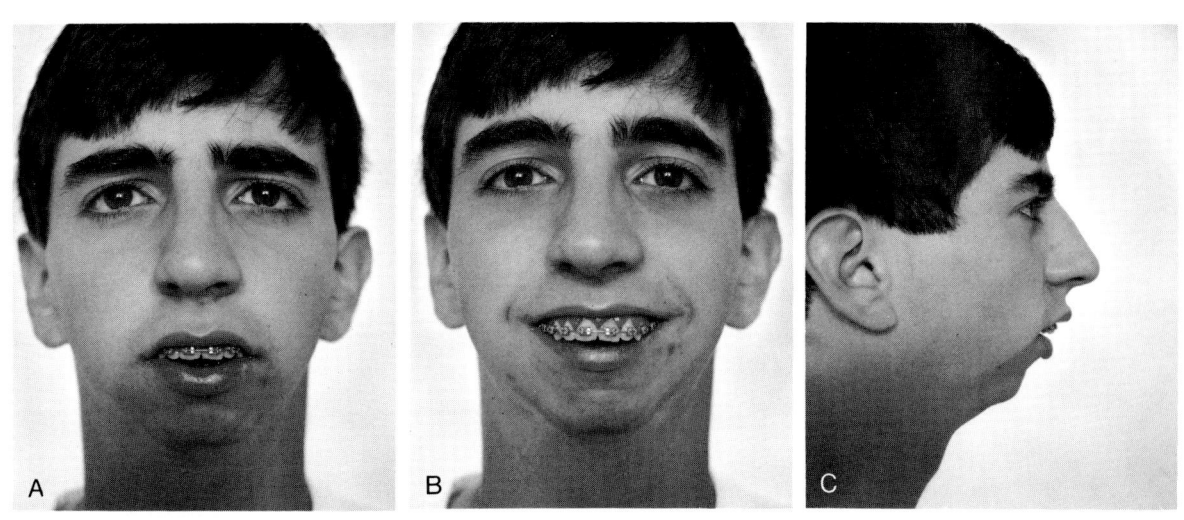

FIGURE 57–24. FACIAL VIEWS OF CASE 3. *A*, Full face. *B*, Smiling. *C*, Profile. Note the extremely small mandible and chin, apparent in all views.

CASE 3, R.S.

This 17-year-old boy was first seen in consultation with a chief complaint of difficulty chewing food and concern over his facial appearance (Fig. 57–24). Mandibular hypoplasia was noted in infancy which became more severe with growth. Partial bilateral temporomandibular joint ankylosis was believed to be the cause. The patient was later worked up for rheumatoid arthritis. At age 3, he developed pain and swelling of both knees which required orthopedic splinting. All tests for juvenile rheumatoid arthritis

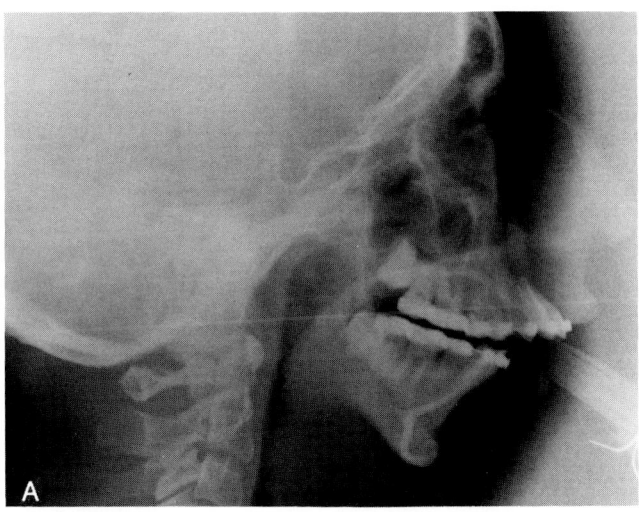

FIGURE 57–25. RADIOGRAPHS OF CASE 3. *A*, Cephalometric radiograph. *B*, Panoramic radiograph. The mandible is small in appearance.

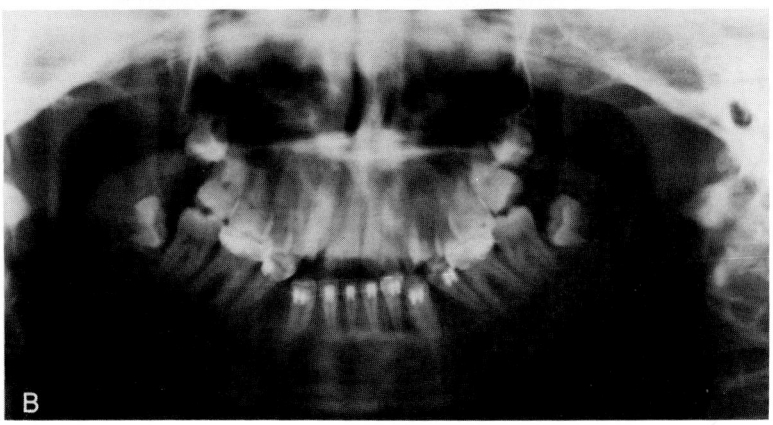

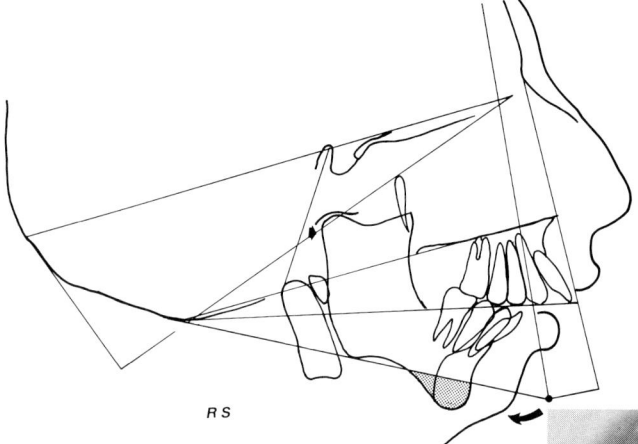

FIGURE 57-26. Cephalometric analysis of Case 3. The Delaire cephalometric analysis clearly demonstrates the deficient mandibular ramus and body. The chin is also severely retruded but vertically long, as shown by the arrow and stippled area. The maxillary position is normal except for some posterior shortening in the molar region. The condyles and glenoid fossas can be seen to be anteriorly positioned.

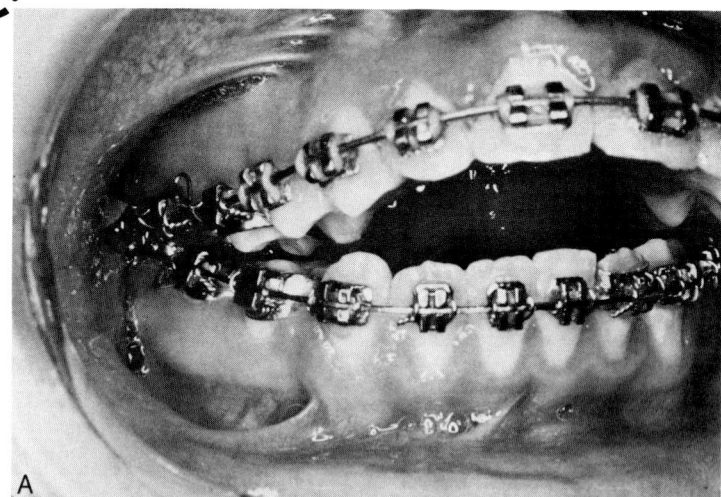

FIGURE 57-27. Presurgical occlusion of case 3. The presurgical orthodontic treatment has worsened the Class II malocclusion and the open bite.

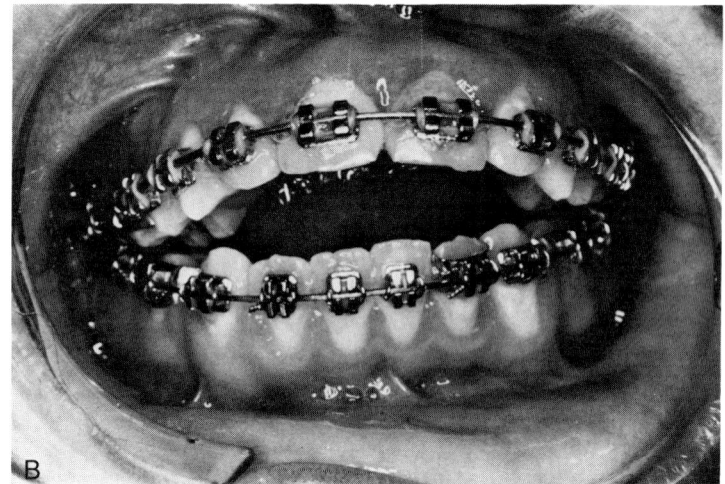

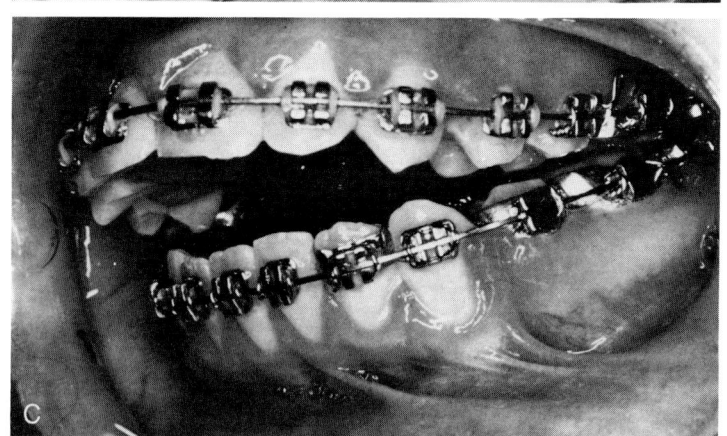

were negative. However, there is a positive family history for rheumatoid arthritis, and this may well represent a seronegative form. Clinical and radiographic examinations revealed the following (Fig. 57-25):

1. Short mandibular ramus syndrome
2. High-angle mandibular deficiency
3. Compensatory posterior maxillary hypoplasia
4. Class II, Division 1 malocclusion—apertognathia
5. Bilateral temporomandibular joint internal derangements with advanced degenerative joint changes

The Delaire analysis clearly shows the deficient mandibular ramus and body. There is a severely retruded but vertically long chin. Maxillary position is fine except for some posterior vertical deficiency, most likely secondary to the mandibular deformity (Fig. 57-26).

Full-banded edgewise appliance therapy was started in January of 1984. Mandibular first premolars were extracted. The maximum interincisal opening was 45 mm, with extreme limitation of lateral excursive movements of the mandible. He demonstrated mild gingivitis secondary to chronic oral breathing and poor oral hygiene (Fig. 57-27).

On July 20, 1986, the following procedures were performed (Fig. 57-28):

1. Bilateral extraoral and mandibular inverted L ramus osteotomies with interpositional autogenous corticocancellous iliac crest bone grafts and rigid plate fixation
2. A Tessier transoral genioplasty with a "jumping" bone flap was performed. The combined advancement of the mandible and chin was 34 mm. The bone flap was stabilized with a threaded stainless steel wire.
3. Skeletal fixation consisting of two malar buttress slings, two piriform aperture slings, and two circumandibular slings
4. Intermaxillary fixation with a surgical stabilizing splint and overcorrection posteriorly extending from the second premolars to the second molars

Intermaxillary fixation was released on September 28, 1986, and the skeletal fixation suspension wires were removed on October 6, 1986. The patient continued active orthodontic therapy until August of 1987, whereupon retainer therapy was implemented. Shortly thereafter, he underwent a free gingival graft to the mandibular incisors. He has demonstrated a stable Class I molar and cuspid occlusion postoperatively (Figs. 57-29 and 57-30). The overjet is 1 to 2 mm secondary to a tooth size discrepancy as a result of extracting mandibular first premolars and a nonextraction maxillary approach. The interincisal opening was 42 mm, with no change in the lateral range of motion from that noted preoperatively. In general, he has demonstrated excellent stability (Fig. 57-31).

FIGURE 57-28. SURGERY OF CASE 3. *A*, Proposed osteotomies. *B*, Completed osteotomies. The mandible is to be advanced and the ramus elongated by inverted L osteotomies together with a sliding genioplasty. The mandibular defects are bone grafted by corticocancellous blocks and fixated with AO plates. The chin is completely advanced by a Tessier type "jumping" bone flap and fixed with a K wire.

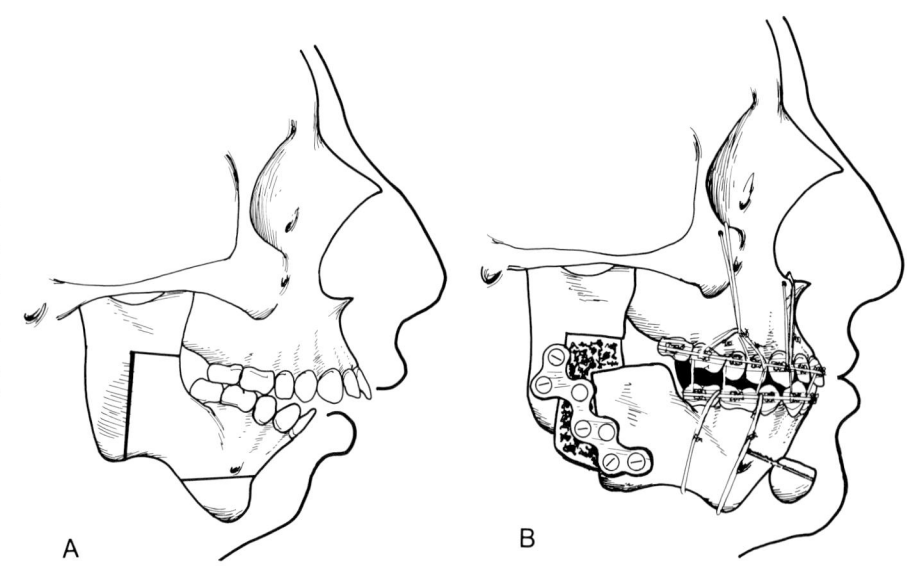

2016 / VI — ORTHOGNATHIC SURGERY

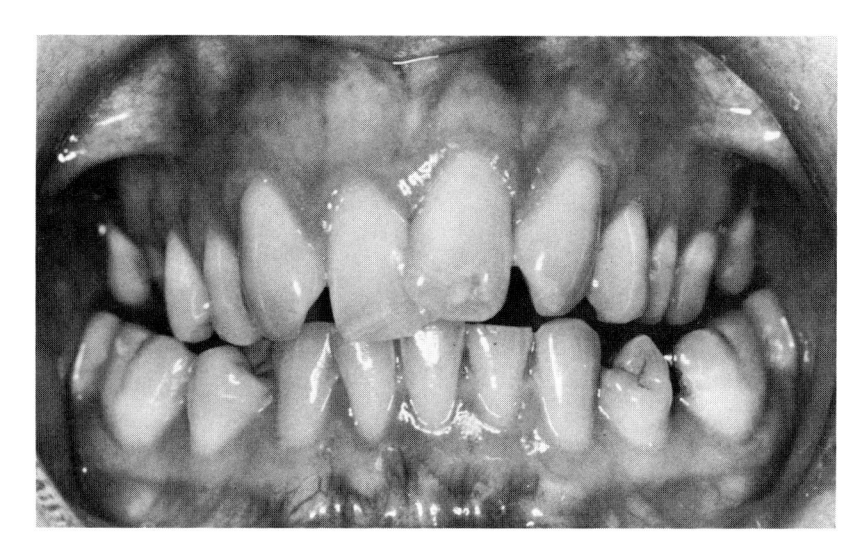

FIGURE 57-33. Preoperative occlusion of Case 4.

2. Bilateral temporomandibular joint internal derangement with advanced degenerative joint disease
3. Transverse maxillary deficiency
4. Microstomia
5. Congenitally missing maxillary lateral incisors
6. Missing maxillary and mandibular third molars and second mandibular premolars
7. Repaired cleft palate
8. Mandibular deficiency, with notable ramus hypoplasia (Fig. 57-34)

The skeletal deformity is further defined by a Delaire cephalometric analysis (Fig. 57-35). The Delaire analysis graphically demonstrates a short mandibular ramus with resultant posterior rotation of the mandibular body and chin. Orthodontic therapy was started using the edgewise technique to align the individual arches in prepara-

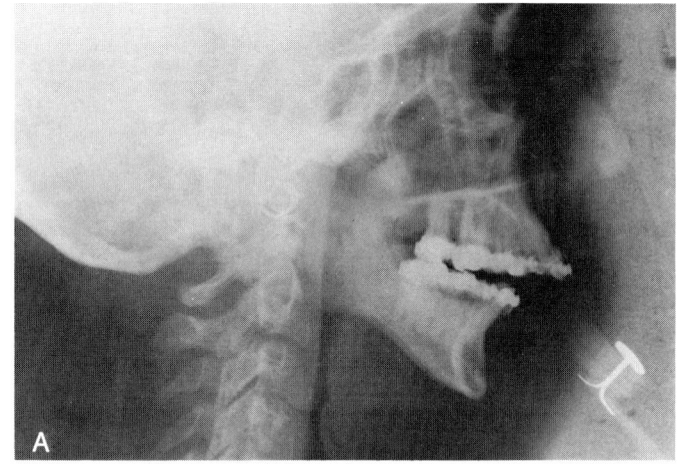

FIGURE 57-34. INITIAL RADIOGRAPHS OF CASE 4. *A*, Cephalometric radiograph. *B*, Panoramic radiograph.

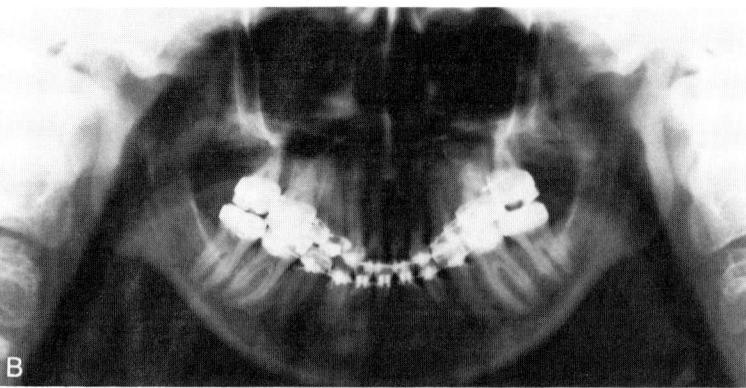

FIGURE 57-35. Cephalometric analysis of Case 4. The Delaire analysis demonstrates the short ramus and body of the mandible as indicated by the arrows. There is some anterior maxillary vertical excess indicated by the solid areas.

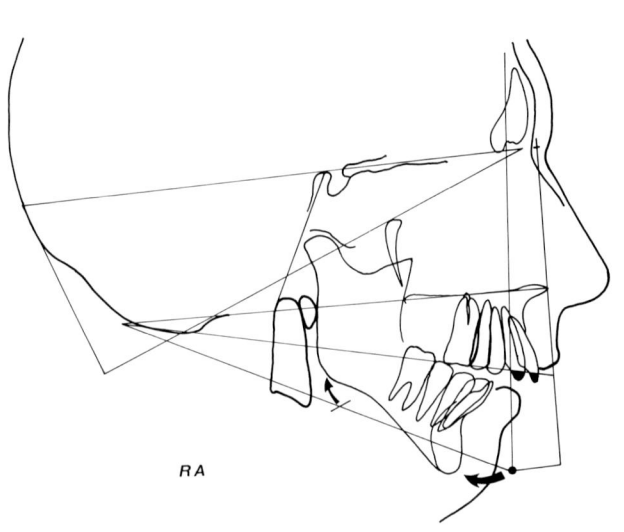

tion for surgery. Following the orthodontic preparation, surgery was performed. The skeletal deformity was corrected in both the maxilla and mandible, lengthening the ramus. The following procedures were performed (Fig. 57-36):

1. Bilateral extraoral inverted L ramus osteotomies with autogenous iliac crest bone grafts and rigid plate fixation
2. Le Fort I three-segment maxillary ostectomies and osteotomies with superior and anterior repositioning and reconstruction of the nasal floor with an autogenous iliac crest bone graft
3. Submucous septoplasty
4. Repair of the oronasal fistula
5. Nasolabial muscle reconstruction
6. Skeletal fixation with infraorbital slings, maxillary K wires, and circumandibular wires
7. Intermaxillary fixation with a surgical stabilizing splint

Immediately upon discharge, the panoramic radiograph indicated incomplete seating of the left mandibular condyle. The patient was returned to surgery on July 28, 1986. Both extraoral wounds were reopened. The bone plates were released and the proximal segments were repositioned superiorly with fixation utilizing rigid bone plates.

The patient's remaining postoperative course was essentially uneventful. Intermaxillary fixation was released on September 18, 1986. The patient continued active orthodontic therapy was removal of all appliances on December 28, 1987 (Figs. 57-37 and 57-38). She has continued to demonstrate excellent stability with no evidence of temporomandibular joint dysfunction (Fig. 57-39).

FIGURE 57-36. OSTEOTOMIES OF CASE 4. *A*, Proposed osteotomies. *B*, Completed osteotomies. The maxilla will be shortened anteriorly by a Le Fort I approach and the mandible lengthened by inverted L osteotomies. The mandibular defects were bone grafted and fixed by AO plates.

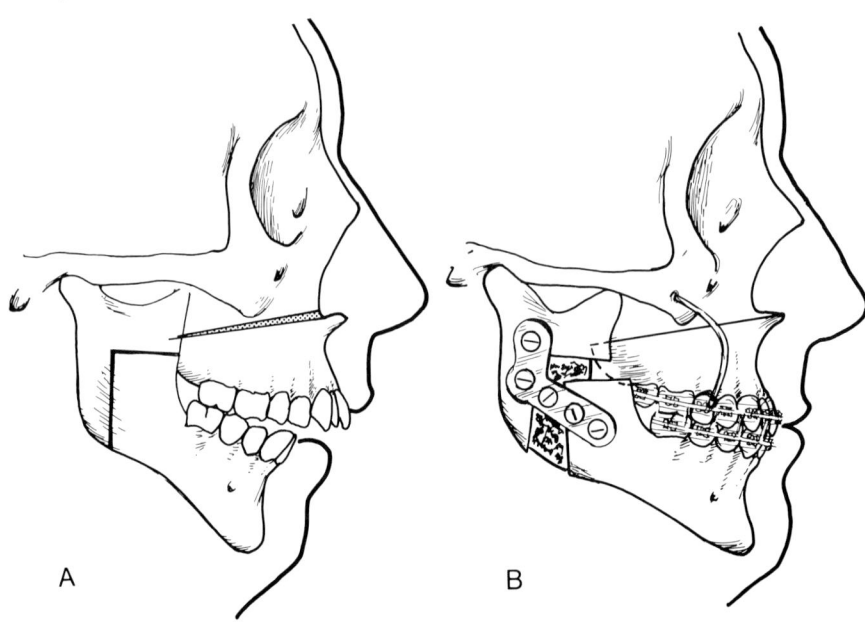

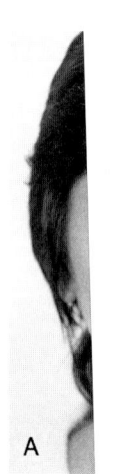

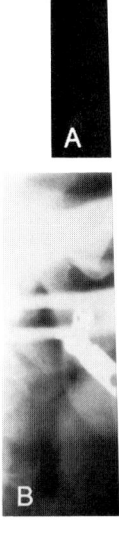

gnathia, myxedema, adenotonsillar hypertrophy, elongated and thickened soft palate and uvula, deviated nasal septum, macroglossia, and neoplasm.[8,27,72]

The mechanisms of obstruction are not yet fully understood. The patency of the upper airway is controlled partially by the central nervous system and is maintained by adjustment of muscular tone of the pharyngeal muscles. The forces that contribute to the tendency toward collapse during inspiration are (1) the surrounding atmospheric pressure (a constant), (2) the weight of the soft tissue of the neck (varies in individuals), (3) the local compliance of the airway walls (varies depending on fatty infiltration, edema, and other factors), and (4) the negative pressure inside the lumen of the airway during inspiration. Normally, airflow varies inversely with resistance and directly with the pressure developed between the alveoli and the airway opening. Guilleminault has shown that a decrease in muscle tone and/or neck fat increases resistance.[20] This "Bernoulli" effect also contributes to collapse: If the volume of airflow is constant, the velocity of air at the constriction decreases. Thus, if there is a narrowing of the airway at one point, the tendency to collapse increases during inspiration.

DIAGNOSING OBSTRUCTIVE SLEEP APNEA

Since sleep apnea has a multisystemic effect upon a patient's well-being, a team approach is necessary to diagnose and treat it. Because of this, sleep-wake centers have evolved. A sleep disorder center may have any or all of the following specialists: neurologist, otolaryngologist, cardiologist, psychologist, nutritionist, orthodontist, oral and maxillofacial surgeon, and a technical support staff. This multidisciplinary approach provides insight into the many factors that are ultimately responsible for sleep apnea.

Polysomnography (PSG) (multiphysiologic sleep recording) is the benchmark for determining whether sleep apnea exists. A number of physiologic variables are monitored during sleep and yield information regarding the patient's sleep-wake state and cardiac and respiratory function.

The basic components of PSG measurement include polygraphic recordings by means of the electroencephalogram (EEG), electro-oculogram (EOG), and chin electromyogram (EMG). Recordings of nasal and oral airflow, oxygen saturation, end-tidal carbon dioxide values, thoracic and abdominal respiratory movements, leg muscle activity, penile tumescence, and esophageal acidity are all measured (Fig. 58–3).

The following factors are usually noted during a typical sleep study: (1) number and length of apneas, (2) sleep latency, (3) time to first REM period, if any, (4) sleep stages, and (5) number of sleep arousals. In normal patients positive findings such as hypoventilation and apneas alone do not justify diagnosis of obstructive apnea. The frequency of events is of utmost importance in the final diagnosis. Therefore, the apnea index (AI) was developed to measure the severity of apnea. By definition, the apnea index is the total number of apneic episodes during sleep divided by the sleep time in minutes and multiplied by 60. Studies have shown that an AI of up to 5 is within normal limits, and anything greater than 5 is abnormal. Sleep-related hypopneas have been documented in most patients during sleep studies. This often compounds the problem, so an apnea-hypopnea index (AHI) has been developed and, as with AI, an AHI of up to 5 is normal in the adult.[19] In addition to PSG, another examination in a typical sleep study is the multiple sleep latency test (MSLT), which provides an objective evaluation of excessive daytime sleepiness.[19]

The otolaryngologist at the center evaluates the patient for any head and neck pathology, usually with the aid of an endoscope for determining the site of the obstruction. The otolaryngologist may be able to perform a Müller maneuver. This procedure has been shown by Sher et al to be highly diagnostic.[58] In the

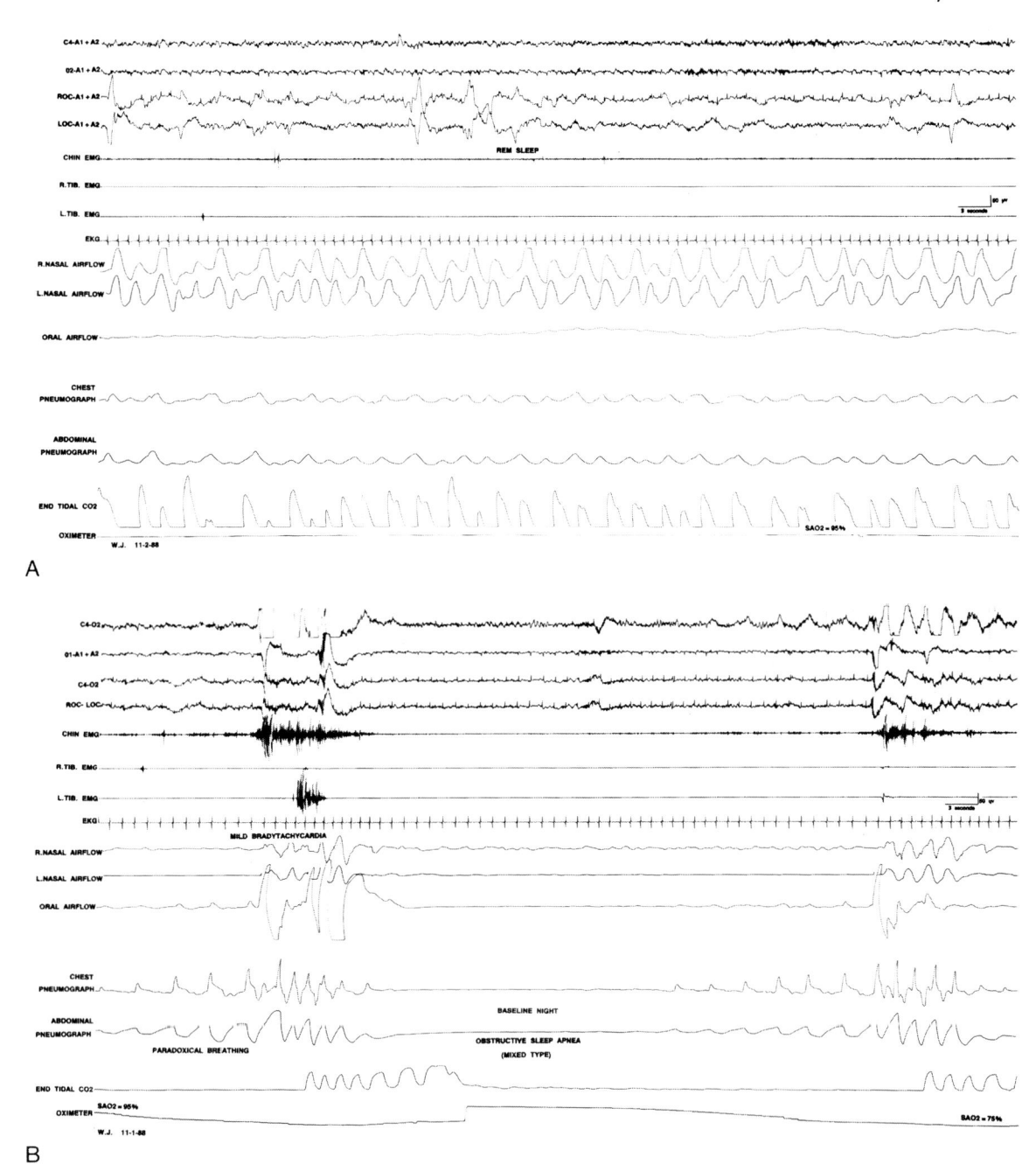

FIGURE 58-3. POLYSOMNOGRAPHY (PSG). MULTIPHYSIOLOGIC PARAMETRIC TESTS UTILIZED TO DOCUMENT SLEEP APNEA. *A*, Normal PSG examination results. Note regular airflow and EKG, minimal muscular activity, and adequate oxygen saturation. *B*, Abnormal PSG. Note cardiac dysrythmias and interrupted airflow with hyperactive muscular activity consistent with snoring and airway obstruction; also note oxygen desaturation after obstructive episodes.

maneuver, the patient is instructed to occlude the nasal airway by gently squeezing the external nares with two fingers and to make a vigorous inspiration with the mouth closed. This provides general information about the degree of obstruction at specific points along the pharyngeal airway and the propensity for dynamic occlusion of the pharyngeal airway during sleep.[10] The degree of obstruction at two levels, the soft palate and base of the tongue, is measured from 1+ (minimal movement) to 4+ (total collapse of the airway). This should be done in both upright and supine positions.

Electromyography and nasopharyngeal endoscopy have illustrated mechanisms of upper airway obstruction such as decreased activity in muscles of the upper airway, pharyngeal collapse, and active contraction of the velopharyngeal sphincter muscles.[10,20,69] Brouillette and coworkers used fluoroscopy for the same purpose of establishing obstructive sites, and others used somnofluoroscopy to predict treatment success.[4,68]

During examination, the soft palate may be found to be an obstructing factor. Performing a Müller maneuver helps identify other areas of collapse, and a lateral cephalograph can provide considerable additional information. A uvulopalatopharyngoplasty (UPPP) is designed to eliminate the mucosal and muscular redundancy in the velopharynx. In this procedure the oropharynx is enlarged to two dimensions, effectively elevating the palate away from the posterior pharyngeal wall (Fig. 58–4).[29]

Computed tomography offers another mechanism to evaluate the airway of the OSA patient.[3,12,25,38,64] Crumley studied the cross-sectional dimension of the airway with cine scans, providing a dynamic view of the airway during various phases of respiration in sleeping patients.[9]

The patency of the human airway has also been evaluated through the use of cephalometrics. Initial airway evaluations utilizing this technique focused on normal growth and development in the nasopharyngeal region.[53] Further study of the nasopharyngeal area centered on measurements of the soft palate, pharyngeal wall, and tongue position.

Earlier investigations focused primarily on speech-related problems. In a dissertation written in 1949, Hixon presented an extensive analysis of morphology and function of the oronasal and pharyngeal areas.[26] He measured lateral cephalometric radiographs of persons with normal and nasal speech taken during rest and phonation of various vowels. Pharyngeal growth examination, velopharyngeal valving competence, tongue height, growth of the soft palate, posterior pharyngeal wall movement, and soft palate function were other areas evaluated using cephalometrics to give a better understanding of pharyngeal growth and function.[23,30,41,48,61,70]

In the 1960s, work by Wildman, Engman, Bushy, Schweiger, and Chierici used cephalometrics to study craniofacial soft tissue anatomy as it related to skeletal

Effects of UPPP

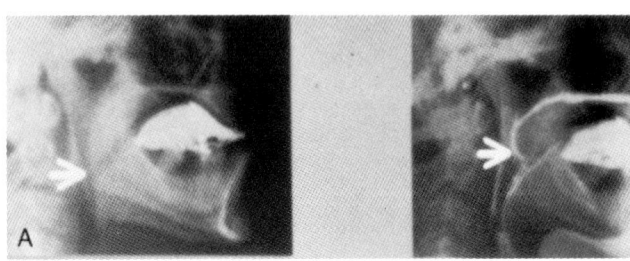

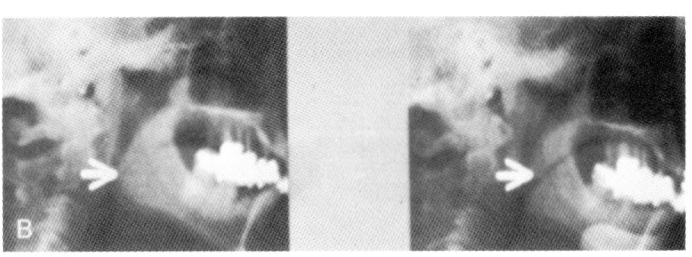

FIGURE 58–4. THE POSTOPERATIVE EFFECTS OF UVULOPALATOPHARYNGOPLASTY (UPPP) AS SEEN ON CEPHALOMETRIC RADIOGRAPHS. Note in these two UPPP patients how the operation has shortened as well as thickened their uvulas. There appear to be minimal changes in their anteroposterior pharyngeal airway widths.

landmarks.[7,13,57,71] Nasopharyngeal dimension and adenoidal tissue evaluation were studied in the 1970s to examine the effect of adenoidal and tonsillar size on respiration and craniofacial and nasopharyngeal development.[14,24,36,37,46]

With the development of sleep-wake centers came a considerable increase in cephalometric literature on the airway and OSA. Hyoid bone position, soft palate length, mandibular body length and position, and soft tissue dimensions (e.g., tongue, soft palate, adenoids, tonsils) have all been evaluated and found to play significant roles in OSA.[10,22,28,39,50,51] Recently, Djupesland evaluated 25 OSA patients and 10 controls cephalometrically.[11] Findings indicated an increased soft palate length and thickness, closer contact between the tongue and soft palate, a more inferiorly positioned hyoid bone, and a reduced nasopharyngeal and oropharyngeal airway space anteroposteriorly in OSA patients.

Laniado assessed the craniofacial soft tissue characteristics of an adult patient population with documented OSA, and for the first time indices of apnea severity were correlated with craniofacial morphology.[33]

Recently, Trieger has proposed that the typical middle-aged, obese male with OSA may have yet a different etiology, unrelated to any skeletal abnormality of the jaws. On cephalometric radiography, the oral and hypopharyngeal airway spaces appear not only narrowed but also clouded, suggesting some infiltrative process. The increased thickness of the posterior pharyngeal wall has been well documented by cephalometric studies.[33,43] The nature of this thickening, previously assumed to be due to fat deposits, is found on histologic examination to be lymphedema. This suggests some interference with lymphatic drainage of the nasopharynx, oropharynx, and hypopharynx which normally flows into the superior vena cava and then into the right atrium of the heart. Lymphedema would imply an increased hydrostatic pressure leading to a transudation of colloid and protein coming out of the capillaries and into the adjacent tissues. This edema suffuses the tissues of the head and neck and narrows the airway. A significant number of patients with OSA have been shown to have right atrial and ventricular dysfunction with a decreased ejection fraction and evidence of hypokinesis (66 per cent) despite enlargement (55 per cent).[6] The right atrium is also seen to be enlarged and to be the major source of an observed increase in a recently described hormone—atrial natriuretic peptide or factor (ANF). This peptide follows a circadian rhythm similar to that of cortisol and renin. Its effects are to produce a diuretic and natriuretic action in the kidney in response to an increased pressure and stretch of the right atrium.

Krieger et al have shown that ANF is markedly increased during sleep in patients with OSA.[32] The introduction of continuous positive airway pressure (CPAP) reverses both the diuresis and the sodium excretion rapidly. CPAP is believed also to decrease cardiac preload and, in effect, unburden the heart. Thus the ANF serum levels may serve as a helpful guide to the effectiveness of treatment of OSA.

One may speculate on what initiates the train of events leading to OSA. In the orthognathic patient it may well be related to the initial hypoxemia associated with the decrease in ventilation secondary to significant obesity. With hypoxemia there is an increased tension in the vasculature of the lungs (mainly mid-sized vessels) and pulmonary artery leading to pulmonary hypertension. The right ventricle hypertrophies to compensate, as does the right atrium. This impedes the forward flow of blood and lymph into the heart and causes lymphedema of the pharyngeal airway. The entire process is greatly facilitated in the presence of any contributing anatomic abnormality such as enlarged tonsils or subglottic or sublingual masses, which may encroach on the airway. In the nonobese patient with a significant anatomic obstruction of the airway, a similar chain of events is created because respiratory exchange is diminished and hypoxemia ensues.

There are data to show that weight loss can provide significant benefit for the patient with OSA. Perhaps this improves ventilation and decreases the workload of the heart, with a secondary gain of better forward flow of blood and lymph, thus opening up the airway. Further studies may prescribe methods of enhancing heart function, in addition to an aggressive program of weight control to help manage the patient with OSA. Various surgical methods directed only toward removing an obvious anatomic factor contributing to obstruction have not been as uniformly successful as anticipated.[34] Persistence of OSA is significantly associated with nocturnal premature death, undoubtedly related to hyposaturation and lethal cardiac dysrhythmias.[65]

TREATMENT OF OBSTRUCTIVE SLEEP APNEA

Treatment of the sleep apnea patient is directed toward identifying the locus (loci) of obstruction. An obvious example is hypertrophic tonsils obstructing the airway, for which a tonsillectomy is recommended. Most often, however, the diagnosis is not that simple. There are often multiple factors involved, e.g., obesity and a compromised airway secondary to retrognathia, or any combination of factors. Most patients with OSA do not have readily identifiable pathology on standard otolaryngologic examination.[58] Rojewski et al reported that in an evaluation of 200 patients with OSA, only three patients were found to have an anatomic problem that could be surgically corrected.[52]

The treatment of the OSA patient can be subdivided into medical and surgical modalities of therapy.[66] Since the pathogenesis of sleep-disordered breathing has not been fully elucidated, therapy in most cases continues to be difficult because the etiology remains obscure. Thus the application of medical and surgical treatment modalities can further be divided into general measures recommended for the management of all cases of sleep-disordered breathing and specific measures recommended for particular disorders.[55]

Medical modalities include treatment by a reduction of the risk factors that can precipitate apneic episodes, e.g., avoidance of alcohol or other central nervous system depressants. Inhalation therapy, with continuous positive airway pressure, and airway patency devices are helpful.[52,66] Surgical treatment techniques include adenoid and tonsil removal if they are enlarged. To correct skeletal deformities that compromise the oropharyngeal airway, tracheostomy, UPPP, maxillomandibular surgery, anterior superior suspension of the hyoid bone, and hyoidoplasty may be undertaken.

Prior to initiating any form of treatment, all patients should undergo a complete and thorough history, physical examination, and laboratory workup. From this a definitive diagnosis can often be reached. Various therapeutic recommendations and modifications are inherent in treatment of the OSA patient.[66] Overall, successful treatment of the OSA patient requires continual follow-up and reassessment of the whole patient and not just the upper airway complication. A multidisciplinary approach achieves the best results.

The results of the UPPP treatment remain variable.[10,17] Only 50 per cent of patients respond with nearly total remission of their symptoms.[16] Failures appear to be related to airway narrowing in the hypopharynx in addition to the oropharynx. Investigators agree that the variability of results may be determined by the anatomic site of airway constriction. Patients showing the greatest benefit with the UPPP are those in whom the Müller maneuver suggests occlusion only at the level of the velopharyngeal sphincter. Patients with multiple sites of obstruction were less relieved by surgery alone.[10] Therefore, patients with hypopharyngeal obstruction such as a large tongue base, an omega-shaped epiglottis, and redundant ariepiglottic folds did not benefit from UPPP.[16] According to Sher and coworkers, the ideal patient for UPPP is one with a 3 to 4+ collapse at the level of the soft palate and no collapse in the lower pharynx.[58]

Another treatment modality is CPAP (Fig. 58–5). This provides pressurized air

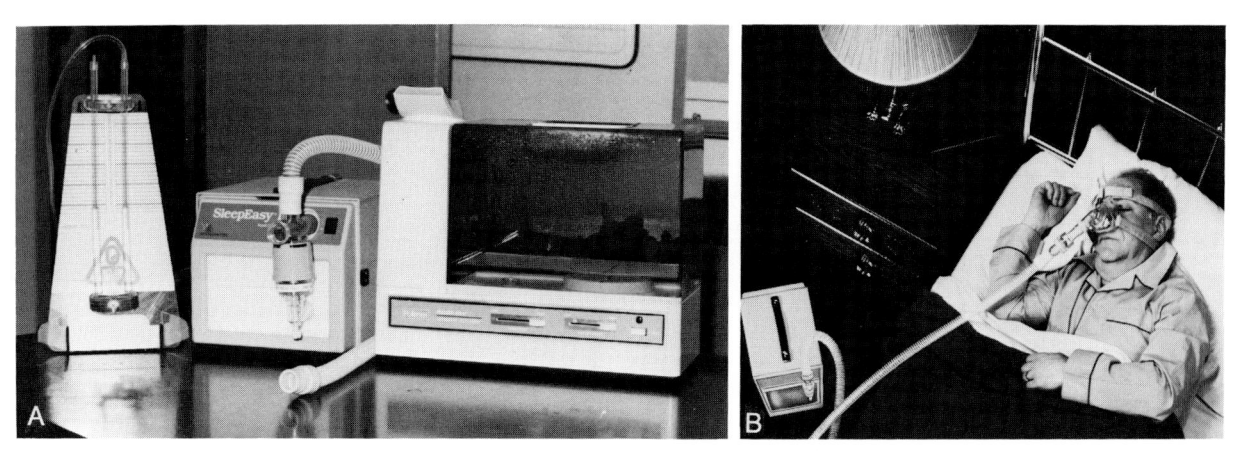

FIGURE 58–5. CONTINUOUS POSITIVE AIR PRESSURE (CPAP). *A*, CPAP machine. *B*, CPAP mask is worn throughout the night by patient. Proper airflow must be determined during preliminary tests.

through a face mask to keep the airway open. The minimum pressure at zero flow required to maintain upper airway patency ranges from 4 to 15 cm of H_2O.[47,54,63]

In a cephalometric study comparing pre- and post-treatment effects of UPPP and CPAP, Moore noted the following: (1) the skeletal and soft tissue craniofacial features of these two groups were statistically the same in all 70 variables measured prior to treatment.[43] Moreover, he found that the post-treatment effects were very comparable. The irony of these findings tends to further obscure the underlying etiologic factor(s) of OSA.

Weight loss is usually recommended to a majority of patients. In Laniado's study correlating numerous variables to apnea severity indices, body mass index (BMI) was consistently the most highly correlated variable when it was entered into the equation.[33] Subjectively, all patients feel that their apnea is less severe after they have lost weight. As a primary form of therapy, however, it is not uniformly effective.[60]

Tracheostomy is usually the last resort in order to establish a definitive airway. On occasion, it may be the most effective and most urgent treatment, especially if the patient is developing frequent, life-threatening dysrhythmias in association with hypoxic episodes. It bypasses the occlusion of the upper airway which occurs during sleep and establishes a more direct patent airway.[16] This continues to be the only consistently effective treatment, except for patients in whom clinically distinct upper airway abnormalities can be identified and corrected, i.e., adenotonsillar hypertrophy, tumor impinging on the airway, and micrognathia.[29] Permanent tracheostomy, however, is associated with a number of potential complications and significant psychosocial problems.[8]

Other alternatives for patients, particularly those with a skeletal abnormality such as retrognathia or micrognathia, are maxillofacial surgery, orthognathic surgery, or intraoral appliance therapy. These procedures can aid in increasing the pharyngeal diameter and correcting the posterior and inferior displacement of the tongue into the pharyngeal cavity. Initially, an orthodontic repositioning appliance such as a modified Herbst is used to open the airway (Fig. 58–6). The widening of the pharynx in an anteroposterior dimension is confirmed cephalometrically, and sleep studies are repeated in 3 to 6 months if there is any improvement. If the results are encouraging and the patient is amenable to surgery, a surgical advancement of the jaw(s) can be performed. OSA has been treated by orthodontic appliances, maxillofacial surgery, or a combination of these procedures.[21,42,49,59] With orthodontic appliances alone it was found that an anterior repositioning of the mandible caused the genioglossus muscle to come forward, the tongue to acquire a more proper posture, and the hypopharyngeal space to open.[21,59] Elimination of wedging of the soft palate against the nasopharyngeal wall was also achieved in a

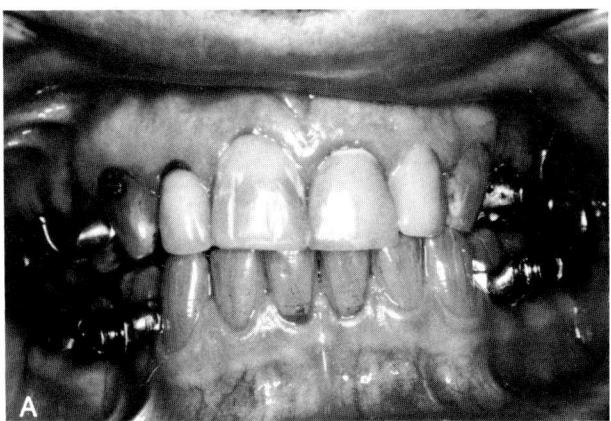

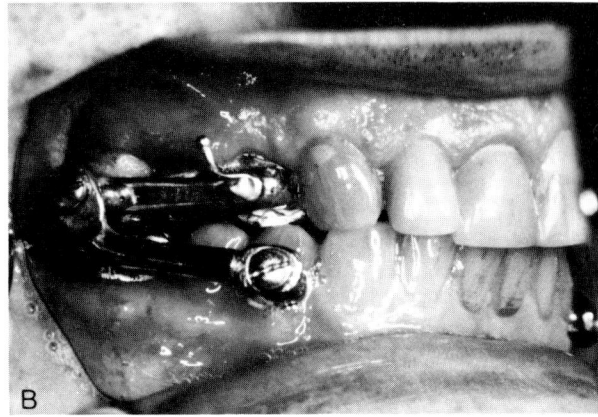

FIGURE 58-6. MODIFIED HERBST APPLIANCE USED IN OSA PATIENTS WITH LOWER PHARYNGEAL AIRWAY OBSTRUCTION. *A*, Lateral intraoral view of Herbst appliance. *B*, Frontal intraoral view of Herbst appliance. The patient places himself into the appliance before sleep by inserting the lower appliance attachment into the upper attachment. The patient then affixes anterior vertical elastics from the upper hook to the lower anterior screw. The patient is therefore fixated in a protrusive closed position.

study of 16 patients using a Herbst appliance. Pancherz found a distinct improvement in 15 patients with snoring and sleep, while one patient could not tolerate the appliance.[44]

Orthodontic appliances have also been used to help predict the success of surgical mandibular advancements.[1,42] Meir-Ewert and Brosig used a protracting device called the Esmarch prosthesis to pull the mandible 3 to 5 mm forward during sleep on 26 OSA patients.[42] Thirteen were excluded because of a poor-fitting appliance or resolution of the sleep apnea by other forms of therapy (e.g., weight reduction) prior to appliance treatment. However, following all-night PSGs with and without the appliance on the remaining 13 individuals, an average improvement of 61 per cent AI 32 per cent in apnea length, and 75 per cent in apnea time was found. Also, snoring was reduced in all patients and disappeared completely in some. Even though micrognathia has been cited in the literature as a common etiology of OSA, few cases of sleep apnea associated with mandibular retrognathism have been reported. Valero and Alroy in 1965 reported a case of a 55-year-old Arab man with sleep apnea and mandibular retrognathism secondary to a traumatic injury at age 3.[67] A tracheostomy was performed and the sleep apnea symptoms disappeared. Blokzijl reported two patients with sleep apnea and mandibular retrognathism who were treated with tracheostomies with good results.[2] Lugaresi et al and Imes et al documented one case each of patients presenting with sleep apnea and mandibular retrognathism who were treated successfully by tracheostomy.[27,40]

In 1970, Piecuch reported on the use of costochondral rib grafts to the temporomandibular joint areas of a 5-year-old girl who presented with mandibular hypoplasia and upper airway obstruction, manifested by apneic periods during sleep. The grafts were successful and the respiratory problems were alleviated following surgery. This finding suggested the possibility that mandibular retrognathia may be a contributing factor in some cases of sleep apnea.

In 1980, Bear and Priest reported on a 35-year-old black male with excessive sleepiness, retrognathic mandible, and short fat neck.[45] Sleep apnea secondary to upper airway obstruction was diagnosed. After the patient refused a tracheostomy, an acrylic occlusal splint was fabricated to protrude the mandible in order to determine whether surgical advancement would have lasting and positive effects on the patient's sleep apnea. An objective measurable improvement in apneic spells was noted; therefore surgical advancement of the mandible was performed. Following surgery the patient had no further problems with excessive daytime sleepiness and no apparent nightly apnea episodes.

OUR PERSPECTIVE

The remainder of this chapter focuses on how sleep apnea patients are evaluated. Case reports are presented to illustrate diagnostic dilemmas that many sleep apnea patients present. In the past 7 years our dental department has been an active participant in our sleep-wake disorders team. In that time, we have evaluated and have acquired cephalometric radiographs on nearly 500 sleep apnea patients.

Radiographic Technique

Three cephalometric radiographs are obtained after placing 1.5 cc of barium sulfate into each nostril and 0.5 cc in the oral cavity (3.5 cc total). This barium sulfate nasal lavage facilitates evaluating and measuring the oral and pharyngeal airways. Three cephalographs are obtained:

1. A normal lateral view in centric occlusion
2. A lateral view in which the mandible is protruded to its maximum extent
3. A posteroanterior projection

Patients are instructed not to swallow or breathe during exposure of all radiographs.

Cephalographs should be obtained in a standardized fashion with a fixed cathode-to-object distance of 60 inches (5 feet) and a constant object-to-film distance. All of our measurements were taken at a 13 cm object-to-film distance. The lateral and PA cephalographs should then be traced and measured. Our cephalometric analysis uses 25 linear and angular skeletal measurements and 22 linear and angular airway soft tissue measurements (Figs. 58–7 and 58–8).

Established normative standards for the lateral projection have proven to be useful in evaluating these patients (Tables 58–1 and 58–2). The posteroanterior projection provides additional information on the mediolateral dimensions of the airway. When it is interpreted along with the lateral cephalograph, the analysis is multidimensional (Fig. 58–9). The protrusive lateral cephalograph is used to assess any dimensional changes to the anteroposterior width of the airway when

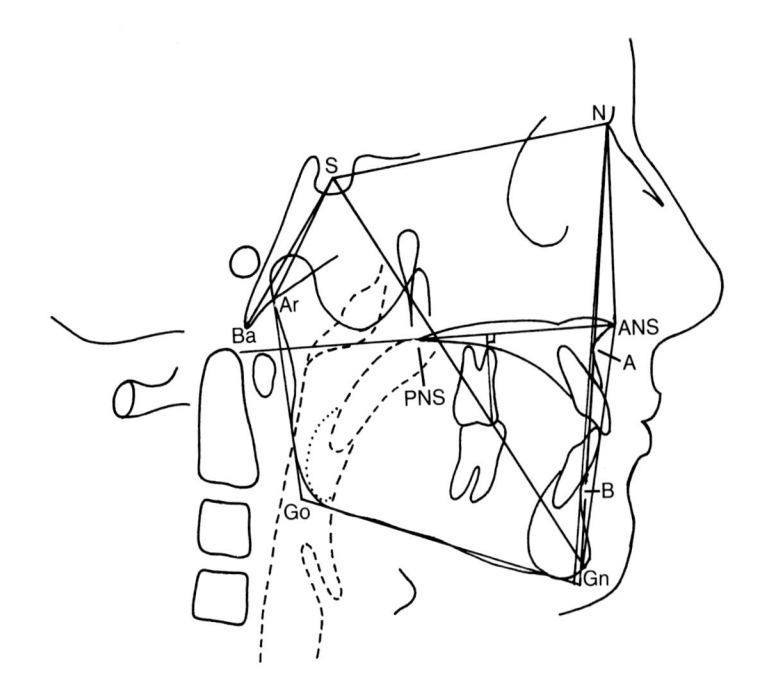

FIGURE 58–7. Skeletal cephalometric measurements for assessment of OSA. Normative data for the above measurements can be found in Table 58–1.

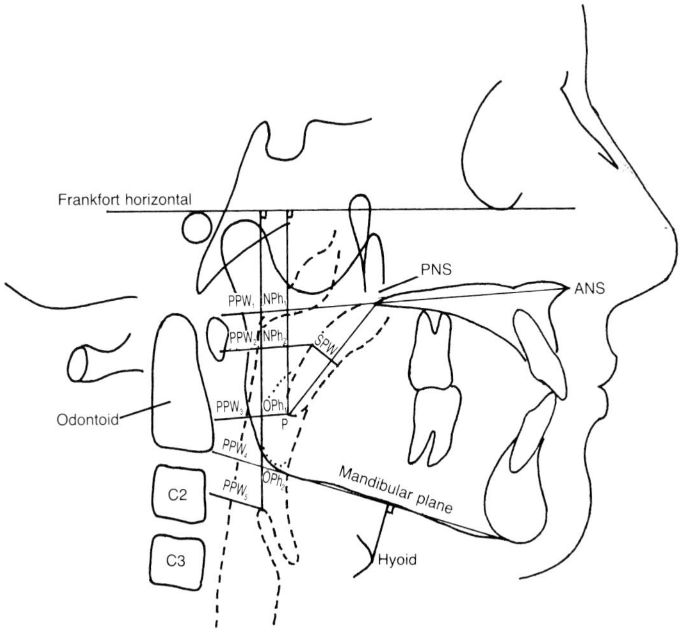

2032 / VII — ORTHOGNATHIC SURGERY

FIGURE 58-8. Soft tissue cephalometric measurements for assessment of OSA. Normative data for the above measurements can be found in Table 58-2.

mandible is advanced. The information from this projection may suggest a possible treatment approach. However, this should not stand alone but should be compared to a direct-view nasopharyngoscopic examination by the otolaryngologist.

At a regularly scheduled treatment planning conference, a discussion of findings with other members from the team generates an appropriate treatment plan for each patient reviewed. When the treatment course of the first 250 patients screened is radiographically reviewed, one notes some interesting trends. Adults

TABLE 58-1. NONAPNEIC POPULATION CEPHALOMETRIC SKELETAL MEASUREMENTS

Measurements	Males Means	SD	Females Means	SD
SNA	83.56°	(3.70)	82.40°	(3.30)
SNB	80.60°	(3.90)	78.50°	(3.95)
ANB	3.20°	(2.30)	3.80°	(2.30)
SNPg	82.00°	(3.70)	79.00°	(3.00)
NAPg	2.38°	(2.20)	3.08°	(2.39)
N-ANS	57.20 mm	(3.90)	50.80 mm	(3.10)
ANS-Gn	73.60 mm	(5.00)	70.40 mm	(6.00)
NS/ANS-PNS	7.30°	(2.50)	7.60°	(3.20)
NS	77.40 mm	(3.89)	71.67 mm	(3.59)
Go-Gn-H	23.30°	(4.50)	23.60°	(6.30)
6-PP	25.50 mm	(3.60)	23.60 mm	(5.80)
G0-Gn/SN	28.90°	(3.70)	33.30°	(4.60)
Go-Gn/FH	25.30°	(4.00)	24.60°	(6.30)
Go-Gn/ANS-PNS	23.00°	(4.50)	25.60°	(4.20)
Go-Gn	84.60 mm	(3.40)	78.50 mm	(5.80)
ANS-PNS	59.10 mm	(3.20)	51.30 mm	(4.20)
S-Gn/FH	62.20°	(3.85)	59.50°	(5.50)
N-Ba/ANS-PNS	26.60°	(3.70)	30.60°	(12.80)
NSBa	126.90°	(4.50)	132.30°	(3.25)
SBa	53.12 mm	(2.00)	46.75 mm	(2.20)
NSAr	121.10°	(4.50)	127.10°	(2.10)
SAr	40.60 mm	(3.60)	32.60 mm	(5.30)
SarGo	142.40°	(6.10)	139.30°	(7.95)
ArGoGn	124.20°	(5.50)	126.00°	(6.50)
ArGo	57.50 mm	(11.00)	48.75 mm	(5.50)

SD = Standard deviations.

TABLE 58-2. NONAPNEIC POPULATION SOFT TISSUE CEPHALOMETRIC MEASUREMENTS

Measurements	Males Means	SD	Females Means	SD
Ptm-ad1	31.00 mm	(5.50)	27.50 mm	(5.35)
Ptm-ad2	27.60 mm	(9.10)	25.60 mm	(4.05)
PAS	12.45 mm	(9.10)	11.75 mm	(4.05)
PNS-P	44.15 mm	(13.30)	47.10 mm	(2.35)
ANS-PNS-P	126.20°	(7.10)	130.60°	(5.50)
SPW	11.65 mm	(1.60)	11.60 mm	(1.80)
NPh1	30.60 mm	(5.20)	28.70 mm	(4.50)
PPW1	11.60 mm	(3.70)	11.60 mm	(1.20)
NPh2	10.50 mm	(4.00)	8.30 mm	(2.50)
PPW2	9.85 mm	(3.70)	8.40 mm	(1.70)
OPh1	10.90 mm	(3.70)	8.30 mm	(5.30)
PPW3	4.40 mm	(2.50)	4.25 mm	(1.70)
OPh2	11.90 mm	(3.90)	9.70 mm	(6.50)
PPW4	5.10 mm	(2.90)	4.25 mm	(1.50)
HPh1	16.90 mm	(6.50)	11.00 mm	(7.30)
PPW5	4.40 mm	(.70)	4.30 mm	(1.25)
HPh2	18.70 mm	(3.70)	22.60 mm	(7.40)
PPW6	5.20 mm	(1.10)	5.20 mm	(1.00)
MP-H	17.00 mm	(5.30)	15.40 mm	(7.20)
P-NPh1	37.35 mm	(7.10)	35.50 mm	(3.30)
EP	57.10 mm	(6.50)	49.75 mm	(7.70)
Ep-P	19.70 mm	(5.70)	14.25 mm	(7.70)

SD = Standard deviations.

with OSA tend to have convex profile, long anterior upper and lower facial height, low-set hyoid bone, steep mandibular plane, large Y axis, obtuse cranial base, obtuse gonial angle, and constricted posterior airway space. The UPPP and CPAP populations are virtually no different in the soft tissue and skeletal cephalometric values, but when these groups are compared to the nonapneic group the differences are localized primarily in the soft tissue airway and not the skeleton. The UPPP and CPAP groups tend to show increased posterior pharyngeal wall thickness as well as a low-set hyoid bone. The patients treated with the protrusive/surgical approach tend to have maxillomandibular retrognathism and excessive vertical facial height secondary to increases in the mandibular plane angle. Other

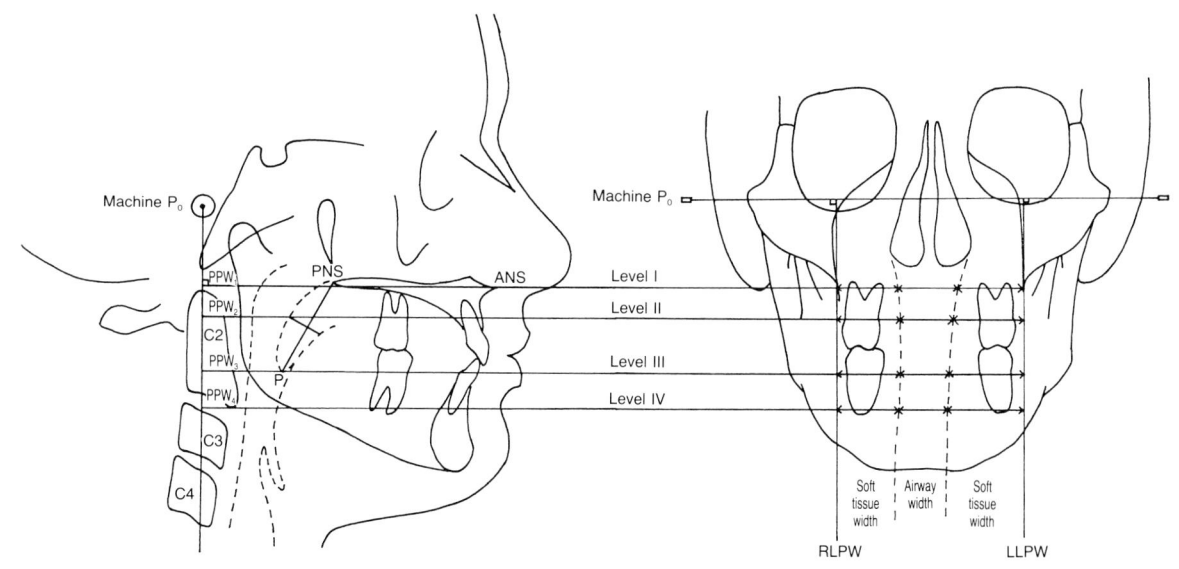

FIGURE 58-9. Analysis of anteroposterior cephalometric radiograph.

abnormal features in this group are (1) low-set hyoid and (2) smaller posterior pharyngeal airway space (particularly at the base of the tongue) secondary to a thickened posterior pharyngeal wall and compounded by a retruded lower jaw.

CASE REPORTS

CASE REPORT 1

L.L., a 46-year-old white male, was referred by the sleep-wake disorders center for evaluation of his sleep apnea. Past medical history was significant for an aspirin allergy, left eye blindness since childhood, and surgical removal of a pilonidal cyst 20 years before. Past dental history was significant for multiple dental restorations.

The patient complained of daytime somnolence ("lethargy") during the past 12 to 15 years. He reported snoring 95 per cent of the time during sleep. Initial PSG studies suggested a moderate OSA pattern. Physical examination revealed a tall, mildly obese male with notable mandibular retrognathism and a Class II dental malocclusion (Fig. 58–10). The radiographic survey documented a lower airway constriction at the base of tongue which improved markedly upon mandibular protrusion. These findings were also substantiated by nasoendoscopic examination. A modified Herbst appliance was fabricated and fit into the patient's dentition so that he would be able to fixate his mandible into a protruded posture. After 3 months, repeat PSGs documented improvement only when the appliance was activated. The patient agreed to surgical correction of his problem. He underwent 6 months of presurgical orthodontic therapy. A bilateral sagittal split osteotomy advancement of the mandible was performed.

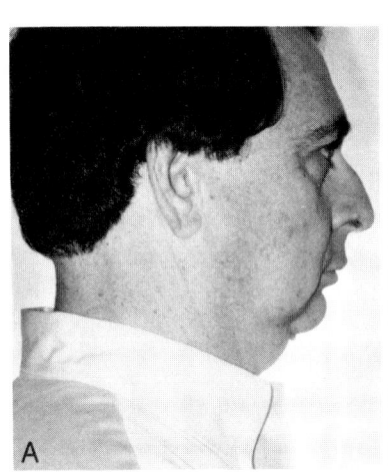

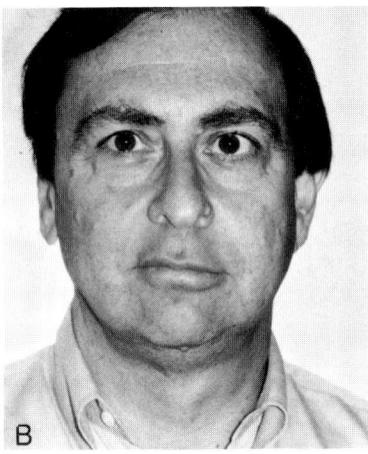

FIGURE 58–10. Preoperative extraoral photographs of Case 1.

FIGURE 58–11. Postoperative extraoral photographs of Case 1.

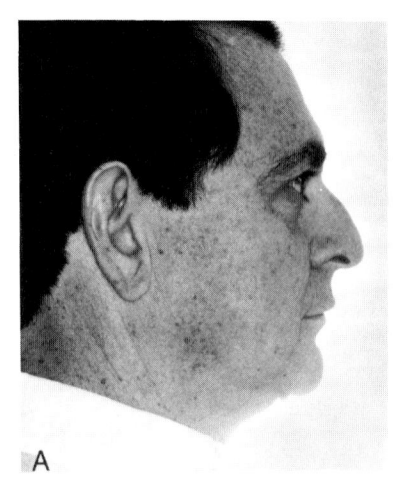

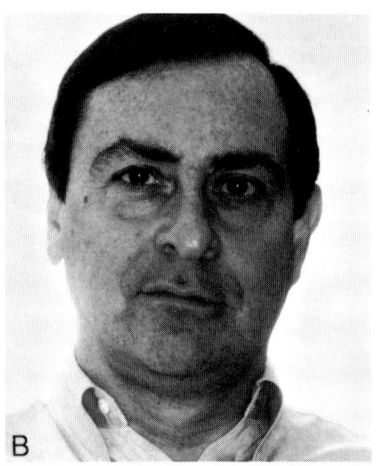

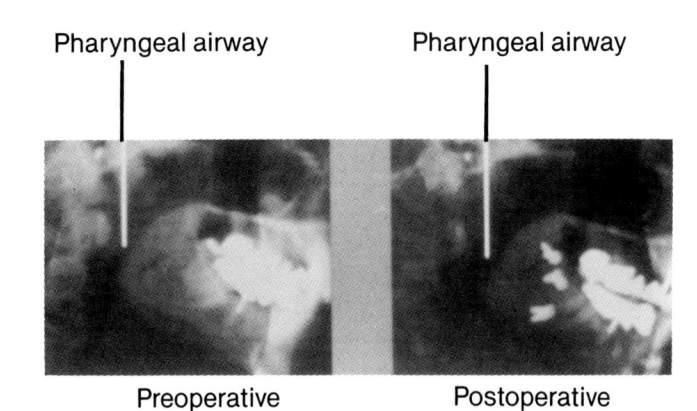

FIGURE 58-12. Pre- and postoperative cephalometric results of Case 1. Note marked improvement in the anteroposterior dimension of the pharyngeal airway in patient L.L.

Four months later the braces were removed and retainers placed. Two and a half years later postsurgical PSG studies and cephalometric evaluation documented remarkable stability and a favorable response (Figs. 58-11 and 58-12).

COMMENT

This patient represents a straightforward documentation of an OSA whose etiologic mechanism clearly was secondary to his mandibular retrognathia and associated lower airway obstruction. Very few OSA patients follow such a scenario in our experience, and only 5 per cent even qualify for preliminary appliance therapy.

CASE REPORT 2

R.W., a 42-year-old Caucasian male, was referred for evaluation of his sleep apnea. Past medical history was unremarkable. Past dental history included routine dental restorations, periodontal therapy, and orthodontic therapy during adolescence. This patient reported an 18-month history of a snoring problem that had worsened in the past 3 months. Polysomnographic evaluation demonstrated a moderate to severe obstructive apnea (AI = 18.8 and AHI = 30.5).

Physical examination revealed an individual with only minimal obesity and average build. His facial profile was convex with mandibular retrognathia. He had a Class I dental and Class II skeletal relationship.

The radiographic survey demonstrated a markedly constricted pharyngeal airway in the AP plane. The airway width improved noticeably when he protruded his mandible. The patient was fit with a modified Herbst appliance so that he could fixate his mandible in a forward position during sleep. After 4 months of wearing his appliance, repeat PSGs were performed with and without the appliance in place. The studies documented marked improvement in both AI and AHI; however, there was no difference between the studies. A follow-up nasoendoscopic study revealed that the patient was obstructed in the upper airway at the level of the soft palate, whereas the initial study had suggested an upper and a lower obstruction pattern.

The patient was referred for a UPPP to eliminate the upper airway constriction. Four months after palatal surgery; PSG studies showed virtual elimination of the apneic episodes with an AI of 0.8 and an AHI of 4.03.

COMMENT

Considering his recent history of snoring, the patient most likely presented in the early stages of OSA. There were no definitive etiologic factors identified. Preliminary evaluation and cephalometric analysis suggested that orthognathic surgery may have been necessary to successfully treat the patient. The follow-up PSGs clearly demonstrated that the appliance was useful, since the apnea was eliminated. Unexpectedly the apnea did not reappear when the protrusive component was eliminated.

The use of the protrusive appliance appears to eliminate certain factors, i.e., mandibular retropositioning and a constricted airway. Once the obstructive cycle was interrupted, it was obvious that precipitating factors were still localized in the upper airway and the patient would benefit in the long term from a UPPP procedure. Three and one-half year postoperative follow-up suggests good stability in results.

19. Guilleminault C: Sleeping and breathing. *In* Sleeping and Waking Disorders: Indications and Techniques. Menlo Park, CA, Addison-Wesley Publishing Co, 1982, pp 155–182.
20. Guilleminault C, Dement WC: Sleep apnea syndrome and its related sleep disorders. *In* Williams RL, Koracan I (eds): Sleep Disorders: Diagnosis and Treatment. New York, John Wiley, 1978, pp 9–28.
21. Guilleminault C: Diagnosis, pathogenesis, and treatment of the sleep apnea syndromes. Ergeb Inn Med Kinderheilkd 52:1–57, 1984.
22. Guilleminault C, Riley R, Powell N: OSA and abnormal cephalometric measurements. Chest 86:793, 1984.
23. Hagerty RF, Hill MJ, Pettit HS, Kane JJ: Posterior pharyngeal wall movement in normals. J Speech Hearing Res 1:203–210, 1958.
24. Handelman CS, Osborne G: Growth of the nasopharynx and adenoid development from one to eighteen years. Angle Orthod 46:243–259, 1976.
25. Haponik EF, Smith PL, Bohlman ME, et al: Computerized tomography in obstructive sleep apnea. Am Rev Respir Dis 127:221, 1983.
26. Hixon EH: An x-ray study comparing oral and pharyngeal structures of individuals with nasal voices and individuals with superior voices. M.S. Thesis, State University of Iowa, 1949.
27. Imes NK, Orr WC, Smith RO, Rogers RM: Retrognathia and sleep apnea: A life-threatening condition masquerading as narcolepsy. JAMA 237:1596, 1977.
28. Jamieson A, Guilleminault C, Partinen M, Quera-Salva MA: OSA patients have craniomandibular abnormalities. Sleep 9:469, 1986.
29. Katsantonis GP, Walsh JK, Schweiger PK, Friedman WH: Further evaluation of UPPP in the treatment of OSAS. Otolaryngol Head and Neck Surg 93:244, 1985.
30. King EW: A roentgenographic study of pharyngeal growth. Angle Orthod 22:23, 1952.
31. Kravath RE, Pollak CP, Borowiecki B: Hypoventilation during sleep in children who have lymphoid airway obstruction treated by nasopharyngeal tube and T and A. Pediatrics 59:865, 1977.
32. Krieger J, Lahsl L, Wilcox R, et al: Atrial natriuretic factor release during sleep in obstructive sleep apnea before and during nasal CPAP. Am Rev Respir Dis 137:57, 1988.
33. Laniado N: Cephalometric Analysis of Adult Obstructive Sleep Apnea. Postgraduate Thesis, Einstein/Montefiore, 1988.
34. Ledereich PS, Thorpy MJ, Glovinsky PB, et al: Five and ten year follow-up of symptoms in patients with obstructive sleep apnea: The Monterfiore long-term follow up study. Sleep Res 17:264, 1987.
35. Leithner C, Frass M, Packer R, et al: Mechanical ventilation with positive end-expiratory pressure decreases release of alpha-atrial natriuretic peptide. Crit Care Med 15(5):484–488, 1987.
36. Linder-Aronson S: Adenoids: Their effect on mode of breathing and nasal airflow and their relationship to characteristics of the facial skeleton and dentition. Acta Otolaryngol Suppl 265, 1970.
37. Linder-Aronson S, Henrikson CC: Radiocephalometric analysis of anteroposterior nasopharyngeal dimensions in 6- to 12-year-old mouth breathers compared with nose breathers. Otol Rhin Laryngol 35:19–29, 1973.
38. Lowe AA, Caccagra G, Montovani M, et al: Three-dimensional CT reconstructions of tongue and airway in adult subjects with OSA. Am J Orthod Dentofac Orthop 90:364–374, 1986.
39. Lowe AA, Santamaria JD, Fleetham JA, Price C: Facial morphology and OSA. Am J Orthod Dentofac Orthop 90:364, 1986.
40. Lugaresi E, et al: Effects of tracheotomy in two cases of hypersomnia with periodic breathing. J Neurol Neurosurg Psychiatry 36:15–26, 1973.
41. McKee TL: A cephalometric radiographic study of tongue positions in individuals with cleft palate deformity. Angle Orthod 26:99–109, 1956.
42. Meir-Ewert K, Brasig B: Prosthetic treatment of obstructive sleep apnea. Sleep Res 15:197, 1986.
43. Moore M: Cephalometric Evaluation of UPPP and CPAP in OSA patients. Postgraduate Thesis, Einstein/Montefiore, 1989.
44. Pancherz H: The Herbst appliance—its biologic effects and clinical use. Am J Orthod Dentofac Orthop 87:1–20, 1985.
45. Piecuch JF: Costochondral grafts to temporomandibular joints. Presented at Annual Meeting of the American Association of Oral and Maxillofacial Surgeons, Chicago, September, 1978.
46. Poole MN, Engel GA, Chaconas SJ: Nasopharyngeal cephalometrics. Oral Surg 49:266, 1980.
47. Rapaport DM, Sorkin B, Garay SM, et al: Reversal of the "pickwickian syndrome" by long-term use of nocturnal nasal airway pressure. N Engl J Med 307:931, 1982.
48. Ricketts RM: The cranial base and soft structures in cleft palate speech and breathing. Plast Reconstr Surg 14:47, 1954.
49. Rider E: Removable Herbst appliance for treatment of OSA. J Clin Orthod 22(4):256–257, 1988.
50. Riley R, Guilleminault C, Herran J, Powell N: Cephalometric analysis and flow volume loops in OSA patients. Sleep 6:303–311, 1983.
51. Rivlin J, Hoffstein V, Kalbfleisch J, et al: Upper airway morphology in patients with idiopathic OSA. Am Rev Respir Dis 129:355, 1984.
52. Rojewski TE, Schuller DE, Clark RW, et al: Videoendoscopic determination of the mechanism of obstruction in obstructive sleep apnea. Otolaryngol Head Neck Surg 92:127, 1984.
53. Rosenberger HC: Growth and development of the nasorespiratory area in childhood. Ann Otol Rhinol Laryngol 43:495–522, 1934.
54. Sanders MH, Moore SE, Eveslase J: CPAP via nasal mask: A treatment for occlusive apnea. Chest 83:144, 1983.
55. Santiago TV, Trontell MC: Therapy of sleep apnea syndromes. *In* Breathing Disorders of Sleep. Montefiore Medical Center, NY, 1986, pp 197–204.

56. Schafer E: Upper airway obstruction and sleep disorders in children with craniofacial anomalies. Clin Plast Surg 9:555, 1982.
57. Schweiger JW: Cranial base angle, amount of palatal tissue, and nasopharyngeal depth in individuals with clefts. Cleft Palate J 3:115, 1966.
58. Sher AE, Thorpy MJ, Shprintzen RJ, et al: Predictive value of Muller maneuver in selection of patients for uvulopalatopharyngoplasty. Laryngoscope 95:1483, 1985.
59. Soll BA, George PT: Treatment of obstructive sleep apnea with a nocturnal airway-patency appliance (letter). N Engl J Med 313(6):386–387, 1985.
60. Strohl KP, Sullivan CE, Saunders NA: Sleep apnea syndromes. *In* Saunders NA, Sullivan CE (eds): Sleep and Breathing. New York, Marcel Dekker, 1984.
61. Subtelny J: A cephalometric study of the growth of the soft palate. Plast Reconstr Surg 19:49–62, 1957.
62. Sullivan CE, Issa FG, Berthon-Jones M, Saunders NA: Pathophysiology of sleep apnea. *In* Saunders NA, Sullivan CE (eds): Sleep and Breathing. New York, Marcel Dekker, 1984.
63. Sullivan CE, Issa FG, Berthon-Jones M, Eves L: Reversal of OSA by CPAP applied through the nares. Lancet 1:862, 1981.
64. Suratt PM, Dee P, Atkinson RL, et al: Fluoroscopic and computed tomographic features of the pharyngeal airway in obstructive sleep apnea. Am Rev Respir Dis 127:487, 1983.
65. Thorpy MJ, Ledereich PS, Glovinsky PB, et al: Survival of patients with sleep apnea. Sleep Res 16:444, 1987.
66. Thorpy MJ, Ledereich P: Medical treatment of OSAS. Handbook of Sleep Disorders, Einstein/Montefiore, 1989.
67. Valero A, Alroy G: Hypoventilation in acquired micrognathia. Arch Intern Med 115:307–310, 1965.
68. Walsh JK, Kantsantonis GP: Somnofluoroscopy as a predictor of UPP efficacy. Sleep Res 13:21, 1984.
69. Weitzman ED, Pollack CP, Borowiecki B, et al: The hypersomnia sleep apnea syndrome: Site and mechanism of upper airway obstruction. *In* Guilleminault C, Dement WC (eds): Sleep Apnea Syndromes. New York, Alan R. Liss, 1978, pp 235–248.
70. Wildman AJ: A study of the relation between nasal emission and the apparent form and function of certain structures associated with nasopharyngeal closure in cleft palate individuals. M.S.D. Thesis, Northwestern University Dental School, 1954.
71. Wildman AJ: Analysis of tongue, soft palate, and pharyngeal wall movement. Am J Orthod 47:439–461, 1961.
72. Zorick F, Roth T, Kramer M, Flessa H: Exacerbation of upper-airway sleep apnea by lymphocytic lymphoma. Chest 77:689, 1980.

spouse or other family member. The diagnosis is established by nocturnal polysomnography.

The pathologic complications of OSA primarily involve the cardiopulmonary and central nervous systems. Sleep disruption produces excessive daytime hypersomnia and behavioral changes, which may lead to occupational or social disability or both. Hypersomnia or daytime fatigue can be a disabling symptom. Mild daytime sleepiness can be normal, but severe daytime fatigue resulting in sleep during ordinary activities is obviously disrupting and abnormal. Causes of sleepiness due to OSA can usually be differentiated from narcolepsy and other medical problems by adequate medical examination and polysomnography.[12,13]

The most serious problem caused by OSA is hypoxemia, which may lead to frank cardiopulmonary disease. The severity of nocturnal hypoxemia depends on the awake baseline oxygenation and pulmonary function, but hypoxemia can be greatly worsened during rapid eye movement (REM) sleep. Obesity appears to aggravate poor nocturnal oxygenation, probably owing to hypoventilation and reduced functional reserve capacity. Pulmonary and systemic hypertension results from hypoxemia. It has been shown that more snorers have hypertension than do age- and weight-matched nonsnoring control subjects. This finding may be due in part to hypercapnia and hypoxemia. Chronic hypoxemia leads to erythrocytosis and cor pulmonale. In other words, OSA may lead to congestive heart failure.[14-16]

Further cardiac progression may lead to life-threatening arrhythmias and may result in death. Therefore, when major complications of OSA occur, immediate intervention is indicated. In addition to treating erythrocytosis and heart failure, the primary problem of OSA must be promptly addressed.[17-19] A primary approach to the problem of sleep apnea involves nasal continuous positive airway pressure (CPAP) or upper airway surgery, that is, maxillomandibular advancement and uvulopalatopharyngoplasty (UPPP).

In addition to the cardiopulmonary sequelae, behavioral changes, such as depression, irritability, intellectual deterioration, and impotence, are associated with OSA. These are most likely related to sleep deprivation but may also result from cerebral hypoxemia.[20,21]

The diagnosis and treatment of OSA commonly involve a multidisciplinary team. The team may include a neurologist, otolaryngologist, cardiologist, psychiatrist, pulmonologist, orthodontist, nutritionist, oral and maxillofacial surgeon, and other technical staff. All individuals with OSA should be routinely screened by an oral and maxillofacial surgeon for orthognathic or craniofacial deformities as part of a complete physical examination data base.

POLYSOMNOGRAPHY

Polysomnography consists of continuous recording of the electroencephalogram, electro-oculogram, chin electromyogram, nasal-oral air flow, thoracic and abdominal respiratory effort, oxyhemoglobin saturation, and anterior tibialis electromyograms, along with infrared videotaping obtained during the patient's normal sleeping time. Each recording is analyzed by hand for total sleep time, sleep stages, arousals, cardiac events, respiratory parameters, nocturnal myoclonus, and oxyhemoglobin desaturation. Data are manually entered into a computer for generation of a report. OSA is defined as an event in which air flow ceases, with continued inspiratory effort for 10 or more seconds. Partial apnea (hypopnea) is defined as an event in which air flow is substantially reduced for 10 or more seconds, resulting in desaturation or arousal or both. The respiratory disturbance index (RDI) is defined as the number of apneas and partial apneas per hour of sleep.[6]

MEDICAL THERAPY

Upper airway obstruction is a phenomenon of passive obstruction with inspiration. Therefore, nasal CPAP provides positive pressure to the oropharynx and acts as a pneumatic splint. The success rate of 70 to 80 per cent for nasal CPAP has been thought to be the best nontracheostomy therapy available. The problem is that about 20 per cent of patients cannot tolerate the device. Complaints of suffocation, dry nose, and poor sleep have been reported. In addition, CPAP requires compliance of the patient and periodic monitoring for adjustment.[22]

Medical pharmacology has offered little benefit to OSA. Only a few agents have been used: oxygen, protriptyline, and progesterone. Protriptyline is a nonsedating tricyclic antidepressant that appears to relieve upper airway obstruction during sleep in occasional patients. Tricyclic antidepressants have been used in narcolepsy-cataplexy syndromes with good results and have been tried in sleep apnea. The results of progesterone therapy are questionable; however, it seems to help patients with primary alveolar hypoventilation or central apneas.[23-25]

SURGICAL THERAPY

Surgery is recommended for those with significant OSA (an RDI greater than 20), orthognathic or craniofacial deformities, abnormal hyoid position, or narrowed posterior airway space and for those unable to tolerate or respond to CPAP.

In the past, tracheostomy has been the most common surgical treatment. Surgeons interested in OSA have been recently challenged to develop a surgical procedure that rivals the success and predictability of tracheostomy but that does not have its inherent morbidity. Patients with OSA have been found to have craniofacial abnormalities that may influence pharyngeal patency.[26] This fact is expecially relevant, since patients in whom UPPP has failed have been successfully treated with maxillofacial surgery. Severe mandibular hypoplasia and macroglossia may obstruct the oropharyngeal and hypopharyngeal airway during supine sleep. In such cases, palatal reduction is of no benefit. Therefore, multiple surgical procedures, designed to increase the posterior airway space, as described in the literature,[27] have been devised. Maxillomandibular advancement surgery has been used with some success as an isolated procedure or in combination with adjunctive procedures, such as septoplasty, turbinectomy, geniotomy advancement, glossectomy, and UPPP. It has been shown that orthognathic surgery increases the airway space and improves OSA; however, the following procedures have been beneficial as isolated surgical modalities.[28]

Septoplasty

Rarely is the presence of specific pathologic tissue responsible for obstructive airway disease, but if so, removal is often curative. OSA occurs during sleep, when pharyngeal tone is relaxed and no single obstructive abnormality is present. In

FIGURE 59-1. Example of septal deviation and bone spur associated with obstructive sleep apnea (OSA).

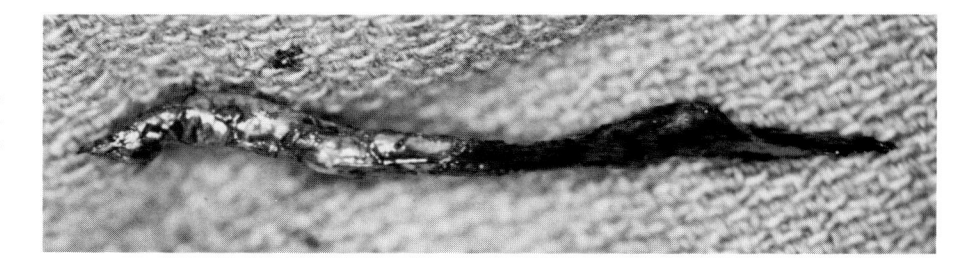

these situations, minor septal deviations increase negative pharyngeal pressure and result in collapse. Nasal obstruction induces or worsens apnea, and several reports have shown that correction of nasal obstruction by septoplasty and submucosal resection has resulted in amelioration or cure of the apnea[29,30] (Fig. 59-1).

Tracheostomy

In the past, tracheostomy has been the most successful surgical treatment; however, tracheostomy is not without postoperative complications and psychosocial difficulties. It requires compliance and cooperation in cleaning and caring for the stoma, which can be complicated by infection, bleeding, malodorous secretions, and granulation tissue with subsequent obstruction. Patients with OSA deserve an effective alternative.[31,32]

Despite the drawbacks, specific indications for tracheostomy exist: (1) severe OSA with impaired function, (2) temporary airway management in conjunction with other surgery, (3) severe pulmonary hypertension or cor pulmonale, (4) life-threatening arrhythmias, and (5) high motivation for "cure" in a patient who can be expected to comply with tracheostomy maintenance.

Uvulopalatopharyngoplasty (UPPP)

Uvulopharyngoplasty has been beneficial in some cases of OSA. The procedure was originally designed to treat snoring and was subsequently applied to airway obstruction. The technique is extremely variable among surgeons, but the intent is to shorten the soft palate, widen the lateral dimension, and open the posterior airway space (Fig. 59-2). The procedure lasts about 45 minutes to 1 hour but can be associated with severe pain, swelling, reflux, and, rarely, mortality. The elimination of loud snoring is most often successful.[33]

Uvulopharyngoplasty results demonstrate a significant improvement in OSA, as measured by the RDI, but the true cure rate is very low. The procedure has been reported to have decreased the RDI to less than 50 per cent of the preoperative value in 56 per cent of patients. Mean data for large series have shown a reduction from an RDI of 60 to an RDI of 30. Although this is a major change in the RDI, it still represents significant sleep apnea and its associated medical problems. Experience at our institution has shown that with UPPP only 7 per cent of patients with OSA experience resolution, 70 per cent improved, and 23 per cent do not improve or worsen. The combination or staging of this procedure with other surgical techniques appears to be synergistic. UPPP is not frequently used with hyoid suspension or mandibular osteotomies, and the cure rate is greatly increased.

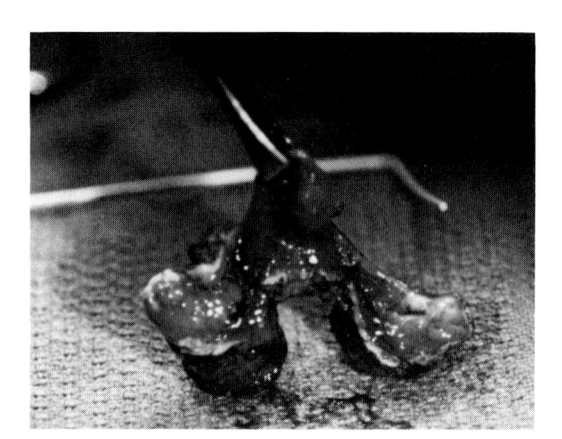

FIGURE 59-2. Large uvula and tonsillar tissue removed during uvulopalatopharyngoplasty (UPPP).

Although results are poor, when UPPP is used as the single modality it should not be abandoned for treatment of sleep apnea. Accurate diagnosis and careful selection of patients can increase effectiveness.[34-36]

PRESURGICAL WORKUP FOR MAXILLOMANDIBULAR ADVANCEMENT IN OBSTRUCTIVE SLEEP APNEA

Abnormalities of the aerodigestive tract may also produce airway obstruction and therefore warrant an evaluation by an otorhinolaryngologist. Frequently, hypertrophied tonsils, adenoids, nasal septal deviations, and polyps are the cause of obstruction.[37,38] Most patients with OSA, however, do not have clearly identifiable pathology on standard otolaryngologic examination. Rojewski reported that in the evaluation of 200 patients with OSA only 3 patients had a single anatomic problem that could be surgically corrected.[39] Occasionally, more serious obstructive masses, such as nasopharyngeal tumors, may be the cause. These cases require a complete head and neck examination with nasopharyngoscopy. Endoscopy is the best clinical method to evaluate the upper airway and to rule out the presence of a tumor. It is also used to visualize the most narrow area of obstruction or flaccid collapse by means of the Müller maneuver. With this maneuver, the scope is kept in place while the patient is asked to attempt inspiration with the nose occluded. The pharynx should resist collapse upon inspiration unless an obstruction is present or an abnormality in the pharyngeal musculature and connective tissue exists. UPPP is thought to be indicated when the location of collapse is in the area of the soft palate. A search for maxillofacial deformities should be pursued if the otorhinolaryngologic evaluation is normal. Cephalometric radiographs are not a conclusive study of the upper airway but are useful because they correlate with volumetric computerized tomography.[40]

All individuals with OSA should be routinely screened by an oral and maxillofacial surgeon for orthognathic or craniofacial deformities after documentation of their disease by nocturnal polysomnography. This screening is part of a complete physical examination data base for patients with sleep apnea and is recommended, since many with sleep apneas have abnormal facial morphology, which may be responsible for their airway obstruction during sleep. Jamieson and colleagues cephalometrically evaluated 155 patients with OSA and compared them with 41 orthodontic patients who did not have sleep apnea and with normal published data. Of the sleep apnea group, 150 had at least two significantly abnormal landmarks. The common findings were decreased cranial base flexure angle, retrognathism, and a low-positioned hyoid.[26] A further detailed description of the orthognathic relationship has been described by Lowe and co-workers.[41] They identified retroposition of the maxilla and mandible, a steep mandibular plane, proclined incisors, large gonial angle, increased facial heights, anterior open bites, and large tongues in 25 male adults with sleep apnea. Many of these abnormalities may reduce the upper airway and cause obstruction.[42] Cephalometric abnormalities of some degree have so often been identified in OSA that orthognathic screening by an oral and maxillofacial surgeon is warranted as part of the complete diagnostic workup.

The purpose of the initial oral and maxillofacial consultation should be to acquaint the patient and surgeon. It should inform the patient of surgical alternatives to nasal CPAP and provide a variety of surgical options. The decision for orthognathic surgery should not be made hastily, but only after thorough consultation. The surgeon should evaluate the results of the sleep study and confirm the presence of OSA. The severity of the disease should be considered in relation to the frequency of events (RDI) and the degree of oxygen desaturation (both total number of events below 90 per cent saturation and lowest saturation value). This

2048 / VII — ORTHOGNATHIC SURGERY

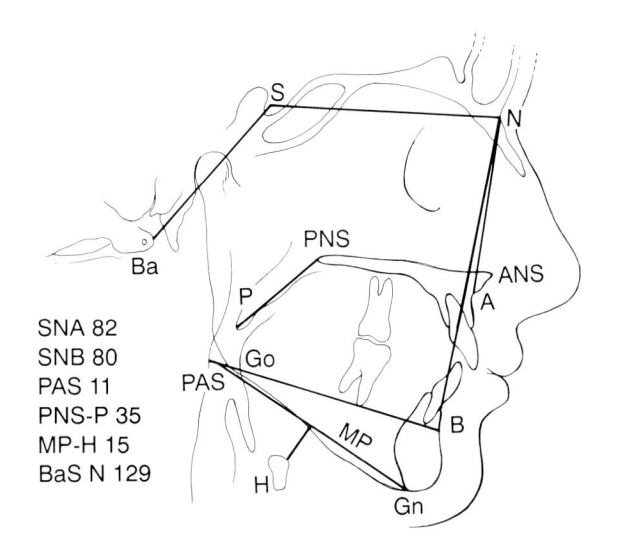

SNA 82
SNB 80
PAS 11
PNS-P 35
MP-H 15
BaS N 129

FIGURE 59-3. The cephalometric radiograph is a brief screening method to evaluate anatomic causes of airway obstruction. Hyoid position and posterior airway space should be measured in a standard method, as described by Riley and colleagues.[44]

first visit is a good opportunity to explain the cephalometric radiograph and demonstrate the posterior airway space. The cephalometric radiograph is viewed as a limited screening tool and should be used briefly to evaluate a few key points (Fig. 59-3). Patients can easily see the hour-glass configuration at the base of the tongue and understand how it is occluded during sleep. They should be made to understand that orthognathic surgery is commonly performed and that it now has application in OSA. They should realize that complications may occur and that the results are never 100 per cent satisfactory. Generally, a cure can be expected in 60 to 80 per cent of patients. In the absence of other medical disease, heart disease, pulmonary dysfunction, obesity, and old age, the success rate may be higher.

During the initial consultation, the oral and maxillofacial surgeon should quickly screen the cephalometric radiograph for gross abnormalities.[27] One should examine both hard and soft tissue, including hyoid position, soft palate, and posterior airway space. Frequently, the SNA and SNB are normal, but the surgeon should identify any other cause of obstruction, such as a low hyoid, narrow posterior airway, or long soft palate. Previous studies have demonstrated significant cure rates in OSA patients with normal SNA and SNB values.[6] Cranial base flexure angle and cranial base length are more often abnormal.[28] Individually, these may seem minor, but in the presence of other factors during sleep, the combination can result in airway obstruction.

It appears that maxillomandibular advancement surgery produces a significant increase in the posterior airway space and in the cure rate for patients with sleep apnea, both those with normal cephalometric values and those with abnormal values. The success of maxillomandibular advancement is far greater than that of UPPP.[28] Therefore, the decision for surgery may begin with a consideration of orthognathic surgery. The surgical objective is to increase the posterior airway by moving the jaws as far forward as possible rather than normalizing facial esthetics or the masticatory system.

Once the decision for maxillofacial surgery is made, one must evaluate the surgical morbidity and risk for the individual. This evaluation involves a comprehensive surgical risk assessment, including a detailed history and physical examination, cardiology consultation with a graded exercise tolerance test (GXT), and pulmonary consultation with a pulmonary function text (PFT). These subsystems are important to evaluate because the sequelae of OSA often result in cardiopulmonary dysfunction.[19] In addition, the incidence of cardiopulmonary disease increases with age, and therefore, cardiac status must be evaluated prior to elective surgery. Cardiologists and pulmonologists are readily aware of the problems associated with the OSA patient, and the solution of their input prior to the development of postoperative complications is wise. If coronary artery disease is present according to the history or the GXT, it should be treated prior to surgery. This treatment may consist of coronary artery bypass grafting or medical management. In many cases, such patients are poor candidates for orthognathic surgery. Similarly, pulmonary dysfunction should be documented. Chronic obstructive pulmonary disease (COPD) produces a low baseline saturation level and exaggerates the severity of OSA. Patients having severe OSA with concomitant COPD do not respond well to surgical intervention. Generally, individuals with a forced expiratory volume of less than 70 per cent of predicted values should not undergo surgery. Occasionally, medically compromised persons may undergo maxillomandibular advancement, but this is the exception rather than the rule, and the decision should be based upon the individual situation. In such situations, consultation with the appropriate specialists is vitally important.

Once the decision to perform maxillomandibular advancement surgery is made, a second presurgical visit is scheduled. During this visit, the surgeon should obtain dental impressions and facebow registrations. Facebow transfers are not essential but do provide accuracy as well as excellent records for future reference. The teeth should be closely examined and their usefulness determined. If the teeth are adequate and have good function, presurgical orthodontics may be recommended. It is important to point out to the patient that without orthodontics a malocclusion will probably exist after surgery. Orthodontics can assist in allowing the mandible to be maximally advanced. This approach may require alteration of the presurgical goals from an orthodontic standpoint. Acceptance of a slight maxillary proclination and linqual version of the mandibular dentition allows the mandible to be moved several millimeters farther. This factor is important because more space is available for the tongue, with a larger posterior airway space. If the teeth are inadequate and have poor function, they should be maintained and used for surgical manipulation of the maxilla and mandible. This step can be done without orthodontics, and the final masticatory function can be rehabilitated prosthetically. The patient should be thoroughly counseled in regard to surgical and dental complications resulting from surgery. These include malocclusion, temporomandibular joint (TMJ) dysfunction, altered facial esthetics, inferior alveolar nerve dysfunction, ozena, anesthetic problems, cardiopulmonary complications, and poor results.

On the basis of our experience at the University of Alabama, we have found it is difficult to advance a maxilla beyond 12 mm and maintain stable bony support. It is also difficult to hold the maxilla stable in three dimensions while rigid fixation is achieved. Therefore, model surgery is performed with these difficulties in mind. With the models accurately mounted in centric relation, a final interocclusal

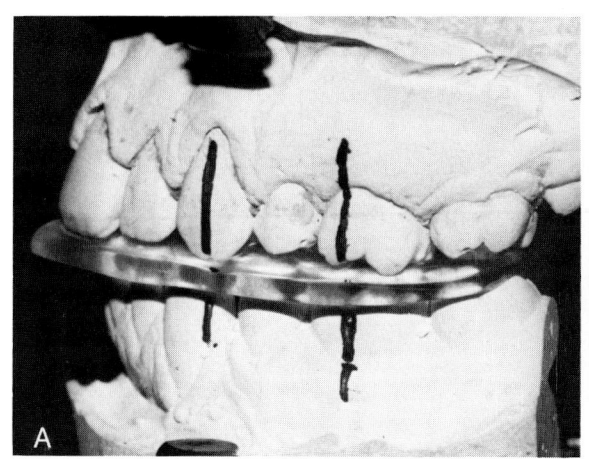

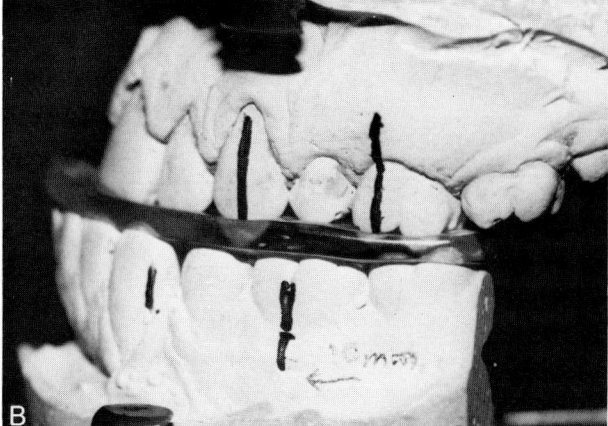

FIGURE 59–4. *A*, Maxillary and mandibular casts are mounted in centric relation to reference marks, and the final occlusal splint is made. *B*, The mandible is then advanced approximately 12 mm bilaterally, and an advancement splint is constructed.

acrylic splint is first made. This splint will actually be used after the advancement splint, but accurate detail is more critical to ensure the exact occlusal relationship. The mandibular advancement splint is then made by advancing the mandibular dental model about 1 cm parallel to the occlusal plane, with dental midlines aligned. This alignment must also be accurate, but minor occlusal abnormalities can be compensated for later by the final splint (Fig. 59–4). The net effect of the model surgery is to allow the mandible to be advanced an arbitrary amount of at least 1 cm and to be rigidly fixed. After the mandible is advanced and fixed into a prognathic position, the maxilla can be advanced and held stable by the mandible in intermaxillary fixation. At the conclusion of the surgery, both jaws are advanced and kept in the proper occlusal relationship while the same plane of occlusion and the facial midline are maintained. Although malocclusions still occur with this method, careful model surgery tends to reduce their frequency and severity.

SURGICAL TECHNIQUE

The technique of maxillomandibular advancement for OSA is similar to that of any orthognathic procedure. However, several differences between this procedure and others exist and have not yet been adequately studied. Areas of difference include the vascular supply in an older age group, bone healing, predictability, stability, and adjunctive procedures and their consequences on speech, vascularity, and healing. Many patients who undergo maxillomandibular advancement surgery have experienced failure with UPPP. Scar formation in the palate may prevent maxillary advancement or impede blood supply. Advancement of the maxilla by a Le Fort I osteotomy may theoretically excessively advance the soft palate and produce hypernasal speech. In a review of more than 50 cases, these potential complications have not been observed when a UPPP was performed either before or simultaneously with maxillomandibular advancement surgery.[28]

Since this patient population includes obese patients with cardiopulmonary disease and airway compromise, it behooves the surgeon to take every reasonable precaution. Patients with OSA may require elective tracheostomy during the perioperative period to ensure a patent airway. This is particularly true if adjunctive procedures such as glossectomy and UPPP are simultaneously performed. Such an aggressive approach is not routinely recommended unless the disease is extremely severe (an RDI greater than 60), and the patient has a long soft palate and maxillofacial deformity. Even then, it is best to stage the procedures unless the patient is not willing to undergo multiple surgeries.

As in the presurgical model surgery, the mandible is advanced first. This step is recommended, since the amount of advancement is arbitrary and not based on the normal functional and esthetic position of the incisor. A standard mucoperiosteal incision and sagittal split osteotomy are done, allowing the mandible to be advanced at least 1 cm. The mandibular advancement splint is used to orient the distal segment and maintain the proper plane of occlusion. Temporary maxillomandibular fixation is then achieved. The mandible should be rigidly fixed with three 2.7-mm bicortical screws in an L pattern, producing a prognathic profile (Fig. 59–5). Maxillomandibular fixation is then removed, and evidence of immediate condylar relapse is evaluated.

At this point, the surgeon's attention is turned to the maxilla. Since enough soft tissue mobilization to allow an advancement of at least 1 cm is required in older patients, it is judicious to preserve the vascularity. Experience indicates that the maxilla can be further advanced with the palatine arteries intact when a high Le Fort osteotomy is performed. These arteries are maintained if possible. In addition, the preservation of a broad-based vascular flap posterior to the zygomatic buttress is also advisable. The vestibular mucosal incision begins high on the zy-

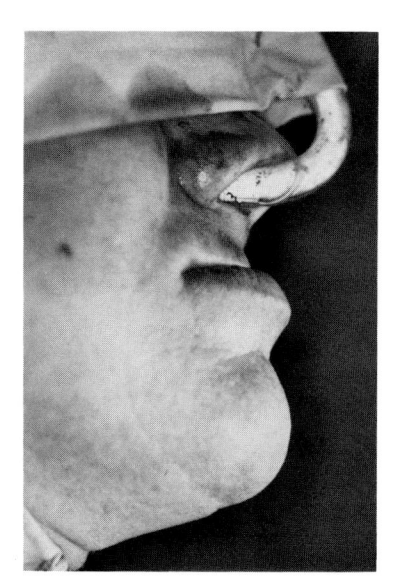

FIGURE 59-5. The mandible is surgically advanced about 10 to 12 mm into a prognathic profile and rigidly fixed with three bicortical screws bilaterally.

goma but not posteriorly and extends anteriorly a few millimeters above the mucogingival junction. The area posterior to the zygomatic buttress is approached by tunneling. A modified stepped Le Fort osteotomy is recommended to prevent the maxillary impaction that naturally occurs when the maxilla is moved along an oblique cut. In addition, this procedure allows the placement of a bone graft or alloplastic implant. When stabilization is provided by miniplates, bone grafting is not necessary.[28] The maxilla must be aggressively mobilized and the palatine arteries preserved if feasible. This goal may require the dissection of the vessels free from the bone toward the maxillary artery. During the downfracture of the maxilla, the septum and inferior turbinates must be evaluated for deviation and obstruction. If necessary, a septoplasty can be performed and the turbinates partially reduced. The maxilla is then placed back into the original occlusal relationship or into the final splint (Fig. 59-6). If the maxilla cannot be advanced far enough to fit the predetermined position by the mandible, it must be further mobilized. If it is still impossible to advance the maxilla fully, then the mandible must be repositioned; however, this has not been experienced. Temporary maxillomandibular fixation is applied, and the maxillomandibular unit is then rotated upward until proper bone contact is achieved. This technique helps hold the maxilla forward and facilitates proper fixation while ensuring preservation of the normal plane of occlusion. Four miniplates are placed bilaterally at the pyriform aperture and at the zygomatic buttress. This technique provides adequate fixation without relapse.

FIGURE 59-6. The maxilla is then advanced by a high Le Fort I osteotomy into the proper occlusal relationship and rigidly fixed with four miniplates.

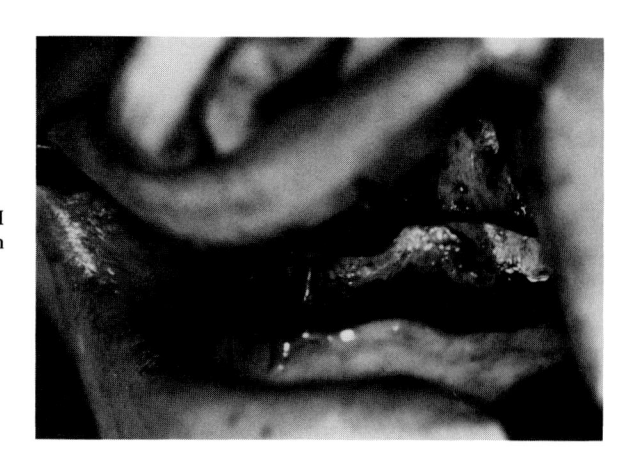

The mucosal incision is closed with a running suture and with perhaps a slight **V-Y** closure. No alar base cinch is recommended so that alar valve opening will occur.

After the Le Fort I and sagittal split osteotomies of the mandible are accomplished, a geniotomy is performed. The geniotomy–tongue advancement is designed to advance the genial tubercle and anterior digastric muscles (Fig. 59–7). This procedure differs from an esthetic genioplasty. Its purpose is to pull the geniohyoid and genioglossus muscles forward and thereby increase the posterior airway space. This pulling forward can be done with hyoid suspension and fascial grafts, but since the digastric and geniohyoid muscles act as an anatomic and functional suspension for the hyoid bone, the position of the bone can be altered by moving the chin anteriorly. A high osteotomy is required which may damage the teeth or result in a symphysis fracture. In a series of 50 patients, one symphysis fracture has occurred.[28]

When the patient will not esthetically tolerate excessive chin advancement, an inferior mandibular osteotomy with hyoid myotomy suspension is indicated.[43] This technique allows significant advancement of the genial tubercle but does not

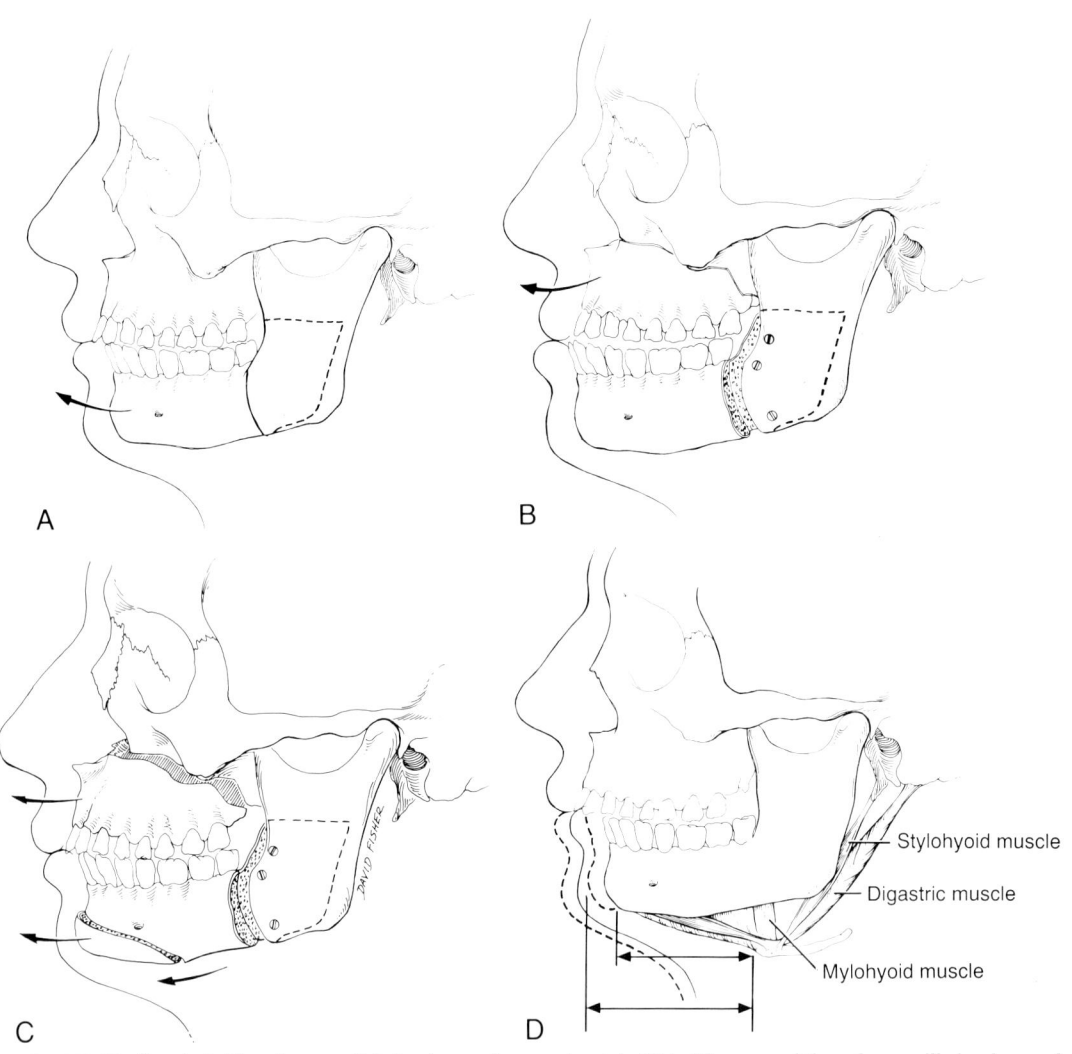

FIGURE 59–7. *A, B,* First the mandible is advanced approximately 10 to 12 mm, and then the maxilla is advanced into the proper occlusal relationship. *C, D,* Geniotomy tongue advancement allows anterior repositioning of the genial tubercles and the anterior belly of the digastrics. This procedure may functionally suspend the hyoid and support the tongue.

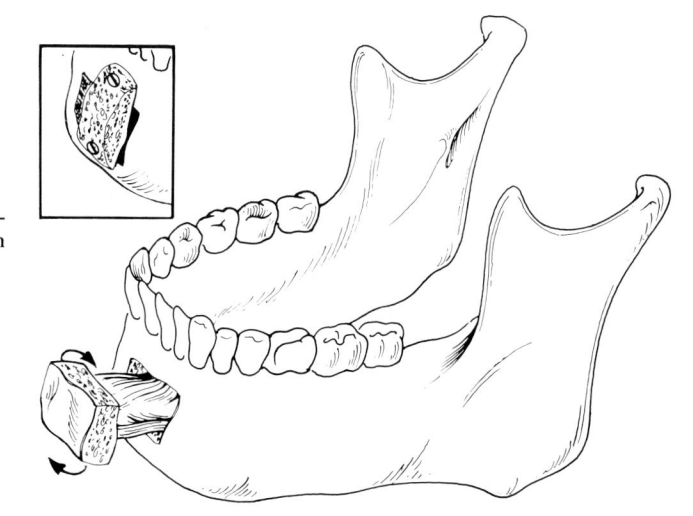

FIGURE 59-8. Inferior mandibular osteotomy allows advancement of the genial tubercle only and does not alter chin esthetics or increase the risk of fracture.

alter the digastric muscle or chin point (Fig. 59-8) and is also less likely to result in fracture of the mandible.

In most instances, the Le Fort I and sagittal split osteotomies, as well as a geniotomy-tongue advancement, can be done with a routine nasoendotracheal tube. It has been noted that excessive swelling can occur as late as 3 days after surgery, and extubation the morning after surgery may be premature. The surgeon may choose to keep the endotracheal tube in place and the patient on positive end-expiratory pressure (PEEP) for an extended period, as deemed necessary. Routine postoperative care within the surgical intensive care unit includes ventilator support. This support is necessary to prevent apnea while allowing administration of narcotics so the patient will be comfortable and tolerate the tube more readily. Almost all patients tolerate PEEP (+5 cm H_2O), intermittent mandatory ventilation (IMV; 4 per minute), and 40 percent inspired oxygen well. These settings can be adjusted as indicated. During the period of intubation, the patient is kept in wire maxillomandibular fixation, which appears to reduce the incidence of malocclusion. Training elastics with arch bars or orthodontics are also useful.

RESULTS OF MAXILLOMANDIBULAR ADVANCEMENT SURGERY

Ninety-six per cent of patients benefit from maxillomandibular advancement surgery (Table 59-1).[28] This finding is subjectively supported by a reduction in the patients' symptoms, such as daytime fatigue, snoring, and respiratory disturbance, and objectively demonstrated by a significant mean decrease in the RDI from 63 to 15.

A surgical success or cure has been defined as a reduction in the RDI to less than 10.[28] Other researchers have used an RDI of 20 with a 50 per cent improvement.[43] Ten is a stricter definition of cure and is closer to normal. A reduction of RDI to 10 or less was achieved in 65.1 per cent of our patients (see Table 59-1).

TABLE 59-1. RESULTS OF MAXILLOMANDIBULAR ADVANCEMENT SURGERY

Subjective improvement	96.0%
Objective improvement	96.0%
Cure	65.1%

2054 / VII—ORTHOGNATHIC SURGERY

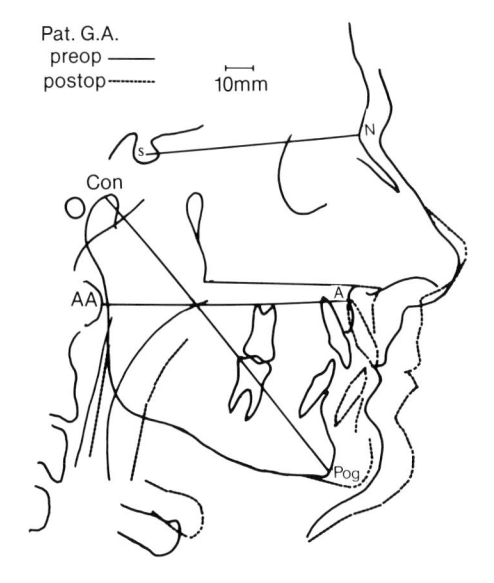

FIGURE 59-9. Presurgical *(solid line)* and postsurgical *(dashed line)* cephalometric tracings demonstrate a significant increase in the posterior airway space.

The posterior airway space consistently increases with maxillomandibular advancement, but the increase does not always correlate with remission of sleep apnea (Fig. 59-9). Hyoid position was also variable and did not correlate with success. Of the 10 surgical failures, the maxilla and mandible were advanced a mean of 7.9 mm and 11.3 mm, respectively. The posterior airway space increased by a mean of 9.0 mm (range of 0 to 14 mm). This figure was not much different from that of the successful group (Tables 59-2 and 59-3). Weight loss for the failure group was 5.1 per cent, versus 6.0 per cent for the successful group—an insignificant difference. There was no statistically significant difference in cephalometric measurements between the two groups.

TABLE 59-2. DATA FROM 19 PATIENTS WITH OBSTRUCTIVE SLEEP APNEA CURED BY MAXILLOMANDIBULAR OSTEOTOMY

PATIENT	ADJUNCTIVE PROCEDURE			DESAT. 90 Pre	DESAT. 90 Post	RDI Pre	RDI Post	ADVANCE Maxillary (mm)	ADVANCE Mandibular (mm)	PAS mm	HYOID mm
1	A		C	392	0	61	5	6	16	10	+7
2	A		C	300	0	77	2	9	20	7	NA
3	A	B		127	3	102	6	3	14	2	-1
4		B	C	592	69	94	6	8	13	8	-9
5	A	B		30	18	11	3	2	10	3	-4
6	A	B		36	1	37	1	4	10	7	-7
7			C	388	1	93	8	10	12	5	-6
8	A	B		31	0	48	8	3	15	10	-1
9				169	9	102	5	8	11	5	0
10	A		C	0	0	22	3	5	11	0	-9
11	A		C	350	3	76	1	10	9	12	-11
12	A	B		102	22	48	6	8	10	8	-6
13	A			246	0	84	8	10	16	7	-5
14			C	234	29	45	10	8	9	3	-6
15	A	B		51	0	32	6	10	17	10	-7
16	A			1	0	36	2	9	12	4	-1
17				208	7	54	4	4	5	5	-10
18	A			154	48	35	7	5	18	8	-6
19	A			35	0	42	5	10	13	5	-3
Mean				181	11	58	5.0	7	13	6	-5

Desat. 90 = number of desaturations below 90 per cent oxyhemoglobin; RDI = respiratory disturbance index; PAS = posterior airway space; A = geniotomy; B = partial glossectomy; C = uvulopalatopharyngoplasty.

TABLE 59-3. DATA FROM 10 PATIENTS WITH OBSTRUCTIVE SLEEP APNEA NOT CURED BUT IMPROVED BY MAXILLOMANDIBULAR OSTEOTOMY

PATIENT	ADJUNCTIVE PROCEDURE	DESAT. 90 Pre	DESAT. 90 Post	RDI Pre	RDI Post	ADVANCE Maxillary (mm)	ADVANCE Mandibular (mm)	PAS mm	HYOID mm
1	A	361	226	69	49	5	6	0	−3
2		2	12	10	23	10	11	+9	+12
3		213	10	36	18	8	11	+9	+3
4		834	114	82	23	9	9	+11	NA
5		554	298	50	20	8	8	+7	−6
6	A B	283	149	92	50	8	12	+14	−7
7	A	553	320	104	56	5	17	+9	NA
8	A	112	0	70	32	10	17	+5	−7
9	A	112	20	50	21	7	13	3	−5
10	A	370	172	79	82	5	9	1	−2
Mean		339	132	64	37	7.5	11.3	6.8	−1.1

Desat. 90 = number of desaturations below 90 per cent oxyhemoglobin; RDI = respiratory disturbance index; PAS = posterior airway space; A = geniotomy; B = partial glossectomy; C = uvulopalatopharyngoplasty.

TABLE 59-4. COMPLICATIONS AND CONVALESCENCE DATA

Hospital stay	7.8 days
Surgical intensive care unit	2.4 days
Estimated blood loss	800 ml
Malocclusion	44% of patients
Perioperative cardiac complications	12%
2 Cardiac arrests	
1 Dysrhythmia	

Complications and convalescence were major concerns for this older population. These patients were in a high-risk group for cardiac disease because of their obesity, hypertension, and hypoxemia. However, there were no perioperative complications resulting in permanent myocardial or central nervous system damage (Table 59-4). No unfavorable soft tissue facial change occurred as a result of the maxillomandibular advancement (Fig. 59-10). Malocclusion following surgery occurred in 44 per cent of patients, but this was easily treated with minor occlusal equilibration or prosthetics.

DISCUSSION AND RECOMMENDATIONS

Attempts have been made to localize the site of functional obstruction of the upper airway in OSA using various radiographic techniques,[44] fiberoptic pharyngoscopy-endoscopy,[45] computerized tomography, cine computerized tomography, and clinical examination.[46] Results of these studies show that there is rarely a single anatomic site of occlusion, but rather multiple levels of upper airway obstruction during episodes of hypopnea and apnea.

Early investigations concentrated on the relationship between OSA and obesity. Recent studies show that an improvement in OSA occurs with weight loss, but this weight loss is often very difficult to achieve and maintain. Furthermore, OSA also occurs in nonobese patients.[47]

Electromyographic studies have demonstrated the importance of genioglossus muscle activity in maintaining upper airway patency in normal individuals.[48] However, in comparison studies, genioglossus function was not found to be significantly abnormal in patients with sleep apnea.[49] Therefore, it appears that neuromuscular dysfunction involving this muscle is not a cause of OSA.

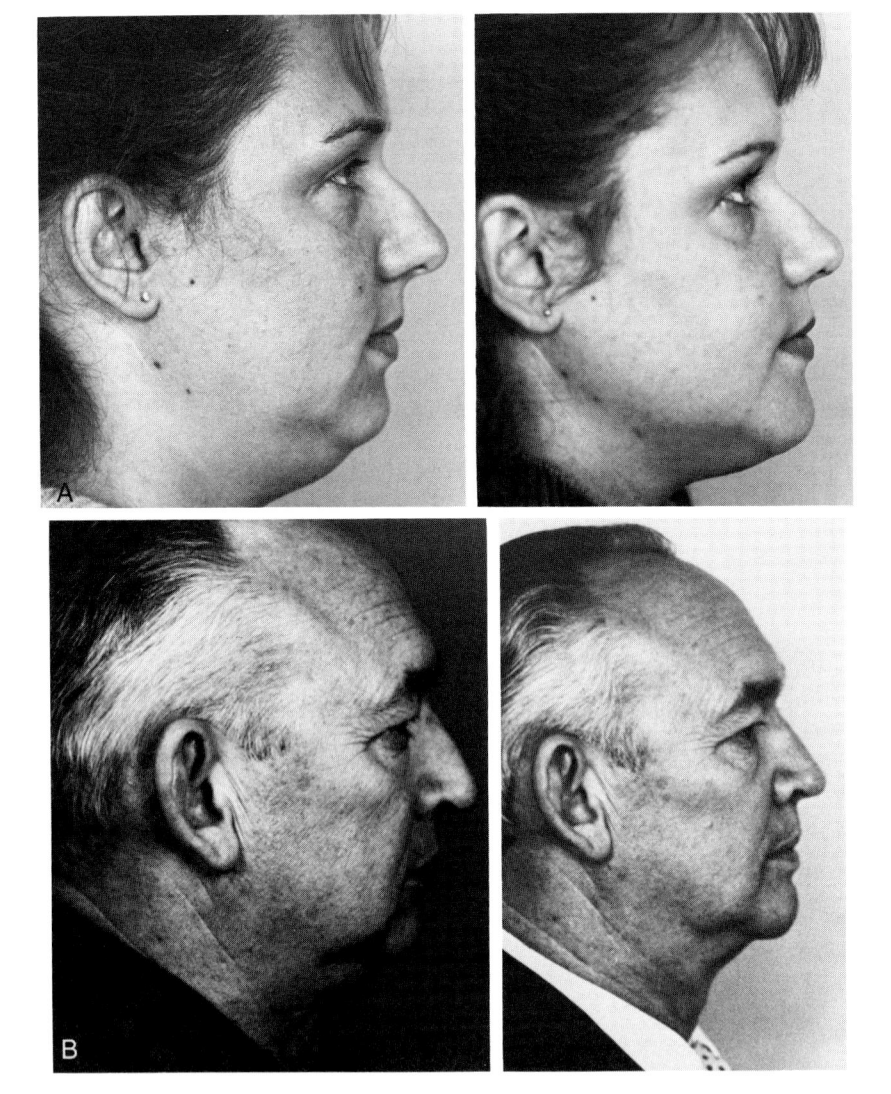

FIGURE 59-10. Presurgical *(A)* and postsurgical *(B)* clinical photographs show no unfavorable soft tissue facial change.

Cephalometric soft tissue analysis of the posterior airway space shows an elongated and widened soft palate as one of the most consistently abnormal features in patients with OSA.[33,42] This finding led to the great interest in UPPP as a surgical treatment. Isolated UPPP, however, has produced improvement in fewer than half of the patients and has cured only a small percentage.[50] Recent data suggest that, at best, only a subgroup of patients with extensive collapse of the velopharyngeal area can expect substantial improvement following UPPP.[51] However, orthognathic surgery has been successful in limited case reports for several years.[52] This has prompted researchers to consider other causes of obstruction such as jaw deformities.

The importance of nasal breathing during sleep has been well documented.[53] Occlusion of the nasal airway by septal deviation or other factors is also thought to be significant in some patients and leads to increased negative pressure in the pharynx. Other obstructions of the airway, such as hypertrophied lymphoid tissue or tumor, have contributed to sleep apnea in some patients. It is thought that the etiology of the OSA syndrome can vary from patient to patient and is likely to be multifactorial in most people. Isolated procedures, such as geniotomy with advancement of the genioglossus muscle,[33] hyoid suspension, septoplasty, tonsillectomy and adenoidectomy, and UPPP have, therefore, failed to cure OSA consistently in all patients.[43]

Many nonsurgical treatments for OSA have also been tried. These include weight reduction, oxygen supplementation, nasotracheal intubation, changing of sleep position, jaw- and tongue-positioning devices, and medications such as protriptyline and medroxyprogesterone acetate. In most cases, these methods yield only limited improvement or are so problematic that few patients can comply with the treatment. The most successful nonsurgical technique has been nasal CPAP.[22] Although this device has helped a great number of people, it is often poorly tolerated and is, at times, ineffective. Nasopharyngeal obstructions may be present, preventing its usage.

Tracheostomy is described as a consistently successful surgical treatment for OSA syndrome.[54,55] This procedure is curative, as it effectively bypasses the possible sites of obstruction. It should be reserved for only the most refractory of cases because morbidity is very high. Since orthognathic surgery is routinely performed with minimal morbidity in young, healthy people, it seems logical to provide this technique for individuals with OSA. Ideally, orthognathic surgery could replace tracheostomy, but the application warrants evaluation in this different age group. Although this surgery has been recommended, many issues remain unresolved, such as the stability of the advancement, the amount of advancement necessary, the complication rate, and the cure rate.

Maxillomandibular advancement surgery fails to cure 35 per cent of patients when one uses the RDI as a method of evaluation. Many of these patients in whom the surgery fails, however, have partial or mixed respiratory disturbances. Essentially all patients have an obstructive apnea index (eliminating partial and mixed apneas) of zero following advancement surgery. These results may be similar to those one could expect with tracheostomy. Follow-up sleep studies are generally not performed after tracheostomy, which totally bypasses the pharyngeal obstruction. There are many ways to evaluate abnormal respirations, and RDI alone is inadequate. It is recommended that RDI, total number of desaturations, lowest desaturation value, total time desaturated, and number of obstructive events be recorded. If the obstructive events are eliminated or greatly reduced, the surgical advancement of the jaws has been successful.

It is difficult to compare results with others in the literature because the criteria for success are poorly defined. "Success" and "cure" are not interchangeable terms. A surgical cure should yield a sleep study similar to that of a normal individual without sleep apnea (an RDI of less than 5). An RDI of less than 10 is considered a success. Although more researchers use RDI than hypoxemia as a measure of disease severity, all agree that hypoxemia is a critical problem. This factor further confounds the issue because in some cases patients are not cured in terms of RDI, but postoperative polysomnography demonstrates no desaturation values below 90 per cent. In this situation, persistent apnea, even without significant desaturation, is considered a surgical failure. Conversely, some obese patients have successful reductions in RDI but, because of the presumed influence of obesity on nocturnal ventilation, continue to have sleep-related hypoxemia. It is, therefore, helpful to consider both values when assessing results. Some researchers consider a surgical success to be an RDI less than 20 because this correlates with decreased patient mortality.[2] Some seem to think that the relative percentage of improvement is important, while others are concerned about the degree of sleep disturbance that occurs with RDIs above 5 or 10. However surgical success is defined, it should correlate with the pathophysiology of the disease and the resolution of morbidity and mortality.

In a comparison of our success and failure groups, there was no statistically significant difference in the demographics, severity of disease, weight change, surgical treatment (in terms of amount of maxillomandibular advancement), or cephalometric changes. In addition, no anatomic obstruction could be identified on the cephalometric radiograph. The reason for our failures is not known. Retrospectively, it is also impossible to predict which patient will be cured. One may suspect that those in the failure group have more underlying cardiopulmonary disease, and this factor is now being evaluated.

When one analyzes success versus failure on the basis of procedures, it appears that success was nearly 100 per cent when maxillomandibular advancement was done following or simultaneous with UPPP. Although maxillomandibular advancement without UPPP does yield success, no failures occurred when both procedures were combined (see Table 59–2). Furthermore, the success rate appears to increase when any adjunctive procedure is added, such as geniotomy–tongue advancement procedures. This finding seems to support the concept that multiple levels of obstruction exist, which is probably why UPPP and septoplasty, when done alone, frequently result in failure. Maxillomandibular advancement surgery is more often successful than UPPP alone, but it, too, is not always successful in causing remission of OSA.

Considering the complication and convalescence factors of maxillomandibular advancement surgery for an older population, such surgery should be indicated only if a high therapeutic index exists. The increased incidence of perioperative cardiac events and the longer hospital stay are not inconsistent with any group of medically compromised patients in whom other modes of therapy have failed (Table 59–4). Staging multiple procedures may be inconvenient for some patients, but by doing so one may eliminate subsets of obstruction with a graduated rate of surgical morbidity. Although septoplasty and UPPP are associated with complications, they are occasionally beneficial and may identify those individuals in whom more aggressive surgery is indicated.

REFERENCES

1. Partinen M, Jamieson A, Guilleminault C: Long term outcome for obstructive sleep apnea syndrome patients. Chest *94*:1200, 1988.
2. He J, Kryger MH, Zorick FJ, et al: Mortality and apnea index in obstructive sleep apnea. Chest *94*:9, 1988.
3. Findley LJ, Bonnie RJ: Sleep apnea and auto crashes. Chest *94*:225, 1988.
4. Aelianus C: Varius History: Book IX. London, Thomas Dung, 1666, Chapter 13, p 177.
5. Kryger MH: Sleep apnea: From the needles of Dionysius to continuous positive airway pressure. Arch Intern Med *143*:2301, 1983.
6. Guilleminault C, van den Hoed J, Mittler M: Clinical overview of sleep apnea syndromes. In Guilleminault C, Dement WC (eds): Sleep Apnea Syndromes. New York, Alan R. Liss, Inc., 1978.
7. Bliwise D, Carskadon M, Carey E, Dement W: Longitudinal development of sleep-related respiratory disturbance in adult humans. J Gerontol *39*:290, 1984.
8. Block AJ, Boysen PG, Wynne JW, et al: Sleep apnea, hypopnea and oxygen desaturation in normal subjects—strong male predominance. N Engl J Med *300*:513, 1979.
9. Block AJ, Wynne JW, Boysen PG: Sleep-disordered breathing and nocturnal oxygen desaturation in postmenopausal women. Am J Med *69*:75, 1980.
10. Lugaresi E, Coccagna G, Mantovani M: Hypersomnia with periodic apneas In Weizman EH (ed): Advances in Sleep Research. Vol 4. Jamaica, NY, Spectrum Publishers, 1978.
11. Lavie P: Sleep disturbances in industry workers. Sleep Res *9*:209, 1980.
12. Mitler MM, van den Hoed J, Carskadon MA, et al: REM sleep episodes during multiple sleep latency test in narcoleptic patients. Electroencephalogr Clin Neurophysiol *46*:478, 1979.
13. Reynolds CF III, Coble PA, Kupfer DJ, Holzer BC: Application of the multiple sleep latency test in disorders of excessive sleepiness. Electroencephalogr Clin Neurophysiol *53*:443, 1982.
14. Tilkian AG, Guilleminault C, Schroeder JS, et al: Hemodynamics in sleep-induced apnea. Studies during wakefulness and sleep. Ann Intern Med *85*:714, 1976.
15. Fletcher EC, DeBehnke RD, Lovoi MS, Gorin AB: Undiagnosed sleep apnea in patients with essential hypertension. Ann Intern Med *103*:190, 1985.
16. Kales A, Bixler ED, Cadieux RJ, et al: Sleep apnea in a hypertensive population. Lancet *2*:1005, 1984.
17. Bartall HZ, Tye KH, Roper P, et al: Atrial flutter associated with obstructive apnea syndrome. A case report. Arch Intern Med *140*:121, 1980.
18. Deedwania PC, Swiryn S, Dhingra RC, Rosen KM: Nocturnal atrioventricular block as a manifestation of sleep apnea syndrome. Chest *76*:319, 1979.
19. Tilkian AG, Guilleminault C, Schroeder JS, et al: Sleep-induced apnea syndrome. Prevalence of cardiac arrhythmias and their reversal after tracheostomy. Am J Med *63*:348, 1977.
20. Berrettini WH: Paranoid psychosis and sleep apnea syndrome. Am J Psychiatry *137*:493, 1980.
21. Santamaria J, Prior J, Fleetham JA: Hypothalamic-pituitary-testicular dysfunction in obstructive sleep apnea. Am Rev Respir Dis 131, 1985.
22. Sullivan CE, Berthon-Jones M, Issa FG, Eves L: Reversal of obstructive sleep apnea by continuous positive airway pressure applied through the nares. Lancet *1*:862, 1981.

23. Martin RJ, Sanders MH, Gray BA, et al: Acute and long-term ventilatory effects of hyperoxia in the adult sleep apnea syndrome. Am Rev Respir Dis 125:175, 1982.
24. Lyons HA, Huang CT: Therapeutic use of progesterone in alveolar hypoventilation associated with obesity. Am J Med 44:881, 1968.
25. Clark RW, Schmidt HS, Schaal SF, et al: Sleep apnea: Treatment with protriptyline. Neurology 29:1287, 1979.
26. Jamieson A, Guilleminault C, Partinen M, Quera-Salva MA: Obstructive sleep apneic patients have craniomandibular abnormalities. Sleep 9:469, 1986.
27. Riley RW, Powell N, Guilleminault C: Current surgical concepts for treating obstructive sleep apnea syndrome. J Oral Maxillofac Surg 45:149, 1987.
28. Waite PD, Wooten V, Lachner J, Guyette RF: Maxillomandibular advancement surgery in 23 patients with obstructive sleep apnea syndrome. J Oral Maxillofac Surg 47:1256, 1989.
29. Sukerman S, Healy GB: Sleep apnea syndrome associated with upper airway obstruction. Laryngoscope 89:878, 1979.
30. Heimer D, Scharf SM, Lieberman A, Lavie P: Sleep apnea syndrome treated by repair of deviated nasal septum. Chest 84:184, 1983.
31. Conway WA, Victor LD, Magilligan DJ Jr, et al: Adverse effects of tracheostomy for sleep apnea. JAMA 246:347, 1981.
32. Ikematsu T: Study of snoring, 4th report. Therapy (in japanese). J Jpn Oto-Rhino-Laryngol 64:434, 1964.
33. FuiJita S, Conway W, Zorick F, Roth T: Surgical correction of anatomic abnormalities in obstructive sleep apnea syndrome: Uvulopalatopharyngoplasty. Otolaryngol Head Neck Surg 89:923, 1981.
34. Kramer M, Anand VK, Schoen L, Draper E: Death associated with uvulopalatopharyngoplasty: A case report. Sleep Res 14:180, 1985.
35. Samelson CF: Sequelae and complications of palatopharyngoplasty: Impact on vocal trill. Sleep 7:83, 1984.
36. Sher AE, Thorpy MJ, Spielman AJ, et al: Predictive value of Müller maneuver in selection of patients for uvulopalatopharyngoplasty. Laryngoscope 95:1483, 1985.
37. Menashe VD, Farrehi C, Miller M: Hypoventilation and cor pulmonale due to chronic upper airway obstruction. J Pediatr 67:198, 1965.
38. Noonan JA: Reversible cor pulmonale due to hypertrophied tonsils and adenoids: Studies in two cases. Circulation (Suppl II) 32:164, 1965.
39. Rojewski TE, Schuller DE, Clark RW, et al: Videoendoscopic determination of the mechanism of obstruction in obstructive sleep apnea. Otolaryngol Head Neck Surg 92:127, 1984.
40. Riley RW, Guilleminault C, Herran J, et al: Cephalometric analysis and flow volume loops in obstructive sleep apnea patients. Sleep 6:303, 1983.
41. Lowe AA, Santamaria JD, Fleetham FA, Price C: Facial morphology and obstructive sleep apnea. Am J Orthod Dentofacial Orthop 90:484, 1986.
42. DeBerry-Borowrecki, Kukwa A, Blanks RH: Cephalometric analysis for diagnosis and treatment of obstructive sleep apnea. Laryngoscope 98:226, 1988.
43. Riley RW, Powell NB, Guilleminault C: Inferior mandibular osteotomy and hyoid myotomy suspension for obstructive sleep apnea: A review of 55 patients. J Oral Maxillofac Surg 47:159, 1989.
44. Riley R, Guilleminault C, Herran F, Powell N: Cephalometric analysis and flow-volume loops in obstructive sleep apnea patients. Sleep 6:303, 1983.
45. Guilleminault C, Hill MW, Simmons FB, Dement WC: Obstructive sleep apnea: Electromyographic and fiberoptic studies. Exp Neurol 62:48, 1978.
46. Stein MG, Gamsu G, deGeer G, et al: Cine CT in obstructive sleep apnea. AJR 148:1069, 1987.
47. Rubinstein I, Colapinto N, Rotstein LE, et al: Improvement in upper airway function after weight loss in patients with obstructive sleep apnea. Am Rev Respir Dis 138:1192, 1988.
48. Remmers JE, de Groot WJ, Sauerland EK, Anch AM: Pathogensis of upper airway occlusion during sleep. J Appl Physiol 44:931, 1978.
49. Sauerland EK, Orr WC, Hairston LE: EMG patterns of oropharyngeal muscles during respiration in wakefulness and sleep. Electromyogr Clin Neurophysiol 21:307, 1981.
50. Riley R, Guilleminault C, Powell N, Simmons B: Palatopharyngoplasty failure, cephalometric roentgenograms, and obstructive sleep apnea. Otolaryngol Head Neck Surg 93:240, 1985.
51. Macaluso RA, Reams C, Vrabec D, et al: Uvulopalatopharyngoplasty: Postoperative management and evaluation of results. Ann Otol Rhinol Laryngol 98:502, 1989.
52. Kuo PC, West RA, Bloomquist DS, McNiel RW: The effect of mandibular osteotomy in three patients with hypersomnia sleep apnea. Oral Surg Oral Med Oral Pathol 48:385, 1979.
53. Nahmias TS, Karetzky MS: Treatment of the obstructive sleep apnea syndrome using a nasopharyngeal tube. Chest 94:1142, 1988.
54. Guilleminault C, Simmons FB, Motta J: Obstructive sleep apnea syndrome and tracheostomy: Long-term follow-up experience. Arch Intern Med 141:985, 1981.
55. Tilkian AG, Guilleminault C, Schroeder JS, et al: Sleep induced apnea syndrome: Prevalence of cardiac arrhythmias and their reversal after tracheostomy. Am J Med 63:348, 1977.

60 SURGICAL MANAGEMENT OF SKELETAL OPEN BITE

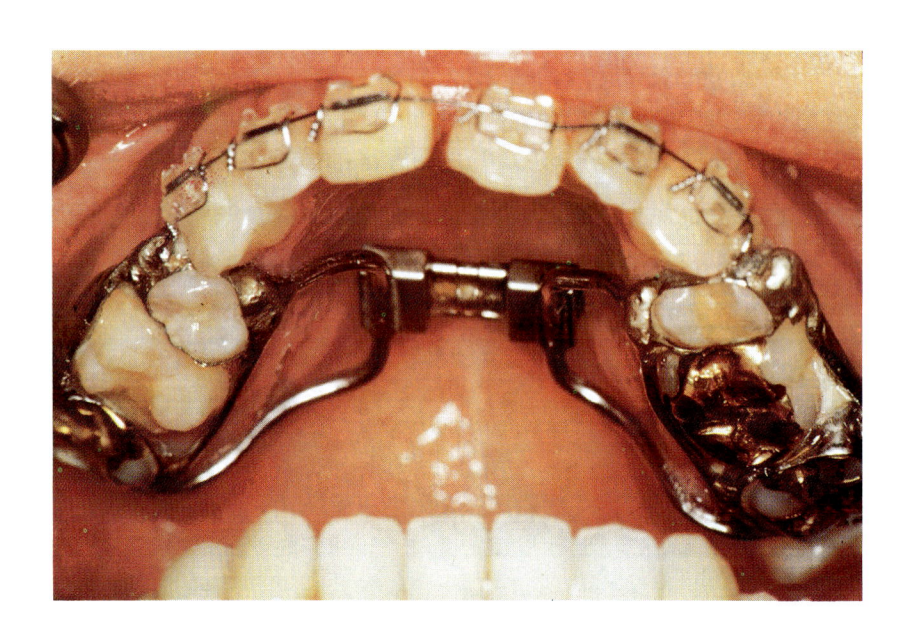

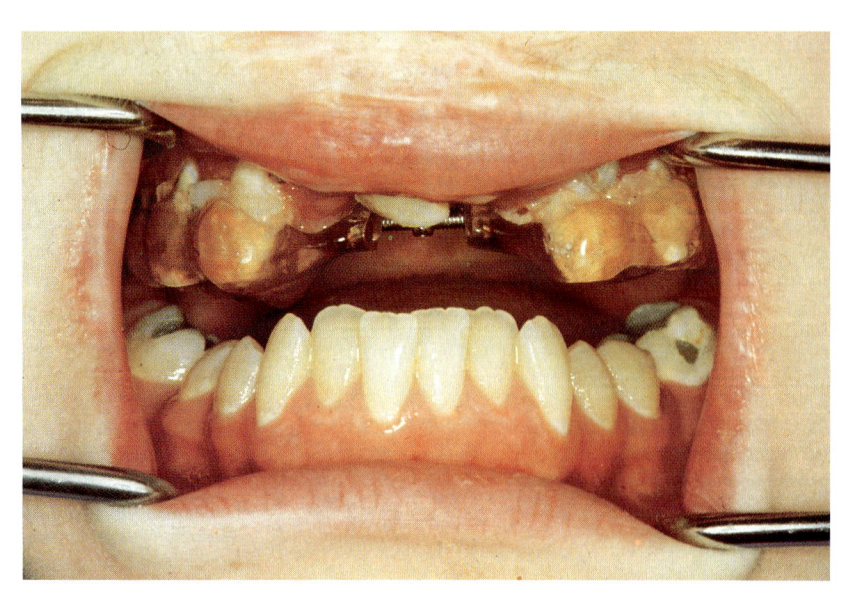

ETIOLOGY
  Functional Aspects
  Developmental Aspects
SURGICAL TREATMENT
  Surgical Planning
  Procedure Order
  Surgical Techniques
CASE EXAMPLES

60

ULRICH JOOS

Skeletal open bite is characterized by a noticeable vertical disproportion of the face with typical changes in the soft tissue and bone. What strikes the eye is the elongated lower face (Fig. 60-1*A* and *B*) with lip incompetence and protruding tongue, which gives the face a slightly moronic appearance. These soft tissue changes are directly related to skeletal deviations of the face: increased anterior facial height caused by an excessive mandibular angle, a disproportionately short maxilla with crossbite, and the major characteristic, dental open bite. In the cephalometric radiograph, these skeletal changes manifest themselves in an anterior rotation of the maxilla with simultaneous posterior rotation of the mandible.

There is hardly a deformity that has caused more frustration to orthodontists and oral surgeons. Several suggestions for therapy have been made in past years; some have been tried, and every now and then failures have been reported. Recently, attempts have been undertaken to regard open bite as an independent clinical entity, something that has even led to the name "open bite syndrome."[1]

In my opinion, a serious error has been made in turning a symptom of various possible syndromes into a syndrome itself. In the following discussion, I should like to try to connect open bite to various syndromes that result from aberrant growth processes and then to suggest treatment options based on the requirements of the individual case.

ETIOLOGY

Functional Aspects

A number of theories exist concerning the etiology of skeletal open bite. What they all have in common is that they attach considerable importance to functional

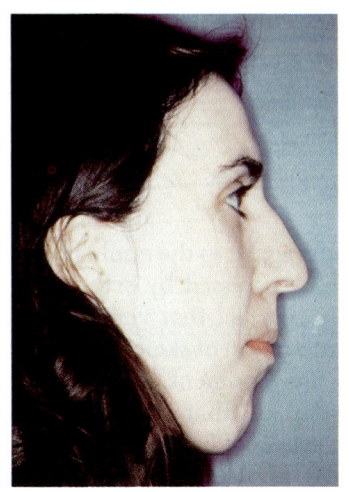

FIGURE 60-1. *A,* Typical long face associated with skeletal open bite. *B,* Open bite with contact only between molars.

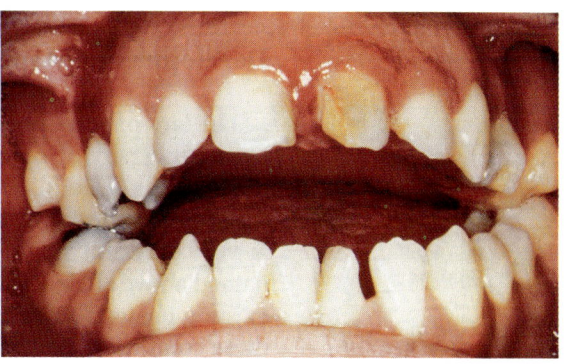

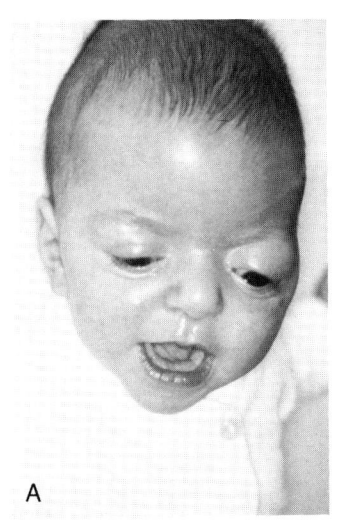

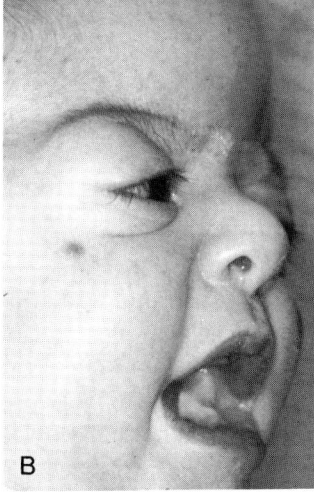

FIGURE 60-4. *A, B,* Apert's syndrome: exophthalmos, maxillary retrusion, and short, high skull.

From the seventh to eighth week on, the chondral bowl is gradually transformed into bone through endochondral ossification. This development corresponds to Carnegy Stages 18, 19, and 20. Interference with the endochrondral ossification in the base of the skull at this early stage causes the severe malformations we see in Apert's syndrome or Crouzon's disease (Fig. 60-4*A* and *B*). Such a disturbance might be impaired chondroblast activity, which prohibits the cells from dividing further, thereby keeping the chondral base of the skull from growing. This would explain the typical signs of Apert's syndrome or Crouzon's disease: upright cranial base, retroinclination of the entire front of the skull and the face, protuberance in the back of the head, and changes in the angle of the skull base (Fig. 60-5*A* and *B*). The clinical manifestations are typical of skeletal open bite, but only in this respect do the deformities overlap (Fig. 60-6*A* and *B*).

The treatment we prefer within the first 6 months after birth is radical osteoclastic surgery modified after Powiertowsky.[10] The method entails removing all of the bones from the coronal suture to behind the sphenofrontal suture (Fig. 60-7).

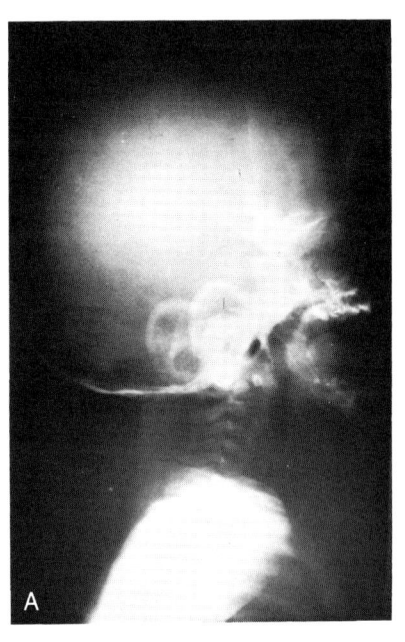

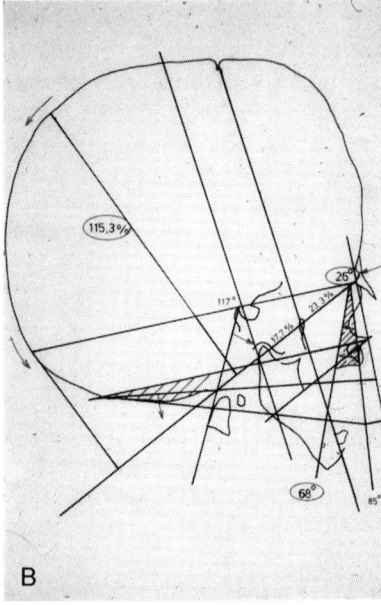

FIGURE 60-5. *A, B,* Cephalometric signs in Apert's syndrome or Crouzon's disease: high skull, maxillary retrusion, and change in the angle of the cranial base.

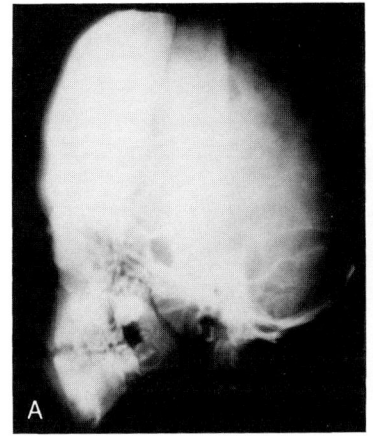

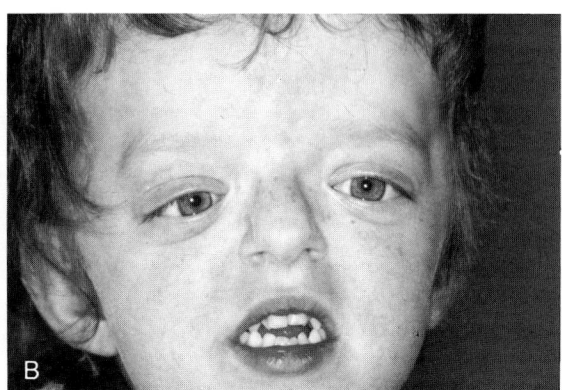

FIGURE 60-6. *A, B,* Severe skeletal open bite in Crouzon's disease.

This procedure not only allows the brain to develop spontaneously but also considerably improves the shape of the cranium and the facial skeleton (Fig. 60–8A and B). The advantage of this early operation is that a completely new calvarium can form according to the requirements stipulated by nature and not by the surgeon. For children older than 1 year, we prefer a classic craniotomy with Le Fort III osteotomy, in which the bone fragments are fixed in the desired position with miniplates (Fig. 60–9A to F).

The ala minor ossis sphenoidalis forms laterally from the ala temporalis, and the sphenoid bone and labyrinth develop from the ala temporalis. In the labyrinth itself, the pars squamosa results from desmal ossification. Thus, the glenoid cavity

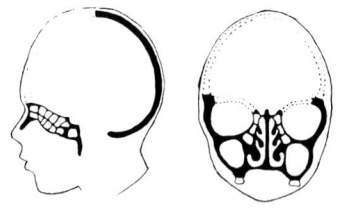

FIGURE 60-7. Radical osteoclastic surgery. (Modified from Powiertowsky, H.: Surgery of Craniosynostosis in Advanced Cases. In Advances and Technical Standards in Neurosurgery. New York, Springer-Verlag, 1974, p. 191.)

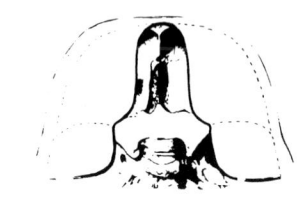

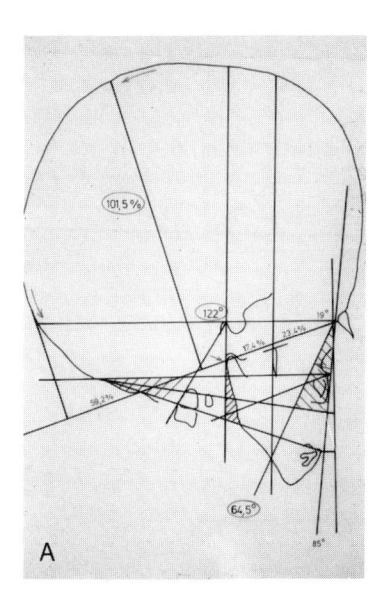

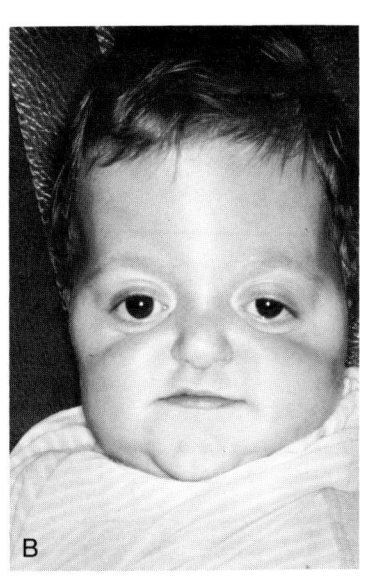

FIGURE 60-8. *A, B,* Three months after radical osteoclastic surgery: improvement in cranial proportions and in cephalometric analysis. Same patient as in Figures 60–4 and 60–5.

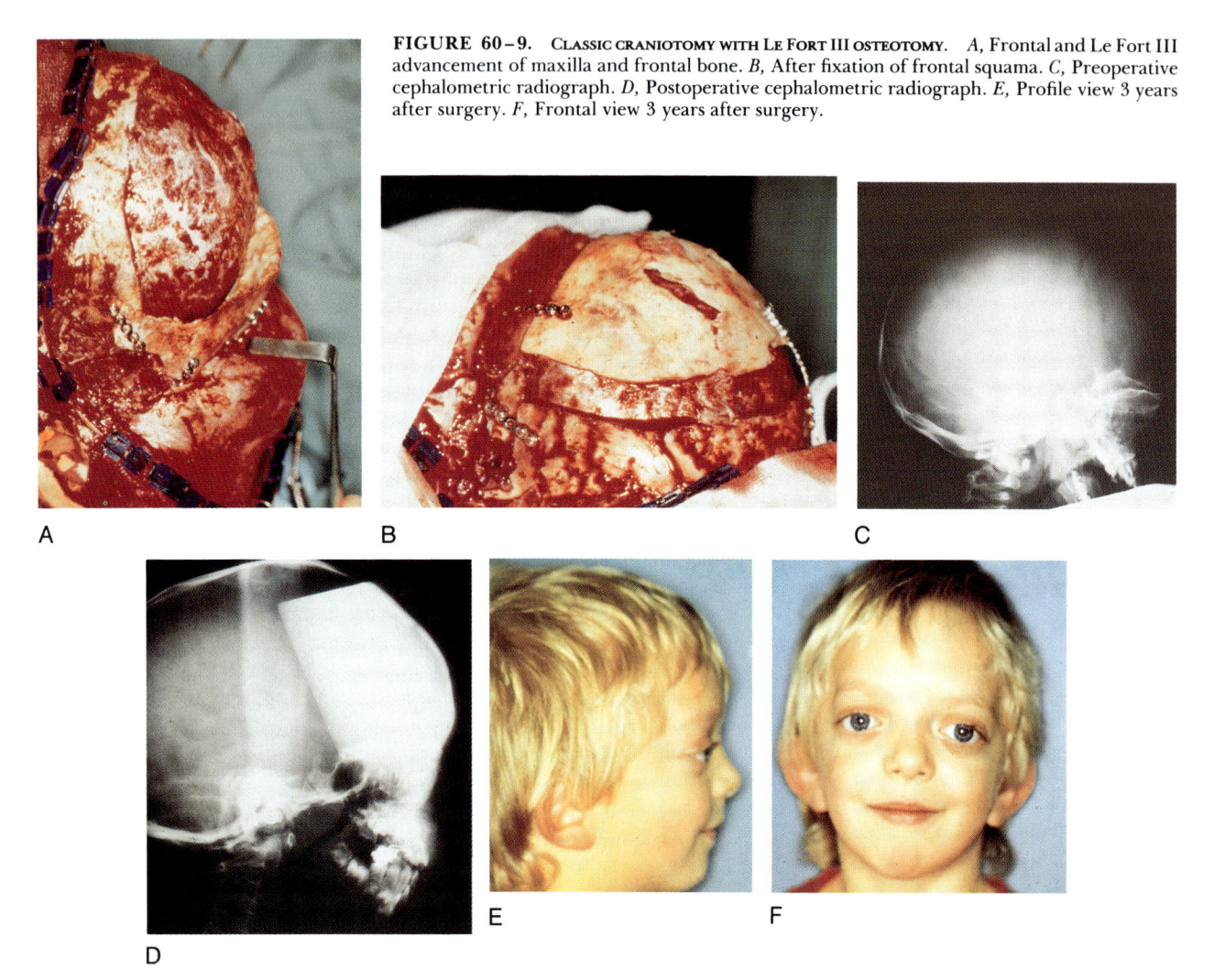

FIGURE 60–9. CLASSIC CRANIOTOMY WITH LE FORT III OSTEOTOMY. *A*, Frontal and Le Fort III advancement of maxilla and frontal bone. *B*, After fixation of frontal squama. *C*, Preoperative cephalometric radiograph. *D*, Postoperative cephalometric radiograph. *E*, Profile view 3 years after surgery. *F*, Frontal view 3 years after surgery.

that forms here has two parts: a chondral and a desmal. This means that the chondrobase defines the position of the temporomandibular joint vertically, sagittally, and transversely. If this development is disturbed in an early stage, conditions such as Goldenhar's syndrome result, with a severely shortened mandibular ramus. The treatment in this case consists of osteotomy in both jaws to achieve normal length of the ascending mandibular ramus and to correct the asymmetry.

The cartilaginous nasal capsule, the ethmoid bone, the nasal septum, and the crista galli grow out of the ethmoid region (Fig. 60–10). The development of nasal cartilage is necessary for the further forward development of the frontal skull base.

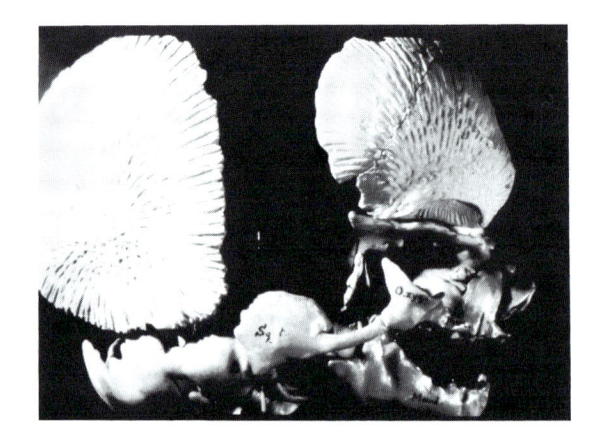

FIGURE 60–10. Embryonic skull showing cartilaginous nasal skeleton and ethmoid bone.

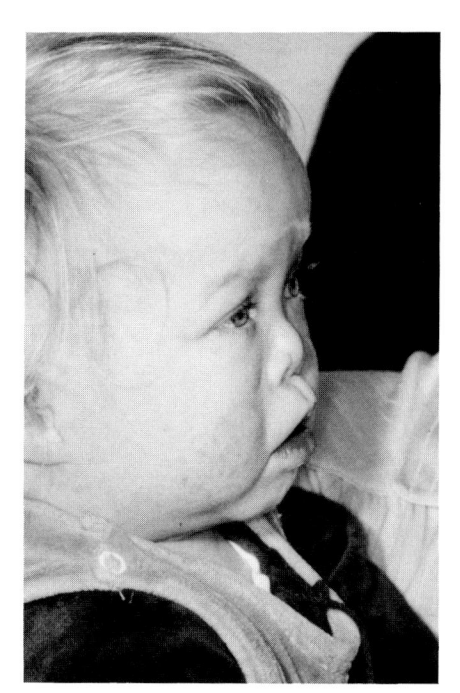

FIGURE 60-11. Binder's syndrome with microrhinia, saddle nose, and abnormally short skull in the sagittal direction.

Again, since this is embryonic cartilage, its growth is governed by endogenous factors. This region is crucial for the sagittal and vertical development of the face. Early disturbances bring about the typical symptoms of a Binder or microrhinia syndrome (Fig. 60-11), marked by an upright anterior base, a change in the angle of the base of the skull, occipital protuberance, and, in particular, deficient maxillary and nasal growth. The clinical manifestation is the same as that of skeletal open bite. Therapy, however, must also incorporate the anterior skull base. The surgical procedure is Le Fort II osteotomy with simultaneous sagittal splitting of the mandible and fixation with miniplates (Fig. 60-12A to F).

Sutural Growth of the Calvarium. Desmal osteogenesis in the calvarium takes place parallel to endochondral bone formation. After the cartilaginous cranial base has formed, the skull cap and the midface retain their membranous character. Very early, in the seventh to eighth week of embryonic growth (Carnegy Stage 18), the first bone centers develop and gradually become larger. For a long time, there was a lack of agreement regarding how these bone centers continue to grow. It was assumed that the osteoblasts divide under endogenic influence, causing the bone center to split. In this way, the sutures would gradually ossify (Fig. 60-13), which would mean that they represent a primary growth center. According to the general opinion today, however, the sutures constitute a secondary growth center. The difference lies in the fact that a secondary growth center is chiefly subjected to functional influences to which the bony structures adapt (Fig. 60-14). The mobility of the sutures is therefore crucial for growth. Studies conducted by Enlow,[11] Björk,[12] Brodie,[13] Moss,[14] and, most recently, Delaire,[15] have clarified the growth processes that take place at the sutures. In a mesenchymal tissue that is at the point of mineralizing, ossification centers appear with osteons. If there is static quiescence, ossification takes place, and a periosteum forms on the surface in two typical positions—an inner osteogenic-cellular layer and above that a fibrous vascular layer (Fig. 60-15). If, during the formation of bone centers, movement occurs, not only does ossification take place but also a new suture forms. The initially three-layered suture during the embryonal period becomes five layered after the embryonal stage because the fibrous layers lie on top of one another. The appearance of the suture is also affected by mobility. The shape of a suture reveals how forceful the movement was at this site (Fig. 60-16A and B). This membranous suture is nothing more than a specialized periosteum in which appositional bone growth takes place. For this, the displacement of the bone centers is decisive.

2068 / VII — ORTHOGNATHIC SURGERY

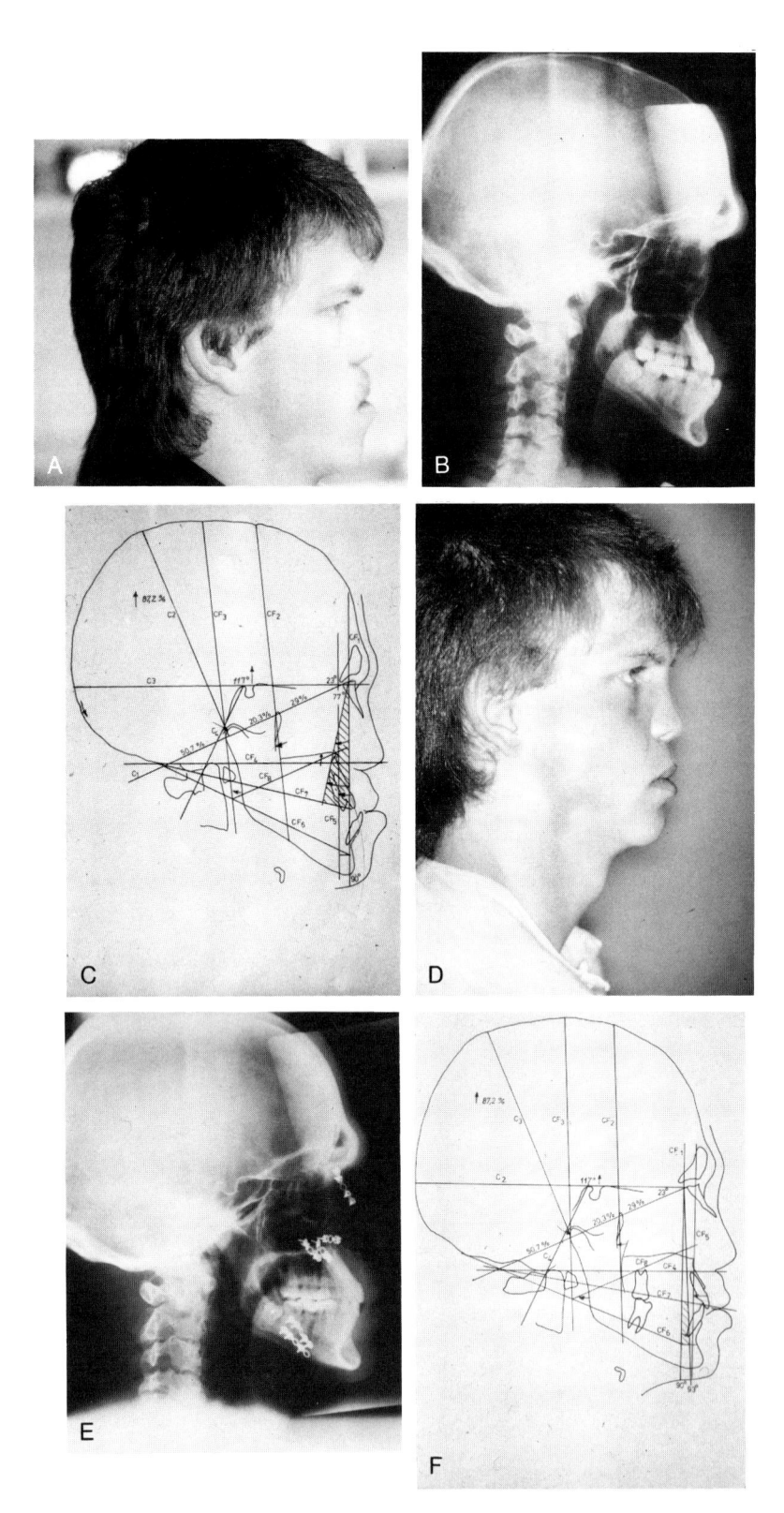

FIGURE 60–12. BINDER'S SYNDROME IN ADULTHOOD. *A*, Lateral image showing maxillary and nasal retrusion and saddle nose. *B*, Preoperative radiograph; note the absence of the anterior spina nasalis. *C*, Cephalometric analysis; note extreme midfacial retroposition and signs of craniostenosis. *D*, After simultaneous Le Fort II osteotomy and sagittal split of the horizontal mandibular ramus. *E*, Postoperative cephalometric radiograph. *F*, Postoperative cephalometric evaluation; note the unchanged abnormality of neurocranium. The facial bone formation is normal.

FIGURE 60-13. Old notion of calvarial growth as a primary growth center. Successive bone growth is endogenically governed.

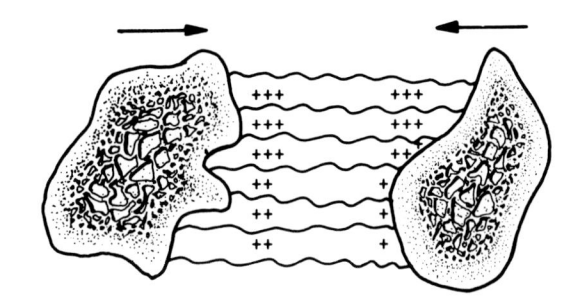

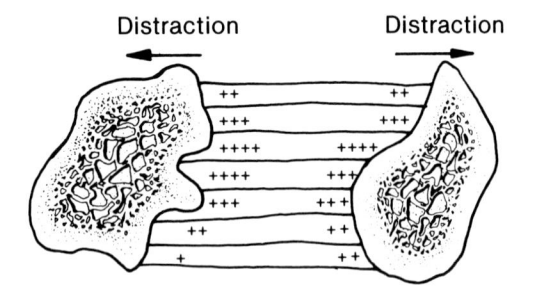

FIGURE 60-14. New notion of calvarial growth as a secondary growth center. Functional influences cause suture distraction, inducing appositional reactive bone growth at the suture site.

FIGURE 60-15. Normal morphology of a sagittal suture. The periosteum is drawn into the suture.

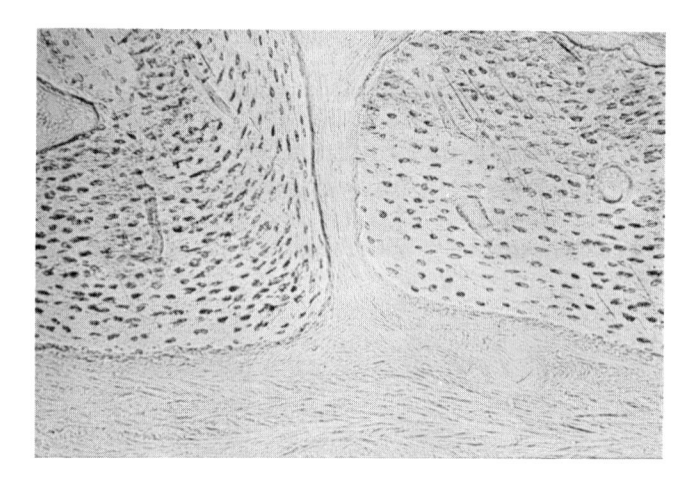

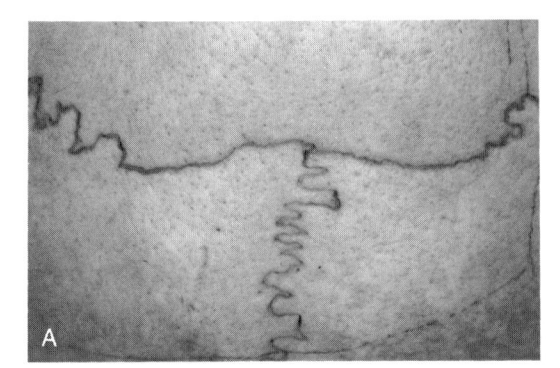

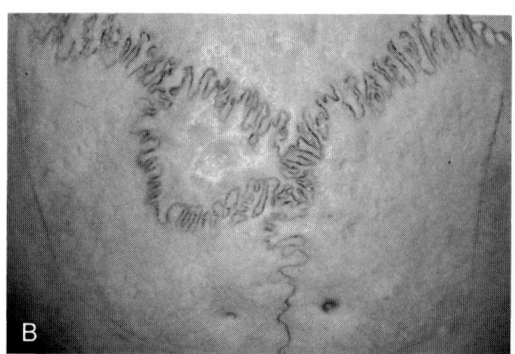

FIGURE 60-16. *A, B,* Various manifestations of sutures on the adult skull, frontal and occipital views. The pronounced digitations display the force of the movements that took place here.

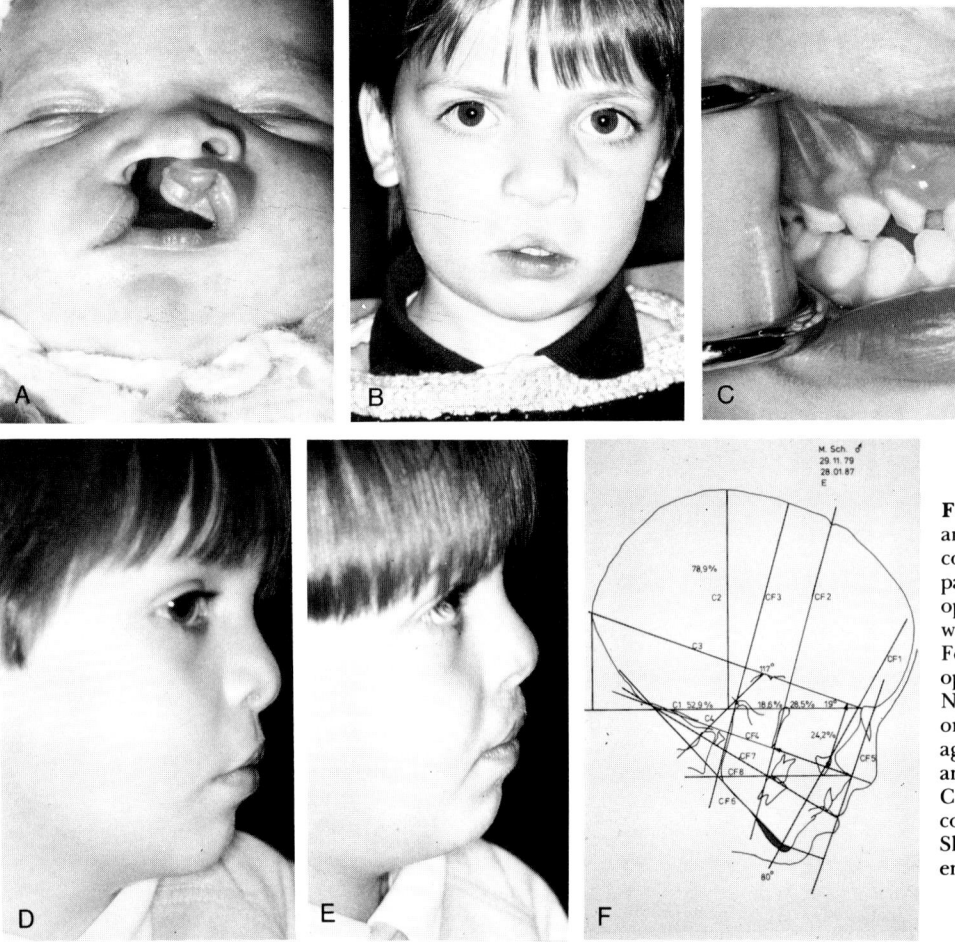

FIGURE 60-26. *A,* Bilateral cleft lip and palate. On the right the defect is complete, while on the left the cleft lip is partially bridged with skin. Simultaneous operation and muscle reconstruction were accomplished in the midface. *B,* Four years after surgery. Normal development of midface and nose is seen. *C,* Normal formation of maxilla without any orthodontic treatment; child is 6 years of age. *D, E,* Clinical aspect at age 6. Nose and midface development is normal. *F,* Cephalometric analysis at age 6 after reconstruction of the midface muscles. Skull development is normal in the presence of cleft lip and palate.

Although we still do not know exactly what mechanisms cause deformities, by being familiar with the growth processes in the skull we nevertheless have the chance to detect them in sufficient time to treat them. In my opinion, the "wait-and-see" policy of postponing corrective surgery after growth has terminated is no longer tenable. Our efforts should be concentrated on recognizing disturbances, especially functional ones, as early as possible to treat them appropriately. Only by performing "functional operations" will we be able to restore normal growth and function.

SURGICAL TREATMENT

There is a plethora of surgical procedures to correct open bite, yet none of them has produced completely satisfactory results. For this reason, the treatment of open bite is regarded as being extraordinarily difficult by oral surgeons[26] and orthodontists[27] alike. Surgeons are not making an exaggerated claim when they say that any form of open bite can be closed surgically and that for this purpose several treatment options are available. The problem associated with treating open bite, however, is the high incidence of relapse, even after technically unproblematic operations. Therefore, the decisive point in managing skeletal open bite is not so much the method itself, but rather the careful diagnostic evaluation on which to base the selection of the appropriate surgical technique.

The first surgical procedure to correct open bite was introduced by Hullihen[28] in 1849. The techniques used at that time were limited to the confines of the mandible and the mandibular body.[29,30] Because of the high rate of complications—in particular, damage to nerves—the osteotomy site was gradually shifted from the horizontal mandibular ramus to the ascending ramus of the maxilla. The most commonly used methods were those developed by Limberg,[31] Caldwell and Lettermann,[32] and then Obwegeser[33] and Dal Pont.[34] In these cases, the ascending ramus of the jaw is severed vertically, sagittally, and in stages to achieve closure of the open bite. Because of the large number of early relapses after these operations, the osteotomy procedure was then carried out in the alveolar process of the maxilla[35,36] as well as the mandible.[37] These techniques were perfected to close the open bite by total maxillary osteotomy[38,39] as well as by dividing the maxilla into three segments.[40,41]

Opinions varied with regard to the value of osteotomies in the horizontal ramus of the mandible. Most surgeons avoided such procedures, accusing them of being complicated, of delaying bone healing, and of being difficult to execute, especially in the area of the mandibular angle.[42-44]

The numerous variations of osteotomy in the ascending ramus of the mandible are usually successful in correcting open bite. The chance of relapse, however, is considerable, as has been shown by Manz and Hadjianghelou,[45] who found a vertical recurrence in 50 per cent of their patients. Mandibular procedures shorten the anterior height of the face while at the same time lengthening the posterior height. This lengthening stretches the pterygomasseteric sling, which is apparently responsible for the relapse. Additional operative procedures such as stripping have not brought about satisfactory results.

Anterior segmental osteotomies, as suggested by Köle, are claimed to be very stable.[46-48] The esthetic results, however, are not always satisfactory. My own studies have shown that a high incidence of relapse is associated with this technique (see Selection of Surgical Technique, p. 2080).

The results of Schuchardt's[36] posterior maxillary osteotomy have also met with mixed reception in the literature. Follow-up examinations by Obwegeser,[26] Nwoku,[49] and Martis[50] revealed a high incidence of early relapse. Höltje and Lendrodt,[51] Stoker and Epker,[52] and Schwenzer,[53] on the other hand, reported stable results. Stability after total maxillary osteotomy has also been reported.[48,54,55]

Thanks to surgical advances, bimaxillary osteotomies are now being performed to correct open bite with concomitant sagittal discrepancy. The procedure combines all the types of osteotomy described above. To date, there have been no conclusive results regarding the rate of relapse.

Attempts have been made to increase stability when treating open bite by applying modern osteosynthesis methods known from their use in traumatology of the maxilla and the midface.[56-58] It has been shown, however, that even accurately positioned plates and screws could not rule out the possibility of relapse.

The foregoing comments intend to demonstrate just how complex and difficult the treatment of skeletal open bite is and to stress the importance of exact diagnostic evaluation and careful therapeutic planning in minimizing the incidence of relapse.

Surgical Planning

Surgical correction of open bite requires painstaking planning based on the evaluation of various documentation records. In addition to clinical evaluation and photographic documentation, the lateral and anteroposterior cephalometric radiographs must be carefully analyzed. After prediction of the profile development has been accomplished, a model analysis is done to study the occlusal relationships and to construct the appropriate splints (see Chapter 7).

CLINICAL EVALUATION

Various factors must be incorporated into the clinical evaluation of open bite: the relationship between the lips and nose, especially the nasolabial angle, the shape and thickness of the lips, and the interlabial gap when the lip muscles are relaxed; the relationship of the upper lip to the teeth and gingiva; the height of the lower third of the face; and the prominence of the chin. Along with these esthetic features, the orofacial functions, such as tongue dyskinesias (particularly tongue pressure), must be taken into account. If so-called bad habits can be observed, such as thumb sucking, the open bite is probably dentoalveolar and not skeletal. The intraoral inspection comprises the assessment of the vertical discrepancy and overjet. Oral hygiene and the condition of the teeth must also be considered, as well as the dental relationship in the molar region.

CEPHALOMETRIC ANALYSIS

Apart from the clinical examinations and model analysis, a lateral cephalometric radiograph study is indispensable. Jarabak,[59] in contrast to the authors named above, tried to divide skeletal open bite into several subgroups on the basis of cephalometric analyses. For a reference line, he chose the Frankfort horizontal and determined the angle of the maxillary plane, which he defined from the spina nasalis in relation to the Frankfort horizontal. In this way, Jarabak was able to distinguish between three types of open bite:

1. *Open bite caused by an elongated posterior maxilla.* Jarabak[59] found a dorsally open angle between the maxillary plane and the Frankfort horizontal. This means that the molars were farther from the Frankfort horizontal than were the incisors, which he regarded as one of the causes of skeletal open bite. Furthermore, in Jarabak's opinion, the vertical height in the area of the upper incisors is too short, which in turn promotes open bite.

2. *Open bite caused by a steep mandibular angle.* This group comprised Angle Class III patients with skeletal open bite. Here Jarabak[59] detected a skeletal deficit in the region of the maxilla and concluded that this was caused by a posterior rotation of the maxilla relative to the cranial base or by such a skeletal relationship between the mandible and maxilla. He found that the mandibular body was often longer than the anterior cranial base. Furthermore, Jarabak observed that in this group the maxillary plane was parallel to the Frankfort horizontal and concluded that this type of open bite was purely mandibular.

3. *Open bite caused by changes in the maxilla and mandible.* In this group, Jarabak[59] found that the mandible and the maxilla were built into the front of the cranial skeleton. At the same time, the mandible was positioned posterior to the cranial base, and the maxillary plane formed an angle of 12 degrees to the Frankfort horizontal.

Jarabak's[59] classification of open bite based on cephalometric analyses was a major improvement over the previous, more symptom-oriented divisions. It also provides evidence that open bite is a symptom that can be traced back to a number of causes, which is why it is incorrect to speak of an open bite syndrome.

By taking embryonic developmental aspects into consideration when analyzing open bite, a direct relationship can be established between the stage of the patient's development during which the disorder had its onset and the degree of severity of the deformity. If the disorder occurred in utero, such as craniosynostosis, the most severe form of open bite will result. If the disturbance occurs after the cranial suture has closed, that is, at the age of 4 years, it will have only functional consequences for cranial and facial growth. Accordingly, changes will be observed only in the maxillomandibular or dentoalveolar region, whereas alterations resulting from early embryonic disturbances are manifest in the craniofacial area.

Before surgical treatment of open bite can be planned, the type and degree of the deformity must be determined in the cephalometric analysis. The more severe

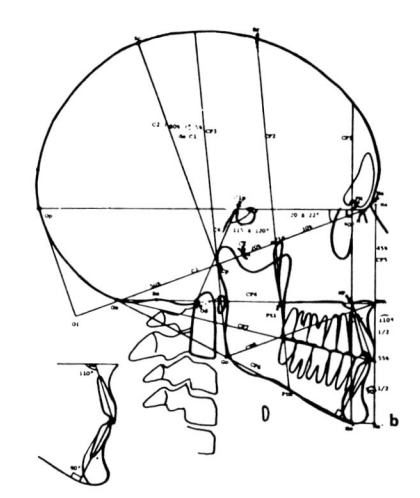

FIGURE 60-27. Delaire analysis including cranial and facial parts, as well as parts of the cervical vertebrae.

the deformity is—that is, the earlier it occurred—the more difficult it is to treat. The conventional cephalometric analyses are usually not sufficient to determine these early craniofacial disturbances. Delaire[60] therefore designed a cephalometric analysis that gives precise information on the bony structures of the entire skull and adjacent soft tissue and hence on the etiology and pathology of dentofacial malformations (Fig. 60-27). The advantage of the Delaire analysis over other cephalometric evaluations is that it demonstrates the architecture of the entire skull, including areas that are not affected by the deformity. Important for the Delaire analysis is the selection of reference points. These must be points that remain stable during growth. When dealing with a skull that is still growing, the selection of reference points is always a problem, and the presence of a severe deformity compounds this problem. If reference points are chosen that lie within the deformity, essential parts of this deformity will be easily overlooked. For this reason, the Delaire analysis uses reference points located on the skull outside the confines of the deformity. An angle frequently used is the SNA angle,[61] which is useful for making decisions for orthodontic treatment. However, when used in treating deformities, this angle can falsify the results. There are two reasons for this:

1. Enlow[11] demonstrated that during growth the N point moves in a cranioventral direction. This means that the movements of the maxilla cannot be covered with the SNA angle. The normal forward rotation of the maxilla is 10 degrees.

2. The A point is not located on the maxilla but on the premaxilla. Consequently, in cases of cleft lip and palate, for example, this angle is not able to provide information on the position of the maxilla, but only the premaxilla (Fig. 60-28). It is absolutely incorrect to maintain that the maxilla in the presence of cleft lip and palate is in an anterior position. Only the premaxilla is in an anterior position; the maxilla is retruded. Frequently, the large SNA angle leads to the therapeutic decision that the premaxilla has to be moved posteriorly for the maxilla to be set in the "correct" position. This conclusion is erroneous, since to achieve satisfactory occlusion, the forward advancement of the maxilla is necessary and not the distal movement of the premaxilla. The same applies to the reference point of the nasal spine used to evaluate vertical discrepancies. The shape and location of the nasal spine are subject to functional factors (Fig. 60-29). If the malformation is caused by functional disturbances, the nasal spine cannot be used to evaluate vertical disproportions.

The Delaire analysis consists of two parts, which must be considered separately:

1. Evaluation of craniofacial balance. Reference lines are an objective, reproducible mechanism for evaluating the craniofacial balance in each particular case based on the relationship of the facial structures to the norms. The individual facial

2078 / VII—ORTHOGNATHIC SURGERY

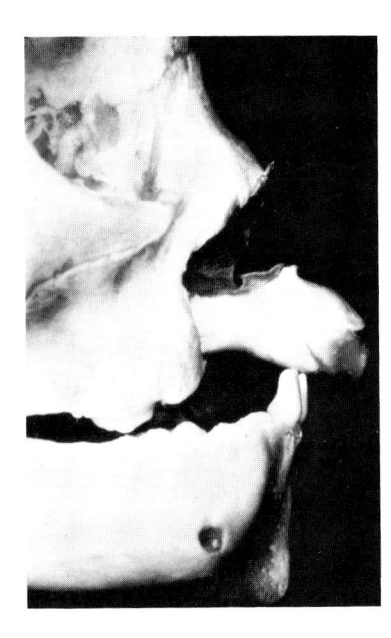

FIGURE 60-28. Skeleton showing a bilateral cleft lip and palate. Point A is located at a considerable distance from the maxilla, so that no information can be gained regarding the position of the upper jaw.

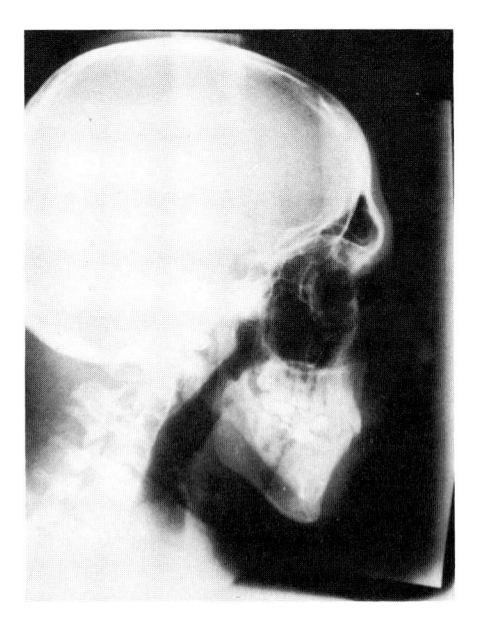

FIGURE 60-29. Upright nasal spine as a normal anatomic variation.

structures can also be put in relation to one another, since relations are measured and not absolute distances and angles.

2. Analysis of bony structures, including the extent of the ossification, the state of the bone surface, outer contours, and adjacent soft tissue. The skull and facial skeleton are evaluated, as well as the upper cervical vertebral column. These three areas must be balanced for stability to be achieved.

Soft Tissue Analysis

The profile analysis we developed entails determining various soft tissue points as established by Burstone,[62] Lines,[63] and Schwarz[64] in the cephalometric radiograph. For this analysis, we use six linear measurements and three angle measurements (Fig. 60-30A and B). A prediction of the profile for the particular surgical techniques can be made by simulating the expected dental and skeletal postoperative changes on the cephalometric radiograph and on the model. The new profile can be drawn, taking into account the relationship between bone and soft tissue change for the specific surgical method. Soft tissue advancement varies, depending on the surgical procedure. In an Obwegeser[33]–Dal Pont[34] operation, the soft tissue advancement is 88 per cent of the bone advancement at the pogonion, 72 per cent at the labrale inferius, and as much as 17 per cent at the labrale superius. In segmental osteotomy in the maxilla, there is an 81 per cent soft tissue adaptation to advanced bone at the SN, 59 per cent at the labrale superius, and 28 per cent at the labrale inferius. In genioplasties with advancement and vertical reduction, on the other hand, we were able to determine that at ME the soft tissue advanced 112 per cent of the bone advancement. This means that by rotating the chin forward and up, a more than sufficient soft tissue drape can be produced. By contrast, after simple chin reduction, the soft tissue advancement was only 33 per cent of the bone

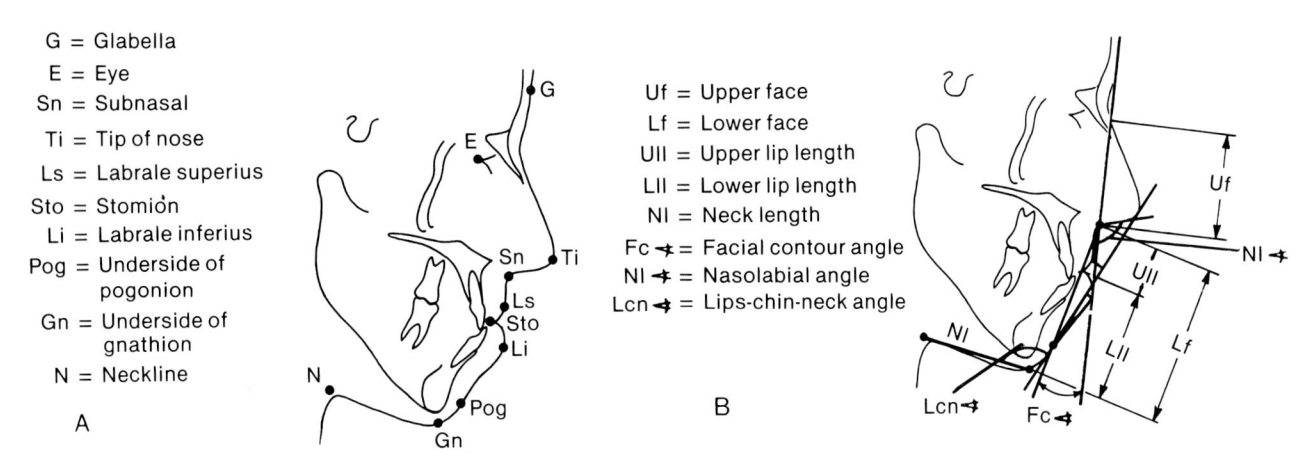

FIGURE 60–30. THE PROFILE ANALYSIS USED AT OUR INSTITUTION. *A,* Reference points. *B,* Angle and linear measurements.

advancement. With the aid of this soft tissue analysis, a more or less exact prediction of the later esthetic changes in the face occurring as a result of the surgically induced osseous changes can be made. Today, such predictions can be made by computer by first simulating the operation and then drawing the profile according to the relationship between hard tissue and soft tissue.

Procedure Order

After the facial esthetics have been clinically evaluated and the cephalogram and soft tissue analyses have been made, the records are transferred to a semi-adjustable articulator, and a model simulation is carried out. The goal is to achieve optimal dental occlusion. The treatment plan is then made on the basis of this information, including the timing of the individual treatment steps.

ORTHODONTIC TREATMENT

As was already mentioned, the opinions and concepts concerning the treatment of open bite vary considerably. Subtelny and Sakuda[27] summarized their findings by saying that the orthodontic treatment of open bite poses serious difficulties and that in many cases treatment is even impossible. Sassouni and Nanda[65] observed that a Class II open bite can be successfully treated by orthodontic measures but that for Class III cases surgical management must be instituted.

The coordination of orthodontic and surgical treatment requires careful timing. In our institution, the orthodontic treatment is usually performed and, when possible, completed before surgical correction is initiated. In cases of extreme open bite, the maxillary and mandibular planes first have to be surgically aligned before orthodontic treatment can commence. The orthodontic treatment we use aims at leveling the dental arches in the maxilla and mandible so that they are well aligned after surgical repositioning. Performing such treatment before surgery facilitates the positioning of the fragments into the new bite situation. After the orthodontic treatment, only the detailed finishing work should be undertaken.

Orthodontic treatment chiefly consists of preparing for the subsequent operation. Arch lengths are shortened by extraction, crowding is corrected, arches are formed, and teeth are inclined. Particularly with respect to this last task, the surgical procedure to be used must be taken into consideration. If the sagittal split ramus osteotomy technique is going to be employed for correction of open bite, the axial inclination of the teeth must be toward the labial to keep them from tipping too far lingually when the anterior mandible has been repositioned posteriorly and superiorly. Extrusion and intrusion of teeth should not be done by orthodontic mechanics, as this frequently produces unstable results and increases the risk of postoperative dental relapse. Ideally, a retention phase of 3 months should be observed between the orthodontic therapy and the surgery.

The correction of vertical and sagittal discrepancies is reserved for surgery and should not be undertaken by preoperative orthodontics.

SELECTION OF SURGICAL TECHNIQUE

Modern surgical methods have made it possible to alter the facial skeleton to almost any degree. Many techniques are applicable that observe the surgical principles with regard to soft tissue drape, adequate blood supply, and bone segment fixation. The possible complications should be one of the top considerations when selecting a particular surgical technique, especially since such operations are elective.[66] Complications include all undesirable results that occur during the operation, in the immediate postoperative phase, and in the follow-up period. In 363 patients operated on for orthodontic reasons between 1979 and 1982, the complications of the surgical techniques were investigated. One hundred and fifty-seven patients presented with an Angle Class II occlusion and 166 with an Angle Class III occlusion. The most frequently performed operation was sagittal split osteotomy in the ascending ramus according to the Obwegeser–Dal Pont method, followed by segmental osteotomy and sagittal splitting in the horizontal ramus. We have been using Delaire's modification of this method since 1976. The incidence of surgical complications was highest (13 per cent) when the Obwegeser–Dal Pont method was used, followed by segmental osteotomy, though in the latter the complications were confined to tooth injury (Fig. 60–31). Relapse was evaluated in the lateral cephalometric radiograph. The ANB angle served as a parameter for the sagittal direction, and the anterior facial height was the parameter for the vertical direction. The majority of the cases classified as relapse showed no occlusal changes in the surgical outcome at the time of follow-up. This means that dental compensatory mechanisms were able to balance out skeletal relapse. A vertical relapse rate of almost 60 per cent was observed after a prognathic open bite had been corrected by using the Obwegeser–Dal Pont technique. By contrast, no vertical relapse occurred in the Delaire group. The sagittal relapse in the Obwegeser group accounted for 18 per cent, and in the Delaire group, 19 per cent, of the surgical changes. Among the Le Fort osteotomies to correct maxillary retrusion, a sagittal relapse of 20 per cent was observed, and a 50 per cent relapse occurred in cases of cleft lip and palate. Even after segmental osteotomies of Angle Class II$_1$ and II$_2$, a vertical relapse of 28 per cent and a sagittal relapse of 10 per cent were seen. On the basis of these complication rates, we made a distinction between the various methods according to indication. The Obwegeser–Dal Pont method is the most appropriate osteotomy for treating Angle Class III open bite when a horizontal growth pattern can be determined cephalometrically. To avoid aseptic necrosis,

Operation	Number	Complications	Relapse sagittal	Relapse vertical
Obwegeser–Dalpont	100	13%	18%	60%
Sagittal Splitting horizontal Ramus	51	3%	19%	2%
Le–Fort I	25	4%	20–50% (CLP)	0%
Köle, Maxil.	119	12%	10%	28%
Köle, Mandib.	73	12%	10%	28%
Chinplasty	39	4%	0%	0%

FIGURE 60–31. Complication and relapse rates after surgery for malocclusion. (1979–1982, N = 363)

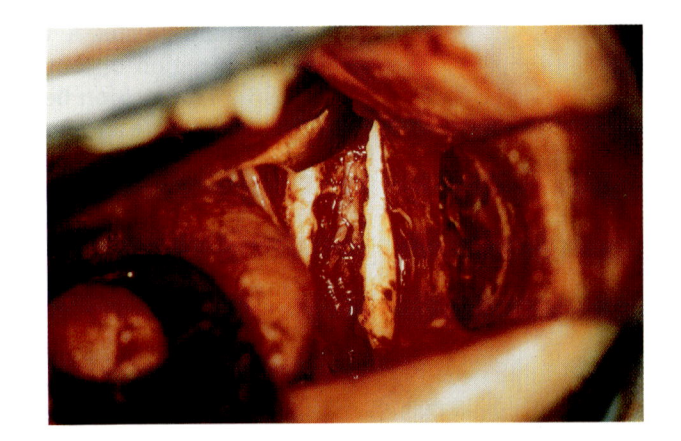

FIGURE 60-32. Vestibular lamella pedicled on the periosteum in the Obwegeser–Dal Pont operation.

the buccal bone lamella should remain pedicled to the periosteum, which can be achieved by using an incision that extends toward the tongue (Fig. 60-32). For Angle Class III and II open bite with vertical growth pattern, we prefer our modification of the Delaire method, since it has the lowest rate of vertical relapse and the lowest complication rates. Segment displacements appear to be applicable only in cases in which the maxillary and mandibular planes are consistent with the norm as determined cephalometrically and in which the overjet or overbite cannot be corrected by orthodontic treatment. Le Fort I osteotomy is used to treat vertical maxillary hyperplasia or anteroposterior maxillary deficiency with dental symmetry and no open bite gap. For treatment of cleft lip and palate deformities with marked retroinclination and hypoplasia of the maxilla, we prefer segmental osteotomy in front of the zygomatic buttress with large bone grafts,[67,68] the advantage being that the very small maxilla can be enlarged and supported with the aid of a bone graft against the zygomatic buttress. Furthermore, the distance from the soft palate to the posterior wall of the pharynx is barely changed, so that speech is not impaired. We consider bimaxillary surgery for treatment of overjet in excess of 10 mm. These techniques can be combined, depending on the growth pattern.

This indication scheme was successfully used for 424 patients with dysgnathia who were treated in our institution between 1983 and 1987.

Surgical Techniques

The following methods have been successfully used at our institution in cases in which it can be ruled out preoperatively that cranial causes are not responsible for the open bite, in which instance other surgical techniques are then required.

SEGMENTAL OSTEOTOMY

Köle Modification of Segmental Osteotomy. Segmental osteotomy of the maxilla or mandible or both, as modified by Köle,[69] is recommended when cephalometric radiographs show that the maxillary and mandibular planes are aligned. Segmental osteotomy should be used only to treat variations in the alveolar process. The technique is best suited for protrusion and retrusion of the alveolar processes in the maxilla and mandible. It is advisable to rotate the segments, particularly when a small apical base makes orthodontic treatment difficult or impossible. In the case of open bite caused by thumb sucking, a subtotal osteotomy can be performed to close the gaps, as we have described elsewhere.[69a]

Indications. The indications are cephalometrically confirmed aligned planes, narrow apical base, and variations in the dentoalveolar region.

Zisser Segmental Osteotomy. We use a special type of segmental osteotomy modified after Zisser[67] for retrusive hypoplastic maxilla, particularly in the case of

2088 / VII — ORTHOGNATHIC SURGERY

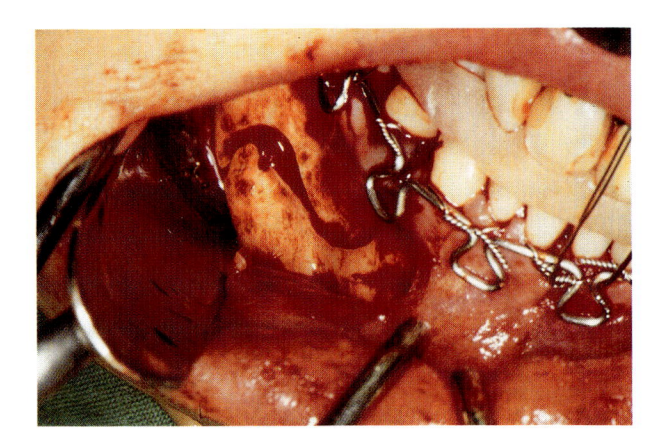

FIGURE 60-46. Vestibular incision. Only the cortical bone is cut.

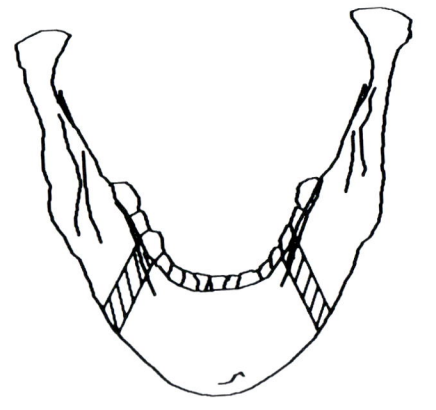

FIGURE 60-47. Schematic illustration of lingual separation. With a round drill, osteotomy of the lingual cortical plate is performed while the soft tissue is protected.

The buccal cortical bone is gradually severed with a thin spherical cutter just up to the area of the spongiosa (Fig. 60-46). If the mandible is moved back at the same time, an osteotomy is carried out both in the alveolar process and in the mandibular body. Finally, an incision is made lingually, parallel to the teeth at a distance of 5 mm from the marginal periodontium. The mucoperiosteal flap is elevated as far as the inferior mandibular border. While the soft tissue is protected, the lingual osteotomy is carried out with a round drill, if necessary, with concomitant ostectomy of the cortical bone only (Fig. 60-47). Sagittal splitting should not be performed until after the contralateral side has been prepared, since after splitting, the anterior segment would only be pedicled on the neurovascular bundle (Fig. 60-48). When the two sides have been prepared, a sagittal split is performed with a mallet and osteotome. An assistant must hold the anterior chin segment in place

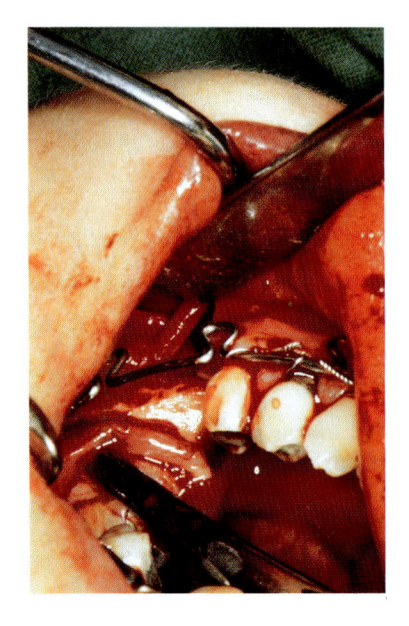

FIGURE 60-48. The inferior alveolar nerve as viewed after osteotomy with mallet and osteotome.

FIGURE 60-49. Maxillomandibular fixation after advancement and adjustment of the anterior segment.

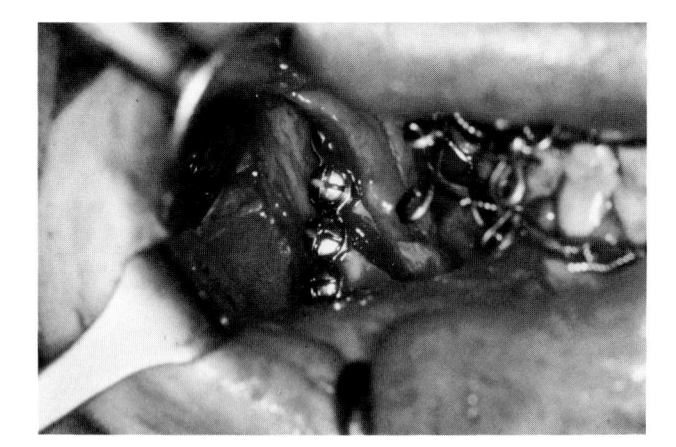

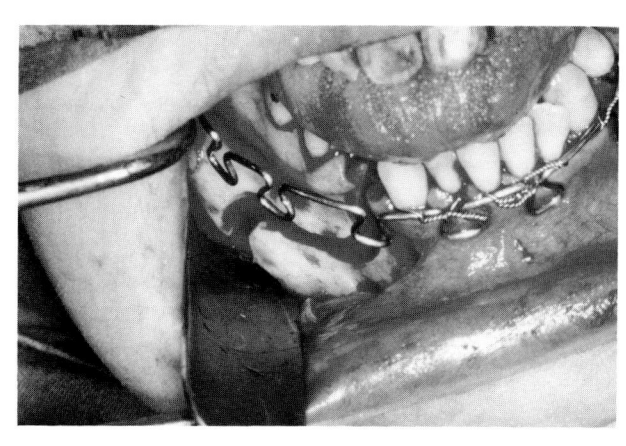

FIGURE 60-50. Fixation with a monocortical mini bone plate.

with his or her hand. After osteotomy and mobilization of the segment, a Schuchardt splint is applied to the distal molars to prevent undesired movements of the anterior segment. Then the mucosa is lingually closed with resorbable sutures, and the anterior mandibular segment is immobilized by means of maxillomandibular fixation (Fig. 60-49). Slight transverse movements of the distal segment can be carried out so that an Angle Class I occlusion can be achieved if this is deemed necessary. After maxillomandibular fixation, a monocortical osteosynthesis plate is applied on the left and right (Fig. 60-50). The intraoral wound is closed in a routine manner. The maxillomandibular fixation can be released 2 to 3 weeks later if the fragments have been stabilized with miniplates. The teeth-bearing mandibular splint should be left in place for approximately 6 weeks.

Indications. Indications are Angle Class III open bite, Angle Class II open bite, Angle Class III open bite with interdental spacing, and Angle Class I open bite.

GENIOPLASTY

Reduction of the anterior vertical height by means of genioplasty is often a valuable adjunctive procedure for treating skeletal open bite. The technique can be used to correct the lack of proportion between the length of the lips and the height of the lower face, which Ballard[5] (see Etiology, discussed previously) considered the most important criterion for surgical reduction in cases of open bite. At the same time, the anterior closure of the oral functional space is achieved, thereby correcting the tongue dyskinesias.[72]

The calculations of the anterior vertical height and the ideal position of the ME are based on the Delaire analysis. The distance N — spina is 45 per cent, and spina — Me is 55 per cent. The corrected position of the spina nasalis according to the Delaire analysis is used. The magnitude of the vertical reduction and the sagittal repositioning is derived from these values.

Several surgical procedures can be used. Apart from the simple chin advancement with height reduction, the technique described by Delaire and by us[69a] is

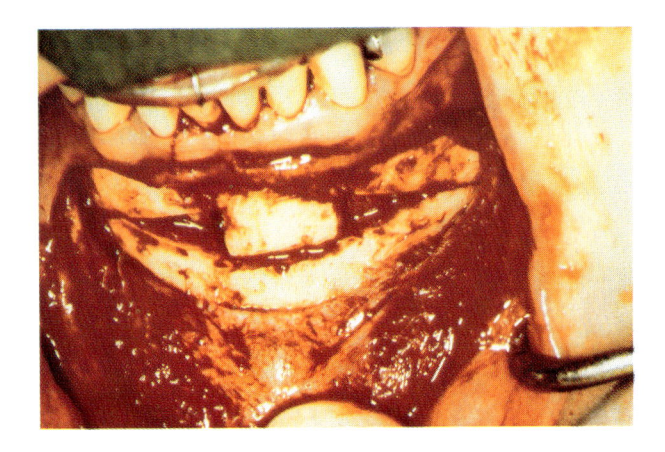

FIGURE 60–51. Osteotomy to reposition the chin while reducing the facial height and moving the chin anteriorly with the muscles maintained attached.

highly recommended. The technique has the advantage of being able to reposition the chin anteriorly and superiorly while the muscles remain attached to the bony chin (Fig. 60–51). In this way, the muscle insertions are also moved anteriorly and superiorly, which relaxes the entire periapical region. Follow-up examinations have demonstrated that a soft tissue augmentation is 112 per cent of the amount the bone is moved forward.

The application of this technique in early childhood, after the lower canines have erupted, is often sufficient to close the open bite, either alone or with adjunctive orthodontic measures. A combination with other surgical procedures is particularly beneficial. In a mild open bite case with Class III malocclusion, an Obwegeser–Dal Pont operation with genioplasty is recommended as a relapse-preventing measure. The vertical height of the bony chin should be reduced the same amount as the open bite. Again, it is important to move perioral muscle insertions superiorly to relax the orolabial region.[72] If necessary, this procedure can be combined with a midline ostectomy to reduce the mandible transversely.[69a]

In extreme cases of open bite in early childhood, before eruption of the lower canines, we use a soft tissue genioplasty. After a vestibular incision has been made, the muscles and periosteum around the chin are dissected distally and lingually with the inserted muscles (Fig. 60–52A and B). After this type of mobilization, a bone hole is drilled under the root tips of 31 and 41. The submental muscles with periosteum are then repositioned superiorly and secured with thick, nonresorbable sutures (Fig. 60–53A and B). These measures also reduce the tension of the perioral muscles. Although open bite can often be closed without orthodontic treatment, adjunctive functional orthodontic treatment is almost always indicated. In some cases, a bony genioplasty must be carried out at a later time.

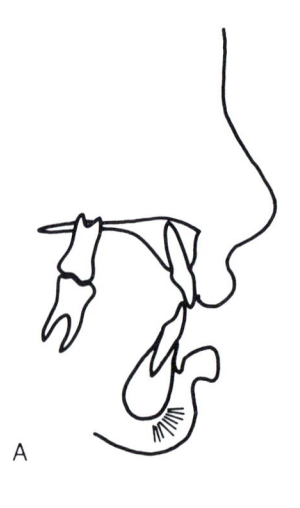

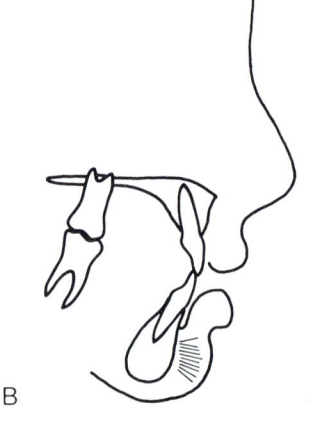

FIGURE 60–52. *A, B,* Schematic illustration of soft tissue genioplasty. The lip muscles are moved superiorly with the attached periosteum.

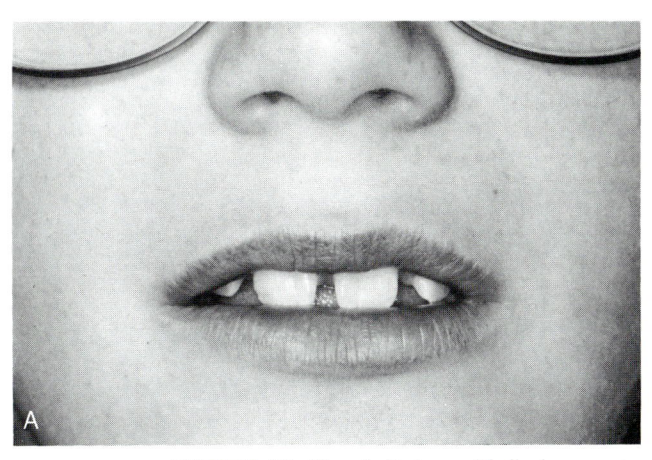

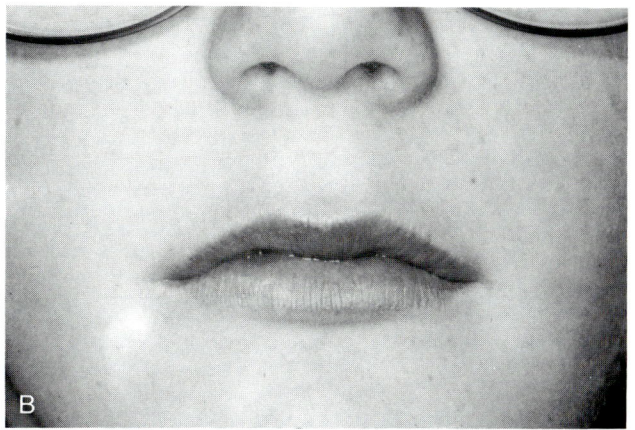

FIGURE 60-53. *A*, Patient with lip incompetence, preoperative view. *B*, After soft tissue genioplasty, lip closure without strain.

BIMAXILLARY OPERATIONS

In extreme cases of open bite, in concert with a Class II or III dysgnathia, it is often not sufficient to carry out corrective measures in one jaw only. Another problem is that when only one jaw is surgically repositioned, the oral space is severely reduced, which produces orolabial and lingual malfunctioning and thus raises the risk of relapse. At our institution, we use bimaxillary operation for excessive overjet (10 mm and more). In most cases, it is necessary to balance out the sagittal discrepancy with the maxilla and the vertical discrepancy with the mandible after careful analysis of each case. We were not able to observe the vertical overdevelopment of the maxilla that is described in the literature, so that we saw no reason to raise the entire maxilla. This discrepancy is probably the result of different interpretations of the cephalometric radiographs.

If the cephalometric evaluation has ruled out a cranial cause of the deformity, we perform all of the foregoing techniques in one session. After careful surgical simulation, temporary and permanent splints are made in the semi-adjustable articulator. During the operation, the maxilla is repositioned first, correctly positioned via an interim splint, and then fixed to the midface with four mini ASIF plates (Fig. 60-54*A* and *B*). Then the mandible is repositioned and stabilized. Our follow-up examinations of 70 patients after bimaxillary operations confirmed that this procedure produces stable results. The exclusion of a cranial cause of the condition is the prerequisite for selecting this technique. Partial relapse could be

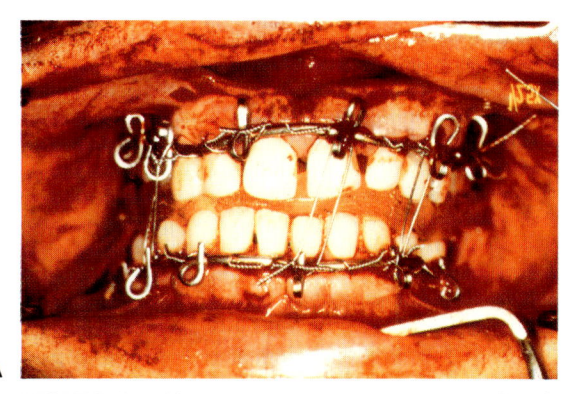

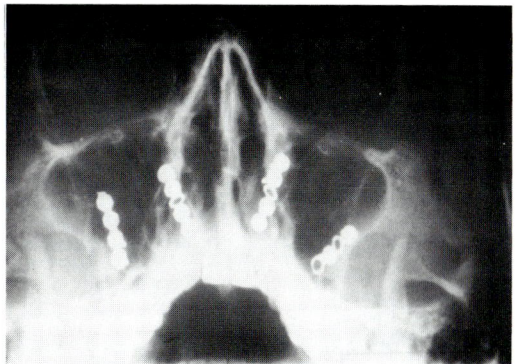

FIGURE 60-54. BIMAXILLARY OSTEOTOMY. *A*, Splint after maxillary osteotomy with intermaxillary immobilization. *B*, Fixation with four miniplates—two positioned paranasally and two at the zygomatic buttress.

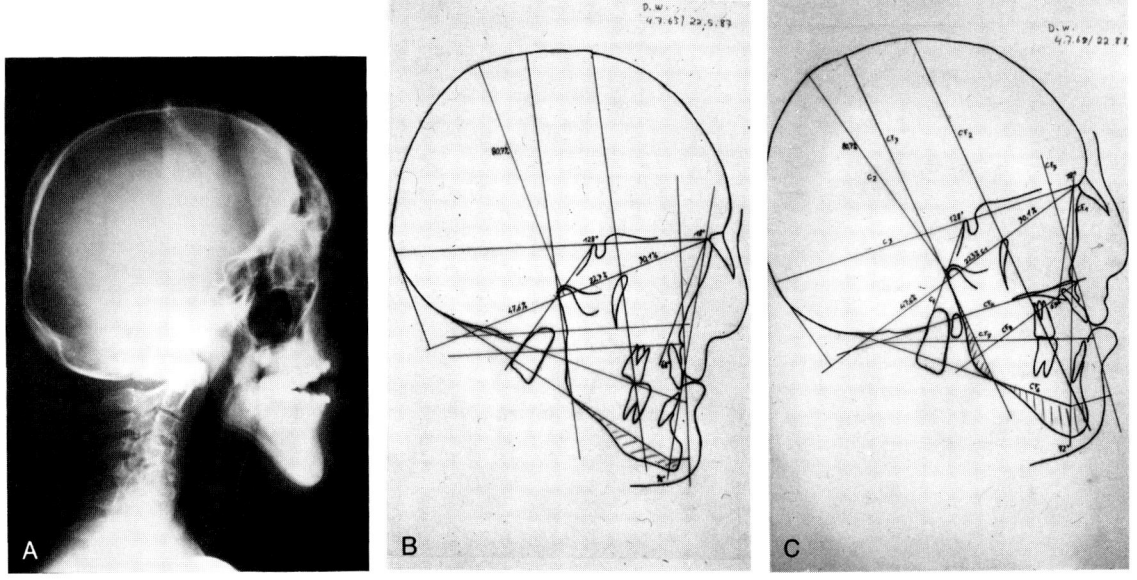

FIGURE 60-55. BILATERAL CLEFT LIP AND PALATE WITH EXTREME OPEN BITE. *A,* Original radiograph. *B,* Cephalometric analysis, preoperative: changed angle of skull base, vertical midface too short, and extreme maxillary retrusion. *C,* Cephalometric analysis, postoperative: unchanged base and partial relapse.

observed in only four patients, all of whom had had extreme cranial or facial deformities: Two patients had craniosynostoses, and two had cleft lip and palate, which had been operated on several times (Fig. 60-55A to C). In such cases, it seems necessary to extend the operation cranially, as in a Le Fort II or III osteotomy, on the one hand, and to carry out muscular reconstruction prior to the skeletal operation to achieve stable results. The follow-up study underscores the importance of careful preoperative diagnostic evaluation in covering all the factors involved in the malformation.

Indications. The indications for this procedure are excessive overjet (10 mm or more) and extreme open bite.

CASE EXAMPLES

CASE 1: SKELETAL OPEN BITE WITH CLASS II MALOCCLUSION

PROBLEM LIST

Esthetics

Frontal: forced lip closure, prominent lower third of face, retruded chin (Fig. 60-56A).

Profile: large lower third of face, backward profile, forced lip closure (Fig. 60-56B).

Occlusion: crowding and rotation of teeth in both jaws and anterior open bite with contact only between molars and second premolars (Fig. 60-56C and D).

Cephalometric Analysis: normal neurocranium and skull base, maxilla in ventral position, inadequate vertical height (Fig. 60-56E and F).

TREATMENT PLAN

Orthodontic Treatment: coordinate jaws and correct axial position of the teeth; align and tip lower anterior teeth toward the labial.

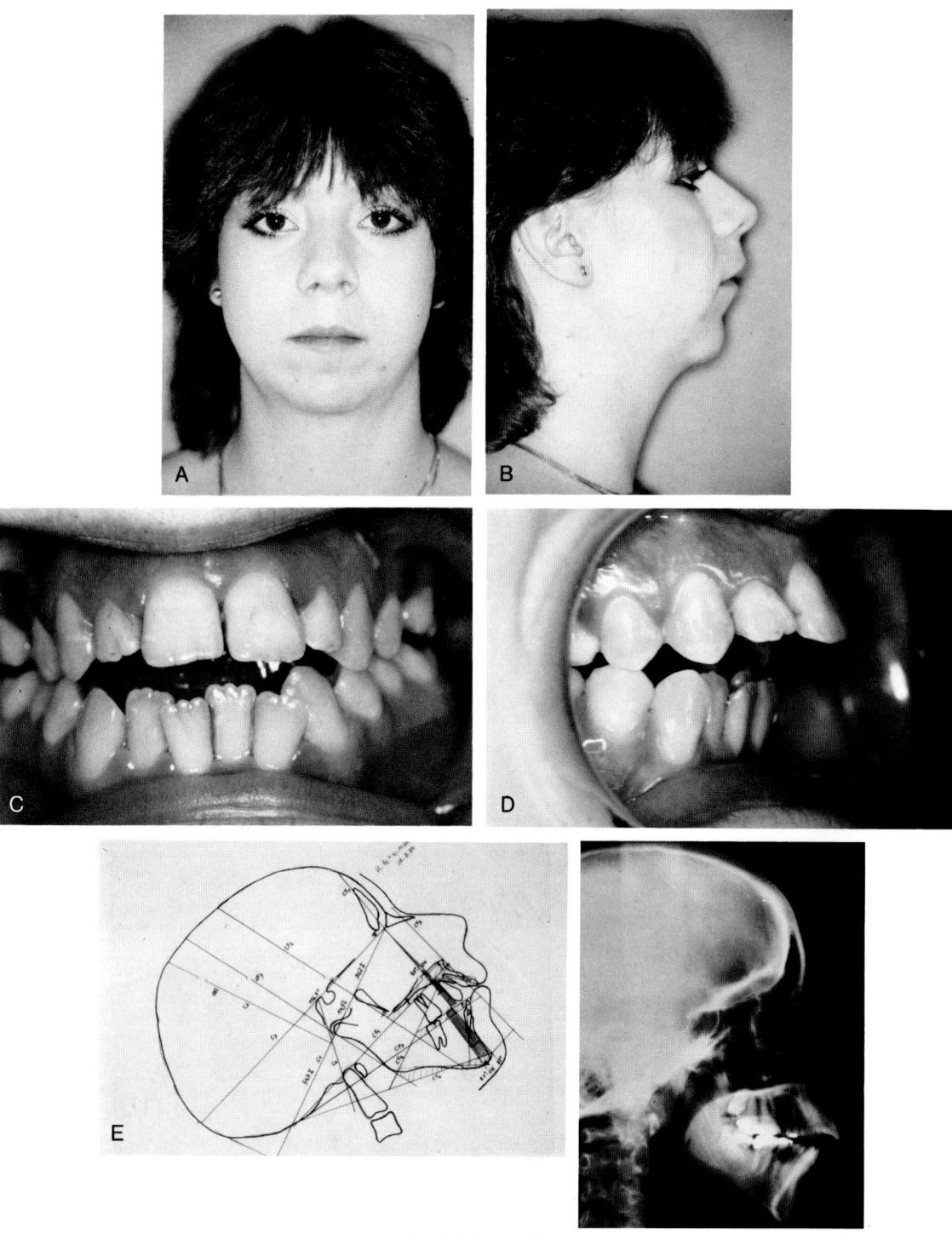

FIGURE 60–56.

Illustration continued on following page

Surgical Treatment: close the open bite with sagittal splitting in the horizontal mandibular ramus and subsequent genioplasty to reduce the anterior vertical facial height.

COMMENTS

Esthetics are postoperatively satisfactory, though the face is still in the ventral position (Fig. 60–56G to K).

Occlusion: narrow maxilla with crowding, broad mandible with anterior teeth tipped lingually, circular open bite with contact only between molars (Fig. 60–58C).

TREATMENT PLAN

Orthodontic Treatment: accomplish transverse expansion of the maxilla, align the jaws, partially correct the position of the mandibular anterior teeth (Fig. 60–58D to F).

Surgical Treatment: extract one molar and close the open bite by means of the sagittal split technique in the horizontal ramus (Fig. 60–57G to K).

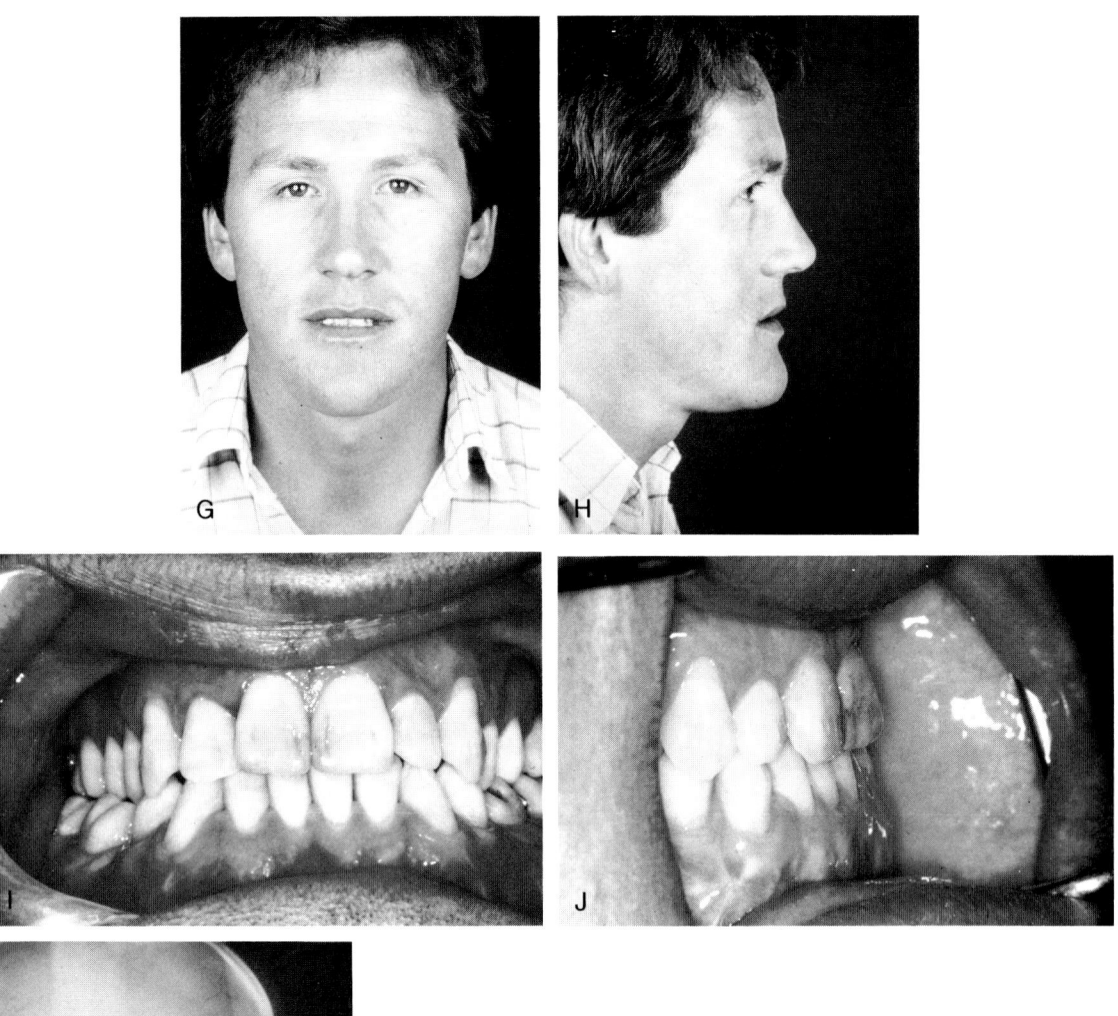

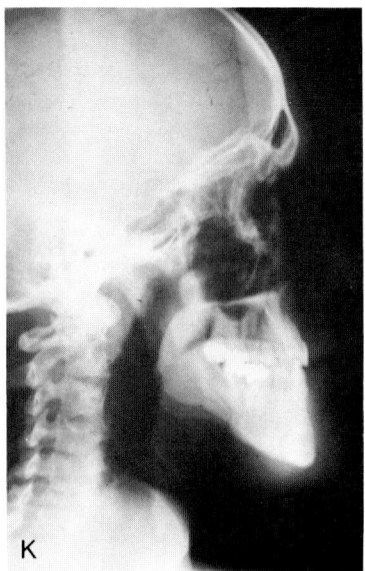

FIGURE 60–57 *Continued.*

CASE 3: CLASS III MALOCCLUSION WITH SLIGHT OPEN BITE

Problem List

Esthetics

Frontal: strong chin; large, prominent lower face; paranasal deficiency (Fig. 60–58A).

Profile: large, strong chin; slight retroposition of midface (Fig. 60–58B).

Occlusion: narrow maxilla with crowding, mandibular teeth crowded and retroclined (Fig. 60–58C and D).

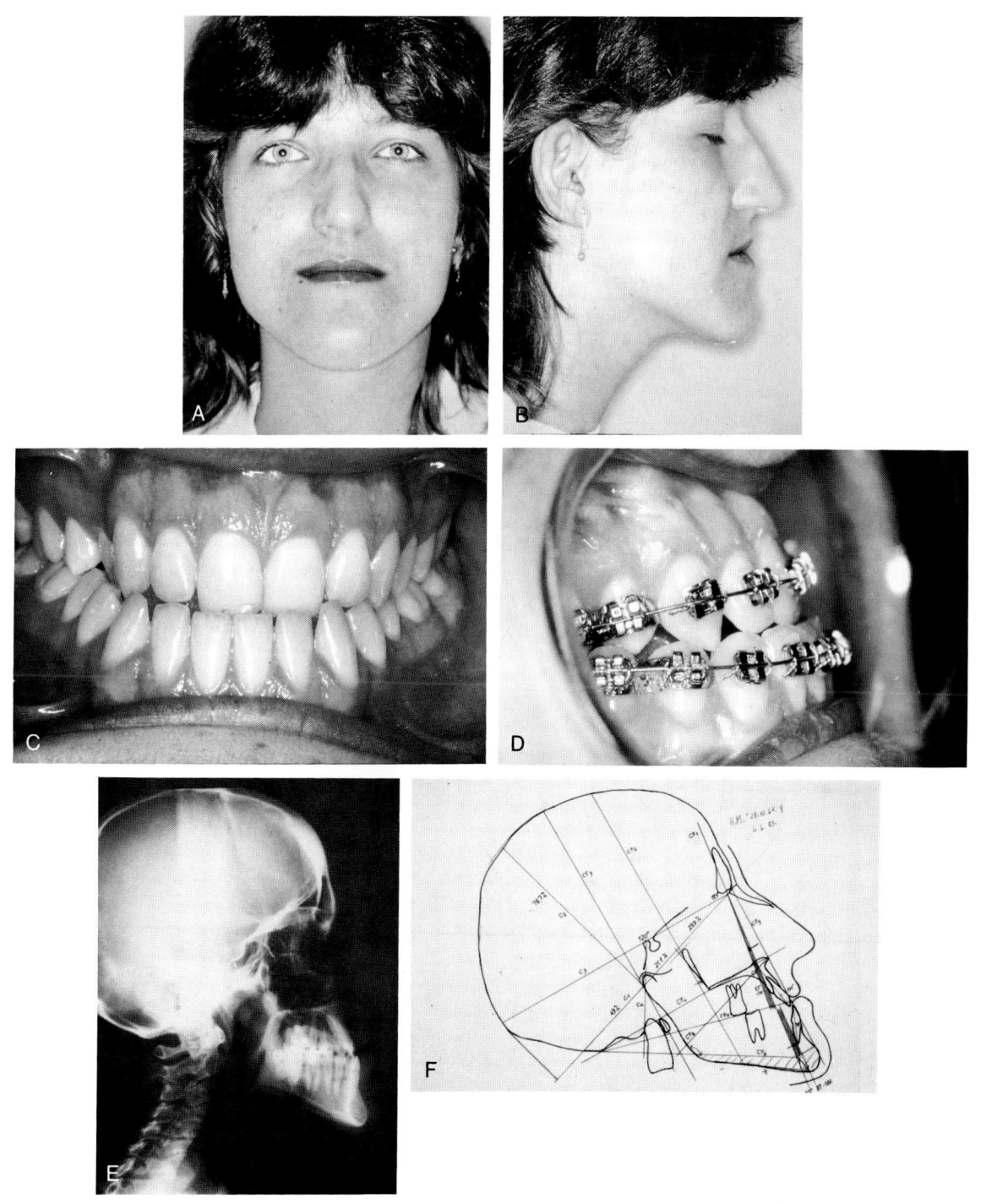

FIGURE 60–58. *Illustration continued on following page*

Cephalometric Analysis: slight maxillary retrusion with mandibular prognathism, normal neurocranium and skull base (Fig. 60–58*E* and *F*).

TREATMENT PLAN

Orthodontic Treatment: coordinate arches, adjust axial inclination of teeth.

Surgical Treatment: genioplasty to reduce the anterior facial height with simultaneous sagittal split in ascending mandibular ramus, correction of malocclusion.

COMMENTS

Postoperatively, face is symmetric but still somewhat too long (Fig. 60–58*G* to *L*).

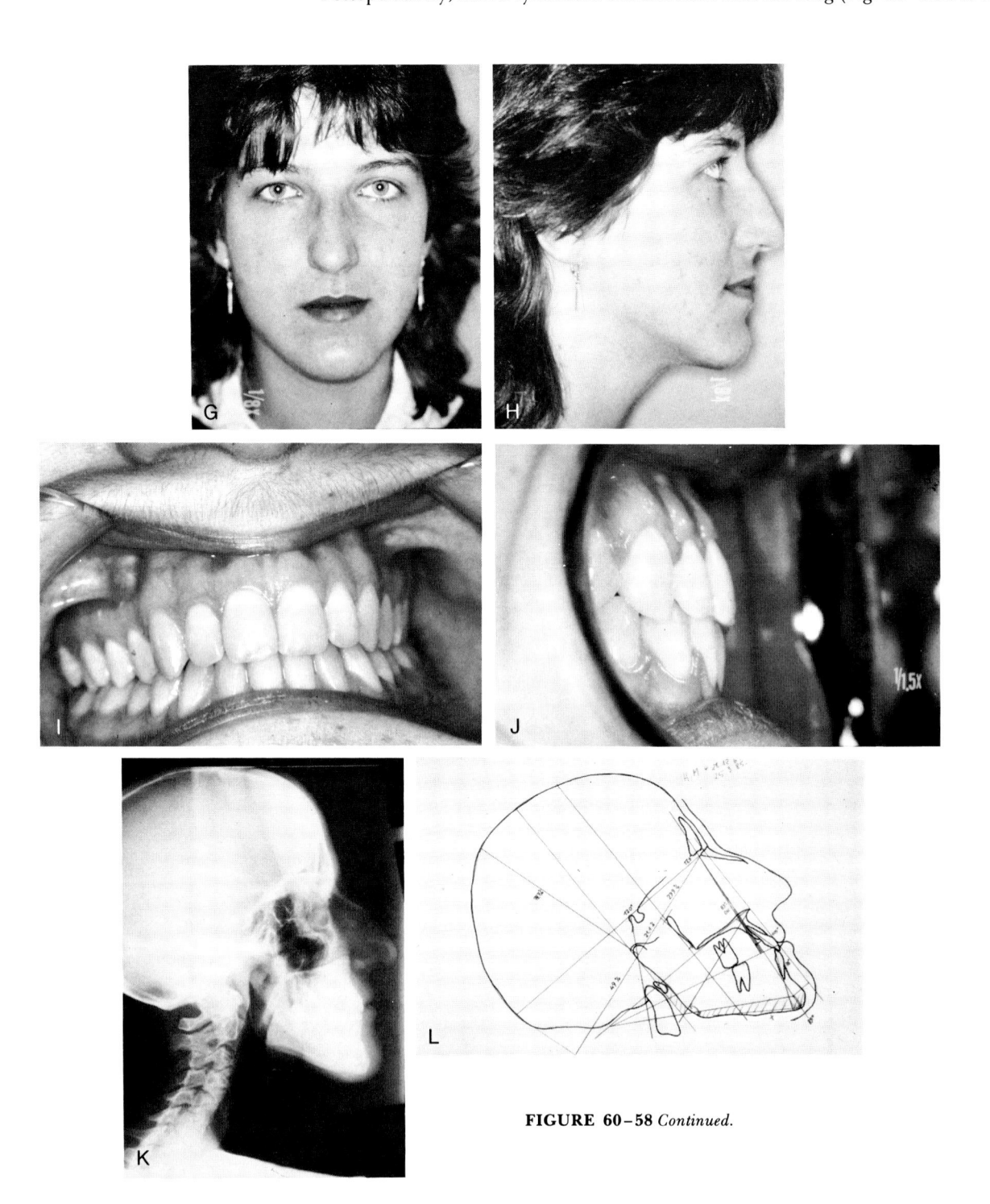

FIGURE 60–58 *Continued.*

CASE 4: SEVERE CLASS III MALOCCLUSION WITH SKELETAL OPEN BITE

Problem List

Esthetics

Frontal: strong lower face with protruding chin; thin, sunken face; lip closure only possible when forced (Fig. 60–59A).

Profile: strong chin, retroposition of face (Fig. 60–59B).

Occlusion: narrow mandible, crowding in both arches, teeth in lower jaw inclined lingually (Fig. 60–59C and D).

Cephalometric Analysis: normal neurocranium and skull base; maxillary retrusion and mandibular prognathism (Fig. 60–59E to G).

Treatment Plan

Orthodontic Treatment: align and level dental arches, correct axial inclination of teeth.

Surgical Treatment: bimaxillary operation with segmental advancement of the maxilla, because the maxilla was hypoplastic, and sagittal split of the horizontal ramus.

Comments

The maxilla was both retruded and hypoplastic. It was therefore advisable to enlarge the maxilla by means of segmental osteotomy and bone grafting. Sagittal split was performed in the mandibular ramus to close the open bite (Fig. 60–59H to M).

CASE 5: CLASS III MALOCCLUSION WITH SKELETAL OPEN BITE

Problem List

Esthetics

Frontal: strong face, protruding chin, long lower third of face (Fig. 60–60A).

Profile: prominent nasolabial fold, maxillary retrusion, long lower face (Fig. 60–60B).

Occlusion: narrow maxilla, broad mandible, crowding of teeth in both arches (Fig. 60–60C to E).

Cephalometric Analysis: normal neurocranium and skull base; maxillary retrusion with extreme mandibular prognathism, normal vertical maxillary height (Fig. 60–60F and G).

Treatment Plan

Orthodontic Treatment: align jaws, correct inclination of lower anterior teeth.

Surgical Treatment: bimaxillary surgery with advancement of maxilla by Le Fort I osteotomy, closure of open bite by means of sagittal split osteotomy of horizontal ramus (Fig. 60–60H to M).

CASE 6: CLASS II SKELETAL OPEN BITE

Problem List

Esthetics: retruded chin, large nasolabial angle, forced lip closure; intraoral open bite with contact only between molars; slight crowding in both arches; crossbite in upper left segment from 3 to 7 degrees (Fig. 60–61A to E).

Treatment Plan

Orthodontic Treatment: align arches and close open bite.

Surgical Treatment: subtotal segmental osteotomy of the left maxilla with transverse rapid expansion (Fig. 60–61F to H).

Comments

The open bite could be closed by orthodontic means after transverse expansion. No further surgical measures were necessary (Fig. 60–61I to N).

Text continued on page 2106

2100 / VII — ORTHOGNATHIC SURGERY

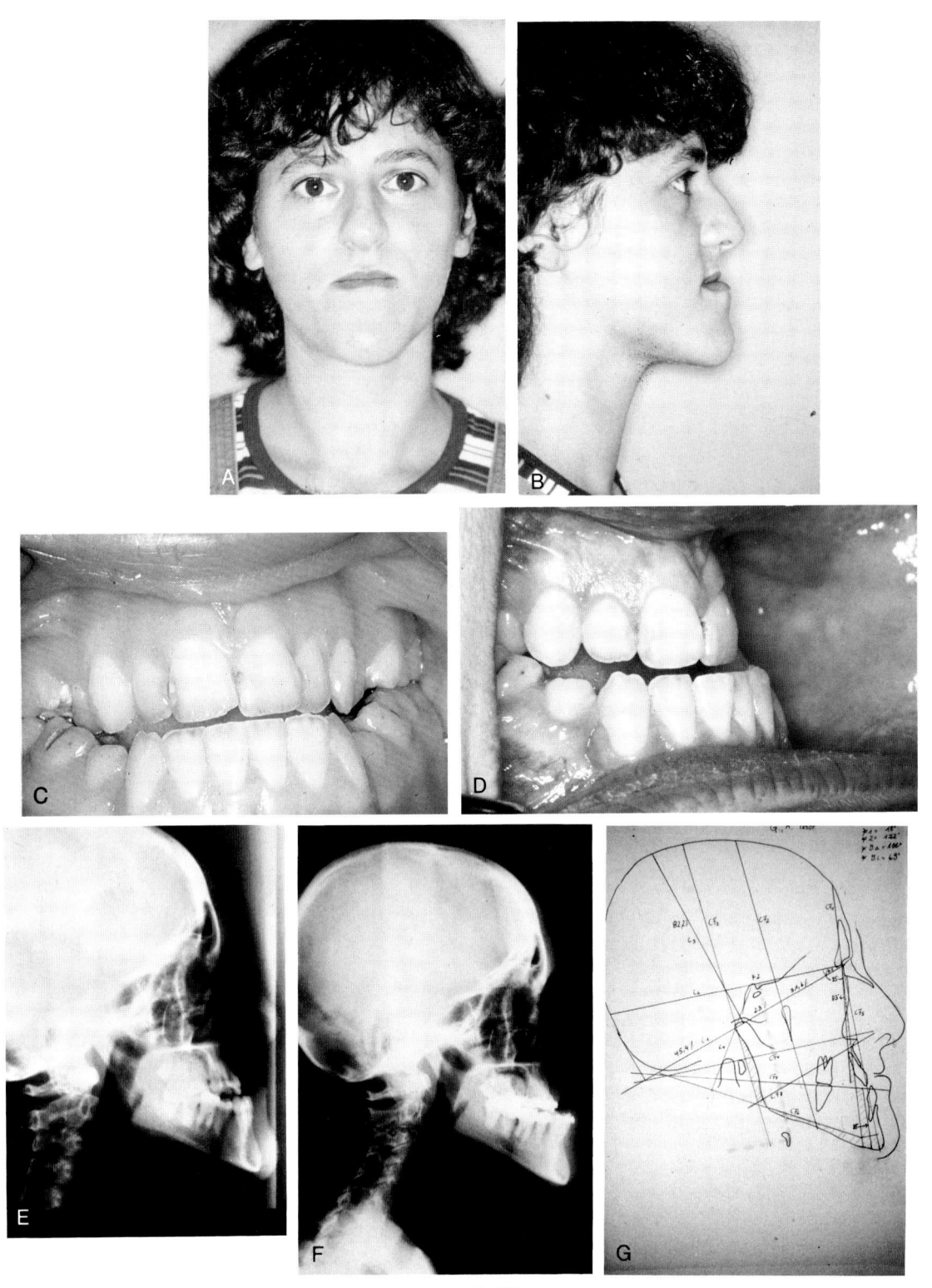

FIGURE 60-59.

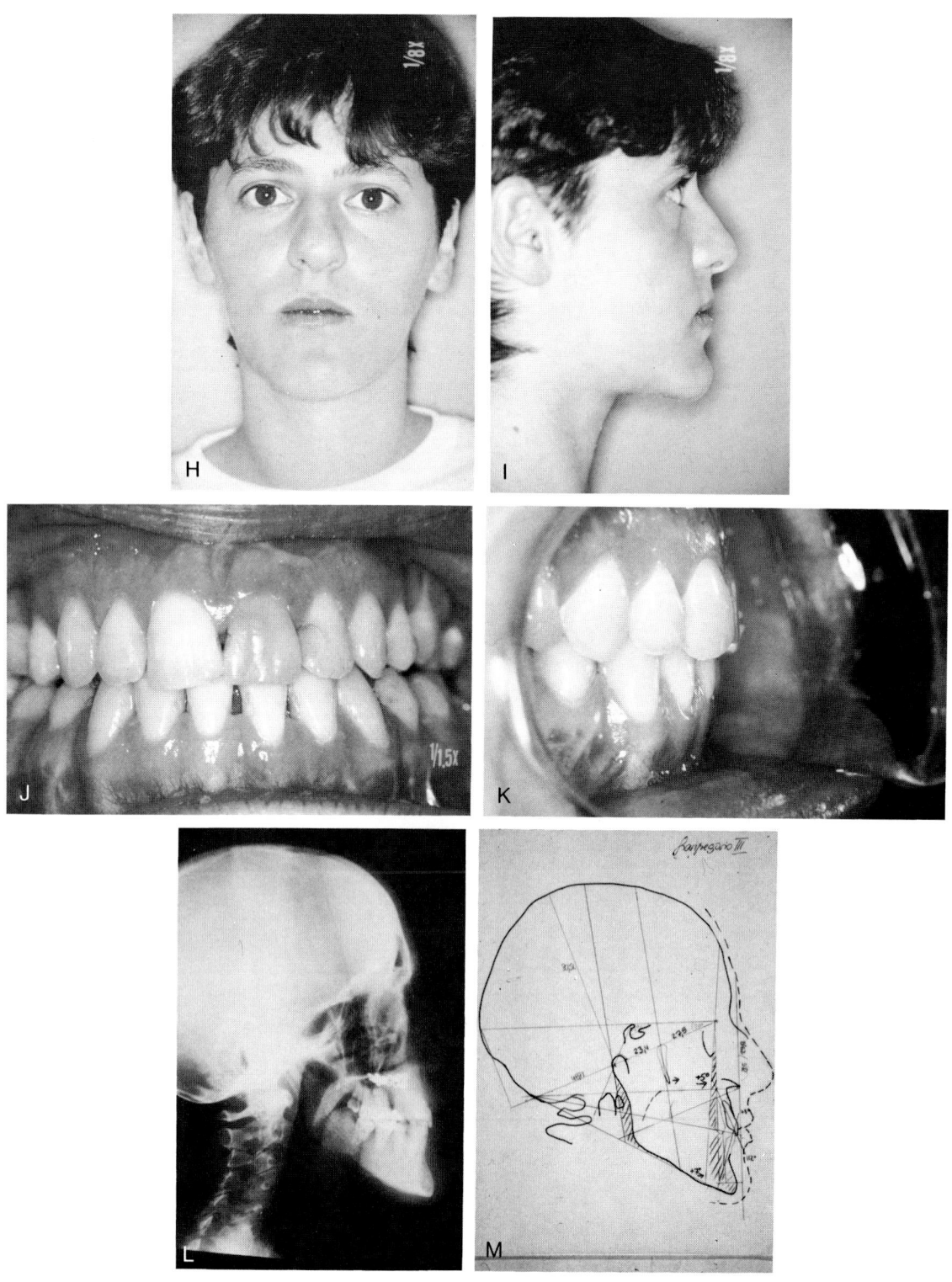

FIGURE 60-59 *Continued.*

2102 / VII — ORTHOGNATHIC SURGERY

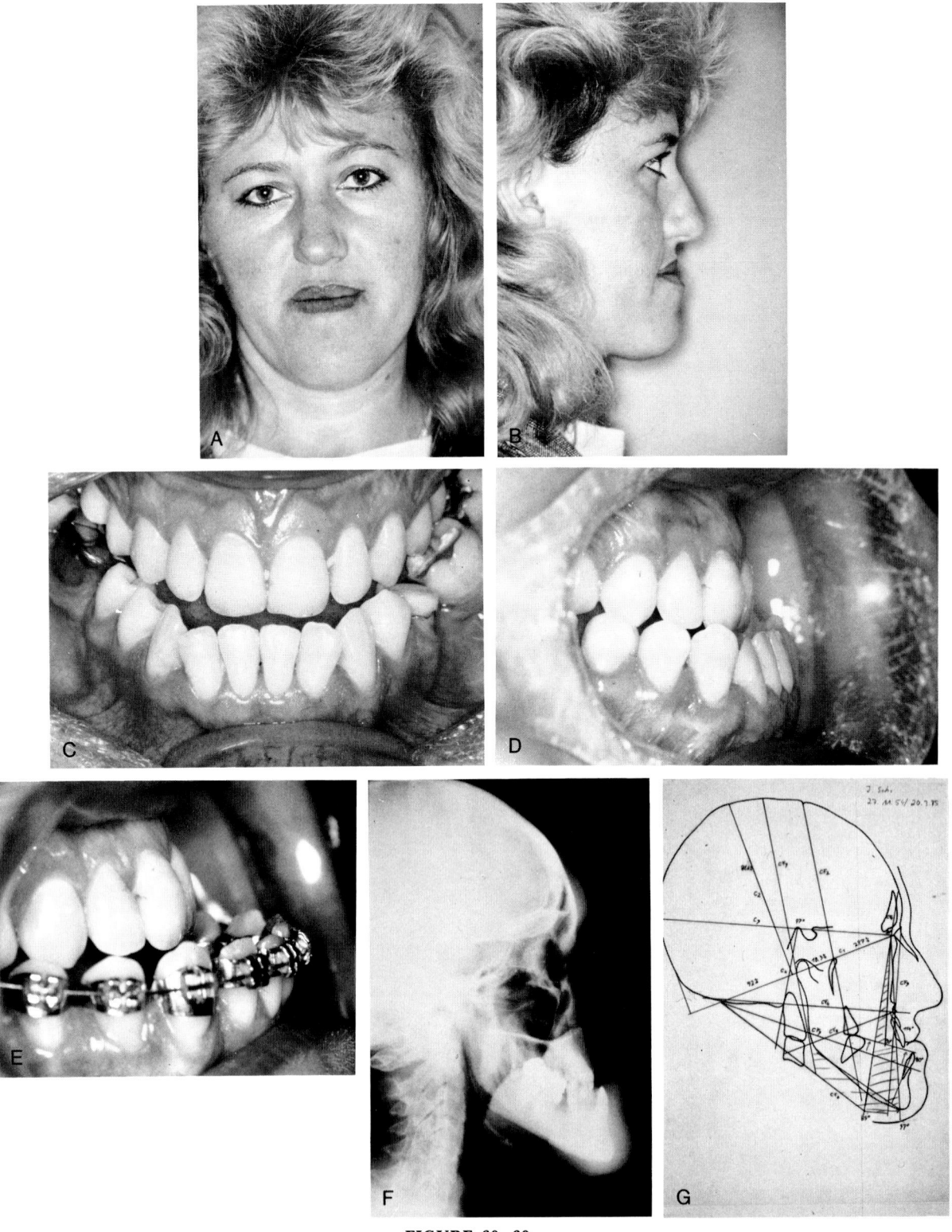

FIGURE 60-60.

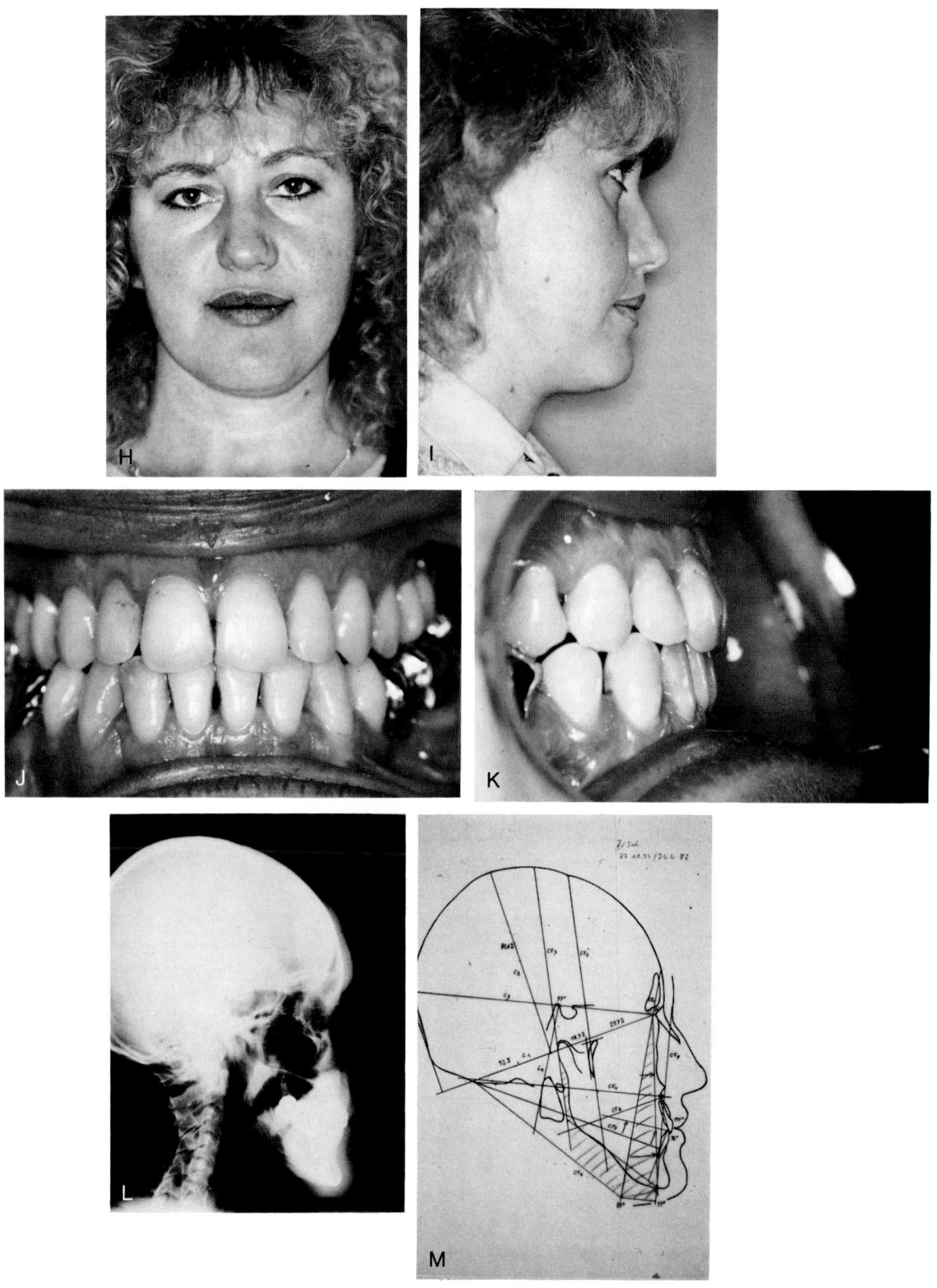

60 — SURGICAL MANAGEMENT OF SKELETAL OPEN BITE BY RAMUS OSTEOTOMIES / **2103**

FIGURE 60–60 *Continued.*

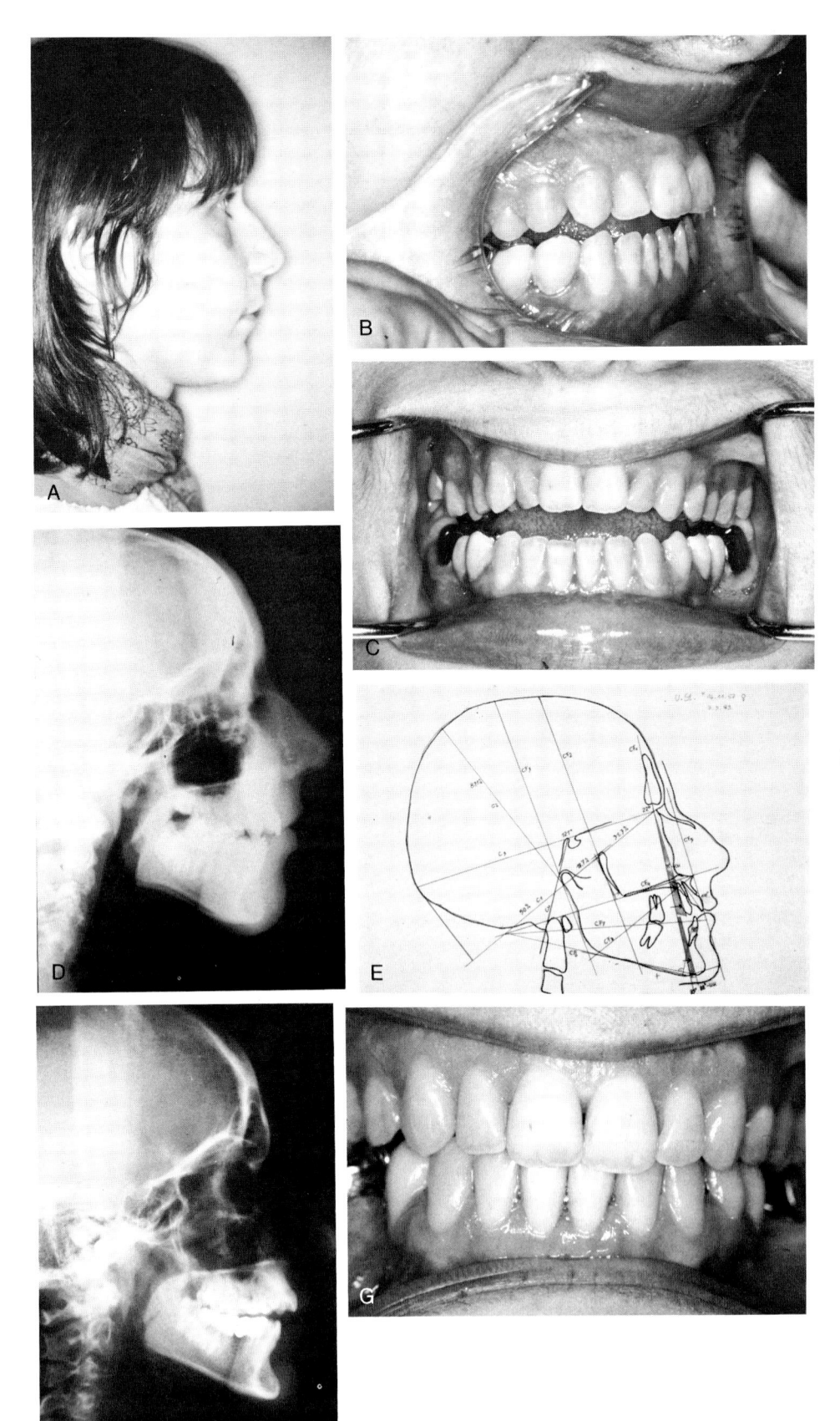

FIGURE 60–61.

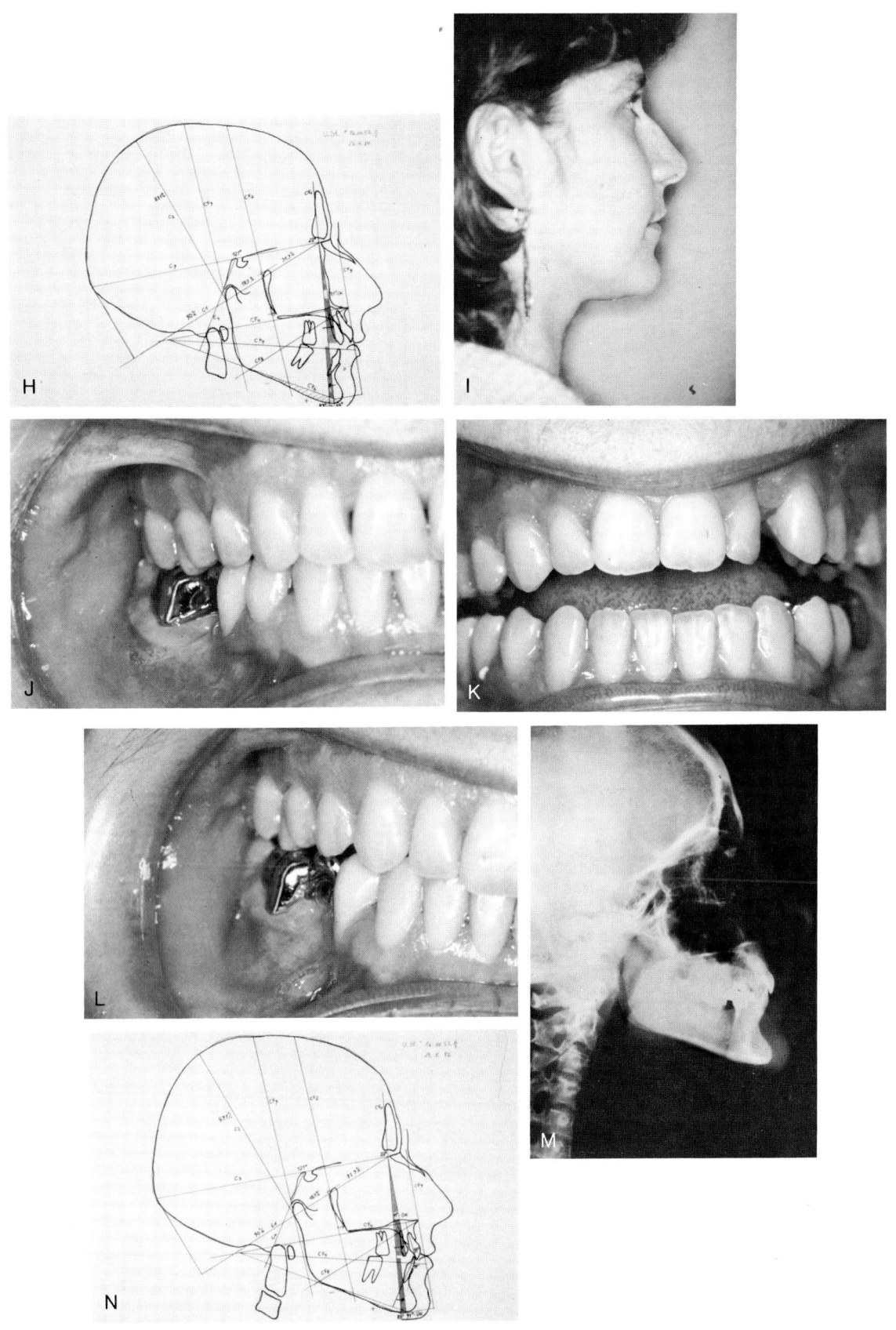

FIGURE 60–61 *Continued.*

2106 / VII — ORTHOGNATHIC SURGERY

CASE 7: CLASS II MALOCCLUSION WITH SKELETAL OPEN BITE

PROBLEM LIST

Esthetics: long lower face with open bite, lip incompetence, tongue positioned between teeth (Fig. 60–62A and B).

Occlusion: open bite with contact only between the molars (Fig. 60–62C).

Cephalometric Analysis: vertical maxillary deficiency, mandibular retrognathism, open bite (Fig. 60–62D and E).

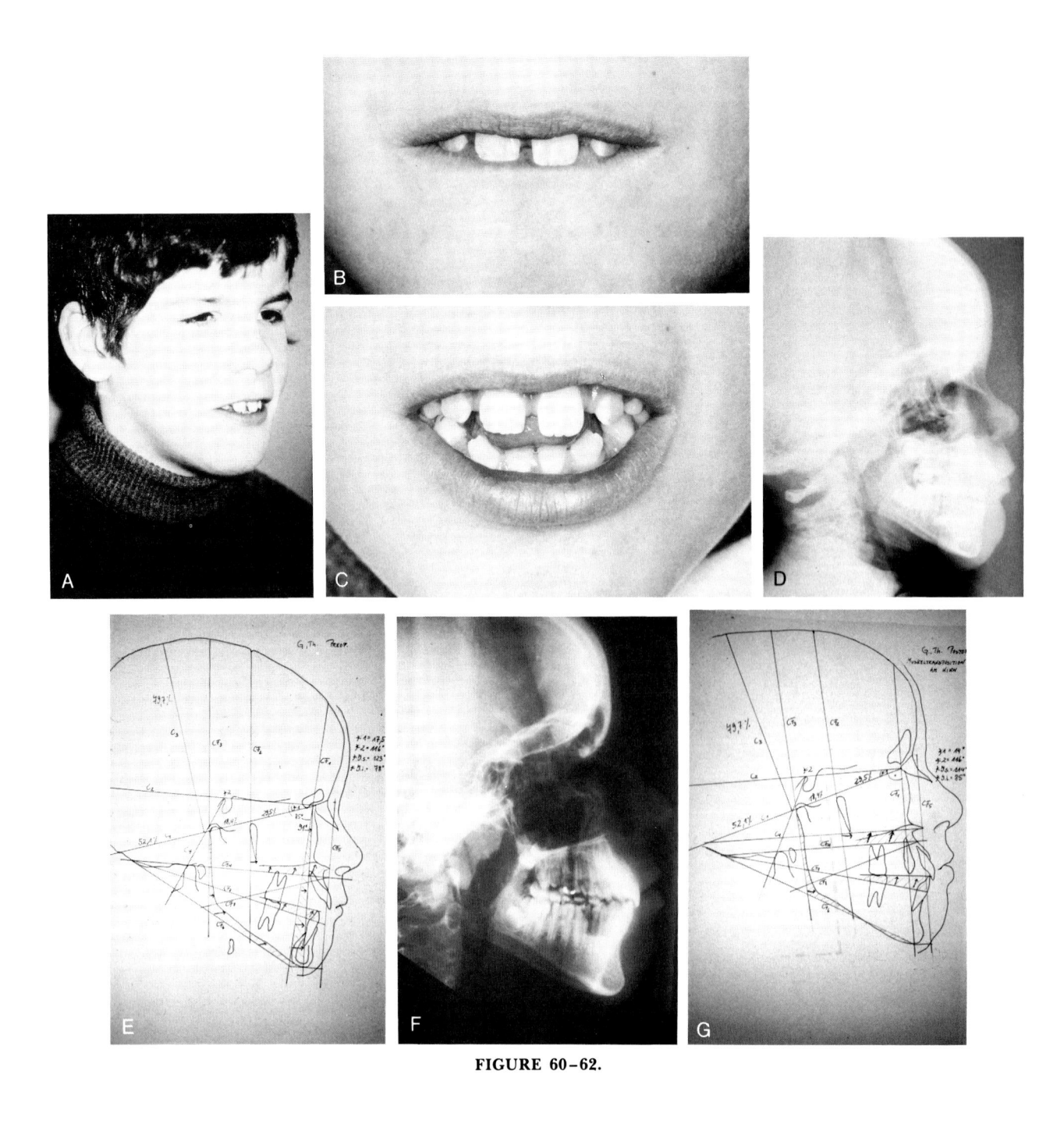

FIGURE 60–62.

TREATMENT PLAN

Orthodontic Treatment: unsuccessful attempt to close the open bite.

Surgical Treatment: moving the chin muscles with soft tissue superiorly; subsequent orthodontic treatment (Fig. 60–62F and G).

COMMENTS

Superior repositioning of the muscles with soft tissue resulted in a spontaneous closure of the open bite. Orthodontic measures were taken to align and level the dental arches.

REFERENCES

1. Epker BN, Fish LC: Surgical-orthodontic correction of open-bite deformity. Am J Orthod 71:278, 1977.
2. Rakosi T: Ätiologie und diagnostische Beurteilung des offenen Bisses. Fortschr Kieferorthop 43:68, 1982.
3. Fränkel R, Fränkel C: Funktionelle Aspekte des skelettalen offenen Bisses. Fortschr Kieferorthop 43:8, 1982.
4. Angle EH: Treatment of Malocclusion of the Teeth: Angle's System. 7th ed. Philadelphia, SS White, 1907.
5. Ballard CF: Variations of posture and behavior of the lips and tongue which determine the position of the labial segments: The implications in orthodontics, prosthetics and speech. Trans Eur Orthod Soc 67: 1965.
6. Linder-Aronson S: Der offene Biss in Relation zum Atmungsfunktion. Fortschr Kieferorthop 44:1, 1983.
7. Jonas I, Mann W, Schlenter W: Hals-Nasen-Ohrenärztliche Befunde beim offenen Biss. Fortschr Kieferorthop 43:127, 1982.
8. Janson M: Basal offener Biss—ein funktionelles Risiko? Fortschr Kieferorthop 43:42, 1982.
9. Stark: Embryologie. 3rd ed. Stuttgart, Georg Thieme Verlag, 1975.
10. Powiertowsky H: Surgery of craniosynostosis in advanced cases. *In* Advances and Technical Standards in Neurosurgery. New York, Springer Verlag, 1974, p 191.
11. Enlow DW: Handbook of Facial Growth. Philadelphia, WB Saunders Company, 1975.
12. Bjork A, Schieller V: Postnatal growth and development of the maxillary complex. *In* James A, McNamara Jr (eds): Factors Affecting the Growth of the Midface. Ann Arbor, MI, University of Michigan, 1976, p 61.
13. Brodie AG: On the growth pattern of the human head. Am J Anat 68:209, 1941.
14. Moss ML, Salentijn L: The primary role of functional matrices in facial growth. Am J Orthod 55:566, 1969.
15. Delaire J: La croissance des os de la vonte du crane. Principes généreaux. Rev Stomatol 62:518, 1961.
16. Joos U, Gilsbach J, Werkmeister R: The development of the midface in premature craniosynostosis treated by radical osteoclastic bone removal. Presented at the 4th International Hamburger Symposium on Kraniofaziale Anomalien und Lippen-Kiefer-Gaumenspalten, Hamburg, 1987.
17. Latham RA: An appraisal of the early maxillary growth mechanism. *In* James A, McNamara Jr (eds): Factors Affecting the Growth of the Midface. Ann Arbor, MI, University of Michigan, 1976, p 169.
18. Moss ML: The role of the nasal septal cartilage in midfacial growth. *In* James A, McNamara Jr (eds): Factors Affecting the Growth of the Midface. Ann Arbor, MI, University of Michigan, 1976, p 196.
19. Delaire J: Considerations sur la croissance faciale. Déductions therapeutiques. Rev Stomatol 72:57, 1971.
20. Scott JH: The cartilage of the nasal septum. Br Dent J 95:37, 1953.
21. Delaire J, Feve R, Chateau JP, et al: Anatomie et physiologie des muscles et du frein de la lèvre supérieure. Rev Stomatol 78:93, 1977.
22. Joos U, Friedburg M: Darstellung des Verlaufs der mimischen Muskulatur in der Kernspintomographie. Fortschr Kiefer Gesichtschir 32:125, 1987.
23. Sarnat BG: Growth of bones as revealed by implant markers in animals. Am J Phys Anthrop 29:225, 1968.
24. Delaire J: La cheilo-rhinoplastie primaire pour fente labio-maxillaire congénitale unilaterale. Rev Stomatol 76:193, 1975.
25. Joos U: The importance of muscular reconstruction in the treatment of cleft lip and palate. Scand J Plast Reconstr Surg 21:109, 1987.
26. Obwegeser H: Der offene Biss in chirurgischer Sicht. Schweiz Monatsschr Zahnheilk 74:668, 1964.
27. Subtelny D, Sakuda M: Open-bite: Diagnostics and treatment. Am J Orthodont 50:337, 1964.
28. Hullihen SP: Case of elongation of under jaw and distortion of face and neck, caused by burn, successfully treated. Am J Dent Sci 9:157, 1849.
29. Lane WA: Cleft Palate and Hare Lips. London, London Medical Publishing Company, 1906.

Before the osteotomy is performed, the panoramic radiograph of the ramus should also be reviewed to verify the location of the mandibular foramen. The bone cut is made with a Stryker oscillating saw using a rounded, angled blade that can make a cut 6 to 7 mm deep. The cut should begin 6 to 7 mm from the posterior border (Fig. 61–6G). When the posterior border is curved medially, it may be difficult to visualize directly. One way to identify the posterior border is to feel it with the saw blade or the curved tip of a small instrument, such as a Freer elevator. Another, but less reliable, aid in locating the foramen is the small protuberance of bone typically found on the lateral surface opposite the foramen. Once the cut is made into the lateral cortex, it is prudent to recheck distance from the posterior border by feeling the cut with the end of a curved Freer elevator or nerve hook. Since the inferior alveolar nerve is medial to the ramus before it enters the foramen, even if the blade cuts into the groove, the neurovascular bundle should not be injured if the oscillating saw blade protrudes through the bone only a couple of millimeters. Once this initial cut has been made, it may be extended in both directions without fear of damage to the neurovascular bundle. The osteotomy is carried superior and slightly anterior to the midportion of the sigmoid notch. The Bauer retractor protects the masseteric artery and nerve. If the planned retrusion is small (up to 5 mm), the inferior cut can be carried parallel and slightly anterior to the posterior border. If the planned retrusion is greater, the osteotomy is angled progressively in an anterior direction (Fig. 61–6G). If the cut is curved forward greatly, the blade should be removed from the bone cut posterior to the mandibular nerve to establish the new direction. Trying to curve the bone cut without removing the blade generally results in a broken blade or an inadequate amount of forward angulation. If the proximal segment is not free, the cut usually has not extended into the sigmoid notch, or, more commonly, through the inferior border.

As the osteotomy is completed, the proximal segment is usually displaced laterally slightly, signaling completion of the cut. The segment is displaced further laterally by pulling the mandible forward and inserting a periosteal elevator between the segment and the ramus (Fig. 61–6H). The elevator is used to move the segment laterally and to stabilize it while portions of the medial pterygoid muscle and periosteum are stripped from the most anterior part of the medial surface, leaving muscle attached along the posterior border. The amount of periosteum and muscle reflected from the proximal segment is largely a function of the degree of anticipated overlap and width of the proximal segment. The goal is to obtain an overlapping surface with little change in the sagittal rotation in the proximal segment while maintaining an adequate pedicle of medial pterygoid muscle. The gently curved or angled osteotomy maintains about a 1-cm-wide bony segment at the angle. It is important to leave the full length of the muscle attachment along the posterior border (Fig. 61–6I), especially to prevent even a few millimeters of "sag" of the condyle. The muscle fibers near the posterior border, especially inferiorly and including the stylomandibular ligament, are tenaciously attached and are less likely to be inadvertently stripped from the proximal segment than are more anterior fibers. The proximal segment is placed lateral to the ramus.

The wound is gently packed with a moist gauze sponge, and a similar procedure is performed on the other side. After the second osteotomy is completed, the mouth is irrigated, the throat pack is removed, and the mandible is placed in its predetermined position. If a coronoidotomy is required because of a large retrusion of the mandible, a periosteal elevator is passed to the sigmoid notch on the medial aspect of the ramus. With the soft tissue thus protected by the elevator, the coronoid is easily sectioned with a drill or reciprocating saw at the level of the sigmoid notch and allowed to retract with the temporalis muscle. The teeth are fixed in occlusion with maxillomandibular wires, and the extent of contact between the proximal and distal segments of the rami is observed (Fig. 61–6J). There is usually some degree of interference of the two segments, which prevents good lateral approximation. Any interference is almost always at the posterosuperior aspect of the distal segment. The interference should be removed with a large rotary cutting instrument by beveling the lateral surface of the osteotomy site of the distal segment and/or the medial surface of the proximal segment. The medial soft tissues are protected from the rotary cutting instrument with a wide periosteal elevator to avoid bleeding. Sometimes a substantial portion of the sigmoid notch area of the distal segment must be removed to achieve good approximation of the two segments. Either vacuum drains or, more often, pressure dressings are placed over the lateral border of the ascending ramus to minimize hematoma formation. If drains are used, they exit through small punch incisions in the skin anterior to the angle of the mandible. Short-term, high-dose steroid therapy is also used to minimize swelling. The proximal segments are examined again to ensure that they are lateral to and approximate the rami. The wound is irrigated and closed in standard fashion.

Rigid Fixation

Rigid fixation is uncommonly used with IVRO. There seem to be several reasons. First, the use of MMF gives predictably good results. Second, the inconvenience of MMF may often be limited to as little as 3 to 4 weeks when other factors that tend to cause relapse are controlled. Further, there are disadvantages to rigid fixation, including technical difficulty, longer operating time, a cheek incision, and less precision in obtaining the planned occlusion. Nonetheless, rigid fixation does have advantages. It is an obvious convenience for patients when MMF can be avoided entirely or for, at most, 7 to 10 days. Early mobilization of the jaw also seems to speed the rehabilitation process, at least for range of motion. Rigid fixation of the mandible also reduces the relapse tendency and, in the case of combined maxillary and mandibular fixation, provides support for a maxilla that for various reasons may have only semirigid fixation. If a maxilla as well as a mandible is not firmly fixated, the relapsing force of the mandible during MMF is not dissipated into the maxilla only as orthodontic movement of the teeth. Rather, this force may be dissipated primarily as skeletal movement of the maxilla and mandible.

Perhaps the best current indications for rigid fixation with IVRO are large retrusions, reduction of the edentulous prognathic mandible, and combined maxillary and mandibular surgery. With large retrusions, the relapse tendency is greater, and rigid fixation would likely provide more stability. For the edentulous mandible, elimination of the use of uncomfortable splints for MMF is a significant advantage. Furthermore, small errors in seating the condyle with rigid fixation have no occlusal consequence, since dentures must be constructed subsequently. The problem of minor occlusal discrepancy resulting from imprecise seating of the condyle can also be eliminated or minimized with combined maxillary and mandibular surgery. Especially if wire osteosynthesis is used in the maxilla, about 10 days of MMF allows minor movement of the maxilla as the jaw muscles seat the condyle. Thus, skeletal movement of the maxilla occurs, but the occlusion is unchanged. When bone plates provide only semirigid fixation, as when maxillary bone contact is poor, a short period of MMF also allows for some adjustment of the maxilla and perhaps the teeth, with the maintenance of a more predictable occlusion.

Either screw fixation[45] or bone plate fixation[22] may be used, although screw fixation is limited to retrusions with larger overlap of the segments. In either case, however, a small cheek incision is required with current instrumentation. Furthermore, plates must be used when (5 to 6 mm or less) retrusion of the mandible is minimal, as is often the case. If the retrusion is greater, more overlap of bone is present, and either bicortical screw fixation or plates may be used.

For small retrusions, the mandible is secured in position with MMF. Interferences between the proximal and distal segments are removed to permit passive approximation of the segments. A T-shaped bone plate is bent to lie passively when the proximal segment is positioned lateral to the distal segment. The top of the T is secured to the proximal segment with two bicortical self-tapping screws. An instrument such as a bone plate–holding forceps is used to position the bone plate and proximal segment. Proper positioning involves seating the condyle and rotating the segment in the sagittal plane until it approximates its original position. The remaining two bicortical screws are placed in the distal segment, taking care to avoid the inferior alveolar nerve (Fig. 61–7). The MMF is released, and reproducibility of the occlusion is determined. If occlusion is not as desired, the proximal segment should be repositioned. It probably is wise to maintain MMF for 7 to 10 days, even in single-jaw osteotomies.

For larger retrusions, for which there is more overlap of the segments, self-tapping bicortical screws can be placed through a cheek incision. After removing interferences to permit passive positioning of the proximal segment lateral to the ramus, an instrument is used to position the segment. A single bicortical screw is placed inferiorly below the inferior alveolar nerve. The positioning instrument can be removed and two additional bicortical screws placed, again avoiding the inferior alveolar nerve (Fig. 61–8). The remainder of the procedure is as described above.

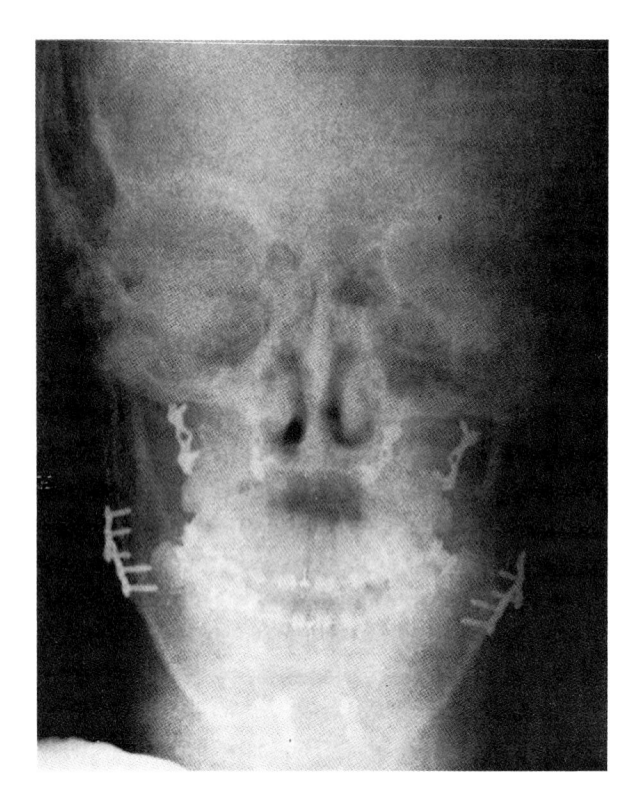

FIGURE 61–7. Anteroposterior (AP) cephalometric radiograph showing use of bone plates with IVRO. (From Kraut RA: Stabilization of the intraoral vertical osteotomy using small bone plates. J Oral Maxillofac Surg 46:908, 1988; with permission.)

FIGURE 61–8. PA radiograph of mandible showing rigid fixation for edentulous mandible with 10-mm retrusion. One year after operation. Three bicortical screws 2 mm in diameter were used on each side.

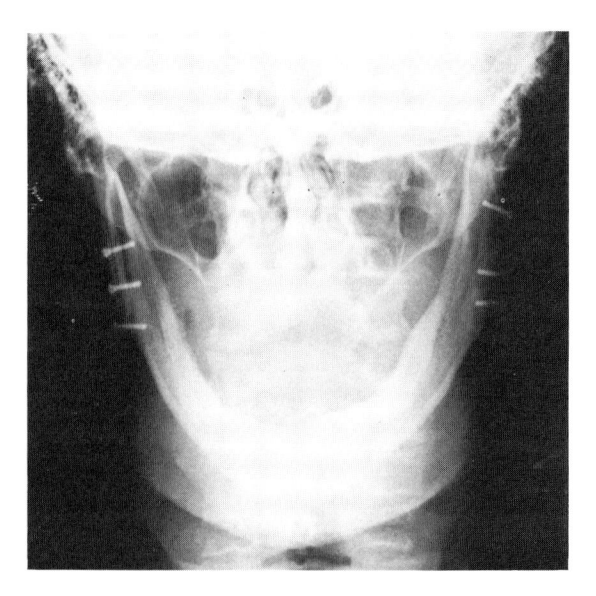

LARGE RETRUSIONS

Large retrusions (greater than 1 cm) can be performed well with the intraoral approach. The coronoid process must be sectioned to prevent interference with the condyle when the mandible is retruded. Cephalometric prediction tracings of the repositioned mandible permit design of the osteotomy to achieve maximal overlap of the segments and minimal clockwise rotation of the proximal segment. The bone cut inferior to the mandibular foramen should curve forward (see Fig. 61–6G). All but the most posterior and inferior portions of the medial pterygoid muscle are detached. This maneuver minimizes opening or clockwise rotation of the proximal segment when the mandible is retruded against the muscle, reducing relapse tendency. The broad overlap of the segments also makes screw fixation easier.

Inverted-L Osteotomy

The intraoral inverted-L osteotomy is an alternative to IVRO, especially for correction of extreme mandibular prognathism when coronoidotomy would be required. A theoretical advantage of this procedure is that both the temporalis and the pterygoid muscles remain attached to the proximal segments, except for the deep tendon of the temporalis muscle, which may be cut. Consequently, the vector of the anterior, superior, and medial pull of the muscles tends to maintain the preoperative spatial relationship of the proximal segment and to hold the condyle in the glenoid fossa. The temporalis and medial pterygoid muscles also stabilize the proximal segment. Carefully executed cephalometric prediction analyses to simulate the planned movements with acetate overlay tracings should be performed to maximize the chance that the horizontal osteotomies of the proximal and distal segments will be juxtaposed or overlap rather than create a gap.

SURGICAL TECHNIQUE

The procedure for the inverted-L, osteotomy (Fig. 61–9A to D) is the same as that for IVRO except for the osteotomy superior to the mandibular foramen. Instead of continuing the vertical cut to the sigmoid notch, the cut ends above the mandibular foramen. The horizontal cut can be made with either a reciprocating saw or a fine fissure bur, taking care to protect the medial soft tissues. If the mandible is cut too close to the sigmoid notch, it is easy to fracture into the sigmoid notch, especially if injudicious force is exerted on the proximal segment during separation. A fracture converts the inverted L into an IVRO with coronoidotomy. The remainder of the procedure is as described for IVRO, including use of rigid fixation.

SAGITTAL SPLIT RAMUS OSTEOTOMY

Indications

The general indications for SSRO are the same as for IVRO in the treatment of mandibular excess. The perceived advantage of a greater area of bone contact between the proximal and distal segments, resulting in more rapid healing and thus stability, has not been borne out by studies.[35,48] The use of rigid fixation, however, is easier and certainly has a wider use with SSRO than with IVRO. The substantially higher incidence of damage to the inferior alveolar nerve is the chief argument against selection of SSRO over IVRO. Nerve damage is an especially important consideration in adults, since nerves in older patients have a diminished capacity for recovering from injury.[25,31] Biologic considerations and evaluation of the surgical site for SSRO are discussed in Chapter 64.

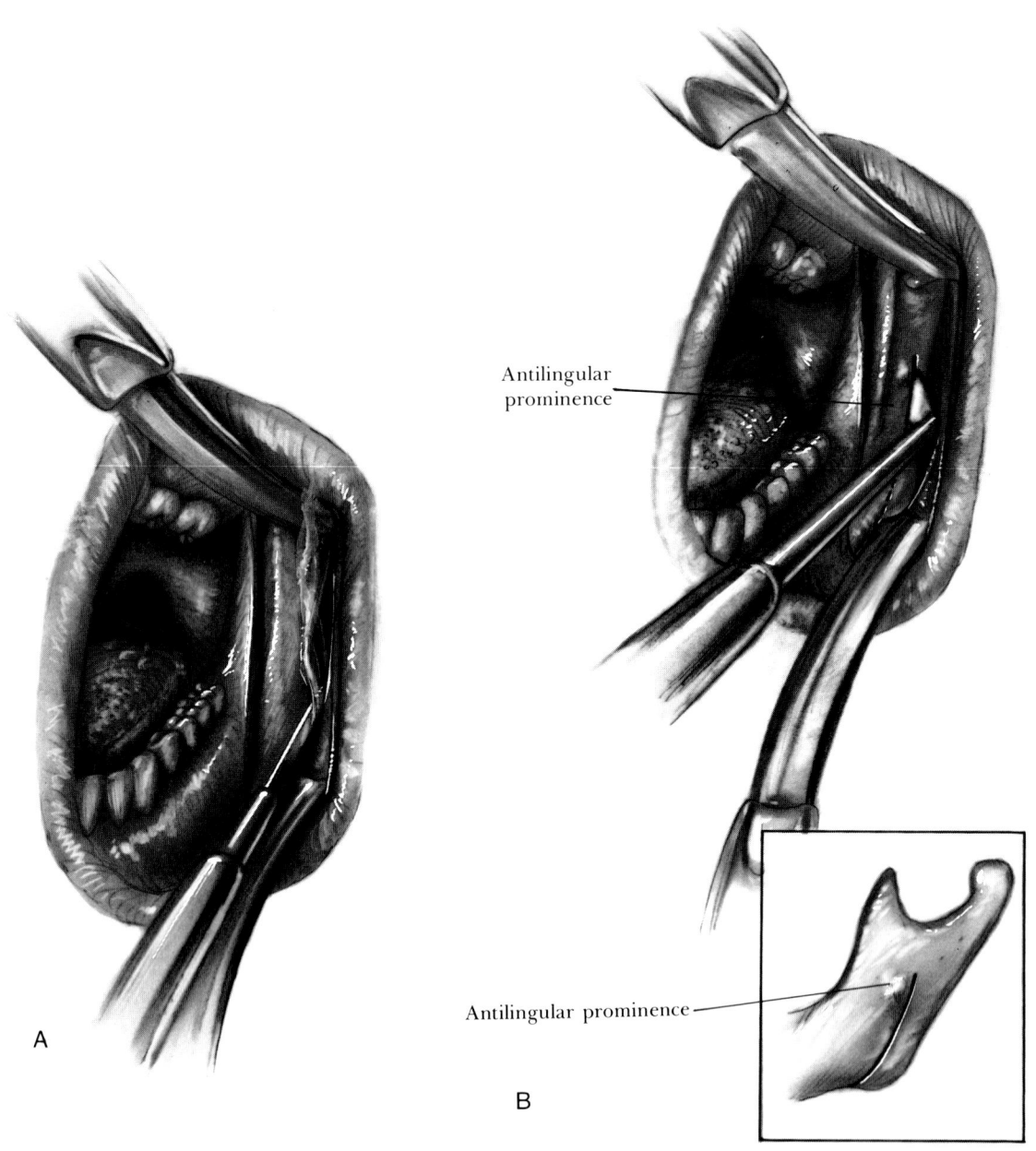

FIGURE 61-9. SURGICAL TECHNIQUE FOR CORRECTION OF MANDIBULAR EXCESS BY INTRAORAL "INVERTED-L" OSTEOTOMY. *A*, Bauer retractors are positioned in the sigmoid and antegonial notches. The periosteal sheath posterior to the vertical ramus is incised to expose the medial pterygoid-masseter muscle sling to facilitate subsequent retrusion of the distal segment. *B*, The vertical portion of the osteotomy is made with a rounded oscillating saw blade. The line of the osteotomy extends inferiorly to the antegonial notch from a point 2 to 4 mm superior and immediately posterior to the antilingular prominence. *C*, A periosteal elevator is positioned on the medial aspect of the ramus opposite the planned horizontal osteotomy to protect the neurovascular bundle and lingual soft tissues. A horizontal osteotomy is made with either a reciprocating saw blade or a laminectomy bur with the anterior aspect of the ascending ramus. Posteriorly, the horizontal osteotomy is made approximately 2 to 4 mm above the antilingular prominence. *D*, The proximal segment is elevated laterally. The medial pterygoid muscle is detached as necessary from the medial aspect of the proximal and distal segments to facilitate retrusion of the distal segment. (From Bell WH, Proffit WR, White RP Jr: Surgical Correction of Dentofacial Deformities. Vol II. Philadelphia, WB Saunders Company, 1985, pp 896–897; with permission.)

61 — MANDIBULAR PROGNATHISM / 2123

Antilingular prominence

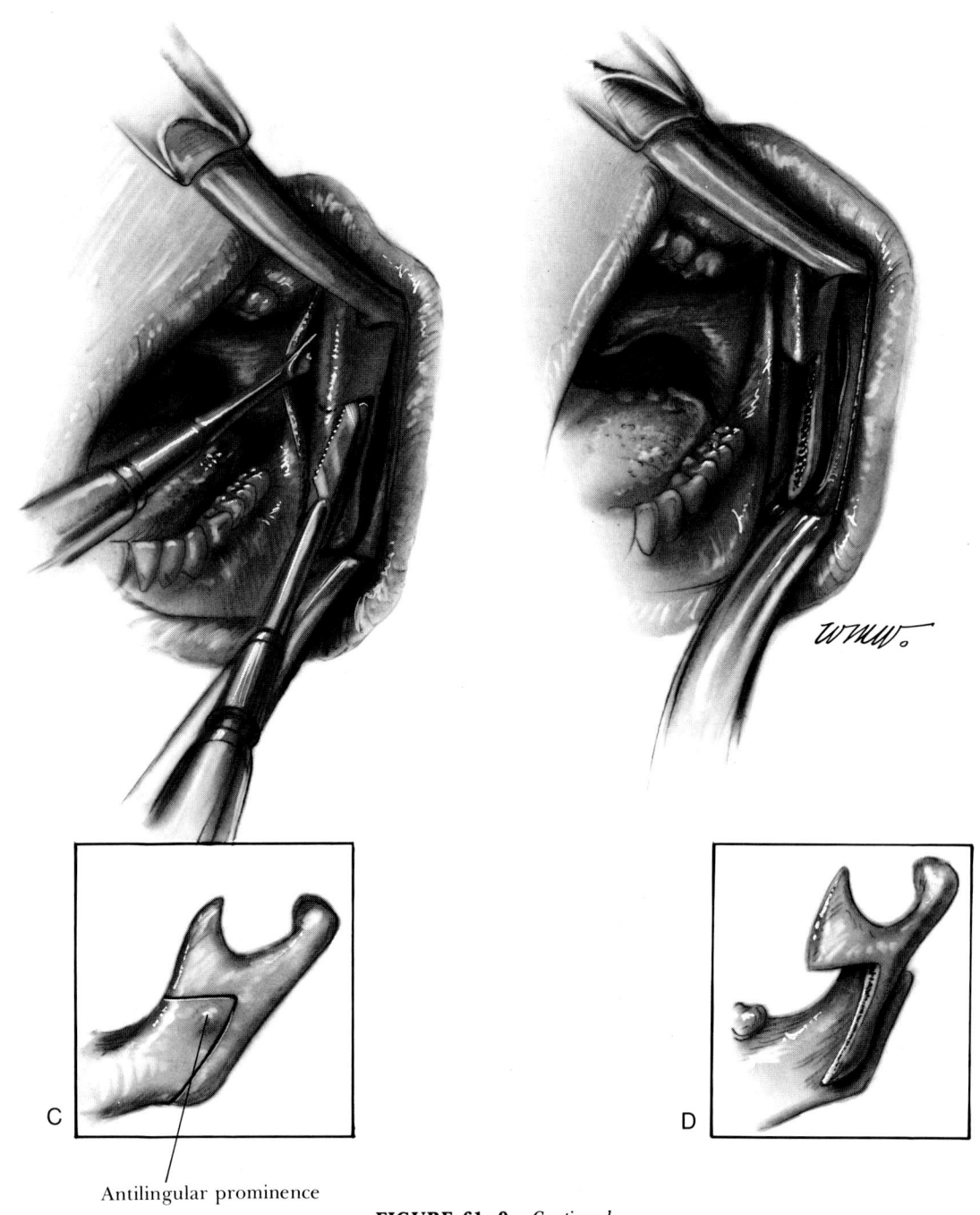

FIGURE 61-9. *Continued*

Surgical Technique

When the patient is ready for operation, a bite block is placed between the teeth on the contralateral side of the mouth. Epinephrine, 1 : 100,000, is infiltrated along the lateral oblique ridge and medial aspect of the ramus superior to the mandibular foramen. An incision through mucosa and periosteum is made over the oblique ridge, starting at the level of the occlusal plane, and is continued forward for about 3 cm close to the mucogingival junction (Fig. 61–10A). This practice reduces the possibility of the development of a scar band that may later serve as a food trap in the sulcus. A notched ramus retractor is placed over the oblique ridge, and considerable pressure is exerted over the notched end as the retractor is moved superiorly (Fig. 61–10B). This measure strips soft tissues away from the periosteum and moves the buccal nerve superiorly and, at the same time, minimizes herniation of the buccal fat pad into the wound. A curved Kocher clamp is placed at the most superior portion of the incision, to serve as a retractor (Fig. 61–10C). The periosteum and temporalis tendon are incised vertically along the anterior border of the ramus, and the incision is carried inferiorly along the oblique ridge to the anterior wound margin. The periosteum is carefully reflected from the medial aspect of the mandible between the mandibular foramen and sigmoid notch (Fig. 61–10D). There is frequently a medial ridge along the anterior border, and care must be exercised with an elevator to avoid perforating the periosteum as it is reflected from bone posterior to the ridge. The periosteal reflection is extended to the posterior ramus and from the sigmoid notch to the lingula. Either a periosteal elevator or a ribbon retractor may be used to retract the medial tissues superior to the lingula (Fig. 61–10E). A stiff ribbon retractor, slightly curved on the end, may be rotated with the inferior portion contacting bone superior to the lingula, thereby protecting the neurovascular bundle from the bur during the medial bone cut. If there is a ridge on the medial aspect of the ramus that obscures vision of the posterior aspect of the medial ramus, a large watermelon-shaped bur is used to reduce the ridge where the cut is to be made, in order to provide better vision. The location of the cut is determined by the location of the neurovascular bundle inferiorly and by the thickness of the anterior border of the ramus. The cut should be started low enough on the anterior border of the ramus so that there clearly are medial and lateral plates. A laminectomy or similar bur is placed parallel to the occlusal plane against the medial aspect of the mandible, with the end of the bur about 5 mm posterior to the neurovascular bundle. The drill is activated, and the cut is extended through the medial cortex, but not into the lateral cortex. A long fissure bur is then used to make a series of drill holes into the anterior border of the ramus and lateral oblique ridge extending inferiorly from the medial cut (Fig. 61–10F). These holes are placed a few millimeters apart and at the level of the medial aspect of the lateral cortex. Holes are placed about as far as the distal aspect of the first molar and then connected using the fissure bur. The medial retractor and the Kocher clamp are removed. The anterior portion of the periosteal incision is reflected along the lateral border of the mandible from the most anterior aspect of the wound, posteriorly to the angle of the mandible, and inferiorly to the inferior border. A Hargis or channel retractor is placed in the wound, with the tip engaging the inferior border. A fissure bur is used to make the vertical cut (Fig. 61–10G). This vertical cut is usually made at about the mesial aspect of the second molar. The cut is progressively deepened until bleeding marrow is seen. Because the inferior alveolar nerve and neurovascular bundle are immediately deep to the cortical bone, the cut should stop as soon as bleeding bone is seen. A special inferior border saw blade is attached to the reciprocating Stryker saw and is used to cut into or through the inferior border, extending posteriorly from the vertical bone cut for 1 to 1.5 cm (Fig. 61–10H). The medial ramus retractor is replaced, and a fine osteotome is used to separate the medial and lateral cortical plates from the anterior border to the area posterior to the lingula, taking

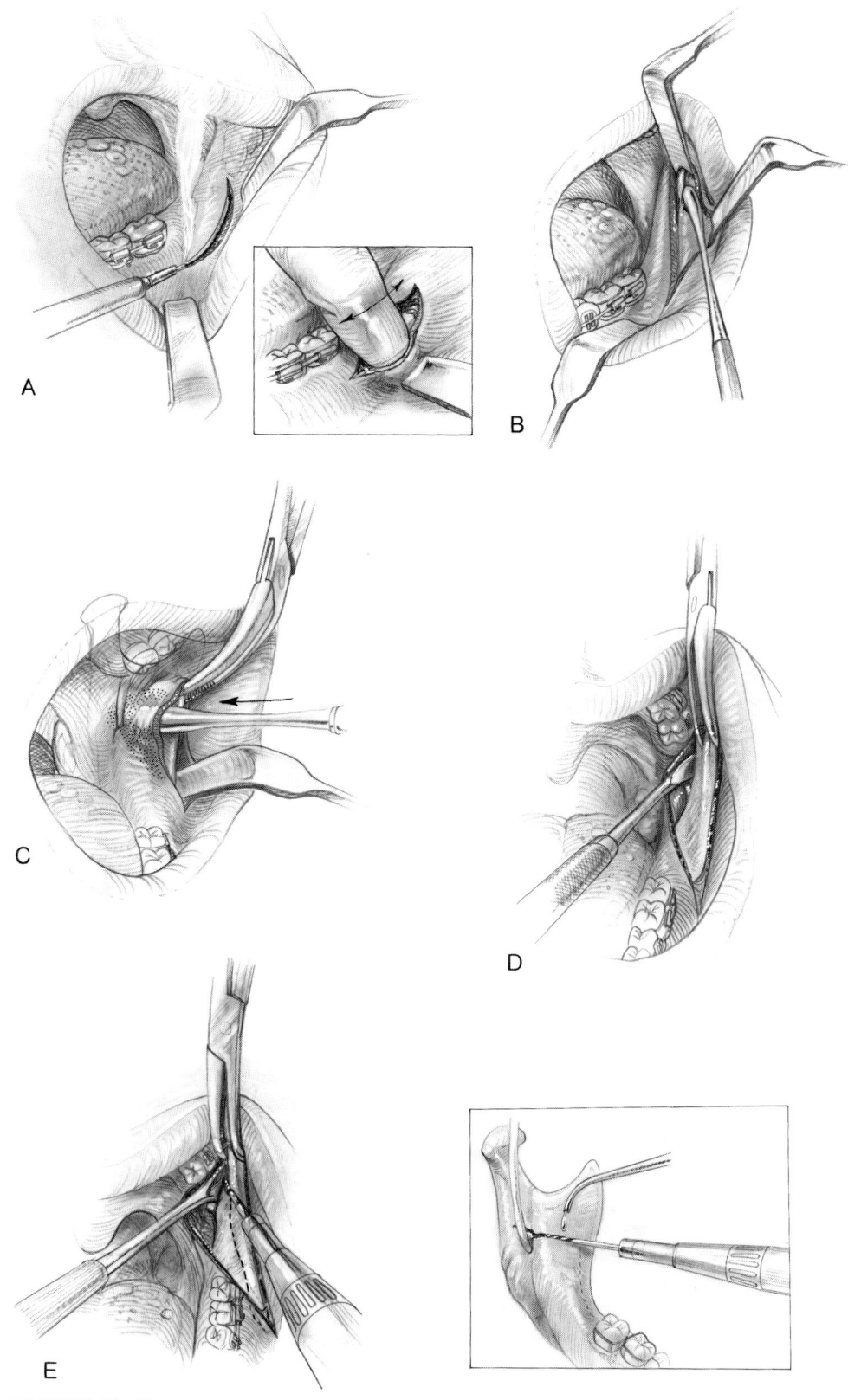

FIGURE 61–10. SURGICAL TECHNIQUE FOR CORRECTION OF MANDIBULAR EXCESS BY SAGITTAL SPLIT RAMUS OSTEOTOMY (SSRO). *A*, Mucosal incision is made over the external oblique ridge. *B*, A notched retractor against the coronoid. An elevator helps reflect the temporalis tendon. *C, D*, Periosteum is reflected from the anterior and medial aspects of the ramus superior to the lingula. *E*, A laminectomy bur cuts through the medial cortical plate, as shown in the inset.

Illustration continued on following page

The Smith sagittal split separator is placed in the inferior aspect of the anterior lateral cut, and synchronized levering is started with the wedge osteotome and the Smith superior ramus separator, observing for uniform movement of the proximal or lateral segment throughout the entire length of the osteotomy (Fig. 61–10K). If movement is not uniform, the Epker or splitting osteotome should be used again in any area of decreased movement. After uniform movement is obtained, the split or separation is completed, and the neurovascular bundle is identified within the wound. Care should be taken not to allow the tip of the suction to brush against the nerve. If a portion of the neurovascular bundle is entrapped in the mandibular canal of the proximal segment, it must be carefully teased from the proximal segment with curettes. In some cases, a fine interdental osteotome must be used to remove obstructing portions of the inferior alveolar canal. Sometimes the inferior portion of the split in the angle region is incomplete because the cortex bends but does not break. In these instances, osteotomes are placed below the visualized inferior alveolar nerve, and the cut is completed, often with the osteotome directed slightly to the medial side (Fig. 61–10L). The proximal segment is grasped with a Kocher clamp and the distal segment with the other hand, and the two segments are moved anteriorly and posteriorly to verify complete separation (Fig. 61–10M). The medial aspect of the proximal segment is examined for any sharp spicules of bone. If sharp spicules are present, they are removed with a bone file or bur (Fig. 61–10M). The medial pterygoid muscle attachments are separated from the proximal and distal segments. The deep temporalis tendon attached to the distal segment is identified and cut with a knife or scissor. The other side is cut in a similar manner. The mouth is irrigated thoroughly. The throat pack is removed, and the posterior pharynx is suctioned to remove blood and fluids. The mandible is placed in the planned occlusion with the maxilla. MMF is used to maintain the mandible in the proper occlusion.

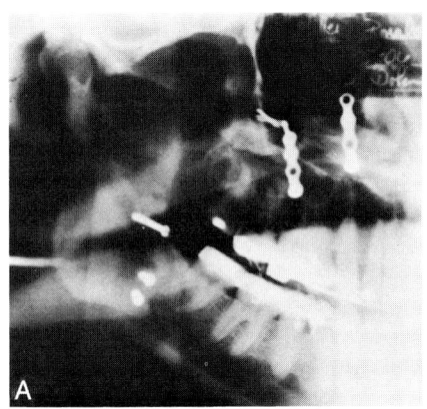

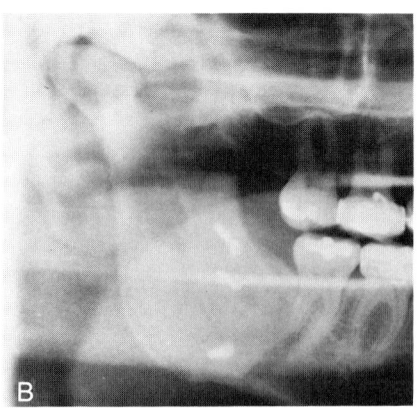

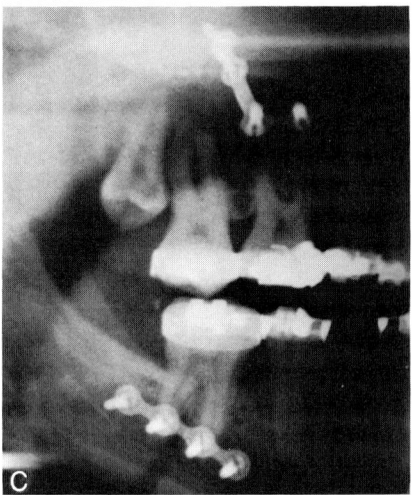

FIGURE 61–11. *A*, Orthopantomograph showing bicortical screws placed transorally with SSRO. *B*, Orthopantomograph showing bicortical screws placed through a cheek incision for SSRO. *C*, Orthopantomograph showing bone plate fixation. (*A* courtesy of B.C. Terry; *C* courtesy of B.C. Rubens.)

The proximal segment is seated firmly in the glenoid fossa, and the degree of overlap is noted. The overlapping bone is removed with either a bone bur or a saw.

If semirigid fixation is to be used, the goals are to prevent rotation of the proximal segment in the sagittal plane, especially counterclockwise rotation, and to allow the masseter, temporalis, and lateral pterygoid muscles attached to the proximal segment to seat the condyle in the glenoid fossa. Use of a slightly loose inferior border wire or a modified bone plate[28] is a good technique to accomplish this purpose.

If rigid fixation is to be used, either screws or plates will fixate the segments. Care is taken to eliminate possible areas of compression when the two segments are approximated and to note the location of the inferior alveolar nerve. The proximal segment is positioned with the condyle seated and the segment rotated in the sagittal plane to approximate the original position. Self-tapping screws may be placed either transorally or transcutaneously (Fig. 61–11A and B). The proximal segment is passively positioned medially against the distal segment. If bone plates are used, the plates must be bent to maintain this passivity. The proximal segment is rotated forward into the mouth for easier access for attachment of the bone plate to the segment. The proximal segment and bone plate are then correctly positioned and secured while two screws are placed in the distal segment (Fig. 61–11C). The reproducibility of the occlusion is examined, and adjustments are made as indicated.

MAXILLOMANDIBULAR FIXATION

The distal segment of the mandible has a strong tendency for opening or clockwise rotation during MMF after surgical procedures in which the ramus is cut, such as IVRO or SSRO (Fig. 61–12). The rotation is apparently secondary to force exerted by the pterygomasseteric sling, although the suprahyoid muscles may have a minor role. With the ramus no longer intact, the molar teeth become a fulcrum. This situation produces a skeletal change consisting of superior movement of the proximal end of the distal segment of the mandible and inferior movement of the chin.[2,21,49] The accompanying change is mild intrusion of the molars and more marked extrusion of the mandibular and maxillary incisor teeth during MMF, providing that these teeth are incorporated into the MMF. It is important to take this force into account when designing MMF. One simple way to counteract this force is to stabilize the mandibular arch bar or wire with a circum-mandibular wire

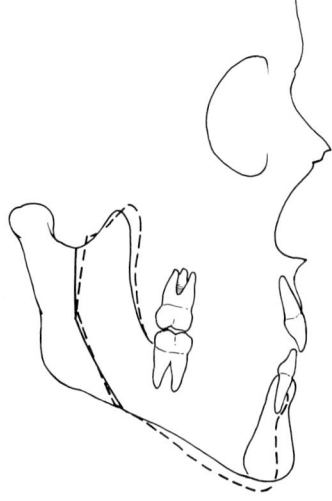

FIGURE 61–12. Clockwise rotation of the distal segment and extrusion of teeth seen after bilateral ramus osteotomy, with maxillomandibular fixation (MMF) as the only fixation technique.

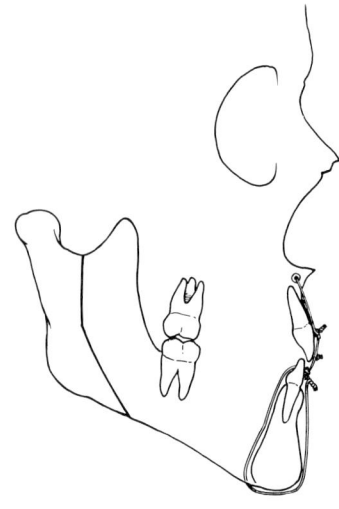

FIGURE 61–13. Placement of wires in the maxilla and mandible for skeletal fixation. This procedure minimizes clockwise rotation of the distal segment.

placed in the symphysis area. A piriform aperture or nasal spine wire serves the same purpose for the maxillary arch bar or wire, that is, transferring this force to bone rather than to the anterior teeth (Fig. 61–13). With anterior skeletal wires, the fulcrum is transferred toward the incisal region. Although there is still superior movement of the proximal end of the distal segment, inferior movement of the chin is minimal. Whatever means of fixation is employed, it is important to understand this tendency for increasing anterior facial height and decreasing posterior facial height and to make appropriate adjustments in the fixation of appliances.

It is almost always wise to construct a thin occlusal splint to guide the mandible into the desired occlusion at the time of surgery. This is especially true if there are any occlusal interferences or if intercuspation of teeth is not good. A splint that does not include the anterior teeth greatly improves speech.

Traditionally, 6 to 8 weeks of MMF has been advocated after IVRO. Recent experience (WH Bell, personal communication, 1989) suggests that 3 to 4 weeks of MMF is sufficient when the mandible is retruded 5 to 6 mm or less. A firm bony union of the overlapping proximal and distal segments is not possible in such a short time, yet the occlusion remains stable. This finding implies that with small retrusions, when there is a minimal change in the position of the mandible, the muscles of mastication do not have a great tendency to displace the segments. Training elastics are used for 2 to 4 weeks after release of MMF and further reduce the stress and strain across the osteotomy site during jaw function. Thus, even though the bony union may not be able to resist great force, it seems sufficiently strong to permit movement of the jaw without loss of the usual degree of stability. For larger retrusions, however, the equilibrium of the muscles of mastication is more disturbed. Thus, in these instances, it seems prudent to maintain the more traditional 6 to 8 weeks of MMF or to use rigid fixation. Until more is known about rigid fixation with IVRO, especially the extent to which it leads to less precise occlusal results, we tend to favor MMF.

If the period of MMF is as long as 6 to 8 weeks and there are minor vertical discrepancies of the teeth, the splint is removed about 2 weeks before MMF is to be discontinued. MMF is immediately reapplied with tight elastics for the remainder of the period of fixation. With elastic MMF, the teeth can be extruded into a better occlusion. If intercuspation is not good and the occlusion is unstable, the occlusal splint should be maintained for the entire period of intermaxillary fixation. After the MMF is released, a single light training elastic is applied in both canine regions for 7 to 28 days. This permits jaw movement, assists closing into the proper occlusion, and reduces stress and strain at the osteotomy site. The elastics are removed for meals and hygiene. If the occlusion is unstable, the orthodontist should become involved in the management of the unstable occlusion immediately. For further guidelines on the use of training elastics and their effects after small mandibular movements, see Chapter 24.

REHABILITATION OF JAW FUNCTION

The goal of rehabilitation is to achieve a good range of motion, adequate bite force, freedom from pain during function, and ability to masticate food well.

The rehabilitation process begins with mobilization of the jaw. This occurs immediately after operation when rigid fixation is used or upon release of MMF, with or without rigid fixation. Both opening and excursive movements are important in achieving good range of motion. Devices that force opening are occasionally used but are not required for good opening.[44,46] It is also possible that the increased load of forced opening might damage articular cartilage in the first 8 to 9 months after mobilization.[44] Six months or longer after IVRO, opening averages about 50 mm[46] without any specific rehabilitation program. There seems to be slightly less vertical opening with SSRO 6 months or more after mobilization of the jaw,[44] but it may be as low as 35 mm.[46] Bite force changes after IVRO and SSRO are largely unknown. Our impression is that patients rarely perceive a decrease in bite force, or at least not enough to interfere with function. With adequate range of motion and bite force, occlusion and pain are the principal factors affecting ability to masticate food well. If pain is present during function, the temporomandibular joint is the chief source. Temporomandibular joint pain, however, is uncommon.[32,43] Internal derangements and condylar position after IVRO or SSRO, both of which can affect joint pain, are addressed later in this chapter. In summary, rehabilitation of range of motion after IVRO or SSRO seems to be good, although it is better with IVRO. Furthermore, the rehabilitation of range of motion does not require special efforts except in uncommon circumstances. This and other goals of rehabilitation are almost always achieved with either operation.

MINIMIZING COMPLICATIONS

Vertical Ramus and Sagittal Split Ramus Osteotomies

NERVE INJURY

The only difference of consequence in complication rates between sagittal split and vertical ramus techniques is the incidence of dysfunction of the inferior alveolar nerve. With the SSRO, the incidence of hypoesthesia or anesthesia is greater[11,54,56,59] than that experienced with the IVRO technique.[1,12,13,59] Surgical experience with the IVRO technique has reduced the already low incidence of inferior alveolar nerve injury to less than 1 per cent (HD Hall, unpublished data, 1989).[59] Moreover, physical damage to the nerve with IVRO procedures appears to be less severe, on the average, than with SSRO, although current technical refinements have also reduced nerve damage after sagittal split ramus procedures. Nonetheless, even experienced surgeons report a 2 to 3.5 per cent incidence of nerve transection[51,52] and up to 85 per cent incidence of long-term dysfunction[25,31,53] with SSRO. In contrast, with IVRO both nerve transection and long-term dysfunction are rare.

The principal cause of nerve trauma with the IVRO procedure is cutting too close to the mandibular foramen and bruising the mandibular nerve or, rarely, transecting it. Cutting too close to the mandibular foramen can usually be avoided by using the posterior border of the ramus as a landmark for the cut. The mandibular foramen is rarely less than 7 mm from the posterior border. A lateral radiograph of the ramus provides additional help in relating the foramen to the border. By using the posterior border of the mandible as a landmark, the cut can be placed to provide for a maximal width of the proximal segment with minimal risk of damage to the inferior alveolar nerve. The risk can be further diminished by use of a saw blade that is only slightly longer than the ramus is thick or by rotating the blade toward the direction of the cut until it is barely protruding through the medial cortex. Even if the neurovascular bundle is near the osteotomy, an oscillating blade would likely cause at most only transitory neuropathy. Rigid fixation is an uncommon cause of inferior alveolar nerve trauma. Visualizing the course of the inferior alveolar nerve from a radiograph and locating the screws posterior and/or inferior to it virtually eliminate the problem. One self-tapping bicortical screw may be placed superior to the mandibular foramen when there is a large retrusion. Finally, a rare cause of inferior alveolar nerve trauma is "trapping" of the proximal segment medial to the ramus.

Although the incidence and severity of nerve damage with SSRO can be reduced by good surgical technique, they remain greater than any of us would wish. Rigid fixation may also cause nerve trauma both by compressing the inferior alveolar nerve and by drilling into the nerve. Both problems may be almost eliminated with care, and the incidence of neuropathy is not appreciably higher after rigid fixation than with MMF alone. Visualizing the course of the nerve from a radiograph and by direct inspection, as well as examining for possible areas of nerve compression, minimizes chances of neurotrauma.

Unfavorable Osteotomy

Only rarely does an unfavorable osteotomy occur with IVRO. If the inferior cut extends to the posterior border rather than the inferior border, the proximal segment is too short. More important, it may have little or no medial pterygoid muscle to hold it in position, with consequent anterior and inferior displacement of the condyle. An unfavorable cut may also injure the inferior alveolar nerve. The unfavorable cut can be avoided by visualizing the entire lateral ramus well, especially near the angle.

An unfavorable osteotomy is more likely to occur with SSRO than IVRO but still is relatively uncommon.

BLEEDING

Intraoperative bleeding is occasionally a nuisance but almost never a problem with either IVRO or SSRO. The bleeding that occurs during IVRO is usually from one or more branches of the maxillary artery just medial to the ramus osteotomy. Bleeding generally can be controlled in a few minutes by placing the proximal segment in its usual position and proceeding with some other aspect of the procedure. Alternatively, the distal segment can be retracted forward in an attempt to visualize the bleeding vessel. Sometimes the vessel can be readily identified and cauterized if it is not near the inferior alveolar nerve. Bleeding during SSRO, on the other hand, is almost always diffuse bleeding that occurs immediately after the split. This bleeding, which can be profuse, often diminishes spontaneously after several minutes but may persist. Bleeding from the inferior alveolar, maxillary, or facial artery is uncommon for the experienced surgeon.

Bleeding can be minimized during IVRO by avoiding deep cuts into the medial soft tissues with the saw blade while performing the osteotomy. The thickness of the ramus is easily assessed by the submentovertex radiograph. If the saw blade is substantially deeper than the bone is thick, the instrument can be rotated toward the direction of the cut to avoid deep medial penetration. Another common source of bleeding occurs during the trimming of the proximal and distal segments near the superior margins to gain better lateral approximation after retrusion. The medial tissues should be protected from the rotary cutting instrument with a retractor or wide periosteal elevator.

Probably the two most common causes of preventable bleeding during SSRO are cutting branches of the maxillary artery during reflection of the medial tissues and tearing or cutting the inferior alveolar artery. Careful subperiosteal reflection on the medial aspect of the ramus and use of retractors to protect the soft tissues during osteotomy virtually eliminate bleeding from branches of the maxillary artery. Avoiding use of chisels or other sharp instruments in the vicinity of the inferior alveolar nerve and vessels, except under direct vision, and care in completing the split minimize damage to the inferior alveolar artery.

CONDYLAR POSITION

The condyle is displaced in a downward and forward direction after vertical ramus osteotomy.[34,42,55,58] The displacement is apparently secondary to pull by the external pterygoid muscle, which moves the condyle anteriorly and inferiorly along the anterior slope of the glenoid fossa. The only other muscle attached to the proximal segment is the medial pterygoid. It opposes the lateral pterygoid muscle by its vertical component of force, which seats the condyle. Thus, the more the medial pterygoid muscle is detached from the proximal segment, the greater is the sag of the condyle in an anterior and inferior direction. Conversely, if the medial pterygoid muscle and stylomandibular ligament remain attached along the posterior border of the proximal segment, as is recommended, even though the more anterior fibers have been detached, there is little, if any, sag of the condyle (Fig. 61–14A to C). When much of the inferior portion of the medial pterygoid muscle is detached, there is mild-[34,42] to-moderate[30] sag (Fig. 61–15). When the entire muscle is detached, as was done during the early development of the IVRO[12] the condyle can sag to the articular eminence and occasionally even more anteriorly as a dislocation. There is a variable tendency for the condyle to model[16] (Fig. 61–16A and B) as well as move in a superior and posterior direction[34,42] in the weeks and

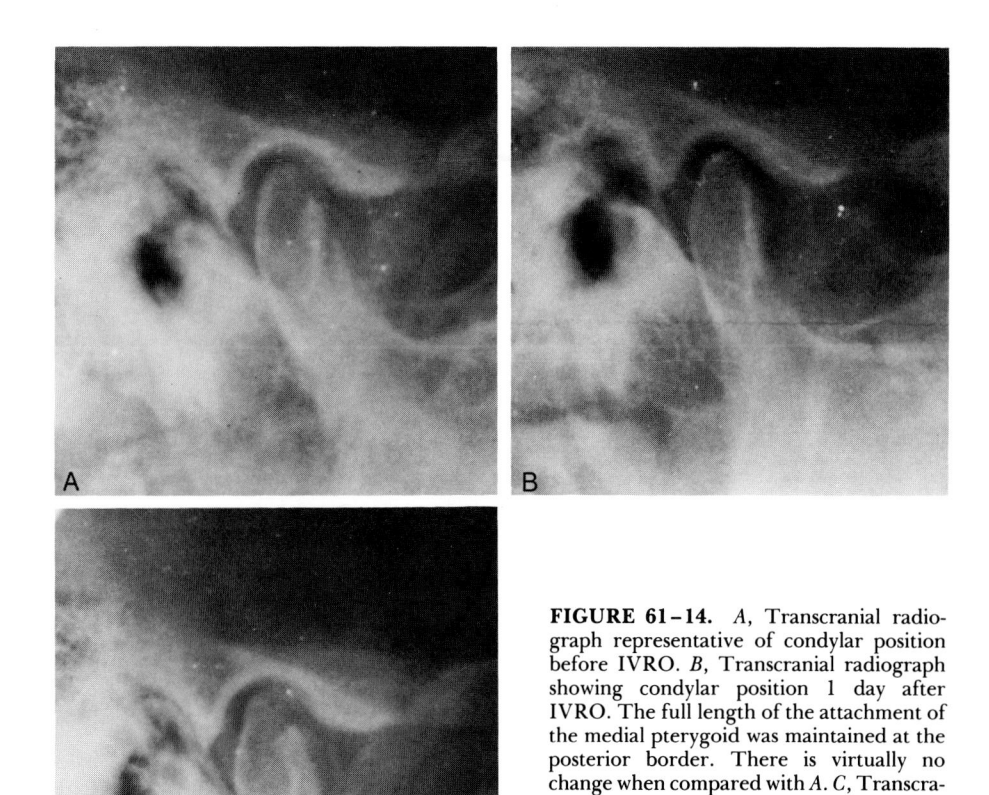

FIGURE 61–14. *A*, Transcranial radiograph representative of condylar position before IVRO. *B*, Transcranial radiograph showing condylar position 1 day after IVRO. The full length of the attachment of the medial pterygoid was maintained at the posterior border. There is virtually no change when compared with *A*. *C*, Transcranial radiograph showing condylar position 6 weeks after IVRO. Comparison of condylar position with that in *A* shows no discernible change. (Courtesy of J.W. Nickerson, Jr.)

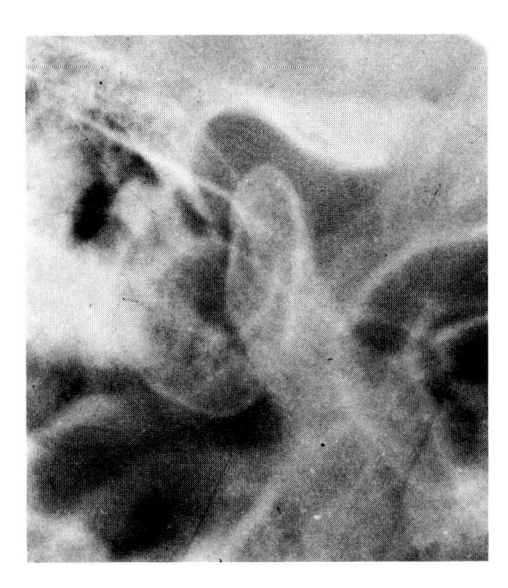

FIGURE 61–15. Moderate "sag" of condyle when about 80 per cent of the inferior portion of the medial pterygoid muscle was detached. Detachment was done on purpose as part of a modified IVRO (condylotomy) procedure for reducing painful anterior dislocation of the disk. Transcranial radiograph taken after 4 weeks of MMF.

months after operation. New bone formation also occurs in the depth of the glenoid fossa.[7] Similar modeling changes of the condyle also occur after SSRO, but both the condylar displacement and the modeling changes are less pronounced.[8] Minimal sag of the condyle after SSRO is not surprising, since the temporalis and masseter muscles tend to seat the condyle. There is probably similar minimal change with the inverted-L osteotomy, since the temporalis as well as the medial pterygoid muscles remain attached, but this has not been documented. There is also a variable degree of rotation and lateral or medial displacement of the condyle when the segments are overlapped with retrusion. The degree of change appears small.[23,43] Rigid fixation also appears to cause minimal condylar displacment after either IVRO or SSRO.[22,23,43]

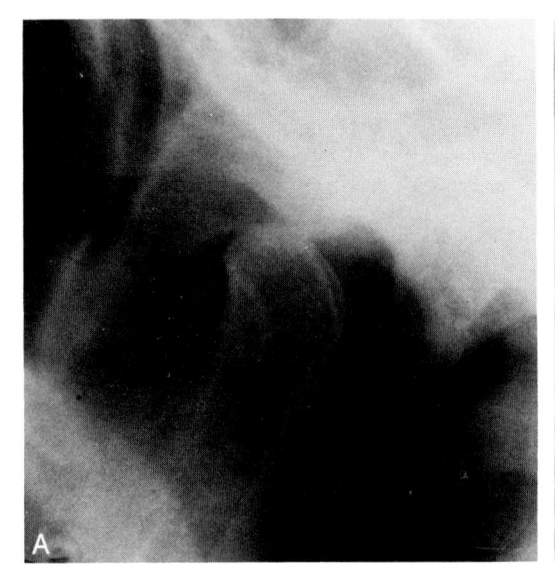

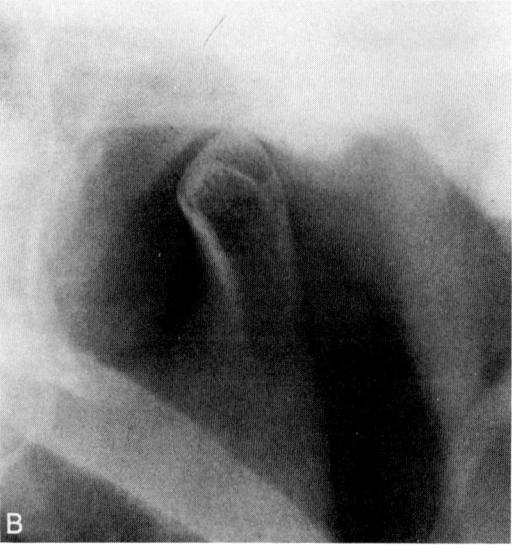

FIGURE 61–16. *A*, Small amount of modeling 5 years after purposeful "sag" induced by modified IVRO (condylotomy). Note secondary contour on the posterior and superior part of the condyle. Transpharyngeal radiograph taken with patient's mouth open. *B*, Moderately extensive modeling of condyle 5 years after modified condylotomy. Note secondary contours of bone on posterosuperior and even anterior surfaces of the condyle. Transpharyngeal radiograph taken with patient's mouth open. (Courtesy of J.W. Nickerson, Jr.)

STABILITY

There is evidence that at least six factors influence stability: (1) amount of retrusion, (2) displacement of the condyle, (3) clockwise rotation of the proximal segment, (4) rigid fixation, (5) skeletal fixation when MMF is used, and (6) growth. The degree of mandibular retrusion at operation directly affects the tendency for anterior relapse.[10,20,34,38] That is, the greater the retrusion, the greater the relapse tendency. Excessive lengthening of the pterygomasseteric sling likely accounts for this tendency. Anterior and inferior displacement of the condyle after IVRO occurs because of stripping of most or all of the medial pterygoid muscle attachment from bone. Both posterior relapse and an anterior open bite often occur immediately after release of fixation when there is pronounced condylar sag.[12] Peterssen and Willmar-Hogeman,[34] however, showed no correlation of condylar displacement and relapse when the displacement was small (about 3 mm). After SSRO, when the proximal segment is rotated clockwise and fixed, forward relapse increases.[10] During healing, the proximal segment rotates counterclockwise toward the original position with forward movement of the mandible. The same phenomenon also seems to occur with IVRO. Skeletal fixation during MMF also provides for improved stability.[21,49] Using bone for fixation, in addition to the teeth, substantially reduces the opening or clockwise rotation of the distal segment during MMF for both IVRO and SSRO. In contrast, if only dental fixation is used during MMF, a variable degree of clockwise rotation of the distal segment occurs with increase in anterior facial height, decrease in posterior facial height, intrusion of posterior teeth, and extrusion of the anterior teeth. If skeletal fixation is used with MMF, only posterior facial height changes appreciably, the result of slight intrusion of the molars. The type of fixation for the bony segments is another factor affecting the extent of relapse. Rigid fixation with SSRO decreases the extent of relapse when compared with semirigid wire osteosynthesis.[32] Too few data on rigid fixation with IVRO[22,32] are available to determine whether it improves stability by reducing or eliminating the demonstrated instability of the osteotomy site.[19,41] The paucity of reports on rigid fixation with IVRO probably reflects both the technical difficulty of the procedure and the good results obtained with skeletal fixation and MMF. Growth can also be a component of anterior relapse, especially in males, who not infrequently exhibit mandibular growth even into their twenties. Although females are less likely to exhibit late growth, such growth can occur. For the majority of patients, these relapse tendencies appear to be relatively small and often occur without change in occlusion.

Other factors that would seem to affect relapse either have not been shown to influence stability appreciably or do so only in the more extreme circumstances or perhaps when other factors affecting relapse tendency are present. For example, bony union of the segments is influenced by a variety of factors, but with the exception of rigid fixation, it is not clear under what circumstances these other factors do make a difference in stability. Decortication of bone and closeness of contact of overlapping segments have been shown to enhance bony union[39,40] but have not yet been correlated with stability. Intuitively, the size of the area of overlap of the segments would seem to affect stability, but this factor has also not been shown to be important, at least within rather wide limits.[35,48] A stable, intercuspating occlusion would also seem to promote stability, but there is no direct evidence that this is the case. The common occurrence of a stable, unchanging occlusion in the presence of skeletal relapse[33,36] implies movement of the teeth.

Biomechanical or muscular limitations are ill defined. Large retrusions and attempts to close large open bites with either IVRO or SSRO are two examples in which the biomechanical limits for good stability may be exceeded. As a general rule, it is probably wise to avoid all but mild lengthening of muscles or altering appreciably the direction of action of the muscles with repositioning of the distal segment. In the case of mandibular excess, the lever arm of the mandible is shortened with retrusion, increasing mechanical advantage while incising or biting. On the other hand, muscle fiber length of the pterygomasseteric sling is lengthened with retrusion. This fact probably accounts for the greater relapse tendency with large retrusions and/or closure of anterior open bites.

Biomechanical influences are important considerations for the surgeon as he or she plans any surgical procedure designed to correct facial disharmonies. With a knowledge of relapse propensities and careful simulation of the planned surgical change by cephalometric prediction studies, the surgeon can design a procedure to maximize esthetics, function, and stability. Maxillary surgery in concert with mandibular ramus surgery is frequently necessary to achieve these objectives in treating the spectrum of problems associated with mandibular prognathism.

INTERNAL DERANGEMENTS OF THE TEMPOROMANDIBULAR JOINT

The incidence of internal derangements of the temporomandibular joint has not been defined for mandibular excess, in contrast to the high incidence associated with mandibular deficiency open bite and mandibular asymmetry.[24] Two observations suggest that the incidence of internal derangements with symmetric mandibular excess is low, perhaps even lower than for the general population. First, arthrosis of the condyle, which is highly correlated with internal derangements,[29] is uncommon in this condition. Second, temporomandibular joint pain is uncommon either before or after operation for mandibular excess. Thus, the best estimate at present is that internal derangements of the temporomandibular joints are no more common in patients with mandibular excess than in the general population and may even be less common.

The incidence of temporomandibular joint dysfunction and pain after IVRO or SSRO with rigid fixation is low.[32,43] Our perception is that it is especially low for IVRO when muscle pedicles position and stabilize the condylar segment. Support for this impression is gained from the high rate of success for treatment of painful internal derangements, utilizing a modified IVRO technique (condylotomy).[30] This low incidence may also be true for SSRO when semirigid fixation is used (see Chapter 24).

RECOMMENDATIONS

The strengths of the IVRO procedure for treatment of mandibular excess are its technical simplicity, speed of operation, virtual absence of damage to the inferior alveolar nerve, and more rapid and complete rehabilitation of range of motion. The single advantage of SSRO lies in the greater ease with which rigid fixation can be applied. There is little difference between the outcomes of these two operations, with one exception. The SSRO procedure has a substantially higher incidence of damage to the inferior alveolar nerve, a proportion of which is permanent. For this reason especially, we recommend IVRO for the treatment of mandibular excess.

Postsurgical Occlusal Problems

In addition to complications or problems related to the surgical intervention itself, three types of occlusal problems are noted in patients who have had combined surgical and orthodontic treatment of mandibular excess. These are as follows:

1. Class II malocclusions or mandibular asymmetry can appear soon after function has resumed. In a few instances, it has been noted that soon after patients begin to function following removal of the wafer and stabilizing arch wires, the mandible drops back unilaterally or bilaterally. This complication can result if the surgeon fails to ascertain that the condyle was seated in the temporal fossa after completion of the osteotomy. This is not an inevitable complication when the condyle is anteriorly and inferiorly displaced but happens often enough[12] that the condyle should be properly positioned. When the condyle is anteriorly and inferiorly displaced, healing will occur with a shortened ramus, and the mandible will drop posteriorly with release of MMF. To avoid this possibility, the medial pterygoid and masseter muscles should be left attached to the proximal segment for IVRO and SSRO, respectively. The muscle pedicle will seat the condyle well in the fossa. Occasionally, the condyle may not appear well seated on the radiograph taken immediately after the operation, but a repeat radiograph taken during the next day or two usually shows the condyle to be well positioned in the fossa. Increased muscle tone is a likely explanation for this change. If the proximal segment is to be rigidly fixed, great care should be taken to ensure that the condyle is well seated before placing the screw fixation. The position of the condyle should also be checked with a radiograph immediately after rigid fixation. If it is not well seated, a procedure to reposition the condyle is indicated. The problem of a poorly seated condyle is related usually to surgical technique.

2. There may be a relapse toward renewed mandibular excess. This complication can be brought about in two ways: first, by renewed mandibular growth after the operation, and second, by change in mandibular position or change in relative position of the jaw segments. The surgical procedures to correct mandibular excess have little or no effect on growth potential of the mandible. The earlier the age at which the surgical procedure is performed, especially in males, the greater the chance of difficulties due to continued growth. Although growth is usually complete, or nearly so, by 15 or 16 years in females and 17 or 18 years in males, occasionally growth continues into the twenties. Tooth position can be controlled to an extent with Class III elastics used postsurgically, but if much skeletal growth occurs, anterior crossbite and chin prominence inevitably return. If the patient begins to function too soon or is allowed to begin function without removing occlusal interferences, new postural adaptive positions of the mandible may be seen; these initially simulate skeletal relapse and can lead to frank skeletal changes in the short term. When the wafer splint is removed after intermaxillary fixation, it is important that the patient have a solid place to bite in centric relation or that active orthodontic treatment, including use of interarch elastics, be in progress.

3. Lateral open bite can develop several months after surgery, frequently in the early stages of retention following removal of orthodontic appliances. Six to 12 months after treatment of mandibular excess, it is not uncommon to find that incisor and molar teeth occlude in centric relation but that premolars do not. Occasionally, a posterior open bite develops, so that only the incisors are in function. The cause of this open bite is obscure. It may be related to a tendency for premolar teeth that have been extruded in the final stages of orthodontic treatment to re-intrude slightly. It may also be influenced by resting posture of the tongue; if the tongue is carried between the teeth at rest, an open bite is likely to be observed. If a total posterior open bite develops (a complication that occurs rarely), lateral spreading of the tongue between the teeth is the most likely cause, and further treatment, including surgical reduction of the tongue, may be needed. An open bite affecting only the premolars is of less clinical consequence and can be corrected with bonded orthodontic brackets and extrusion of the teeth with light elastics. If such retreatment is needed, the brackets should be left in place and light elastics continued at night for 2 to 3 months after the teeth have been brought back into occlusion.

REFERENCES

1. Akin RK, Walters PJ: Experience with the intraoral vertical subcondylar osteotomy. J Oral Surg 33:343, 1975.
2. Åstrand P, Ridell A: Positional changes of the mandible and the upper and lower anterior teeth after oblique sliding osteotomy of the mandibular rami. Scand J Plast Reconstr Surg 7:120, 1973.
3. Bell WH, Schendel SA: Biologic basis for modification of the sagittal ramus split operation. J Oral Surg 34:362, 1977.
4. Bell WH, Kennedy JW: Biological basis for vertical ramus osteotomies—a study of bone healing and revascularization in adult rhesus monkeys. J Oral Surg 34:215, 1976.
5. Boyne PJ: Osseous healing after oblique osteotomy of the mandibular ramus. J Oral Surg 24:125, 1966.
6. DalPont G: Retromolar osteotomy for correction of prognathism. J Oral Surg 19:42, 1961.
7. Eckerdal O, Sund G, Åstrand P: Skeletal remodelling in the temporomandibular joint after oblique sliding osteotomy of the mandibular rami. Int J Oral Maxillofac Surg 15:233, 1986.
8. Edlund J, Hansson T, Petersson A, Willmar K: Sagittal splitting of the mandibular ramus. Scand J Plast Reconstr Surg 13:437, 1979.
9. Epker BN: Modifications in the sagittal osteotomy of the mandible. J Oral Surg 35:157, 1977.
10. Franco JE, Van Sickles JE, Thrash WJ: Factors contributing to relapse in rigidly fixed mandibular setbacks. J Oral Maxillofac Surg 47:451, 1989.
11. Guernsey LH, DeChamplain RW: Sequelae and complications of intraoral sagittal osteotomy in the mandibular rami. Oral Surg 32:176, 1971.
12. Hall HD, Chase DC, Payor LG: Evaluation and refinement of the intraoral vertical subcondylar osteotomy. J Oral Surg 33:333, 1975.
13. Hall HD, McKenna SJ: Further refinement and evaluation of intraoral vertical ramus osteotomy. J Oral Maxillofac Surg 45:684, 1987.
14. Hayward J, Richardson ER, Malhotra SK: The mandibular foramen: Its anteroposterior position. Oral Surg 44:837, 1977.
15. Hebert JM, Kent JN, Hinds EC: Correction of prognathism by an intraoral vertical subcondylar osteotomy. J Oral Surg 28:651, 1970.
16. Hollender L, Ridell A: Radiography of the temporomandibular joint after oblique sliding osteotomy of the mandibular rami. Scand J Dent Res 82:466, 1974.
17. Hullihen SP: Case of elongation of the underjaw and distortion of the face and neck, caused by a burn, successfully treated. Am J Dent Sci 9:157, 1849.
18. Hunsuck EE: Modified intraoral splitting technique for correction of mandibular prognathism. J Oral Surg 26:250, 1968.
19. Isaacson RJ, Kopytov OS, Bevis RR, Waite DE: Movement of the proximal and distal segments after mandibular ramus osteotomies. J Oral Surg 36:263, 1978.
20. Kobayashi T, Watanabe I, Veda K, Nakajiana T: Stability of the mandible after sagittal ramus osteotomy for correction of prognathism. J Oral Maxillofac Surg 44:693, 1986.
21. Komori E, Aigase K, Sugisaki M, Tanabe H: Skeletal fixation versus skeletal relapse. Am J Orthod Dentofac Orthop 92:412, 1987.
22. Kraut RA: Stabilization of the intraoral vertical osteotomy using small bone plates. J Oral Maxillofac Surg 46:908, 1988.
23. Kundert M, Hadjianghelou O: Condylar displacement after sagittal splitting of the mandibular rami. J Craniomaxillofac Surg 8:278, 1980.
24. Link JJ, Nickerson JW: TMJ internal derangement in an orthognathic population (abstract). J Oral Maxillofac Surg 47[Suppl 1]:87, 1989.
25. MacIntosh RB: Experience with the sagittal osteotomy of the mandibular ramus: A 13 year review. J Maxillofac Surg 9:151, 1981.
26. Moose SM: Correction of abnormal mandibular protrusion by intraoral operation. J Oral Surg 3:304, 1945.
27. Moose SM: Surgical correction of mandibular prognathism by intraoral subcondylar osteotomy. J Oral Surg 22:197, 1964.
28. Nickerson JW Jr: Stabilization of the proximal segment in sagittal split osteotomy: A new technique. J Oral Maxillofac Surg 41:683, 1983.
29. Nickerson JW Jr, Boering G: Natural course of osteoathrosis as it relates to internal derangements of the temporo-mandibular joint. Oral Maxillofac Clin North Am 1:27, 1989.
30. Nickerson JW, Veaco NS: Condylotomy in surgery of the temporomandibular joint. Oral Maxillofac Clin North Am 4:303, 1989.
31. Nishioka GJ, Zysset MK, Van Sickles JE: Neurosensory disturbance with rigid fixation of the bilateral sagittal split osteotomy. J Oral Maxillofac Surg 45:20, 1987.
32. Paulus GW, Steinhäuser EW: A comparative study of wire osteosynthesis versus bone screws in the treatment of mandibular prognathism. Oral Surg 54:2, 1982.
33. Peppersack WJ, Chausse, JM: Long-term follow-up of sagittal splitting technique for correction of mandibular prognathism. J Maxillofac Surg 6:117, 1978.
34. Peterssen A, Willmar-Hogeman K: Radiographic changes of the temporomandibular joint after oblique sliding osteotomy of the mandibular rami. Int J Oral Maxillofac Surg 18:27, 1989.
35. Phillips C, Zaytoun HS Jr, Thomas PM, Terry BC: Skeletal alterations following TOVRO or BSSO procedures. Int J Adult Orthod Orthog Surg 3:203, 1986.
36. Reitzik M: Surgically corrected mandibular prognathism, a cephalometric analysis of 50 cases. Am J Orthod 66:82, 1974.
37. Reitzik M: The surgical correction of mandibular prognathism using rigid internal fixation—a

report of a new technique together with its long-term stability. Ann R Coll Surg Engl 70:380, 1988.
38. Reitzik M: Skeletal and dental changes after surgical correction of mandibular prognathism. J Oral Surg 38:109, 1980.
39. Reitzik M, Schoorl W: Bone repair in the mandible: A histologic and biometric comparison between rigid and semirigid fixation. J Oral Maxillofac Surg 41:215, 1983.
40. Reitzik M: Cortex-to-cortex healing after mandibular osteotomy. J Oral Maxillofac Surg 41:658, 1983.
41. Rosenquist B, Selvik G, Rune B, Petersson A: Stability of the osteotomy site after oblique sliding osteotomy of the mandibular rami. A stereometric and plain radiographic study. J Craniomaxillofac Surg 15:14, 1987.
42. Rosenquist B, Rune B, Petersson A, Selvik G: Condylar displacement after oblique sliding osteotomy of the mandibular rami. A stereometric and plain radiographic study. J Craniomaxillofac Surg 16:301, 1988.
43. Spitzer WJ, Steinhäuser EW: Condylar position following ramus osteotomy and functional osteosynthesis, a clinical function-analytic and computer tomographic study. Int J Oral Maxillofac Surg 16:257, 1987.
44. Stacy GC: Recovery of oral opening following sagittal ramus ostectomy for mandibular prognathism. J Oral Maxillofac Surg 45:487, 1987.
45. Steinhäuser EW: Bone screw and plates in orthognathic surgery. Int J Oral Surg 11:209, 1982.
46. Storum KA, Bell WH: Hypomobility after maxillary and mandibular osteotomies. Oral Surg 57:7, 1984.
47. Thoma KH: Oral Surgery. St Louis, CV Mosby, 1948.
48. Tornes K: Osteotomy length and postoperative stability in vertical subcondylar ramus osteotomy. Acta Odontol Scand 47:81, 1989.
49. Tornes K, Wisth PJ: Stability after vertical subcondylar ramus osteotomy for correction of mandibular prognathism. Int J Oral Maxillofac Surg 17:242, 1988.
50. Trauner R, Obwegeser H: The surgical correction of mandibular prognathism and retrognathia with consideration of genioplasty. Part 1. Surgical procedures to correct mandibular prognathism and reshaping of the chin. Oral Surg 10:677, 1957.
51. Turvey T: Intraoperative complications of sagittal osteotomy of the mandibular ramus: Incidence and management. J Oral Maxillofac Surg 43:504, 1985.
52. Van Merkesteyn JPR, Groot RH, Van Leeuwaarden R, Kroon FHM: Intra-operative complications in sagittal and vertical ramus osteotomies. Int J Oral Maxillofac Surg 16:665, 1987.
53. Walter JM Jr, Gregg JM: Analysis of postsurgical neurologic alteration in the trigeminal nerve. J Oral Surg 37:410, 1979.
56. Wang JH, Waite DE: Evaluation of the surgical procedure of sagittal split osteotomy of the mandibular ramus. Oral Surg 38:167, 1974.
55. Ware WH, Taylor RC: Condylar repositioning following osteotomies for correction of mandibular prognathism. Am J Orthod 54:50, 1968.
56. White RP Jr, Peters PB, Costich ER, Page HL: Evaluation of sagittal split ramus osteotomy in 17 patients. J Oral Surg 27:851, 1969.
57. Winstanly RP: Subcondylar osteotomy of the mandible and the intraoral approach. Br J Oral Surg 6:134, 1968.
58. Wisth PJ, Tornes K: Radiographic changes in the temporomandibular joint subsequent to vertical ramus osteotomy. Int J Oral Surg 4:242, 1975.
59. Zaytoun HS Jr, Phillips C, Terry BC: Long-term neurosensory deficits following transoral vertical ramus and sagittal split osteotomies for mandibular prognathism. J Oral Maxillofac Surg 44:193, 1986.

II. Orthodontic Considerations

RONALD R. HATHAWAY

INCIDENCE
ETIOLOGY
PATIENT EVALUATION AND
TREATMENT OBJECTIVES

TREATMENT PRINCIPLES
CASE REPORTS

Historically, there has been no shortage of broad generalizations concerning the patient with dentofacial deformity of mandibular excess. In the nineteenth century, when physical qualities had been associated with psychological qualities, Lavater wrote "A face is dull when the lower part is bigger than one of the two upper parts."[60] It is interesting that the term "progenia" was first used by the psychiatrist Meier, who somehow believed that an excessively large mandible was a symptom of disability and epilepsy.[61]

Fortunately, the modern orthodontist and oral surgeon have greatly benefited from numerous advances in the science of surgical orthodontics. Thus, state-of-the-art practice by today's clinician is more exacting than ever. Improvements that greatly enhance the ability to treat with predictability the person with a dentofacial problem are continually reported in the literature.

INCIDENCE

Dentofacial deformity in the lower third of the face resulting from excess mandibular growth is not as common as mandibular deficiency. According to Rakosi and associates, the frequency of a Class III malocclusion is approximately 1 to 3 per cent, depending on age and geographic variation.[62] However, it is inaccurate to classify all Class III malocclusions as "prognathic," indicating that they all have a component of mandibular excess. In an effort to identify specific skeletal and dental relationships of adults who have a Class III malocclusion, Ellis and McNamara[63] analyzed cephalometric tracings of 302 adult patients who had a Class III molar and cuspid relationship. In this study, pure mandibular skeletal protrusion, commonly cited as the principal anomaly in Class III malocclusion, was no more common than was pure maxillary skeletal retrusion (19.2 per cent versus 19.5 per cent). Still, 65 to 67 per cent of the entire sample of patients exhibited some retrusive component to the maxilla, and although this was associated with mandibular skeletal protrusion in 30.1 per cent of the cases, it was also associated with a normal mandibular skeletal position in 19.5 per cent of the cases. Thus, the importance of a differential diagnosis in recognizing a patient's dental and skeletal compensations, as related to overall facial imbalance, must be taken into consideration, with the emphasis that the Class III malocclusion is not a single clinical entity.

ETIOLOGY

The etiology of mandibular excess has been studied extensively over the past 50 years. Enlarged tonsils, inability to breathe nasally, congenital anatomic defects, hormonal and endocrine imbalances, pituitary gland disease, posture, trauma, premature loss of first molars, and irregular eruption of the permanent incisors or loss of the primary incisors have all been cited,[62,64-67] but not conclusively proved. The primary determinant of absolute mandibular excess, however, is disparate

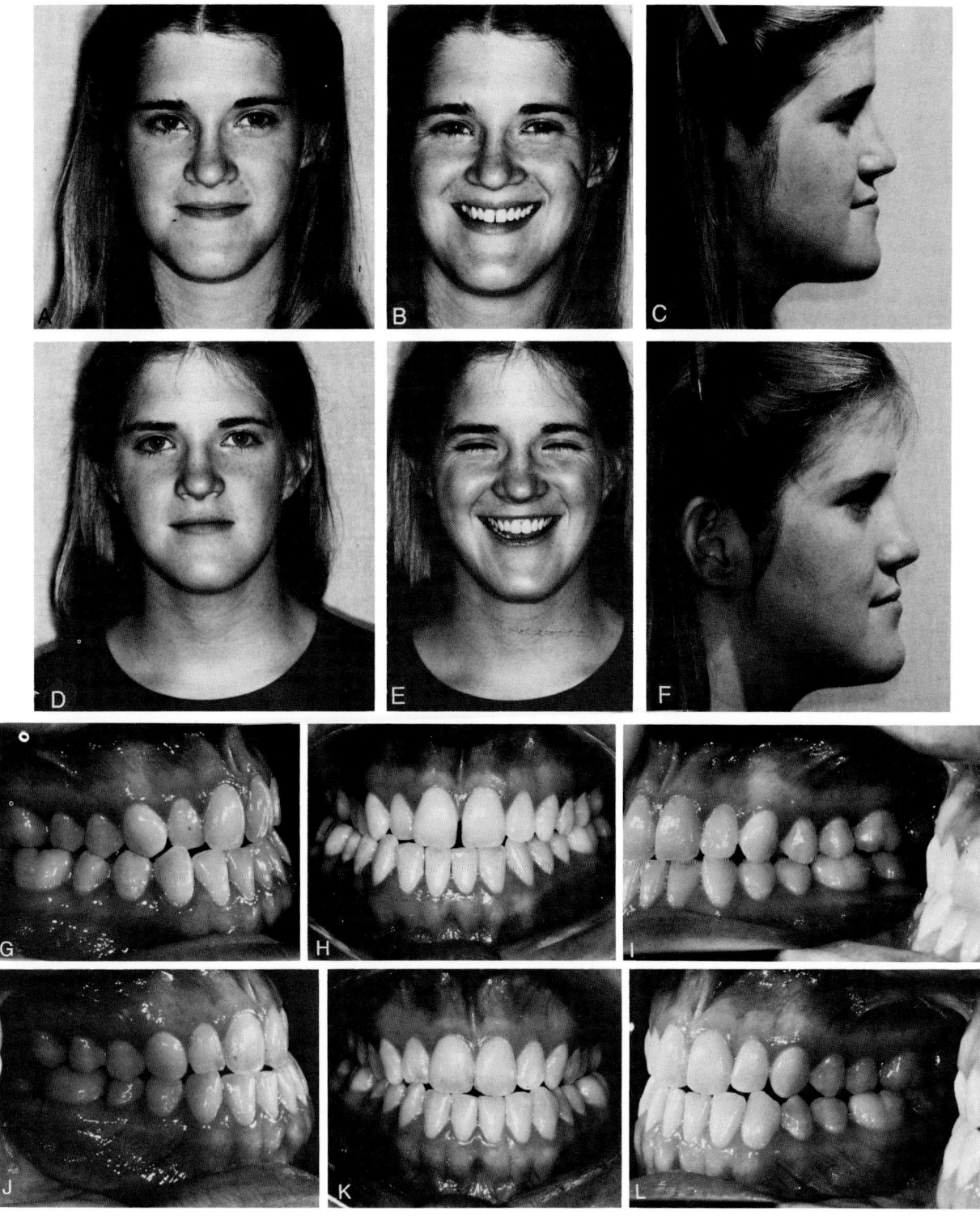

FIGURE 61-17. Facial appearance of a young patient with mild mandibular asymmery of her right side (*A–C*) and facial appearance of her identical twin sister with mandibular asymmetry toward her left side (*D–F*). *G–I*, Occlusion of patient in *A–C*. *J–L*, Occlusion of patient in *D–F*. When comparing patients, note the dental crossbite and midline shift on contralateral sides.

vertical and horizontal growth in the lower third of the face compared with the upper face.

The genetic nature of this problem has been studied by Suzuki.[68] He surveyed 1362 persons in 242 Japanese families in which mandibular excess occurred more frequently. In those families with a history of prognathism, 34.3 per cent of the family members exhibited prognathism, and in families with no history, only 7.5 per cent had the trait. Forty per cent of the children of parents who were prognathic also had the trait. If only one parent was affected, only 20.2 per cent of the children were affected. Therefore, it was Suzuki's conclusion that this deformity involved a complicated hereditary mechanism. In addition to the prognathic component in these patients, quite often there is a variable degree of mandibular asymmetry, which, even in identical twins (Fig. 61–17A to L), is not always expressed in the same direction.

In an article by Worms and colleagues,[69] it was stated that dental compensations were concurrent with deviations from harmonious skeletal jaw base relationships and that teeth alter their normal vertical lengths and axial inclinations to maintain functional relationships. They stated that in the case of absolute mandibular excess the lower incisors usually are lingually inclined and that the maxillary incisors frequently are labially inclined. In addition, as the malocclusion increases in severity, spacing in the maxillary anterior dentition quite often becomes obvious, and the amount of anterior dental crossbite is almost always less than the skeletal imbalance present. They also stated most emphatically that recognition and removal of dental compensations are essential for proper surgical corrections. Rakosi and Schulli[70] stated that "mouth breathing, especially in patients with enlarged tonsils, can promote development of a prominent mandible. The tongues of mouth breathers are often flat, and this anteriorly displaced flat tongue causes a widened mandibular arch and a narrow maxillary arch with a high palate." Again, in these cases there is usually an extreme lingual tipping of the mandibular incisors as well as a labial tipping of the maxillary incisors.

On occasion, the initial signs of a true progressive mandibular prognathism can be observed in infancy.[62] According to Rakosi, the sequential development of mandibular excess may be observed in the first months of life as follows:

1. The primary maxillary centrals erupt in a lingual relationship to the mandibular incisors, and there is no overjet.
2. The primary lateral incisors erupt into a normal relationship while the central incisors remain in crossbite.
3. Some weeks later there is a full incisor crossbite.
4. The tongue flattens as it drops away from palatal contact and assumes a more forward position, pressing against the lower incisors.
5. The child continues to protract the mandible habitually into a protruded functional and morphologic relationship.

PATIENT EVALUATION AND TREATMENT OBJECTIVES

The Growing Patient

Recognition of the type of mandibular excess (relative or absolute) and growth pattern is essential for proper planning and timing of treatment. Clinically, there appear to be many types of mandibular excess with variable facial growth propensities. Many of these types are *relative* to a vertical or an anteroposterior maxillary deficiency and are not true mandibular prognathism.[71] Although the esthetic problem of patients with this type of deficiency appears to be manifested in the mandible, which is often implicated as the etiologic site, the disharmonic jaw relationship has frequently occurred before puberty and is related to the maxilla or to a vertical discrepancy. Unlike *true* mandibular prognathism, however, growth after puberty usually remains relatively proportionate. In *true mandibular prognathism,* however, disharmonic sagittal and vertical growth and the consequent jaw disharmony are anticipated and usually manifested during and after the pubertal growth spurt. Disproportionate maxillomandibular growth associated with true mandibular prognathism is best demonstrated by sequential cephalometric monitoring of facial growth, and a constellation of factors must be considered. The degree of anterior crossbite frequently has little to do with the diagnosis and predictability of growth. Typically, such studies reveal progressive lingual inclination of mandibular teeth and crowding of the lower anterior arch, progressive increase of the gonial angle (increasing more obliquely), Class III malocclusion, progressive increase of mandibular length and magnitude of the mandibular plane angle, and decrease in the anteroposterior dimension of the mandibular symphysis and ramus. Schulhof and coworkers[72] have identified four cephalometric "predictor measurements" to distinguish between normal growth and abnormal growth manifested by persons with true mandibular prognathism. These aberrant measurements include decreased cranial base flexure (and decreased growth from basion to nasion), anterior ramus position, anterior porion location, and a Class III molar relationship. When such findings are revealed by sequential cephalometric monitoring, extractions for orthodontic purposes and surgical intervention are usually deferred until completion of the pubertal growth spurt. As a general rule, the decision to intervene surgically in cases of mandibular growth excess should be predicated on prior evaluation of several cephalometric films, taken over a 12- to 18-month period, demonstrating negligible growth. Exceptions to this rule are discussed in the treatment section below, but when the clinician initially observes a severe sagittal skeletal discrepancy in a young, growing patient, there is usually a greater period of growth remaining, and the prognosis for orthopedic-orthodontic correction alone is poor.

The Adult Patient

Evaluating the Face

The most obvious manifestation of mandibular excess is a prominent lower third of the face when viewed sagittally. In addition, if the patient is truly prognathic, there is often a more obtuse neck-chin angle (greater than 120 degrees) and a taut soft tissue appearance in the mandibular inferior border and submental region. On the other hand, pronounced flattening in the zygomatic-molar area and paranasal areas usually indicates a significant component of midface deficiency that may or may not coexist with the mandibular excess. The upper lip in profile may also alert the clinician to what degree, if any, there is a combined problem of maxillary deficiency, which might initially be assessed from a short, flattened appearance of the upper lip and an acute nasolabial angle. However, from the frontal perspective, the patient with absolute mandibular excess appears to have a broad, flattened lower third of the face and a small chin button. Sometimes because of dentoalveolar compensations, the labiomental fold may appear softened, along with a thin lower lip. In addition, if the mandibular excess is severe, lip incompetence may be observed.

The Functional Examination

ASYMMETRIES

It is not unusual to note asymmetry of the lower third of the face in these cases. Upon examining the patient, great care must be taken to avoid a posturing effect of essentially completed in those patients who have problems of excessive growth, especially mandibular prognathism. Furthermore, there seems to be a lack of evidence to indicate that mandibular setback procedures performed early will attenuate further excessive growth.[83] It appears that many, if not most, of these patients tend to outgrow their surgical correction. However, in cases in which the psychosocial impact of the deformity on the growing patient is great, early surgery may be desirable. Finally, the clinician should adopt a cautious approach to performing a gap arthroplasty or "condylar shave" to attenuate future growth when the temporomandibular joint apparatus is functioning normally.

In summary, different types of Class III malocclusions are found in growing patients. Even with a similar skeletal problem, variations exist not only in the form and/or constitution of skeletal parts of the face but also in the direction, velocity, and timing of growth changes. Individual reactions to chin cap therapy are quite different. For instance, redirection of mandibular growth at the chin seems to be favorably controlled by the chin cap, but control over growth velocity seems to be slight. Since it is essential for diagnosis and treatment to predict exact variations in growth when this appliance is used, it is recommended that records be taken as early as possible. Although the effect on mandibular growth by a chin cap may still be unresolved, chin cap therapy can sometimes be effective, but this is unpredictable. Finally, it is clear that further investigation is needed to gain more practical direction for the efficacy of chin cap use on growing patients.

Orthodontic Treatment of the Adult Patient with Mandibular Excess

The Nonsurgical Option

The first option to consider is orthodontic treatment alone. The patient's dentofacial problem may be one of a mild-to-moderate sagittal discrepancy with no severe vertical components. In such limited treatment cases, the amount of soft tissue improvement may be insignificant compared with that which would be achieved through surgical means. Therefore, in presenting the treatment alternatives, it is important to address the patient's chief complaint. A frank discussion of treatment objectives in terms of esthetics, function, and stability allows the patient to make an informed decision of the risks and benefits of alternative treatment plans, which is more likely to yield results that meet the patient's expectations.

When orthodontics is the sole means of treatment for mandibular excess, extraction is very likely. If the lower first bicuspids are extracted, the reverse overjet can often be corrected, but a molar Class III occlusal relationship remains — something less than desirable according to some orthodontic philosophies. However, with minor post-treatment equilibration techniques, functional interferences may be eliminated and stability improved. Another consideration is to extract maxillary second bicuspids and mandibular first bicuspids, in which case a Class I molar and canine relationship may be achieved. The final option may be to extract two mandibular incisors, especially when maxillary lateral incisors are congenitally missing. However, with problems due to an absolute mandibular excess there is always the danger from extraction techniques of creating a poor Holdaway ratio, wherein the mandibular incisors appear to be overretracted in relation to the facial plane and the chin (pogonion) remains very prominent.

Another factor to consider is any late growth, which can be quite difficult to predict but which does occur in some cases even into adulthood.[83] With anticipated growth, the chances for successful surgical treatment will be greatly compromised if extractions have been performed and the anterior segments retracted. Finally, in the case of the brachycephalic patient without dental crowding, it is conceivable that nonextraction orthodontic therapy alone can open the bite sufficiently to cause a rotation of the chin down and back, thus camouflaging the mandibular prominence and aiding in correcting the Class III malocclusions.

Presurgical Orthodontics

ELIMINATING DENTAL COMPENSATIONS

In addition to the basic surgical orthodontic treatment principles, there are a few additional goals to be achieved for the patient with mandibular excess. First, in eliminating or reducing dental compensations for the skeletal deformity, it is usually necessary to procline the uprighted, lingually positioned mandibular incisors and to upright the flared maxillary incisors. This practice obviously increases the negative overjet, and the patient should be prepared for this, bearing in mind that surgery will ultimately resolve this increased sagittal discrepancy. The total amount of incisor flaring prior to surgery should closely approximate the final desired results. If the orthodontist wishes to build in a safety factor to offset postsurgical forward displacement of a mandible, it is suggested that the maxillary incisor crowns be torqued labially 10 to 12 degrees in excess, thereby creating a 2-mm overjet that can be corrected by uprighting these maxillary teeth postsurgically. The presurgical advancement of the lower incisors can frequently be accomplished without extraction, provided that these movements occur within the biologic limitations of the attached gingiva and the supporting alveolar bone. If this is not possible, periodontal corrective therapy in the form of free gingival grafting should be performed first. Some useful mechanics for proclining the mandibular incisors include open coil springs; utility arches with molar tip-back bends and anterior torque; continuous arch wires with stops at the mesial aspects of the molar tubes so that the anterior aspect of the wire will lie 1 to 2 mm forward of the incisors prior to bracket engagement; any type of bite-opening wire when it is forward of the incisors prior to bracket engagement; any type of bite-opening wire when it is desirable to reduce the curve of Spee prior to surgery; and Class II elastic wear (which should always be of brief duration and used in conjunction with stable rectangular arch wires to prevent upper molar extrusion).

When severe crowding exists, extraction therapy is required to decompensate the anterior occlusion fully. In the mandibular arch, the extraction of second bicuspids usually allows the molars to translate forward as the orthodontist permits the loss of anchorage to occur, thereby increasing the Class III molar relationship prior to surgery. In the maxillary arch, first bicuspids may be removed to alleviate anterior crowding and/or to retract the incisors maximally. In addition, if a two-jaw surgical plan dictates maxillary advancement procedures, it may be desirable to obtain maximal retraction of the upper incisors through first bicuspid extractions. However, when no maxillary surgery is to be performed, retracting the upper incisors could create an obtuse nasolabial angle and compromise good facial esthetics. Thus, extraction of maxillary second bicuspids may become the treatment of choice.

In a very real sense, the two-jaw approach to the correction of severe mandibular excess does make the orthodontist's job easier. This allows full decompensation of the incisor positions, whereas in the isolated mandibular setback procedure, it may be necessary to flare the lower incisors excessively, limit the magnitude of the surgical setback, or tolerate a positive overjet.

ESTABLISHING ARCH COMPATIBILITY

Correcting Transverse Problems. The next goal for the orthodontist is to establish arch compatibility, which, at the time of surgery, permits an optimal canine and molar occlusion, eliminates crossbites, and allows the dental midlines to be coincident. The transverse discrepancy commonly seen consists of a differentially tapered maxillary arch and relative crossbite with the greatest constriction at the intercanine region. With the extraction of maxillary first bicuspids, the canine will be posteriorly retracted during space closure into a wider portion of the dental arch, thus facilitating a small increased intercanine width. The orthodontist is cautioned, however, not to be overzealous in attempting to "round out" this anterior segment with expanded, broad-shaped arch wires, when canine stability will be compromised. As a general rule, the canines in each quadrant will relapse toward their original position when they are bodily expanded more than a few millimeters. Similarly, in an attempt to offset canines orthodontically, fenestrations of the labral plate of the alveolar bone and gingival recession can occur with aggressive orthodontic forces.

When there are no vertical or sagittal problems in the maxillary arch and the degree of mandibular excess is not severe enough to warrant consideration of maxillary advancement procedures, a surgically assisted expansion of the maxilla with a palatal expansion device may solve the absolute transverse problem. If the above procedure is employed, it may be performed very early in the course of orthodontic treatment once initial leveling has been accomplished. The expansion appliance can incorporate a posterior "fan-type" hinge, with the expansion screw placed anteriorly to obtain a maximal anterior effect. One advantage of early sequencing with surgically assisted expansion is that it allows for a period of observation and, it is hoped, stabilization of the results before the mandibular setback procedure. There are situations, however, in which the intercanine width is so severely reduced that orthodontics, or even surgically assisted expansion, will not facilitate maxillary-mandibular canine compatibility, and then segmental osteotomies to expand the canines may be the only realistic option. In addition, if the mandibular arch is extremely broad, a symphyseal sectioning procedure may be considered; however, the chance of postsurgical morbidity and the tendency for torquing of condyles along with a reduced intercondylar distance must be addressed in formulating the plan. Given this predicament, there may be some reasons for leaving or even orthodontically tipping the mandibular posterior dentition into linguoversion, as the arch is extremely broad and this plan would eliminate more radical surgery.

When the crossbite is relative in nature, crossbite elastics may be used to correct compensatory dental tipping most commonly expressed in the mandibular buccal segments. It should be noted that with expansion there will be a mild-to-moderate bite-opening effect. Therefore, in cases in which there is a reduced lower anterior vertical facial height and only a dental crossbite, it may be advisable to correct the transverse problem after surgery.

Tooth Size Discrepancies. Another consideration in achieving arch compatibility includes formulating a plan to deal with tooth size discrepancies. Quite often, even without performing a Bolton analysis, it will be obvious that the maxillary incisors are small, in which case coil springs can maintain medial and distal spaces for esthetic bonding. Such bonding also has functional benefits by permitting proper positioning of the dental midlines and good canine function. When the maxillary lateral incisors are severely deformed and have a poor long-term prognosis, they may be extracted in place of maxillary bicuspids, in which case the canine will function in the lateral incisor position and the first bicuspid becomes canine. Usually, some reduction of the lingual cusp at the first bicuspid is required in this situation. However, if the potential occlusal interferences are great enough, then it may be desirable to extract the first bicuspids and retract the canines, leaving space for a bridge to replace the lateral incisor. Finally, in cases such as the above, interproximal reduction in the opposing arch or, sometimes, extraction of a single mandibular incisor may be used to achieve arch compatibility. If such methods are to be properly considered in the treatment plan, a diagnostic wax setup should be done.

Sequencing of Treatment for Vertical Problems. Perhaps the most cognitively difficult goal in the surgical orthodontic treatment plan involves the sequencing of treatment of vertical problems. Decisions must be made whether to intrude or extrude anterior and posterior segments orthodontically and at what times during treatment these movements are to be accomplished. Another factor is consideration of whether or not it is more feasible to use surgery to facilitate these goals. Mandibular excess with concomitant vertical maxillary excess frequently shows excessive tooth–to–upper lip relationship and an open bite. Soft tissue measurements also confirm an increase in anterior facial height. It is necessary to differentiate true vertical maxillary excess from vertical macrogenia, in which case a simple inferior border recontouring procedure may be the treatment of choice. The orthodontic mechanics in this situation should attempt to maximize the open bite prior to surgery, which attenuates the opening tendency after surgery. In most cases, Class II mechanics can be employed; however, a segmented arch technique must be used when a moderate-to-severe vertical step is present in the maxillary occlusal plane, usually seen abruptly distal to the canine or lateral incisor. If the step is distal to the incisor, the job of the surgeon may be made easier, as the canine–first bicuspid interdental space technically is a more difficult osteotomy site. When the vertical discrepancies are amenable to orthodontic leveling, the orthodontist attempts to intrude the incisors (slightly extruding posterior teeth) and may employ a Burstone-type intrusion arch inserted into the molar headgear tubes and ligated to the anterior segment overlying the anterior segmental wire. The location for ligating this overlay wire is important, as tying this intrusion arch in at the midline effects lingual root torquing, whereas tying distal to the long axis of the canine effects some degree of labial root torquing. In addition, when the osteotomy for the anterior segment is planned, adequate spacing must be present at the osteotomy site to facilitate the surgical cut.

When mandibular excess with a decreased lower anterior facial height is present, there may be a problem of vertical maxillary deficiency, and usually a steep curve of Spee is found in the lower arch and *should not* be corrected prior to surgery. This accentuated curve can be more conveniently and efficiently leveled postsurgically with continuous TMA arch wires or NiTi bite-opening wires (ORMCO Corp., Glendora, CA) to erupt the bicuspids. In some cases in which there is severe supraeruption of the lower incisors, a subapical osteotomy may be considered at the time of setback procedures.

Surgical Orthodontic Teamwork

This phase of treatment requires real teamwork, and the surgeon and orthodontist need to be in constant communication. In the months preceding the planned surgery, it is the orthodontist's responsibility to obtain study casts, which may be cut and/or hand articulated. This practice ensures that occlusal interferences have been eliminated, thereby allowing surgical manipulation to the full extent desired. Occasionally, slight molar cusp reduction prior to surgery promotes a better fit and leads to greater stability by decreasing the potential for an open bite to rebound following surgery. Any such equilibration should, however, be minor and is not intended as a substitute for proper banding of the second molars from the start of orthodontic treatment. Another reason for obtaining study models prior to surgery is to ensure that adequate intercanine width is available to achieve proper canine function. Few factors are more frustrating for the surgeon at the time of their procedures than to encounter canine interferences that prevent adequate closure of the bite. Ultimately, this problem will fall back in the hands of the orthodontist when he or she attempts to finalize a functional occlusion.

All extraction sites should be completely closed at the time of surgery and figure-eight tied shut with ligature wire, unless an interdental osteotomy is planned, in which case 2 to 3 mm of space should be adequate. In addition to study models, it is necessary to obtain a panoramic film and/or supplemental periapical films to confirm that the roots of the teeth are adequately divergent and that space exists for the planned osteotomy cuts. A lateral cephalometric film should be taken and used in the final prediction tracing that will be correlated with the model surgery. In addition, a presurgical posteroanterior film is required when asymmetries exist. Finally, the models should be mounted on a semi-adjustable articulator whenever maxillary osteotomies or a subapical body osteotomy is planned.

Postsurgical Management

POSTOPERATIVE VISITS

With wire osteosynthesis and rigid internal fixation, the bony segments may be fairly stable as early as 3 or 4 weeks after surgery. The decision about when to commence postsurgical orthodontics is up to the surgeon, which in turn depends on satisfactory healing and may need to be postponed. However, the patient should always be seen by the orthodontist within a 24- to 48-hour period following splint removal. At the first postsurgical orthodontic appointment, the stabilizing arch wires are removed, as newly created dental interferences must be corrected expeditiously to prevent unseating of the condyles. In addition, at this first appointment loose bands and brackets should be repaired. Working arch wires, that is, 0.016 stainless steel, should be placed. These wires allow flexibility for light vertical elastics (3/8 inch, 2 ounces, in the form of either a zigzag or a box pattern), which permits the occlusion to settle while simultaneously serving as training elastics to override the proprioceptive tendency toward centric occlusion. If it is also necessary to maintain anterior torque control, a TMA rectangular wire may be used. If slight asymmetries exist, the box elastics may assume a Class II or Class III vector, and crossbite elastics may be used to correct any remaining transverse problems. With postsurgical elastic wear, weekly and sometimes even daily appointments should be made to monitor progress and identify any untoward movements. After 3 to 4 weeks, the patient may omit elastic wear while eating, and vertical steps can be placed in the arch wires to promote intercuspation. When extended elastic wear (beyond 2 months) is required, it is always a good idea to replace the lighter working arch wires with heavier rectangular ones to prevent unwanted molar extrusion.

STABILITY FACTORS

Proffit and associates[84] have reviewed data on patients treated with a variety of mandibular setback approaches, including transoral vertical ramus osteotomies, bilateral sagittal split osteotomies with wire osteosynthesis and maxillomandibular fixation, and bilateral sagittal split osteotomies with rigid internal fixation via bone screws. It was concluded that with any of these procedures, clinically significant repositioning of the chin takes place. The greatest forward repositioning of the chin was found to occur with bilateral sagittal split osteotomies when rigid internal fixation was used. Therefore, these clinicians recommended modifications in the surgical technique that seek to reduce the forceful seating of the condyles and the posterior movement of the ramus segment in this procedure.

ORTHODONTIC RETENTION

Retention appliances should be so constructed to inhibit any relapse tendencies in the direction of the original malocclusion. Thus, a positioner designed to inhibit molar extrusion and facilitate small amounts of incisor elongation may be prescribed where an open bite previously existed. When extractions have been performed, a Hawley retainer should include circumferential wires that wrap around the distal molar. Under no circumstances should crossover wires be incorporated into the retainer when opening the bite would be undesirable. Finally, a fixed lingual retainer (bonded appliance) may be affixed for the patient with esthetic concerns, but only after the vertical dimensions have been stabilized and the patient has been instructed in the need for meticulous oral hygiene. The utilization of this fixed type of retainer to prevent interdental spacing can be a good plan, especially when midsymphyseal procedures have been performed.

CASE REPORTS

CASE 1 (Fig. 61–18)

When initially seen by her orthodontist, D. H., a 26-year-old woman, was primarily concerned with getting her teeth and jaws aligned as well as eliminating the click and pop in her jaw on the right side. Clinical examination revealed the following additional information.

PROBLEM LIST

Esthetic Analysis

FRONTAL (Fig. 61–18*A* and *B*). The patient's mandibular skeletal midline appeared to be shifted about 4 mm to the right, and the nose was broad and flat. In addition, when the patient smiled, there appeared to be a slight vertical maxillary asymmetry, the right side being approximately 3 mm longer than the left side.

PROFILE (Fig. 61–18*C*). When viewed in this aspect, the asymmetric mandible appeared prognathic. The forehead was flattened, and there was a small, upturned nose with an acute nasolabial angle. The upper lip appeared flat, and the lower lip was everted. The chin appeared to be contour deficient, and although the throat was long, the neck-chin angle was good. In addition, this patient appeared to have mild midface deficiency in the zygomatic-orbital region; however, there was a component of slight maxillary dentoalveolar protrusion.

Cephalometric Analysis (Fig. 61–18*I*)

D. H. was bimaxillary protrusive with excessive effective mandibular length. Her mandibular plane angle was slightly decreased, and the maxillary incisors were flared and bodily forward. The lower incisors were only slightly flared and bodily forward. She had an increased lower anterior facial height. The anteroposterior measurements, 6 to 9, relate to McNamara's cephalometric analysis.

Anteroposterior Proportions

1. SnV-ULP = +7
2. SnV-LLP = +10
3. SnV-Po′ = +2
4. NLA = 99°
5. ULD = 67°
6. Mandibular length (Co-Gn) = 139
7. Maxillary length (Co–point A) = 90
8. Maxillomandibular differential = 49
9. $\underline{1}$–Point A = 9

Vertical Proportions

1. $\underline{1}$-Stm$_s$ = 3.5
2. G-Sn = 75/Sn-Me′ = 76
3. Sn-Stm$_s$ = 26.5/Stm$_i$-Me′ = 49
4. ILG = 1

Incisor Position

1. $\underline{1}$-HP = 125°
2. $\underline{1}$-PP = 119.5°
3. $\underline{1}$-GoMe = 102°

Occlusal Analysis (Fig. 61–18*J–N*)

DENTAL ARCH FORM. There was a relative maxillary consriction, although this arch appeared tapered, with flattening in the area of the left buccal segment. The mandibular arch was broad anteriorly and tapered bilaterally in the molar segments.

DENTAL ALIGNMENT. There was 5 mm of arch length discrepancy in the maxillary arch, which was confined to the anterior teeth. The left lateral incisor was displaced lingually, and the left cuspid was displaced buccally. In the mandibular arch, a 2-mm arch length discrepancy was presnt and was confined to the bicuspid areas. These incisors appeared to be in good alignment; however, the second bicuspids were rotated and buccally displaced. The mandibular right second bicuspid had received endodontic therapy, and a poorly contoured amalgam restoration was present.

DENTAL OCCLUSION. D. H. had an end-to-end occlusion anteriorly where the maxillary left incisor was in dental crossbite. The molars on the left side were in a Class III relationship, and there was 0 mm overjet and 0 mm overbite. On the right side, the molars were in Class I relationship, and the crossbite extended from the second bicuspid to the lateral incisor.

TREATMENT PLAN

Presurgical Orthodontics

1. Extract all four third molars and both maxillary first bicuspids

2154 / VII — ORTHOGNATHIC SURGERY

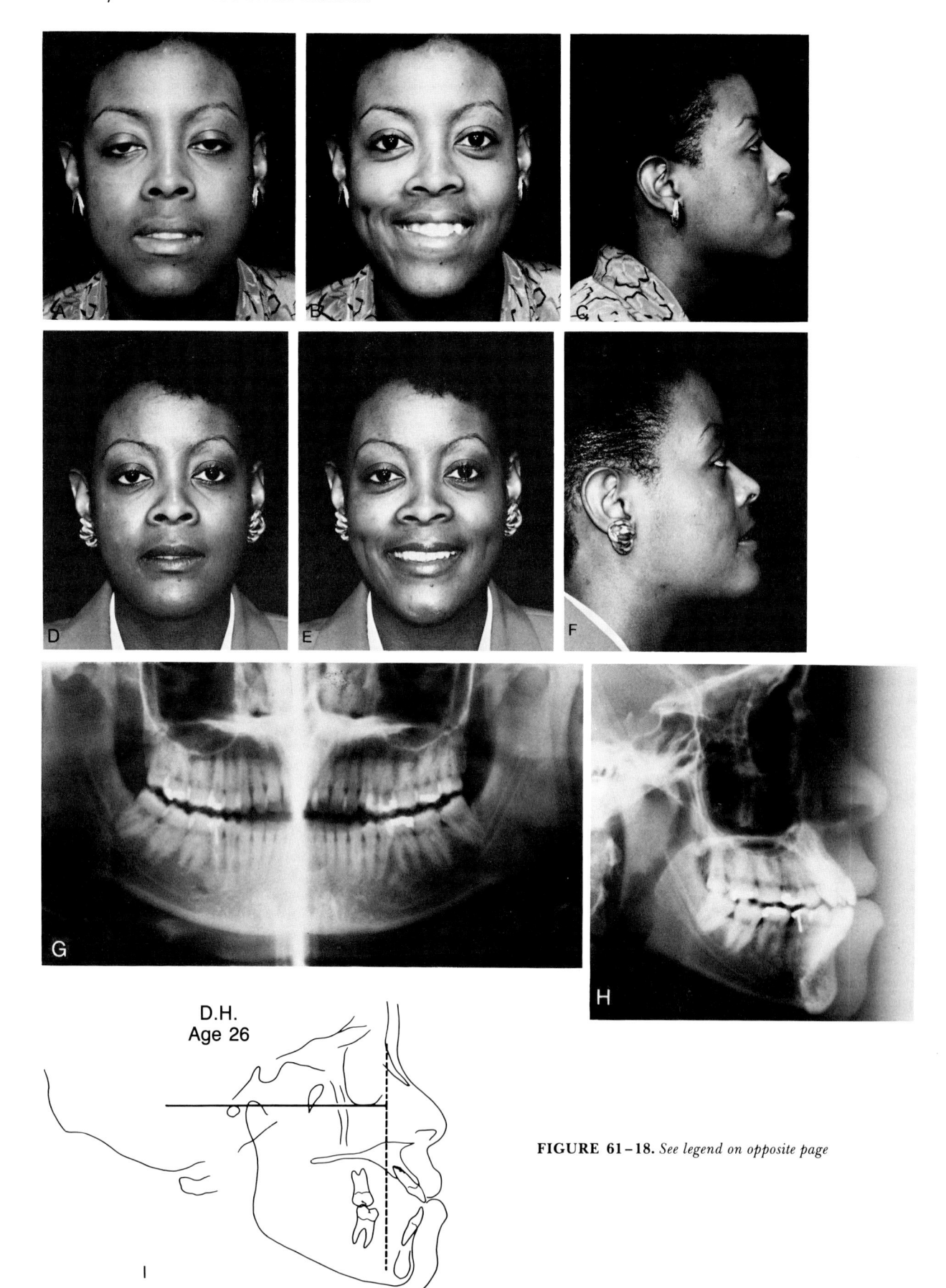

FIGURE 61–18. *See legend on opposite page*

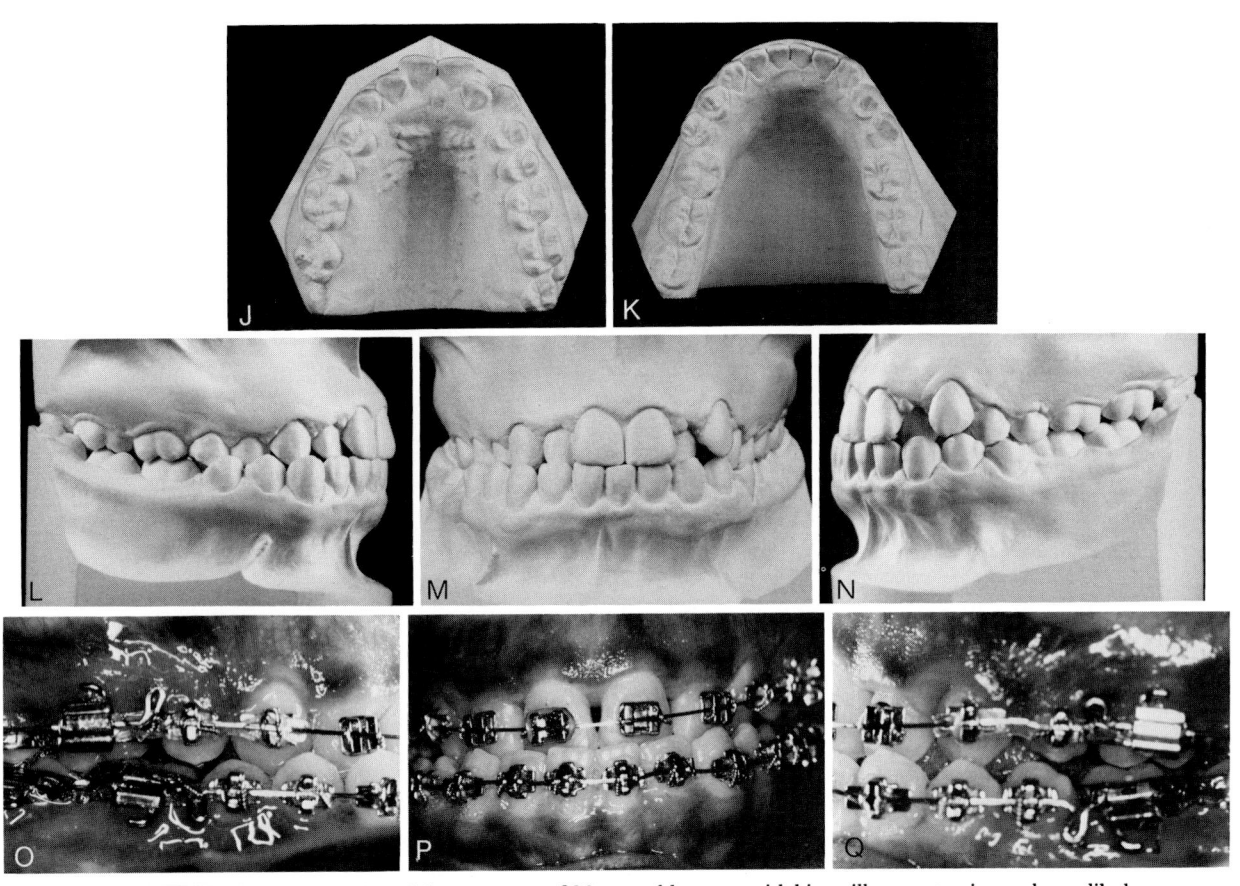

FIGURE 61-18. *A-C*, Facial appearance of 26-year-old woman with bimaxillary protrusion and mandibular excess as shown prior to orthodontic treatment. *D-F*, Appearance of patient after combined surgical orthodontic treatment. *G-I*, Radiographic and cephalometric appearance prior to initiating orthodontic treatment. Note maxillary protrusiveness in combination with mandibular excess and proclined incisors. *J-N*, Pretreatment occlusion in Class III molar relationship and crossbite due to relative maxillary constriction. *O-Q*, Presurgical occlusion following extraction of maxillary first bicuspids and closure of spaces.

Illustration continued on following page

2. Level, align, and correct rotations in the maxillary arch
3. Close maxillary extraction spaces until maxillary incisors are decompensated
4. Air-rotor slenderize in the mandibular bicuspid region
5. Level, align, and correct mandibular rotations
6. Insert stabilizing arch wires prior to surgery

Surgical Treatment

1. Three-segment Le Fort I osteotomy to expand and impact maxilla approximately 3 mm
2. Asymmetric mandibular setback, approximately 6 mm
3. Alar base cinch (suture to narrow width)
4. Chin implant

Postsurgical Orthodontics

1. Box elastics on the left and right sides after surgery to help interdigitate the teeth.
2. Class III elastics on the left and Class II elastics on the right for a brief period while detailing the occlusion.

Active Treatment and Follow-up

Ths patient initially presented with a midopening click in the left temporomandibular joint and reported that her joints popped when she yawned and that she had occasional mild pain. Mild mucogingival defects were present in some of the cuspid and incisor regions prior to treatment; however, this patient maintained excellent hygiene throughout treatment. The maxillary arch wires used on this patient consisted of a 0.0175 Wildcat wire for 3 months for initial alignment and rotation correction, a 0.016 stainless steel wire for the next 2 months to continue leveling and alignment,

2156 / VII—ORTHOGNATHIC SURGERY

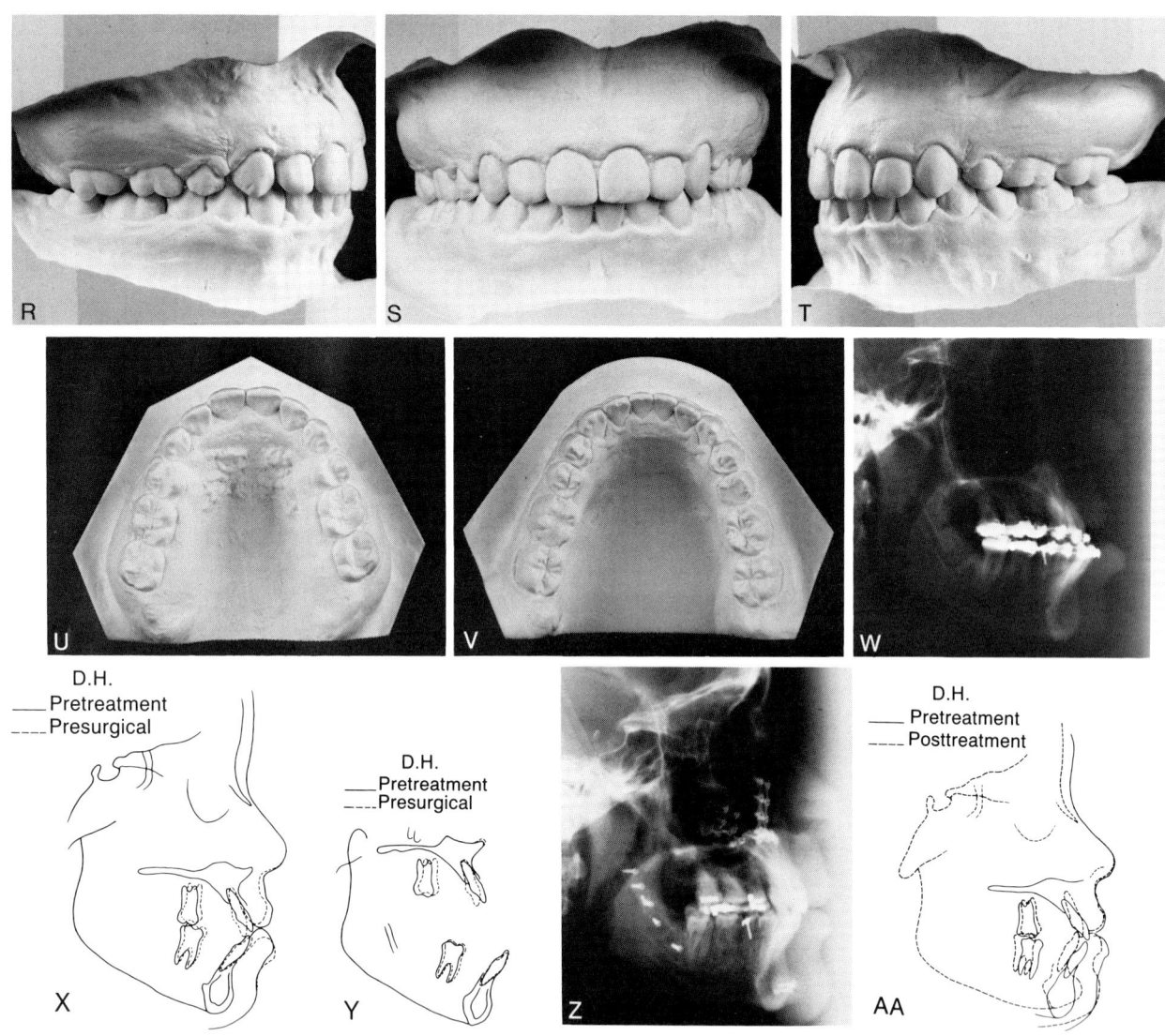

FIGURE 61–18. *Continued* *R–V*, Final occlusion following surgical orthodontic treatment. *W–Y*, Presurgical cephalogram and tracings indicating retraction of maxillary incisors and reciprocal mesial movement of maxillary first molars after extraction and space closure. *Z, A′*, Postsurgical cephalogram indicating rigid maxillary fixation and cephalometric tracings noting major changes in mandible and lip-chin soft tissue contour. (Surgeon: Larry M. Wolford, Dallas; orthodontist: Chris Nevant, Plano, TX.)

and a 0.016 × 0.022 stainless steel arch wire, which was used for 4 months to retract the incisors in the maxillary arch using power chains. After surgery, the maxillary arch was quickly releveled with a 0.017 × 0.025 TMA wire, which accomplished most of the final positioning. In the mandible, a 0.0175 Wildcat wire (GAC International Inc., Central Islip, NY) was used for 2 months for initial alignment, which was followed by a 0.016 stainless steel wire for 2 months. A 0.017 × 0.025 TMA wire was then used for 2 months for leveling, and the arch was stabilized with a 0.017 × 0.025 stainless steel wire.

During surgery the anterior maxilla was impacted 3 mm, the anterior portion of the posterior segment 1.5 mm, and the posterior maxilla 3 mm, and expansion was accomplished to correct the transverse discrepancy. The mandible was set back in an asymmetric fashion with mandibular ramus osteotomies to achieve a Class I cuspid and Class II molar relationship. A 7-mm Proplast chin implant was placed to create an esthetically pleasing soft tissue chin contour.

D. H. is extremely pleased with the results of treatment and regrets only not being treated earlier. The tooth-lip relationship is ideal, and the chin implant helps to produce a balanced profile (Fig. 61–18*F*). She continues to have an inconsistent click in her left temporomandibular joint; however, it is currently asymptomatic.

CASE 2 (Fig. 61-19)

A. S., a 32-year-old man, initially contacted his orthodontist with the desire to improve facial esthetics and to obtain "a better bite." A functional examination revealed essentially normal temporomandibular joints that were symptom free.

PROBLEM LIST
Esthetic Analysis

FRONTAL (Fig. 61-19 A and B). A S.'s face appeared brachycephalic in spite of satisfactory lower facial height. The clinical examination corroborated the appearance of hypotonic perioral musculature in the photographs taken while he was at rest.

PROFILE (Fig. 61-19C). The face appeared very concave and was protrusive in the mandible. The lip posture was relaxed when the lips were together. The maxillary malar hypoplasia and flattened upper lip were pronounced in profile.

Cephalometric Analysis (Fig. 61-19I)

Tracings confirmed an absolute mandibular excess of considerable magnitude; however, the sagittal position of the maxilla was essentially normal. The mandibular plane angle was acceptable, while the anteriormost mandibular incisors were in good position. The other incisors appeared retroclined. The anteroposterior measurements, 6 to 9, relate to McNamara's cephalometric analysis.

Anteroposterior Proportions

1. SnV-ULP = +5
2. SnV-LLP = +13
3. SnV-Po' = +12
4. NLA = 89°
5. ULD = 70°
6. Mandibular length (Co-Gn) = 149
7. Maxillary length (Co-pointA) = 92
8. Maxillomandibular differential = 57
9. $\underline{1}$-Point A = 9

Vertical Proportions

1. $\underline{1}$-Stm$_s$ = 4
2. G-Sn = 75.5/Sn-Me' = 75
3. Sn-Stm$_s$ = 24/Stm$_i$-Me' = 49
4. ILG = 2

Incisor Position

1. $\underline{1}$-HP = 125°
2. $\underline{1}$-PP = 132°
3. $\underline{1}$-GoMe = 93°

Occlusal Analysis (Fig. 61-19J-N)

DENTAL ARCH FORM. The maxillary arch was ovoid with greater curvature in the right cuspid-bicuspid segment. The lower arch appeared asymmetrically tapered, with the crowns of the right buccal segment in linguoversion.

DENTAL ALIGNMENT. The maxillary arch had 2 mm of arch length discrepancy, the cuspids were asymmetrically related to the midsagittal plane, and the right second molar was rotated buccally. There appeared to be a 3- to 4-mm arch length discrepancy confined to the mandibular anterior segment.

DENTAL OCCLUSION. The molars were in a severe Class III relationship bilaterally, which was of greater magnitude on the nonedentulous side. An overbite of 3.5 mm existed, and the overjet was −2 mm. The right segment was in full crossbite, and the left segment was in an end-to-end relationship. A. S. occluded primarily on the left and right second molars.

TREATMENT PLAN
Presurgical Orthodontics

1. Extract impacted maxillary left third molar
2. Align maxillary and mandibular arches with light Wildcat wires initially
3. Proceed with 0.016 NiTi wires in both arches
4. Place 0.016 × 0.022 surgical wires

Surgical Treatment

1. Bilateral intraoral vertical ramus osteotomies with mandibular setback
2. High Le Fort I osteotomy with 5-mm advancement
3. Infraorbital suspension
4. Intermaxillary fixation

2158 / VII — ORTHOGNATHIC SURGERY

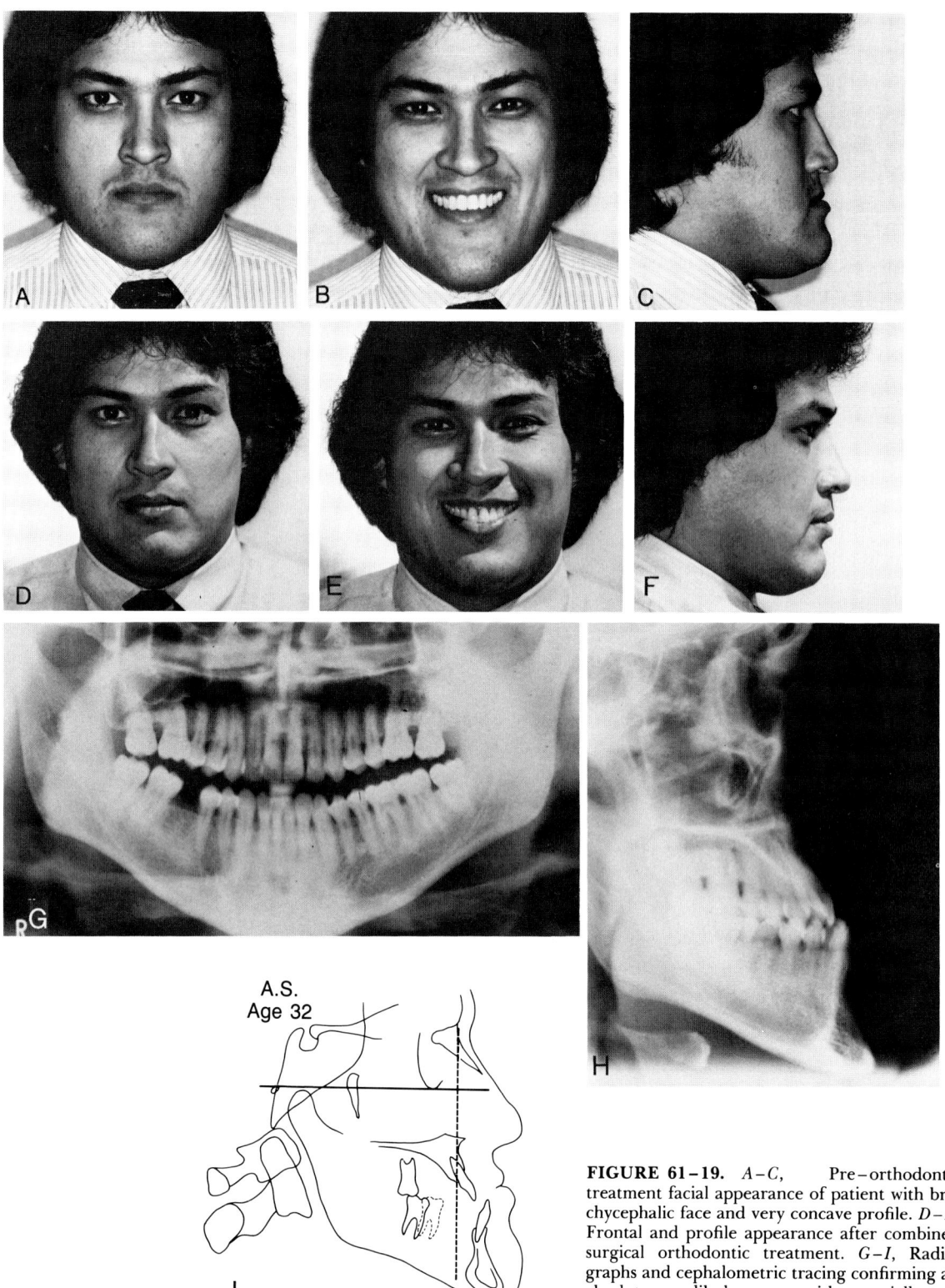

FIGURE 61–19. *A–C,* Pre–orthodontic treatment facial appearance of patient with brachycephalic face and very concave profile. *D–F,* Frontal and profile appearance after combined surgical orthodontic treatment. *G–I,* Radiographs and cephalometric tracing confirming an absolute mandibular excess with essentially normal sagittal position of the maxilla.

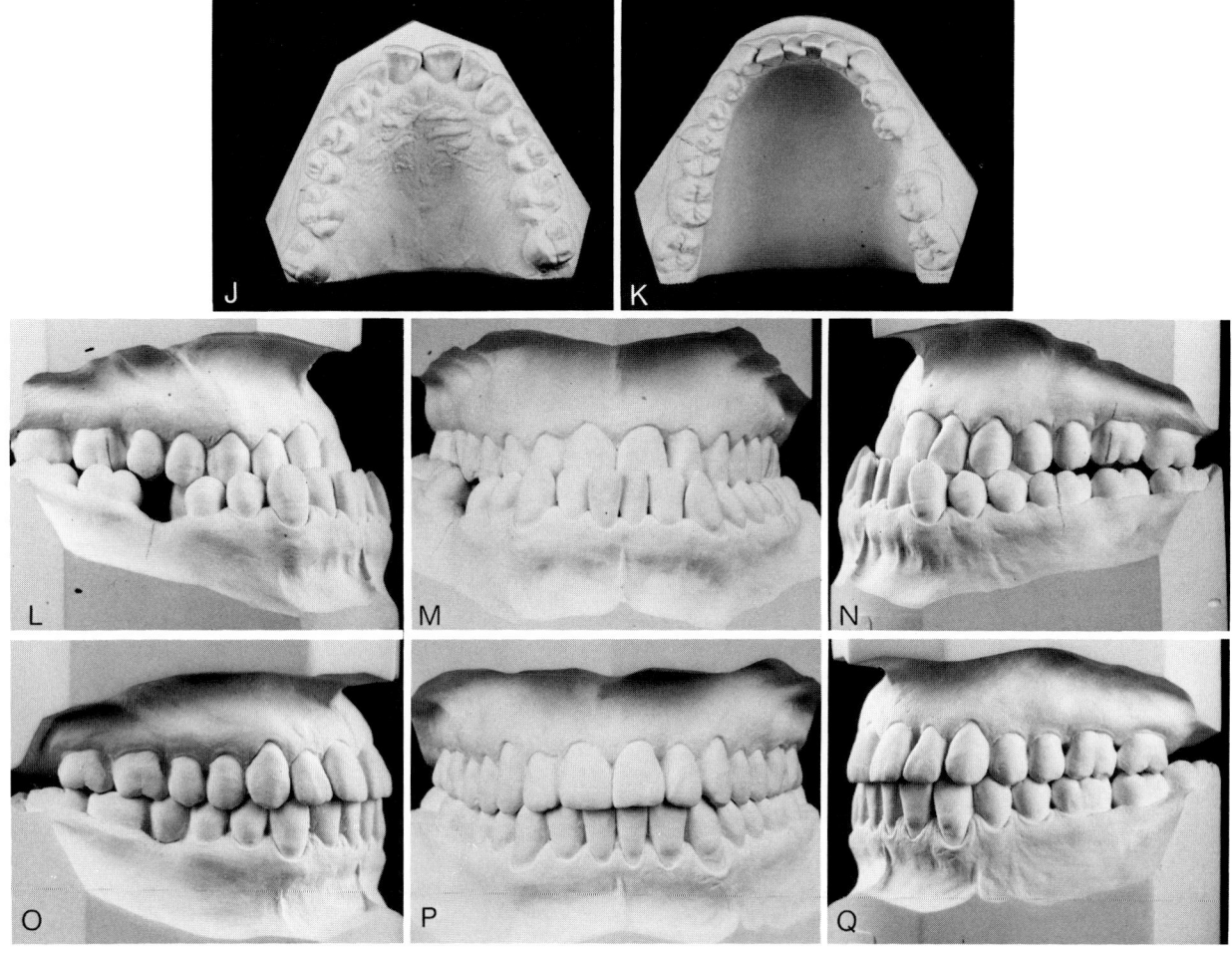

FIGURE 61-19. *Continued* *J-N*, Pre-orthodontic treatment occlusion with severe Class III molar relationship on the left side, negative overjet, and functioning occlusion primarily on the left second molar. *O-S*, Final occlusion after combined surgical orthodontics and prosthetic replacement of missing mandibular right first molar. *T-W*, Radiographs and cephalometric tracings after surgical orthodontic treatment, showing improved facial balance, a more orthognathic profile, and a very pleasing masculine chin contour. *X*, Post-treatment occlusion with prosthetic placement of a bicuspid-sized pontic. (Surgeon: Douglas P. Sinn, Dallas; orthodontist: Patrick Ohlenforst, Irving, TX.)

Illustration continued on following page

Postsurgical Orthodontics

1. Place up-down elastics initially to facilitate maximal intracuspation
2. Bilaterally place light posterior Class II elastics for 2 months, with patient in 0.016 stainless steel arch wires
3. Detail and finish occlusion
4. Deband and deliver positioner
5. Stabilize with a maxillary Hawley retainer and a mandibular fixed lingual wire (bonded cuspid to cuspid)

ACTIVE TREATMENT AND FOLLOW-UP

After a period of adequate stabilization, A. S. saw his prosthodontist for a three-unit gold bridge to replace the absent mandibular right first molar. The use of a bicuspid-sized pontic permitted satisfactory intracuspation. Throughout all phases of treatment, A. S. had received oral hygiene therapy, which was monitored at 6-month intervals to minimize the exacerbation of mucogingival problems anticipated from the initial recordings of gingival pocket depths. This patient at present has good facial balance. With a more orthognathic profile, he has retained a very pleasing and masculine chin contour. The lips and perioral musculature appear more symmetric and esthetic both in repose and during animation (Fig. 61-19*D* and *E*).

2160 / VII—ORTHOGNATHIC SURGERY

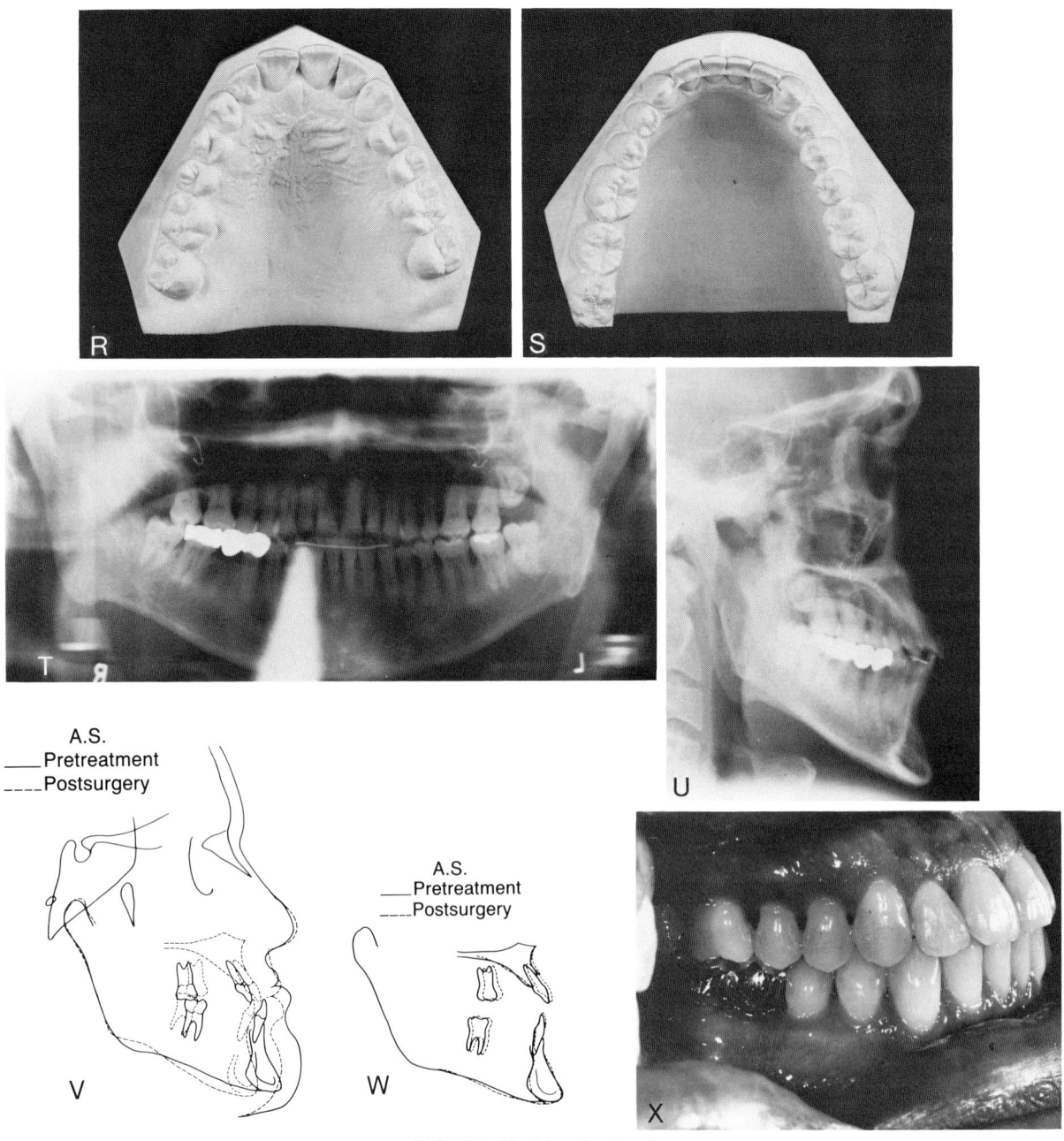

FIGURE 61-19. *Continued*

CASE 3 (Fig. 61–20)

This 44-year-old man initially sought the services of his oral surgeon for correction of his anterior open bite, which he recalled having ever since his earliest teenage years. He reported no previous treatment with braces; however, he thought that he may have worn a palatal expansion appliance at around age 15. J. K.'s main concerns at the time of the initial examination were directed toward functional rehabilitation of his bite.

PROBLEM LIST

Esthetic Analysis

FRONTAL (Fig. 61–20A). The patient appeared to have a dolichocephalic type of facial pattern combined with mandibular asymmetry expressed as deviation of the mandibular skeletal midline to the patient's left side. At the time of the initial examination, the patient was told that it would not be necessary to remove the mustache but that as presurgical orthodontics was completed, it might become necessary to do so in order that the face might be reassessed. The right side of the face was flat, and the left side (which was the short side) appeared to be concave. It is interesting that there was no obvious manifestation of canting of the maxillary occlusal plane when the patient occluded on a tongue blade. The patient had inadequate incisal display upon animation, with only 3 mm of the incisors showing. He also had approximately 6 mm of lip incompetence, which was masked by his mustache. There was a severe mucogingival defect on the labial radicular surface of the maxillary right cuspid, with fenestration and loss of bone. The maxillary dental midline in relation to the midsagittal plane of the face was deviated 1 mm to the right, and the mandibular dental midline to this plane deviated 5 mm to the left.

PROFILE (Fig. 61–20C). Anteroposteriorly, J. K.'s nose appeared to be somewhat large, although this, too, was obscured by his mustache. There was a steep mandibular plane angle, excessive lower anterior facial height, and a contour-deficient chin.

Cephalometric Analysis (Fig. 61–20J)

The tracing revealed a mildly retrusive maxilla, posterior vertical excess, an excessive effective mandibular length (indicating a true prognathism), and a steep mandibular plane angle. The anteriormost maxillary incisors were mildly proclined. The anteroposterior measurements, 6 to 9, relate to McNamara's cephalometric analysis.

Anteroposterior Proportions

1. SnV-ULP = +1
2. SnV-LLP = −1
3. SNV-Po' = +13
4. NLA = 100°
5. ULD = 81°
6. Mandibular length (Co-Gn) = 140
7. Maxillary length (Co–pointA) = 92
8. Maxillomandibular differential = 48
9. $\underline{1}$–Point A = 6

Vertical Proportions

1. $\underline{1}$-Stm_s = 0.5
2. G-Sn = 78/Sn-Me' = 88
3. Sn-Stm_s = 29/Stm_i-Me' = 53
4. ILG = 5.5

Incisor Position

1. $\underline{1}$-HP = 114°
2. $\overline{1}$-PP = 110.5°
3. $\overline{1}$-GoMe = 92°

Occlusal Analysis (Fig. 61–20K–O)

DENTAL ARCH FORM. The maxillary arch was very tapered and extremely constricted in the bicuspid–first molar segments. The mandibular arch was very broad in form and rounded in the anterior segment.

DENTAL ALIGNMENT. The crowding and irregularity of the incisors were more pronounced in the maxillary arch, where there appeared to be an excessive curve of Spee. In the mandibular arch, there was very mild anterior crowding and a reverse curve of Spee.

DENTAL OCCLUSION. The molars were in a Class II relationship bilaterally and in crossbite on both sides because of an absolute transverse skeletal discrepancy in the maxilla.

TREATMENT PLAN

Presurgical Orthodontics (Fig. 61–20P and Q)

1. Extract both maxillary cuspids

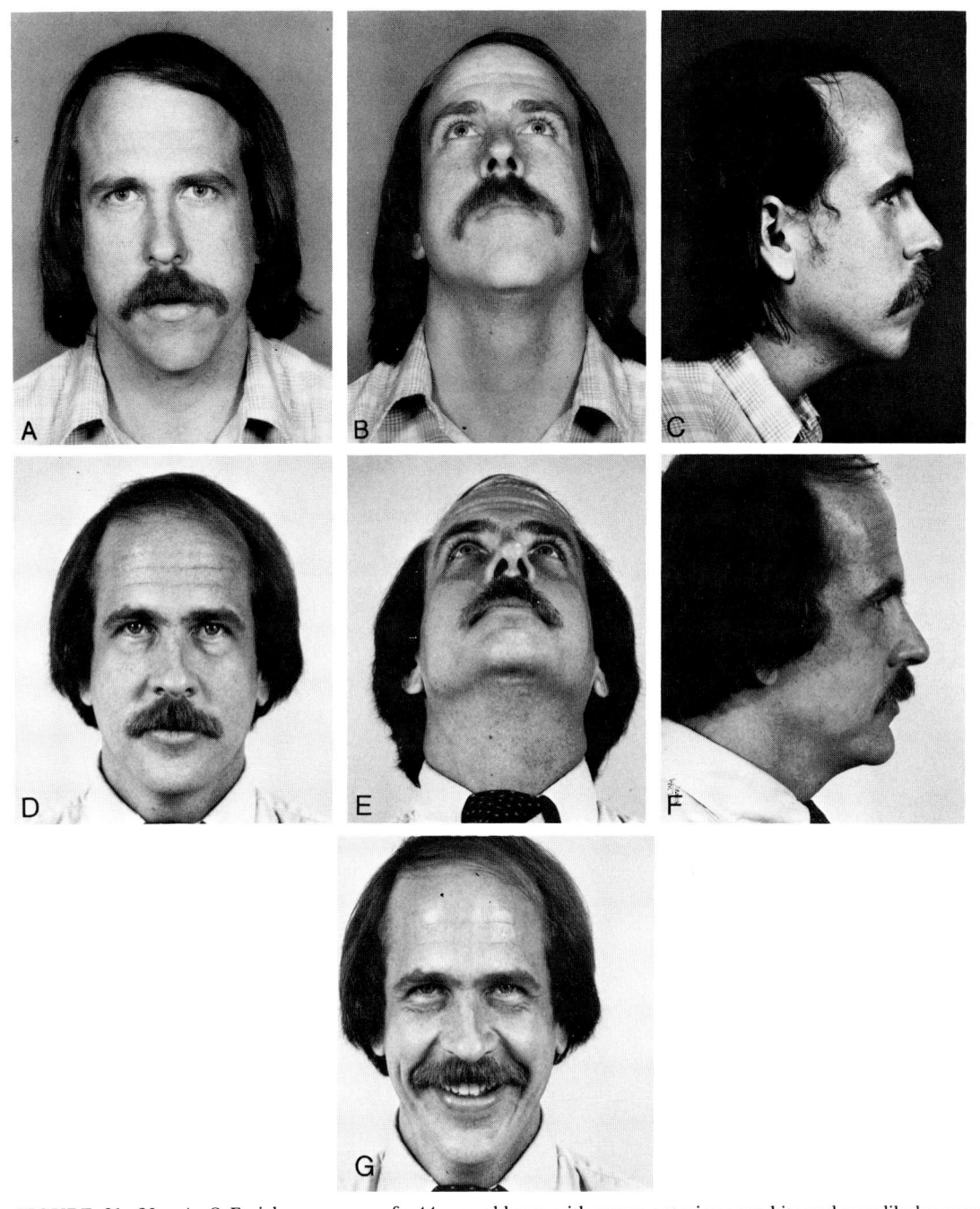

FIGURE 61–20. *A–C,* Facial appearance of a 44-year-old man with severe anterior open bite and mandibular excess prior to the initiation of orthodontic therapy. *D–G,* Facial appearance after surgical orthodontics, which dramatically improved function and esthetics. *H–J,* Pre–orthodontic treatment radiographs and cephalometric tracing revealing a mildly retrusive maxilla, a long effective mandibular length, and a steep mandibular plane angle. *K–O,* Occlusion prior to initiating orthodontic treatment showing a very tapered maxillary arch due to an absolute transverse skeletal discrepancy, a Class II left-side molar relationship due to asymmetry, a counterclockwise rotation of the mandible, and mild crowding in the mandibular incisor segment. *P, Q,* Presurgical photographs of the occlusion showing partial closure of the maxillary cuspid extraction sites and complete closure of the mandibular first bicuspid extraction sites. *R–V,* Final occlusion. *W–Y,* Postoperative cephalogram and tracings reveal that the lips, which are now competent, remain full and show the extent to which the maxillary and mandibular molars were brought forward in orthodontic closure of the spaces. (Surgeon: William H. Bell, Dallas; orthodontist: Thomas Creekmore, Houston.)

    2. Extract both mandibular first bicuspids
    3. Level and align, completely closing mandibular extraction sites on rectangular wires with closing loops
    4. Level and align the maxillary arch, maintaining the incisor segment in its present plane, leaving spaces distal to the lateral incisors for osteotomy sites

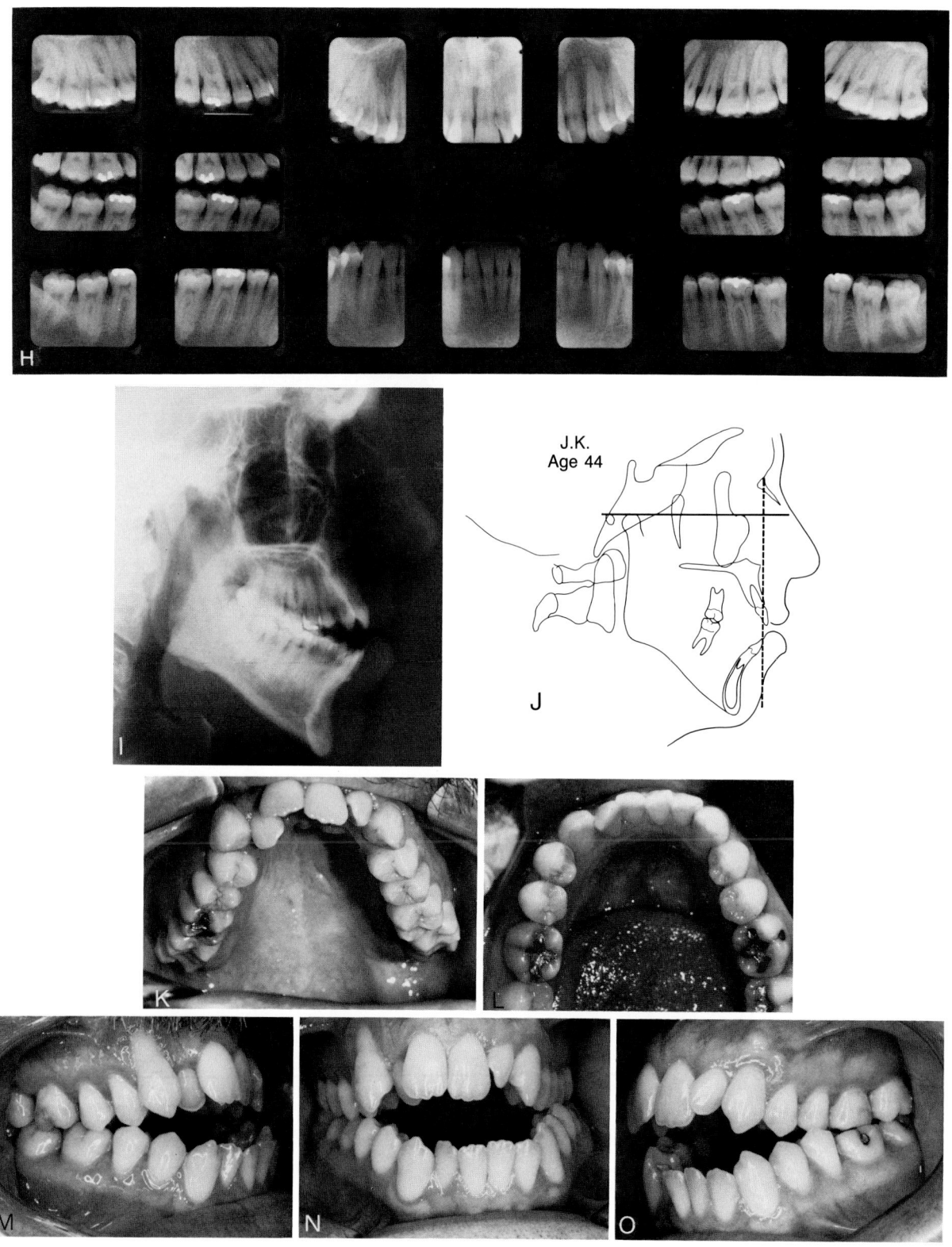

FIGURE 61–20. *Continued*

Illustration continued on following page

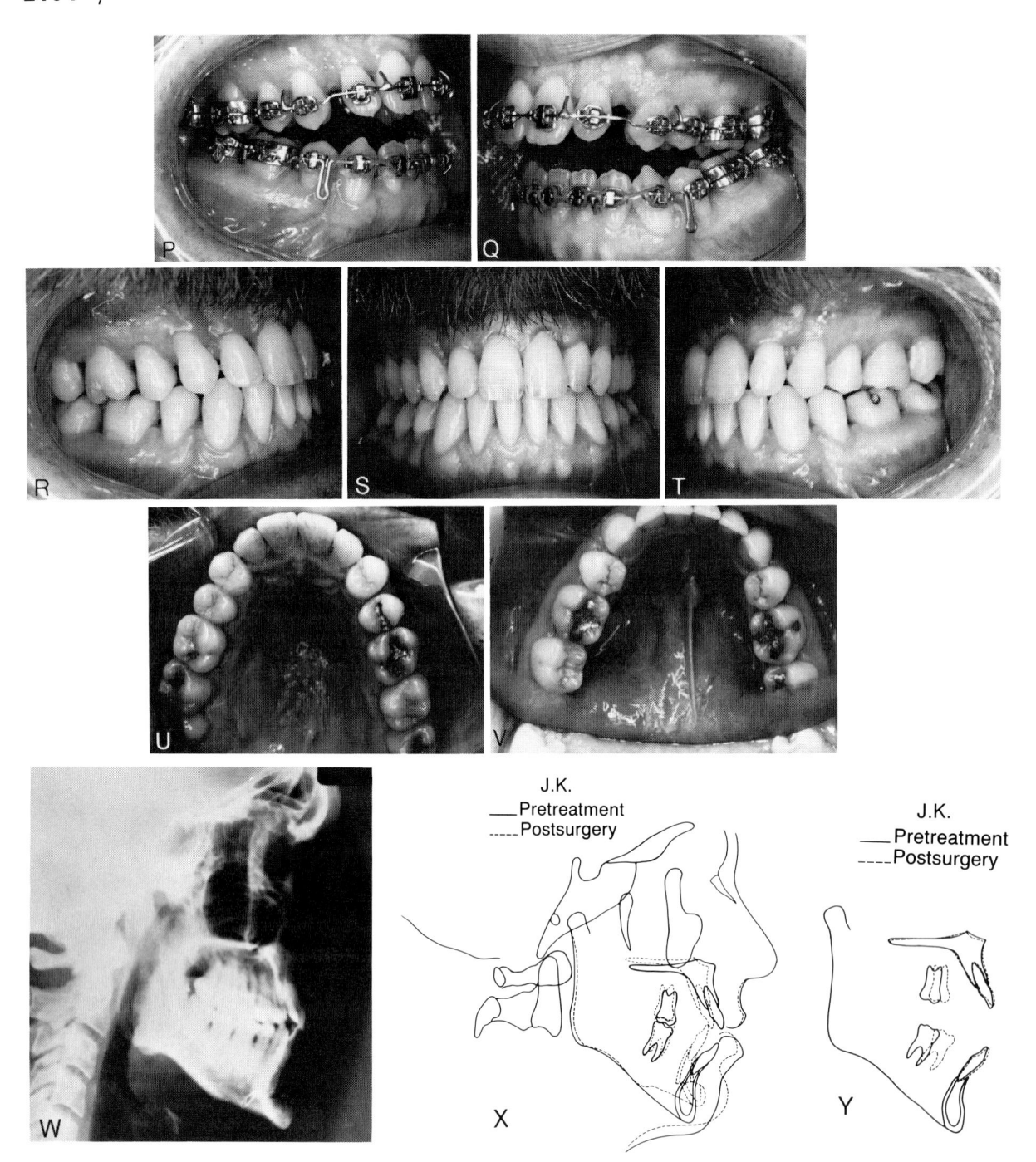

FIGURE 61–20. *Continued*

Surgical Treatment

1. Maxillary three-piece Le Fort I osteotomy
2. Right intraoral vertical ramus osteotomy
3. Left sagittal split ramus osteotomy
4. Osteotomy of the inferior border of the mandible
5. Occlusal splint
6. Skeletal fixation

Postsurgical Orthodontics

1. Anterior vertical elastics to maintain the closure of the bite
2. Posterior box elastics to obtain maximal intercuspation
3. Removal of surgical wires and finishing and detailing the occlusion on continuous arch wires

ACTIVE TREATMENT AND FOLLOW-UP

During surgery, the posterior portion of the maxilla was raised approximately 8 to 9 mm, and a transverse genioplasty was performed. J. K. 's postoperative progress went exactly as planned, and his functional and esthetic results are excellent. The facial proportionality and symmetry have dramatically improved. J. K. initially presented with mild-to-moderate gingivitis and was followed throughout surgical orthodontic treatment at his dentist's office for maintenance therapy. Maxillary and mandibular Hawley retainers were used to stabilize the occlusion.

CASE 4 (Fig. 61–21)

J. C., a 28-year-old woman, was initially seen in consultation with her orthodontist. Study parameters showed the typical dentofacial features of absolute mandibular prognathism and vertical maxillary excess and were the basis for the following problem list.

PROBLEM LIST

Esthetic Analysis

FRONTAL. This aspect was characterized by a symmetric long face, narrow nasal alar bones, deficiency in paranasal areas, excessive exposure of gingiva when smiling (3 mm), 6 mm of tooth exposure with lips in repose, and a 7-mm interlabial gap (Fig. 61–21A and B).

PROFILE. This view revealed an acute nasolabial angle, dorsal nasal hump, prominent chin, flattened labiomental sulcus, flattening in paranasal areas (Fig. 61–21C).

Cephalometric Analysis (Fig. 61–21G)

The tracing revealed a vertical maxillary excess with typical Class III skeletal pattern, moderate chin prominence, excessive effective mandibular length, oblique gonial angle, and retroclined mandibular incisors. The anteroposterior measurements, 6 to 9, relate to McNamara's cephalometric analysis.

Anteroposterior Proportions

1. SnV-ULP = +1
2. SnV-LLP = +1
3. SnV-Po' = +1
4. NLA = 99°
5. ULD = 67°
6. Mandibular length (Co-Gn) = 132
7. Maxillary length (Co–pointA) = 87
8. Maxillomandibular differential = 45
9. $\underline{1}$–Point A = 8

Vertical Proportions

1. $\underline{1}$-Stm_s = 5.5
2. G-Sn = 68/Sn-Me' = 74.5
3. Sn-Stm_s = 21/Stm_i-Me' = 48
4. ILG = 5.5

Incisor Position

1. $\underline{1}$-HP = 105°
2. $\underline{1}$-PP = 100.5°
3. $\underline{1}$-GoMe = 71°

Occlusal Analysis

DENTAL ARCH FORM. The maxillary and mandibular arches were normally tapered and V shaped. A study of the lateral widths of the two arches showed that the maxillary arch was constricted 5 mm. (The analysis was based on the occlusal relationship that was achieved when the models were hand articulated into a simulated, corrected Class I cuspid and molar relationship.)

DENTAL ALIGNMENT. There was minimal crowding of labially inclined maxillary anterior teeth and retroclined mandibular anterior teeth.

DENTAL OCCLUSION. There was a Class III cuspid and molar relationship and an overjet of −8 mm. The entire lower dentition was positioned anterior to the upper dentition (Fig. 61–21K and L).

TREATMENT PLAN

Presurgical Orthodontics

1. Decompensate the dentition without extraction
2. Complete bonding and banding
3. Align and level maxillary and mandibular arches

2166 / VII — ORTHOGNATHIC SURGERY

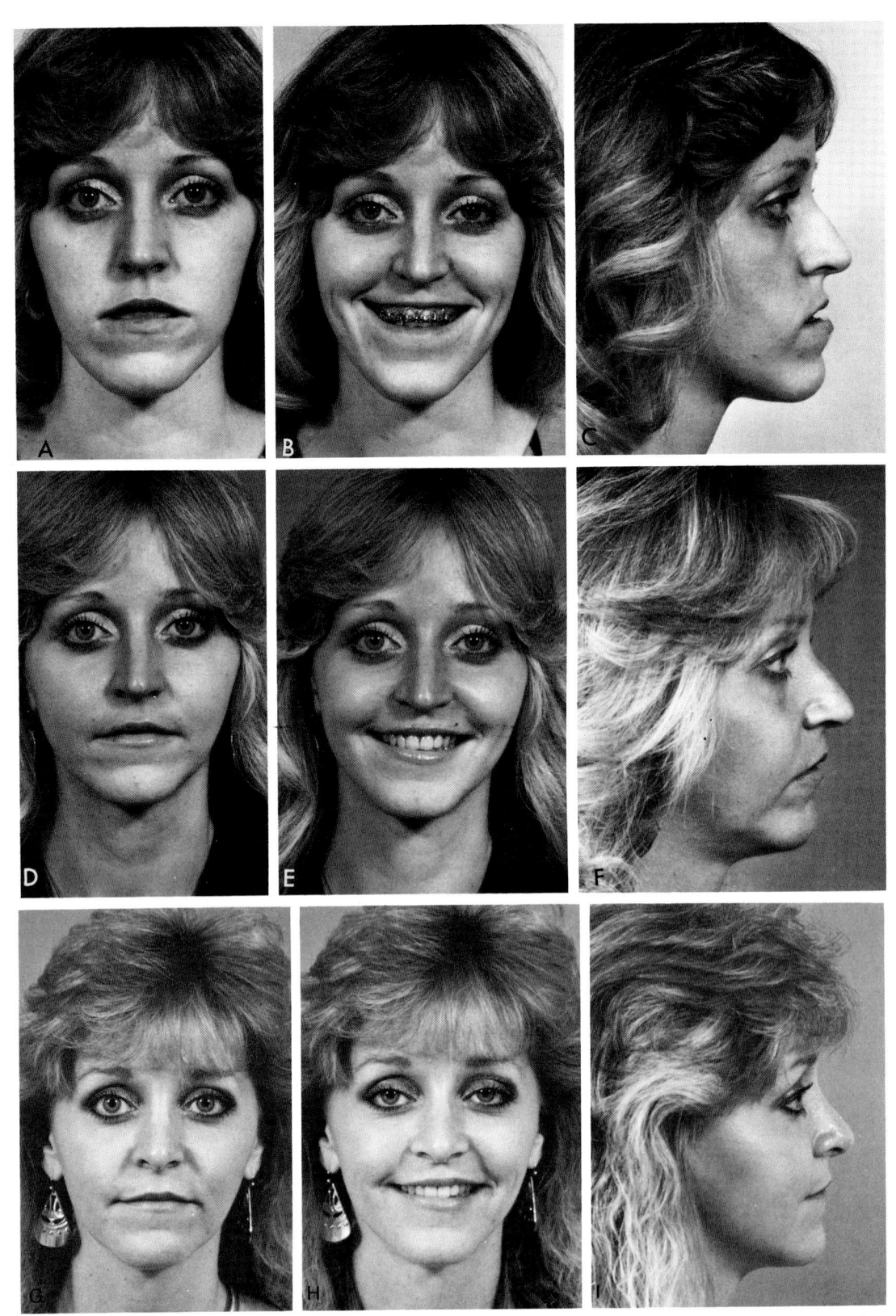

FIGURE 61-21. *A-C*, Facial appearance of 28-year-old woman with vertical maxillary excess and absolute mandibular excess before surgery. *D-F*, Appearance after surgical orthodontic treatment. *G-I*, Appearance 5 years after rhinoplasty.

FIGURE 61-21. *Continued* *J*, Cephalometric tracing before orthodontic treatment, showing vertical maxillary excess, mandibular excess, and typical dental compensations: retroinclination of mandibular anterior teeth and proclination of maxillary anterior teeth. *K*, Cephalometric tracing after presurgical orthodontic treatment designed to decompensate the dentition. *L*, Positional changes of teeth by presurgical orthodontic decompensation of dentition. *M*, Composite cephalometric tracings before (*solid line*) and after (*broken line*) surgical treatment.
Illustration continued on following page

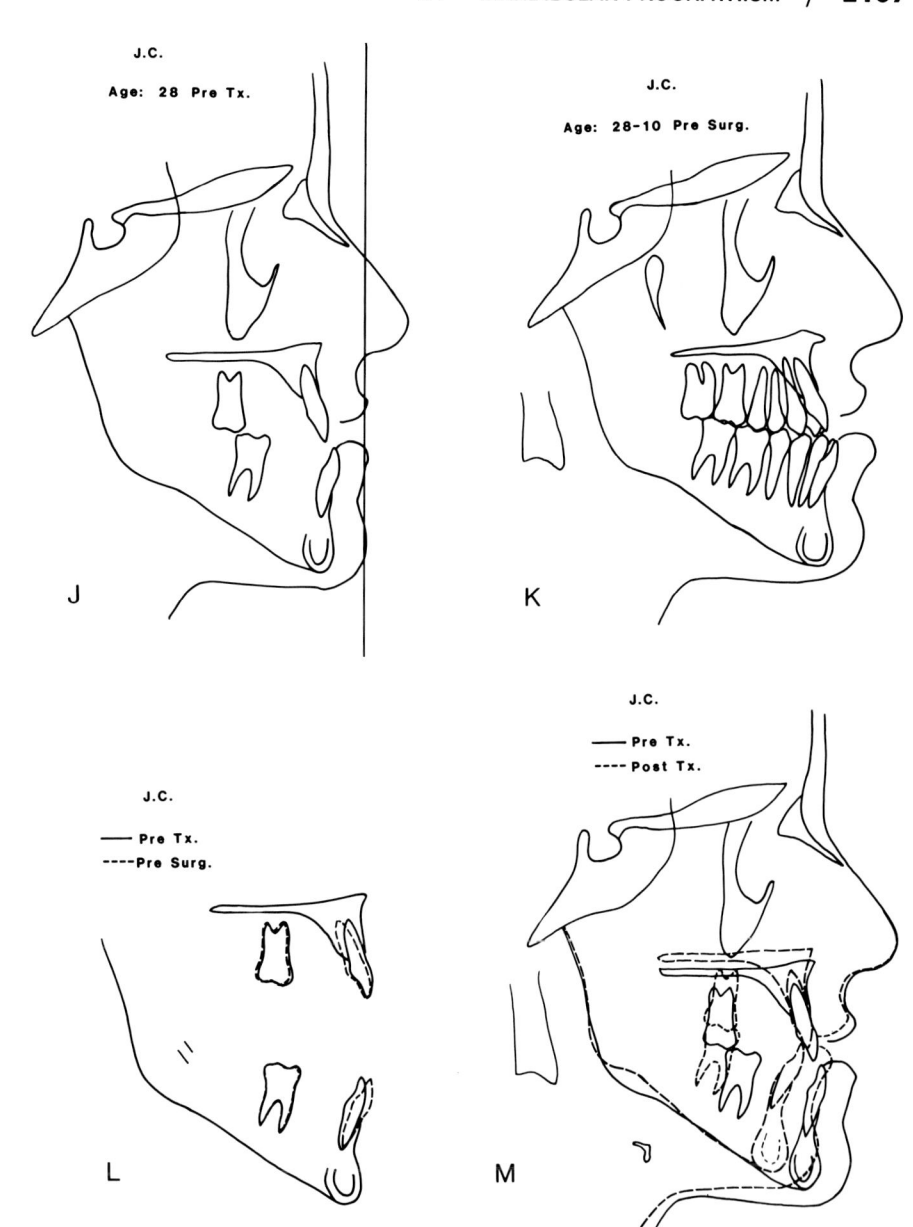

4. Correct crowding of lower anterior teeth and increase underjet by tipping the lower incisors forward into a more favorable position (see Fig. 61–21*I*)

Surgical Treatment (Fig. 61–21*Q* and *R*)

1. Two-segment Le Fort I osteotomy to (a) reposition the maxilla 4 mm superiorly to achieve an esthetic lip-tooth relationship and a symmetric esthetic smile and to facilitate the widening of nasal alar bases; and (b) widen the maxilla 3 mm to achieve transverse harmony with the mandible (osteotomy in the right lateral incisor-canine interdental space).

2. Posterior repositioning of the mandible 8 mm by bilateral intraoral vertical ramus osteotomies to achieve maxillomandibular harmony and produce a Class I cuspid and molar relationship

3. Secondary rhinoplasty to reduce dorsal nasal hump and raise nasal tip

4. Advancement genioplasty

Postsurgical Orthodontics

1. Occlusal and muscular rehabilitation
2. Final interdigitation of teeth with vertical elastics (light wire in maxillary arch; heavy rectangular wire in mandibular arch)
3. Occlusal adjustment
4. Retention with maxillary and mandibular Hawley retainers

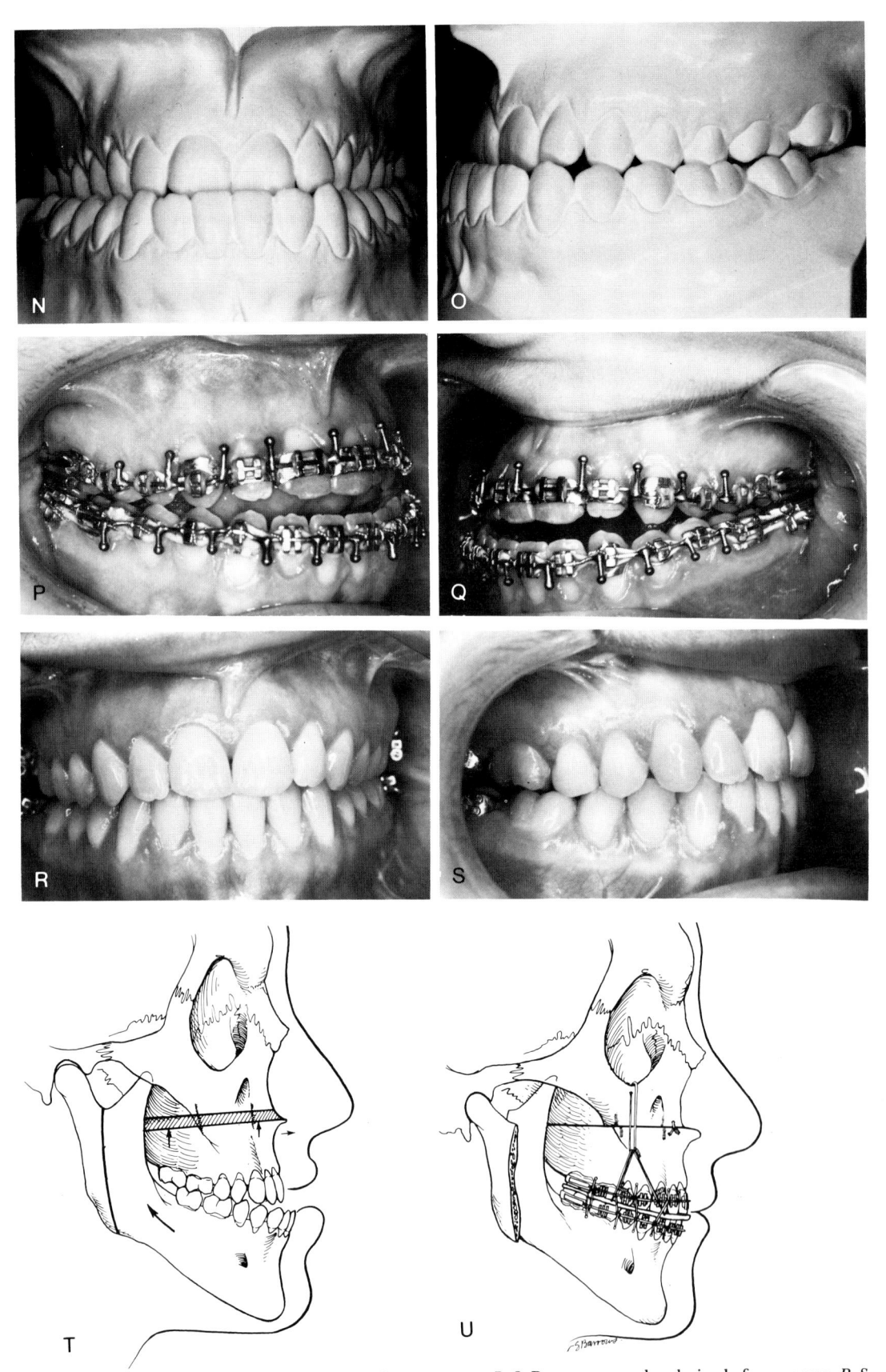

FIGURE 61–21. *Continued* N, O, Occlusion before treatment. P, Q, Decompensated occlusion before surgery. R, S, Occlusion after surgical orthodontic treatment. T, Plan of surgery: Two-segment Le Fort I osteotomy to reposition maxilla superiorly (anterior maxilla, 3 mm; posterior maxilla, 5 mm) to reduce incisor exposure and interlabial gap and widen maxilla; IVROs to retract mandible and achieve maxillomandibular harmony. Arrows indicate planned positional movement of jaws and chin; solid lines indicate planned osteotomies; cross-hatched area indicates planned ostectomies. U, Postoperative results: Repositioned maxilla fixed with interosseous wires and infraorbital rim suspension wires ligated to interocclusal splint. Nonrigid skeletal fixation achieved with infraorbital rim suspension wires and circum-mandibular wires ligated to interocclusal splint. (Surgeon: William H. Bell, Dallas; orthodontist: George D. Richie, Wichita Falls, TX. From Bell WH, Proffit WR, White RP Jr: Surgical Correction of Dentofacial Deformities. Vol III. Philadelphia, WB Saunders Company, 1985, pp 122–125; with permission.)

Active Treatment and Follow-up

The preoperative phase of orthodontic correction was accomplished within 10 months with an edgewise orthodontic appliance (Fig. 61–21M and N). After the dentition was decompensated and the arches were properly aligned and leveled, the maxilla was superiorly repositioned 4 mm and the mandible was retracted 8 mm (Fig. 61–21Q and R). The maxilla was widened 3 mm to correct the transverse maxillary deficiency. Final alignment of the incisors and interdigitation of the teeth were completed in another 4 months by orthodontics. Post-treatment dental symmetry, normal overbite and overjet, and restoration of normal functional movements of the mandible were obtained after 16 months of combined surgical and orthodontic treatment (Fig. 61–21O). Occlusal and skeletal stability has been maintained over a 2-year postoperative follow-up. A secondary rhinoplasty in combination with a small advancement genioplasty created positive subtle changes.

REFERENCES

60. Launter JK: Nachgelassene Schriften v. Band (Hundert physiognomische Regeln mit vielen Kupfern). Zurich, 1802.
61. Meier L: Uber Crania progeniaen. Arch Psychiatrie Nerv Krank vol 1, 1968.
62. Rakosi T: Treatment of Class III malocclusions. In Graber TM, Rakosi T, Petrovic AG: Dentofacial Orthopedics with Functional Appliances. St Louis, CV Mosby, 1985, pp 392–393.
63. Ellis EE, McNamara JA: Components of adult Class III malocclusion. J Oral Maxillofac Surg 42:295, 1984.
64. Gold JK: A new approach to the treatment of mandibular prognathism. Am J Orthod 35:893, 1949.
65. Davidov S, Geseva N, Donceva T, Devhova L: Incidence of Prognathism in Bulgaria. Danl Abstr G:240, 1961.
66. Montelsone L, Duuigneaud JD: Prognathism. J Oral Surg 21:190, 1963.
67. Newman, GB: Prevalence of malocclusion in children six to fourteen years of age and treatment in preventable cases. J Am Dent Assoc 52:566, 1956.
68. Suzuki S: Studies on the so called reverse occlusion. J Nihon Univ Sch Dent 5:51, 1961.
69. Worms FN, Isaacson RJ, Speidel TM: Surgical orthodontic treatment planning: Profile analysis and mandibular surgery. Angle Orthod 1:24, 1976.
70. Rakosi T, Schulli W: Class III anomalies: A coordinated approach to skeletal, dental and soft tissue problems. J Oral Surg 39:860–870, 1981.
71. Bell WH, Proffit WR, White RP (eds): Surgical Correction of Dentofacial Deformities. Philadelphia, WB Saunders Company, 1980.
72. Schulhof RJ, Nakamura S, Williamson E: Prediction of abnormal growth in Class III malocclusions. Am J Orthod 71:421, 1977.
73. Egermark-Erikson I, Carlsson GE, Magnusson T: A long-term epidemiological study of the relationship between occlusal factors and mandibular dysfunction in children and adolescents. J Dent Res 66:67–71, 1987.
74. Epker B, Fish L (eds): Dentofacial Deformities. Vol 1. St Louis, CV Mosby, 1986.
75. Jacobson A: Update on the Wits Appraisal. Angle Orthod 58:3, 205, 1988.
76. McNamara JA: A method of cephalometric evaluation. Am J Orthod 86:449, 1984.
77. Thompson JR: Abnormal function of the stomatognathic system and its orthodontic implications. Am J Orthod 48:758, 1962.
78. Hickham JH: Maxillary protraction therapy: Diagnosis and treatment. J Clin Orthod 25:102, 1991.
79. Nanda R: Biochemical and clinical considerations of a modified protraction headgear. Am J Orthod 78:125, 1980.
80. Graber LW: Chin cap therapy for mandibular prognathism. Am J Orthod 72:23, 1977.
81. Petit H: Adaptation following accelerated face mask therapy. In McNamara JA, Ribbens K, Howe R (eds): Clinical Alteration of the Growing Face. Monograph 14, Craniofacial Growth Series, Center for Human Growth and Development. Ann Arbor, MI, The University of Michigan, 1983.
82. Vig KWL: Orthodontic perspectives in craniofacial dysmorphology. In Vig KWL, Burdi AR (eds): Craniofacial Morphogenesis and Dysmorphologies. Monograph 21, Craniofacial Growth Series, Center for Human Growth and Development. Ann Arbor MI, The University of Michigan, 1986.
83. Behrents RG: Atlas of Growth in the Aging Craniofacial Skeleton. Monograph 20, Craniofacial Growth Series, Center for Human Growth and Development, Ann Arbor, MI, The University of Michigan, 1985.
84. Kokich V, Shapiro P: The effects of LeFort I osteotomies on the craniofacial growth of juvenile Macaca nemestrina. In McNamara JA, Jr, Carlson DS, Ribbens KA (eds): The Effect of Surgical Intervention on Craniofacial Growth. Monograph 12, Craniofacial Growth Series, Center for Human Growth and Development. Ann Arbor, MI, The University of Michigan, 1982.
85. Proffit WR, Phillips C, Dann C, Turvey TA: Stability after surgical-orthodontic correction of skeletal Class III malocclusion. I. Mandibular setback. Int J Adult Orthod Orthog Surg 6:7, 1991.

62 SOFT TISSUE CHANGES ASSOCIATED WITH ORTHOGNATHIC SURGERY

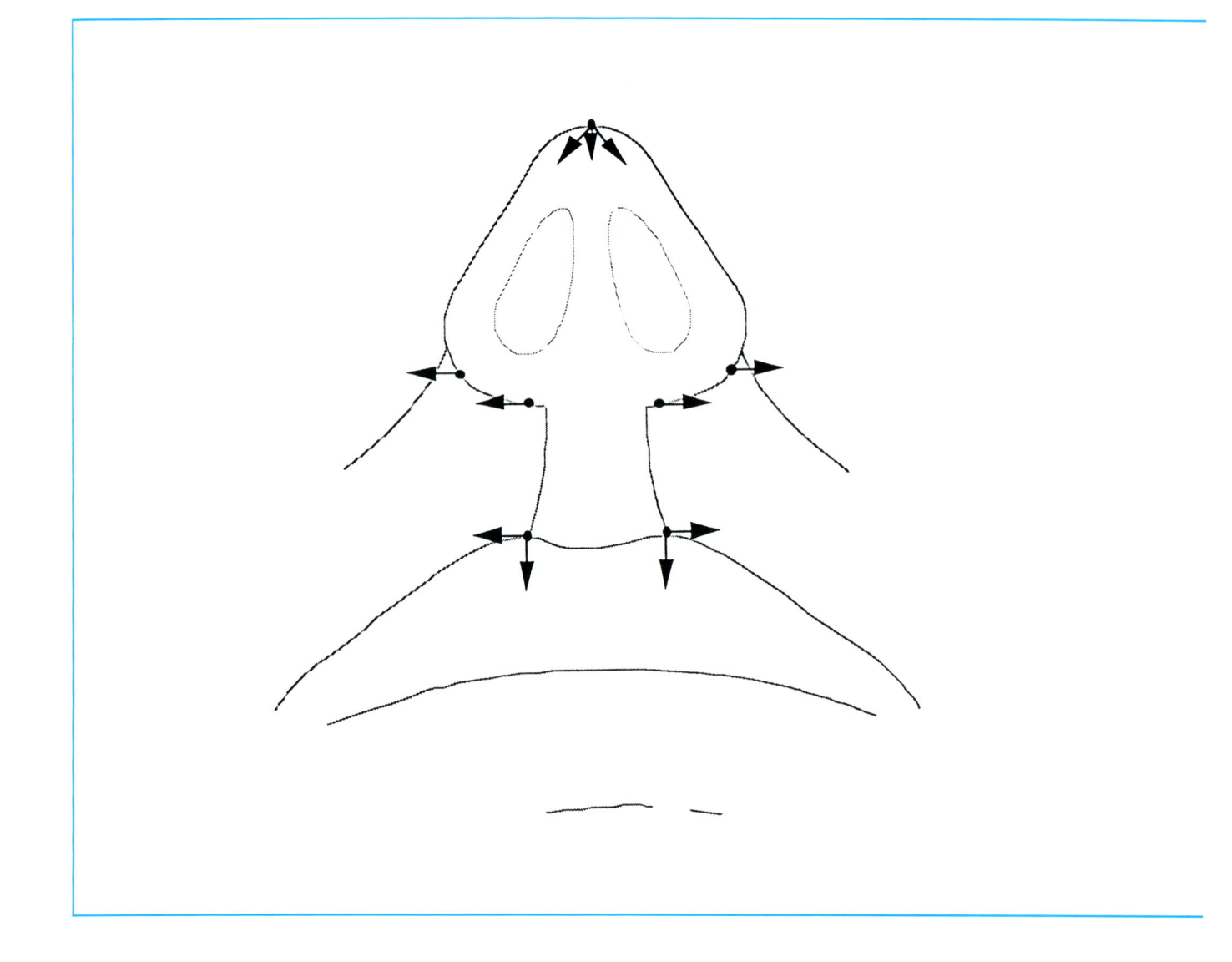

62

HISTORICAL PERSPECTIVE
ESTHETICS IN SOCIETY
FACIAL PROPORTIONS (CANONS)
ANATOMY
   Nose and Septum
   Upper and Lower Lip
   Chin
GENERAL CONSIDERATIONS
ORTHODONTIC CONSIDERATIONS
CEPHALOMETRIC CONSIDERATIONS
SOFT TISSUE CONSIDERATIONS
ORTHODONTIC INCISOR RETRACTION
MAXILLARY SURGICAL PROCEDURES
   Nasal Effects
   Anterior Segmental Setback
   Advancement
   Impaction
   Functional Considerations
   Downgraft
   Setback
   Combined Vectors of Maxillary Repositioning

MANDIBULAR SURGICAL PROCEDURES
   Anterior Segmental Setback
   Advancement (Sagittal)
   Setback (Sagittal and VRO)
   Autorotation
GENIAL SEGMENT SURGICAL PROCEDURES
   Advancement
   Alloplastic
   Setback (Horizontal Reduction)
   Vertical
POOR SURGICAL ESTHETIC RESULTS AND TECHNIQUES OF SOFT TISSUE CONTROL
   Maxilla
   Mandible
   Chin
SECONDARY REVISION OF POOR SURGICAL RESULTS
SIMULTANEOUS NASAL AND ORTHOGNATHIC SURGERY

NORMAN J. BETTS
RAYMOND J. FONSECA

The prime objective of orthognathic maxillofacial surgery is the harmonious relationship of the skeletal-dental components of the facial complex. A secondary and very important objective is the concomitant achievement of pleasing soft tissue esthetics. In order to achieve the latter, surgical treatment goals must maximize soft tissue esthetics. This requires that the clinician be aware of the soft tissue response to osseous surgery so that effective treatment strategies may be developed.[65] Well-planned cooperative treatment between the orthodontist and the surgeon should allow the correction of functional deficiencies while maximizing the soft tissue esthetic outcome.[29]

This chapter will address the soft tissue changes associated with orthognathic surgical procedures and their different vectors of movement. The techniques used in attempting to control these soft tissue changes will be presented and evaluated. The intent is to help the clinician to understand, control, and maximize to the patient's advantage the soft tissue changes related to orthodontically and surgically induced change.

HISTORICAL PERSPECTIVE

Concern with prediction and control of soft tissue changes originated in the orthodontic literature. As orthognathic surgical procedures evolved, a primary objective of treatment was correction of functional deficits. Often this was done at the expense of soft tissue and esthetic concerns. As these procedures became commonplace, concern over their effects upon the perioral soft tissues developed. Early studies produced average ratios relating specific hard and soft tissue landmarks. These ratios were of use in predicting the response of the soft tissues to the various skeletal and dental changes. However, they are averages and investigators observed that individual variability was large. This indicated that several factors may contribute to the soft tissue response. Consequently, more sophisticated statistical tools such as the multiple stepwise regression were employed with variable success to identify these factors and develop prediction equations.

In an attempt to control the soft tissue changes to the patient's and surgeon's advantage, emphasis shifted to the handling of the soft tissues, and techniques such as the alar cinch and V-Y closure were developed.

ESTHETICS IN SOCIETY

Physical appearance is of great importance in our society.[20,36,43] The appearance of one's face is the most important element of physical attractiveness. One's perception of oneself and the perceptions of others are both essential to self-esteem. Consequently, the presence of a dentofacial abnormality can be distressing both socially and psychologically.[8] Conversely, the correction of a dentofacial deformity can have significant effects upon self-esteem and personality.

Patients visualize themselves and others primarily from the frontal aspect. During the study of the soft tissue and esthetic changes associated with orthognathic surgery, frontal face esthetics have historically been less emphasized than profile esthetics. This is unfortunate; more emphasis on frontal esthetics is indicated in future investigations.[18,54,55]

FACIAL PROPORTIONS (CANONS)

The key to successful correction of dentofacial deformities is the preoperative identification of deformities. It must then be discerned whether the abnormality is a hard or soft tissue deformity. One successful technique used to identify abnormalities is to compare the patient's full face and profile to established facial canons. This allows the examiner to readily identify areas of deformity. For quantification of these deformities the radiographic and intraoral evaluations, as well as analysis of mounted dental casts, is crucial. During the clinical examination of facial proportions, the patient should be seated in a straight chair with the head in its natural position and the soft tissues in repose.

Full Facial Examination

The evaluation proceeds from a general assessment of balance among the various facial features to assessment of specific relations between them. After gross asymmetries are identified, the general balance between the upper, middle, and lower thirds is evaluated. The upper third is defined as the hairline to glabella, the middle third as glabella to subnasale, and the lower third as subnasale to menton (Figs. 62–1A,B and 62–3A,B). During assessment of the upper third, hair loss (e.g., male pattern baldness) must be taken into account. The important structures in the middle third are the eyes, cheeks, and nose. If marked exposure of inferior sclera is noted, infraorbital hypoplasia or exophthalmos may be present. The inter–inner canthal distance should be equal to the greatest alar width (Fig. 62–1C). An abnormality in this relation may indicate orbital hypertelorism, telecanthism, or a narrow or wide alar base width. In cases of ocular and/or orbital asymmetry or deformity, the pupillary heights, interpupillary distance, and inner and outer canthal distances should be measured. The cheek area is the widest portion of the face. The location of the prominence of the cheek should be 10 mm lateral and 15 to 20 mm inferior to the lateral canthus. The buccal area of the cheek should be flat or within the confines of a tangent from the cheekbone to the angle

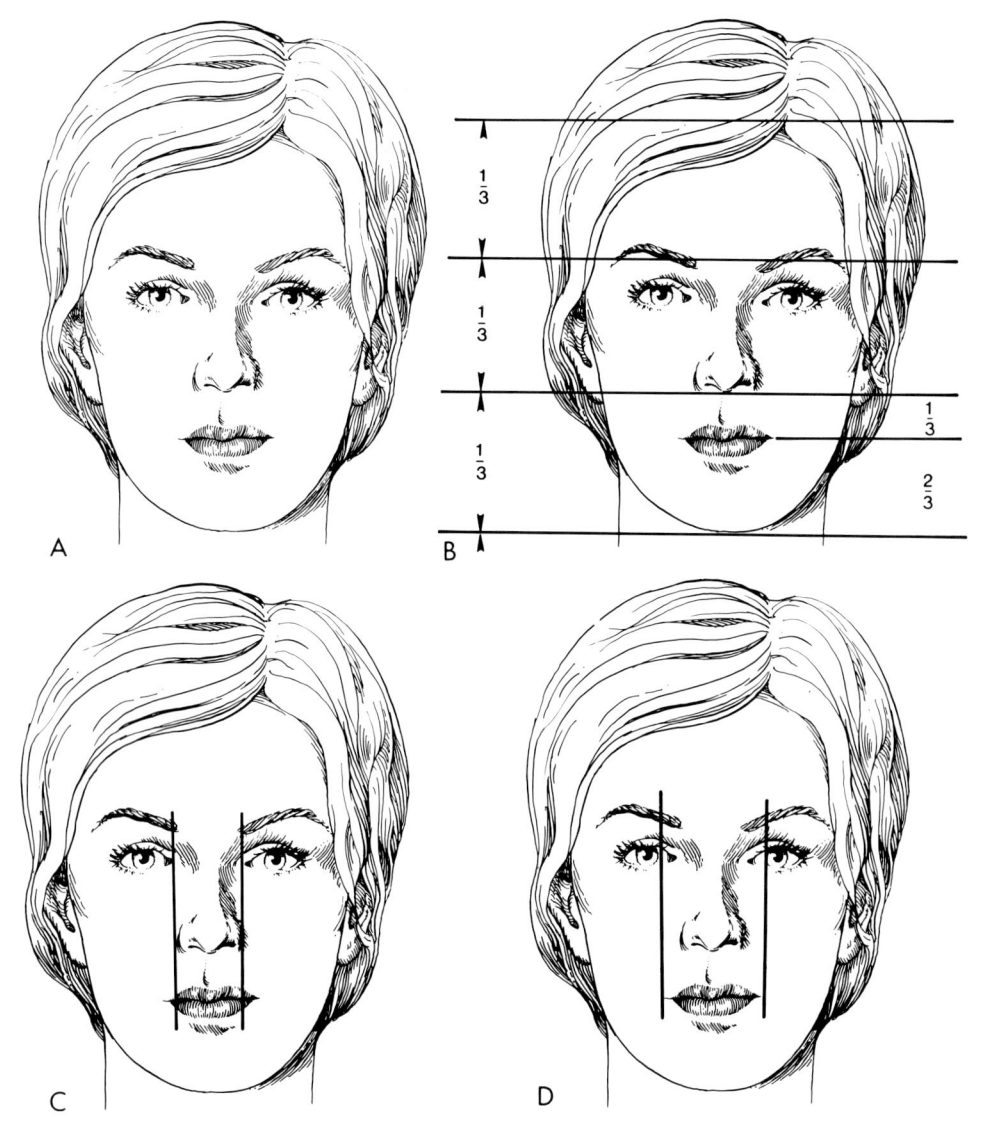

FIGURE 62–1. Normal facial proportions in the full-face examination. *A*, patient in "natural head position" facing the examiner. *B*, The thirds of the face are roughly equal in vertical dimension. Note that this lower third can be divided into an upper one-third and a lower two-thirds. *C*, Inter-inner canthal distance is about equal to nasal alar base width. *D*, The oral aperture is as wide as the distance from right to left medial limbus. (Adapted from Proffit WR, Epker BN, Ackerman JL: Systematic description of dentofacial deformities: The data base. *In* Bell WH, Proffit WR, and White RP (eds): Surgical Correction of Dentofacial Deformities. Philadelphia, WB Saunders, 1980, p 116.)

of the mandible. Cheek projection is best evaluated from above. The nasal structures must be evaluated for symmetry and balance with the rest of the face. A view of the patient from below is helpful in evaluating dorsal nasal symmetry, and alar width and symmetry. The lower third contains the upper and lower lips, the oral aperture, and the chin. The lower third can be divided vertically into an upper one third and a lower two thirds (Figs. 62–1*B* and 62–3*B*). Although the assessment of upper lip length is important, the relationship of the upper incisor to the upper lip and lower lip is essential to the treatment planning process. The width of the oral aperture is approximately equal to the distance between the right and left medial limbus (Fig. 62–1*D*). Interlabial gap and lip competence should be assessed. A prominent and everted lower lip should be evaluated to determine if it is caused by contact with dentoalveolar structures or true hypertrophy. The chin should be assessed for symmetry, vertical relations, morphology, and hyperactivity of the mentalis muscle. Lastly, the mandibular angles are assessed with regard to both their transverse and vertical symmetry and their fullness.

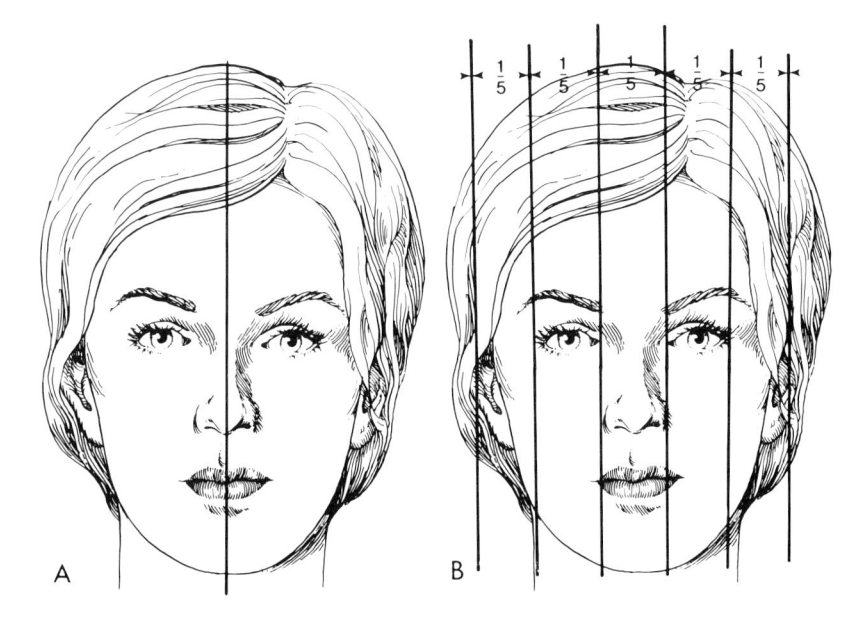

FIGURE 62–2. Evaluation of facial symmetry. A, Right-left symmetry is checked by holding an object so that it bisects the glabella, nasal tip, upper lip, and chin. B, The face is divided into fifths. (Adapted from Proffit WR, Epker BN, Ackerman JL: Systematic description of dentofacial deformities: The data base. In Bell WH, Proffit WR, and White RP (eds): Surgical Correction of Dentofacial Deformities. Philadelphia, WB Saunders, 1980, p 120.)

Facial Symmetry

Right to left symmetry is best checked by holding an object (dental floss held between two fingers) so that it bisects the glabella, nasal tip, upper lip, and chin (Fig. 62–2A). The soft tissues and dental midlines are evaluated in relation to this object. Most faces have some slight asymmetry, and this can be assessed by dividing the face into fifths (Fig. 62–2B).

Profile Examination

The facial thirds are assessed again from the profile view. The facial elements are evaluated for both anteroposterior and vertical abnormalities. In the middle third, the infraorbital rim should be 0 to 2 mm before, and the lateral orbital rim located 8 to 12 mm behind, the anterior projection of the globe. The cheek prominence is located 1.5 to 2.0 cm lateral and 2.0 cm inferior to the lateral canthus of the eye, and the paranasal areas should be slightly convex. The nasolabial and nasocolumellar proportions must also be evaluated, as well as the labiomental fold, submental length, neck-to-chin proportion, and submental cervical morphology of the lower third of the face (Fig. 62–3A,B).

When evaluating patients from different racial and ethnic groups, the examiner must keep in mind that different canons and interrelationships of the facial elements may apply. A more extensive description of esthetic evaluation of the face can be found in other texts.[77]

ANATOMY

Nose and Septum

SKELETAL

The external landmarks of the nose are the radix, dorsum, supratip depression, tip, and columella. Other important structures are the columellar-lobular junction, the ala, the alar groove, and the nasolabial angle (Fig. 62–4A,B). The basilar view of the nose reveals the (1) tip, (2) lobule, (3) columella, (4) ala, (5) alar-facial

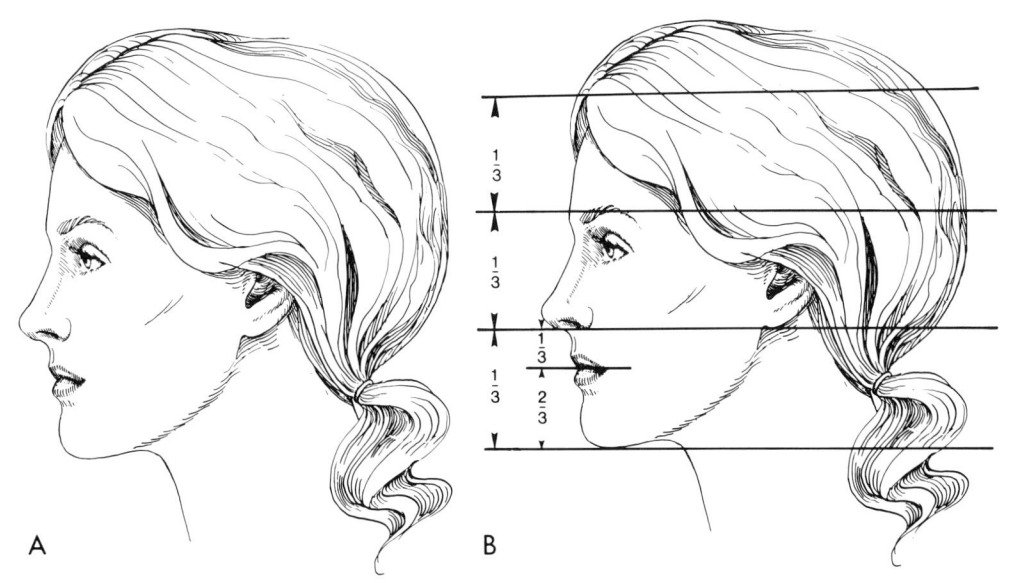

FIGURE 62-3. Normal facial dimensions in the profile examination. *A,* Head in "natural head position" with the visual axis parallel to the floor. *B,* Thirds of the face are equal, and the lower third is broken into an upper one-third and a lower two-thirds. (Adapted from Proffit WR, Epker BN, Ackerman JL: Systematic description of dentofacial deformities: The data base. *In* Bell WH, Proffit WR, and White RP (eds): Surgical Correction of Dentofacial Deformities. Philadelphia, WB Saunders, 1980, p 120.)

junction, (6) inner border of the ala, (7) outer border of the ala, (8) nostril, and (9) foot of the ala (Fig. 62–5). The height of the nasal base is made up of the height of the lobule (one third) plus the height of the columella (two thirds) (Fig. 62–5).

The internal nasal anatomy consists of cartilaginous and skeletal components. The osseous components of the nose include the nasal bones, the vomer, the perpendicular plate of the ethmoid, the maxilla, and the anterior nasal spine. The cartilaginous portion of the external nose is situated anterior to the piriform aperture. The upper cartilages are the paired lateral nasal cartilages and overlap the nasal bones by approximately 9 mm in the midline and 4 mm laterally. The nasal septum projects from between the upper lateral cartilages in the inferior one third of the nose. The alar (lowest lateral) cartilages are responsible for the structure and support of the tip lobule and consist of the medial and lateral crura. There is a lateral sesamoid cartilage complex that extends the lateral support of the lateral

FIGURE 62-4. The external nasal anatomy. *A,* The full face view. *B,* The profile view.

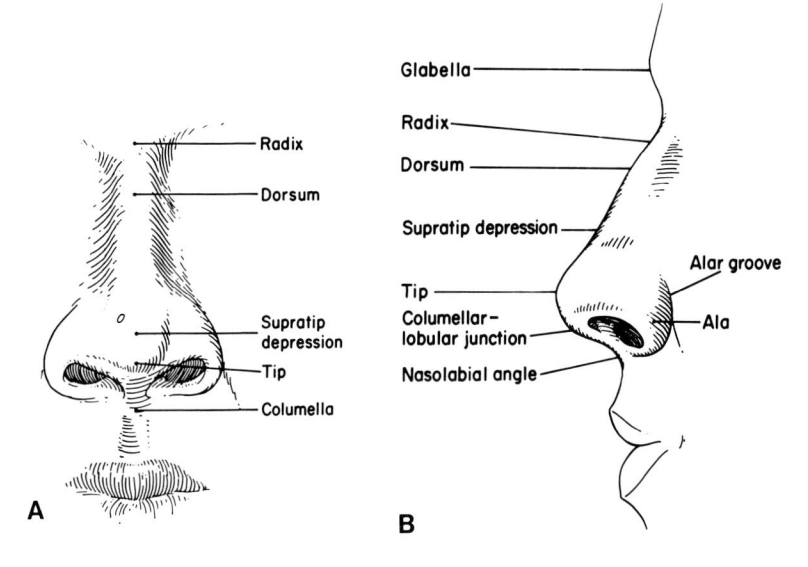

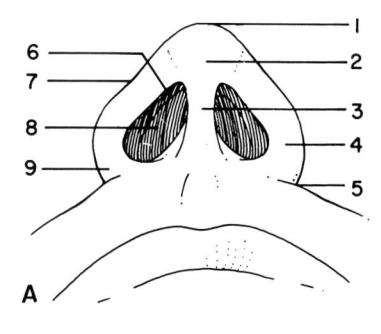

FIGURE 62-5. The structures of the nasal base from a basilar view. (1) tip, (2) lobule, (3) columella, (4) ala, (5) alar-facial junction, (6) inner border of the ala, (7) outer border of the ala, (8) nostril, and (9) foot of the ala. The height of the nasal base is made up of the height of the lobule (one third) plus the height of the columella (two thirds).

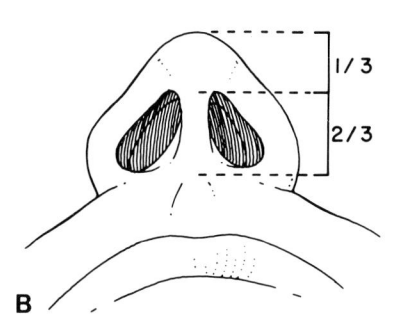

crus to the piriform rim. The medial crura parallel each other in the midline and curve laterally, resting on the anterior nasal spine (Fig. 62-6). The cartilaginous portion of the nasal septum is quadrangular and articulates with the vomer posteriorly. The free margin of the cartilaginous septum is separated from the columella by the juxtaposition of two mucocutaneous flaps called the membranous septum.[48,82] (Fig. 62-7).

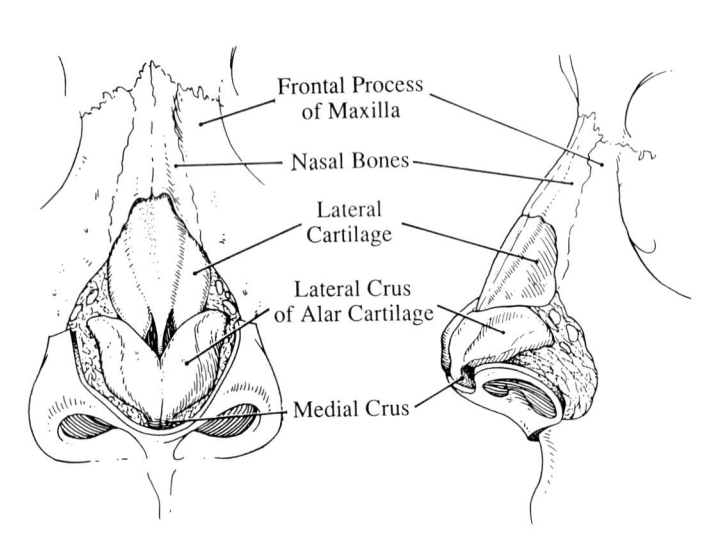

FIGURE 62-6. The bony and cartilaginous structures of the external nose.

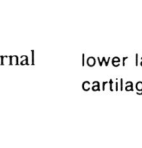

FIGURE 62-7. The bony and cartilaginous structures of the internal nose.

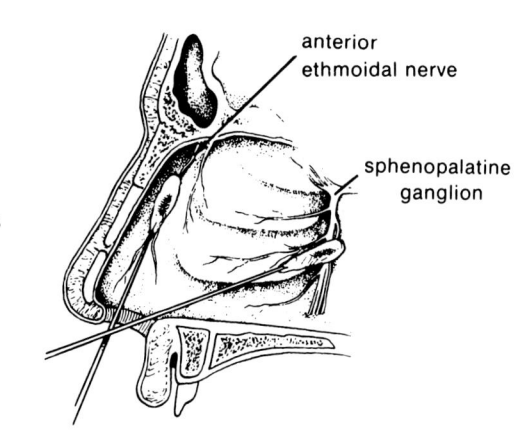

FIGURE 62-8. Innervation of the internal nose with cotton-cocaine swabs in place.

Nerves

The nerves of sensation to the external nose are the branches of the ophthalmic and maxillary divisions of the trigeminal nerve. The ophthalmic division of the trigeminal nerve supplies sensation to the soft tissues over and under the nasal bones and over the lobule, the anterior third of the nasal septum, and the anterior lateral walls of the internal nose. This is accomplished through the terminal branches of the nasociliary nerve and through the infratrochlear and anterior ethmoidal nerves. The maxillary nerve branches supply sensation to the soft tissues of the lower lateral nose, the posterior two thirds of the nasal septum, and the posterior two thirds of the lateral nasal walls. The sensory supply to the external nose is from the infraorbital nerve through its terminal branches, the external nasal and the superior palpebral nerves. The internal nasal structures are supplied by branches from the nasopalatine, greater palatine, and anterior superior alveolar nerves (Fig. 62-8). The motor nerves to the muscles of the nose are from the buccal branches of the facial nerve.[81,82]

Vasculature

The nose is highly vascular, possessing arterial contributions from both the internal and external carotid systems. The external nose and anterior septum are supplied from the external carotid system through the facial artery and its branches. The superior septum and orbital area are supplied through the internal carotid system by the ethmoidal branches of the ophthalmic artery. The superior labial branch of the facial artery supplies the columella, the lateral nasal branch of the facial artery supplies the ala and dorsum of the nose, and the angular artery supplies the upper nasal skin. The rest of the external nose is supplied by the dorsal nasal branch of the ophthalmic artery, the infraorbital branch of the maxillary artery, and the external nasal branches of the anterior ethmoidal artery (Fig. 62-9). The anterior portion of the septum is supplied by the septal branch of the

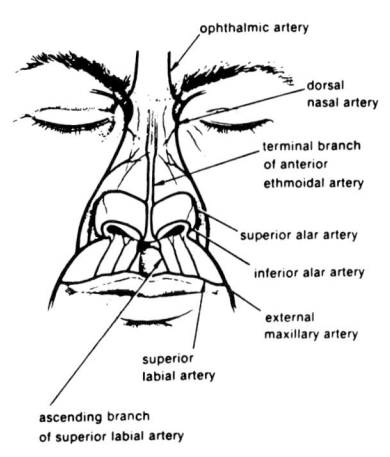

FIGURE 62-9. The vascular supply of the external nose.

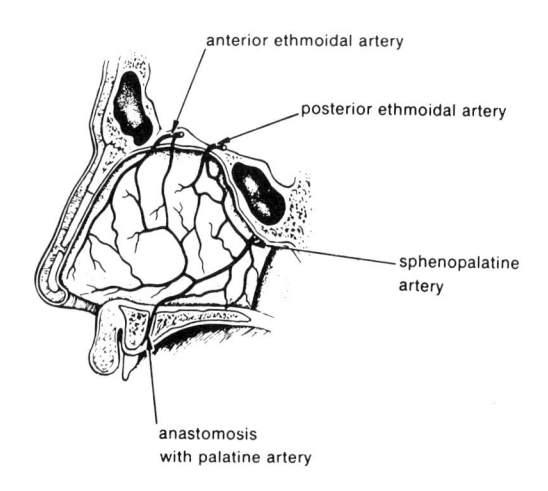

FIGURE 62-10. The vascular supply of the septum.

facial artery. A large plexus is formed here with contributions from the septal branch of the superior labial artery, the palatine artery, and the posterior septal artery and is a common site of nosebleed. The rest of the septum is supplied by the medial nasal branches of the anterior ethmoidal artery, the medial nasal branch of the posterior ethmoidal artery, and branches of the sphenopalatine artery (Fig. 62-10). The lateral nasal walls are supplied by the ethmoid branches of the ophthalmic artery and the terminal branches of the sphenopalatine artery and the posterior lateral nasal and descending palatine arteries.[81,82]

MUSCLES

The importance of the facial muscles in the appearance of the face was addressed by Schendel and Delaire.[67] They noted that the facial muscles are the most obvious feature of the patient. The three functions of the facial muscles are to animate the superficial and deep mobile elements of the face, support and unite the hard and soft tissues, and influence the growth of the facial skeleton.

The major muscles of the nasolabial region are the procerus, nasalis, dilator naris, depressor septi, levator labii superioris alaque nasi, levator labii superioris, levator anguli oris, and the zygomaticus major and minor. The procerus draws the skin of the forehead downward producing transverse wrinkles at the root of the nose. The nasalis muscle is divided into the pars transversa and the pars alaris and along with the dilator naris and depressor septi muscle dilates the nasal aperture. During this action the nose is flattened and widened, the alar cartilage is drawn downward and outward and the lower end of the septum moves downward. A portion of the levator labii superioris alaeque nasi raises the ala of the nose[48,81] (Fig. 62-11). The remaining muscles of the face will be discussed in the following sections.

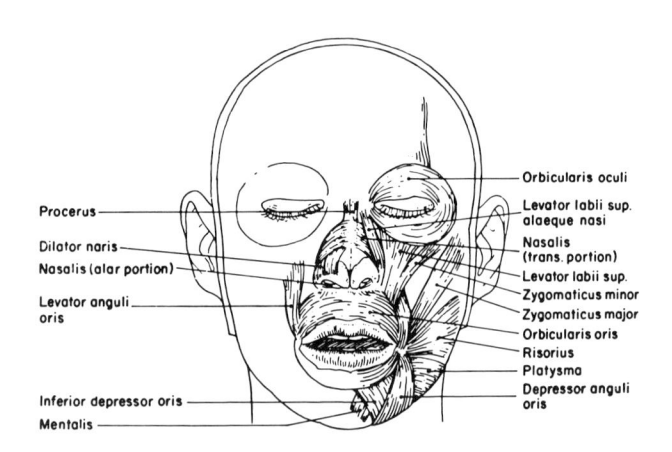

FIGURE 62-11. The muscles of the face.

Upper and Lower Lip

SKELETAL

The skeletal support of the upper and lower lips is comprised of the maxilla, the mandible, and the dentition.

NERVES

The motor innervation of the upper and lower lips comes from buccal, mandibular, and marginal mandibular branches of the facial nerve. The sensory innervation comes from the maxillary and mandibular divisions of the trigeminal nerves.

VASCULATURE

A large portion of the blood supply to the upper and lower lips comes from the facial artery and its branches, the inferior and superior labial arteries. However, the vascular anastomoses of the face are extensive, so that if the blood supply from one artery is compromised the involved tissue will receive perfusion from another source.

MUSCLES

The orbicularis oris muscle is a sphincter muscle that constitutes the bulk of the upper and lower lips. Three muscles enter the upper lip from above and are its principal elevators: the levator labii superioris alaeque nasi, the levator labii superioris, and the zygomaticus major. The corners of the mouth are affected by the levator anguli oris, which elevates the lip and draws it medially, the zygomaticus major, which turns the angle of the mouth upward and outward, the risorius, which widens the mouth, and the depressor anguli oris, which depresses the corner of the mouth. The depressor labii inferioris muscle inserts into the skin of the lower lip and draws the lower lip downward and laterally[81] (Fig. 62-11).

Chin

SKELETAL

The greatest anteroposterior thickness of the mandible at the midline of the mandibular symphysis in adults varies from 10 to 20 mm. This may limit the amount of advancement possible with a genioplasty.

The height of the mandibular symphysis from the incisal edge to menton is an important anatomic consideration. However, the average length of the mandibular teeth is more important, since to assure tooth vitality the vertical position of the horizontal osteotomy must be 4 to 5 mm below the tooth apices. The average length of the mandibular central incisor is 21.4 mm, that of the mandibular lateral incisor length is 23.2 mm, and that of the length of the mandibular canine is 25.4 mm. The remaining vertical height of bone between the tooth apices and the inferior border of the mandible dictates the amount of bone that can be removed.[34]

NERVES

The mental nerves are a continuation of the inferior alveolar nerve and its course curves anterior and inferior to the mental foramen. The nerve then courses posteriorly and superiorly, exiting the foramen bilaterally near the apices of the mandibular first and second premolars. Care must be taken to allow for this anterior and inferior extension of the nerve when planning osteotomy cuts. The mental nerve separates into several bundles as it exits the foramen, and they often lie superficially in the lower buccal vestibule. The mandibular canal continues anteriorly as a narrow canal that carries the incisive nerve to the mandibular anterior teeth. The skin in the submental region and along the inferior border of the mandible is innervated by the cervical nerves.[34] The muscles of the chin are innervated largely by the mandibular and marginal mandibular branches of the facial nerve.[81]

VASCULATURE

The bony mandibular symphysis receives its blood supply internally from the inferior alveolar artery and its extension, the incisive artery. The periosteum and muscle attachments also provide a large percentage of the blood supply to the mandible. The entire vascular needs of the mandible can be met without the contribution of the inferior alveolar artery.[34]

MUSCLES

The normal soft tissue thickness over the osseous chin is 10 to 12 mm.[17] Three groups of muscles that attach on the lingual aspect of the mandibular symphysis must be considered. The paired genioglossus muscles attach at the superior aspect of the genial tubercle. The paired geniohyoid muscles attach just below. The paired anterior digastric muscles attach on the inferior border in the digastric fossa. Depending upon the height of an osteotomy, various amounts of lingual musculature will be severed. The mentalis, depressor anguli oris, depressor labii inferioris, and platysma have sites of origin or insertion on the anterior and lateral aspects of the mandible. Differential incision placement and exposure of the genial segment involve severing or detaching different muscle groups[81] (Fig. 62-11).

GENERAL CONSIDERATIONS

There is a plethora of literature on the subject of soft tissue changes associated with orthognathic surgery. Each investigation that has attempted to identify or quantify the soft tissue changes associated with orthognathic surgery has its merits and flaws. Since there have been no standardized quantitative or qualitative criteria used in these studies, it is difficult to assess their usefulness in helping the surgeon identify and understand the soft tissue changes associated with osseous surgery. In an attempt to make some objective comparisons between methodologically different studies, a set of characteristics for the theoretically ideal study of the soft tissue changes associated with orthognathic surgery were identified (Table 62-1). The evaluation of individual investigations against these criteria should help the reader to assess their usefulness and validity. This technique for assessing the previous literature is helpful and should be considered for use in other areas of scientific investigation.[9]

Most of the studies dealing with this subject provide ratios of soft to hard tissue movement. Ratios are averages and describe the relationship of only two specific points. It is highly improbable that consistently accurate predictions of soft tissue change can be made with only simple correlations. The complex behavior of the anatomic structures comprising the facial soft tissue drape is much more realistically described by the interaction of several factors within the skeletal framework. This may explain some of the extreme variability that many authors have encountered.[18,31,42,57,65] Therefore, at best, ratios merely serve to give a general appreciation of the expected outcome.[65] It would be ideal if prediction equations could be formulated that could account for all of this variability and still be accurate and individualized.

The multiple regression and stepwise regression analysis are commonly used methods for understanding the nature of the complex interplay of various factors in determining the soft tissue response to surgery.[65] Some authors have stated that ratios are just as efficacious in predicting the soft tissue response to osseous surgery as are these sophisticated statistical tests.[42,65] This may be due to several factors,

TABLE 62-1. THEORETICAL IDEAL CHARACTERISTICS OF A STUDY TO INVESTIGATE THE SOFT TISSUE CHANGES ASSOCIATED WITH ORTHOGNATHIC SURGERY

1. Prospective
2. Adequate sample size
3. Randomized treatments (if treatments differ within the sample)
4. Nongrowing patients
5. No previous trauma to the osseous structures of the face
6. Exclusion of patients with congenital defects or syndromes (e.g., cleft patients)
7. Elimination of the confounding effects of pre- and postoperative orthodontic tooth movement [42,65]
8. Constant presence or absence of orthodontic appliances
9. Same cephalostat used for all cephalograms with identical source-subject and subject-film distances
10. Soft tissues in repose for all cephalograms[4]
11. Superimposition of cephalograms on the nearest osseous structure not affected by surgery or on a stable reference line[10,65]
12. Use of a tracing template to assist in landmark identification[10,56,65,70]
13. Evaluation of both profile and full facial soft tissue changes, or 3D analysis
14. No concomitant or prior soft tissue surgery
15. Exclusion of segmental surgical procedures
16. One vector of movement (or grouped in study)[70]
17. No concomitant osseous surgery on another portion of the facial skeleton[42]
18. Homogeneity of the soft tissue incisions and closure techniques[35,42,55,65,73,77]
19. No hard tissue contouring (e.g., recontouring of ANS)
20. Use of rigid osseous fixation
21. Uniform follow-up intervals
22. Follow-up time of at least 6 months (1 year is preferable)
23. Error analysis of measurement and landmark identification

such as lack of inclusion of important variables (method of soft tissue closure and osseous contouring) into their data base; use of a mixed sample population (race, age, or gender); use of a small number of patients; and inability to limit the sample to specific vectors of osseous movement.[9,42,57,65]

Recent investigations have shown improved predictive ability when patients were grouped by vector specific movement of the osseous segments.[9,70]

ORTHODONTIC CONSIDERATIONS

When a jaw imbalance is present, the force of the facial musculature on the teeth influences their position, causing dental compensation. If such a case is approached surgically, the teeth will dictate the surgical positioning of the jaws. If the teeth are in compensated positions, the surgery will correct only that portion of the jaw imbalance not compensated for by the teeth. Consequently, in order to achieve a full correction of the jaw imbalance, it is necessary to remove the dental compensations and properly relate the teeth to their respective jaws before surgery. When the teeth are appropriately related to their respective jaws just before surgery, the jaw-to-jaw discrepancy will appear clinically more severe and the patient will "look worse."[56,60]

When ratio studies are evaluated, it becomes apparent that the incisor teeth do not always accurately reflect the osseous movement. This may be due to postoperative orthodontic tooth movement. The molar teeth or bony landmarks such as anterior nasal spine (ANS) undergo less postoperative change and may more accurately describe the osseous surgical movement. Therefore, these landmarks should produce a more accurate ratio or prediction.[65]

A patient with an open-bite tendency should be carefully evaluated by the orthodontist and the surgeon, who should decide whether segmental orthodontic mechanics are indicated. If teeth are extruded to close a skeletal open bite, they may rebound after the removal of orthodontic appliances, leading to a relapse of the open bite.

CEPHALOMETRIC CONSIDERATIONS

The use of a standardized cephalometric technique is essential to the study of this subject. The components of a standardized cephalometric technique are (1) use of the same cephalometer, with the same source-subject and subject film distances, and (2) patient positioning in natural head position with the teeth in occlusion and soft tissues in repose. Relaxed soft tissues may be difficult to achieve and reproduce. Relaxed lip posture is especially difficult to achieve in patients with excessive lip incompetence. These patients often distort the labiomental fold by contracting the mentalis muscle to seal their lips. If the lips are not in repose when the cephalogram is taken, accurate treatment planning of the soft tissues is impossible. In order to acquire the required treatment planning information, two cephalograms may be needed: the first with the teeth in occlusion and the second with the teeth disoccluded and the mandible in rest position, to demonstrate relaxed lip position.[3] Obviously, the cephalogram obtained from the standardized cephalometric technique must allow visualization of the complete soft tissue profile.

To minimize measurement error during cephalometric analysis, superimposition must occur on landmarks or planes approximating the structures being evaluated. This superimposition should be on landmarks not modified or changed during the surgical procedure.[10,65] Another contributing factor to measurement error is orthodontic tooth movement during the period of study. Orthodontic changes can be minimized by obtaining the preoperative cephalogram within one month of the planned surgical procedure[42,65] and performing minimal postoperative orthodontics.[65] It is also important that there be a constant presence or absence of orthodontic appliances during the study period. The presence of orthodontic appliances influences lip posture, and their placement or removal will change the soft tissue drape.[9]

Landmark identification is simplified and becomes more accurate when templates are used.[10,65,70] This is especially valid for soft tissue landmarks.[56] Soft tissue landmarks are often arbitrary (deepest or most prominent points) and located on gently curving contours. These landmarks can therefore move vertically over the surface of the tissue after surgically induced change.[57,60] If tracing templates are used, these points can be accurately reproduced.

The nasolabial proportion (angle) should be evaluated preoperatively because it is believed to be an important diagnostic criterion for total maxillary advancement.[18]

SOFT TISSUE CONSIDERATIONS

The ability to predict the hard and soft tissue changes before an orthognathic surgical procedure is critical to the treatment planning process. With the refinement of surgical procedures and the advent of rigid fixation techniques, the surgeon is able to accurately move and retain the osseous components in a planned position. However, the soft tissues are another matter. This is because the change in soft tissue morphology after combined orthodontic and surgical therapy is dependent on several factors. These include surgical procedure,[35,42,47,54,65,73,77] method of wound closure,[35,42,54,65,73,77] the new spatial arrangement of the skeletal and dental element,[73] the adaptive qualities of the soft tissues,[73] growth,[47,71] orthodontic vectors of tooth movement,[47,73] lip thickness,[18,23,42,47,63,70] lip tonus,[65] lip area, lip contact (competence), lip strength, interlabial gap, amount of overjet, amount of fatty tissue and musculature, and postoperative edema.[47]

Because of swelling, tissue redistribution, and functional adaptation, long-term follow-up is needed to assess soft tissue changes after surgical procedures. Most authors suggest that the soft tissues stabilize after a 6-month time period.[18,23,24,47,73] Other authors suggest that a period of at least 12 months is required.[56,80]

Surgical technique and method of wound closure have been shown to affect soft tissue relationships.[35,42,53,54,65,73,77] For example, the horizontal incision in the upper labial vestibule, commonly used to gain access to the maxilla for the Le Fort I osteotomy, causes shortening of the lip with loss of vermilion and a decrease in lip thickness.[35] However, the use of vertical incisions with a tunneling approach and palatal flap for the same surgical procedure produces minimal postoperative lip changes.[73] In a recent study investigating the soft tissue response to maxillary surgery, it appeared that soft tissue changes were consistent and that they may be affected more by the type and position of the soft tissue incision and methods used in closure than by the surgically induced hard tissue change.[9]

Changes in facial esthetics and occlusion following orthognathic surgery are highly dependent on the stability achieved following surgery.

It has been shown by many authors that thin lips move more predictably than do thick lips.[18,23,42,47,63,70] Two theories have been advanced to explain this observation. First, the actual bulk of a thick lip may have a tendency to absorb a large amount of bony advancement without a perceptible change in soft tissue contour. Secondly, "dead space" under the lip may absorb the first portion of a bony advancement before the soft tissue is affected (e.g., severe maxillary retrognathia).[18,23,42,47,63,70]

One of the major obstacles to quantification of the soft tissue changes associated with orthognathic surgery has been the inability of a two-dimensional analyses such as a cephalogram or photograph to accurately describe the three-dimensional structures of the face.[9] For example, Sakima and Sachdeva[65] stated that lip morphology may be best described by considering the volumetric redistribution of the soft tissues and that this cannot be measured on the lateral cephalogram. For accurate quantification of a three-dimensional object, at least two two-dimensional analyses oriented at 90 degrees to each other are required. The ideal analysis would be measurement of the three-dimensional structure itself, and the next best option would be measurement of a nondistorted, three-dimensional model.[9]

The soft tissue of the face is relatively incompressible, and the morphologic changes seen in the lip as a result of surgery may be attributed to soft tissue redistribution.[65,78] Several investigators have documented minimal postsurgical change in the area of the upper lip, lower lip, and chin, with return to preoperative values.[19,65,78] The new three-dimensional imaging techniques may be useful for the evaluation and quantification of this soft tissue redistribution after orthognathic surgical procedures have been performed.

The general trend noted in the literature is that the horizontal changes in the soft tissues are often predictable, whereas the vertical changes are unpredictable. This may be due to smaller movements in the vertical plane and the use of soft and hard tissue landmarks better suited for horizontal assessment. Hard tissue change is less predictable and less stable in the vertical dimension.

The cephalometric landmarks shown in Figure 62–12 will be used to describe the relationships between the soft and hard tissue changes presented in the rest of this chapter.

ORTHODONTIC INCISOR RETRACTION

The majority of studies investigating the effect of orthodontic treatment on the perioral soft tissues have dealt with maxillary and mandibular incisor retraction. Early studies in the orthodontic literature stressed that the soft tissue profile was closely related to the skeletal and dental structures.[59] In a subsequent paper,

2184 / VII—MANDIBULAR DEFICIENCY

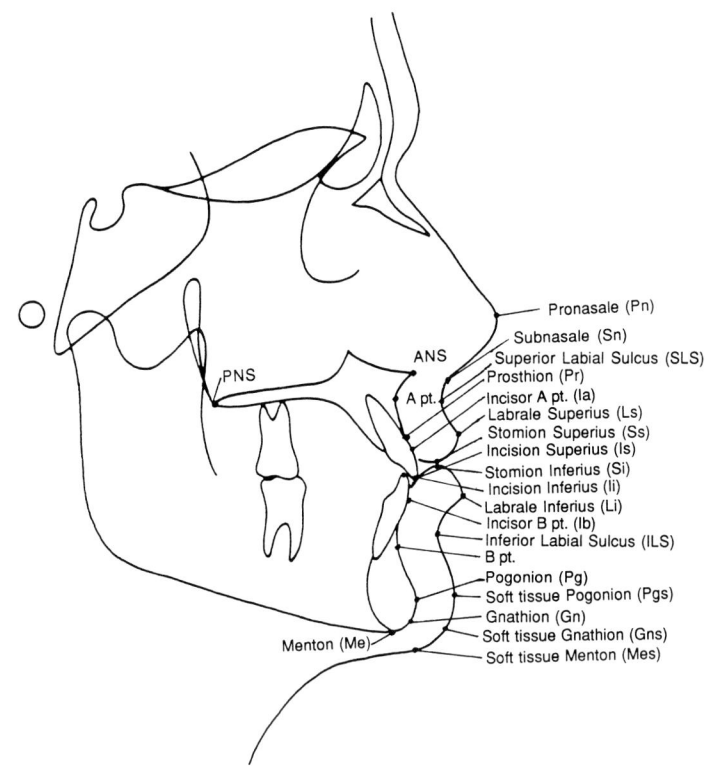

FIGURE 62-12. The hard and soft tissue cephalometric landmarks utilized for the evaluation of the hard and soft tissue changes associated with orthognathic surgical procedures. These landmarks are referenced in Tables 62-2 to 62-15.

Subtelny[71] indicated that not all parts of the soft tissue profile directly follow the underlying skeletal profile. Burstone[12] agreed and suggested that a direct relationship between hard and soft tissue changes may not always exist because of variation in the thickness of the soft tissues covering the face. The effects of growth and development, large ANB differences, positional relationship of the upper incisor on the lower lip (overbite and overjet), and adipose tissue are other factors that confuse the issue and may contribute to the great individual variability observed.[10]

The changes in the soft tissues associated with orthodontic incisor movements are seen in Table 62-2.

TABLE 62-2. SOFT TISSUE CHANGES ASSOCIATED WITH ORTHODONTIC TOOTH MOVEMENT

Superior sulcus(H)	−0.89:1	Upper incisor retraction	Bloom (1961)*
Upper lip(H)	−0.87:1	Upper incisor retraction	
Lower sulcus(H)	−0.87:1	Lower incisor retraction	
Lower lip(H)	−0.93:1	Lower incisor retraction	
Lower lip(H)	−0.82:1	Upper incisor retraction	
Upper lip(H)	−0.34:1	Upper incisor retraction	Rudee (1964)*
Lower lip(H)	−1.56:1	Lower incisor retraction	
Lower lip(H)	−1:1	Upper incisor retraction	
Upper, Lower lip(H)	−/+0.75-.9:1	Incisor protrustion or retraction	Robinson (1972)*
Upper lip(H)	−0.5:1	Ls: Ia Upper incisor retraction	Hershey (1972)
Lower lip (H)	−1.22:1	Li: Ib lower incisor retraction	
Upper lip(H)	−0.5:1	Maxillary incisor retraction	Proffit, Epker (1980)
Increased nasolabial angle			
No nasal change			
Upper lip(H)	−0.63:1	Ls: Upper incisor retraction	Rains (1982)

* Includes growing patients.

Review of the literature indicates that with incisor retraction, the upper lip rotates backward around subnasale,[54] with an associated reduction in the prominence of the lips relative to their adjacent sulci.[31] Also, upper lip thickness increases with maxillary incisor retraction (1 mm with 3 mm of incisor retraction,[58] 1 mm with 1.5 mm of incisor retraction[2]). Correlation analysis discloses that upper lip response not only is related to the upper incisor retraction but also is related to lower incisor movement, mandibular rotation, and the lower lip. This confirms that the lips have effect upon each other.

The lower lip moves less predictably with retraction of the incisors than does the upper lip.[31] Several theories have been advanced to explain this phenomenon. Hershey[31] has theorized that this is because the lower lip is much more self-supporting and not so dependent on underlying incisor support. Other investigators[31,64] believe that this may be due to the fact that both the upper and lower incisors affect the lower lip positioning (note the $-1:1$ effect of upper incisor retraction to lower lip retraction). They believe that the upper teeth, not the lower, establish the curve of the lower lip. Therefore, if the upper incisor is retracted more than the lower incisor, the lower lip may displace more posteriorly than the lower incisor ($-1.56:1,$[64] $-1.22:1$[31]). Another theory is that many factors contribute to the final position of the lower lip. This theory is supported by correlation analysis that indicates that mandibular rotation has a greater influence upon lower lip response than incisor movement. Stepwise regression analysis lends further support to this theory by revealing that there is a complex interaction between dental movement, mandibular rotation, and the perioral soft tissues as well as a complex relationship within the soft tissues themselves.

MAXILLARY SURGICAL PROCEDURES

It has been observed by previous investigators that the majority of the soft tissue change after the Le Fort I surgery is expressed in the nasal and labial structures.[48-50]

Nasal Effects

Movement of the maxilla does affect the nasal dorsum.[18,24,42,48-50,55] However, the lower portion of the nose is significantly affected by maxillary surgery. The general trend is a widening of the greatest alar width and alar base width in all patients regardless of the vector of surgical maxillary movement. An associated shortening of the columella height, alar height, and nasal tip protrusion is seen, and the nasolabial angle is decreased or remains constant in most cases[9] (Fig. 62-13).

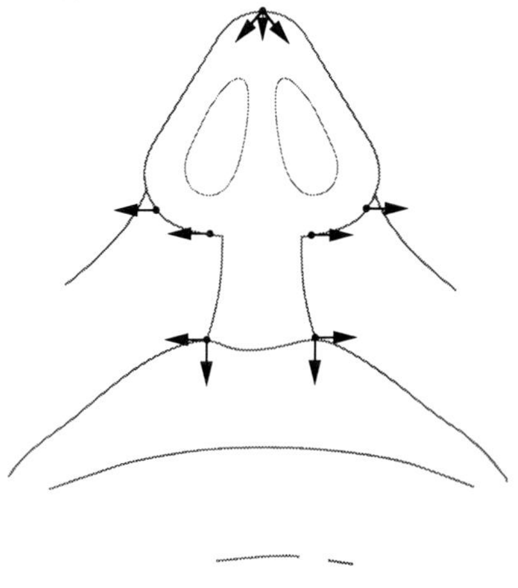

FIGURE 62-13. The general trends of postoperative changes in the nasal and labial soft tissues expressed in a nonvector format (the arrows are not specific for length, but are specific for direction). Generally, the alar base of the nose widens and the nasal tip decreases in height in relation to the adjacent soft tissues. The philtral columns of the lip widen and lengthen, and the nasolabial angle decreases. (Adapted from Betts NJ: Changes in the nasal and labial soft tissues after surgical repositioning of the maxilla. MS Thesis in Oral and Maxillofacial Surgery. University of Michigan, 1990.)

TABLE 62-3. NASAL EFFECTS OF MAXILLARY SURGERY

DIRECTION OF MAXILLARY MOVEMENT	ALAR BASES	NASAL TIP	SUPRATIP DEPRESSION	DORSAL HUMP	NASOLABIAL ANGLE
Superior	Increase	Increase	Increase	Decrease	Decrease
Anterior	Increase	Increase	Increase	Decrease	Decrease
Inferior	Inferior	Decrease	Decrease	Increase	Increase
Posterior	None	Decrease	Decrease	Increase	Increase

Adapted from O'Ryan F, Schendel, S, and Carlotti A: Nasal anatomy and maxillary surgery. III. Surgical techniques for correction of nasal deformities in patients undergoing maxillary surgery. Int J Adult Orthod Orthogn Surg 4(3):158, 1989, by permission of Quintessence Publishing Co.

Different movements of the maxilla have distinct effects upon the nasal and labial morphology (Table 62-3). Superior repositioning of the maxilla causes elevation of the nasal tip,[7,29] widening of the alar bases,[7,29] and a decrease in the nasolabial angle.[7] Maxillary inferior repositioning produces loss of nasal tip support with a possible "polybeak" deformity, downward repositioning of the columella and alar bases, thinning of the lip, and an increase in the nasolabial angle. Maxillary advancement has the greatest effect on the nose and upper lip. This movement precipitates advancement of the upper lip, subnasale and nose, thinning of the lip,[35] widening of the alar bases, and an increase in the supratip break if the anterior nasal spine is left intact.[48-50] Pronasale moves horizontally in the following manner: It advances slightly when the maxilla is intruded, advances slightly more when the maxilla is intruded and advanced, or remains in the same place when the maxilla is intruded and retracted.[57] The nasal tip advances approximately one half the distance of subnasale.[24] The explanation of this may be widening at the alar base, which reduces the nasal tip protrusion.[9]

Preoperative alar base width of the nose is important in final postsurgical outcome. Narrow noses were observed to widen more at the alar base than did broad noses.[9,53] Another factor that is important to nasal change is rotation of the maxilla (palatal plane).[11,65] A steepening of the occlusal plane raises the nasal tip and a flattening of the occlusal plane decreases the superior movement of pronasale.[11,42]

UPPER LIP

The upper lip is also significantly effected by maxillary surgery. However, the upper lip is attched to the nose and this prevents a 1:1 soft tissue change.[39] The upper lip widens and lengthens at the philtral columns after maxillary surgery.[9] If a V-Y or double V-Y closure is not done at the time of surgery, shortening of the upper lip and loss of exposed vermilion can occur.[35]

Anterior Segmental Setback

The soft tissue changes associated with the maxillary segmental setback osteotomy include an increase in the nasolabial angle because of posterior lip rotation around subnasale,[5,6,38,39] lengthening of the upper lip, decrease in interlabial gap,[38] and uncurling and retraction of the lower lip with associated decrease in the depth of the inferior labial sulcus[6] (Table 62-4).

Advancement

Maxillary advancement had the most effect on the nose and upper lip. This movement precipitates advancement of the upper lip, subnasale, and nose,[42,48-50]

TABLE 62-4. SOFT TISSUE CHANGES ASSOCIATED WITH ANTERIOR SEGMENTAL SETBACK OSTEOTOMY

Increased nasolabial angle			
Upper lip(H)	−0.68:1	Ls:Ia	Bell, Dann (1973)
Upper lip(H)	−0.5:1	Ls:Is	Lines (1974)
Upper lip(H)	−0.67:1		
Increased NL angle			
Lower lip(H)	−0.3:1		Proffit, Epker (1980)
Upper lip(H)	−0.43:1	Ls:Is	
Nasolabial angle	12.2 degrees	Increase	Lew, Loh (1989)

slight shortening of the upper lip, thinning of the lip (approximately 2 mm),[25,48-50,70] widening of the alar bases,[48-50] and deepening of the supratip depression if the anterior nasal spine is left intact.[14,24,48-50,63] A progressive increase in the horizontal soft tissue displacement is seen from the tip of the nose to the free end of the upper lip.[42] A concomitant decrease in nasolabial angle is observed with only slight changes in the lower lip.[18,54] Leaving the ANS intact has a favorable effect on the forward displacement of the upper lip and especially the base of the nose (subnasale).[23] The ratios derived from previous investigations can be found in Table 62-5.

Note should be taken of the significant difference between the ratio of horizontal change of upper incisor to vermilion border of the upper lip in previous studies (0.6:1)[23,24,42] and the ratio reported by Carlotti et al[14] (0.9:1). The upper lip also lengthens rather than shortens.[14,23] This improvement is due to the use of the alar cinch suture and V-Y closure (nasolabial muscle reconstruction) during the surgical procedure. This ratio reduces with larger advancements because of soft tissue

TABLE 62-5. SOFT TISSUE CHANGES ASSOCIATED WITH MAXILLARY ADVANCEMENT

Upper lip(H)	0.67:1	Ls: Is Cleft pts. removed ANS	Lines (1974)
Upper lip(H)	0.5:1	Ls: Is	Dann, Fonseca (1976)
Upper lip(V)	0.3:1	Ls Is	
Nasolabial angle	−1.2deg:1	NLA: Is	
Nasal tip(H)	0.28:1	Pn: Is	
Nasal base(H)	0.57:1	Sn: A pt.	Freihofer (1976)
Upper lip(H)	0.56:1	Ls: Is Cleft pts	
Nasal base(H)	0.57:1	Sn: A pt.	Freihofer (1977)
Nasal tip(H)	0.28:1	Pn: A pt. Cleft pts	
Upper lip(H)	0.5:1		Proffit, Epker (1980)
Nasal tip(H)	0.17:1	Pn: Ia	Radney (1981)
Upper lip(H)	0.5:1	Ls: Is	
Nasal tip(H)	0.17:1	Pn: Ia	Mansour (1983)
Nasal base(H)	0.24:1	Sn: Ia	
Upper labial sulcus(H)	0.52:1	SLS: Ia	
Upper lip(H)	0.62:1	Ls: Ia	
Upper lip(H)	0.5:1	Ss: A pt.	Bundgaard (1986)
Upper lip(V)	−0.3:1	Ss: A pt.	
Upper labial sulcus(H)	0.8:1	SLS: A pt. Alar cinch, V-Y	Carlotti (1986)
Upper lip(H)	0.9:1	Ls: Is	
Upper lip(H)	0.82:1	Ls: Is	Rosen (1988)
Upper lip(V)	−0.32:1	Ss: Is	
Nasal base(H)	0.51:1	Sn: A pt.	
Nasal base(H)	0.3:1	Sn: A pt. (thick lip)	Stella (1989)
Nasal base(H)	0.46:1	Sn: A pt. (thin lip)	

stretching.[14] If the ANS is left intact, the nasolabial angle may remain relatively unchanged. This is because as the nasal tip raises slightly, subnasale migrates forward along with the upper lip.[77]

Impaction

Superior repositioning of the maxilla causes elevation of the nasal tip,[24,48-50] widening of the alar bases (2 to 4 mm),[48-50,53,63] and decrease in the nasolabial angle.[48-50] These nasal changes occur without change in angulation of the upper lip[42,57] (Table 62-6). The upper lip closely follows the movement of the maxillary incisor in the horizontal plane. This occurs because the lip is supported forward on the incisor, which is more anteriorly located than previous support of the lip, the lip support area of the alveolus.[57,80] The lip follows superiorly approximately 40 per cent of the vertical maxillary change. This lip shortening is accentuated with advancement, impaction surgery.[63] The amount of vertical soft tissue change increases progressively from the nasal tip to stomion superius, with loss of vermilion if a V-Y closure is not used.[42,57] However, Phillips[53] found that the vermilion borders of the upper and lower lips decreased slightly in the lateral portion of the lip, even with a V-Y closure. Interestingly, when superimposition is done on maxillary landmarks, the soft tissues of the lip migrate downward in relation to the maxilla. This may be due to the connection of the upper lip to the nose.[42,65]

It is important to be able to predict how much the lip shortens with maxillary impaction, so that an accurate postoperative tooth-to-lip ratio can be achieved.[42,57]

Functional Considerations

Recent studies have suggested that nasal air flow is actually improved after maxillary impaction surgery, with an increase in percentage of nasal respiration.[28,40,76]

TABLE 62-6. SOFT TISSUE CHANGES ASSOCIATED WITH MAXILLARY IMPACTION

Upper lip(V)	−0.38:1	Ls: Incisor (VME)	Schendel (1976)
Upper lip(V)	−0.51:1	Ls: Incisor (Bimax)	
Upper lip(V)	−0.4:1	Ss: Is	Radney (1981)
Upper lip(V)	−0.3:1	Ls: Is	
Upper labial sulcus(V)	−0.25:1	SLS: Is	
Nose(V)	−0.2:1	Sn: Is	
Nose(V)	−0.16:1	Pn: Is (ANS removed)	
Upper labial sulcus(H)	0.76:1	SLS: Ia	Mansour (1983)
Upper lip(H)	0.89:1	Ls: Ia	
Nose(V)	−0.15:1	Pn: Pr	
Nasal base(V)	−0.28:1	Sn: Pr	
Upper lip(V)	−0.31:1	Ls: Pr	
Upper lip(V)	−0.42:1	SLS: Is	
Upper labial sulcus(V)	0.12:1	SLS: ANS	Sakima (1987)
Upper lip(V)	−0.06:1	Ls: ANS	
Upper lip(V)	−0.41:1	Ss: ANS	
FULL FACE			
Greatest alar width	Ave=3.4mm	Full facial photographs	Phillip (1986)
Alar base width	Ave=2.7mm		
Decreased vermilion more lateral	Ave=1mm	V-Y	

TABLE 62-7. SOFT TISSUE CHANGES ASSOCIATED WITH MAXILLARY SETBACK

Upper lip(H)	−0.76:1	Ls: Incisor (VME)	Schendel (1976)
Upper lip(H)	−0.66:1	Ls: Incisor (Bimax)	
Upper lip(H)	−0.67:1	Ls: Is	Radney (1981)
Upper labial sulcus(H)	−0.33:1	SLS: Is	
Nose(H)	−0.33:1	Sn: Is	
Nasolabial angle	Increase		

Downgraft

There is a paucity of data on the soft tissue effects of maxillary downgrafting procedures. Maxillary inferior repositioning produces loss of nasal tip support with a possible "polybeak" deformity, downward repositioning of the columella and alar bases, thinning of the lip, and increase in the nasolabial angle.[48-50] Lengthening and thinning of the upper lip are also observed.[54]

Setback

Maxillary setback procedures result in loss of nasal tip support because of posterior movement of the ANS and piriform bases.[49] The lip rotates posteriorly and superiorly about subnasale with increasing nasolabial angle[57,68] and thickens slightly[68] (Table 62-7).

Combined Vectors of Maxillary Repositioning

Very few maxillary surgical procedures are pure movements in one direction; most are combinations of the above movements (advancement and impaction, advancement and downgraft, setback and impaction, setback and downgraft). The expected soft tissue changes would be a combination of the expected changes from the pure vectors of movement (Figs. 62-14 to 62-16).

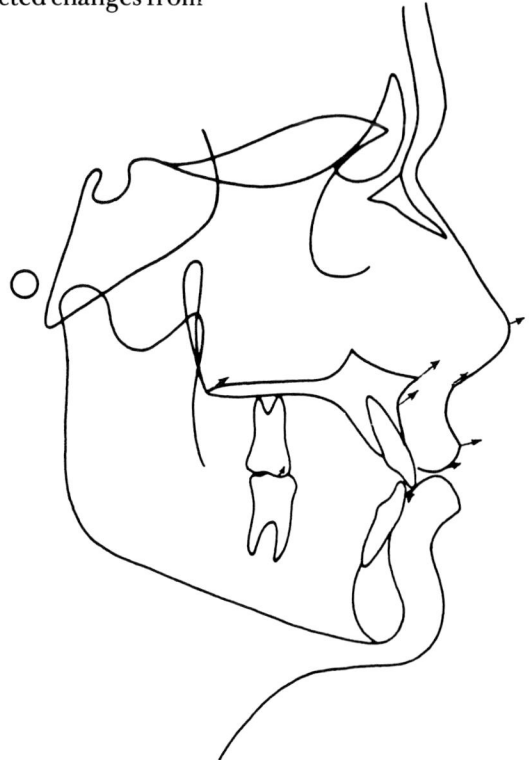

FIGURE 62-14. The average hard and soft tissue changes of the advancement, impaction group in vector format (arrows depict mean direction and mean amount of change). Note that the nasal tip elevates slightly, but subnasale advances more, effectively decreasing nasal tip protrusion. (Adapted from Betts NJ: Changes in the nasal and labial soft tissues after surgical repositioning of the maxilla. MS Thesis in Oral and Maxillofacial Surgery. University of Michigan, 1990.)

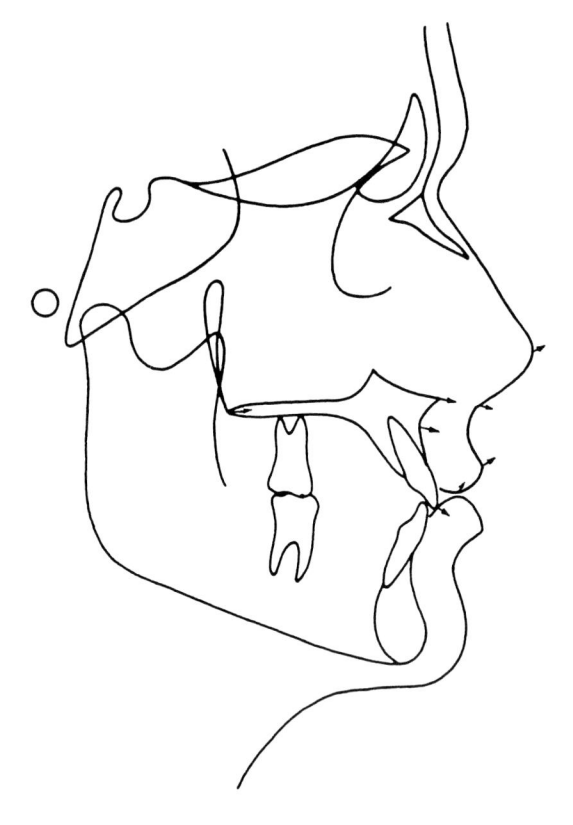

FIGURE 62-15. The average hard and soft tissue changes of the advancement, downgraft group in vector format (arrows depict mean direction and mean amount of change). Note that the nasal tip elevates slightly, but subnasale advances more, effectively decreasing the nasal tip protrusion. (Adapted from Betts NJ: Changes in the nasal and labial soft tissues after surgical repositioning of the maxilla. MS Thesis in Oral and Maxillofacial Surgery. University of Michigan, 1990.)

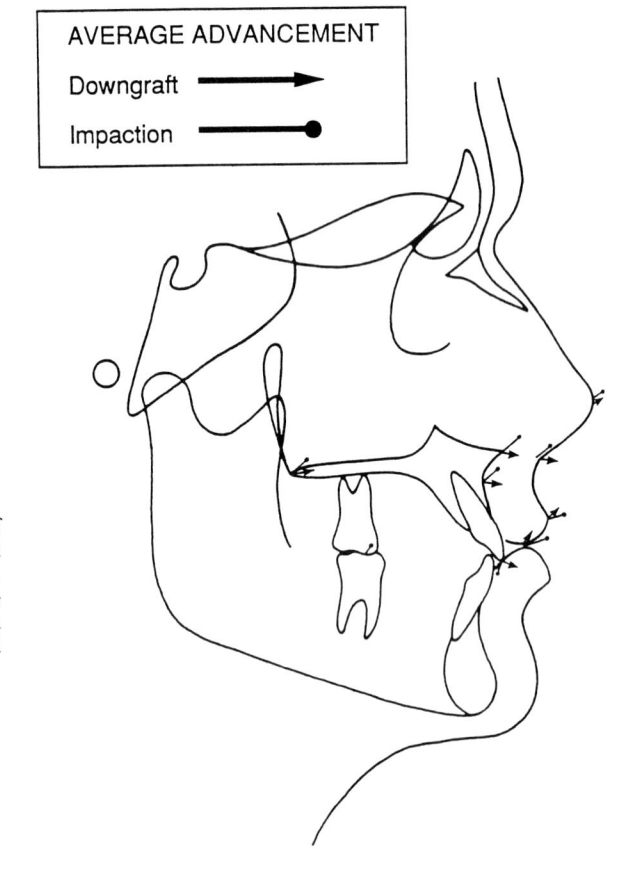

FIGURE 62-16. Overlay of average hard and soft tissue changes of advancement, impaction and advancement, downgraft in vector format (arrows and lines depict mean direction and mean amount of change). Note that subnasale moves in the direction of the anterior nasal spine and A point. (Adapted from Betts NJ: Changes in the nasal and labial soft tissues after surgical repositioning of the maxilla. MS Thesis in Oral and Maxillofacial Surgery. University of Michigan, 1990.)

MANDIBULAR SURGICAL PROCEDURES

Generally the movements of soft tissues of the mandible follow those of the hard tissues closely. The exception is the lower lip. Because of its contact with the upper incisor and upper lip, its movement is often variable and unpredictable.

Anterior Segmental Setback

The upper lip movement follows that of the lower incisor posteriorly, which causes a flattening of the labiomental fold. There is less posterior displacement of the soft tissues as the chin is approached. No effective change is observed at the chin[39] (Table 62-8).

TABLE 62-8. SOFT TISSUE CHANGES ASSOCIATED WITH MANDIBULAR ANTERIOR SEGMENTAL OSTEOTOMY

Lower lip(H)	−0.75:1	Li: li	Lines (1974)
Lower lip(H)	−0.67:1		Proffit, Epker (1980)
Chin(H)	no change		
Lower lip(H)	−0.71:1	Li: li	Lew, Loh (1989)

Advancement (Sagittal)

The soft tissue changes associated with mandibular advancement surgery are limited to the structures below the superior labial sulcus. There is little change in the upper lip[39,46,72] and none above the ANS.[19] The lower lip advancement is variable, and the lip lengthens.[19] The lower labial sulcus and chin adhere to the bony structure of the mandible and follow underlying osseous tissues closely, advancing more than the lower lip. This leads to an opening of the labiomental fold. As with maxillary and genial surgeries, the vertical changes are variable (Table 62-9).

A correlation between the vertical change in menton and the angle and depth of the labiomental fold has been elucidated. As menton moves caudally, the angle opens and the depth decreases.[46]

Facial height is also affected by mandibular advancement. In low Angle class II cases, there is little increase in facial height with advancement, but in high Angle class II cases, a marked increase in facial height occurs with advancement.

The position of the lower lip is affected by the upper incisor as well as the lower incisor. The anterosuperior portion of the upper one half of the lower lip touches the upper incisor in Angle class II non–open-bite cases and is usually folded forward. As the mandible is advanced, the chin and lower labial sulcus come forward while the superior portion of the lower lip does not, since it already has been folded forward by its contact with the upper incisor. This causes an opening

TABLE 62-9. SOFT TISSUE CHANGES ASSOCIATED WITH MANDIBULAR ADVANCEMENT

Lower lip(H)	0.62:1	Li: li	Lines (1971)
Chin(H)	1.1	Pgs: Gn	
Lower lip(H)	0.85:1	Li: li	Talbott (1975)
Lower labial sulcus	1.01:1	ILS: B pt.	
Chin(H)	1.04:1	Pgs: Pg	
Lower lip(H)	0.75:1		Proffit, Epker (1980)
Chin(H)	1:1		
Lower lip(H)	0.38:1	Li: li	Quast (1983)
Lower labial sulcus(H)	0.97:1	ILS: B pt.	
Chin(H)	0.97:1	Pgs: Pg	
Chin(H)	0.97:1	Gns: Gn	
Chin(H)	0.87:1	Mes: Me	
Lower lip(H)	0.56:1	Li: li	Mommaerts (1987)
Lower labial sulcus	1.06:1	ILS: B pt.	
Chin(H)	1.03:1	Pgs: Pg	
Chin(V)	0.93:1	Mes: Me	
Upper lip(H)	−0.02:1	Ls: li	Hernandez (1989)
Lower lip(H)	0.43:1	Li: li	
Lower labial sulcus(H)	0.93:1	ILS: B pt.	
Chin(H)	0.94:1	Pgs: Pg	
Chin(H)	0.95:1	Gns: Gn	
Chin(H)	0.97:1	Mes: Me	
Lower lip(H)	0.26:1	Li: li	Dermaut (1989)
Lower labial sulcus(H)	1.19:1	ILS: B pt.	
Chin(H)	1.1:1	Pgs: Pg	

TABLE 62-10. SOFT TISSUE CHANGES ASSOCIATED WITH MANDIBULAR SETBACK

Lower lip(H)	−0.69 : 1	Li: Pg	Aaronson (1967)
Lower labial sulcus(H)	−0.93 : 1	ILS: Pg	
Lower labial sulcus(H)	approx. −1 : 1	ILS: B pt.	Robinson (1972)
Chin(H)	approx. −1 : 1	Pgs: Pg	
Upper lip(H)	−0.2 : 1	Ls: li	Lines (1974)
Lower lip(H)	−0.75 : 1	Li: li	
Chin(H)	−1 : 1	Pgs: Gn	
Upper lip(H)	−0.2 : 1	Ls: Pg	Hershey (1974)
Lower lip (H)	−0.6 : 1	Li: Pg	
Chin (H)	−0.9 : 1	Pgs: Pg	
Upper lip(H)	−0.2 : 1		Proffit, Epker (1980)
Lower lip (H)	−0.75-.8 : 1		
Chin(H)	−1 : 1		

of the labiomental fold and may explain why the ratio of advancement at labrale inferius to the incisor inferius is reduced.[19,39,54] Consequently during treatment planning, the lower lip must be uprighted to a relatively normal position before it is advanced in order to approximate its true postoperative position.

Setback (Sagittal and VRO)

Mandibular setback surgery has no effects upon subnasale or the tissues located above subnasale. However, a slight posterior displacement of the upper lip, with lengthening,[26,54,78] and a slight increase in the nasolabial proportion (angle) is observed.[1] The soft tissues follow the mandible posteriorly, with the chin following most closely followed by the inferior labial sulcus and the lower lip. The lower lip shortens and becomes more protrusive by curling out, and the labiomental fold deepens and becomes more accentuated[1,26,32,78] (Table 62-10). Vertical changes of the soft tissues of the lips are related to the hard tissue vertical changes. During superior mandibular repositioning, the lower lip becomes shorter, protrusive, and smaller in area. In contrast, with inferior mandibular repositioning, the lower lip becomes longer with increased area.[78] Again, the vertical soft tissue changes correlate poorly with the hard tissue movements.[62]

Autorotation

During autorotation of the mandible, the soft tissues follow the osseous landmarks on approximately a 1 : 1 basis[42,57] except the lower lip, which falls slightly lingual to the arc of rotation.[42,57,68] A slight increase in the labiomental angle is often observed,[42] as well as a slight thickening of the lips as the vertical facial height decreases[39] (Table 62-11).

GENIAL SEGMENT SURGICAL PROCEDURES

Hofer[33] was the first to describe the horizontal genial osteotomy. It was accomplished through an extraoral incision. Later Trauner and Obwegeser[74] advocated the same osteotomy through an intraoral incision. Since then, the symphysis has been exposed both intraorally and extraorally for osteotomy of the inferior border of the mandible to advance, retract, widen, narrow, lengthen, or shorten the chin.[6] Methods of diagnosing genial abnormalities have been described elsewhere.[34]

TABLE 62-11. SOFT TISSUE CHANGES ASSOCIATED WITH MANDIBULAR AUTOROTATION

Chin(V)	−0.8 : 1	Pgs: Gn	Lines (1974)
Chin(H)	1 : 1		
Lower labial sulcus	1 : 1	ILS: B pt.	Radney (1981)
Chin(H)	1 : 1	Pgs: Pg	
Lower li(H)	0.75 : 1	Li: li	Mansour (1983)
Lower labial sulcus(H)	0.9 : 1	ILS: B pt.	
Chin(H)	0.86 : 1	Pgs: Pg	
Lower lip(V)	−0.93 : 1	Si: ls	
Chin(V)	−1.2 : 1	Mes: Me	
Lower lip (V)	−1.03 : 1	Si: Me	Sakima (1987)
Lower lip(V)	−1.48 : 1*	Li: Me	
Inferior labial sulcus(V)	−1.05 : 1	ILS: Me	
Inferior labial sulcus(H)	0.61 : 1	ILS: Me	
Chin(H)	0.79 : 1	Pgs: Me	
Chin(V)	−0.98 : 1	Pgs: Me	

* May represent uprighting of the lower lip due to a loss of contact with the upper incisor.

Early studies describing the soft tissue changes associated with genial surgery had several problems. They included few cases and related short-term results; and the cephalograms were superimposed on the cranial base. Superimposition of the cephalograms should occur upon the areas of the mandible not changed with surgery,[3,34,51] because concomitant maxillary and mandibular surgery may invalidate chin measurements calculated from superimpositions on the cranial base.[27,44,66]

Overall, most of the change seen after genioplasty is in the soft tissue of the chin, and less effect is seen in the labial sulcus and lower lip.[13]

Advancement

BONY

Early attempts at advancement genioplasty utilized nonpedicled free grafts or onlay bone grafts. However, autologous, homologous, or heterologous bone grafts were subsequently observed to involve excessive resorption and low predictability. Because of these findings, the surgical emphases shifted to the horizontal osteotomy of the anterior mandible.

At first a degloving incision was used to expose the anterior mandible.[5,44,74] However, several investigators showed that minimal soft tissue stripping gave a more predictable hard and soft tissue response because of less bone resorption in the advanced segment.[3,6,21,27,51] No bony remodeling of gnathion or menton was observed, but bony resorption could be demonstrated near the osteotomy (the anterosuperior and posteroinferior aspects of the advanced genial segment).[5,27,44,74] However, bony apposition occurred at B point and the inferior border osteotomy.[44] These same studies demonstrated that when the technique of minimal soft tissue stripping was used, the soft tissues followed the hard tissues closely without chin droop.[3,6,27,51,66] There was also a small but negligible effect upon the labiomental sulcus,[27,66] an increased submental length, an improved lower lip-to-tooth relationship,[27] less soft tissue thinning,[66] and an improved neck-chin angle (Table 62-12).

The soft tissue changes following horizontal advancement genioplasty depend upon the magnitude and direction of the positional change of the genial segment, the design of the mucosal and osseous incisions, the amount of soft tissue stripping, and other concomitant jaw movements.[3,5,27,44,74]

The advantages of osseous genial surgery are preservation of the normal chin

TABLE 62-12. SOFT TISSUE CHANGES ASSOCIATED WITH ADVANCEMENT GENIOPLASTY

Chin(H)	0.57:1	Pgs: Pg Ant. Sliding	Bell, Dann (1973)
Chin(H)	0.75:1	Pgs: Pg Horizontal (some Multistep)	McDonnel (1977)
Chin(H)	0.67:1		Proffit, Epker (1980)
Chin(H)	approx. 1:1	Horizonal w/broad soft tissue pedicle IVRO setback	Bell (1981)
Lip(H)	0.44:1	Li: Pg Horizontal	Busquets (1981)
Chin(H)	0.83:1	Pgs: Pg (some w/ostectomy)	
Chin(H)	0.97:1	Pgs: Pg Horizontal w/broad pedicle (IVRO setback)	Scheideman (1981)
Chin(H)	0.85:1	Horizontal w/broad pedicle	Bell (1983)
Chin(H)	0.81:1	Pgs: Pg Advancement only Horizontal sliding with broad pedicle	
Chin(H)	0.93:1	Pgs: Pg Adv. and vertical reduction Horizontal sliding w/broad pedicle Max. impaction	Gallagher (1984)
Chin(H)	0.7:1	Horizontal	Epker (1986)
Chin(H)	0.73:1	Pgs: Pg Overlapping bone flap	Tulasne (1987)
Chin(H)	0.97:1	Pgs: Pg Horizontal w/broad pedicle	Park, Ellis (1989)

contour,[16] improved predictability of the soft tissue response,[6] stability,[6,66] versatility,[6] and preservation of blood supply to osteotomized segments.[16]

Those patients who had both vertical reduction and advancement genioplasties showed slightly larger soft tissue advancement than those who had advancement genioplasty only (0.93:1 vs. 0.81:1). This may be explained by bunching of the soft tissues. When the soft tissues are bunched (vertical reduction more than advancement), the soft tissues advance more than when they are stretched (advancement only).[27]

Since pogonion remodels postsurgery (because of its close proximity to the osteotomy cut), those measures based upon it may be less accurate. This is why some authors resorted to using gnathion and soft tissue gnathion in their investigations.

Tulasne[75] suggested that the overlapping bone flap genioplasty gives a more natural contour to the lower face and a better balance between the lower lip, chin, and submental region than the sliding genioplasty associated with a wedge ostectomy. However, it is associated with a large amount of bony resorption, especially in adolescent patients.

Alloplastic

Early attempts at advancement genioplasty included the use of alloplastic implants (Table 62-13). Unfortunately, long-term follow-up revealed several unforeseen complications. For this reason advancement genioplasty with alloplastic implants has fallen somewhat out of favor. The disadvantages of alloplastic materials include resorption or deformation of the underlying symphyseal bone with possible devitalization of the mandibular anterior teeth,[17,25,52,54,60,61] drift of implant,[5,6,17] extrusion of implant,[17] infection (especially with Proplast)[5,6] and a less predictable soft tissue to hard tissue ratio.[5,6] Also, with these materials one cannot address excessive or reduced chin height.[6]

Resorption of the symphyseal bone is the most often seen complication of alloplastic chin implants. This resorption is most pronounced with Silastic (acrylic)

TABLE 62-13. SOFT TISSUE CHANGES ASSOCIATED WITH ALLOPLASTIC CHIN IMPLANTS

Chin(H)	0.6:1	Pgs: Pg Silicone (unstable/resorption)	Bell, Dann (1973)
Chin(H)	0.9:1	Pgs: Pg Implant Proplast™ (resorption)	Dann, Epker (1977)
Chin(H)	1:1		Proffit, Epker (1980)

implants, less with Proplast, and even less with Interpore. The resorption has been shown to occur whether or not the implant was placed above or below the periosteum.[6,25] This resorption is especially marked when the implant is placed high on the symphysis and placed under tension by the tonicity and activity of the lower lip and mentalis muscle.[6,25,61] Consequently, this resorption may be worse in patients with lip incompetence.[52] Also, the resorption is more pronounced in children and adolescents secondary to their decreased bone density. Fortunately, when the implants are removed, the bone of the anterior mandible returns to near preoperative levels.[52]

Several points can be taken from the previous studies. If alloplastic implants are to be used, they should be placed subperiosteally, low on the inferior border below the mentalis muscle, and over dense cortical bone. Alloplastic implants should not be used in correction of severe deformities but can be used in patients with a mild to moderate deformity.[25,52,61] A periodic radiographic examination of the implant for monitoring of bony resorption is recommended.[25,60]

Setback (Horizontal Reduction)

Early attempts at reduction of horizontal excess of the genial segment of the mandible by bony recontouring caused very little improvement of the soft tissue profile[34] (Table 62-14). Therefore, this technique has been abandoned. The soft tissue changes associated with setback genioplasty are less well correlated with the hard tissue movements than during advancement genioplasty.

Reduction genioplasty is contraindicated in a patient with minimal or no labiomental fold. Flattening of the chin and elimination of the labiomental fold will result.[4] It is also important to realize that setback genioplasty will make undesirable changes in the neck-chin proportion. In a patient with a poor neck-chin proportion, this procedure is contraindicated.

Vertical

AUGMENTATION AND REDUCTION

The soft tissues follow the hard tissues quite closely in vertical augmentation genioplasty. However, this is not the case for the vertical reduction (inferior border ostectomy or sandwich ostectomy) genioplasty.

TABLE 62-14. SOFT TISSUE CHANGES ASSOCIATED WITH SETBACK GENIOPLASTY

Chin(H)	-0.33:1	Pgs: Pg Ant. recontouring; degloving dissection	Hohl, Epker (1976)
Chin(H)	-0.75:1	Interpositional	Wessberg (1980)
Chin(H)	-0.58:1	Pgs: Pg Horizontal w/broad pedicle	Bell (1981)

TABLE 62-15. SOFT TISSUE CHANGES ASSOCIATED WITH VERTICAL AUGMENTATION OR REDUCTION GENIOPLASTY

AUGMENTATION			
Chin(V)	1:1	Interpositional	Wessberg (1980)
REDUCTION			
Chin(V)	−0.25:1	Mes: Me Inf. border Ostectomy degloving dissection	Hohl, Epker (1976)
Chin(V)	−0.26:1	Pgs: Pg Horizontal w/broad pedicle	Park, Ellis (1989)

POOR SURGICAL ESTHETIC RESULTS AND TECHNIQUES OF SOFT TISSUE CONTROL

Maxilla

UNESTHETIC SOFT TISSUE CHANGES

The secondary soft tissue changes found with maxillary surgery include widening of the alar bases,[14,48-50,67] upturning of the nasal tip, flattening and thinning of the upper lip,[14,48-50,67,73] downturning of the commissures of the mouth,[14,48-50,67] and opening of the nasolabial angle. These changes are similar to those found in the aging face and are generally perceived as unesthetic.[48-50] Other potentially unesthetic changes include loss of normal lip pout and a decrease in visible vermilion.[14,67,73]

There are several reasons why the soft tissues of the face are deformed after maxillary surgery. These include a failure to correctly diagnose a deformity, unpredictable movement of the soft tissues in relation to the hard tissues, and inadequate reapproximation of the soft tissues during surgery.[73] A lack of understanding of the preoperative nasal morphology, improper handling of the soft tissues, and failure to appreciate the influence of the magnitude and direction of maxillary movement on the nose can also contribute to unfavorable nasal esthetics.[48-50]

Several investigators suggest that the etiology of these soft tissue changes is attributed to three factors: (1) elevation of the periosteum and muscle attachments adjacent to the nose without adequate replacement, (2) postsurgical edema, and (3) increased bony support in advancement cases.[29,80]

The importance of muscle repositioning following superior impaction of the maxilla was emphasized by many investigators.[14,67,69,80] They state that the muscles detached during stripping of the periosteum required for maxillary surgery shorten and retract laterally. The muscles reattach in this position if they are not reapproximated at the time of surgery. The lateral movement of the muscles and subcutaneous tissues causes the alar base to flare and the upper lip to thin.

The loss of visible vermilion may be due to other causes. These include a rolling-under of the vermilion of the upper lip secondary to incision high in the vestibule with associated scarring and retraction[14,67,80] or inclusion of large amounts of tissue during closure.[80] This loss of vermilion, which is especially unattractive in those individuals with already thin lips,[7] is more pronounced with posterior superior positioning of the maxilla.

Postoperative widening of the alar base after the maxillary Le Fort I procedure may have a favorable outcome in a patient with vertical maxillary hyperplasia and thin, slit-like nares.[77] However, when there is a wide preoperative alar base, these same changes become undesirable,[29,80] especially with anterior or superior repositioning of the maxilla[15] (Fig. 62-17 A-D). Before techniques to control nasal width were developed, Bell[7] suggested that at the time of preoperative assessment, patients with a wide nose should be warned that a rhinoplasty may be indicated.

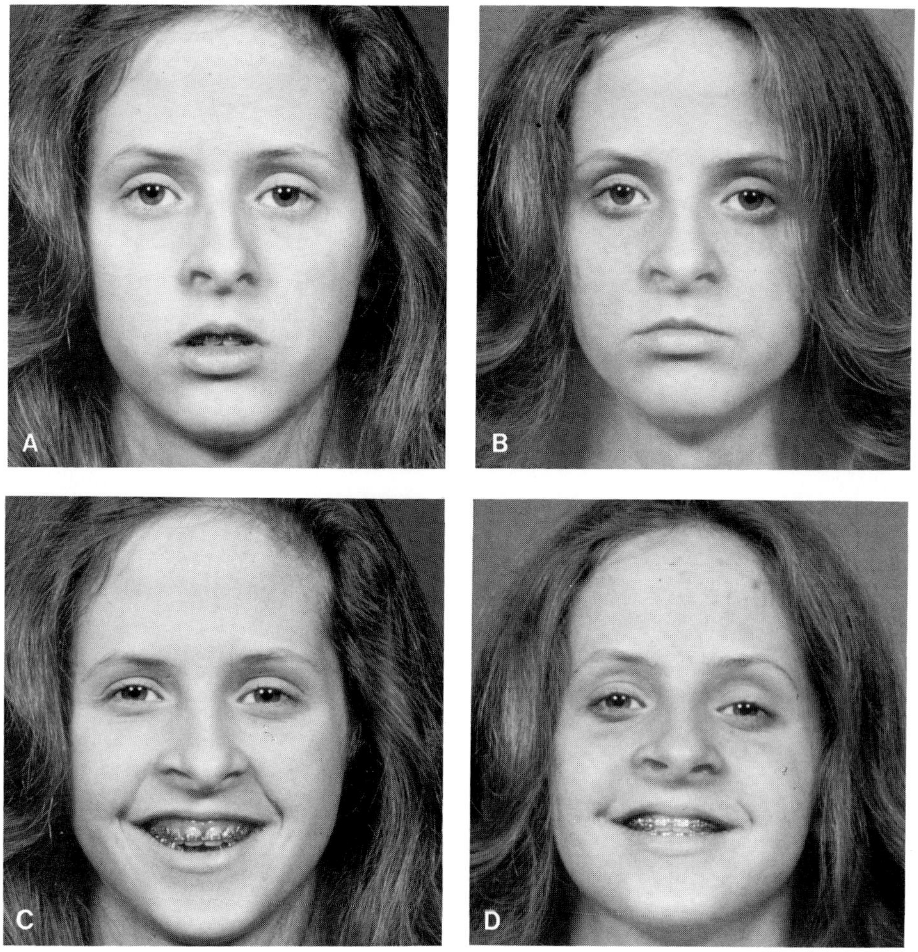

FIGURE 62-17. *A–D*. Unesthetic widening of the alar base and downturning of the corners of the mouth in a patient with an already wide nose. This patient was treated with a maxillary procedure without an alar cinch or V-Y closure. *A*, Preoperative full facial view. *B*, Postoperative full facial view. *C*, Preoperative smiling full facial view. *D*, Postoperative smiling full facial view.

Techniques to control the soft tissues

To control the soft tissue changes associated with maxillary surgery, the surgeon must first be aware of any pre-existing deformity, the anticipated soft tissue adaptation to the surgical procedure being planned, and the importance of the orofacial muscles upon form, function, and esthetics. Once this has occurred, the soft tissues can be manipulated to advantage by the surgeon.[9,69]

Several surgical techniques have been suggested to help control the detrimental soft tissue changes associated with maxillary surgery. They include the V-Y closure, the alar cinch suture, a combination of the alar cinch suture and the V-Y closure, contouring of the anterior nasal spine, septum reduction, and the double V-Y closure.

V-Y Closure

There is always an A-P thinning of the upper lip (especially with maxillary advancement) and a loss of vermilion (especially with maxillary impaction unless a V-Y closure is used) (Fig. 62–18 *A–C*).

The upper lip, when closed in a V-Y manner, follows the hard tissues forward at more nearly a 1:1 ratio, with a prevention of upper lip thinning and loss of the vermilion.[14,69,70,77]

The V-Y closure is accomplished during closure of the maxillary vestibular incision. The mucosa, periosteum, and interposed muscular tissue is engaged by the needle on either side of the incision and sutured in a continuous fashion. The superior aspect of the incision is gradually advanced toward the midline by taking smaller bites of tissue in the upper margin and larger bites in the lower margin. The

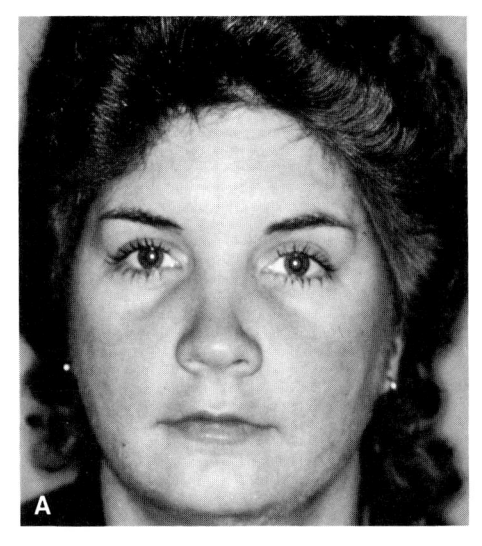

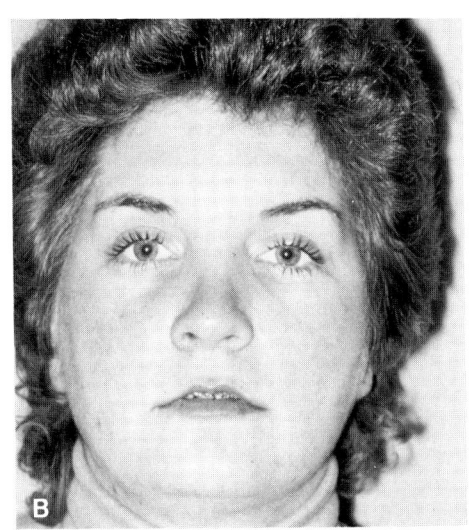

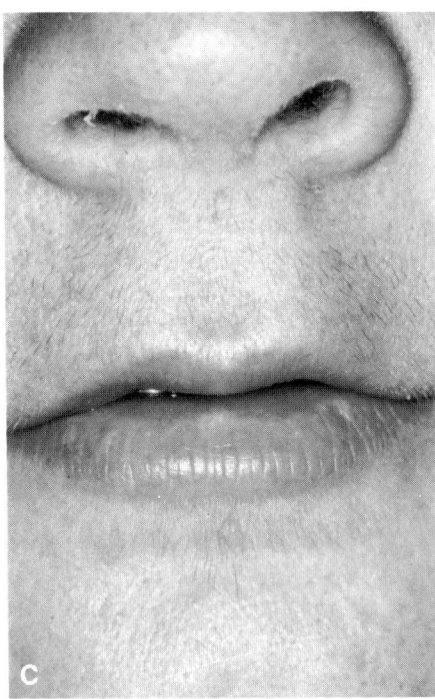

FIGURE 62-18. Unfavorable change in the vermilion of the upper lip following maxillary impaction surgery in a patient with a pre-existing thin vermilion. *A*, Preoperative state. *B*, Postoperative state. *C*, Close-up of the postoperative state. Note that the loss of vermilion is more pronounced in the lateral portions of the lip than in the medial portion.

midline of the lip is retracted anteriorly with a skin hook. After both sides have been closed, there should be approximately 0.5 to 1 cm of excess tissue in the midline; this tissue is then approximated. Often, following this type of closure, the lip will look rather full and short in the midline. Within the next several days, the lip will lengthen and become more normal in appearance[69] (Fig. 62-19).

ALAR CINCH

Collins and Epker[15] identified patients who were likely to develop undesirable nasal esthetic changes as those who had normal or wide frontonasal esthetics before surgery, and would undergo a superior and/or anterior surgical repositioning of the maxilla. These observations led to the development of techniques designed to control the alar width after maxillary surgery. Bell[7] described adjunctive techniques to prevent widening of the alar bases in maxillary impaction cases, including reduction of the anterior extent of the piriform rim, reduction of ANS, and trimming of the height of the anterior nasal floor. A different technique for

FIGURE 62-19. The V-Y closure technique for suturing of the maxillary vestibular incision. The mucosa, periosteum, and interposed muscular tissue is engaged by the needle on either side of the incision and sutured continuously. The superior aspect of the incision is gradually advanced toward the midline by taking smaller bites of tissue in the upper margin and larger bites in the lower margin. The midline of the lip is retracted anteriorly with a skin hook. After both sides have been closed, there should be approximately 0.5 to 1 cm of excess tissue in the midline; this tissue is then approximated.

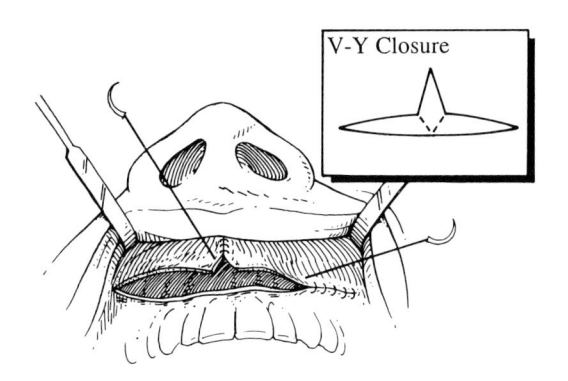

correcting the flat and flaring nose was described by Millard.[45] This served as a model for the later development of the alar cinch techniques (Collins and Epker).[15] The original cinch suture was passed from the fibroadipose tissue on one side of the alar base to the other and was tied to a predetermined width (Fig. 62-20).

This technique was then modified to a figure of 8 suture that was passed from lateral to medial, catching the fibroadipose tissue of the alar base.[29,80] Schendel[67] suggests that the suture should not be passed through the fibroadipose tissue but rather through the transverse nasalis muscles of the nose.

Recent observations have suggested that the alar cinch suture does not control the alar base width[9,41] and may even cause further widening of the alar base.[9] Subsequently, another technique of alar cinch suturing was suggested. In this technique, a hole is placed in the anterior nasal spine and a suture is passed through soft tissues at the base of the nose and back to the ANS. This is done bilaterally with two individual sutures.[77]

Other authors concluded that the alar base cinch suture was inadequate to maintain the alar base width and that a V-Y closure was also indicated with nasolabial muscle reconstruction.[69]

To ensure an esthetic reconstruction of the alar base, a preoperative measurement of the greatest alar width must be taken on the patient and recorded in the chart. This number should be available during surgery so that it can be used as a reference at the time of nasolabial muscle reconstruction. This procedure is often difficult with an nasoendotracheal tube in place, and some surgeons have advocated switching the patient from nasoendotracheal to orotracheal intubation before closure of the circumvestibular incision.

Combination of Alar Cinch and V-Y Closure

Several investigators have indicated that the best control of the alar base in patients having a maxillary impaction, or advancement impaction, could be achieved by using the V-Y closure and the alar cinch suture together.[29,48-50,67,69,77] They quantified the alar base width changes with and without the alar base cinch suture. All patients had a V-Y closure. They found that the alar bases widened in all

FIGURE 62-20. The alar base cinch suture. The suture is passed from the fibroadipose tissue (or transverse nasalis muscle) on one side of the alar base to the other and is tied to a predetermined width.

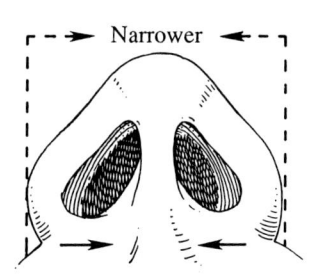

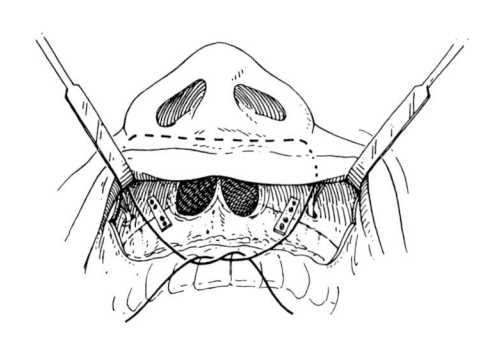

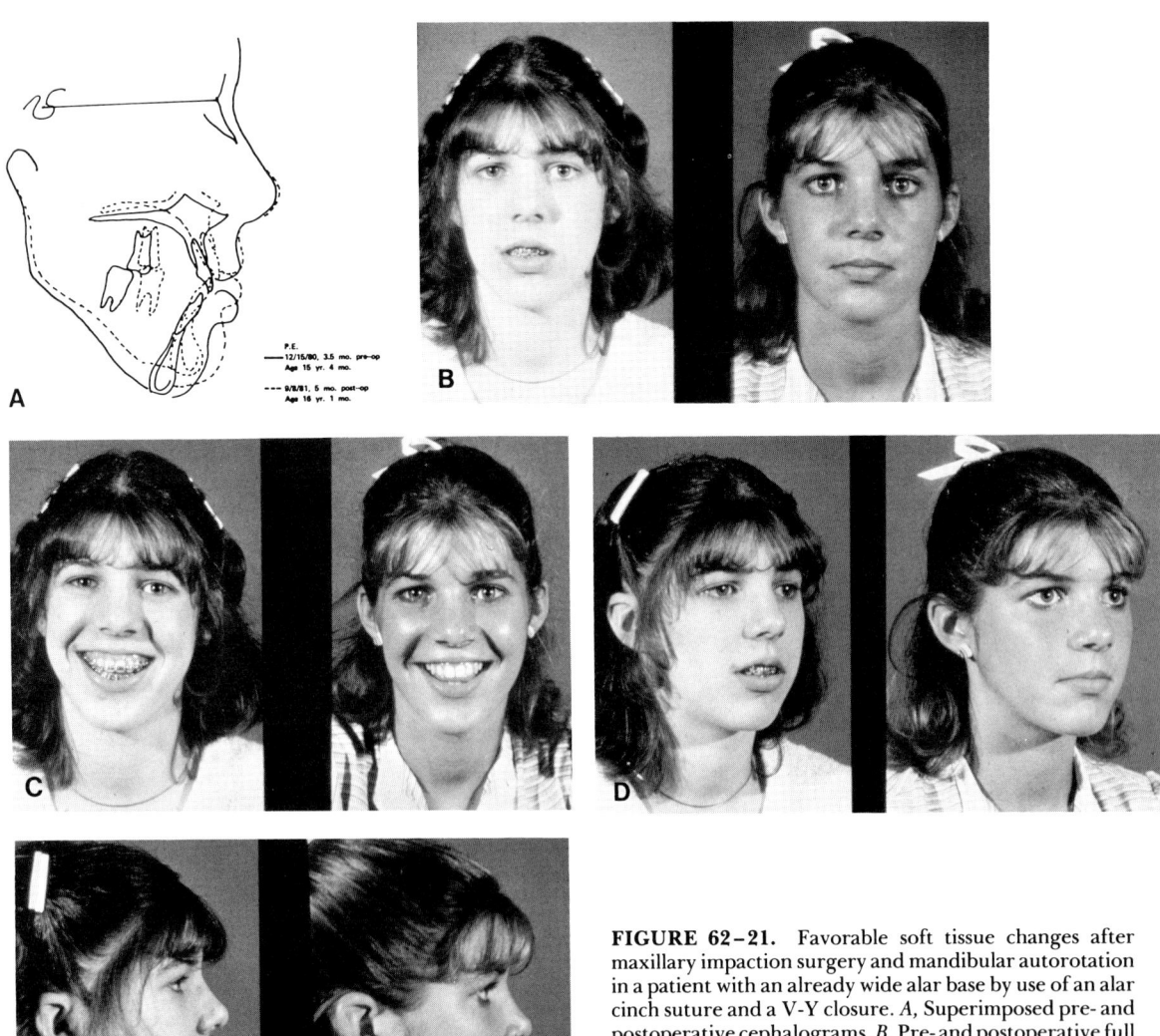

FIGURE 62-21. Favorable soft tissue changes after maxillary impaction surgery and mandibular autorotation in a patient with an already wide alar base by use of an alar cinch suture and a V-Y closure. *A,* Superimposed pre- and postoperative cephalograms. *B,* Pre- and postoperative full facial view. *C,* Pre- and postoperative smiling full facial view. *D,* Pre- and postoperative three-quarter view. *E,* Pre- and postoperative profile view.

patients and there was less widening when the alar cinch suture was used. The alar base widened an average of 2.9 per cent with the alar cinch suture, and 10.8 per cent without it.[29]

The simultaneous placement of an alar cinch suture and a V-Y closure (nasolabial muscle reconstruction) is successful in repositioning of the lip muscles in a predictable manner,[69] in preventing shortening of the lip in impaction cases,[29,69] in maintenance of the normal lip pout,[69] in prevention of loss of vermilion,[14,29,69] in maintaining the anteroposterior thickness of the lip,[29] in preventing widening of the alar base,[14,29,69] and in preventing drooping of the corners of the mouth[69] (Fig. 62-21 *A-E*).

Contouring of the Anterior Nasal Spine (ANS)

Reduction of ANS is indicated in patients undergoing large advancements or impactions of the maxilla who already have good nasal tip projection.[24] The hard

FIGURE 62-22. Reduction of the anterior nasal spine during a maxillary osteotomy. This procedure is indicated in patients undergoing large advancements or impactions of the maxilla who already have good nasal tip projection. This procedure is contraindicated in patients who have poor preoperative nasal tip projection or who are having a maxillary setback procedure.

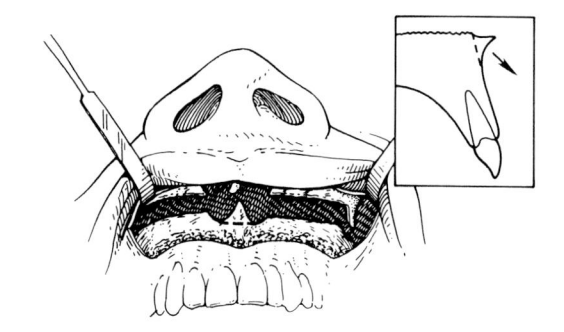

tissue changes in the position of ANS affect primarily the soft tissue landmarks subnasale and pronasale[9] (Fig. 62-22).

This technique should not be used in patients who have poor preoperative nasal tip projection. The nasal tip will rise if ANS is left intact when advancing or impacting the maxilla. Reduction of ANS is also contraindicated in patients who are having a maxillary setback procedure. The result could lead to a "polybeak deformity," or drooping of the columella (Fig. 62-23 A-D).

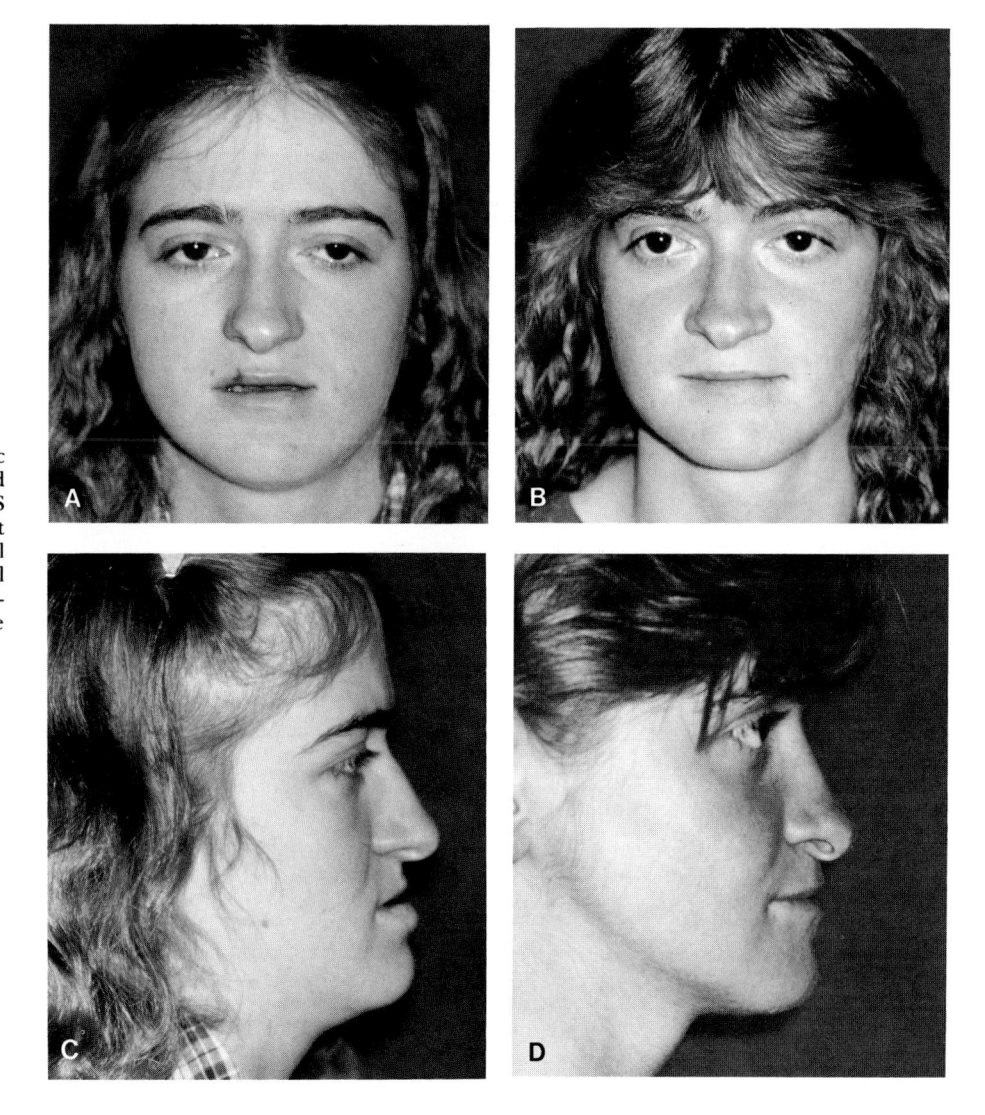

FIGURE 62-23. Poor esthetic outcome in a patient who had overzealous reduction of ANS after a maxillary advancement procedure. A, Preoperative full facial view. B, Postoperative full facial view. C, Preoperative profile view. D, Postoperative profile view.

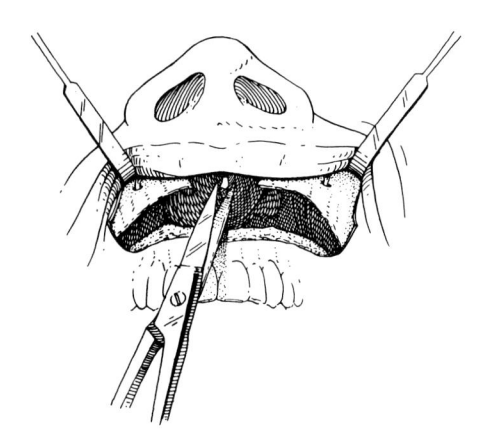

FIGURE 62-24. Septal reduction during maxillary impaction osteotomy. The cartilaginous nasal septum should be reduced during maxillary impactions of greater than 3 mm to prevent postoperative deviation or buckling of the septum. This is done by incising the nasal mucosa and reflecting the septal perichondrium and removing the appropriate amount of cartilage with a scissor or scalpel blade. The same amount of septum should be removed as the maxilla is impacted. This technique can be combined with reduction of the maxillary nasal crest.

SEPTUM REDUCTION

The cartilaginous nasal septum should be reduced during maxillary impactions of greater than 3 mm to prevent postoperative deviation or buckling of the septum.[7,38] This is done by incising the nasal mucosa and reflecting the septal perichondrium and removing the appropriate amount of cartilage with a scissor or scalpel blade (Fig. 62-24). The same amount of septum should be removed as the maxilla is impacted.[77] This technique can be combined with reduction of the maxillary nasal crest.[7] The septum can be reattached to the ANS with suture,[77] or left unsutured. Excessive reduction of the septum can result in either a saddle nose deformity or a polybeak deformity depending upon the location of the overreduction.[77]

DOUBLE V-Y CLOSURE

A new technique of V-Y closure, the double V-Y closure, was first proposed by Lassus[37] for thickening of the thin lip. Hackney et al.[30] compared muscle reorientation using an alar cinch suture in conjunction with a simple closure technique, a single V-Y closure technique, and a double V-Y closure technique. They observed that all three methods of closure yielded a significant increase in alar base width, and the double V-Y closure preserved the vermilion (especially in the lateral portion of the lip) with less variability than the other two techniques of closure. The true indication for this procedure is the patient who has a thin preoperative lateral vermilion.

Mandible

When contemplating a mandibular setback osteotomy the surgeon must carefully assess the patient's submental/cervical morphology. If a patient has a short submental length and existing poor submental/neck proportion, mandibular setback may worsen this, resulting in a "double chin." If this unesthetic side effect is a possibility, the surgeon may elect to combine the mandibular setback procedure with an advancement genioplasty.

Chin

Incorrect planning, vestibular scarring, excessive detachment of soft tissue from the chin, suprahyoid myotomy, improper closure of the soft tissue incision, hematoma formation, genial remodeling, and excessive bone resorption may compromise the results of chin surgery.[27]

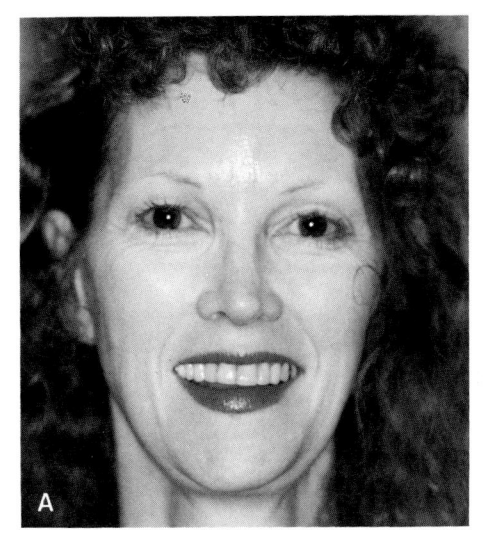

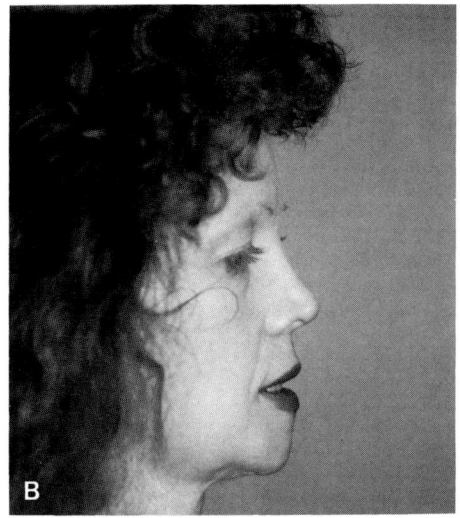

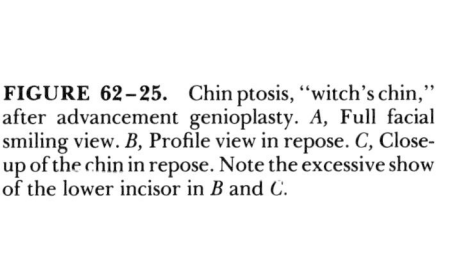

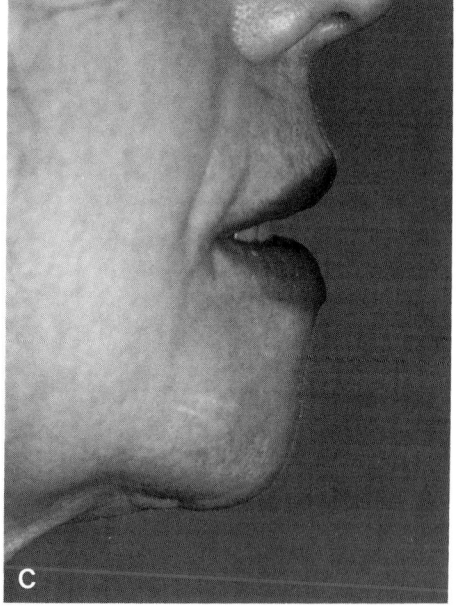

FIGURE 62–25. Chin ptosis, "witch's chin," after advancement genioplasty. *A*, Full facial smiling view. *B*, Profile view in repose. *C*, Close-up of the chin in repose. Note the excessive show of the lower incisor in *B* and *C*.

Bone resorption is related to the amount of soft tissue dissection and therefore is more pronounced in nonpedicled genioplasties.[5] Adolescent patients also have more bone resorption after genioplasty procedures.[75]

Chin ptosis or "witch's chin"[4] (Fig. 62–25 *A–C*) is an unesthetic complication secondary to the degloving dissection of the chin or lack of reattachment of the mentalis muscle at the time of surgery. This may lead to an inferior tissue slide, causing excess interlabial incompetence and exposure of the lower teeth and redundant tissue in the submental area.[6,66,74]

Several investigators have demonstrated that utilization of a procedure that minimizes soft tissue stripping may produce a more predictable hard and soft tissue response in the osteotomized segment.[3,6,21,27,51,66] Therefore, the surgeon should attempt to maintain as much soft tissue pedicle on the labial and lingual aspects of the mandible as possible. In addition to a predictable soft to hard tissue ratio, preservation of the soft tissue pedicle ensures a greater blood supply to the osteotomized segment, less bony resorption, and a decreased risk of infection.[21,34]

During closure the mentalis muscles must be reapproximated to prevent ptosis of the chin. An incision out into the unattached tissues of the lip can help prevent postoperative wound dehiscence and facilitate muscle reapproximation.

A tape chin dressing placed at the end of the surgical procedure is recommended to stabilize the soft tissues and prevent hematoma formation. Different surgeons have recommended different dressing materials and periods of immobilization (5 to 7 days,[16] one week,[27,66,75,79] 7 to 10 days,[4] and 10 to 14 days[34]).

SECONDARY REVISION OF POOR SURGICAL RESULTS

The best method of treatment of a poor soft tissue outcome is prevention. The deformity should be recognized, the soft tissue effects of the surgical procedure should be anticipated, and the correct interceptive procedure should be instituted. However, if a secondary procedure is required, the same techniques described in the preceding sections may be utilized. Revision surgery is more difficult than control of the soft tissues at the time of the original surgery because of scarring and change in normal anatomic relationships.[6,80] Rosen[63] suggests that these secondary procedures be attempted only after the final soft tissue drape has been established and the residual defect has been identified.

Other procedures that can be utilized to revise a poor surgical outcome are submental lipectomy, nasal wedge resection (Weir excisions),[63] and rhinoplasty.

SIMULTANEOUS NASAL AND ORTHOGNATHIC SURGERY

Rhinoplasty procedures and orthognathic surgery can be performed simultaneously. The advantages of simultaneous surgery are improved nasal airway function, facial esthetics, and patient convenience. There are no contraindications to rhinoplastic surgery when mandibular or genial surgery is being performed, as long as rigid fixation is employed for fixation of the mandibular osteotomies. However, when maxillary or two-jaw surgery orthognathic surgery is planned, relative indications and contraindications apply. The relative indications for simultaneous surgery are functional nasal septal deviations, minor defects of alar base or tip morphology, and significant nasal dorsal abnormalities. The relative contraindications are major tip deformities, minor abnormality of tip position, and planned detailed correction of major nasal deformities.

Large dorsal deformities, such as dehumping combined with lateral nasal osteotomies, can easily be corrected with simultaneous surgery because the margin of error is great and the final result is usually much better than the preoperative condition (Fig. 62–26 A–D). On the other hand, the surgical correction of small dorsal deformities should be postponed because the margin of error is small. Surgical procedures designed to alter the nasal tip or alar base should not be attempted because the relationship and position of these two structures is greatly influenced by maxillary surgical procedures, and the final outcome may be unpredictable.

The surgical sequencing should include completion of the maxillary osteotomy with the use of rigid fixation before the rhinoplasty procedure is begun. This is essential in order to provide a stable base for the nasal soft tissues. A stable osseous base allows a more accurate correction of the nasal deformity by rhinoplasty.

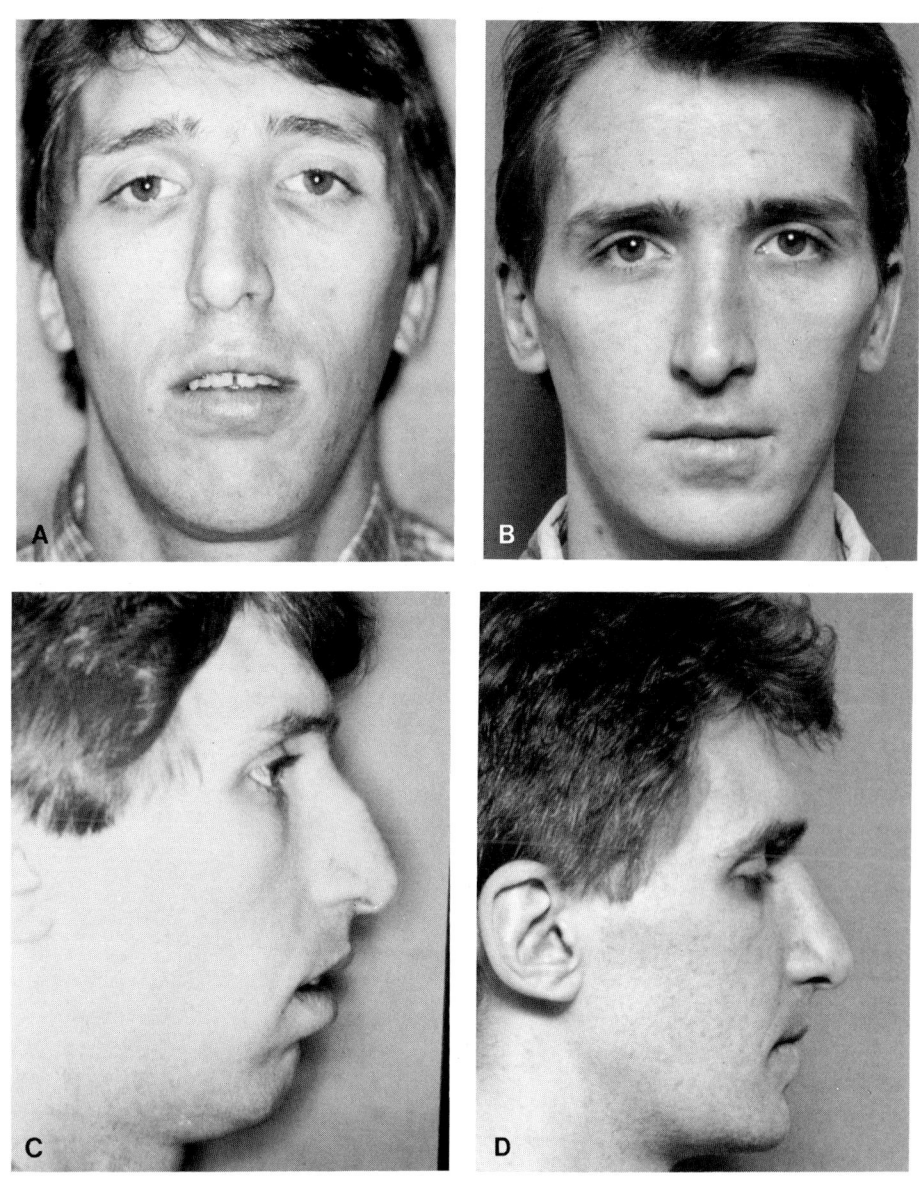

FIGURE 62-26. Patient treated with simultaneous maxillary impaction, mandibular advancement, advancement genioplasty, and dorsal dehumping rhinoplasty. *A,* Preoperative full facial view. *B,* Postoperative full facial view. *C,* Preoperative profile view. *D,* Postoperative profile view.

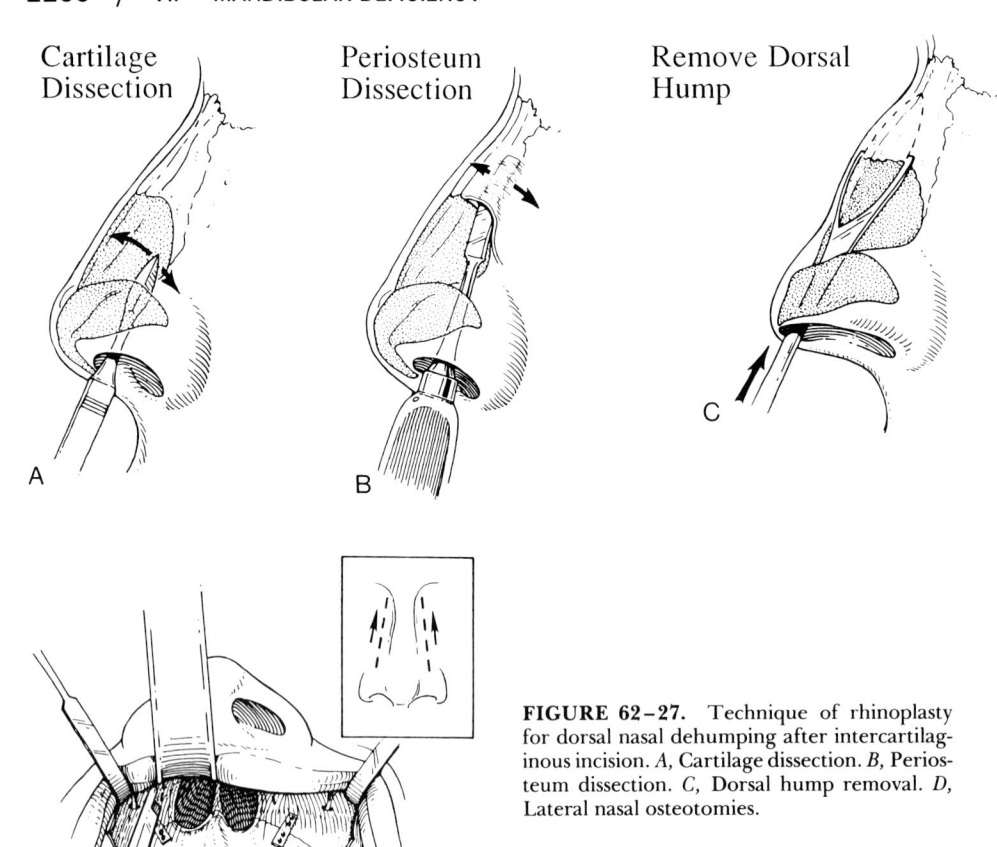

FIGURE 62-27. Technique of rhinoplasty for dorsal nasal dehumping after intercartilaginous incision. *A,* Cartilage dissection. *B,* Periosteum dissection. *C,* Dorsal hump removal. *D,* Lateral nasal osteotomies.

However, closure of the vestibular incision can be delayed until after the lateral nasal osteotomies have been completed. This allows better access and visualization of the osteotomies (Fig. 62-27 A-D).

The performance of simultaneous orthognathic and rhinoplastic procedures increases the anesthetic risk to the patient and necessitates the use of rigid fixation for two reasons. The first is the need to switch from nasoendotracheal intubation to oral-endotracheal intubation while the patient is still under general anesthesia. The second is an increased risk of respiratory obstruction during emergence from anesthesia secondary to manipulation of both the oral and nasal airways. Rigid fixation allows access to the airway without compromising the surgical result and allows the patient to more easily maintain a patent airway.

The most important consideration for simultaneous rhinoplasty and orthognathic surgery is proper patient selection. The surgeon and the patient should have a reasonable expectation of what can be achieved, and the possible need for revision rhinoplasty should be explained to the patient.[50,77]

REFERENCES

1. Aaronson SA: A cephalometric investigation of the surgical correction of mandibular prognathism. Angle Orthod 379(4):251, 1967.
2. Anderson JP, Joondeph DR, Turpin DL: A cephalometric study of profile changes in orthodontically treated cases ten years out of retention. Angle Orthod 43:324, 1973.

3. Bell WH: Correction of mandibular prognathism by mandibular setback and advancement genioplasty. Int J Oral Surg 10:221, 1981.
4. Bell WH, Brammer JA, McBride KL, et al: Reduction genioplasty: Surgical techniques and soft tissue changes. Oral Surg Oral Med Oral Pathol 51:471, 1981.
5. Bell WH, Dann JJ III: Correction of dentofacial deformities by surgery in the anterior part of the jaws: A study of stability and soft tissue changes. Am J Orthod 64:162, 1973.
6. Bell WH, Gallagher DM: The versatility of genioplasty using a broad pedicle. J Oral Maxillofac Surg 41:763, 1983.
7. Bell WH, Proffit WR: Esthetic effects of maxillary osteotomy. In Bell WH, Proffit WR, White RP (eds): Surgical Correction of Dentofacial Deformities. Philadelphia, WB Saunders, 1980, pp 368–370.
8. Berscheid E: An overview of the psychological effects of physical attractiveness. In Luckem CW, Ribbens KA, McNamara JS Jr (eds): Psychological aspects of facial form. Monograph No. 11 Ann Arbor: Center for Human Growth and Development, University of Michigan, 1980.
9. Betts NJ: Changes in the nasal and labial soft tissues after surgical repositioning of the maxilla. MS Thesis in Oral and Maxillofacial Surgery. University of Michigan, 1990.
10. Bloom LA: Perioral profile changes in orthodontic treatment. Am J Orthod 47:371, 1961.
11. Bundgaard M, Melson B, Terp S: Changes during and following total maxillary osteotomy (Le Fort I procedure): A cephalometric study. Europ J Orthod 8:21, 1986.
12. Burstone CJ: Integumental contour and extension patterns. Angle Orthod 29:93, 1959.
13. Busquets CJ, Sassouni V: Changes in the integumental profile of the chin and lower lip after genioplasty. J Oral Surg 39:499, 1981.
14. Carlotti Jr AE, Aschaffensburg PH, Schendel SA: Facial changes associated with surgical advancement of the lip and maxilla. J Oral Maxillofac Surg 44(8):593, 1986.
15. Collins PC, Epker BN: The alar base cinch: A technique for prevention of alar base flaring secondary to maxillary surgery. Oral Surg Oral Med Oral Pathol 53(6):549, 1982.
16. Converse JM, Wood-Smith D: Horizontal osteotomy of the mandible. Plast Reconstr Surg 34:464, 1964.
17. Dann JJ III, Epker BN: Proplast genioplasty: A retrospective study with treatment recommendations. Angle Orthod 47:173, 1977.
18. Dann JJ, Fonseca RJ, Bell WH: Soft tissue changes associated with total maxillary advancement: A preliminary study. J Oral Surg 34(1):19, 1976.
19. Dermaut LR, De Smit AA: Effects of sagittal split advancement osteotomy on facial profiles. Europ J Orthod 11:366, 1989.
20. Dion KE, Berscheid E, Walster E: What is beautiful is good. J Pers Soc Psychol 24:285, 1972.
21. Ellis E, Dechow PC, McNamara JA Jr, et al: Advancement genioplasty with and without soft tissue pedicle: An experimental investigation. J Oral Maxillofac Surg 42:637, 1984.
22. Epker BN, Fish LC: Definitive immediate presurgical planning. In Dentofacial Deformities: Integrated Orthodontic and Surgical Correction, Vol 1. St. Louis, CV Mosby, 1986, pp 103–127.
23. Freihofer HPM Jr: The lip profile after correction of retromaxillism in cleft and non-cleft patients. J Maxillofac Surg 4:136, 1976.
24. Freihofer HPM Jr: Changes in nasal profile after maxillary advancement in cleft and non-cleft patients. J Maxillofac Surg 5:20, 1977.
25. Friedland JA, Coccano PJ, Converse JM: Retrospective cephalometric analysis of mandibular bone absorption under silicone rubber chin implants. Plast Reconstr Surg 57(2):144, 1976.
26. Fromm B, Lundberg M: The soft-tissue facial profile before and after surgical correction of mandibular protrusion. Acta Odontol Scand 28:157, 1970.
27. Gallagher DM, Bell WH, Storum KA: Soft tissue changes associated with advancement genioplasty performed concomitantly with superior repositioning of the maxilla. J Oral Maxillofac Surg 42:238, 1984.
28. Guenther TA, Sather AH, Kern EB: The effect of Le Fort I maxillary impaction on nasal airway resistance. Am J Orthod 85:308, 1984.
29. Guymon M, Crosby DR, Wolford LM: The alar base cinch suture to control nasal width in maxillary osteotomies. Int J Adult Orthod Orthogn Surg 3(2):89, 1988.
30. Hackney FL, Nishioka GJ, Van Sickels JE: Frontal soft tissue morphology with double V-Y closure following Le Fort I osteotomy. J Oral Maxillofac Surg 46:850, 1988.
31. Hershey HG: Incisor tooth retraction and subsequent profile change in postadolescent female patients. Am J Orthod 61(1):45, 1972.
32. Hershey HG, Smith LH: Soft tissue profile change associated with surgical correction of the prognathic mandible. Am J Orthod 65:483, 1974.
33. Hofer O: Operation der prognathic und mikrogenie. Dtsch Zahn Mund Kiererheilkd 9:121, 1942.
34. Hohl TH, Epker BN: Macrogenia: A study of treatment results, with surgical recommendation. Oral Surg Oral Med Oral Pathol 41:545, 1976.
35. Ingersoll SK, Peterson LJ, Weinstein S: Influence of horizontal incision on upper lip morphology. J Dent Res 61:218, 1982 (abstr. No. 360).
36. Kalik MS: Toward an interdisciplinary psychology of appearance. Psychiatry 41:243, 1977.
37. Lassus C: Thickening the thin lips. Plast Reconstr Surg 68:950, 1981.
38. Lew KKK, Loh FC, Yeo JF, et al: Profile changes following anterior subapical osteotomy in Chinese adults with bimaxillary protrusion. Int J Adult Orthod Orthognathic Surg 4(3):189, 1989.
39. Lines PA, Steinhauser EW: Soft tissue changes in relationship to movement of hard tissue structures in orthognathic surgery: A preliminary report. J Oral Surg 32:891, 1974.
40. Lints RR, Spalding PM, Vig PS, et al: The effects of maxillary surgery on nasal respiration. Int J Adult Orthod Orthognath Surg, in press.

41. Mack JA, Vizuette JR, LaBanc J, et al.: Three-dimensional changes of upper lip and nose following maxillary superior repositioning. Abstract presented at 68th Annual Meeting, American Association of Oral and Maxillofacial Surgeons, New Orleans, September 1986.
42. Mansour S, Burstone C, Legan H: An evaluation of soft tissue changes resulting from Le Fort I maxillary surgery. Am J Orthod 84(1):37, 1983.
43. Mathes EW: The effects of physical attractiveness and anxiety on heterosexual attraction over a series of five encounters. J Mar Fam 37:769, 1975.
44. McDonnel JP, McNeil RW, West RA: Advancement genioplasty: A retrospective cephalometric analysis of osseous and soft tissue changes. J Oral Surg 35:640, 1977.
45. Millard DR: The alar cinch in the flat, flaring nose. Plast Reconstr Surg 65:669, 1980.
46. Mommaerts MY, Marxer H: A cephalometric analysis of the long-term, soft tissue profile changes which accompany the advancement of the mandible by sagittal split ramus osteotomies. J Craniomaxillofac Surg 15:127, 1987.
47. O'Reilly MT: Integumental profile changes after surgical orthodontic correction of bimaxillary dentoalveolar protrusion in black patients. Am J Orthod Dentofac Orthop 96(3):242, 1989.
48. O'Ryan F, Schendel S: Nasal anatomy and maxillary surgery. I. Esthetic and anatomic principles. Int J Adult Orthod Orthogn Surg 4(1):27, 1989.
49. O'Ryan F, Schendel S: Nasal anatomy and maxillary surgery. II. Unfavorable nasolabial esthetics following the Le Fort I osteotomy. Int J Adult Orthod Orthogn Surg 4(2):75, 1989.
50. O'Ryan F, Schendel S, Carlotti A: Nasal anatomy and maxillary surgery. III. Surgical techniques for correction of nasal deformities in patients undergoing maxillary surgery. Int J Adult Orthod Orthogn Surg 4(3):157, 1989.
51. Park HS, Ellis E III, Fonseca RJ, et al: A retrospective study of advancement genioplasty. Oral Surg Oral Med Oral Pathol 67:481, 1989.
52. Peled IJ, Wexler MR, Ticher S, et al: Mandibular resorption from silicone chin implants in children. J Oral Maxillofac Surg 44:346, 1986.
53. Phillips C, Devereux JP, Camilla Tulloch JF, et al: Full-face soft tissue response to surgical maxillary intrusion. Int J Adult Orthod Orthogn Surg 1(4):299, 1986.
54. Proffit WR, Epker BN: Treatment planning for dentofacial deformities. In Bell WH, Proffit WR, White RP (eds): Surgical Correction of Dentofacial Deformities. Philadelphia, WB Saunders, 1980, pp 183–187.
55. Proffit WR, Epker BN, Ackerman JL: Systematic description of dentofacial deformities: The data base. In Bell WH, Proffit WR, White RP (eds): Surgical Correction of Dentofacial Deformities. Philadelphia, WB Saunders, 1980, pp 114–122.
56. Quast DC, Biggerstaff RH, Haley JV: The short-term and long-term soft-tissue profile changes accompanying mandibular advancement surgery. Am J Orthod 84:29, 1983.
57. Radney LJ, Jacobs JD: Soft-tissue changes associated with surgical total maxillary intrusion. Am J Orthod 80(2):191, 1981.
58. Rickets RM: Foundation for cephalometric communication. Am J Orthod 46:330, 1960.
59. Riedel RA: An analysis of dentofacial relationships. Am J Orthod 43:103, 1957.
60. Robinson M: Bone resorption under plastic chin implants. Arch Otolaryngol 95:30, 1972.
61. Robinson M, Shuken R: Bone resorption under plastic chin implants. J Oral Surg 27:116, 1969.
62. Robinson SW, Speidel TM, Isaacson RJ, et al: Soft tissue profile change produced by reduction of mandibular prognathism. Angle Orthod 42:227, 1972.
63. Rosen HM: Lip-nasal aesthetics following Le Fort I osteotomy. Plast Reconstr Surg 81(2):171, 1988.
64. Rudee, DA: Proportional profile changes concurrent with orthodontic therapy. Am J Orthod 50:421, 1964.
65. Sakima T, Sachdeva R: Soft tissue response to Le Fort I maxillary impaction surgery. Int J Adult Orthod Orthognath Surg 4(2):221, 1987.
66. Scheideman GB, Legan HL, Bell WH: Soft tissue changes with combined mandibular setback and advancement genioplasty. J Oral Surg 39:505, 1981.
67. Schendel SA, Delaire J: Facial muscles: Form, function, and reconstruction in dentofacial deformities. In Bell WH, Proffit WR, White RP (eds): Surgical Correction of Dentofacial Deformities. Philadelphia, WB Saunders, 1980, pp 259–280.
68. Schendel SA, Eisenfeld JH, Bell WH, et al: Superior repositioning of the maxilla: Stability and soft tissue osseous relations. Am J Orthod 70(6):663, 1976.
69. Schendel SA, Williamson LW: Muscle reorientation following superior repositioning of the maxilla. J Oral Maxillofac Surg 41(4):235, 1983.
70. Stella JP, Streater MR, Epker BN, Sinn DP: Predictability of upper lip soft tissue changes with maxillary advancement. J Oral Maxillofac Surg 47:697, 1989.
71. Subtelny JD: A longitudinal study of the soft tissue facial structures and their profile characteristics, defined in relation to underlying skeletal structures. Am J Orthod 45:481, 1959.
72. Talbott JP: Soft tissue response to mandibular advancement surgery, MS Thesis in Dentistry. University of Kentucky, 1975.
73. Tomlak DJ, Piecuch JF, Weinstein S: Morphologic analysis of upper lip area following maxillary osteotomy via the tunneling approach. Am J Orthod 85(6):488, 1984.
74. Trauner RT, Obwegeser H: The surgical correction of mandibular prognathism and retrognathia with consideration of genioplasty. Part I. Surgical procedures to correct mandibular prognathism and reshaping of the chin. Oral Surg Oral Med Oral Pathol 10:677, 1957.
75. Tulasne JF: The overlapping bone flap genioplasty. J Craniomaxillofac Surg 15:214, 1987.
76. Turvey TA, Hall D, Warren DW: Alterations in nasal airway resistance following repositioning of the maxilla. Am J Orthod 85:109, 1984.

77. Waite PD: Simultaneous orthognathic surgery and rhinoplasty. Oral Maxillofacial Surg Clin North Am p 339–350, 1990.
78. Weinstein S, Harris EF, Archer SY: Lip morphology and area changes associated with surgical correction of mandibular prognathism. J Oral Rehab 9:335, 1982.
79. Wessberg GA, Wolford LM, Epker BN: Interpositional genioplasty for the short face. J Oral Surg 38:584, 1980.
80. Wolford LM: Discussion: Rosen HM: Lip-nasal aesthetics following Le Fort I osteotomy. Plast Reconstr Surg 81(2):180, 1988.
81. Woodburne RT: Essentials of Human Anatomy, 6th ed. New York, Oxford University Press, 1978, pp 196–208.
82. Zide MF: Applied surgical anatomy of the nose. Oral Maxillofacial Surg Clin North Am, p 289–302, 1990.

63 MAXILLARY AND MIDFACE DEFORMITY

Human genetics research starts in the clinic. Patients are a constant stimulus to thoughtful analysis. They present challenges for research and are the driving force behind our science.

—MICHAEL BROWN, M.D., *Nobel Laureate*

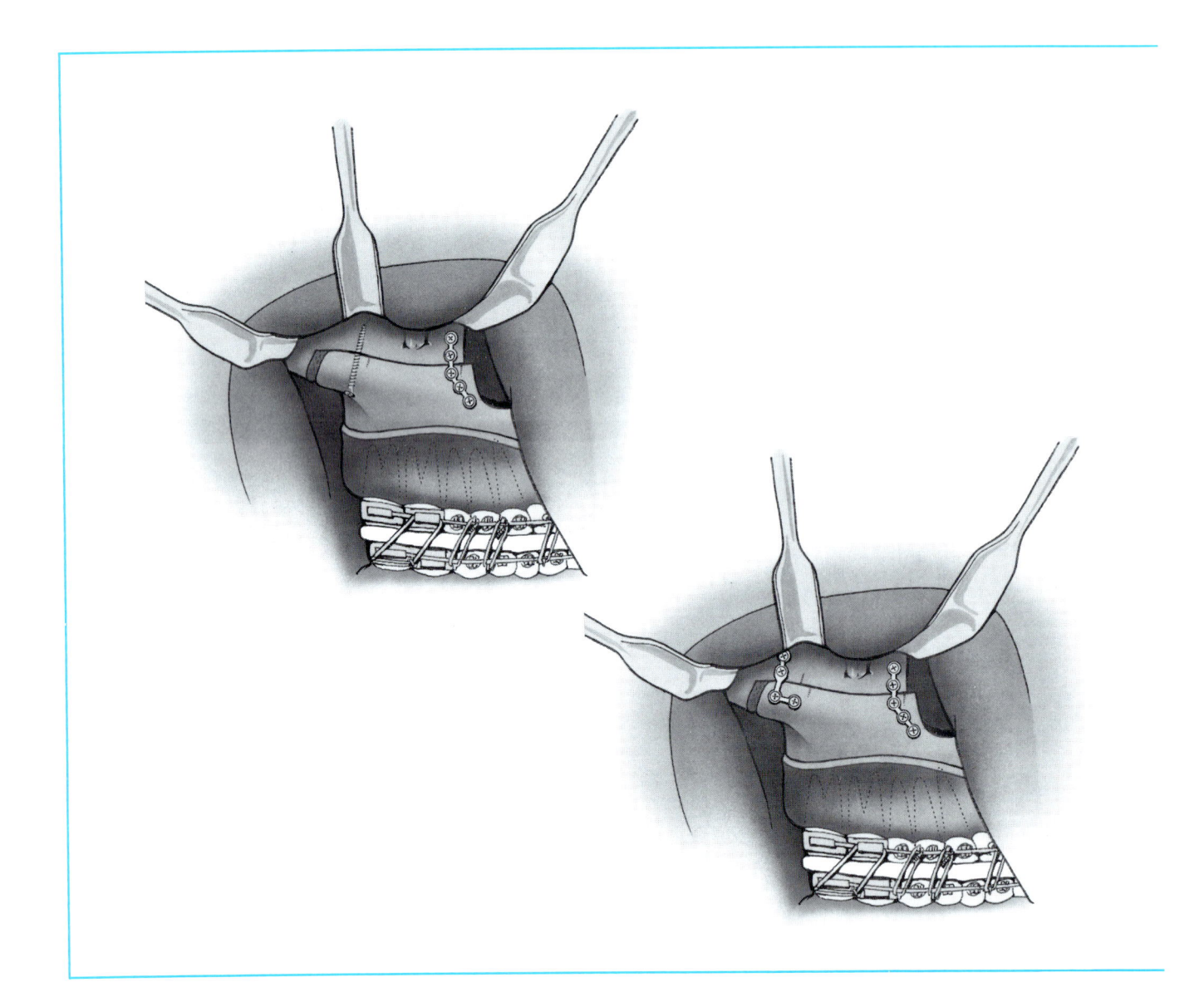

INDIVIDUALIZING THE OSTEOTOMY DESIGN FOR THE LE FORT I DOWNFRACTURE
  Biologic Foundation
  Clinical Application
  Anatomic Basis for Osteotomy Design
  Traditional-Level Le Fort I Osteotomy
  Maxillary Step Osteotomy
  High Le Fort I Osteotomy
  Surgical Technique for Exposure of the Osteotomy Site
  Osteotomy Design for High Le Fort I Osteotomy
  Sectioning the Maxilla
  The Downsliding Technique
  Stabilization of the Maxilla with Rigid Skeletal Fixation
  The Mini Fixation System
  The Micro System of Rigid Fixation
  Anatomic Considerations
  Segmentation of the Maxilla
  Three- and Four-Segment Le Fort I Osteotomy
  Two-Segment Le Fort I Osteotomy
  Inferior Repositioning of the Maxilla
  Neuromuscular Rehabilitation
  Conclusion
CASE REPORTS
  Occlusal Considerations
SPECIAL ADJUNCTIVE CONSIDERATIONS
  Malar Midfacial Augmentation
  Augmentation of the Malar Prominence by Sagittal Osteotomy of the Zygoma and Interpositional Bone Grafting
  Zygomatic Complex Reduction—System for Accurate Bilateral Symmetric Reduction
  Model Surgery for Facial Asymmetry Deformities
  Orthopedic-Assisted Maxillary Advancement in the Cleft Lip and Palate Patient, Using External Headframe Traction
  Orthopedic Correction of Maxillary Deficiency
  The Lip Lift

I. Individualizing the Osteotomy Design for the Le Fort I Downfracture

WILLIAM H. BELL
DAVID DARAB
ZHIHAO YOU

An overview of new and modified techniques of repositioning and stabilizing the maxilla by the Le Fort I downfracture technique is presented in this section. Osteotomy design, anatomic considerations, biologic principles, and techniques of sectioning the maxilla are discussed. In addition, rigid fixation utilizing mini, pan, or micro bone plate systems is described. Case reports are presented that illustrate the use of various osteotomy designs for Le Fort I and other adjunctive surgical procedures in treating patients with dentofacial deformities and mandibular dysfunction.

Today there is a clinical,[2,12,17,21,22,24,37,48,75,96] functional,[2,3,16,21,23,56,70,83,94,95] and biologic[10,11,15,39] foundation for surgical repositioning of the maxilla in many adult and adolescent patients. Restoration of normal jaw function or improved function, optimal facial esthetics, and long-term dental and skeletal stability are essential for successful orthognathic surgery. The key to achieving these objectives is to analyze facial proportions and then to establish and implement esthetic priorities through the use of cephalometric planning and anatomic model surgery studies.[13]

A large proportion of individuals with dentofacial deformities manifest mandibular dysfunction and a variety of problems ranging from painless clicking in the temporomandibular joints to dysfunction and severe, intolerable pain in the joints and muscles. A balanced biomechanical relationship between the masticatory muscles, jaws, temporomandibular joints, and teeth is necessary to achieve normal function after surgical repositioning of the jaws. To attain these objectives, orthognathic surgery techniques combining maxillary, mandibular, and chin surgery with efficient orthodontic treatment and systematic neuromuscular rehabilitation have been developed (see Chapter 46).

The combined surgical and orthodontic approach, when used in concert with small bone plate and screw osteosynthesis and systematic muscular rehabilitation after surgery, increases treatment efficiency and frequently improves jaw function. The simplicity, versatility, and visibility provided by the Le Fort I downfracture technique affords the surgeon great latitude and safety in correcting maxillary deformities.[18] In addition, the ability to reposition the maxilla in all three dimensions of space dramatically increases the efficiency of treatment by the surgeon and orthodontist.

BIOLOGIC FOUNDATION

The delivery of an adequate amount of blood to the tissue capillaries for normal function of the organ is the primary purpose of the vascular system. Successful transposition of the maxillary dento-osseous segments by Le Fort I osteotomy depends on preserving the viability of the segment by proper design of the soft tissue and bony incisions.[7-11,15,19,52,72-74,81,88,106-108] The collateral circulation within the maxilla and its enveloping soft tissues, and the many vascular anastomoses in the maxilla, permit numerous technical modifications of the Le Fort I osteotomy.

Vascular anastomoses between the maxilla and its enveloping soft tissues are crucial in providing compensatory blood supply to dento-osseous segments after the nutrient medullary vascular system is transected. To demonstrate how the blood vessels between the maxilla and its enveloping mucoperiosteum communicate, 25 fresh cadavers were used. Nineteen of the cadavers were studied by means of arterial angiography, ABS (acrylonitrile-butadiene-styrene) casting mold, and Chinese ink perfusion.[107] The microvascular resin casts were made in the other seven cases and observed by scanning electron microscope.[106] The results indicated that the normal blood supply of the maxilla originates centrifugally from the alveolar medullary arterial system (Fig. 63–1A and B).[107] The mucoperiosteal arterial system also gives off many branches that penetrate the cortical bone and supply blood to the maxilla (Fig. 63–2).[106] The vascular connections between the maxilla and its surrounding soft tissues consist of not only capillaries but also arteries and veins, which are arranged in various configurations (Fig. 63–3A and B). The multiple sources of blood supply to the maxilla and the abundant vascular communications between the hard and soft tissues constitute the biologic foundation for maintaining dento-osseous viability despite transection of the medullary blood supply after osteotomies (Fig. 63–4).

Inelastic palatal mucosa may limit the amount of expansion possible by the Le Fort I osteotomy unless technical modifications are made.[14] After this procedure, excessive maxillary expansion and segmentation may devascularize and devitalize the expanded maxilla by stripping the soft tissue pedicle away from the underlying palatal bone. Parasagittal osteotomies, bone grafting, and long-term retention compensate for large lateral movements of the maxilla. When the maxilla is severely constricted, requiring a great deal of widening, dual access to the buccal and palatal areas or specially designed maxillary osteotomies may be advisable to achieve the necessary expansion. These techniques provide access to the buccal and palatal areas, allow extensive lateral movement of the maxilla and lengthening of the maxillary arch without stretching the palatal mucosa, and facilitate closure of the mucosal wound margins over the grafted palatal bony defects.

Modifications in the design of the bony and soft tissue incisions have been made to facilitate movement of the maxilla and to prevent impairment of circulation to

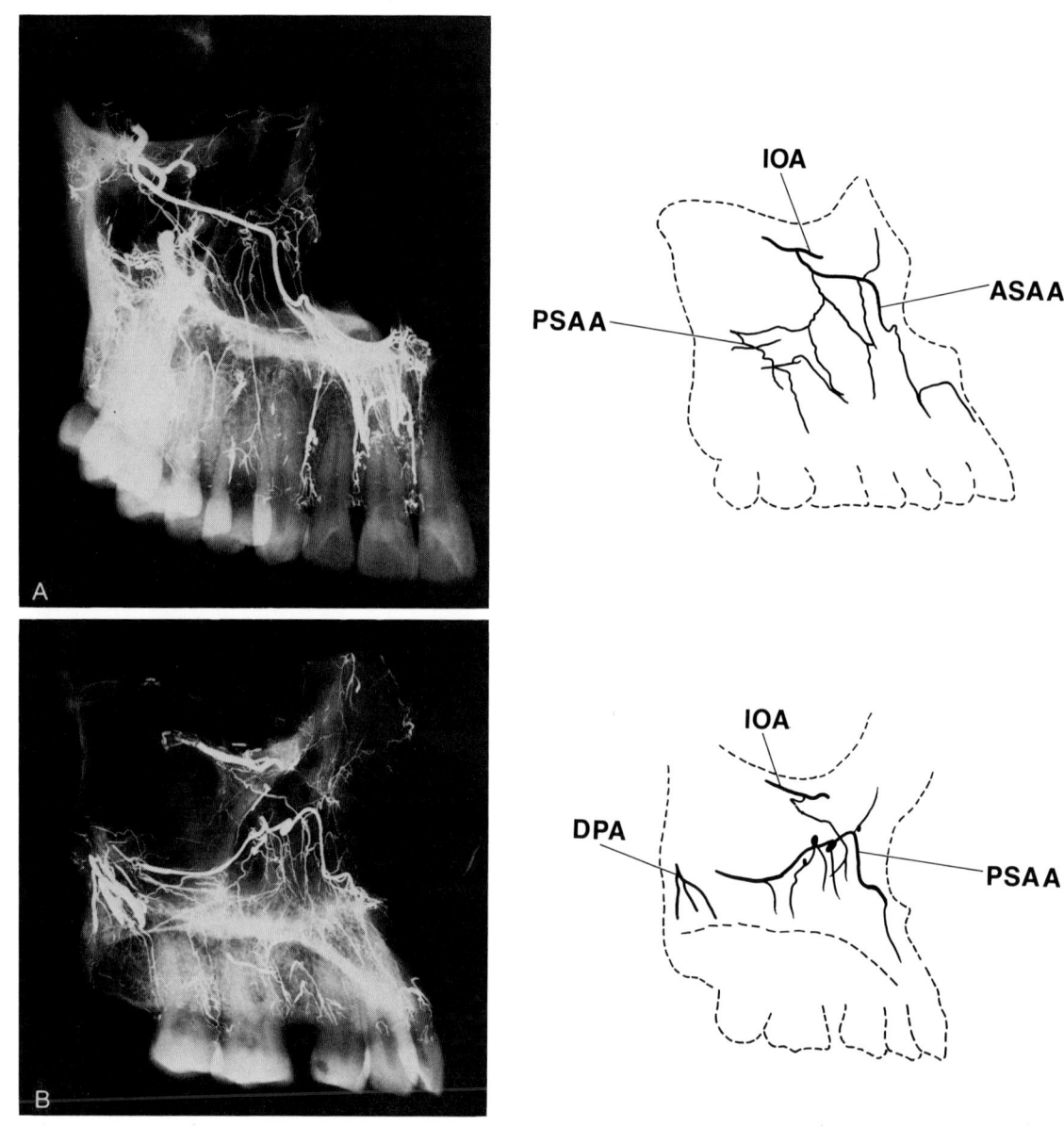

FIGURE 63-1. Representative arterial angiograms, with accompanying diagrams, of nine human cadavers show that the maxillary alveolar arterial system may consist of both anterior and posterior superior alveolar arteries (*A*, four specimens) or of only the posterior superior alveolar artery (*B*, five specimens). In the latter circumstance, the posterior superior alveolar artery enters the maxillary tuberosity, travels forward, and extends to the midline, giving off branches to each tooth and its surrounding tissues. ASAA = Anterior superior alveolar artery; PSAA = posterior superior alveolar artery; IOA = infraorbital artery; DPA = descending palatine artery.

the mobilized maxilla.[20] In an attempt to identify the effects of soft tissue flap design, segmentation of the maxilla, stretching of the vascular pedicle during healing, and transection of the descending palatine vessels, clinically analogous four-piece maxillary osteotomies were performed, using the Le Fort I osteotomy technique, in 14 adult rhesus monkeys. The revascularization and bone healing associated with the operation were studied at various time intervals by microangiographic and histologic techniques (Fig. 63–5*A* and *B*).[18] Transient vascular ischemia, osteonecrosis in the margins of the osteotomized segments, and variations in the osseous union of the segments were observed in the experimental animals.

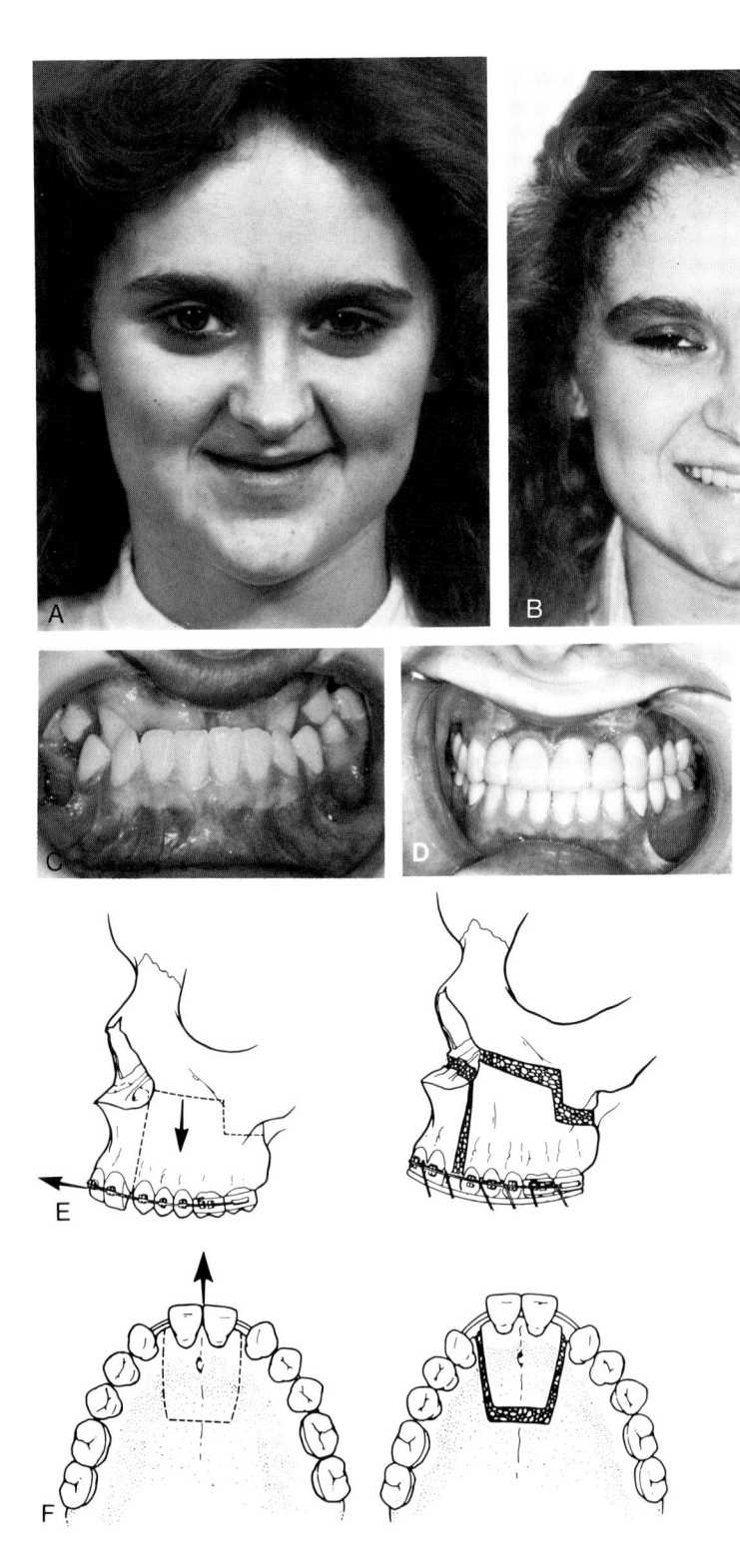

FIGURE 63–9. *A,* Facial appearance of a 15-year-old girl with anteroposterior and vertical maxillary deficiency (relative mandibular excess) before treatment. *B,* Facial appearance after surgical orthodontic treatment. The maxilla was repositioned inferiorly (7 mm) and anteriorly (5 mm) by Le Fort I osteotomy and interpositional bone grafting to improve the smile line, increase the upper lip prominence, reduce the prominence of the mandible, and correct the anterior crossbite. Genioplasty reduced the chin prominence and increased the chin width. *C,* Pretreatment Class III malocclusion. Multiple teeth are congenitally missing, and there are partially edentulous areas in the posterior maxillary and mandibular regions. Occlusion was achieved after presurgical orthodontic alignment and leveling of the maxillary and mandibular arches; 3-mm interdental spaces were left in the canine–central incisor regions. *D,* Postsurgical occlusion after edentulous areas were restored with fixed bridges. The maxilla was repositioned to correct the malocclusion and create 7-mm spaces between the central incisors and canine teeth. *E,* Plan of surgery: Le Fort I osteotomy and interpositional bone graft to reposition the maxilla inferiorly. *F,* The maxilla was segmented by vertical interdental osteotomies in the lateral incisor–canine interspaces to increase arch length and normalize the inclination and position of the central incisors. (*A–C* from Bell WH, Proffit WR, White RP Jr: Surgical Correction of Dentofacial Deformities. Vol III. Philadelphia, WB Saunders Company, 1985, pp 20, 21; with permission.)

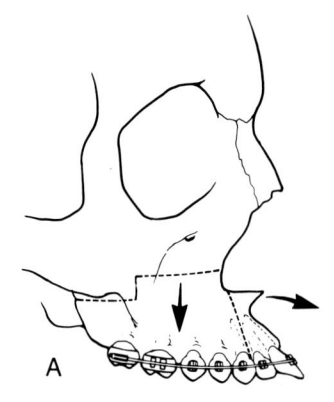

FIGURE 63-10. *A,* Three-segment Le Fort I osteotomy designed to increase the maxillary arch length. Arrows indicate the planned positional movements of the maxilla. The maxilla was repositioned to correct the malocclusion and create 7-mm spaces between the central incisors and the canine teeth; in addition, the maxilla was inferiorly repositioned by Le Fort I osteotomy and interpositional bone graft. *B,* Correction of vertical maxillary deficiency by inferior repositioning of the maxilla by three-segment Le Fort I osteotomy. The maxilla was sectioned between the lateral incisor and canine teeth to facilitate uprighting of the incisors, eliminating the need to extract bicuspid teeth. The inferiorly repositioned maxilla was stabilized by a combination of T-shaped bone grafts for mechanical stability and particulate autogenous marrow for osteogenic purposes.

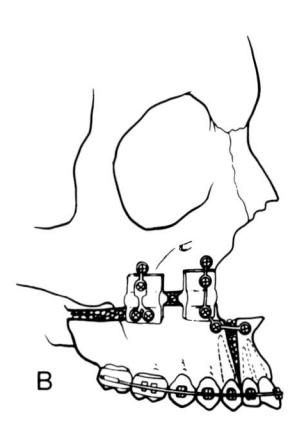

labiobuccal and palatal aspects of the areas where they are planned. Meticulous and precise surgical technique, prudent selection of osteotomy sites, good lighting of the surgical field, careful use of thin, sharp osteotomes, and the use of directly bonded orthodontic appliances are vital adjuncts to safe and successful interdental and subapical osteotomies.

When the objectives are posterior movement of the maxilla, concomitant alteration of the transverse dimension, and segmentation to close spaces created by extraction of the premolar teeth or prematurely lost molar teeth, the entire maxilla may be mobilized and repositioned by Le Fort I osteotomy. This procedure, making possible the simultaneous movement of anterior and posterior maxillary dento-osseous segments, affords maximal versatility. With it, the relationship between the anterior and posterior teeth can be improved, the axial inclination of the anterior teeth altered, and the desired transverse and vertical dimensions achieved. Segmentation of the anterior maxilla to improve the axial inclination of the anterior teeth without ostectomy or extractions may be the treatment of choice in selected cases; the desired anteroposterior position is achieved by Le Fort I osteotomy.

When the maxilla is repositioned posteriorly or superiorly (or both) and narrowed, there is a distinct possibility of telescoping the anterior and posterior portions of the maxilla into the nasal cavity or maxillary antra and causing osseous instability that is difficult to control with interosseous wire fixation. Stability of the repositioned maxilla can be improved by interpositional autogenous bone grafts, suspension wires, skeletal fixation, or small bone plates or by altering the geometric design of the osteotomy. The clinician must foresee the possible consequences of the planned positional changes. On the basis of the probable results of surgery, he or she may opt to alter the geometric design of the osteotomies to avoid undesirable consequences and may plan to telescope the proximal and distal segments to improve the juxtaposition of their margins.

2224 / VII—ORTHOGNATHIC SURGERY

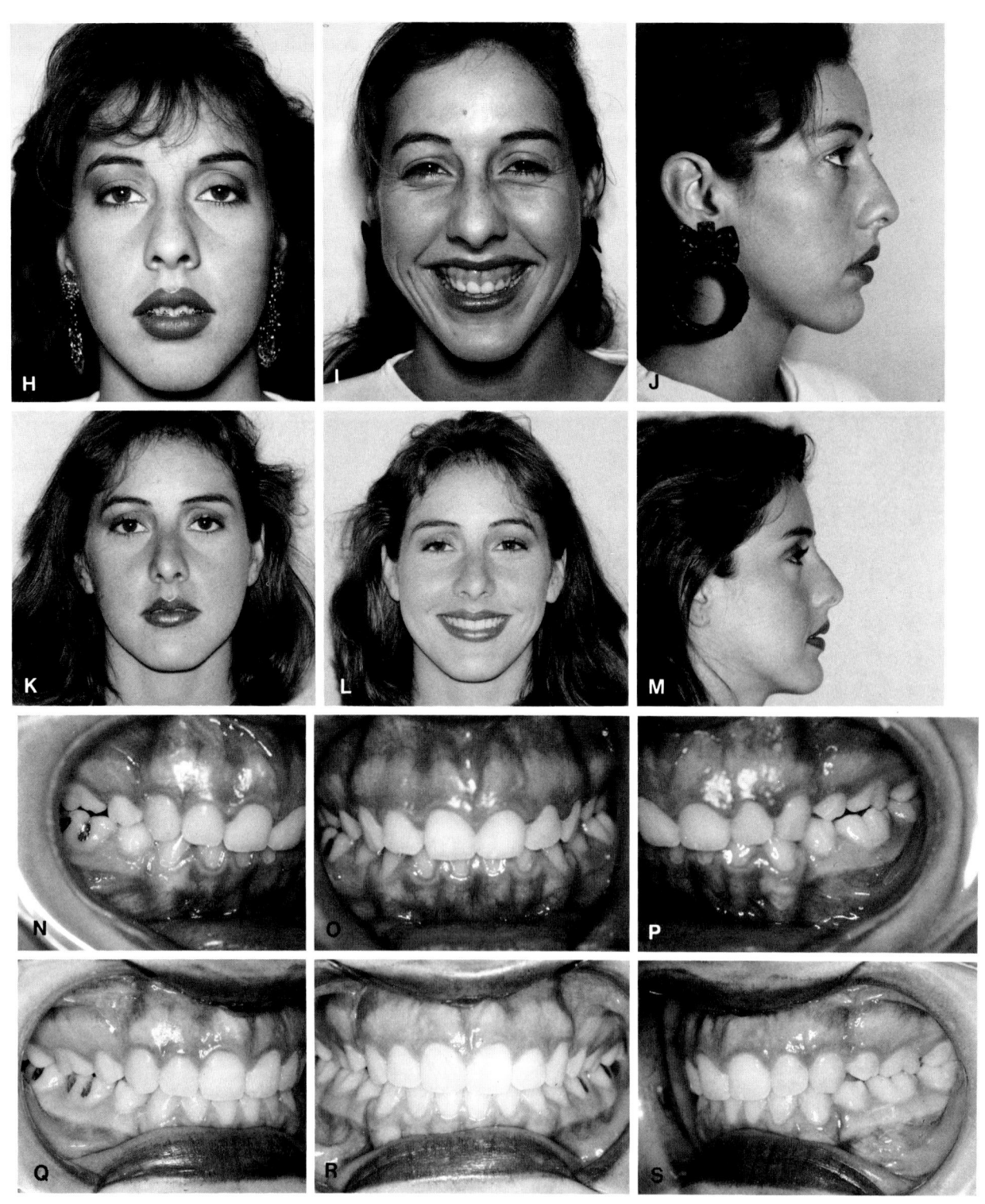

FIGURE 63–11 *Continued.* *H–J*, Facial appearance of a 19-year-old female patient with vertical maxillary excess and relative mandibular deficiency before surgical and orthodontic treatment. *K–M*, Facial appearance 2 years after treatment. *N–P*, Occlusion before treatment. *Q–S*, Occlusion 2 years after surgical and orthodontic treatment.

Illustration continued on following page

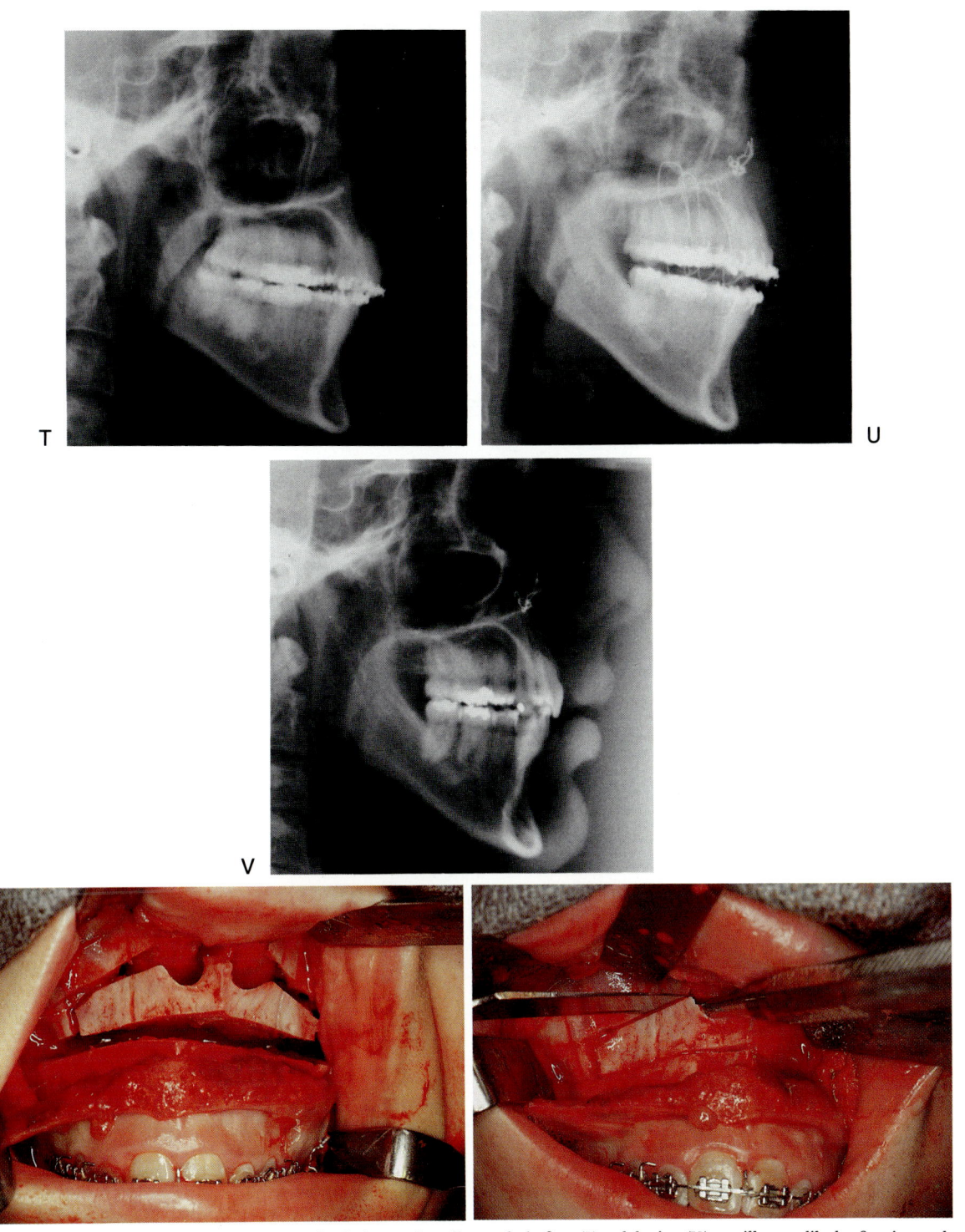

FIGURE 63-11 *Continued.* *T-V,* Cephalometric radiographs before *(T)* and during *(U)* maxillomandibular fixation and 2 years after surgery *(V)*. *W, left* and *right,* Patient with severe vertical hyperplasia treated by Le Fort I osteotomy, which superiorly repositioned the maxilla 9 mm. Ostectomy was made at a low level to maximize the interfacing of the margins with the osteotomy sites. Clinical results were very stable over an 8-year follow-up period.

CASE: R.S.

A 19-year-old woman had received orthodontic treatment over a period of 3 years. Four bicuspid teeth were extracted to facilitate correction of a Class I malocclusion with moderate crowding. The patient related that her facial esthetics became progressively worse, that her lips "sank in," and that her nasal tip drooped during the orthodontic treatment. Clinical (Fig. 63–12D to F) and cephalometric (Fig. 63–12J) analysis revealed anteroposterior maxillary deficiency and anteroposterior and vertical mandibular deficiency. Her chin was in a normal anteroposterior position. She manifested an excellent Class I occlusion, free of temporomandibular joint dysfunction.

PROBLEM LIST

Esthetics

FRONTAL. The facial appearance was compromised after orthodontic treatment. There was a poor vermilion show and a pointed chin.

PROFILE. Anteroposterior maxillary deficiency with retrusive lips was present. The nasal tip projection was poor.

Cephalometric Analysis (Fig. 63–12J)

1. Poor nasal tip projection.
2. Anteroposterior maxillary deficiency.

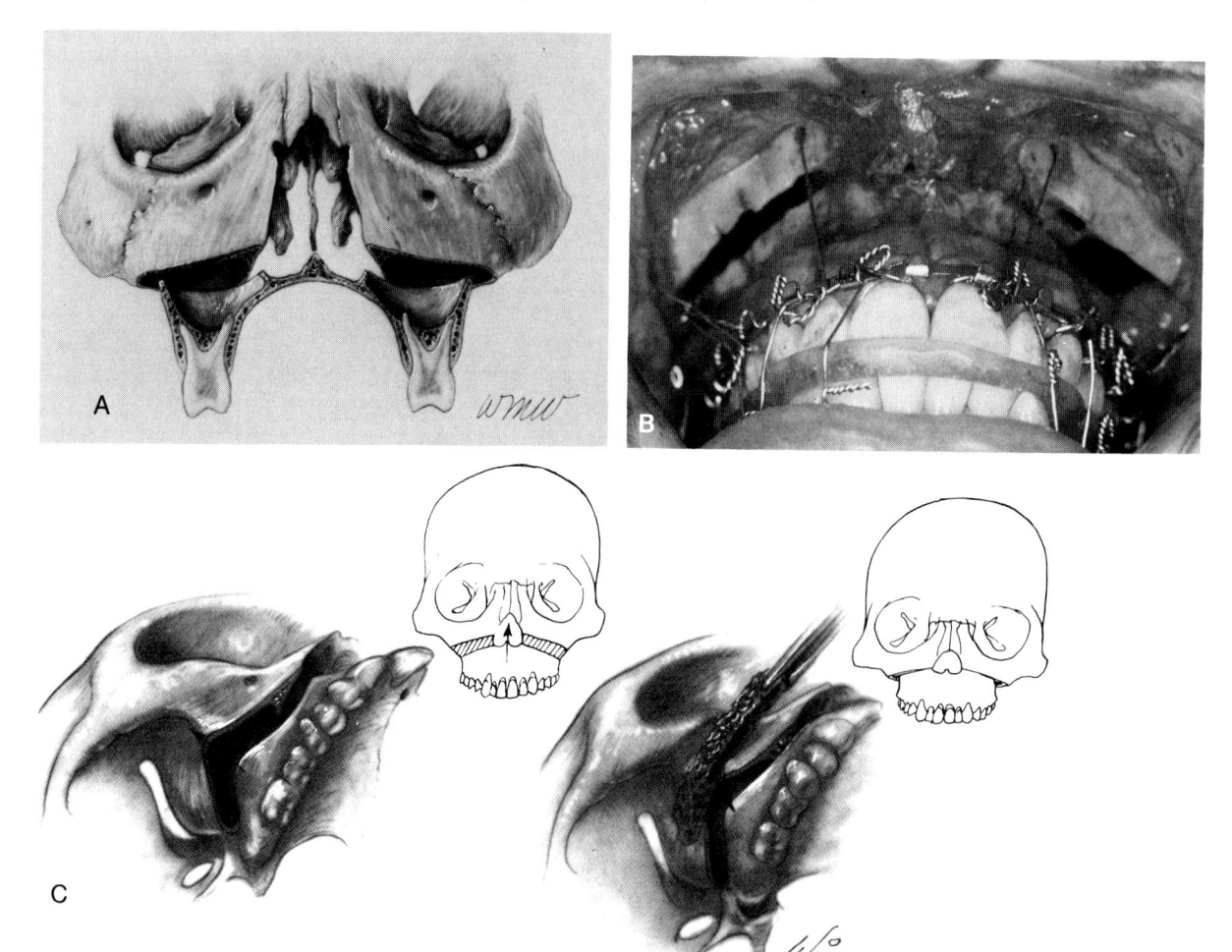

FIGURE 63–12. *A–C,* When osteotomies are made in the superior aspect of the lateral maxilla, where bony walls are angular, the margins of the proximal and distal segments may not be juxtaposed, allowing telescoping of the posterior maxilla into the maxillary antrum and possible osseous instability and difficulty in stabilizing the repositioned maxilla. Improved stability of the repositioned maxilla can be achieved by interpositional autogenous cancellous bone grafts and bone plates and screws. (*C* from Bell WH, Proffit WR, White RP Jr: Surgical Correction of Dentofacial Deformities. Vol II. Philadelphia, WB Saunders Company, 1980, p 1099; with permission.)

Illustration continued on following page

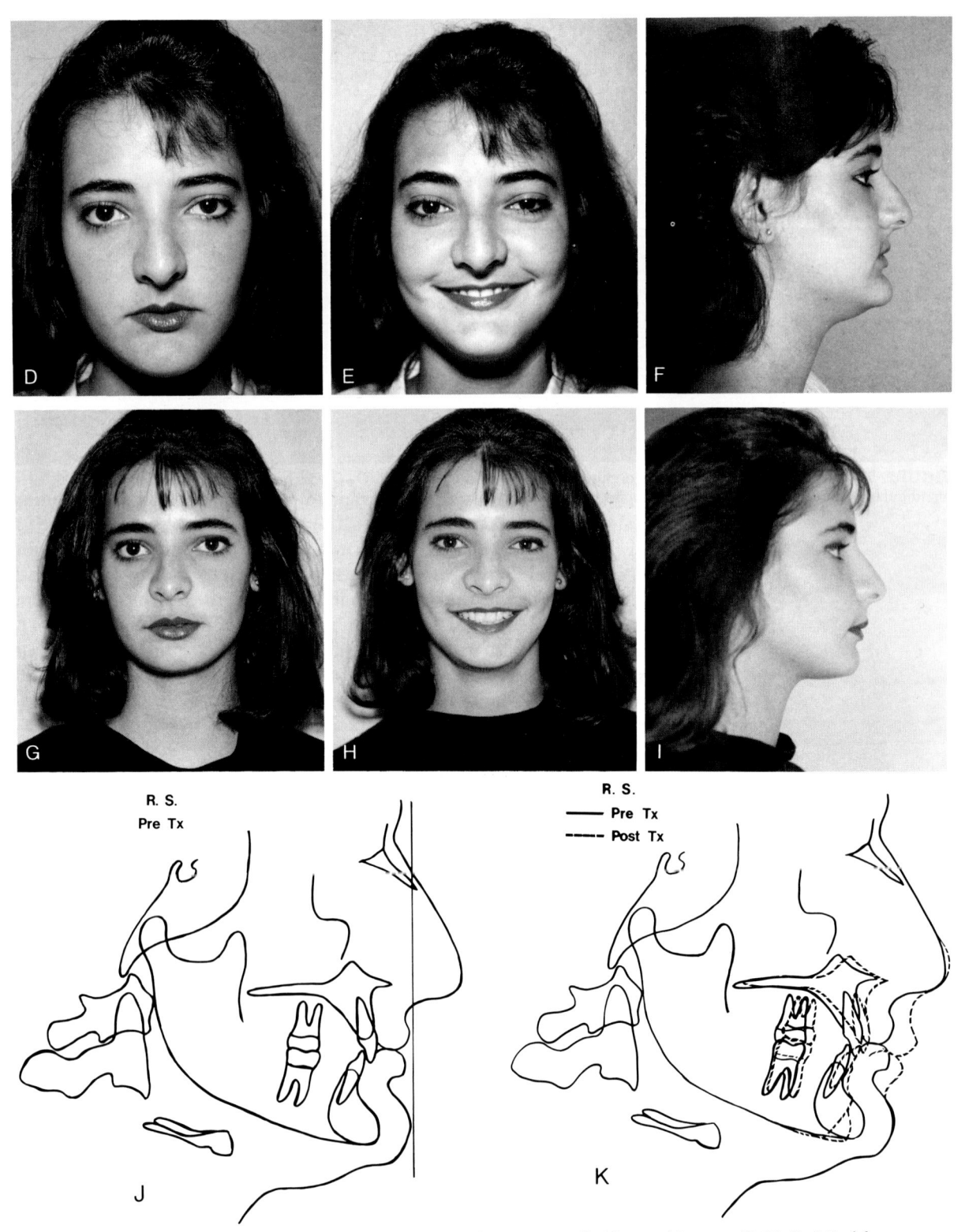

FIGURE 63-12 *Continued.* *D-F*, Presurgical facial appearance of a 19-year-old woman (R.S.). *G-I*, Facial appearance after an 8-mm advancement of the maxilla and mandible and a genioplasty to decrease chin prominence and increase chin height. *J*, Preoperative cephalometric tracing. *K*, Composite cephalometric tracings before surgery *(solid line)* and 9 months after orthognathic surgery *(broken line)*. The improved esthetic balance between the upper lip and nose was achieved by increasing the prominence of the upper lip and decreasing the apparent "nasal prominence."

Illustration continued on following page

ingly, the greater the anterior movement of the maxilla, the greater the reduction in incisor vertical. Clearly, one must be cognizant of this romping effect when designing maxillary osteotomies, or unpredicted changes in vertical dimension could result, compromising esthetics.

It is possible to take advantage of this romping effect with the traditional-level Le Fort I osteotomy when superior and anterior repositioning of the maxilla is desirable. The exact angulation of the lateral maxillary osteotomy must be determined from accurate cephalometric prediction studies and anatomic model surgery (see Chapter 7). From clinical analysis, the magnitude of anterior and superior repositioning of the maxillary incisors is determined. The cuspid and molar roots are identified on the lateral cephalometric radiograph, and a reference mark is placed at a safe level about 5 mm superior to the tooth root apices. The two reference marks are connected with a straight line extending from the piriform aperture to the tuberosity and pterygomaxillary fissure. This line identifies the lateral maxillary osteotomy. A maxillary acetate template is next constructed, with the reference marks and osteotomy outlined. This template is then overlaid on the cephalometric tracing, with the maxillary incisor in its new position. Any alterations in occlusion plane angulation are accomplished at this time. The difference between the osteotomy lines on the cephalometric tracing and on the maxillary template represents the magnitude of superior repositioning along the lateral maxillary wall. This distance is recorded and transferred to the lateral maxilla at the time of surgery, signifying the magnitude of ostectomy necessary to achieve the planned result. It is important to point out that because of the inclination of the lateral maxillary osteotomy, combined with the anterior repositioning, the amount of ostectomy is always less than the magnitude of superior repositioning. It is for this reason that careful cephalometric planning and accurate surgery are necessary to prevent unpredictable changes in the incisor vertical. In addition, at the time of surgery an external reference pin in the nasofrontal region is utilized to measure the amount of vertical and anteroposterior incisor change. The anteroposterior as well as transverse maxillary position is transferred from the model surgery with an intermediate acrylic splint. An intermediate splint is routinely used when combined maxillary and mandibular surgery is performed.

Fixation of the traditional-level Le Fort I osteotomy following maxillary advancement with superior repositioning can be achieved with piriform rim mini plates in combination with posterior mini plates in the zygomaticomaxillary buttress region or with zygomatic suspension wires secured to the buccal tube on the maxillary first molar (Fig. 63–16*A* and *B*). The lack of sufficient bone thickness along the lateral and anterior maxillary walls, frequently encountered in the hypoplastic maxilla, may rarely preclude the use of screw or plate osteosynthesis. Occasionally, planned telescoping of the lateral maxillary walls after superior repositioning enables positional screws to be placed in the anterior region. Additional stability, which may be needed to resist posterior relapse, can be achieved by "sandwiching" corticocancellous bone grafts between the telescoped maxillary segments with positional screws or plates or both.

The traditional-level Le Fort I osteotomy is indicated when a small (5 mm) anterior movement with good bony interfaces is anticipated following maxillary advancement (frequently combined with superoinferior maxillary repositioning). Advantages of the traditional-level Le Fort I osteotomy include (1) speed; (2) the general familiarity with this osteotomy design; (3) simplicity; (4) facility in repositioning the maxilla superiorly and posteriorly; (5) the ease and safety of segmentation; (6) the capacity of the procedure to be combined with Le Fort III osteotomy in selected cases; and (7) its capacity to be combined with lateral maxillary osteotomies to facilitate widening of the maxilla by a rapid maxillary expansion appliance —a secondary Le Fort I osteotomy is made at the same level as the initial lateral maxillary osteotomy. Disadvantages include (1) possible telescoping of repositioned segments; (2) difficulty in obtaining sufficient bone for the application of

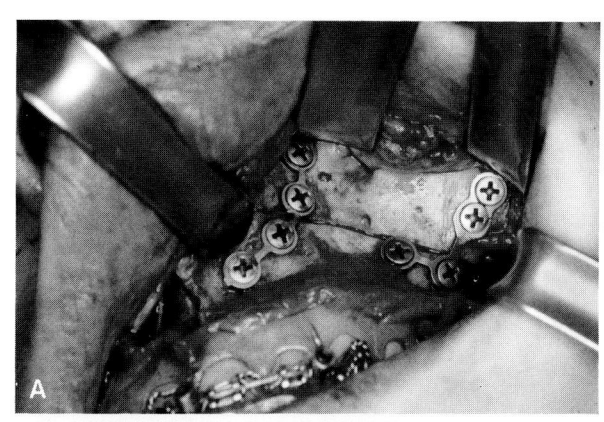

FIGURE 63-16. *A,* Traditional low-level Le Fort I osteotomy stabilized anteriorly and posteriorly by mini plates. *B,* Superiorly repositioned maxilla with excellent interfacing of the margins of the osteotomies, stabilized anteriorly with an L-shaped mini plate and a zygomatic suspension wire secured to a buccal tube on the maxillary first molar.

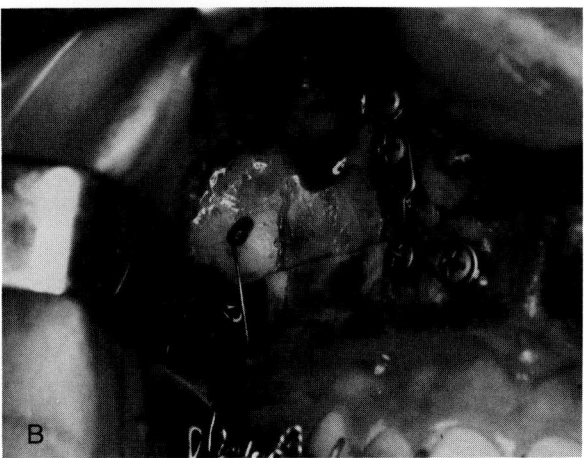

screw and/or plate osteosynthesis in individuals with aberrant anatomy (exceedingly thin anterior maxillary walls); (3) difficulty in positioning corticocancellous bone grafts in the pterygopalatine region; (4) potential for unpredictable changes in the vertical maxillary position; (5) relatively poor augmentation of malar, infraorbital, and paranasal areas; and (6) the possibility that this procedure may not be feasible at an early age because of developing tooth buds contiguous to the planned line of bone sectioning.

MAXILLARY STEP OSTEOTOMY

In an effort to improve the predictability and accuracy of maxillary advancement surgery and eliminate the incline or ramping effects previously described with the traditional Le Fort I osteotomy, the maxillary step osteotomy was designed (Fig. 63-17).[20,24,30,91] In this technique, the lateral maxillary osteotomy is made parallel to the Frankfort horizontal or natural horizontal plane, which places the osteotomy higher into the zygomaticomaxillary buttress where a vertical step is made. A horizontal osteotomy is then continued posteriorly to the pterygoid plates, parallel to the anterior horizontal osteotomy (Fig. 63-17). It is important to keep the anterior and posterior osteotomies parallel to minimize interferences during maxillary repositioning. With this osteotomy design, anterior and superior maxillary repositioning can be easily accomplished by performing an ostectomy along the lateral maxillary walls. Fixation can be achieved with anterior piriform mini plates either alone or combined with posterior zygomatic suspension wires or mini plates.

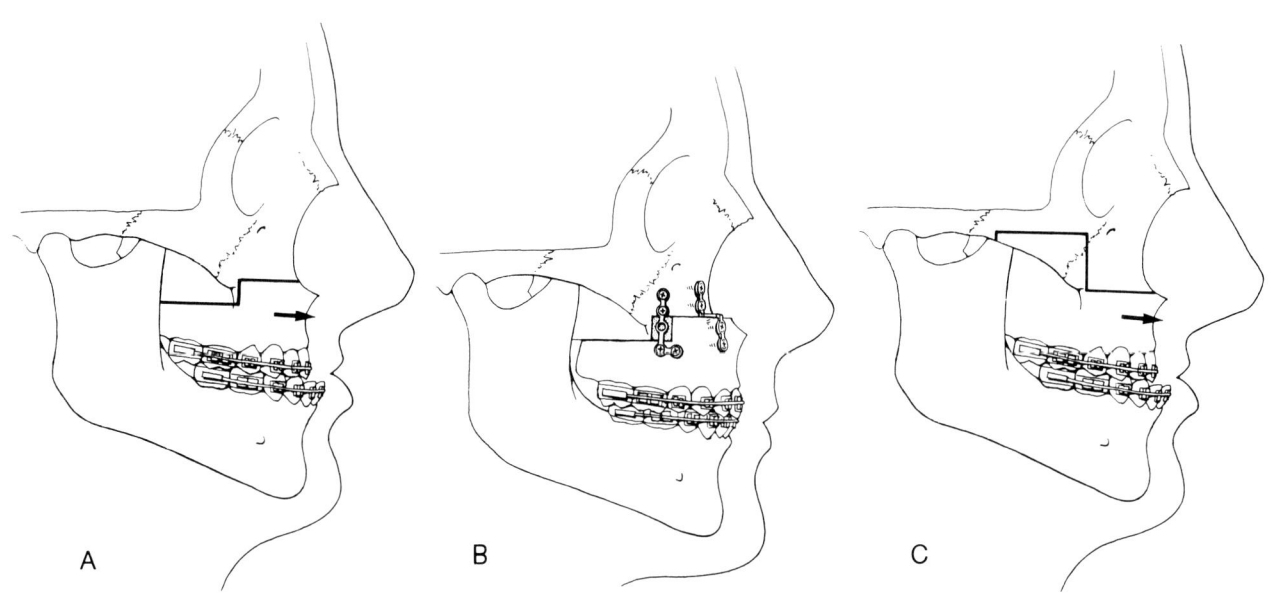

FIGURE 63-17. *A* and *B*, The illustrated deformity manifests anteroposterior maxillary deficiency. Planned surgical movement includes maxillary advancement *(arrow)* by step osteotomy. *A*, The lateral osteotomy is made parallel to the Frankfort horizontal and approximately 5 mm superior to the cuspid. The vertical step is prepared at the zygomaticomaxillary buttress; the posterior horizontal continuation of the osteotomy is made at a level approximately 4 to 5 mm superior to the molar apices and parallel to the anterior cut. *B*, The completed osteotomy cuts. Note the parallel horizontal osteotomies. The osteotomy sites following removal of the bone corresponding to the amount of superior repositioning planned are shown. The repositioned maxilla is stabilized with mini plates anteriorly and posteriorly. *C*, Frontal and lateral views of the superior step osteotomy. The osteotomy is made parallel to the Frankfort horizontal plane. The vertical step in the maxillary buttress region is carried superiorly, and the horizontal continuation is extended posteriorly through the zygomaticomaxillary buttress complex and into the zygomatic arch. The repositioned maxilla is stabilized by metal plate and screw osteosyntheses. Such an osteotomy design may be indicated when the anterior maxillary bony walls are exceedingly thin; augmentation of the anterior maxilla and paranasal area may be necessary.

The design of this osteotomy is dependent on accurate cephalometric prediction studies. The apices of the cuspid and molar roots are first identified. With use of the cephalometric prediction tracing, a line is scribed from low on the piriform rim, superior to the cuspid apex, to the zygomatic buttress parallel to Frankfort horizontal. At the time of surgery, this bone cut is sequentially extended posteriorly until the dense portion of the zygomatic buttress is sectioned. Careful assessment of bone thickness in the planned vertical osteotomy site in the zygomaticomaxillary buttress may be helpful in designing and positioning the osteotomy in denser bone. A vertical step is then extended inferiorly. The inferior extent of this vertical step, together with the horizontal osteotomy extending posterior to the pterygoid plates, must be sufficiently superior to avoid injury to the molar roots. It is important that the anterior and posterior horizontal osteotomies remain parallel to avoid interferences during anterior repositioning of the maxilla. Once the osteotomy has been designed on the prediction tracing, the vertical distance from the cuspid and molar occlusal surfaces is recorded. These measurements are transferred to the lateral maxillary wall at the time of surgery by placing reference marks at the predetermined level above the cuspid adjacent to the piriform aperture and above the molars at the zygomatic buttress. Once the osteotomy design has been transferred to the patient, the Le Fort I downfracture is accomplished in the routine manner. With the cephalometric prediction studies as a guide, the lateral osteotomy is initiated at the piriform rim and extended posteriorly until the thick bone of the zygomatic buttress is sectioned. In this manner, a sufficient quantity of bone is assured for the application of screw and plate osteosynthesis.

Advantages of this osteotomy design include the following: (1) Pure anteroposterior maxillary repositioning can be achieved when a vertical change at the incisor is undesirable; this is made possible by the design principle that makes the horizontal osteotomy parallel to the natural horizontal or the Frankfort horizontal; (2) vertical osteotomy at the zygomatic buttress provides a well-visualized place for corticocancellous bone graft placement and superior augmentation of the paranasal area; and (3) the vertical osteotomy may be extended more superiorly into denser bone in the zygomaticomaxillary buttress, and the vertical osteotomy serves as a stable anteroposterior reference line. Disadvantages include the following: (1) This procedure is technically more difficult; (2) it requires accurate cephalometric prediction studies for predictable results; and (3) insufficient bone along the lateral maxillary wall or the zygomaticomaxillary buttress may preclude the application of screw or plate osteosynthesis.

Stringer and Boyne[91] have designed a superior step osteotomy that also parallels the Frankfort horizontal; the osteotomy is made at a low level anteriorly, courses vertically into the zygomaticomaxillary buttress, and then continues posteriorly into the zygomatic arch (Fig. 63–17C). Such an osteotomy design may be indicated when the anterior maxillary walls are very thin. With this technique, the authors augment the paranasal areas and anteroinferior orbital rim areas with bone implants (Bioss).

HIGH LE FORT I OSTEOTOMY

Esthetic Basis for High Le Fort I Osteotomy

When the nasofrontal projection and position of the globe are normal, the major esthetic components to be addressed are the maxillomandibular disproportion, the zygomatic bone, the infraorbital area, and the paranasal area. Although a combination of the Le Fort I osteotomy and an augmentation procedure is frequently used to correct these deformities, a more ideal approach would be an osteotomy designed to correct the maxillomandibular disproportion and malocclusion, the paranasal area, and the zygomatic deficiency (Figs. 63–18 and 63–19).[1,20,26,27,35,36,46,57,58,60,102] Because the esthetic epicenter of the zygomatic bone is located in an area approximately 2 cm lateral and 1.5 cm inferior to the lateral canthus, the horizontal and posterior extent of such an osteotomy in the zygoma

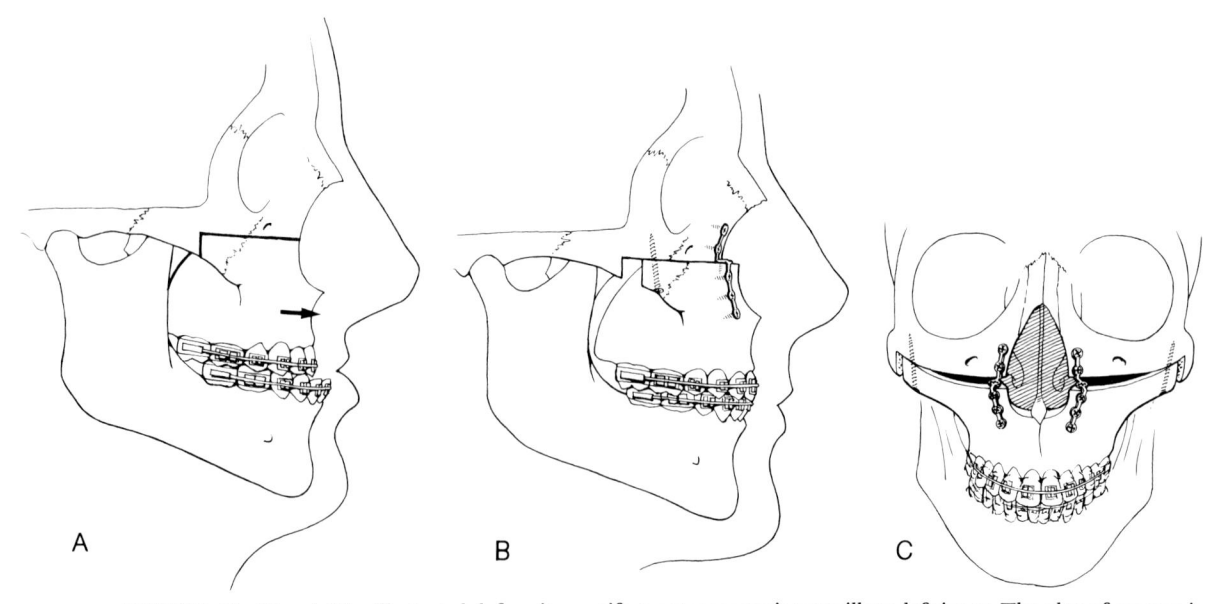

FIGURE 63–18. *A*, The illustrated deformity manifests anteroposterior maxillary deficiency. The plan of surgery is anterior repositioning *(arrow)* by zygomaticomaxillary osteotomy as part of a modified high Le Fort I osteotomy. *B* and *C*, Anteriorly repositioned maxilla stabilized by a 20-mm-long 2-mm-diameter self-tapping positional screw placed in the dense zygomatic pillar. Jaw fixation plates (1.5 mm) and screws may be used in the lateral piriform rim to stabilize the anteriorly repositioned maxilla.

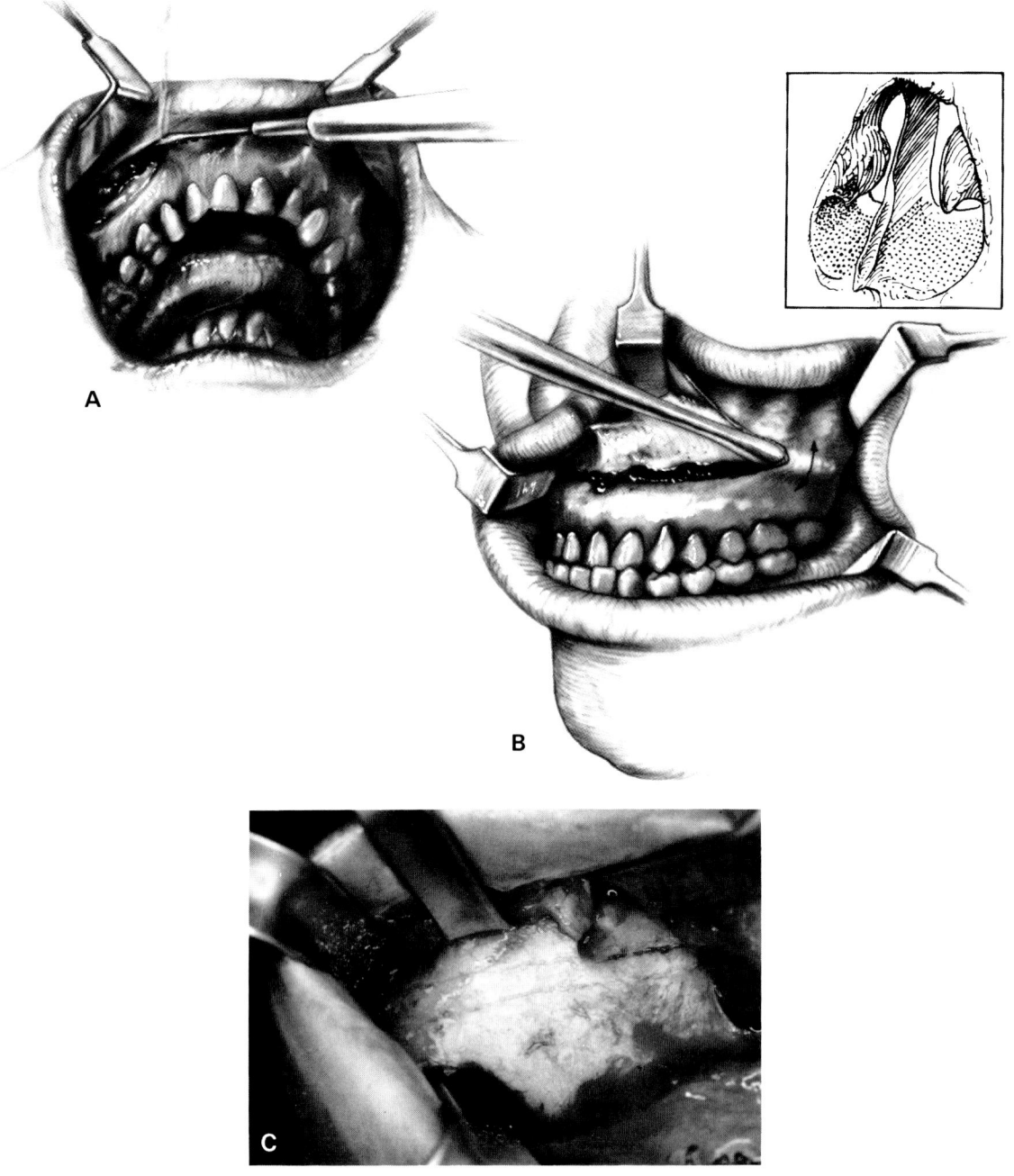

FIGURE 63-20. *A* and *B*, An electrosurgical cutting blade is used to make a horizontal incision in the maxillary vestibule above the mucogingival junction that extends from the second molar region of one side to a similar area on the contralateral side. The margins of the superior flap are raised to expose the lateral walls of the maxilla, the zygomatic crests, the anterior nasal floor, the piriform aperture, and the pterygomaxillary junction. To ensure maximal circulation to the maxillary bone and teeth, the inferior mucoperiosteal tissues are elevated just enough to visualize and palpate the bone encasing the apices of the teeth, the piriform aperture, and the pterygomaxillary junction or to facilitate interdental osteotomies. A right-angle retractor is placed anteriorly to facilitate visualization of the anterolateral portion of the maxilla. A curved Freer elevator is used to detach the mucoperiosteum from the nasal floor, the base of the nasal septum, and the lateral nasal walls superiorly to the base of the inferior turbinate. (Stippling on the inset indicates areas of detached mucoperiosteum.) Since the anteroinferior margin of the piriform rim is usually elevated above the nasal floor, care must be taken to remain in a subperiosteal plane by dissecting inferiorly and posteriorly from the inferior piriform rim. The dissection is carried to the posterior aspect of the hard palate, onto the base of the nasal septum approximately 5 mm above the nasal floor, and then to the base of the inferior turbinate on the lateral nasal wall. The posterolateral portion of the maxilla is visualized by tunneling subperiosteally to the pterygomaxillary suture and then carefully positioning the tip of a curved right-angle retractor at the suture. *C,* The margins of the superior flap are raised to expose the infraorbital nerve and the maxilla immediately lateral and medial to the infraorbital nerve, root of the zygoma, inferior aspect of the zygoma, anterior nasal floor, piriform aperture, and pterygomaxillary junction. (*A* and *B* from Bell WH, Proffit WR, White RP Jr: Surgical Correction of Dentofacial Deformities. Vol II. Philadelphia, WB Saunders Company, 1980, p 1097; with permission.)

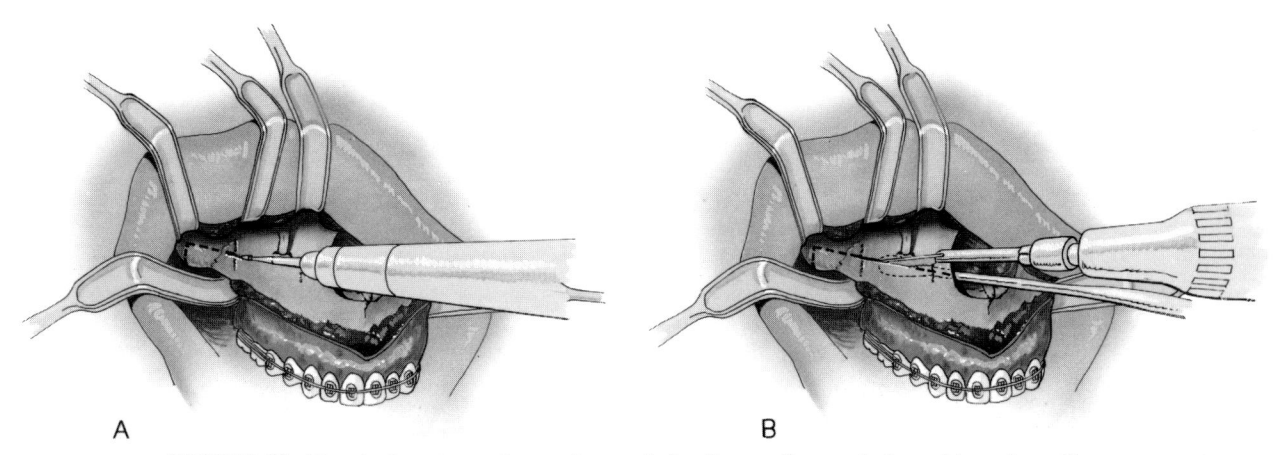

FIGURE 63-21. *A,* Anterior and posterior vertical reference lines and planned lateral maxillary osteotomies are etched into the lateral maxilla at the desired level with a No. 701 fissure bur. *B,* The major portion of the lateral maxilla is sectioned from the contralateral side with a reciprocating saw blade. (Modified from Bell WH, Mannai C, Luhr HG: Art and science of the Le Fort I downfracture. Int J Adult Orthodont Orthognath Surg 3(1):23-52, 1988; with permission.)

omy is designed so that the largest possible bony interface can be created while the bone cut is positioned at a safe distance above the tooth apices in the thicker part of the maxilla. The lateral maxillary osteotomy courses from the piriform aperture at the level of the anterior attachment of the inferior turbinate, extending immediately inferior to the infraorbital foramen and then into the denser bone of the root of the zygoma 5 mm or more above the inferior aspect of the zygoma (Fig. 63-22). The osteotomy design must also be consistent with the esthetic objectives of the planned surgery.

When osteotomies or ostectomies are made in the thick body and root of the zygomas, the margins of the proximal and distal segments are consistently juxtaposed after surgery. The posterior portion of the maxilla is sectioned with a fissure bur to determine sequentially the relative thickness of the zygomaticomaxillary buttress and to provide a stable index and referent for subsequent sectioning of the lateral maxilla and placement of screw and plate osteosynthesis. The degree of penetration of the root of the zygoma and posterior extension of the lateral maxillary osteotomy will vary according to the degree of pneumatization of the antrum and the position of the posterior wall of the antrum. When trial sectioning of the maxilla and zygomaticomaxillary buttress reveals relatively thick bone, the maxillary step osteotomy may be used and is technically easier if the objective is not to

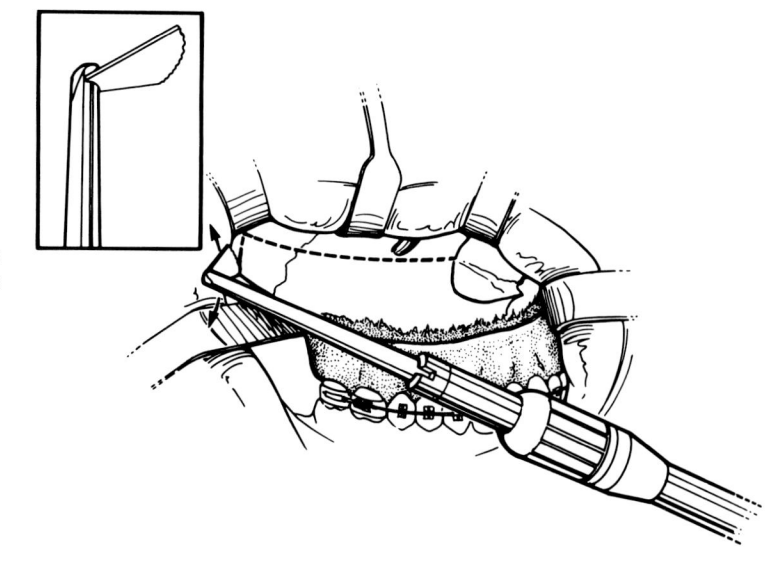

FIGURE 63-22. Vertical through-and-through osteotomy is made with an oscillating saw blade to the inferior and deep aspect of the zygoma.

advance a portion of the malar bone. If the posterior portion of the lateral maxilla and the zygomaticomaxillary buttress are very thin, great care and meticulous technique are exercised to avoid fracturing the root of the zygoma. Even if this should occur, as it has in two patients, the fractured free segment can be repositioned as planned and stabilized to the distal segment with an interosseous wire, circumzygomatic wire, or small bone plate.

The surgeon must be ever flexible and prepared to selectively modify the osteotomy design on the basis of the anatomic and clinical findings at the time of surgery. This is particularly so in those cases in which the anterior maxillary bony walls are exceedingly thin. In such cases, it may not be possible to stabilize the maxilla with bone plates and screws. In addition, there is a greater chance of fracturing the malar complex if high Le Fort I osteotomies are made. The surgeon may elect in such cases to alter the design of the surgical procedure and make the lateral maxillary osteotomies at a lower level. On the other hand, when the anterior maxillary walls are 2 mm thick, or more, the osteotomy design may be individualized, with relatively good assurance that interfacing of the osteotomy sites will be accomplished and stabilization of the repositioned maxilla with bone plates or screws will be feasible. Similar principles also apply in cases of redo surgery in which anatomic relationships may have been altered by a previous surgical procedure. In many of these cases, it will be necessary to repeat the osteotomy at the same level that the Le Fort I osteotomy was initially made, because the previous bone cuts may be incompletely healed and bony dehiscences may be present.

SECTIONING THE MAXILLA

The major portion of the lateral maxilla is sectioned from the contralateral side with a reciprocating saw blade; the osteotomy is then extended anteriorly to the lateral piriform rim. With a periosteal elevator or small malleable retractor passed subperiosteally medial to the lateral nasal wall to protect the nasal mucoperiosteum, the anterior aspect of the lateral nasal wall at the level of the inferior turbinate is sectioned with the reciprocating saw blade (see Fig. 63–21B).

The horizontal osteotomy is extended posteriorly into the dense root of the zygoma and zygomatic arch to the point 6 to 8 mm above the inferior aspect of the zygomatic arch and 6 to 10 mm distal to the zygomaticomaxillary suture line. Then a vertical through-and-through osteotomy is made with an oscillating saw blade to the inferior and deep aspect of the zygoma (Fig. 63–22). With the contents of the infratemporal fossa reflected, the osteotomy is directed inferiorly and medially at a 45-degree angle to the pterygomaxillary junction (Fig. 63–23). Because the bone in this area is generally relatively thin, the osteotomy can usually be made with a finely tapered, curved osteotome. When the bone is thick, however, the posterior vertical osteotomies are made with an oscillating or reciprocating saw blade. Finally, the maxilla is separated from the pterygoid process by malleting an osteotome directed medially and anteriorly into the pterygomaxillary suture (Fig. 63–23).

The midportion of the medial antral wall is sequentially sectioned with a fissure bur and finely tapered osteotome positioned between the margins of the lateral maxillary ostectomy. Sectioning of the medial antral wall is terminated at least 1 cm short of the perpendicular plate of the palatine bone to avoid transecting the descending palatine vessels (Fig. 63–24). The thin antral wall contiguous to the vessels generally fractures when the maxilla is downfractured.

A nasal septal osteotome positioned parallel to the hard palate is malleted toward a finger positioned on the posterior nasal spine to separate the base of the posterior bony nasal septum from the maxilla. Gradually increasing inferior pressure on the anterior aspect of the maxilla facilitates visualization of the nasal surface of the

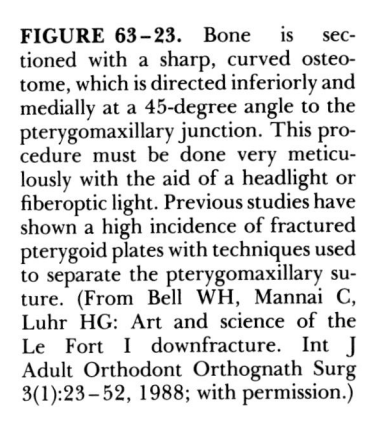

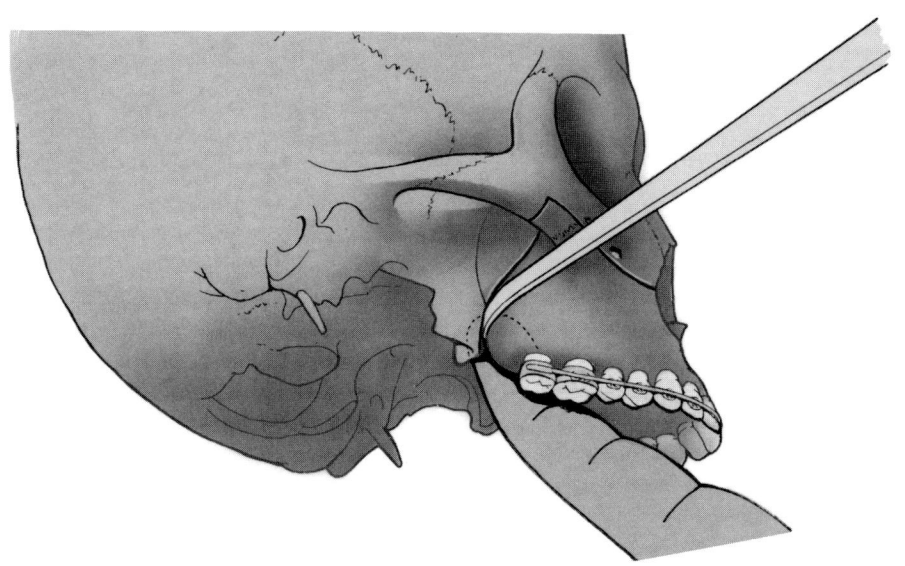

FIGURE 63-23. Bone is sectioned with a sharp, curved osteotome, which is directed inferiorly and medially at a 45-degree angle to the pterygomaxillary junction. This procedure must be done very meticulously with the aid of a headlight or fiberoptic light. Previous studies have shown a high incidence of fractured pterygoid plates with techniques used to separate the pterygomaxillary suture. (From Bell WH, Mannai C, Luhr HG: Art and science of the Le Fort I downfracture. Int J Adult Orthodont Orthognath Surg 3(1):23–52, 1988; with permission.)

maxilla and lateral nasal walls. While the midface structures are stabilized by the assistant, the surgeon uses both hands to hinge the maxilla inferiorly and posteriorly. The assistant simultaneously detaches the remaining mucoperiosteum from the nasal floor and the horizontal plate of the palatine bone to facilitate downfracturing (Fig. 63–25).

The posterior part of the maxilla is separated from its remaining bony attachments by forward pressure of a periosteal elevator or similar instrument against the thick and strong posterior aspect of the horizontal plate of the palatine bone to achieve mobility and movement of the maxilla to the contralateral side (Fig. 63–26). A similar procedure is accomplished on the opposite side.

With the maxilla in the downfractured position, bone interferences in any area can be readily identified and removed under direct visualization. Reduction of the height of the lateral nasal walls is accomplished with rongeurs. Meticulous and sequential reduction of the posterior aspect of the lateral nasal wall and the alveolopalatal junction in the area opposite the second and third molars is accomplished

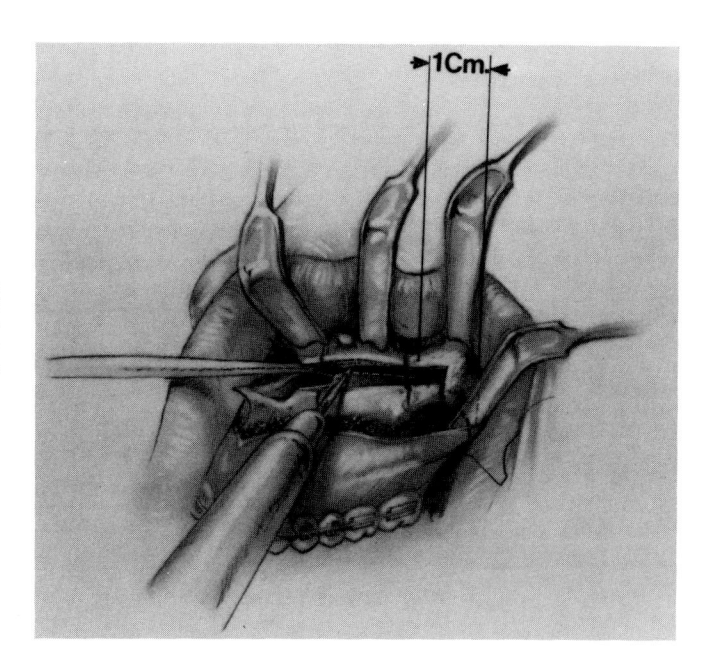

FIGURE 63-24. The midportion of the medial antral wall is sectioned with a finely tapered bur. Sectioning of the medial antral wall is terminated at least 1 cm short of the perpendicular plate of the palatine bone to avoid transecting the descending palatine vessels.

2244 / VII — ORTHOGNATHIC SURGERY

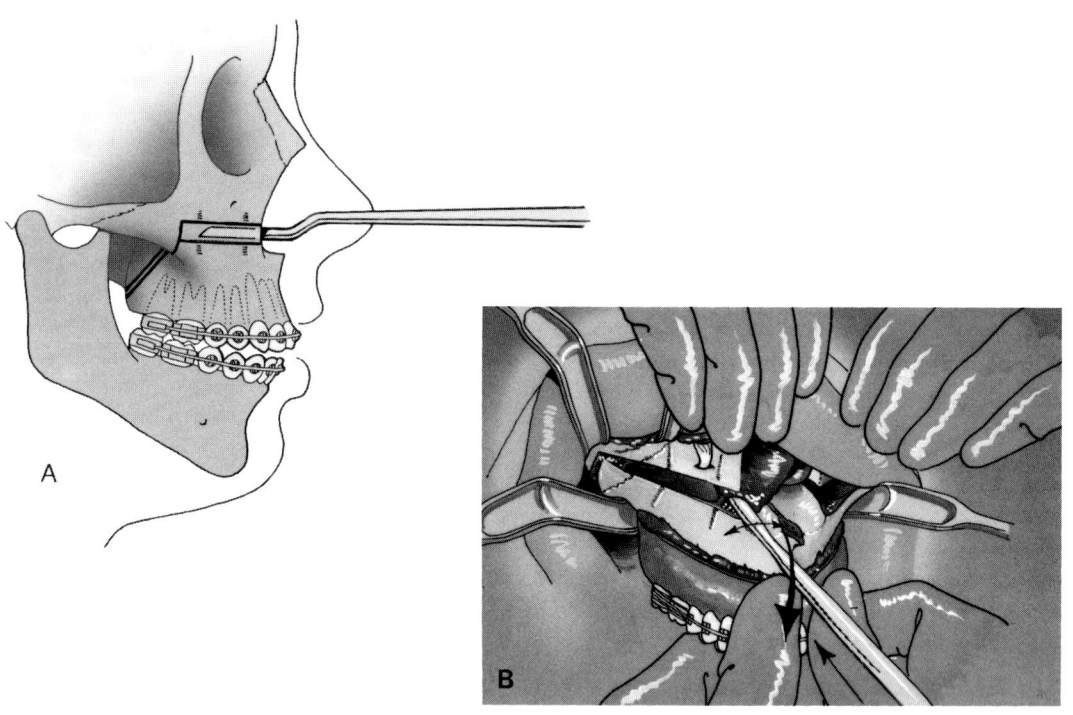

FIGURE 63-25. *A,* Separation of the nasal septum from the maxilla with the osteotome placed parallel to the hard palate. *B,* The maxilla is downfractured; the nasal mucoperiosteum has been detached and retracted away from the nasal surface of the maxilla and the horizontal plate of the palatine bone.

with rongeurs and burs. Finally, osteotomes, burs, and/or Kerrison forceps may be used to expose the descending palatine vessels carefully (Fig. 63-27). After the overlying bone has been excised, an effort is made to preserve the integrity of these vessels whenever feasible. When the planned posterior and superior movements are problematic, the vessels can be sharply transected or cauterized after vascular clips have been placed. With large retractors positioned, the posterior maxillary tuberosity can be removed to facilitate posterior maxillary repositioning (Fig. 63-28*A* and *B*).

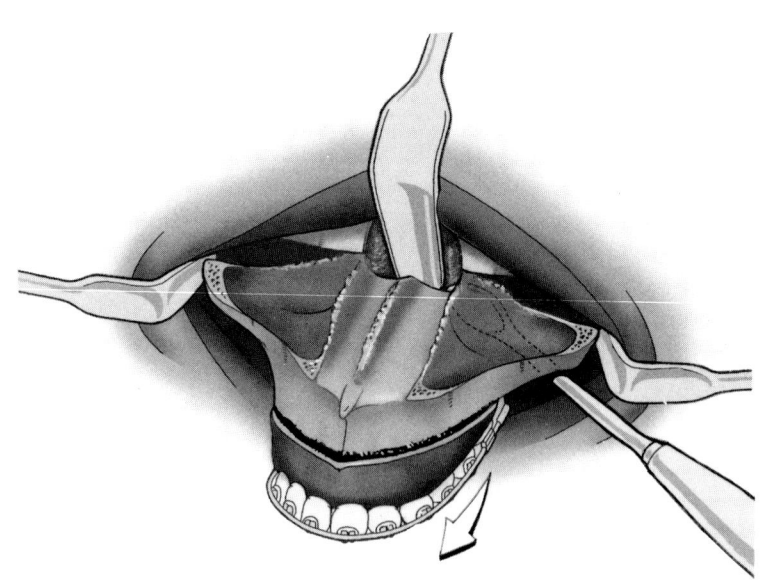

FIGURE 63-26. The mobilized maxilla has been hinged inferiorly on an axis that passes through the condylar heads. The mucoperiosteum has been detached and separated from the nasal surface of the maxilla and the horizontal plate of the palatine bone to facilitate downfracturing. The posterior part of the maxilla is separated from its remaining bony attachments by forward pressure of a periosteal elevator or similar instrument exerted against the thick posterior aspect of the horizontal plate of the palatine bone to achieve mobility. (From Bell WH, Mannai C, Luhr HG: Art and science of the Le Fort I downfracture. Int J Adult Orthodont Orthognath Surg 3(1):23-52, 1988; with permission.)

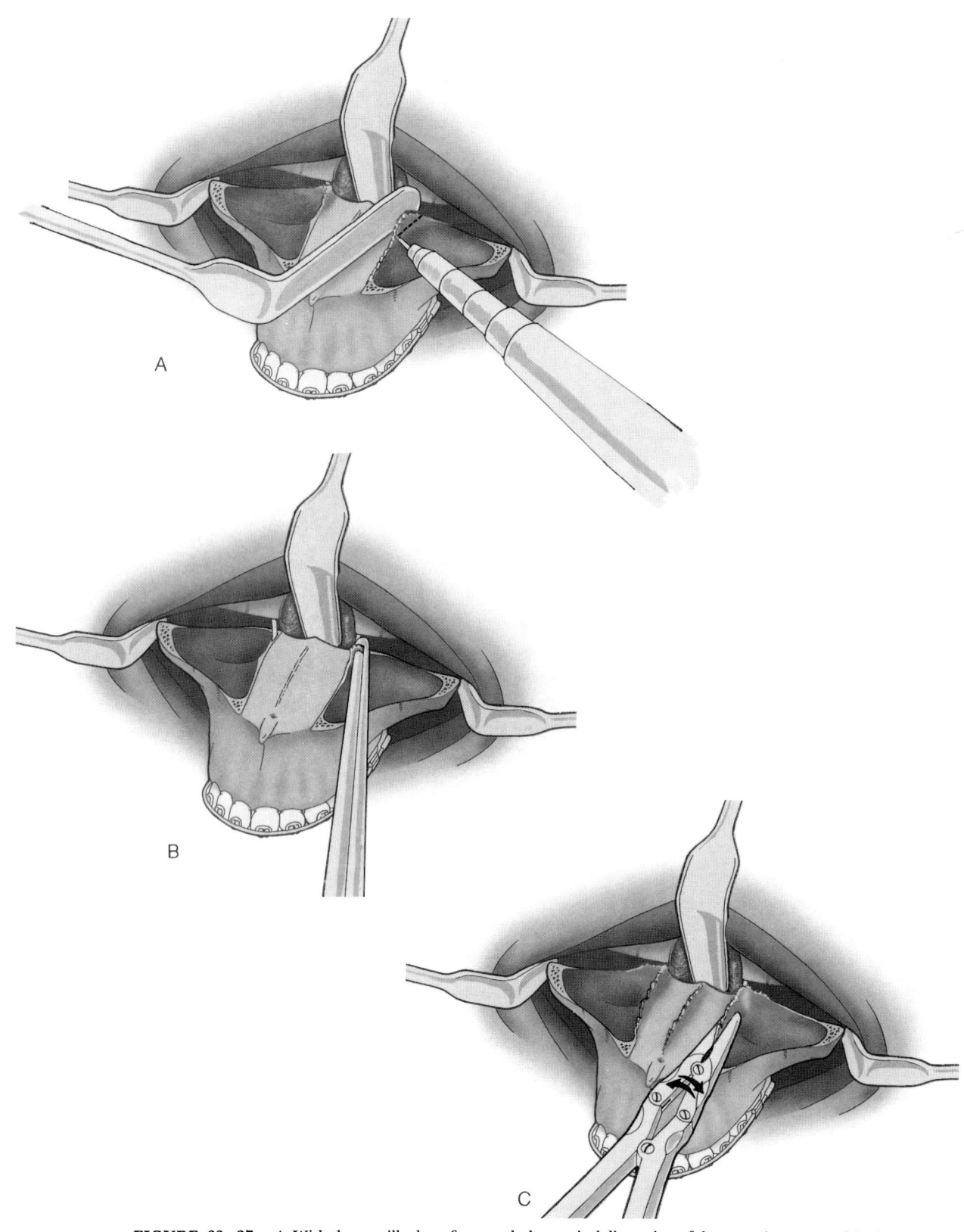

FIGURE 63-27. *A*, With the maxilla downfractured, the vertical dimension of the posterior aspect of the lateral nasal wall and alveolopalatal junction in the area opposite the second and third molars is carefully reduced with a No. 701 fissure bur to expose the descending palatine vessels. Retractors are positioned to protect the contiguous soft tissues and enhance accessibility and visualization; the typical vertical bony prominence of these structures lies lateral to the descending palatine vessels. *B*, Exposure of the descending palatine vessels with Kerrison forceps. *C*, Reduction of the lateral nasal wall and the alveolopalatal junction with rongeurs. (*A* from Bell WH, Mannai C, Luhr HG: Art and science of the Le Fort I downfracture. Int J Adult Orthodont Orthognath Surg 3(1):23–52, 1988; with permission.)

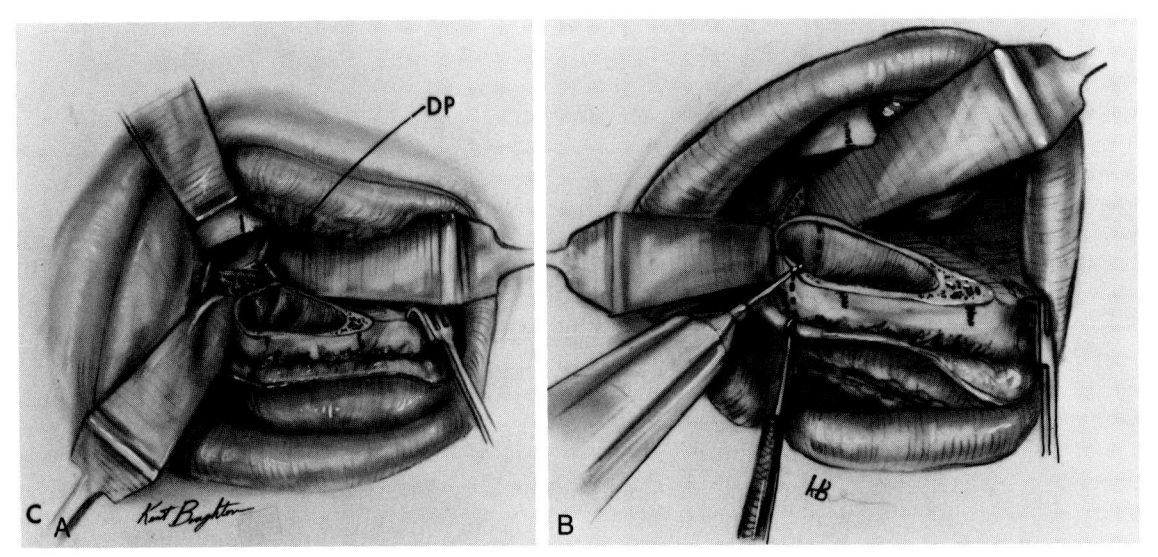

FIGURE 63-28. *A,* The descending palatine (DP) vessels are exposed; curved-out retractors are in place. *B,* With the large, curved-out retractors positioned, the posterior maxillary tuberosity is removed to facilitate posterior repositioning of the maxilla. *C,* Submucosal resection of the cartilaginous nasal septum. (*B* from Bell WH, Mannai C, Luhr HG: Art and science of the Le Fort I downfracture. Int J Adult Orthodont Orthognath Surg 3(1):23–52, 1988; with permission. *C* from Bell WH, Proffit WR, White RP Jr: Surgical Correction of Dentofacial Deformities. Vol II. Philadelphia, WB Saunders Company, 1980, p 1105; with permission.)

The height of the vomer is reduced an amount proportional to the planned superior movement of the maxilla. A midsagittal groove is made in the superior aspect of the maxilla to accommodate the nasal septum and to prevent its lateral displacement. Submucosal resection of the cartilaginous nasal septum (Fig. 63–28C) is accomplished to facilitate superior movement of the repositioned maxilla and to prevent buckling of the septum. The mucoperichondrium enveloping the inferior aspect of the cartilaginous septum is incised and detached bilaterally from the inferolateral aspect of the septum. The height of the cartilage is reduced an amount proportional to the superior movement of the maxilla. The maxilla can now be rotated upward into the planned relationship without buckling the septum. The mucosal margins are then closed with catgut sutures.

After the maxilla is completely mobilized, the interocclusal splint is precisely ligated to the maxilla. The mandibular teeth are indexed into the splint, and maxillomandibular fixation is accomplished with wire ligatures between the vertical lugs attached to the arch wire. The maxillomandibular complex is moved as a unit through the mandibular arc of rotation so that the areas of bone contact can be visualized as the maxilla is positioned upward and forward. Bone is removed from the posterior margins until the mobilized segment can be passively seated in the desired vertical position and the margins of the lateral maxillary osteotomies are juxtaposed. With the condyles held upward and forward against the posterior slopes of the articular eminences, the maxillomandibular complex is repeatedly rotated closed to the desired vertical position (Fig. 63–29). Finally, the maxilla is stabilized in the planned position by appropriate bone plate osteosynthesis (Fig. 63–30A and B).

THE DOWNSLIDING TECHNIQUE

The Le Fort I downsliding technique is a variation of the high Le Fort I osteotomy (Fig. 63–31).[20,82] Patients with a combination of vertical and anteroposterior deficiency may be candidates for this osteotomy design.

Septal cartilage
Vomer
Septal ostectomy

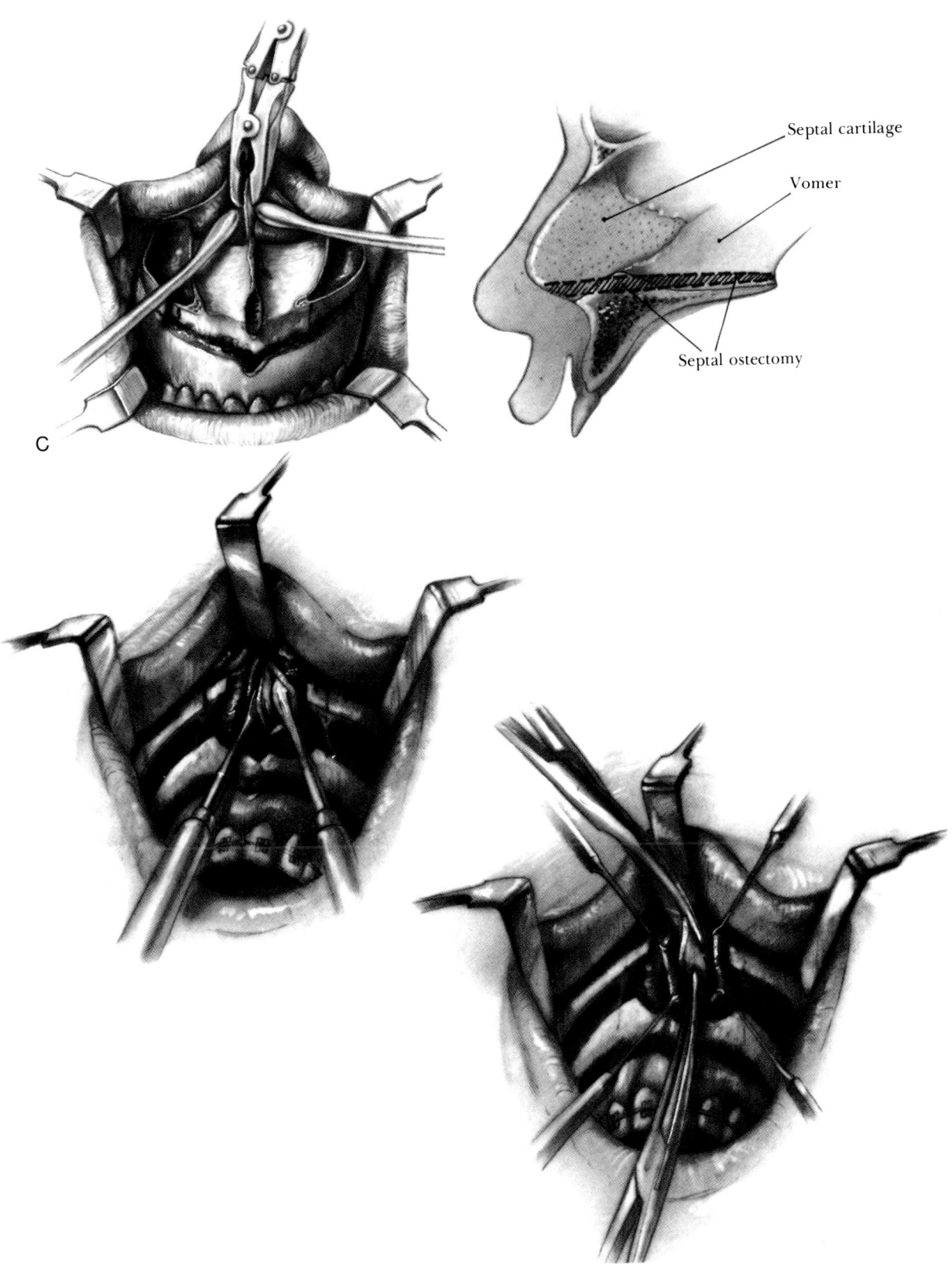

FIGURE 63–28 *Continued*

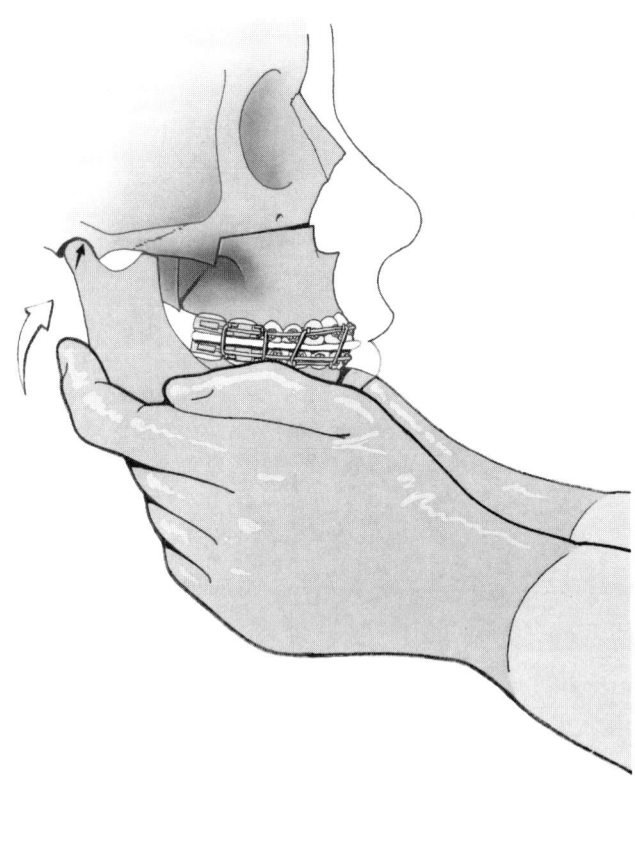

FIGURE 63–29. After the interocclusal splint is precisely ligated to the maxilla, the mandibular teeth are indexed into the splint; maxillomandibular fixation is accomplished with wire ligatures between vertical lugs attached to the arch wire. With the condyles held upward and forward against the posterior slopes of the articular eminences *(curved arrows)*, the maxillomandibular complex is rotated closed to the desired vertical position. The maxilla is stabilized with small bone plates and screws. (From Bell WH, Mannai C, Luhr HG: Art and science of the Le Fort I downfracture. Int J Adult Orthodont Orthognath Surg 3(1):23–52, 1988; with permission.)

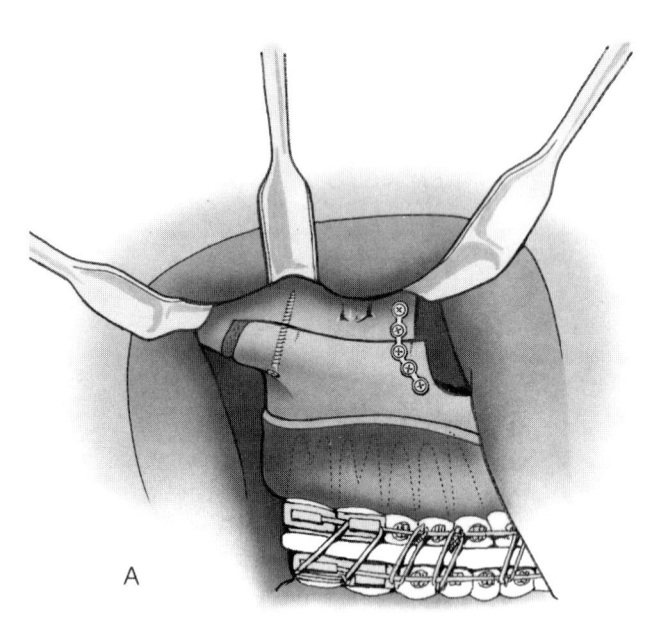

FIGURE 63–30. *A*, Anteriorly repositioned maxilla stabilized with 20-mm-long 2-mm-diameter positional screw in the pillar of the zygoma. A curved mini plate is used to stabilize the anterior part of the maxilla. *B*, Curved mini plates are used to stabilize the anterior and posterior parts of the repositioned maxilla. When the maxilla is anteriorly and *superiorly* repositioned, planned telescoping frequently facilitates stabilization of the distal segment by 2-mm-long positional screws placed obliquely through the root of the zygoma into the dense pillar of the zygoma.

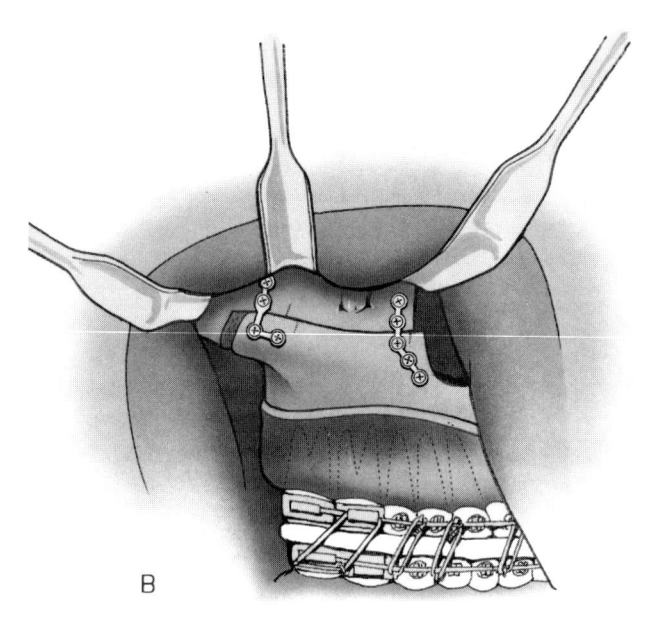

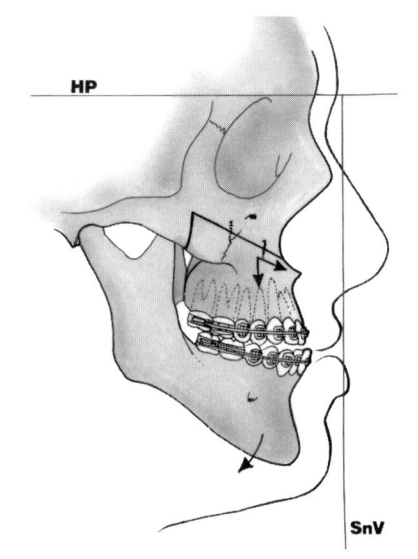

FIGURE 63-31. DOWNSLIDING TECHNIQUE. The osteotomy is angulated to provide an inclined plane that will increase the vertical dimension as the maxilla slides forward *(arrows)*.

When anteroposterior maxillary deficiency is associated with vertical maxillary deficiency, the surgical plan should include maxillary advancement in addition to correction of the vertical discrepancy. In selected cases, both corrections may be achieved by downward and forward sliding movement of the maxilla (Fig. 63–31).[82] The lateral maxillary osteotomy designs are individualized. The osteotomy is angulated to provide an inclined plane that will increase the vertical dimension as the maxilla slides forward. The horizontal length from the piriform rim to the lateral aspect of the zygoma is measured on a lateral cephalogram. From this measurement the downward angulation of the osteotomy and the position of the vertical step are calculated.

Anteriorly, an angulated cut extends from high on the lateral aspect of the zygoma to low on the anterior piriform rim. Posteriorly, the osteotomy is directed inferiorly and medially at a 45-degree angle to the pterygoid plate. As the maxilla is advanced, bony defects are created at the vertical steps. In selected cases of minimal vertical maxillary deficiency, the lip-to-tooth relationship and anteroposterior deficiency can be corrected solely by the Le Fort I downsliding technique. When vertical maxillary deficiency is more severe, the Le Fort I osteotomy is combined with interpositional bone grafting (Fig. 63–32).

FIGURE 63-32. Le Fort I osteotomy and interpositional bone grafting for correction of vertical maxillary deficiency.

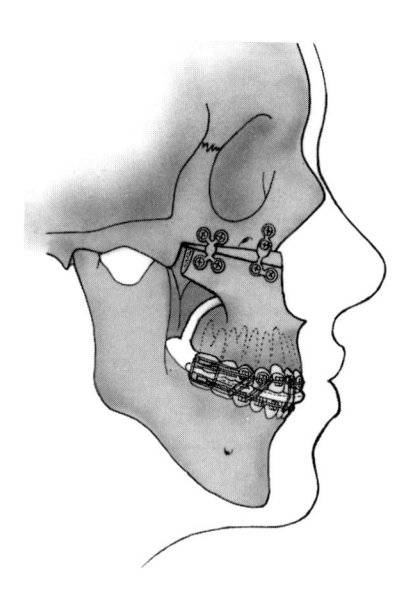

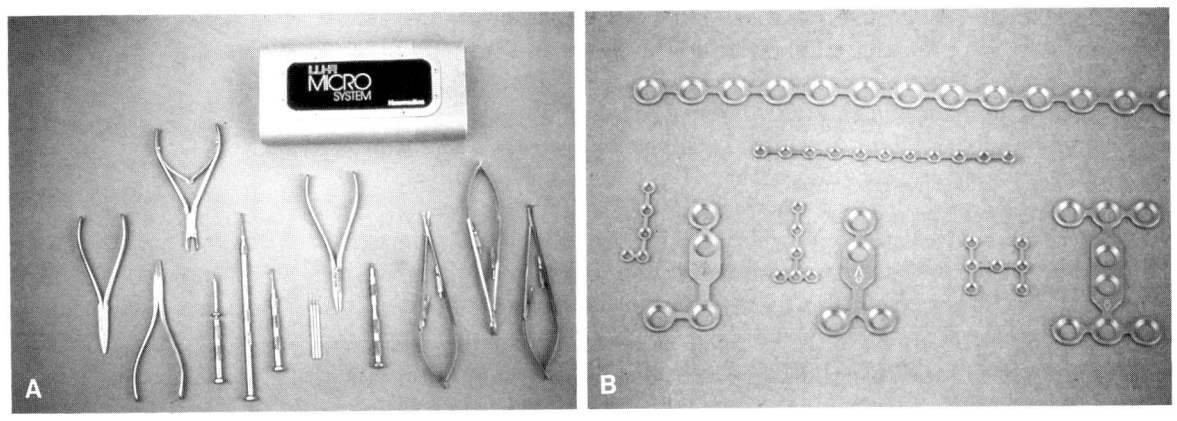

FIGURE 63-36. *A,* Luhr micro system instrumentation. *B,* Comparison between mini and micro system sizes.

The tiny plates and screws designated as "micro" were designed by Hans Luhr for use in special situations. These situations include infant craniofacial surgery, especially when severely comminuted fractures are present, comminuted frontal sinus wall fractures, and other fractures of thin or delicate areas of the facial skeleton like the periorbital area. Luhr did recognize that "Continued clinical experience will probably reveal further indications in maxillofacial, as well as neuro or hand surgery."[88]

The micro system consists of the cobalt-chromium-molybdenum alloy Vitallium, which has been used in skeletal surgery for the past 40 years because of its resistance to corrosion and its superior physical strength. The diameter of screws is 0.8 mm, and the thickness of plates is only 0.5 mm. The number of different types of micro plates has been deliberately kept low (Fig. 63-36A and B). Owing to the special design of the connection bar between the plate holes, each plate can be contoured in all three dimensions (Fig. 63-37A to D). Thereby they can be

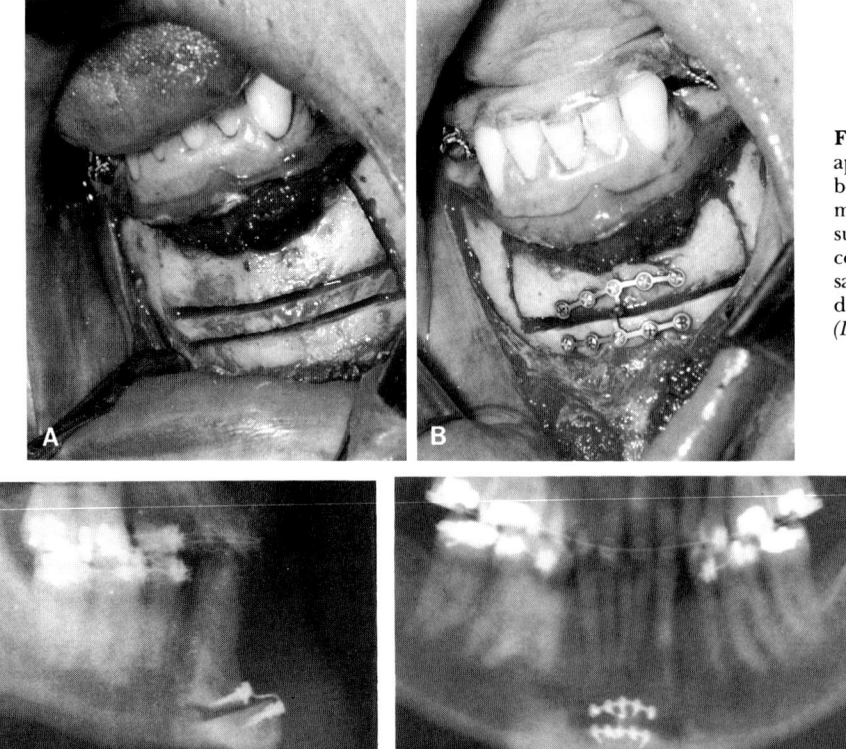

FIGURE 63-37. *A,* Mandibular subapical osteotomy secured at the inferior border with a well-contoured H-pattern micro plate and screw system *(B).* The superior portion of the dentoalveolar complex is controlled by a lingual-occlusal mandibular splint. Cephalometric radiograph *(C)* and panoramic radiograph *(D)* of segment control.

adapted to virtually every complex bone structure. The question concerning the holding power of the self-tapping micro screws has been answered by satisfactory results from torque load tests. Clinical experience has confirmed the excellent holding power of these self-tapping micro screws, which are available in lengths of 2, 3, 4, 5, 6, 8, 10, and 12 mm. The bone is predrilled by a 0.5-mm surgical drill. The use of magnifying spectacles is recommended to achieve the exact placement of micro plates and screws. Three-dimensional stabilization can be achieved with plates as opposed to wires, which act in two dimensions, i.e., against tension forces only. These requirements are fulfilled by a plate and screw system of micro dimension.

The following are indications for the application of the micro system:

1. Superior repositioning of the maxilla at the Le Fort I or "high Le Fort I" level that is not associated with large maxillary sagittal movements, i.e., maxillary advancements or setbacks greater than 2 to 3 mm (Fig. 63–38A to F).
2. Stabilization of small onlay bone grafts.
3. Contiguous osteotomies, such as combined mandibular anterior subapical osteotomy with simultaneous genioplasty (sliding osteotomy of the inferior border of the mandible).
4. Selected segmental osteotomies when no signficant expansion is required (greater than 3 mm).

The following situations are contraindications to the application of the micro system:

1. Bone thickness less than 2 mm.
2. Large sagittal advancements or setbacks of the maxilla.
3. Significant maxillary expansion — contraindicated because palatal mucosal and muscular tension may induce thin plate distortion and bone relapse.
4. Inexperience with the system.

Advantages of this system include extreme ease in plate contouring without templates, excellent pull-out strength of screws, and excellent adaptation of plates to bone contour.

As in the application of any new technique or system, a learning curve exists. Practice with fracture size and mini systems is recommended until the surgeon feels comfortable. Laboratory work with dry facial skeleton or animal laboratory practice or both are strongly suggested.

Our use in 25 selected osteotomies over the past 2 years has been very positive. No immediate, short-term, or long-term complications have occurred in any patients treated to date. It is likely that even further indications in orthognathic, trauma, and reconstructive bone graft surgery will emerge.

More recently, an additional plating system has become available — the pan fixation system (Howmedica) (Fig. 63–39A to C). The plates and screws and instruments are all miniaturized versions of the mini system, but larger than the micro system. The system employs biocompatible Vitallium 1- to 3-mm screws and plates that are 0.5 mm in diameter. The system provides remarkable strength in selected patients. In addition, the plates are easy to contour and readily adapt to even complex bony configurations.

ANATOMIC CONSIDERATIONS

Nasolacrimal Anatomy

Injury to the lacrimal apparatus has been reported following facial trauma, craniofacial surgery, rhinoplasty, nasal antrostomy, and maxillectomy.[28,40,63,76]

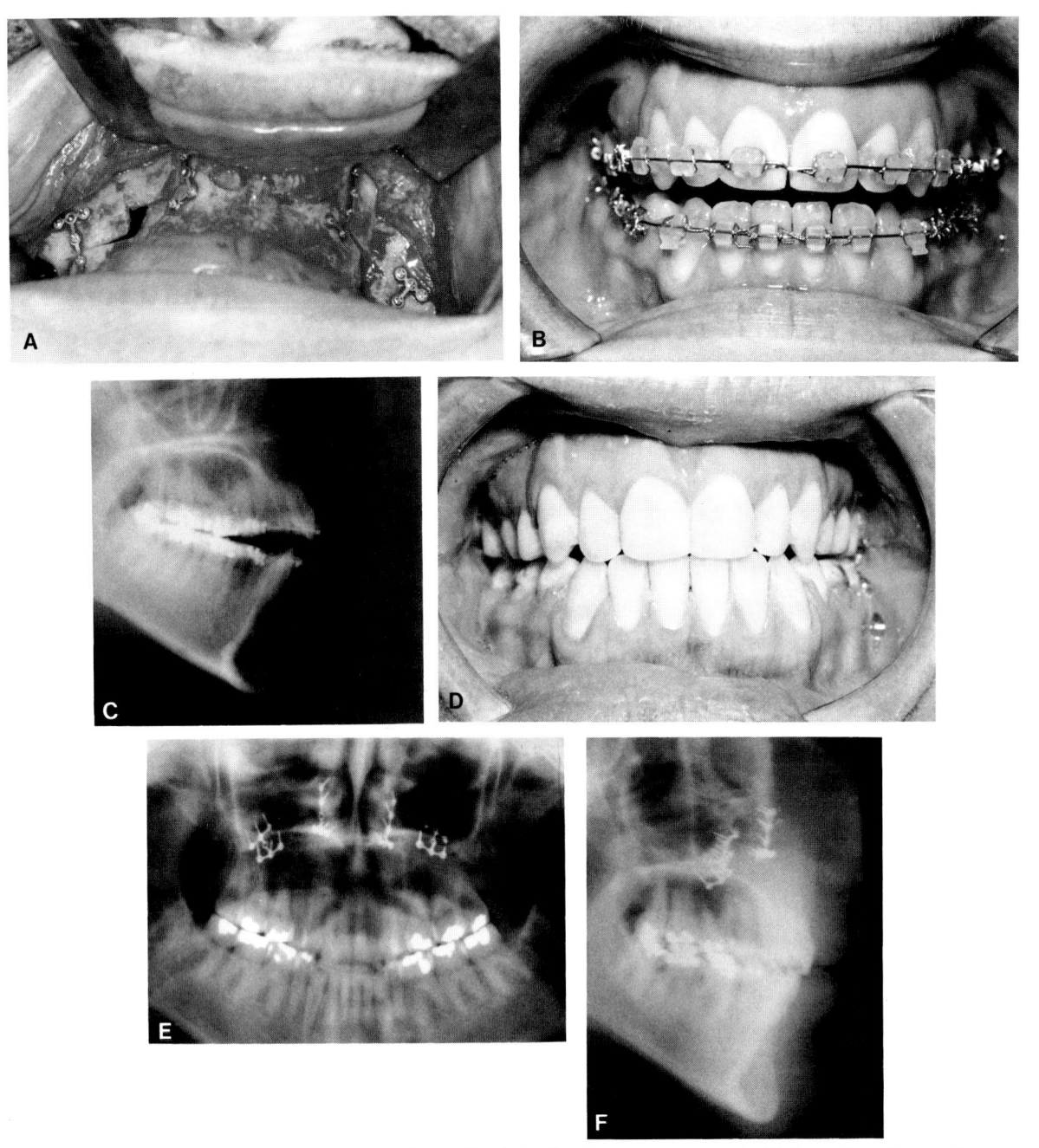

FIGURE 63-38. *A*, Superior repositioning of the maxilla via Le Fort I osteotomy secured with four micro plates and screws. Preoperative occlusion *(B)* and radiograph *(C)*. Postoperative occlusion *(D)* and radiographs *(E* and *F)* at 7 months.

Transient or permanent epiphora secondary to nasolacrimal apparatus injury has been documented occasionally with high Le Fort I osteotomy.[42,58] Although the nasolacrimal system has been the subject of extensive clinical and anatomic studies with respect to ophthalmology and otolaryngology,[31,64] it remains uncertain whether high-level Le Fort I osteotomies jeopardize the integrity of this system. The lacrimal drainage system consists of canaliculi, lacrimal sac, and nasolacrimal duct (Fig. 63-40A and B). The nasolacrimal duct commences from the lacrimal sac, passes within the bony nasolacrimal canal, and empties into the inferior meatus of the nose under the inferior turbinate bone. The canal and meatal portions of the nasolacrimal duct are the two parts of the lacrimal apparatus that are most likely to be damaged by high-level Le Fort I osteotomy.

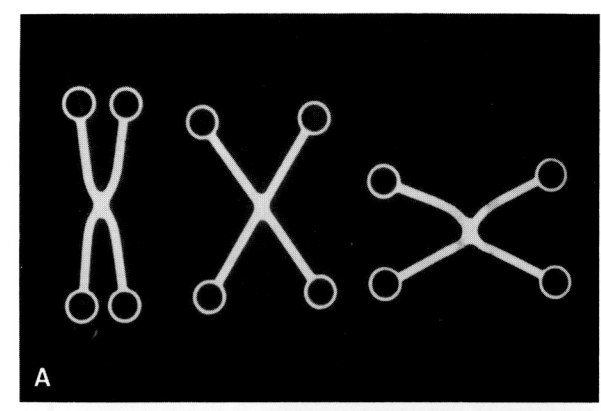

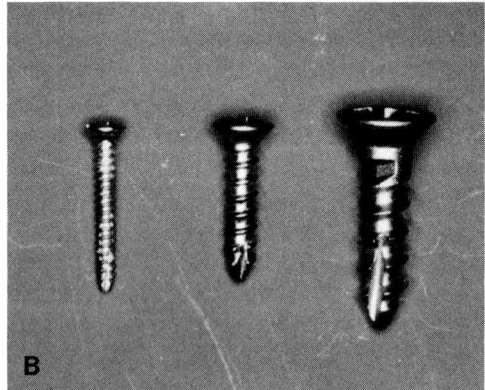

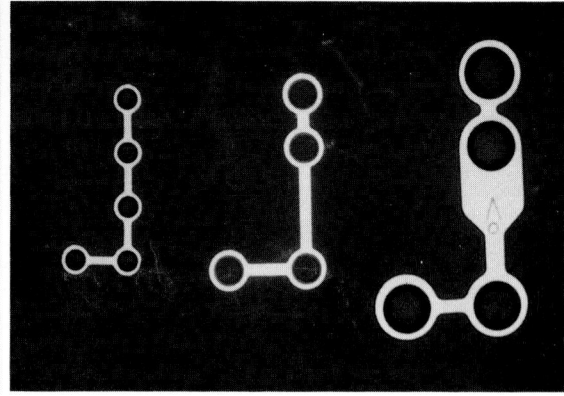

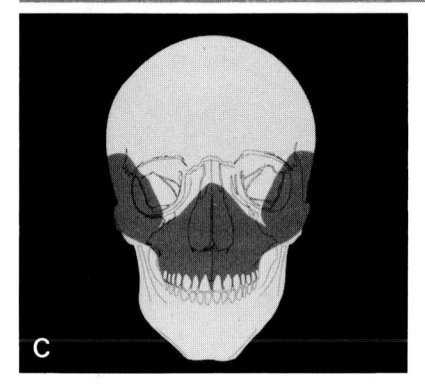

FIGURE 63-39. *A*, Luhr pan fixation instrumentation. *B*, *left* and *right*, Comparison between mini, pan fixation, and micro system sizes. *C*, Anatomic sites where the pan fixation system may be used selectively. The stronger weight-bearing pillars of the facial skeleton are usually stabilized by stronger mini fixation plates. They are particularly useful in the paranasal and infraorbital areas, where the skin may be relatively thin.

The positional relationship between the nasolacrimal canal and high-level Le Fort I osteotomy was studied by You and associates.[105] One hundred intact Indian dry skulls were used in this study (Figs. 63–41 and 63–42). The simulated high Le Fort I osteotomy in all of the 100 skulls was made under the inferior orifice of the nasolacrimal canal, with a mean distance of 5.2 mm and ranging from 0.5 mm to 11.5 mm. The results indicated that the osteotomy, when made just beneath the infraorbital foramen and extending to the piriform rim at the level of the anterior attachment of the inferior turbinate, will usually not jeopardize the nasolacrimal duct within its bony canal (Fig. 63–43).

Once the nasolacrimal duct exits the bony canal, there is a 2- to 5-mm extension into the inferior nasal meatus, termed the meatal portion. Traditional low-level Le Fort I osteotomy is usually accomplished beneath the ostium of the nasolacrimal meatal portion. Demas[32] and Little[65] reported that the distance from the nasal floor to the opening of the nasolacrimal meatal portion ranges from 11 to 17 mm. They considered that this distance was safe for most cases in which the maxilla was to be superiorly repositioned by the traditional Le Fort I osteotomy. In a dissection of 200 nasolacrimal ducts, Schaefer[87] found that the meatal portion of the nasolacrimal duct may empty beneath the inferior turbinate or extend to the nasal floor.

associates,[105] the inferior orifice of the nasolacrimal canal was positioned in an area that extended 2 mm medially and 3.5 mm laterally along a line connecting the lacrimal fossa and the anterior attachment of the inferior turbinate. The line extending from the lacrimal fossa to the anterior attachment of the inferior turbinate on the anterior aspect of the maxilla is a good approximation of the course of the nasolacrimal canal (see Fig. 63–41).

In a review of 54 cases of quadrangular Le Fort I osteotomies, Keller and Sather[58] reported that lateral epiphora for 1 year was noted in one patient. Freihofer and Brouns[42] reported that 4 per cent of their patients sustained lacrimal system disturbance after varied midfacial osteotomies. The incidence of nasolacrimal abnormalities in congenital craniofacial deformities has been reported to be as high as 30 to 40 per cent. Consequently, the incidence of nasolacrimal injuries in such patients may indeed be higher than in patients with dentofacial deformity. To date, no such problems have been observed in our series of patients who have had high-level Le Fort I osteotomies for the correction of dentofacial deformities. If clinicians understand the regional anatomy well, position the osteotomies of the lateral nasal wall precisely, and protect the meatal portion of the nasolacrimal duct carefully, the incidence of permanent injury to nasolacrimal structures will, in all likelihood, be very low.

SEGMENTATION OF THE MAXILLA

At present, about 80 per cent of all patients undergoing orthognathic surgery are treated by the Le Fort I downfracture and various mandibular surgical procedures. Maxillary repositioning is accomplished in approximately 80 per cent of patients treated, by sectioning the maxilla into two, three, and four segments.[22] Many technical modifications of this versatile technique are feasible to facilitate simultaneous anteroposterior, vertical, or horizontal movements of the maxilla. Space closure, arch alignment, leveling, and increased arch length can be accomplished by vertical interdental osteotomies. The design of the osseous and soft tissue incisions is individualized to maintain the largest possible dento-osseous segment and preserve the maximal viable soft tissue pedicle.

THREE- AND FOUR-SEGMENT LE FORT I OSTEOTOMY

Interdental osteotomies are most frequently made in the canine–lateral incisor interspaces, with relatively little risk to the contiguous teeth (Fig. 63–44). The

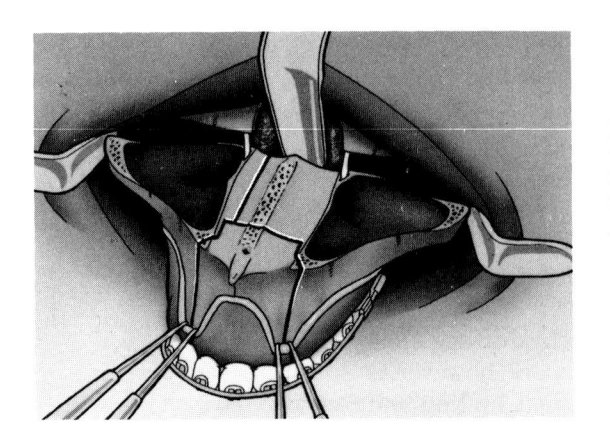

FIGURE 63–44. SECTIONING THE MAXILLA INTO THREE SEGMENTS BY LE FORT I OSTEOTOMY. In the canine–lateral incisor region, there is usually a wider and thicker zone of keratinized gingiva than is normally found in the canine-premolar region, where there is frequently a high frenum attachment and a narrower and thinner band of keratinized gingiva. Consequently, healing of a vertical incision made in this area is usually uncomplicated, and dehiscence of the wound margins is rare. Vertical interdental osteotomies in the lateral incisor–canine interspaces are connected by a U-shaped transpalatal osteotomy distal to the incisive canal; the posterior aspect of the maxilla is sectioned parasagittally.

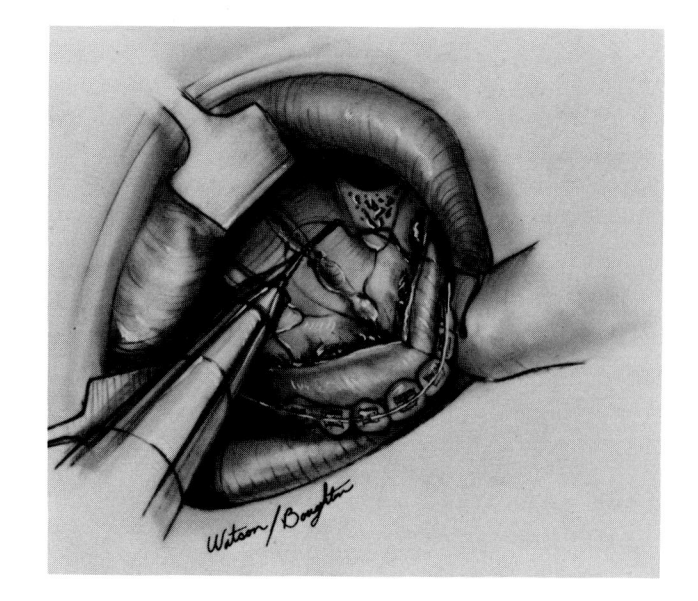

FIGURE 63-45. With the surgeon's finger positioned on the palatal mucosa, a U-shaped transpalatal osteotomy distal to the incisive canal is made to connect the vertical interdental osteotomies in the lateral incisor–canine interspaces. (From Bell WH, Mannai C, Luhr HG: Art and science of the Le Fort I downfracture. Int J Adult Orthodont Orthognath Surg 3(1):23–52, 1988; with permission.)

planned changes must be carefully simulated by correlated model surgery and cephalometric planning studies. Segmentation of the anterior maxilla to improve the axial inclination of the anterior teeth and increase arch length without ostectomy or extractions is the treatment of choice in selected cases (Fig. 63–44). When interdental osteotomies produce large spaces between the teeth, bone grafts or bone substitutes may be placed between the margins of the sectioned bone to stabilize and consolidate the segments and prevent periodontal problems. Hydroxyapatite is not used when teeth are to be orthodontically repositioned into an alveolar graft site after surgery. In such cases, autogenous particulate marrow is routinely used.

Vertical interdental osteotomies in the lateral incisor–canine interspaces are connected by a U-shaped transpalatal osteotomy distal to the incisive canal (Fig. 63–45). This modified osteotomy design provides a broader soft tissue pedicle to the anterior dento-osseous segment. The maxilla can be sectioned parasagittally to increase or decrease the intermolar width and improve interdigitation of the teeth. The mucoperiosteum is elevated to expose the interdental bone at the site of the proposed vertical osteotomy; it is usually retracted so that the crestal alveolar bone in the osteotomy site and the bony prominences overlying the canines and lateral incisors can be identified. The mucoperiosteum is minimally detached from the incisor segment to maximize its soft tissue pedicle. It can be elevated more from the larger posterior segment because the vascular pedicle from the contiguous bone and attached mucoperiosteum is broader. The margins of the mucosa are retracted with skin hooks to allow visualization of the labial osteotomy site and prevent injury to the attached gingiva.

Vertical interdental osteotomies are made with a fissure bur and extended from the anterior aspects of the nasal floor inferiorly to the level of the attached gingiva 3 to 4 mm above the level of the alveolar crestal bone. Superiorly, they are deepened into the spongiosa and extended to intersect with the planned palatal osteotomies. More inferiorly, they are made through the cortical alveolar bone only. When there is minimal bone between closely spaced teeth, the inferior labial cortex is sectioned with a sharp spatula osteotome only. The surgeon's finger is positioned on the palatal mucosa, and a fissure bur is used to connect the vertical interdental osteotomies on the two sides. The integrity of the palatal mucosa along the entire course of the planned osteotomy is preserved by carefully malleting the osteotome against the finger. A finely tapered spatula osteotome is malleted interproximally to fracture first the thicker, incompletely sectioned palate. The interradicular

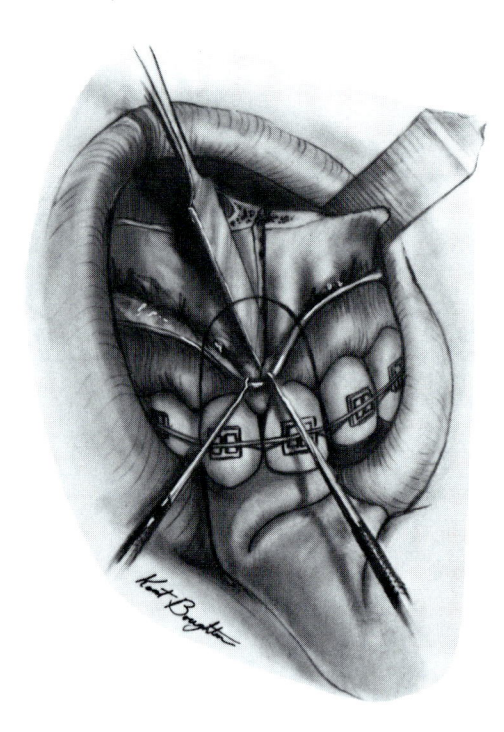

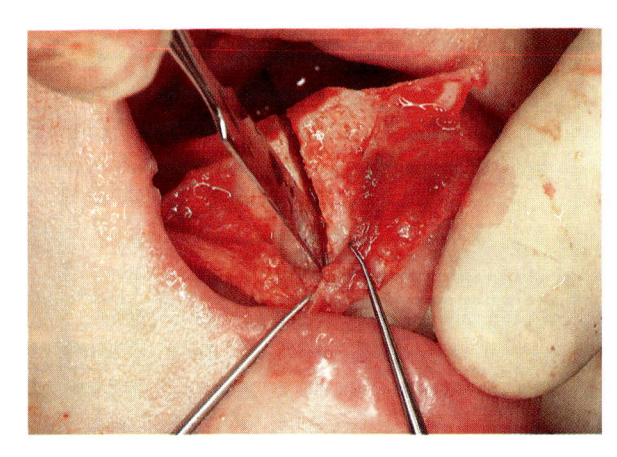

FIGURE 63–46. *Left* and *right*, Finally, a spatula osteotome is malleted into the interseptal area between the lateral incisors and canines to fracture the crestal alveolar bone. (*Left* from Bell WH, Mannai C, Luhr, HG: Art and science of the Le Fort I downfracture. Int J Adult Orthodont Orthognath Surg 3(1):23–52, 1988; with permission.)

sectioning proceeds sequentially superiorly and inferiorly in a stepwise fashion a half chisel at a time, until the osteotome transects the palatal and alveolar bone and its tip makes contact with the parasagittal osteotomy.

Finally, a tapered osteotome is directed into the thin interseptal area between the lateral incisors and canines to fracture the crestal alveolar bone (Fig. 63–46). A finger pressed on the mucosa detects when the osteotome has transected the palatal cortex. The proximal and distal segments must be freely movable with light digital pressure. Sectioning the bone in this manner minimizes detachment of the labial or palatal soft tissue and the removal of crestal alveolar bone.

By widening the maxilla with parasagittal osteotomies, much of the relaxation needed for expansion can be achieved, while a safe soft tissue pedicle to the posterior dento-osseous segments is maintained (Fig. 63–47). If the anterior part of the maxilla is widened, an interdental osteotomy is performed to intersect with the transverse portion of the palatal U-shaped osteotomy. When more widening of the maxilla is desired, bilateral parasagittal osteotomies are made, and a bone graft is placed between the margins of the expanded segments. Indeed, if widening is excessive, multiple osteotomies may be made. Parasagittal incisions through the palatal mucosa may also be made to facilitate large lateral maxillary movements. Such movements are not indicated very often. Particulate marrow or slices of cancellous bone may be placed along the lateral maxillary osteotomies to facilitate consolidation and healing.

TWO-SEGMENT LE FORT I OSTEOTOMY

Increasing the arch length by sectioning the maxilla into two segments can facilitate correction of moderately crowded and rotated incisors (Fig. 63–47). In addition, an ideal Class I canine relationship can be achieved by widening or narrowing the maxilla. The inferior aspect of the expanded maxilla is stabilized with an interocclusal splint; the superior portion may be stabilized adjunctively with a mini bone plate fixed across the interdental osteotomy site. A bone graft may also be placed between the margins of the expanded segments.

When the interocclusal splint is removed, a new arch wire is placed to maintain

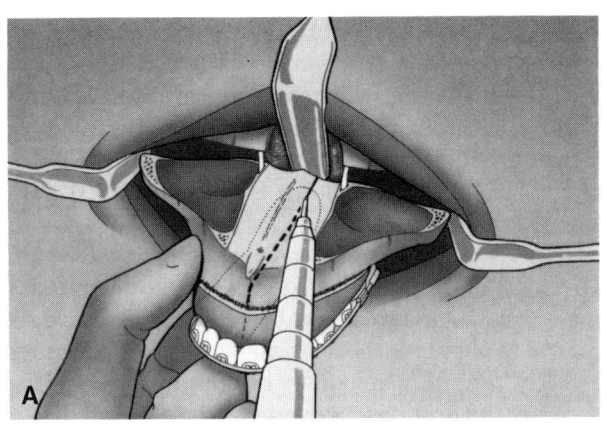

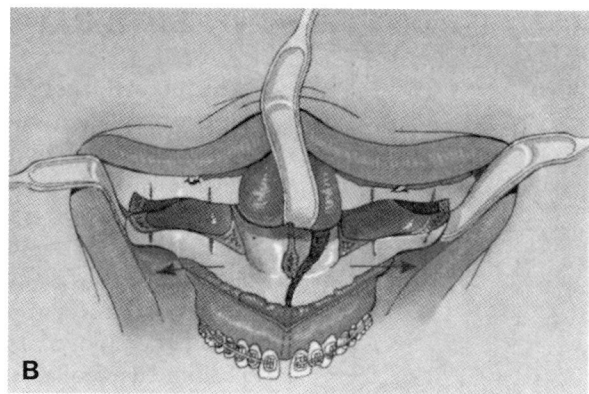

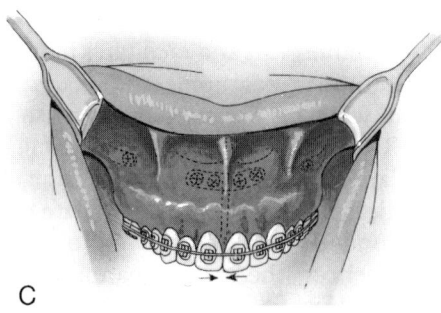

FIGURE 63-47. *A*, Two-segment Le Fort I osteotomy to increase anterior maxillary arch length. The parasagittal palatal bone is sectioned with a No. 703 fissure bur in the area midway between the midpalatal suture and the junction of the horizontal and vertical parts of the maxilla. *B*, Widening the maxilla and increasing anterior arch length by two-segment Le Fort I osteotomy. *C*, After the interocclusal splint is removed, a new arch wire is placed to maintain horizontal osseous stability and facilitate alignment of the anterior teeth by closure of interincisal space. A mini plate can also be passively adapted across the interdental osteotomy site for additional stabilization of the expanded maxilla. (*A* and *B* from Bell WH, Mannai C, Luhr, HG: Art and science of the Le Fort I downfracture. Int J Adult Orthodont Orthognath Surg 3(1):23–52, 1988; with permission.)

horizontal stability and facilitate alignment of the anterior teeth by closure of the interincisal space. If the posterior part of the maxilla is widened significantly, horizontal stability is maintained with a transpalatal arch or acrylic splint. The facility to achieve additional maxillary expansion is another advantage of the transpalatal arch.

Expansion of the downfractured maxilla is accomplished by a parasagittal palatal osteotomy (Fig. 63–47). After the nasal crest of the maxilla is reduced with a bone bur and rongeurs, the osteotomy is angled laterally to an area midway between the midpalatal suture and the junction between the horizontal and vertical parts of the maxilla. The parasagittal osteotomy is made through the maxilla in an area where the bone is very thin, but the palatal mucosa is thick and extensible and resists tearing when the maxilla is expanded (Fig. 63–47). The surgeon's finger is positioned on the palatal mucosa to feel the rotating bur as it transects the palatal cortical bone (see Fig. 63–45). The thick portion of the anterior maxilla is then sequentially sectioned with a fissure bur and by malleting a spatula osteotome into the deeper portion of the midpalatal suture and between the central incisors. The two halves of the expanded maxilla are indexed into and ligated to an interocclusal splint. The downfractured maxilla may also be narrowed after parasagittal osteotomy. The maxilla is then ligated to an interocclusal splint and stabilized with rigid skeletal fixation.

It should be realized that even very rigid plates that are placed beside the piriform aperture and the zygomatic buttress may not necessarily prevent transverse relapse of a parasagittally sectioned maxilla. To maintain the desired width, a prefabricated, strong transpalatal arch or splint should be inserted after surgery. The patient should wear this appliance for at least the first 4 to 6 months after surgery.

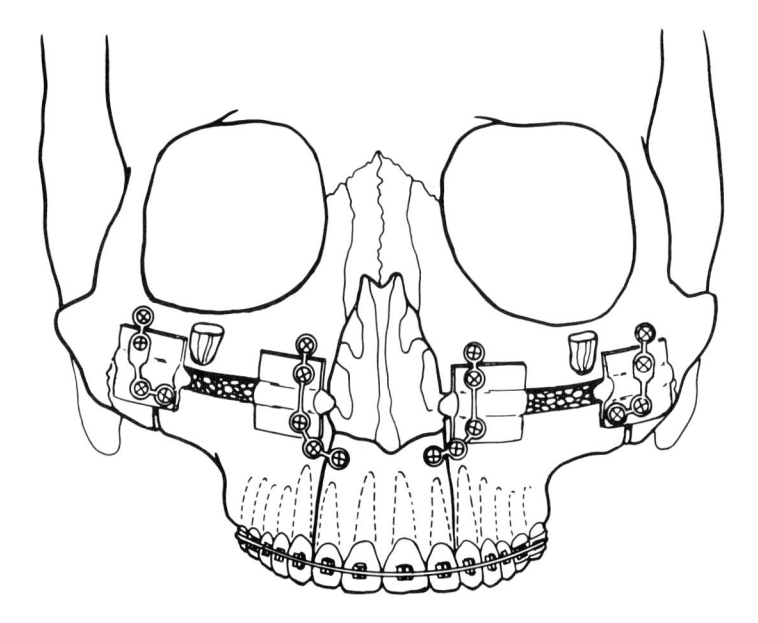

FIGURE 63-51. SURGICAL TECHNIQUE OF THE HIGH LE FORT I OSTEOTOMY WITH VERTICAL STEP OSTEOTOMY IN THE ZYGOMATICOMAXILLARY BUTTRESS. The plan of surgery is the correction of vertical maxillary deficiency and simultaneous uprighting of the maxillary incisor teeth. Interpositional corticocancellous bone grafts are stabilized with positional screws to increase vertical stability. Particulate bone marrow grafts are interposed between the bony margins to increase osteogenesis between the segments.

correction of the vertical discrepancy. In selected cases, both corrections may be achieved by downward and forward sliding movement of the maxilla (Fig. 63-51). The lateral maxillary osteotomy designs are individualized.

NEUROMUSCULAR REHABILITATION

Following the patient's recovery from surgery, several training elastics are placed to facilitate occlusal and neuromuscular rehabilitation.[16] Light vertical training elastics are placed bilaterally between soldered interproximal lugs attached to maxillary and mandibular orthodontic arch wires in the canine-first premolar interspaces. Range-of-motion exercises four or five times per day are usually commenced on the second or third postoperative day.

Appropriate training elastics are placed during the day and night. The type of surgical procedure, compliance by the patient, individual variability, resultant occlusion, and clinical judgment determine the duration of rehabilitation. The objective of occlusal and neuromuscular rehabilitation is to achieve a stable Class I occlusion, adequate interincisal distance, normal protrusive and lateral movements, and a functional position of the condyles (see Chapter 46 for details.)

CONCLUSION

Our present-day Le Fort I osteotomy technique is the harvest of yesterday's research; current clinical results are memorials to the courage, persistence, ingenuity, and research of the surgical pioneers of the Le Fort I downfracture. Recent technical innovations, combined with new individualized Le Fort I osteotomy designs, efficient orthodontic treatment, systematic neuromuscular rehabilitation, improved understanding of surgical anatomy, and rigid skeletal fixation, facilitate the achievement of improved jaw function, long-term dental and skeletal stability, and balanced facial proportions.

REFERENCES

1. Abubakker AO, Sotereanos GC: Modified Le Fort I (maxillary-zygomatic) osteotomy: Rationale, basis, and surgical technique. J Oral Maxillofac Surg 49:1089–1097, 1991.
2. Astrand P: Chewing efficiency before and after surgical correction of developmental deformities of the jaws. Swed Dent J 3:1–11, 1974.
3. Banks P, MacKenzie I: Criteria for condylotomy: A clinical appraisal of 211 cases. Proc R Soc Med 68:601–613, 1975.
4. Bays RO: Rigid stabilization system for maxillary osteotomies. J Oral Maxillofac Surg 43:60–63, 1985.
5. Beals SP, Munro JR: The use of miniplates in craniomaxillofacial surgery. Plast Reconstr Surg 79:33, 1987.
6. Belifante LS, Mitchell DL: Use of alloplastic material in the canine fossa–zygomatic area to improve facial esthetics. J Oral Surg 35:121–125, 1977.
7. Bell WH: Revascularization and bone healing after anterior maxillary osteotomy: A study using adult rhesus monkey. J Oral Surg 27:249–255, 1969.
8. Bell WH: Revascularization and bone healing after posterior maxillary osteotomy. J Oral Surg 29:313–320, 1971.
9. Bell WH: Revascularization and bone healing after maxillary corticotomies. J Oral Surg 30:640–648, 1972.
10. Bell WH: Biological basis for maxillary osteotomies. Am J Phys Anthropol 38:279–289, 1973.
11. Bell WH: Bone healing and revascularization after total maxillary osteotomy. J Oral Surg 33:253–260, 1975.
12. Bell WH: Le Fort I osteotomy for correction of maxillary deformities. J Oral Surg 33:412–426, 1975.
13. Bell WH: Correction of the short-face syndrome–vertical maxillary deficiency: A preliminary report. J Oral Surg 35:110–120, 1977.
14. Bell WH: Surgical-orthodontic correction of horizontal maxillary deficiency. J Oral Surg 37:897, 1979.
15. Bell WH, Fonseca RJ, Kennedy JW, et al: Bone healing and revascularization after total maxillary osteotomy. J Oral Surg 33:235, 1975.
16. Bell WH, Gonyea W, Finn RA, et al: Muscular rehabilitation after orthognathic surgery. Oral Surg 56:229–235, 1983.
17. Bell WH, Jacobs JD: Tridimensional planning for surgical orthodontic treatment of mandibular excess. Am J Orthod 80:263–288, 1981.
18. Bell WH, Kawamura H, Finn RA, Quejada J: Revascularization after Le Fort I osteotomy and transection of the descending palatine vessels. IADR Abstract, 1980.
19. Bell WH, Levy BM: Healing after anterior maxillary osteotomy. J Oral Surg 28:728–734, 1970.
20. Bell WH, Mannai C, Luhr HG: Art and science of the Le Fort I downfracture. Int J Adult Orthod Orthognath Surg 3:23–52, 1988.
21. Bell WH, Proffit WR, White RP (eds): Surgical Correction of Dentofacial Deformities. Vols 1 and 2. Philadelphia, WB Saunders Company, 1980.
22. Bell WH, Sinclair PM, Jacobs JD, et al: Simultaneous repositioning of the maxilla, mandible, and chin. In Bell WH, Profitt WR, White RP (eds): Surgical Correction of Dentofacial Deformities. Vol 3. Philadelphia, WB Saunders Company, 1984, pp 1–226.
23. Bell WH, Yamaguchi Y, Poor MR: Treatment of temporomandibular joint dysfunction by intraoral vertical ramus osteotomy. Int J Adult Orthod Orthognath Surg 5:9, 1990.
24. Bennett MA, Wolford LM: The maxillary step osteotomy and Steinmann pin stabilization. J Oral Maxillofac Surg 43:307–311, 1985.
25. Binder WJ: Submalar augmentation: A procedure to enhance rhytidectomy. Ann Plast Surg 24:200, 1990.
26. Brennan HG: Augmentation malarplasty. Arch Otolaryngol 108:441–444, 1982.
27. Brusati R, Sesenna E, Raffaini M: On the feasibility of intraoral maxillo-malar osteotomy. J Craniomaxillofac Surg 17:110–115, 1989.
28. Cies WA, Bayliss HI: Epiphora following rhinoplasty and Caldwell-Luc procedures. Ophthalmic Surg 7:77, 1976.
29. Converse JM, Horowitz SL, Valauri AJ, et al: The treatment of nasomaxillary hypoplasia: A new pyramidal naso-orbital maxillary osteotomy. Plast Reconstr Surg 45:527, 1970.
30. Darab DJ, Bell WH: Fixation for the modified Le Fort I osteotomy. J Oral Maxillofac Surg 49:904–907, 1991.
31. Della Rocca RC, Nesi FA, Lisman RD: Anatomy of ocular adnexa and orbit. In Smith BC: Ophthalmic Plastic and Reconstructive Surgery. Vol I. St Louis, CV Mosby Company, 1987, pp 15–74.
32. Demas PN, Sotereanos GC: Incidence of nasolacrimal injury and turbinectomy-associated atrophic rhinitis with Le Fort I osteotomies. J Craniomaxillofac Surg 17:116–118, 1989.
33. Drommer R, Luhr HG: The stabilization of osteotomized maxillary segments with Luhr miniplates in secondary cleft surgery. J Maxillofac Surg 9:166, 1981.
34. El Deeb M: Evaluation of local blood flow after total maxillary osteotomy. J Oral Surg 39:249–254, 1981.
35. Epker BN, Wolford LM: Middle-third facial osteotomies: Their use in the correction of acquired and developmental dentofacial and cranial deformities. J Oral Surg 33:491–514, 1975.
36. Epker BN, Wolford IM: Middle-third facial osteotomies: Their use in the correction of congenital dentofacial and craniofacial deformities. J Oral Surg 34:324, 1976.
37. Epker BN, Wolford LM: Dentofacial Deformities: Surgical-Orthodontic Correction. St. Louis, CV Mosby Company, 1980.

38. Farkas G, Kolar JC: Anthropometrics and art in aesthetics of women's faces. Clin Plast Surg 14:599, 1987.
39. Finn RA, Throckmorton GS, Bell WH, et al: Biomechanical considerations in the surgical correction of mandibular deficiency. J Oral Surg 38:257, 1980.
40. Flowers RS, Anderson R: Injury to the lacrimal apparatus during rhinoplasty. Plast Reconstr Surg 42:577, 1968.
41. Freihofer HPM Jr: Results of osteotomies of the facial skeleton in adolescence. J Maxillofac Surg 5:267, 1977.
42. Freihofer HPM Jr, Brouns JJA: Midfacial movement. Oral Maxillofac Surg Clin North Am 2:761–773, 1990.
43. Glassman AS, Mahigian SJ, Medway JM, et al: Conservative surgical orthodontic adult rapid palatal expansion: Sixteen cases. Am J Orthod 86:207, 1984.
44. Harle F: Le Fort I osteotomy (using miniplates) for correction of the long face. Int J Oral Surg 9:427, 1980.
45. Harsha BC, Terry BC: Stabilization of Le Fort I osteotomies utilizing small bone plates. Int J Adult Orthod Orthognath Surg 1:69, 1986.
46. Henderson D, Jackson IT: Naso-maxillary hypoplasia — the Le Fort II osteotomy. Br J Oral Surg 2:77, 1973.
47. Hinderer UT: Malar implants for improvement of the facial appearance. Plast Reconstr Surg 56:157–165, 1975.
48. Hogeman KE: Cited in Willmar K: On Le Fort I osteotomy. Scand J Plast Reconstr Surg 12 [Suppl]:1–68, 1974.
49. Holland GR, Robinson PP: A morphological study on the reinnervation of the teeth after segmental osteotomy in the cat. Int J Oral Surg 15:380–386, 1986.
50. Horster W: Experience with functionally stable plate osteosynthesis after forward displacement of the upper jaw. J Maxillofac Surg 8:176, 1980.
51. Hutchinson D: Tooth survival following various methods of subapical osteotomy. Int J Oral Surg 1:81–86, 1972.
52. Indresano AT, Lundell MI: Blood flow changes in the rabbit maxilla following an anterior osteotomy. J Dent Res 62:743–745, 1983.
53. Johnson JV: Evaluation of teeth vitality after subapical osteotomy. J Oral Surg 27:256–257, 1969.
54. Kaban LB, West B, Conover M, et al: Midface position after Le Fort III advancement. Plast Reconstr Surg 73:758, 1984
55. Kaminishi R, David H: Improved maxillary stability with modified Le Fort I technique. J Oral Maxillofac Surg 41:203–205, 1983.
56. Karabouta I, Martis C: The TMJ dysfunction syndrome before and after sagittal split osteotomy of the rami. J Maxillofac Surg 43:185–188, 1985.
57. Keller EE, Sather AH: Intraoral quadrangular Le Fort II osteotomy. J Oral Maxillofac Surg 45:223–232, 1987.
58. Keller EE, Sather AH: Quadrangular Le Fort I osteotomy. J Oral Maxillofac Surg 48:2–11, 1990.
59. Kohn MW: Evaluation of tooth sensation after segment alveolar osteotomy in 22 patients. J Am Dent Assoc 89:154–156, 1974.
60. Kufner J: Four-year experience with major maxillary osteotomy for retrusion. J Oral Surg 29:549–553, 1971.
61. Kuo PC, Will LA: Surgical-orthodontic treatment of maxillary constriction: State of the art. Oral Maxillofac Surg Clin North Am 2:751–759, 1990.
62. Lang J (Stell PM, translator): Clinical Anatomy of the Nose, Nasal Cavity and Paranasal Sinuses. New York, Thieme Medical Publishers, 1989.
63. Lauritzen C, Lilja J: Nasolacrimal obstruction in craniofacial surgery. Scand J Plast Reconstr Surg 19:269, 1985.
64. Lemke N, Della Rocca RC: Surgery of the Eyelids and Orbit: An Anatomical Approach. Norwalk, CT, Appleton and Lange, 1990, pp 96–135.
65. Little C, Mintz S, Ettinger AC: The distal lacrimal ductal system and traumatic epiphora. Int J Oral Maxillofac Surg 20:31–35, 1991.
66. Luhr HG: Aus Stabilen Osteosynthese bei Unterkieferfrakturen. Dtsch Zahnaerztl Z 23:754, 1968.
67. Luhr HG: Stabile Fixation von Overkiefer-Mittelgesichtsfrakturen durch Mini-Kompressionsplatten. Dtsch Zahnaerztl Z 34:851, 1979.
68. Luhr HG: A micro-system for cranio-maxillofacial skeletal fixation. J Craniomaxillofac Surg 16:312–314, 1988.
69. MacGregor AJ: Histology of a pulp following segmental alveolotomy. Br J Oral Surg 8:292, 1971.
70. Magnusson T, Ahlborg D, Finne K, et al: Changes in temporomandibular joint pain-dysfunction anomalies. Int J Oral Maxillofac Surg 15:707–714, 1986.
71. McCarthy JG, Grayson B, Bookstein F, et al: Le Fort III advancement osteotomy in the growing child. Plast Reconstr Surg 74:343, 1984.
72. Meyer MW, Cavanaugh GP: Blood flow changes after orthognathic surgery: Maxillary and mandibular subapical osteotomy. J Oral Surg 35:495–501, 1976.
73. Nelson RL: Quantitation of blood flow after anterior maxillary osteotomy: Investigation of three surgical approaches. J Oral Surg 36:106–111, 1978.
74. Nelson RL, Path MG, Ogle RG, et al: Quantitation of blood flow after Le Fort I osteotomy. J Oral Surg 35:10–16, 1977.
75. Obwegeser HL: Surgical correction of small or retrodisplaced maxilla: The "dish-face deformity." Plast Reconstr Surg 43:351, 1969.

76. Osguthorpe JD, Calcaterra TC: Nasolacrimal obstruction after maxillary sinus and rhinoplastic surgery. Arch Otolaryngol 105:264, 1979.
77. Pepersack WJ: Tooth vitality after alveolar segmental osteotomy. Maxillofac Surg 1:85, 1973.
78. Phillips JH, Rahn BA: Fixation effects on membranous and endochondral onlay bone-graft resorption. Plast Reconstr Surg 82:872–877, 1988.
79. Pospisil OA: Supra-apical midfacial osteotomies—new surgical techniques and their application. J Craniomaxillofac Surg 16:110–119, 1988.
80. Powell NB, Riley RW, Laub DR: A new approach to evaluation and surgery of the malar complex. Ann Plast Surg 20:206–214, 1988.
81. Quejada JG, Kawamura H, Finn RA, Bell WH: Wound healing associated with segmental total maxillary osteotomy. J Oral Maxillofac Surg 44:366–377, 1986.
82. Reyneke JP, Mosureik CV: Treatment of maxillary deficiency by a Le Fort I downsliding technique. J Oral Maxillofac Surg 43:914–916, 1985.
83. Riley RW, Powell N, Guilleminault C: Current surgical concepts for treating obstructive sleep apnea syndrome. J Oral Maxillofac Surg 45:149–157, 1987.
84. Robinson PP: Reinnervation of teeth following segmental osteotomy in the cat. J Dent Res 59:1741–1749, 1980.
85. Rosen HM: Miniplate fixation of the Le Fort I osteotomies. Discussion by H.G. Luhr. Plast Reconstr Surg 78:748, 1986.
86. Sadao T: A longitudinal study on electrical pulp testing following Le Fort type osteotomy and Le Fort type of fracture. J Maxillofac Surg 3:14, 1975.
87. Schaefer JP: Types of ostia nasolacrimalia in man and their genetic significance. Am J Anat 13:183–192, 1912.
88. Scheideman GB: Wound healing after anterior and posterior subapical osteotomy. J Oral Maxillofac Surg 43:408–416, 1985.
89. Steinhauser EW: Bone screws and plates in orthognathic surgery. Int J Oral Surg 11:209, 1982.
90. Storum KA, Bell WH: The effect of physical rehabilitation on mandibular function after ramus osteotomies. J Oral Maxillofac Surg 44:94–99, 1986.
91. Stringer DE, Boyne PJ: Modification of the maxillary step osteotomy and stabilization with titanium mesh. J Oral Maxillofac Surg 44:487–488, 1986.
92. Sugg GR: Early pulp changes after anterior maxillary osteotomy. J Oral Surg 39:14–20, 1981.
93. Sun D, Bell WH, Mannai C, et al: Long-term evaluation of human teeth after Le Fort I osteotomy: A histologic and developmental study. Oral Surg Oral Med Oral Pathol 65 (4):379–386, 1988.
94. Throckmorton GS, Finn RA, Bell WH: Biomechanics of differences in lower facial height. Am J Orthod 77:410, 1980.
95. Tucker MR, Thomas PM: Temporomandibular pain and dysfunction in the orthodontic surgical patient: Rationale for evaluation and treatment sequencing. Int J Adult Orthod Orthognath Surg 1:11–20, 1986.
96. Turvey TA: Simultaneous mobilization of the maxilla and mandible: Surgical technique and results. J Oral Maxillofac Surg 40:96–99, 1982.
97. Upton LG, Scott RF, Hayward JR: Major maxillomandibular malrelations and temporomandibular joint pain-dysfunction. J Prosthet Dent 51:686–690, 1984.
98. Van Sickels J, Jeter T, Aragon S: Rigid fixation of maxillary osteotomies: A preliminary report and technique article. Oral Surg Oral Med Oral Pathol 60:262–265, 1985.
99. Waite PD, Matukas VJ: Zygomatic augmentation with hydroxylapatite: A preliminary report. J Oral Maxillofac Surg 44:349–352, 1986.
100. Wardrop RW, Wolford LM: Maxillary stability following downgraft and/or advancement procedures with stabilization using rigid fixation and porous block hydroxyapatite implants. J Oral Maxillofac Surg 47:336, 1989.
101. Ware WH: Pulpal response following anterior maxillary osteotomy. Am J Orthod 60:156–164, 1971.
102. Whitaker LA: Aesthetic augmentation of the malar-midface structures. Plast Reconstr Surg 80:337–346, 1987.
103. Whitaker LA: Facial proportions in aesthetic surgery. In Frankas LG, Monro IR (eds): Anthropometric Facial Proportions in Medicine. Springfield, IL, Charles C Thomas, 1987, p 103.
104. Whitaker LA, Morales L, Farkas LC: Aesthetic surgery of the supraorbital ridge and forehead structures. Plast Reconstr Surg 78:23, 1986.
105. You ZH, Bell WH, Finn RA: Anatomy of nasolacrimal canal and high Le Fort I osteotomy. Presented at the 73rd annual meeting of the American Association of Oral and Maxillofacial Surgeons, Chicago, 1991.
106. You ZH, Zhang ZK, Zhang XE, Xia JL: The study of vascular communication between jaw bones and their surrounding tissues by SEM of resin casts. West China J Stomatol 8:235–237, 1990.
107. You ZH, Zhang ZK, Zhang XE, Xia JL: A study of maxillary and mandibular vasculature in relation to orthognathic surgery. Chin J Stomatol 26(5):263–266, 1991.
108. You ZH, Zhang ZK, Zhang XE: Le Fort I osteotomy with descending palatal artery intact and ligated: A study of blood flow and quantitative histology. Contemp Stomatol 5(2):71–74, 1991.
109. Zide BM, Jelks GW: Surgical Anatomy of the Orbit. New York, Raven Press, 1985, pp 34–39.
110. Zide MF, Epker BN: Systematic aesthetic evaluation of the cheeks for cosmetic surgery. Oral Maxillofac Surg Clin North Am 2:351, 1990.
111. Zins JE, Whitaker LA: Membranous versus endochondral bone: Implications for craniofacial reconstruction. Plast Reconstr Surg 72:778, 1983.
112. Zisser GM, Gattlinger B: Histologic investigation of pulpal changes following maxillary and mandibular alveolar osteotomies in the dog. J Oral Maxillofac Surg 40:332–339, 1982.

II. Case Reports

The use of the Le Fort I osteotomy and other adjunctive surgical procedures to treat a varied group of patients with dentofacial deformities is described and illustrated in the following case reports.

Greater efficiency of orthodontic treatment, improved facial esthetics, and greater stability may be achieved by individualizing the osteotomy design through a better understanding of surgical anatomy relating to the various types of midfacial osteotomies and through the use of bone plate and screw osteosynthesis.

OCCLUSAL CONSIDERATIONS

The stability of orthodontic results is often overlooked. The causes of occlusal relapse are poorly understood. Many clinical investigators have concluded that conventional determinants of stability, such as duration or amount of treatment and arch expansion, fail to account for much of the variability. Utley and Harris (Determinants of molar relationships — Stability in orthodontic cases. J Dent Res [Suppl] 67:252, 1988) have studied occlusal stability after orthodontic treatment. Their study examined postretention stability as a function of the number, location, and cross-sectional areas of occlusal stops present at the end of full-banded orthodontic treatment in 110 cases. Study models taken at the time of debanding and again an average of 5 years out of retention were studied. The results indicated that the number of occlusal contacts was higher in stable cases at the end of treatment. The teeth settled into an improved relationship with larger areas of intertooth contact. The authors concluded that with greater numbers of tooth contacts after treatment, there was greater postretention stability. They also considered that "detailing" of a case is specifically under the clinician's control. In addition, it was noted that changes in occlusal contacts were closely related to changes in the jaw relationships after treatment. Although their studies were made on orthodontic patients, the results are probably applicable to the orthognathic patient as well. Therefore, it behooves the surgeon and orthodontist to coordinate their plan of treatment carefully before any orthodontic treatment is started.

Ideal Class I canine transverse relationships, maximal interdigitation, and slight overcorrection of the overbite are essential. To achieve these objectives, it is frequently necessary to section the maxilla into two, three, or four segments. The three-segment Le Fort I osteotomy is particularly useful in achieving the "ideal" occlusion, which will in itself give additional assurance of long-term stability. In nonextraction cases, the maxilla is most frequently sectioned between the lateral incisors and the canine teeth. When first bicuspid extractions are a part of the orthodontic plan, the maxilla is usually divided into three segments in the residual bicuspid extraction sites.

CASE 1 (Fig. 63–52*A* to *V*)

A.S., a 14-year-old student, sought treatment to decrease the prominence of her maxillary incisors, improve her smile line, increase the prominence of her chin, and correct her malocclusion (Fig. 63–52*A* to *C*). In addition, she was concerned about episodic pain and popping in her right temporomandibular joint. She habitually postured her mandible forward to compensate for her retrognathic mandible and Class II malocclusion, which was associated with vertical maxillary hyperplasia. The results of the clinical assessment implicated the disparity between centric relation and centric occlusion as a possible contributing cause of her mandibular dysfunction (Fig. 63–52*M* to *O*).

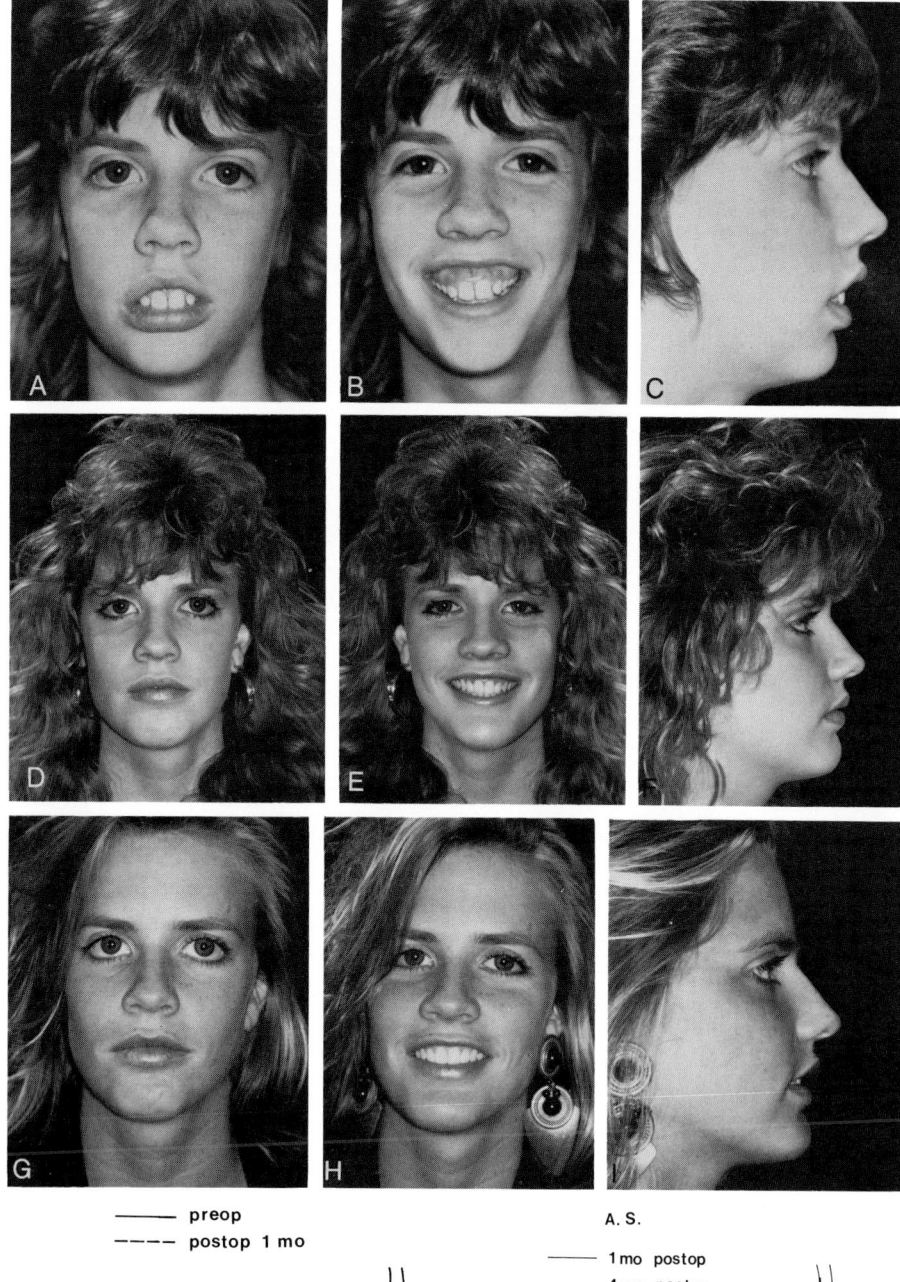

63 — MAXILLARY AND MIDFACE DEFORMITY / **2273**

FIGURE 63-52. *A–C,* Preoperative facial appearance of a 15-year-old patient. *D–F,* Facial appearance 2 years after orthognathic surgery. *G–I,* Facial appearance 6 years after orthognathic surgery. *J,* Pretreatment cephalometric tracing (at age 15 years), with mandible in centric relationship and lips in repose. *K,* Cephalometric tracings before and after (at age 18 years) orthognathic surgery. *L,* Skeletal and dental stability indicated by cephalometric tracings before and 6 years after orthognathic surgery (at age 24 years).
Illustration continued on following page

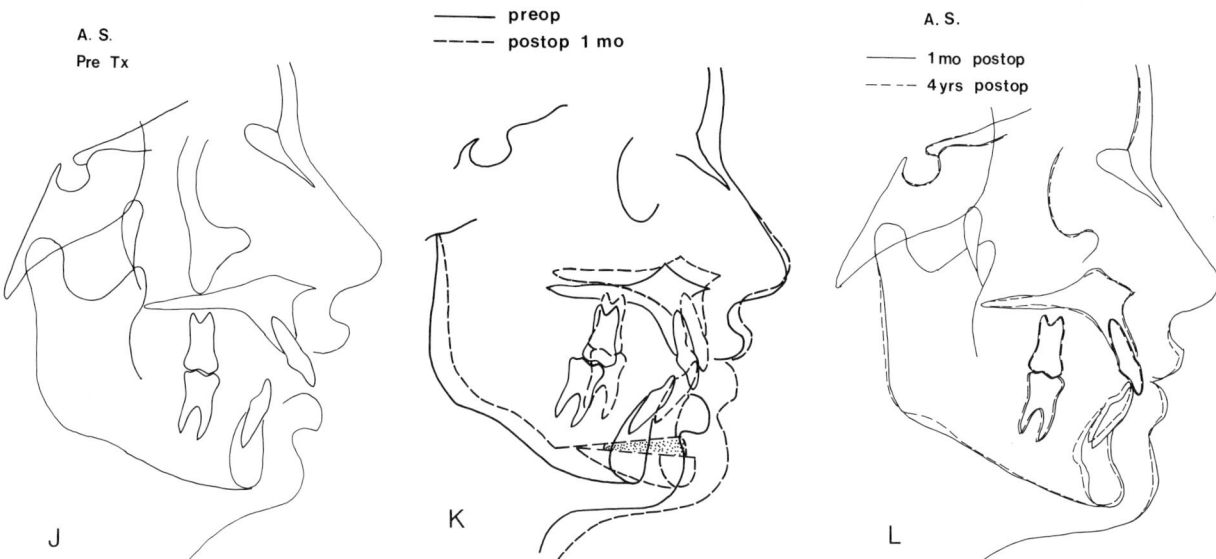

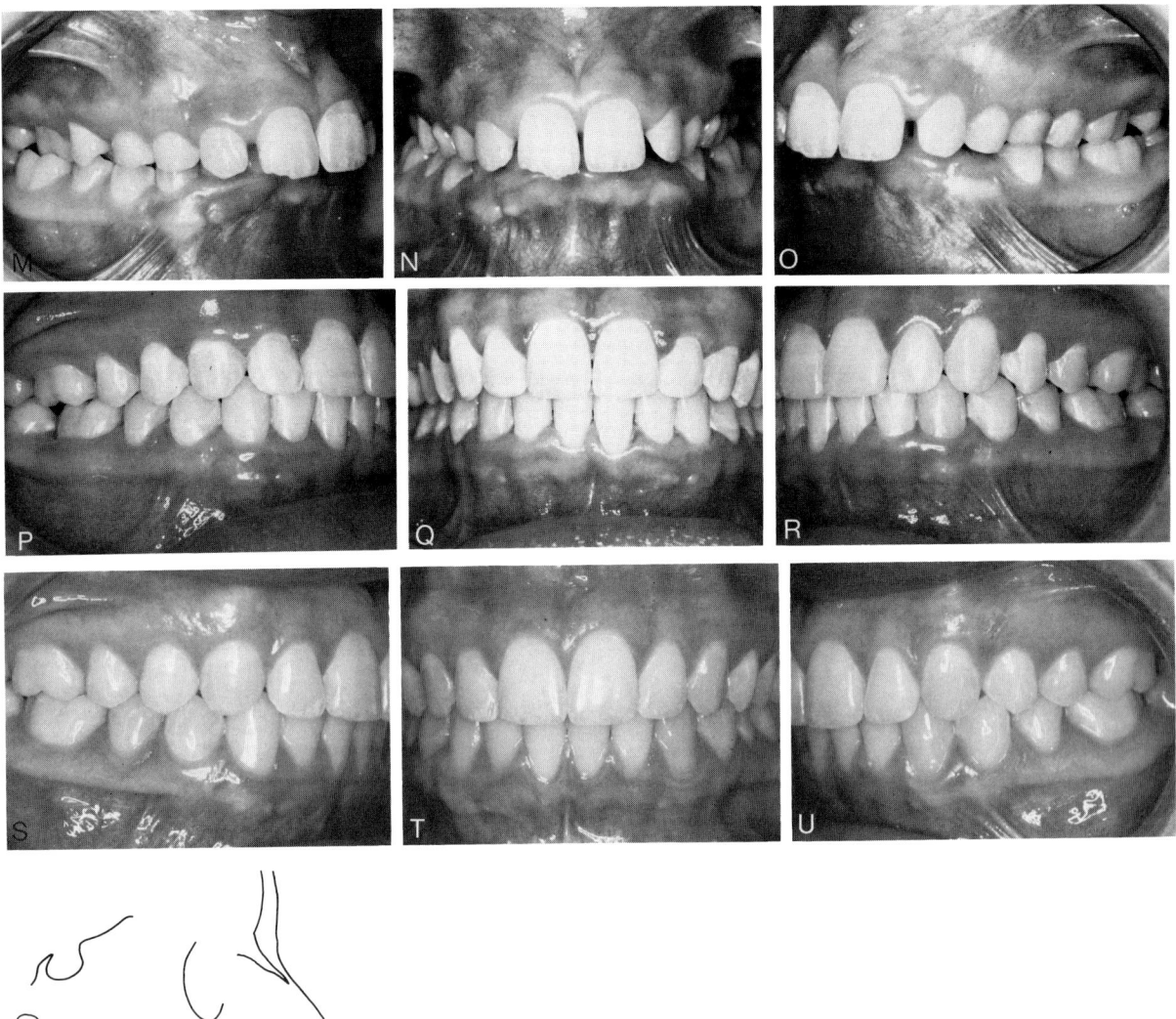

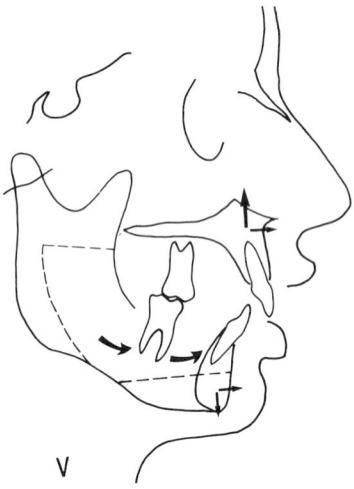

FIGURE 63–52 *Continued.* *M–O*, Presurgical symmetric Class II malocclusion. *P–R*, Class I occlusion after orthognathic surgery and orthodontic treatment. *S–U*, Occlusion 6 years after surgical and orthodontic treatment. *V*, Plan of surgery.

The surgical treatment plan consisted of the following (Fig. 63–52*V*):

1. Two-segment Le Fort I step osteotomy to superiorly reposition the maxilla (7 mm in the anterior and 5 mm in the posterior), to reduce the interlabial gap and amount of incisor exposure, and to widen the maxilla.
2. Bilateral sagittal split ramus osteotomies to advance the mandible 5 mm into a Class I canine and molar relationship.
3. Osteotomy of the inferior border of the mandible with interpositional bone grafting to increase the chin prominence (5 mm) and chin height (5 mm).
4. Submental lipectomy to reduce submental fat and improve the submental-cervical angle.

TREATMENT

Complete leveling and alignment of the maxillary arch, without extractions, were accomplished by extruding the premolars and first molars and proclining the maxillary incisors. The mandibular arch was aligned and partially leveled without extractions. After these objectives were accomplished, there was a 6-mm overjet, and the maxillary and mandibular incisors were in good relationship to their bony bases. The maxillary and mandibular osteotomies and genioplasty were performed simultaneously, and the jaws were stabilized by rigid skeletal fixation.

Concomitant extraction of impacted mandibular third molars and sagittal split ramus osteotomies required stabilization of the mandible with a five-hole curved Vitallium bone plate. The proximal portions of the ramus segments were fixed and stabilized with 12-mm bicortical screws; 8-mm unicortical screws were used to stabilize the distal segments to avoid damage to the roots of the molar teeth. Anteroposterior and vertical facial height proportions were achieved by orthodontic and surgical treatment (Fig. 63–52*J* to *L*). Occlusal and skeletal stability has been maintained over a 6-year postoperative follow-up period (Fig. 63–52*S* to *U*).

CASE 2 (Fig. 63–53*A* to *L*)

B.B., a 31-year-old flight attendant, had a 13-year history of dull pain, clicking, and popping in her right temporomandibular joint and masticatory muscle fatigue. She also complained of persistent nasal congestion and many "choking" episodes when eating solid foods. She habitually postured her mandible forward to compensate for her Class II malocclusion. Long-term symptomatic treatment with several anterior repositioning occlusal splints did not relieve her symptoms. Despite long-term popping and clicking in both temporomandibular joints, laminographic studies of the temporomandibular joints were normal.

Clinical and radiographic examinations showed the typical dentofacial features of absolute mandibular deficiency and mild vertical maxillary hyperplasia (Fig. 63–53*A* and *B*). Profile analysis revealed a mildly obtuse nasolabial angle, bilateral flattening of the paranasal and canine fossa areas, a retrusive upper lip, and less exposure of the vermilion border in the upper lip than in the lower lip.

A Class II malocclusion was associated with mild horizontal maxillary constriction and with a 3-mm maxillary arch length deficiency caused by small lateral incisors. Her Class II malocclusion encouraged forward posturing of the mandible to improve mandibular function (Fig. 63–53*G*). Mandibular advancement to eliminate the centric relation–centric occlusion disparity was considered an essential part of successful treatment from the point of view of function.

A correlative study of the nasolabial relationship, columella length, and upper lip drape was used adjunctively to construct a new SnV reference line that was calculated to achieve harmony between the nose and upper lip and aid in planning for the anteroposterior soft tissue changes. The maxilla was repositioned anteriorly 5 mm, the amount and direction necessary to achieve the desired esthetic result. These movements were accomplished by a two-segment Le Fort I osteotomy, which increased the arch length by creating a 2.5-mm space between the central incisors. The mandible was advanced 10 mm into a satisfactory Class I relationship to compensate for the 5-mm forward movement of the maxilla (Fig. 63–53*L*). The right and left sides of the maxilla were sectioned through the roots of the zygomas to increase the prominence of the zygomas and lateral orbital rims.

COMMENT

Within 2 weeks after surgery, the patient returned to work. Joint popping, clicking, and pain were no longer present. Rigid skeletal fixation facilitated efficient refinement of the postoperative occlusion. Presurgical and postsurgical orthodontics and surgical treatment were accomplished within 12 months. Increasing the arch length in the anterior maxilla facilitated treatment of the malaligned maxillary anterior teeth after surgery. Rigid stabilization of the repositioned maxilla in a Class I canine occlusion was the key to the achievement of this objective. The combined maxillary and mandibular surgical treatment, in concert with orthodontic treatment, achieved the planned anteroposterior facial proportions and functional objectives of treatment. Skeletal and dental stability and esthetic facial proportions have been maintained 6 years postoperatively. Swallowing and functional movements of the mandible were normalized. A gradual elimination of pain and dysfunction was noted during the first 8 weeks after surgery. The patient has remained asymptomatic for more than 6 years.

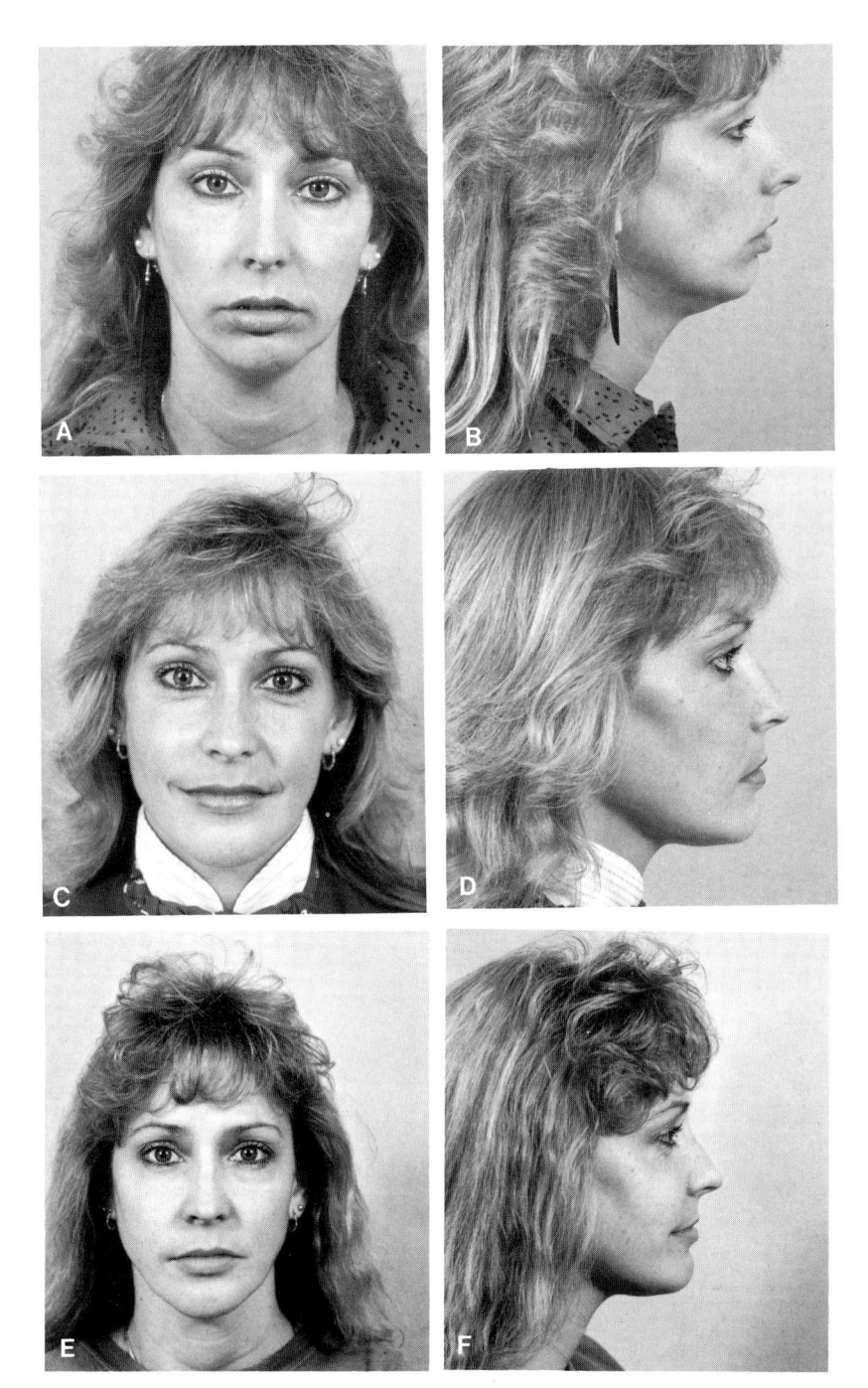

FIGURE 63-53. *A* and *B*, Facial appearance of a 30-year-old female patient with vertical maxillary excess, anterior open bite, and absolute mandibular deficiency before surgical orthodontic treatment. *C* and *D*, Facial appearance after 12 months of treatment. *E* and *F*, Facial appearance 6 years after treatment.

63 — MAXILLARY AND MIDFACE DEFORMITY / **2277**

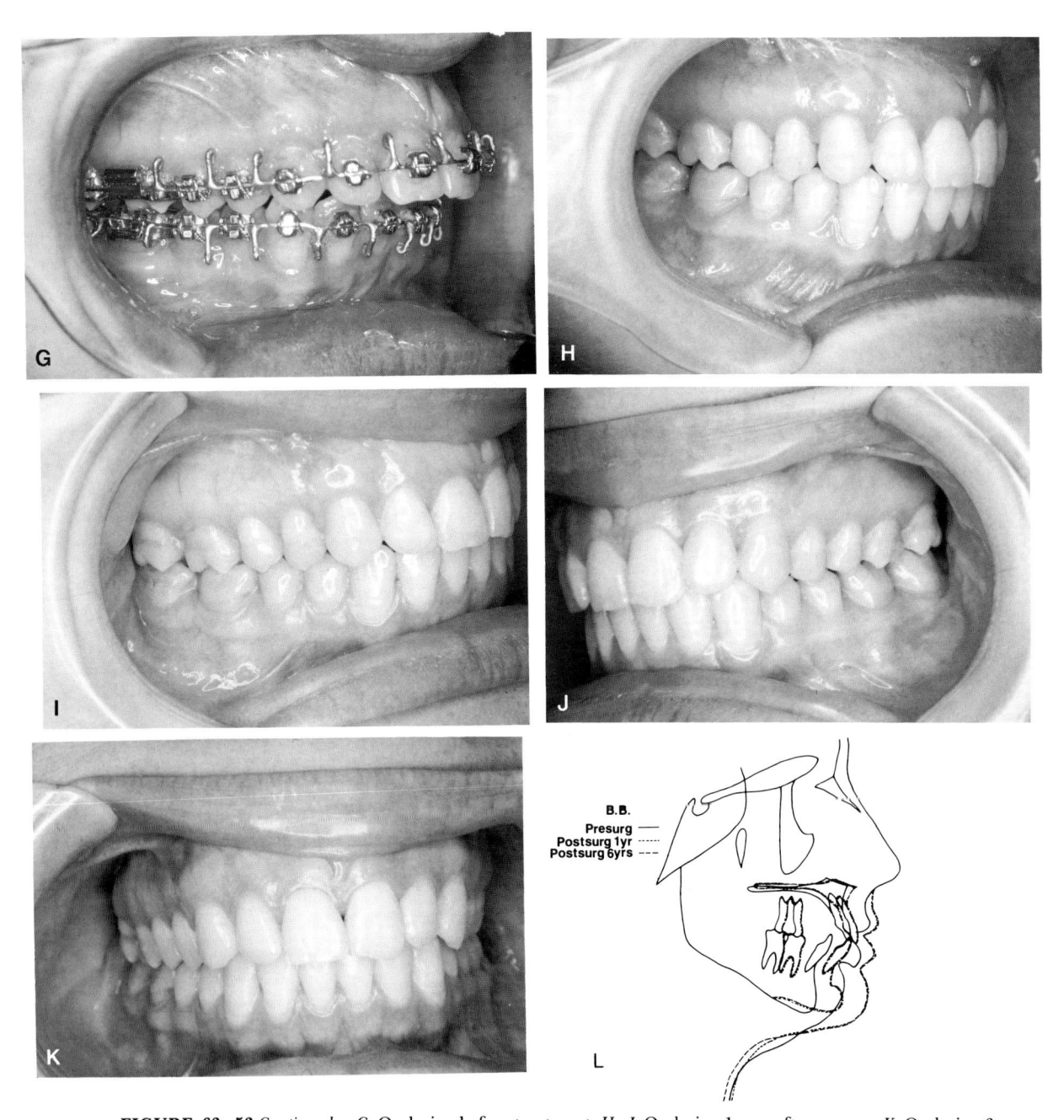

FIGURE 63–53 *Continued.* *G*, Occlusion before treatment. *H–J*, Occlusion 1 year after surgery. *K*, Occlusion 6 years after surgery. *L*, Composite cephalometric tracings before surgery, 1 year after surgery, and 6 years after surgery.

CASE 3 (Fig. 63–54A to O)

P.C., a 19-year-old Latin American woman, was referred for treatment of her asymmetric, long face. She had received many years of orthodontic treatment during adolescence.

PROBLEM LIST: ESTHETICS (FIG. 63–54A TO C)

The patient exhibited a mildly asymmetric, long face with excessive chin prominence and height. Clinical and cephalometric examination (Fig. 63–54G) showed the typical dentofacial features of asymmetric relative mandibular prognathism with mild

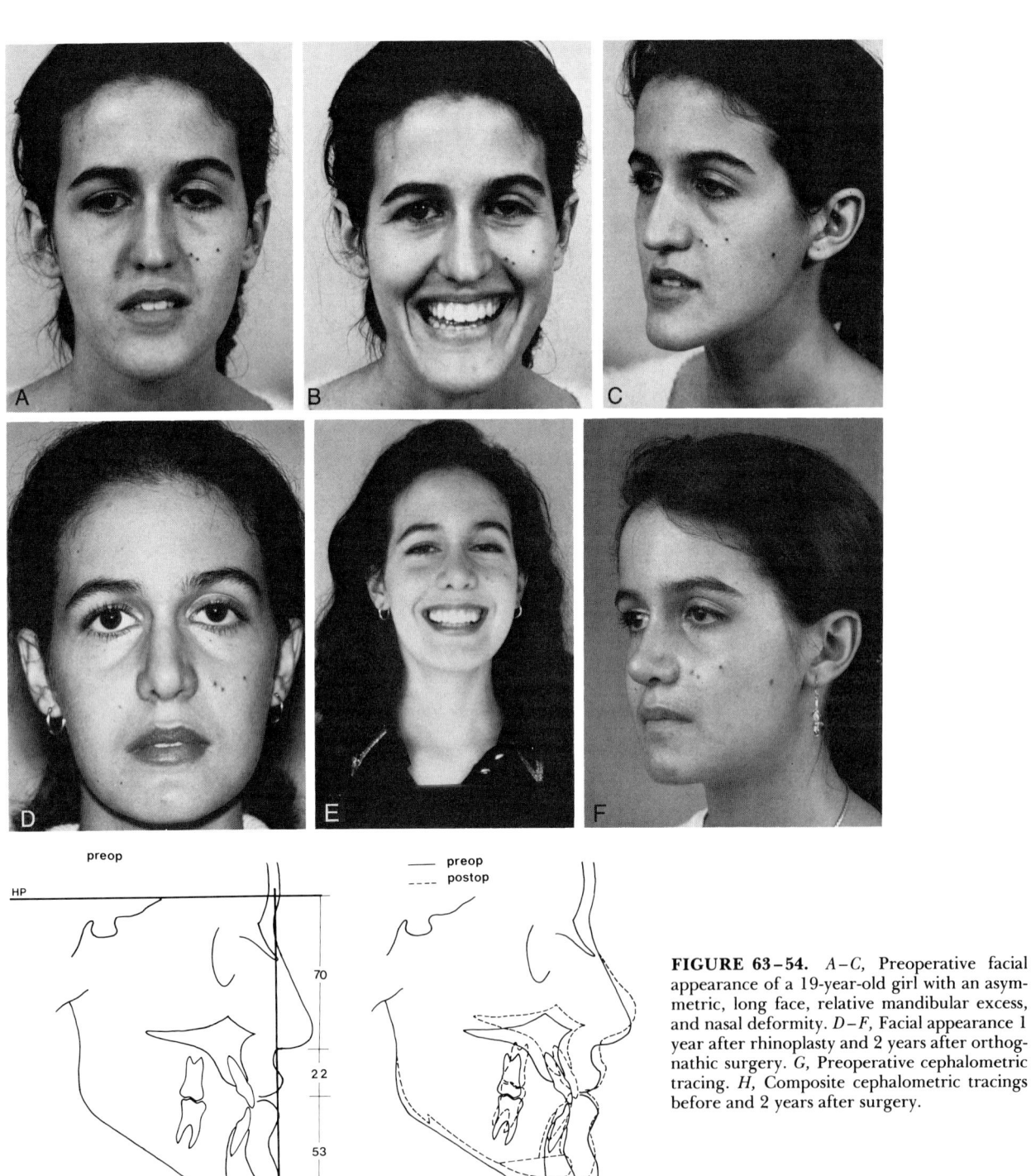

FIGURE 63–54. *A–C,* Preoperative facial appearance of a 19-year-old girl with an asymmetric, long face, relative mandibular excess, and nasal deformity. *D–F,* Facial appearance 1 year after rhinoplasty and 2 years after orthognathic surgery. *G,* Preoperative cephalometric tracing. *H,* Composite cephalometric tracings before and 2 years after surgery.

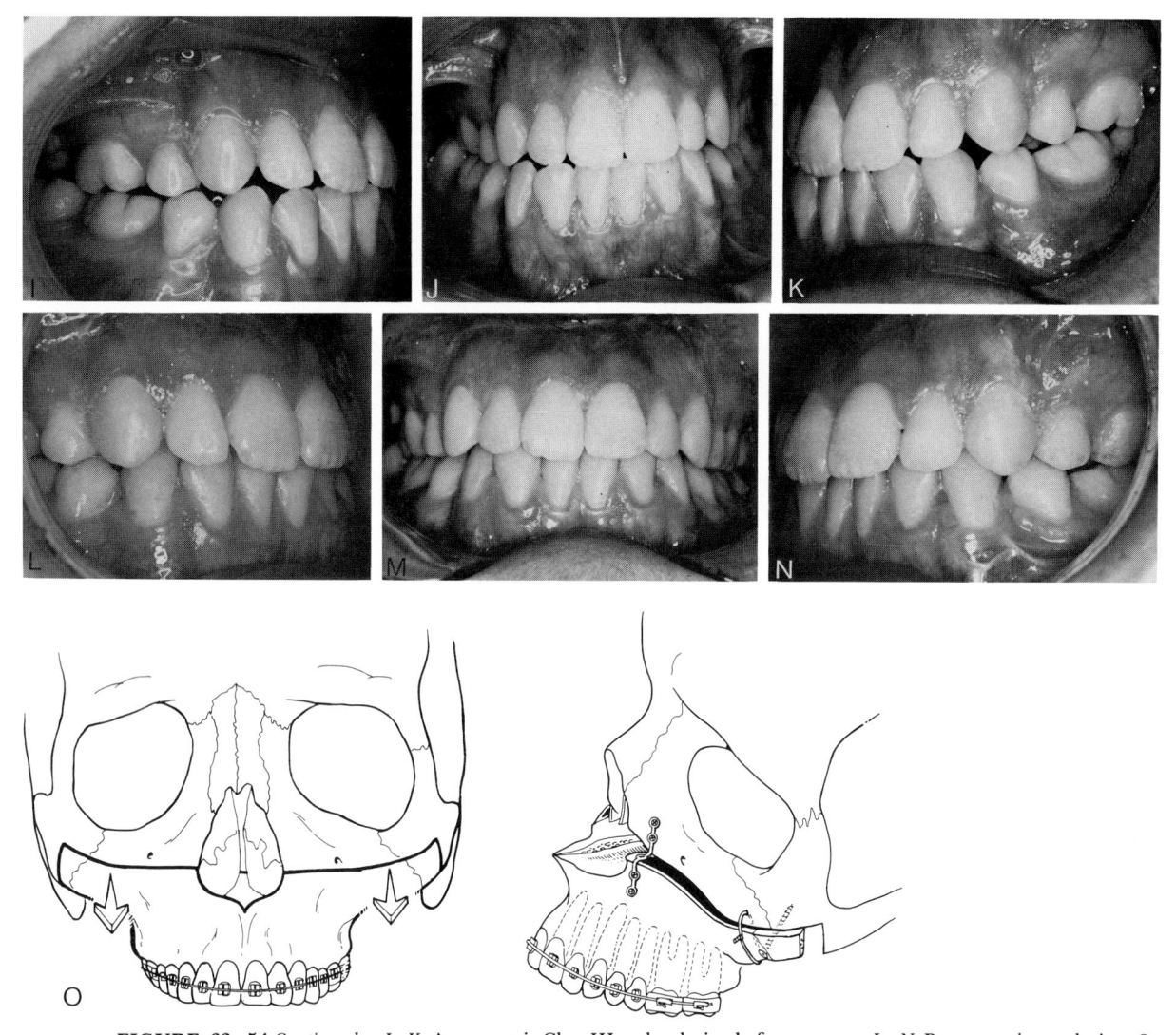

FIGURE 63–54 *Continued.* *I–K,* Asymmetric Class III malocclusion before surgery. *L–N,* Postoperative occlusion. *O,* Plan of surgery: Le Fort I osteotomy to reposition the maxilla superiorly and anteriorly, bilateral IVROs to correct mandibular asymmetry, and straightening genioplasty.

vertical maxillary hyperplasia and lip incompetence. Profile analysis revealed an acute nasolabial and nasocolumellar angle, bilateral flattening of the paranasal and malar regions, and excessive chin prominence and height. The nose was narrow and asymmetric because of a bulbous right lateral cartilage. The patient's prominent nasal dorsum and nasolabial disproportion indicated the need for rhinoplasty after orthognathic surgery.

An asymmetric Class III malocclusion was associated with adequate alignment of the maxillary and mandibular arches. A correlative study of the nasolabial proportions, columellar length, and nasal prominence and projection was used adjunctively to construct a new SnV reference line that was calculated to achieve harmony between the nose and upper lip and aid in planning for the anteroposterior soft tissue changes. In view of the fact that a functional occlusion could be achieved, the patient refused additional orthodontic treatment.

PLAN OF SURGERY (FIG. 63–54O)

Stage I

1. Le Fort I osteotomy to reposition the maxilla superiorly and anteriorly. The maxilla was repositioned anteriorly 6 mm by a high-level Le Fort I osteotomy (through the roots of the zygomas and subjacent to the infraorbital foramina) to increase the malar and paranasal prominence and widen the base of the nose. With the maxilla downfractured, a section of nasal cartilage was excised and preserved in a

freezer for subsequent nasal tip surgery. This secondary nasal septal surgery was accomplished 10 weeks after the definitive orthognathic surgery.

2. Intraoral vertical ramus osteotomies to correct the mandibular asymmetry and achieve the desired Class I occlusion.

3. Reduction of chin height by 6 mm and of chin prominence by 4 mm, by ostectomy of the inferior border of the mandible. The chin was repositioned laterally to achieve chin symmetry.

Stage II (Ten weeks after orthognathic surgery)

The nasal asymmetry and residual nasolabial disproportion were corrected by open rhinoplasty to narrow the lateral nasal cartilages, increase the nasal tip prominence, and reduce the dorsal nasal prominence.

FOLLOW-UP

The maxillary, mandibular, and chin surgical procedures were accomplished simultaneously to shorten the face, increase the malar and paranasal prominence, correct the malocclusion, and widen the nasal ala.

Several months later, rhinoplasty was performed, with the patient under local anesthesia and in an outpatient setting, to reduce the dorsal nasal hump, narrow the right lateral cartilage, and rotate the nasal tip with a preserved autogenous cartilaginous nasal strut previously harvested at the time of Le Fort I osteotomy. A Weir procedure was accomplished on the right side, where asymmetric widening of the nasal alar base occurred after Le Fort I osteotomy. Balanced anteroposterior, vertical, and transverse facial proportions were achieved by orthognathic and nasal surgery (Fig. 63–54D, E, F, and H). The postoperative Class I occlusion has remained stable and functional over a 2-year follow-up period (Fig. 63–54L to N).

SEQUENCING CONSIDERATIONS OF NASAL SURGERY

In this particular patient, surgery was programmed in two stages to facilitate clinical observation of nasal tip changes resulting from superior and anterior repositioning of the maxilla. Such changes cannot be predicted with certainty, despite the fact that in this individual they would usually be calculated to be positive after maxillary surgery.

The nose is evaluated both independently and relative to the upper lip and midface. On the basis of the clinical findings, this patient was deemed to have an independent nasal deformity. If the nasolabial angle is acute (downturned nasal tip), forward maxillary movement can be reasonably expected to raise the nasal tip and have a positive esthetic effect on the nasal and facial proportions. When the nasolabial angle is acute, the columella appears long in its anteroposterior dimension, and the upper lip is retrusive, the maxilla can be repositioned anteriorly to ameliorate undesirable esthetics in the midface and nose. A correlated study of the nasolabial proportions, columella length, and upper lip drape is used adjunctively in planning anteroposterior maxillary changes and nasal tip changes. It is important to know and understand the limitations of nasal surgery—how much change in the nasal proportions can be reasonably expected to occur with the rhinoplasty done some 2 to 6 months after surgical repositioning of the maxilla. The amount of forward maxillary movement will depend on simulated rhinoplasty and the calculated changes that will occur in the nasal tip.

To place the treatment into proper clinical perspective, the orthognathic and nasal surgery analyses and treatment objectives must be coordinated. The limitations of nasal surgery must be understood and carefully coordinated with the changes that can be reasonably expected with both nasal and orthognathic surgical procedures. The amount of forward maxillary movement depends on simulated rhinoplasty and changes that occur in the nasal tip. Free-hand tracings of a "new" upper lip contour are made with cephalometric planning studies aided by a constructed SnV reference line, which is used adjunctively to achieve proportionality between the upper lip and the nose. An overall knowledge of the anticipated soft tissue changes associated with three-dimensional movements of the jaws and teeth is combined with the surgeon's individual artistic sense of facial proportionality and beauty.

Precise predictions of nasal tip changes are not always possible. Even in the best of hands, it may be difficult, if not impossible, to predict the delicate soft tissue changes associated with maxillary advancement and its effect on abnormal tip position. Successful orthognathic and nasal surgery mandates predictability of soft tissue changes associated with orthognathic surgery.

Surgeons—William H. Bell, D.D.S., and Douglas P. Sinn, D.D.S., Dallas, TX
Orthodontist—Jose Carlos Elgoyhen, D.D.S., Buenos Aires, Argentina

CASE 4 (Fig. 63–55A to O)

M.D., a 17-year-old girl, sought treatment to increase the prominence of her upper lip and correct her malocclusion. Prior orthodontic treatment was accomplished in concert with extraction of maxillary and mandibular first bicuspid teeth. Although tooth alignment was satisfactory, there was residual VME, 3-mm overjet, and nasolabial disproportion.

PROBLEM LIST

Esthetics (Fig. 63–55A, B, C, and G)

Clinical and cephalometric analysis disclosed vertical maxillary hyperplasia, anteroposterior maxillary deficiency, absolute mandibular deficiency, and a contour-deficient chin. The patient's maxillary anterior teeth were positioned 5 mm anterior to the mandibular anterior teeth in a Class II relationship. The nose appeared large and relatively disproportionate to the rest of the face.

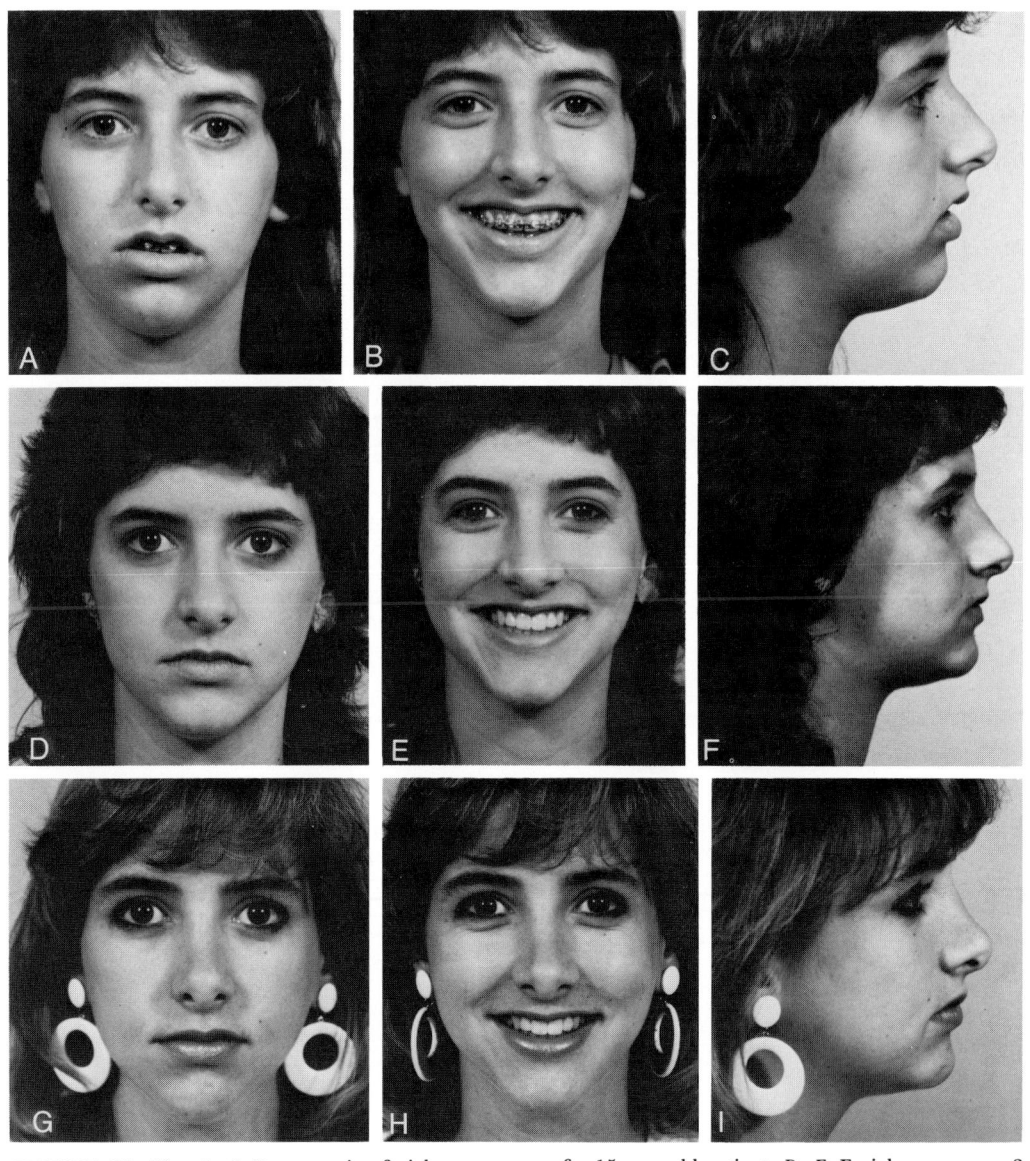

FIGURE 63–55. *A–C*, Preoperative facial appearance of a 15-year-old patient. *D–F*, Facial appearance 2 years after orthognathic surgery. *G–I*, Facial appearance 3 years after nasal surgery and 6 years after orthognathic surgery.

Illustration continued on following page

FIGURE 63–55 *Continued.* *J*, Pretreatment cephalometric tracing (age 15 years) with mandible in centric relationship and lips in repose. *K*, Post–orthognathic surgery cephalometric tracings (at age 18 years). *L*, Skeletal and dental stability indicated by cephalometric tracings taken with the mandible in centric relationship 3 years after rhinoplasty and 6 years after orthognathic surgery. *M*, Presurgical asymmetric Class II malocclusion. *N*, Class I occlusion after orthognathic surgery. *O*, Occlusion 6 years after surgical and orthodontic treatment.

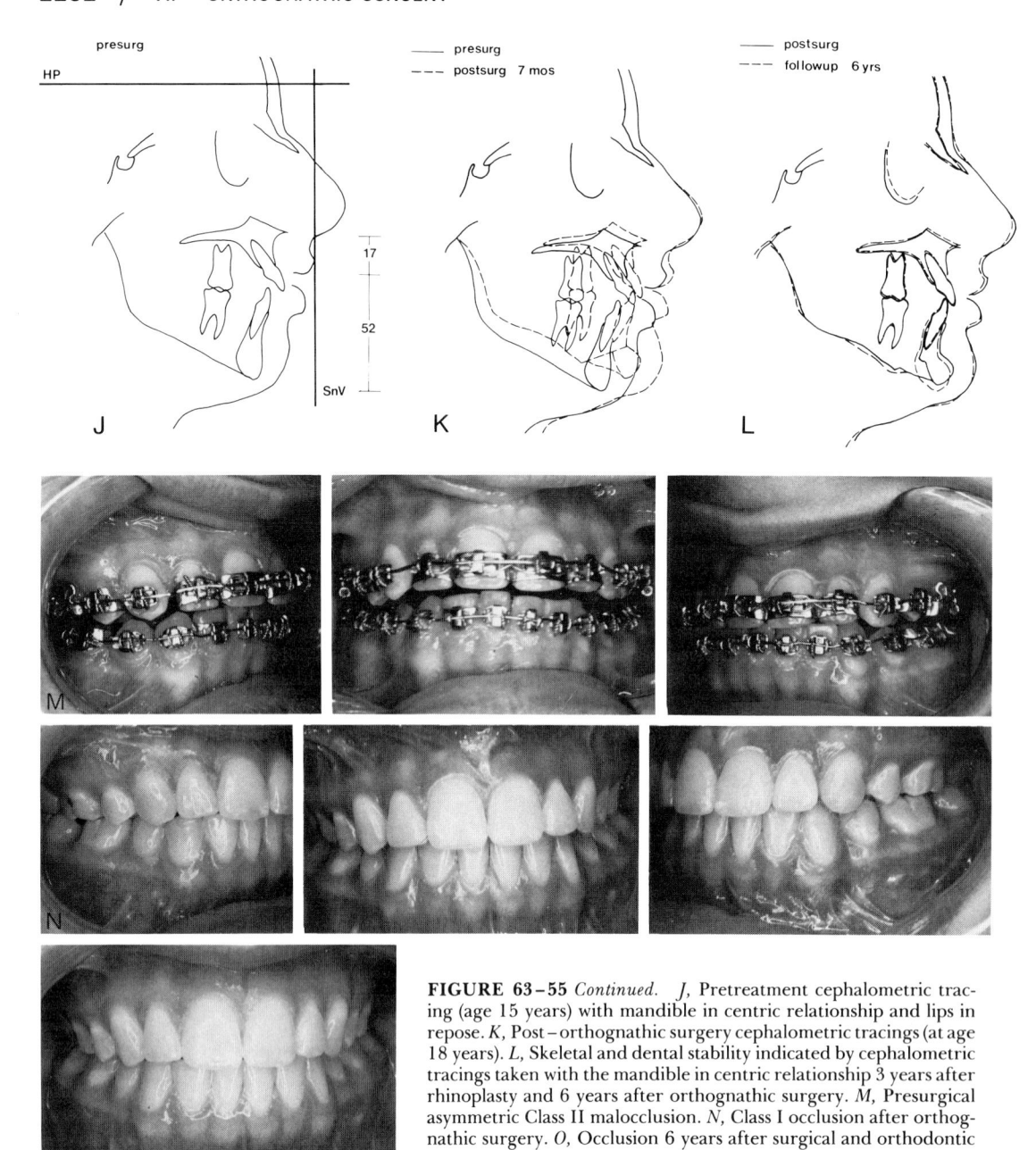

Plan of Treatment

Orthognathic Surgery

1. Le Fort I osteotomy to reduce maxillary height by 3 mm and increase the prominence of the upper lip vermilion by 4 mm (traditional low-level Le Fort I technique).
2. Bilateral sagittal split ramus osteotomies to advance the mandible 6 mm to achieve the desired Class I occlusion.
3. Advancement genioplasty (7 mm) by osteotomy of the inferior border of the mandible.

Follow-up

The maxilla was raised superiorly 3 mm to improve the upper lipline–tooth relationship and was advanced 5 mm to increase the prominence of the upper lip and decrease the nasolabial disproportion. Malar and orbital rim prominence was considered adequate—hence the low-level Le Fort I osteotomy without augmentation was the selected surgical technique. Two years after orthognathic surgery, rhinoplasty was performed to correct the residual nasal deformity. Although the rhinoplasty reduced the sagittal prominence of the nose and rotated the nasal tip, there was some residual columellar prominence after nasal surgery.

CASE 5 (Fig. 63–56A to R)

C.N., a 13-year-old girl, was seen in consultation regarding correction of her malocclusion. She had been under the care of an orthodontist since age 8. Her crowded Class I malocclusion had been treated by orthodontic mechanics facilitated by extraction of maxillary first premolars. The dominant clinical findings were as follows.

ORIGINAL PROBLEM LIST

Esthetic Analysis (Fig. 63–56A to C)

An esthetic analysis revealed a long face with a long and prominent chin; lip incompetence; and excessive exposure of teeth and gingiva when the patient was smiling.

Cephalometric Analysis (Fig. 63–56J)

1. Excessive lower anterior facial height.
2. Retroclined mandibular anterior teeth $\overline{1}$ to MPA, 62°; $\overline{1}$ to NA, 22°, 5 mm; $\overline{1}$ to NB, −4°, 1 mm.

Occlusal Analysis

Occlusal analysis revealed missing maxillary first premolars; slight Class III molar relationship; Class III canine relationship; and lower incisors excessively angled to the lingual aspect and moderately crowded.

A retrospective study of the patient's previous cephalometric radiographs, taken between ages 8 and 12, showed that continued excessive growth of the mandible relative to the maxilla and cranial base had caused a 4-degree reduction in the ANB angle and a 60-mm reduction in convexity. On the basis of this growth tendency and the fact that the patient was late in maturing (she did not reach puberty until age 15), surgical correction was deferred for 12 months upon onset of her menses. In addition, she was only 5 feet tall, in contrast to her mother, who was 5 feet 7 inches tall, and her father, who was 6 feet tall.

The orthodontic plan called for independent treatment of the maxillary and mandibular arches, aligning the maxillary teeth on the maxilla and the mandibular teeth on the mandible by tipping the lingually inclined lower incisors forward, without extractions. Treatment produced a large anterior crossbite. A secondary list of problems was evolved to aid in planning treatment for the patient at age 16 years.

SECONDARY PROBLEM LIST

Esthetic Analysis

FRONTAL. An analysis of the frontal view revealed a short-appearing upper lip; lip incompetence (6 mm), with excessive tooth exposure upon smiling; flattening of the paranasal areas; a narrow nose and long face with a prominent, square, asymmetric chin; and an asymmetric maxillary dental midline.

PROFILE. An analysis of the profile revealed a retrusive upper lip and disharmony between the upper and lower lips, with the lower lip prominent and everted.

Cephalometric Analysis (Fig. 63–56K)

Analysis demonstrated an anteroposterior maxillary deficiency: ANB = −4°; SNA = 78°; SNB = 82°.

Occlusal Analysis (Fig. 63–56O)

DENTAL ARCH FORM. Symmetric, V-shaped maxillary and mandibular arches were present. This analysis was based on the occlusal relationship that was achieved when the models were hand articulated into a simulated corrected Class I canine relationship.

DENTAL ALIGNMENT. The maxilla had missing first premolar teeth, which had been extracted at age 8; the teeth were well aligned because of previous orthodontic treatment. The mandible had a symmetric arch with good alignment of the teeth.

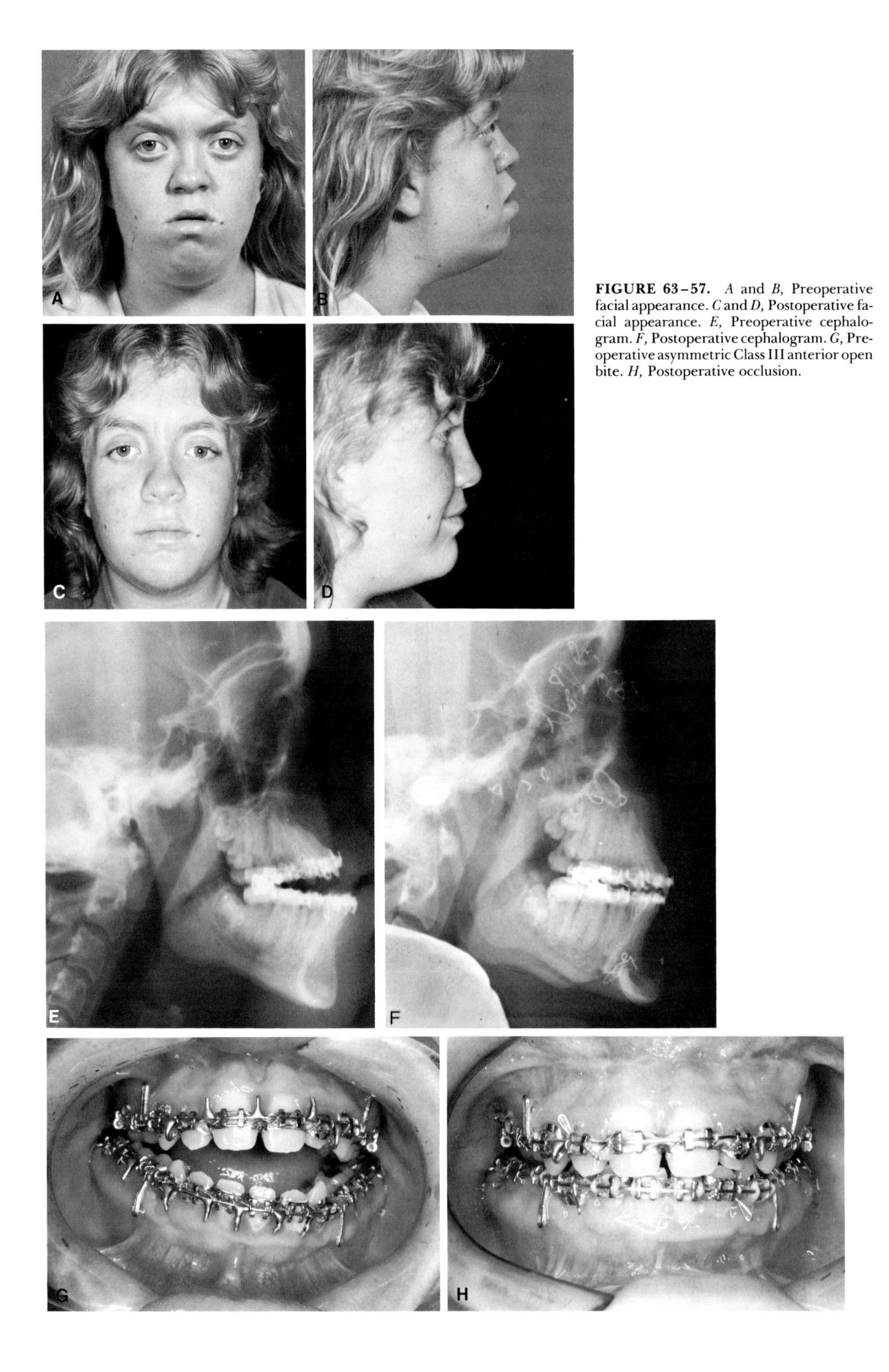

FIGURE 63–57. *A* and *B*, Preoperative facial appearance. *C* and *D*, Postoperative facial appearance. *E*, Preoperative cephalogram. *F*, Postoperative cephalogram. *G*, Preoperative asymmetric Class III anterior open bite. *H*, Postoperative occlusion.

III. Special Adjunctive Considerations

We are what we repeatedly do. Excellence, then, is not an act, but a habit.
— ARISTOTLE

1. MALAR MIDFACIAL AUGMENTATION

WILLIAM H. BELL

Augmentation of the malar bones and of the infraorbital and paranasal areas may be accomplished with alloplastic materials or onlay cortical bone grafts placed simultaneously with Le Fort I osteotomy. Implants are frequently used to augment the zygomas and infraorbital areas. Occasionally, submalar implants are placed to augment the area immediately subjacent to the malar bones. Augmentation of this type is most frequently indicated in low-level Le Fort I osteotomy. Refinements in the contours of the advanced maxilla are made with a combination of Avitene (collagen) and hydroxyapatite or other alloplastic materials.

Malar Midfacial Augmentation with Anatomic Silastic Implants

Cheekbone augmentation is a successful and consistently predictable cosmetic procedure. High cheekbones have always been recognized as a sign of beauty. Flatness of the cheekbones, however, seen in many patients with dentofacial and craniofacial deformities, tends to give an individual an older, expressionless, and sadder look. Simultaneous Le Fort I osteotomy and transoral malar bone augmentation may be done successfully in selected patients.[4,7,12,17,23]

Although individualization of the Le Fort I osteotomy design will frequently achieve desirable soft tissue changes of the midface, there are situations in which adjunctive augmentation is desirable and may be more practical. The patient undergoing low-level Le Fort I osteotomy frequently benefits from such adjunctive augmentation. When these procedures are performed simultaneously, careful, correlated consideration must be given to the soft tissue changes associated with movement of the overlying soft tissue (see Chapter 62).

The zygomatic prominence, also termed the malar eminence, is defined as the part below the lateral canthus that gives the impression of being the most prominent part of the malar complex in any view. The malar midfacial structures in Caucasians frequently benefit from simultaneous low-level Le Fort I osteotomy and augmentation of the malar bones and infraorbital rims. "High cheekbones," historically considered a characteristic of the beautiful face, most often refer to the highlighting of the ledge effect of the malar-midfacial structures produced by greater anterior and lateral projection at the malar eminences. The term does not necessarily refer to more superiorly positioned cheekbones, but rather to greater anterior and lateral projection at the malar eminence.

On occasion, patients may state very clearly their desire for prominent "cheekbones." Selection of the implant size and position will depend on the esthetic judgment of the surgeon and the patient's wishes. In patients with thin soft tissues and a diminutive face, smaller implants are used. On the other hand, larger implants may be indicated in patients with more massive facial morphology and thicker soft tissues.

The malar-midfacial region extends from the nasolabial ridge obliquely across the malar eminence and out onto the zygomatic arch. For surgical planning, the region is divided into the medial zone (paranasal area); the middle zone, comprising the malar eminence (cheekbone); and the lateral zone, comprising the zygomatic arch.[23] Ideally, the middle zone is most prominent in the anterolateral plane. The lateral zone is most prominent in a lateral direction and is the widest point of the face. All three zones and the symmetry of each must be considered when the malar-midfacial region is to be altered.[23] The supraorbital ridges should project 4 to 8 mm anterior to the anterior surface of the cornea; the highlight of the malar eminence should project slightly beyond the cornea.

Preoperative Assessment

Analysis of the patient must be accomplished before surgery. With the patient in the supine position on the operating room table, it is impossible to judge how thick or thin the implant should be and exactly where it should be positioned. Implant size and position depend on esthetic judgment and the individual patient's desires.

Since a lack of agreement on the location of the malar eminence exists, it is difficult to assess what is normal, what is proportionate and esthetic, and what is disproportionate and unesthetic. In short, the surgeon must individualize the plan of treatment on the basis of clinical judgment in addition to objective measurements.

Skin thickness and the magnitude of bony hypoplasia in all three dimensions of space indicate the size of the implant. In the malar-midfacial regions, implants 6 mm thick (medium size) are most commonly used. When the overlying tissues are relatively thick and the bony deficiency is sizable, large implants 8 mm thick will probably be indicated. When, however, the skin is thin and relatively little augmentation is necessary, small implants (4 mm) may be used.

Implant size must be determined prior to surgery, with careful consideration given to the symmetry of the two sides of the face and the possible need for different-sized implants or carving to reduce implant prominence in one of the three zones. This is most likely to be necessary in the medial zone. Generally, this prominence is 10 to 15 mm lateral and 15 to 20 mm inferior to the lateral canthus. In a critical assessment of this prominence, the patient should be viewed from a 45-degree oblique angle and a submental vertex angle. Then, an assessment of the supraorbital and infraorbital rims and of the maxillary anteroposterior and vertical position, as reflected by soft tissue drape, must be considered in establishing the true esthetic position of the lateral prominence of the malar complex. No single measurement, angular or linear, will totally suffice. The final decision on augmentation should be made with the use of onlay sizers that directly simulate the effect of the implant to be used.

Marking of the Implant Site on the Skin — an Option

The infraorbital groove and foramen along the lower orbital rim are carefully observed. The infraorbital groove and foramen are approximately 1 cm below the infraorbital rim and may be marked on the overlying skin with a vertical line. Another major landmark is the malar prominence, determined by palpating the most prominent part of the malar eminence. The proposed implant may be placed on the skin prior to surgery and outlined in proper position over the malar eminence and zygoma just lateral to the infraorbital foramen (Fig. 63–58A). A subperiosteal pocket is created with a periosteal elevator directly beneath the area marked on the skin of the proposed site for the alloplastic implant (Fig. 63–58B). The marking of the implant site on the skin is a rarely used option.

Exposure of the Implant Site

A precise subperiosteal plane of dissection will ensure accurate, reproducible, and symmetric results. The circumvestibular incision used for Le Fort I osteotomy offers excellent accessibility to the malar bones, zygomatic arches, and infraorbital area (Fig. 63–58B).

The soft tissue margins of the circumvestibular incision are easily modified and retracted superiorly with a periosteal elevator, to create a ledge of soft tissue for the implant to rest against. This ledge provides a thickness of tissue so that the implant is not palpable in the upper buccal sulcus and facilitates positioning of the implant.

The subperiosteal dissection is extended superiorly, laterally, and inferiorly across the malar eminence. The infraorbital rim medial and lateral to the infraorbital nerve is meticulously exposed. The thumb and index finger of the hand that is not holding the periosteal elevator are maintained sequentially on the superior and inferior edges of the malar eminence, and then on the zygomatic arch. The periosteal elevator is passed precisely on bone between the thumb and index finger, avoiding straying off the bone edges, so that the implant will duplicate bone extension and rest soundly on the bone itself. The dissection is carried laterally past the zygomaticotemporal suture to the point where the zygomatic arch starts to turn medially or posteriorly. This lateral extension of the pocket is stretched so as to be large enough to receive one of the three different implant sizers (small, medium, and large). All soft tissue is carefully dissected off the bone, allowing the implant to rest directly and passively against bone.

The pocket should be large enough to visualize the implant as it is fed into the pocket with a smooth tissue forceps. The implant is first directed along the zygomatic arch, and then the medial portion is positioned downward and underneath the infraorbital foramen area.

The implant position should be such that the superior aspect curves naturally with the orbital rim and is designed to extend to the infraorbital rim. Once the soft tissue pocket has been created on one side, the distalmost or lateral end of the implant sizer is grasped with a tissue forceps. A long, curved-out Langenbeck retractor is inserted through the full extent of the pocket. The pocket is visually inspected as far as can be seen, to make certain all soft tissue has been removed from bone. This visualization is greatly implemented by the use of a headlight or fiberoptic attachment. Now the implant sizer is inserted to the full lateral extent of the pocket, and held in place passively at its medial end, which is now within the pocket, before the retractor is removed (Fig. 63–58C). The medial end of the implant must rest passively in the medial end of the pocket, without any tendency to buckling or medial shift. If there is any pressure or medial shift, the size of the pocket is inadequate. Further dissection or a smaller sizer is used, depending on the surgeon's esthetic judgment. The inferior edge of the medial portion of the implant should also rest passively against the ledge of soft tissue that was created. The medial edge of the implant should rest just lateral and inferior to the infraorbital nerve and inferior to the infraorbital rim. It should be verified that the implant exerts no pressure against the infraorbital nerve. If necessary, a V-wedge can be removed from the superior surface of the implant to accommodate the infraorbital nerve. When the esthetic result is satisfactory, the implant sizer is replaced by the comparable implant, which is easily stabilized to underlying bone with one positional screw that fixes the implant to the bone (Fig. 63–58D). Great care is exercised to position the implants symmetrically. By direct examination and palpation, the proper position and orientation are assured. Once the implant of desired size is in position, it is anchored to the underlying bone with one or two positional screws that are fixed to the body of the zygoma. Excellent stability of the implant is ensured when the implant becomes enveloped by a connective tissue capsule.

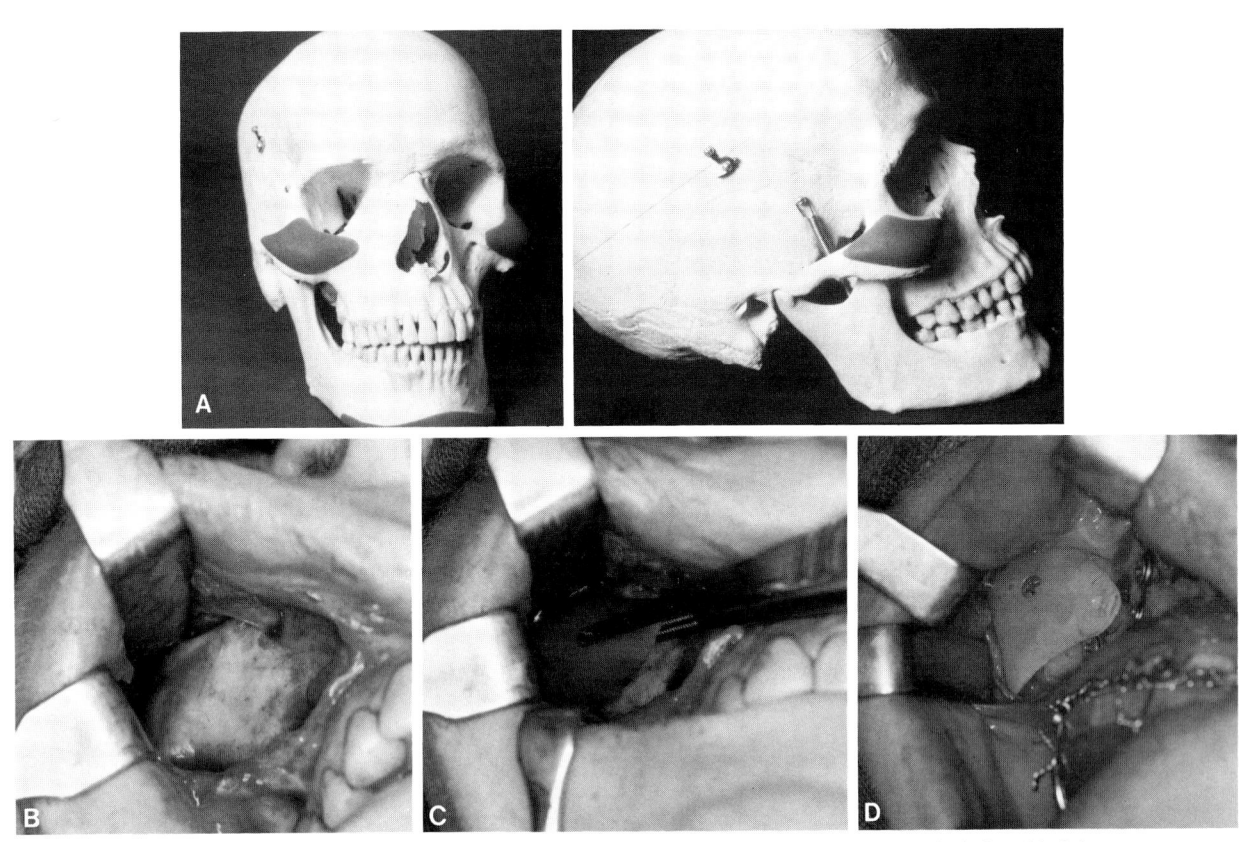

FIGURE 63-58. *A, Left* and *right*, Preformed implant sizers are positioned on the malar bones. *B,* The infraorbital rim, malar eminence, and zygomatic arch are routinely widely exposed by subperiosteal undermining. *C,* The implant sizer is trial fitted, and the implant site is adjusted until the sizer is passively seated. *D,* The McGhan implant is passively seated and stabilized to the malar bone with a 2-mm by 10-mm self-tapping positional screw. *E* and *F,* Preoperative facial appearance of a 15-year-old girl with three-dimensional facial asymmetry. *G* and *H,* Facial appearance after step Le Fort I osteotomy, intraoral and vertical ramus osteotomies, straightening genioplasty, and augmentation of the malar bones. Preformed Silastic implants were placed through circumvestibular incisions following completion of the planned three-segment Le Fort I osteotomy. *I,* Facial appearance of a 35-year-old cleft lip and palate patient with three-dimensional lack of malar bone prominence. *J,* Facial appearance 1 year after intraoral placement of medium-sized Silastic implants on malar bones.

Advantages and Disadvantages of Malar Implants

A "submarine"-style anatomic implant that has become available during recent years is most commonly used for augmentation of the malar bone (Fig. 63–58*E* to *J*). A superior projection fits on the orbital projection of the zygoma. The implants, which are feathered at their periphery, are available in three sizes. Implants may be trimmed to form with a scalpel or scissors to meet the individual patient's requirements. The anatomically designed implants, however, usually provide an accurate contour to the facial structure with minimal alteration.

A disadvantage of the preformed silicone cheek implants is the fact that Silastic has memory; consequently, great care must be exercised intraoperatively to ensure that the implant lies passively on the underlying bone to prevent migration and an unesthetic, asymmetric, and untapered margin. Although it is tempting to squeeze the implant into a small pocket, assuming that this will prevent displacement, an adequate pocket should be developed. On the basis of preliminary clinical assessment, the desired sizer is selected and inserted to be sure that it is seated passively. Implant displacement is inevitable if the implant is squeezed into a pocket that is too small. A small pocket will produce tension, which may cause displacement. The capsule that forms around the implant stabilizes the implant in the desired position. Occasionally, one of the stock sizes has to be carved to produce a custom stabilized

FIGURE 63-58 *Continued*

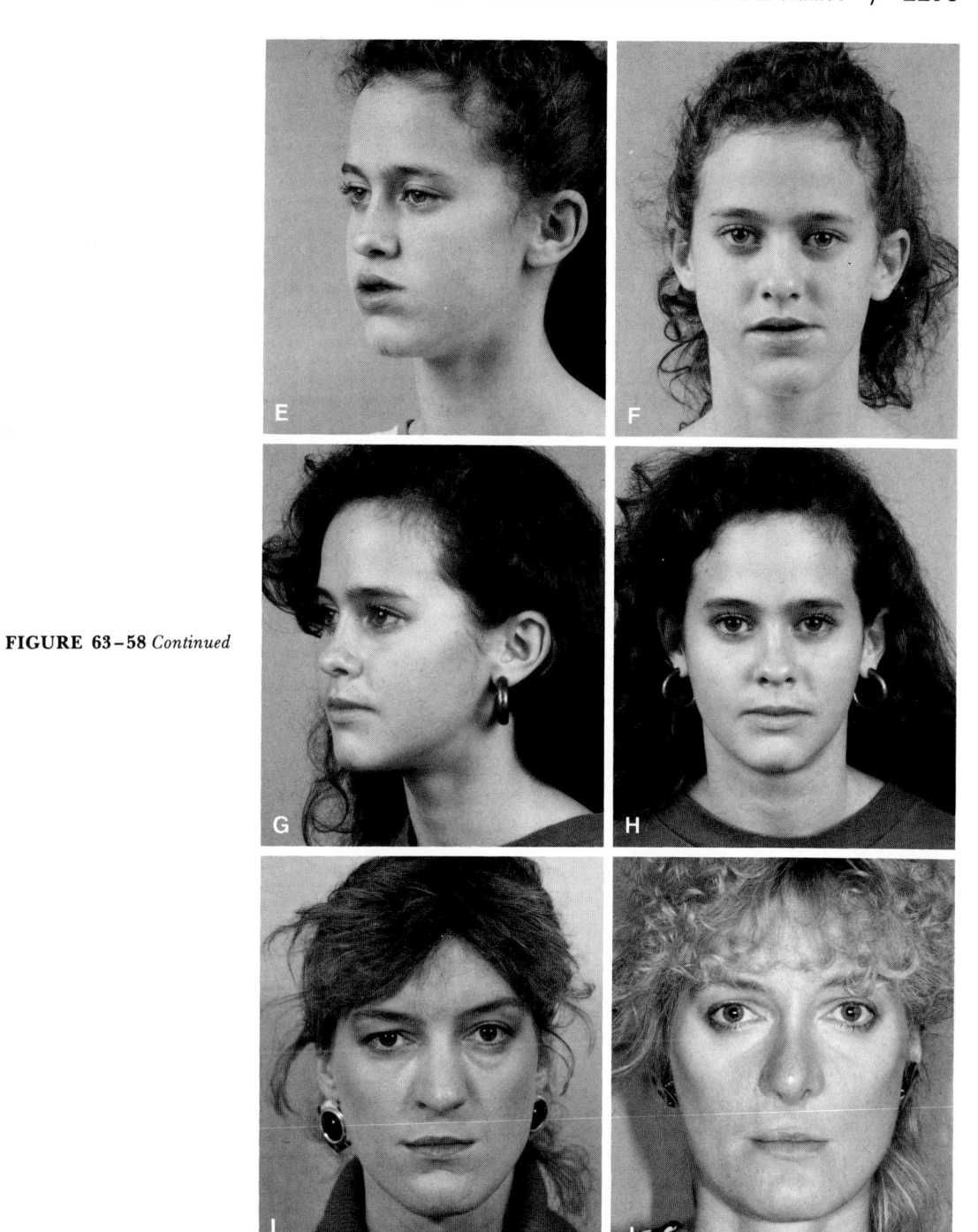

fit. More commonly, however, one of the three available standard sizes (small, medium, or large) will produce the desired effect with minimal or no necessary alterations.

Submalar Augmentation

Fullness of the cheeks is one of the strongest characteristics of youth, suggesting the presence of healthy midfacial soft tissues. Midthird facial deficiency and degeneration of the underlying soft tissues combine to produce morphologic changes and signs of facial aging. Such changes are commonly revealed by the development

2294 / VII — ORTHOGNATHIC SURGERY

of folds and depressions of the cheeks. Patients who prematurely exhibit these signs of aging may be candidates for simultaneous Le Fort I osteotomy and submalar augmentation.[5]

Submalar augmentation in patients with deficient bone structure or severe atrophy of overlying soft tissue helps to restore youthful fullness to the cheeks. Subperiosteal tunneling through circumvestibular incisions provides complete exposure of the anterior surface of the maxilla and lateral zygomatic areas. The areas subjacent to the inferior surface of the zygoma and over the tendinous insertions of the masseter muscle are similarly exposed.

The facial morphology and appropriate anatomic configuration are identified by careful clinical assessment. Sizers may be used adjunctively in choosing the appropriate-sized submalar implant. The submalar implants are made of soft, solid silicone rubber in a three-dimensional anatomic design contoured to accommodate the variation of midfacial bone structure. The implants are individualized for each patient and are carved to form if necessary (frequently unnecessary). The bulk of the implant is placed over the anterior surface of the maxilla. The tapered, posterolateral extension rests on the superior tendinous attachments of the masseter muscle. Alternatively, the posterolateral extension may be wrapped around the zygomatic arch. After the size is selected, the implant is placed on the anterior skin surface and outlined in the desired position. Proper placement of the implant augments the skeletal structure and provides natural contours to the face. The major part of the implant is usually positioned along the inferior edge of the zygoma. When used in conjunction with Le Fort I osteotomy surgery, submalar implants are easily positioned and passively stabilized to the underlying bone with one or two positional screws (Fig. 63–59A to D).

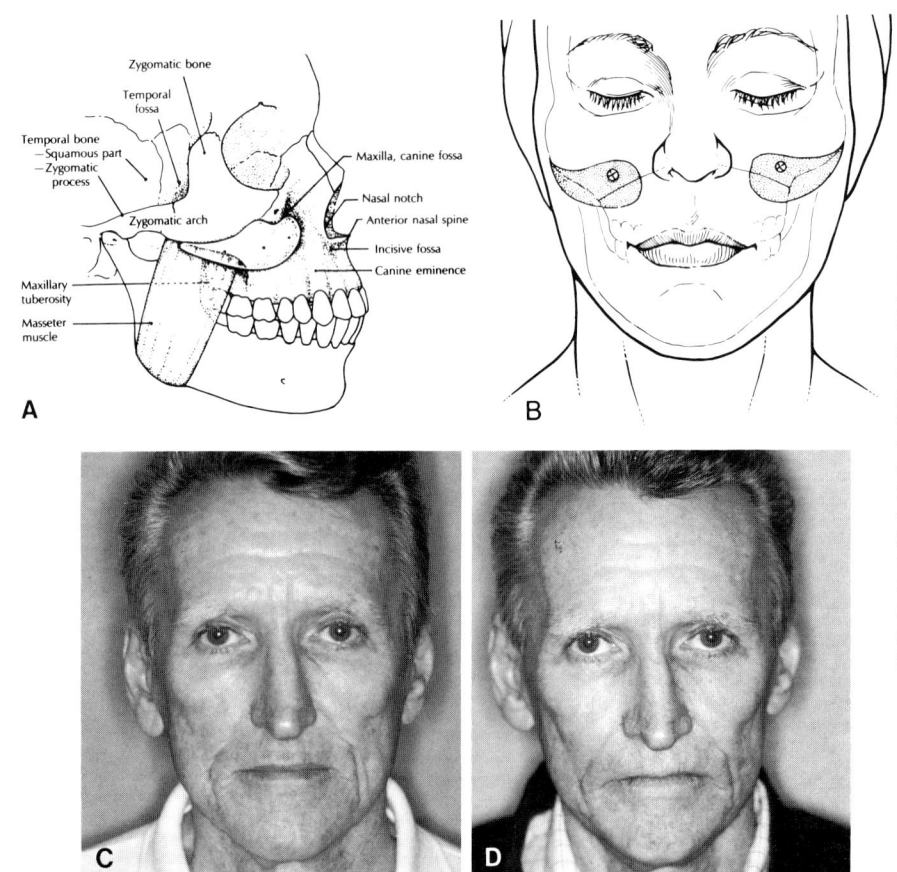

FIGURE 63–59. *A,* The curved lateral portion of the Binder submalar implant extends around the malar eminence to create a "high cheek bone" appearance. The implant is fixed to the underlying bone with a single self-tapping screw. *B,* The implant is inserted and observed for fullness, position, and symmetry. Ideally, the Le Fort I osteotomy is individualized to correct the midfacial deformity. *C* and *D,* Facial appearance of a patient who has the stigmata of anteroposterior maxillary deficiency and was a good candidate for simultaneous Le Fort I osteotomy and submalar augmentation. Facial appearance before (*C*) and after (*D*) Le Fort I osteotomy and placement of the submalar implant.

Augmentation of the Midface with Bone Grafts

Onlay bone grafts have been used widely in the restoration and augmentation of the facial skeleton (Fig. 63–60A to C). Clinical and experimental studies have demonstrated, however, that there is often a significant and unpredictable loss of graft volume because of resorption. This phenomenon has prompted much investigation into the basic biology of onlay bone grafting. Multiple factors that are thought to play a significant role in graft survival have been defined.

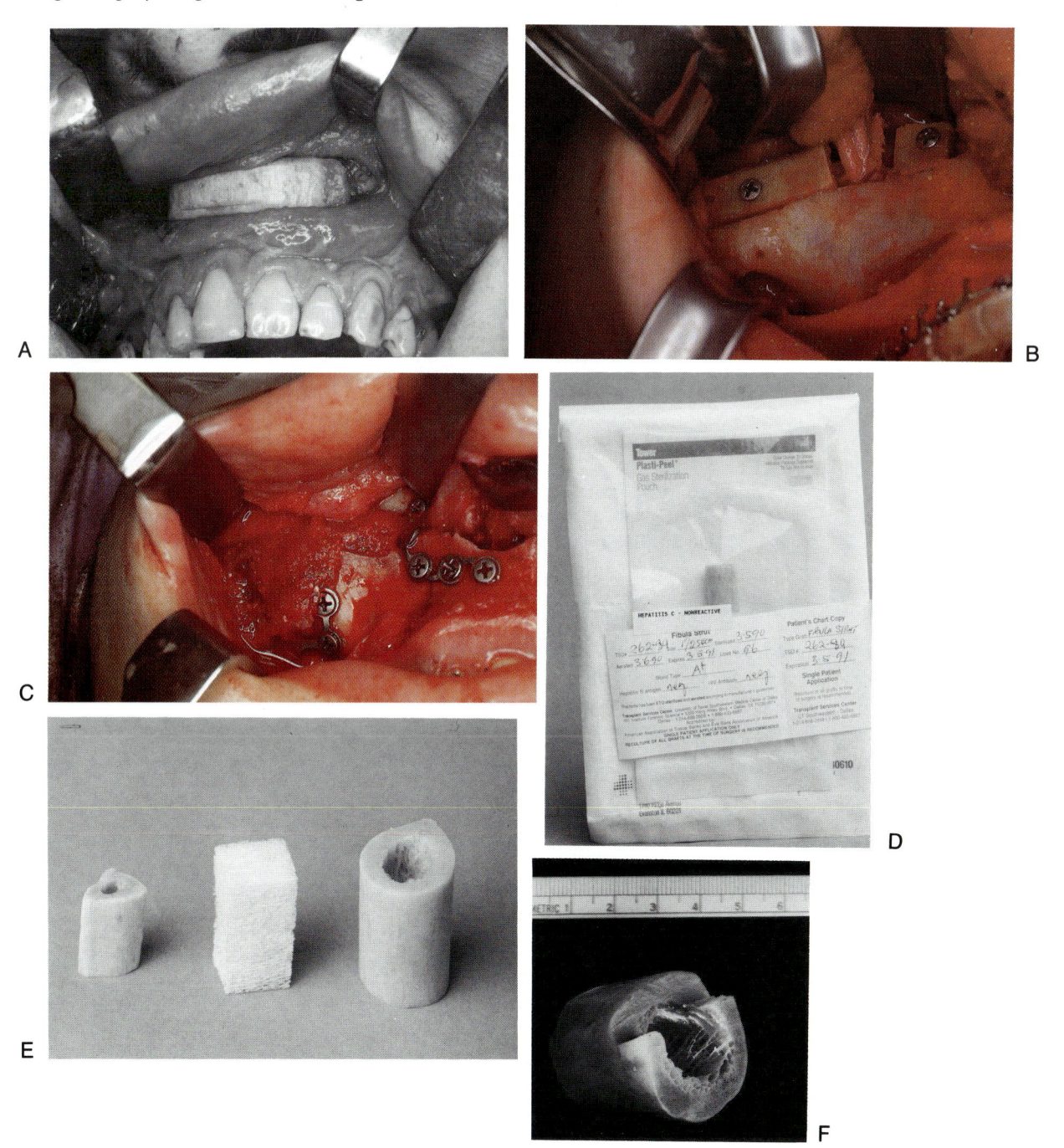

FIGURE 63–60. *A,* Onlay bone graft harvested from the chin and applied to the base of the nose. *B,* Onlay autogenous cortical bone grafts applied to the infraorbital rim and malar bone. *C,* Augmentation of the infraorbital rims and malar bones with cortical onlay grafts stabilized with countersunk lag screws. *D,* Allogeneic bone allograft stored in sterile plastic container. *E,* Various anatomic sources of allogeneic bone implants (left to right): fibula, cancellous plug, and tibia. *F,* Cross-sectional view of tibial allogeneic bone, which was shaped to serve as an onlay implant to the anterior aspect of the maxilla.

Maintenance of Onlay Bone Grafts

Clinical observations and experimental evaluations have identified various factors that may influence the ultimate resorption or incorporation of autogenous bone grafts.[1-3,8-10,14,15,24-26] These include the following: (1) the histologic bony architecture (cancellous or cortical), (2) the presence or absence of periosteum, (3) the graft orientation (position of cancellous, cortical, or periosteal surface in relation to the soft tissue envelope), (4) the recipient bed (irradiation, scarring, soft tissue construction, and infection), (5) the recipient location (resorptive or depository surface), (6) the rate of revascularization (early versus delayed), (7) the graft viability (vascularized and nonvascularized bone grafts), (8) the type of fixation (or lack of fixation), (9) the host's age at the time of grafting, (10) the graft dimensions (length, width, and height), (11) the implantation site (orthotopic or heterotopic), (12) the graft position in relation to mechanical stress (inlay, onlay, or bridging), and (13) the embryonic origin of the graft.

Autogenous bone grafting generally is felt to be the most effective method of restoring onlay osseous defects. There is, however, considerable discussion regarding the optimal anatomic form that the transplant should take. Several recent experimental studies have concluded that autogenous onlay membranous grafts, orthotopically placed, are less resorptive than endochondral grafts, heterotopically placed. The dense architecture (more cortical bone) of onlay membranous bone grafts is postulated to be a critical factor that is responsible for its decreased resorption. In addition, animal and clinical studies indicate that long-term permanence and maintenance of osseous contour are a result of the functional stimulation of osseointegrated implants.

The experimental findings of LaTrenta and colleagues indicated that rigid fixation of bone grafts increased the weight and volume of membranous and endochondral onlay bone grafts when compared with wire fixation. They hypothesized that rigid skeletal fixation served three important functions: (1) complete immobilization of the bone graft, (2) compression, and (3) early consolidation of the graft–recipient bed junction.

The maxillofacial surgeon is called upon frequently to augment deficient bony contour with endochondral or membranous bone. Clinically, cortical or corticocancellous bone is available from a multitude of sources, both autogenous and allogeneic. The common denominator of success has been the dense architecture of the onlay bone graft (cortical bone). Autogenous cortical bone from the cranium, hip, mental symphysis, or mandibular ramus has been used selectively to augment and reconstruct deficient bony contour of the malar bone, infraorbital rims, paranasal areas, and skeletal nasal base. A mixture of particulate hydroxyapatite and Avitene to which a small amount of saline has been added is readily mixed into a material of doughy consistency, which serves well as a contour restoration material and may be used in conjunction with bone grafts.

Bone Allografts for Transplantation*

Allograft bone is obtained from donors who have been found to have a negative medical history for sepsis, communicable disease, cancer, or death from unknown causes. These donors also have a negative serologic test for syphilis (STS), as well as nonreactive serologic testing for human immunodeficiency virus (HIV) antibody, hepatitis B surface antigen (HBsAg), HCV, and human T-cell lymphotropic virus–1 (HTLV–1); further, bacterial cultures from these donors do not exhibit any indication of systemic septic processes.

---

*Transplant Services Center, UT Southwestern Medical Center, Dallas, TX.

Bone is processed by cleaning all extraneous tissue and periosteum following an aseptic surgical extraction. Grafts are cleaned with pyrogen-free deionized water and defatted in three washes of 10 per cent sodium hypochlorite followed by three washes of absolute ethyl alcohol (ETOH). Each wash is followed by three rinses in pyrogen-free deionized water. Bone is air dried and sterilized by exposure to ETOH or gamma irradiation.

The bone, which is stored in sterile plastic containers at room temperature, provides a practical and useful source of bone for onlay grafting (Fig. 63–60D). Over the past 3 years, tibia and fibula onlay grafts have been used selectively in the paranasal, malar, infraorbital, and base of the nose regions (Fig. 63–60E and F). They have been occasionally combined with hydroxyapatite and Avitene or autogenous particulate marrow grafts. Preliminary clinical results with these allografts have been encouraging, although it is premature to conclude what their ultimate fate will be and how they will compare with autogenous cortical onlay cranial, iliac crest, or local bone grafts (taken from the mental symphysis or the ramus of the mandible).

Allogeneic tibia and fibula have been used to selectively augment the bony contour of the midface. Because of the very dense architecture of the cortical onlay bone grafts, bone holes are carefully drilled, tapped, countersunk, and stabilized with long bone screws or plates or both. Reducing onlay cortical bone grafts to the proper size and dimension is considerably more difficult than contouring cancellous bone. Careful selection of the allogeneic graft from a multitude of available sizes and shapes in the bone bank facilitates the process and reduces the amount of graft manipulation at the time of surgery. Templates patterned from posteroanterior and lateral cephalographs, careful presurgical analysis of the patient's face, and the use of Silastic sizers implement graft selection, preparation, and procurement.

REFERENCES

1. Albrektsson T: Repair of bone grafts. A vital microscopic and histological investigation in the rabbit. Scand J Plast Reconstr Surg 14:1, 1980.
2. Antonyshyn O, Colcleugh RG, Anderson C, Path FRC: Growth potential in onlay bone grafts: A comparison of vascularized and free calvarial bone and sutural bone grafts. Plast Reconstr Surg 79:12, 1987.
3. Bassett CL: Clinical implications of cell function in bone grafting. Clin Orthop 87:49, 1972.
4. Belinfante LS, Mitchell DL: Use of alloplastic material in the canine fossa–zygomatic area to improve facial esthetics. J Oral Surg 35:121, 1977.
5. Binder WJ: Submalar augmentation: A procedure to enhance rhytidectomy. Ann Plast Surg 24(3):200, 1990.
6. Binder WJ, Kamer FM, Parkes ML: Mentoplasty—a clinical analysis of alloplastic implants. Laryngoscope 91:383, 1981.
7. Brennan HG: Augmentation malarplasty. Arch Otolaryngol 108:441, 1982.
8. Burchardt H: The biology of bone graft repair. Clin Orthop 174:28, 1983.
9. Gray JC, Elves MW: Early osteogenesis in compact bone isografts: A quantitative study of the contributions of the different graft cells. Calcif Tissue Int 29:225, 1979.
10. Habal MB, Reddi AH: An update on bone grafting and bone substitutes in reconstructive surgery. Adv Plast Reconstr Surg 3:147, 1987.
11. Hauben DJ, van der Meulen JCH: The use of musculoperiosteal flap for correction of craniofacial anomalies: Experimental study. In Williams HB (ed): Transactions of the VIII International Congress of Plastic and Reconstructive Surgery. Quebec, McGill University Press, 1983, p 72.
12. Hinderer UT: Malar implants for improvement of the facial appearance. Plast Reconstr Surg 56:157, 1975.
13. Hurley LA, Stinchfield FE, Bassett AL: The role of soft tissue in osteogenesis. J Bone Joint Surg 41A:1243, 1959.
14. Knize DM: The influence of periosteum and calcitonin on onlay bone graft survival: A roentgenographic study. Plast Reconstr Surg 53:190, 1974.
15. Kusiak, JF, Zins JE, Whitaker LA: The early revascularization of membranous bone. Plast Reconstr Surg 76:510, 1985.
16. Lozano AJ, Cestero HJ Jr, Salyer KE: The early vascularization of onlay bone grafts. Plast Reconstr Surg 58:302, 1976.
17. Powell NB, Riley RW, Laub DR: A new approach to evaluation and surgery of the malar complex. Ann Plast Surg 20:206, 1988.

18. Smith JD, Abramson M: Membranous versus endochondral bone autografts. Arch Otolaryngol 99:203, 1974.
19. Thompson N, Casson JA: Experimental onlay bone grafts to the jaws: A preliminary study in dogs. Plast Reconstr Surg 46:341, 1970.
20. Thorogood PV, Gray JC: The cellular changes during osteogenesis in bone and bone marrow composite autografts. J Anat 120:27, 1975.
21. Waite PD, Matukas VJ: Zygomatic augmentation with hydroxylapatite: A preliminary report. J Oral Maxillofac Surg 44(5):349, 1986.
22. Weiland AJ, Phillips TW, Randolph MA: Bone grafts: A radiologic, histologic, and biomechanical model comparing autografts, allografts, and free vascularized bone grafts. Plast Reconstr Surg 74:368, 1984.
23. Whitaker LA: Aesthetic augmentation of the malar-midface structures. Plast Reconstr Surg 80:337, 1987.
24. Wilkes GH, Kernahan DA, Christenson M: The long-term survival of onlay bone grafts. A comparative study in mature and immature animals. Ann Plast Surg 15:374, 1985.
25. Zins JE, Kusiak JF, Whitaker LA, Enlow DH: The influence of the recipient site on bone grafts to the face. Plast Reconstr Surg 73:371, 1984.
26. Zins JE, Whitaker LA: Membranous versus endochondral bone: Implications for craniofacial reconstruction. Plast Reconstr Surg 72:778, 1983.

2. AUGMENTATION OF THE MALAR PROMINENCE BY SAGITTAL OSTEOTOMY OF THE ZYGOMA AND INTERPOSITIONAL BONE GRAFTING*

MICHAEL G. DONOVAN

Facial beauty and harmony are directly related to correct facial proportions and certain characteristics viewed as desirable by society. The effect of lateral facial prominence in the midface or malar region is one such desirable characteristic. The proportional oval face with prominence in the malar region is a facial feature held in high esteem and used to attract attention in advertisements. Hypoplasia or asymmetry of the malar region may distort the nasal profile and add to the impression of a long, narrow face. The majority of the surgical procedures described in the literature for treatment of transverse midface deficiency with flattening of the malar eminence involve the use of onlayed alloplastic materials.[2,3,7,13,15] Some of the problems noted with the use of these techniques are implant migration, capsule formation, error in positioning, incorrect choice of implant, infection, and the patient's awareness of its presence.[16]

The use of autogenous materials to augment the malar region may avoid some of the problems associated with the use of alloplastic materials. Surgical techniques for malar augmentation and reconstruction utilizing autogenous materials employ costal cartilage,[14] conchal cartilage,[12] rib grafts,[8] iliac bone grafts,[5] and calvarial bone grafts.[10] Disadvantages noted with the use of onlay autogenous materials are graft resorption,[4,6] difficulty in the proper contouring of the graft material, and potential donor site morbidity.

The sagittal osteotomy of the zygoma with interpositional bone grafting, as originally described by Powell,[10] has several advantages when used to correct transverse maxillary deficiency and augment the malar prominence. An alternate surgical technique for the correction of transverse maxillary deficiency and augmentation of the malar region is the sagittal osteotomy of the zygoma with interpositional bone grafting on hydroxyapatite.

---

* The opinions or assertions contained herein are the private views of the author and are not to be construed as official or as reflecting the views of the Department of the Army or the Department of Defense.

Indications

Numerous widely accepted cephalometric analyses are available for evaluating facial proportions in the vertical plane.[2] The cephalometric standards for evaluating the bony skeleton and soft tissues in the transverse plane, particularly in the malar region, are not as well defined.[11] When the patient is evaluated for transverse midface augmentation, the clinical assessment by the surgeon and the patient's desires are crucial in determining the extent of the augmentation.

The most common indication for the treatment of transverse maxillary deficiency is the long face syndrome. The patient who presents with excessive vertical growth, with or without apertognathia, will also frequently display a transverse midface deficiency related to the facial growth pattern. Numerous treatment modalities exist for addressing the narrow vertical facial growth pattern. The corrective surgical procedures may include superior repositioning of the total maxilla or of the posterior maxilla, or a vertical reduction genioplasty.[1,9] When used as an adjunctive procedure, the sagittal osteotomy of the zygoma with interpositonal bone grafting will correct the transverse midface deficiency and add to the overall facial proportions and harmony.

Patients with an asymmetric facial growth pattern may display hypoplasia of the zygomatic complex on the affected side, in conjunction with underdevelopment of the maxillomandibular complex.[2] Unilateral zygomatic augmentation of the affected zygomatic complex in hemifacial microsomia or one of the variants of this facial developmental growth problem can be easily accomplished in conjunction with the maxillary and mandibular surgery. Unilateral augmentation of the affected zygoma that is done when the maxillomandibular disharmony is being corrected will allow for a more complete correction of the patient's developmental problem. The patient who has suffered trauma and who has a less than optimal restoration of the normal lateral projection of the zygomatic buttress can also benefit from this procedure.

Patients seeking facial cosmetic surgery frequently desire "more prominent cheek bones." The sagittal osteotomy of the zygoma with interpositional bone grafting is a short surgical procedure with predictable results that has met with consistent approval by the patient. The biggest disadvantage with the technique has to do with the lack of anteroposterior augmentation of the malar bone.

Surgical Technique

The incision used to expose the zygomatic buttress is similar to that used for the Le Fort I osteotomy. A horizontal incision is made at the depth of the maxillary vestibule. The lateral prominence of the zygomatic buttress is palpated and serves as a landmark for the posterior extension of the incision. The incision is extended anteriorly to the lateral extension of the piriform rim to allow adequate relaxation of the incision and exposure of the entire zygoma. If the zygomatic augmentation is to be done in conjunction with a maxillary procedure, the standard Le Fort I incision will allow for adequate exposure. The incision is carried sharply to bone, and a subperiosteal dissection is utilized to expose the anterior, lateral, and posterior surfaces of the zygoma. A careful subperiosteal dissection will prevent herniation of the buccal fat pad into the operative field.

Once the exposure of the zygoma is completed inferiorly, the dissection is continued superiorly to identify the lateral orbital rim. The dissection is then redirected slightly posteriorly and continued superiorly until the junction of the posterior surface of the lateral orbital rim and the superior surface of the temporal process of the zygoma is exposed. Release of the anterior fibers of the masseter muscle will be required for adequate exposure and will facilitate the placement of a channel retractor on the superior surface of the temporal process of the zygoma

6. Donald PJ, Col A: Cartilage implantation in head and neck surgery: Report of a national survey. Otolaryngol Head Neck Surg 90:85, 1982.
7. Kent JN, Westfall RL, Carlton DM: Chin and zygomaticomaxillary augmentation with Proplast: Long-term follow-up. J Oral Surg 39:912, 1981.
8. Longacre JJ, deStefano GA, Holmstrand K: The early versus late reconstruction of congenital hypoplasias of the facial skeleton and skull. Plast Reconstr Surg 27:489, 1961.
9. McBride KL, Bell WH: Chin surgery. In Bell WH, Profitt WR, White RP (eds): Surgical Correction of Dentofacial Deformities. Philadelphia, WB Saunders Company, 1980, pp 1210–1279.
10. Powell NB, Riley RW: Cranial bone grafting in facial aesthetic and reconstructive contouring. Arch Otolaryngol Head Neck Surg 113:713, 1987.
11. Prendergast M, Schoenrock LD: Malar augmentation. Patient classification and placement. Arch Otolaryngol Head Neck Surg 115:964, 1989.
12. Siemian WR, Samiian MR: Malar augmentation using autogenous composite conchal cartilage and temporalis fascia. Plast Reconstr Surg 80:395, 1988.
13. Silver WE: The use of alloplastic material in contouring the face. Facial Plast Surg 3:81, 1986.
14. Straith CL, Lewis JR: Associated congenital defects of the ears, eyelids, and malar bones (Treacher Collins syndrome). Plast Reconstr Surg 4:204, 1949.
15. Waite PD, Matukas VJ: Zygomatic augmentation with hydroxylapatite: A preliminary report. J Maxillofac Surg 44:349, 1986.
16. Wilkinson TS: Complications in aesthetic malar augmentation. Plast Reconstr Surg 71:643, 1983.

3. ZYGOMATIC COMPLEX REDUCTION — SYSTEM FOR ACCURATE BILATERAL SYMMETRIC REDUCTION

CESAR E. SOLANO

Clinical judgment during surgery in the past has frequently been used to determine the amount of bone to be removed. This practice, however, has sometimes led to increased surgical time and unpredictable, asymmetric results. The achievement of a symmetric reduction has been difficult with these methods. The technique described here achieves a bilateral symmetric reduction of the zygomaticomaxillary complex (ZMC). The principles of this technique can also be applied to mentoplasty when osteotomy of the inferior border of the mandible is not indicated.

The workup for an accurate symmetric bilateral reduction of prominent malar bones involves three-dimensional planning considerations. At present, no surgical technique allows accurate symmetric reduction and contouring of the malar bones. The following technique will facilitate the achievement of predictable results and allows for an esthetic and symmetric reduction of the prominent malar bones.

Technique

A template is first made from an autoclavable material (sheet Silastic), either directly from the patient's face or from a facial moulage. The template determines the three-dimensional extensions of the ostectomy. The same template is used in the right and left zygomatic regions. A standard circumvestibular incision or bicoronal flaps are utilized to achieve adequate surgical access to the ZMC. The template is placed over the ZMC, using the orbital rim as a reference. With a No. 1 round bur, a map is drawn over the ZMC around the template. This map delineates the superoinferior and lateral extension of the area to be surgically reduced. On the basis of a submental cephalometric radiograph and computerized tomographic (CT) scan, the amount of anteroposterior reduction is determined. The amount of reduction required will confirm the clinical impressions that were formed during the precise clinical examination. The template has four perforated holes (A,B,C, and D), which are used as guides for the symmetric placement of the bur. With the tip of the bur at a known determined distance from the base of the handpiece and with the template over the surgical site, the drill bur is placed inside template perforation A. Similar perforations are made in the B,C, and D areas. The perforations of each hole are made until the base of the handpiece contacts the outer cortex. The depth of the bony perforations determines the magnitude of the anteroposterior reduction. Finally, all perforations are connected, and recontouring of the ZMC is accomplished with a barrel-shaped bur.

A 27-year-old man sought treatment to reduce his prominent cheekbones (Fig. 63–69). Clinical examination, photographs, facial moulage, CT scan, and radiographic analyses were used to develop a treatment plan and quantitate the amount of bone to be removed. This technique decreased the risk of asymmetric and unesthetic reduction of the ZMC during surgery.

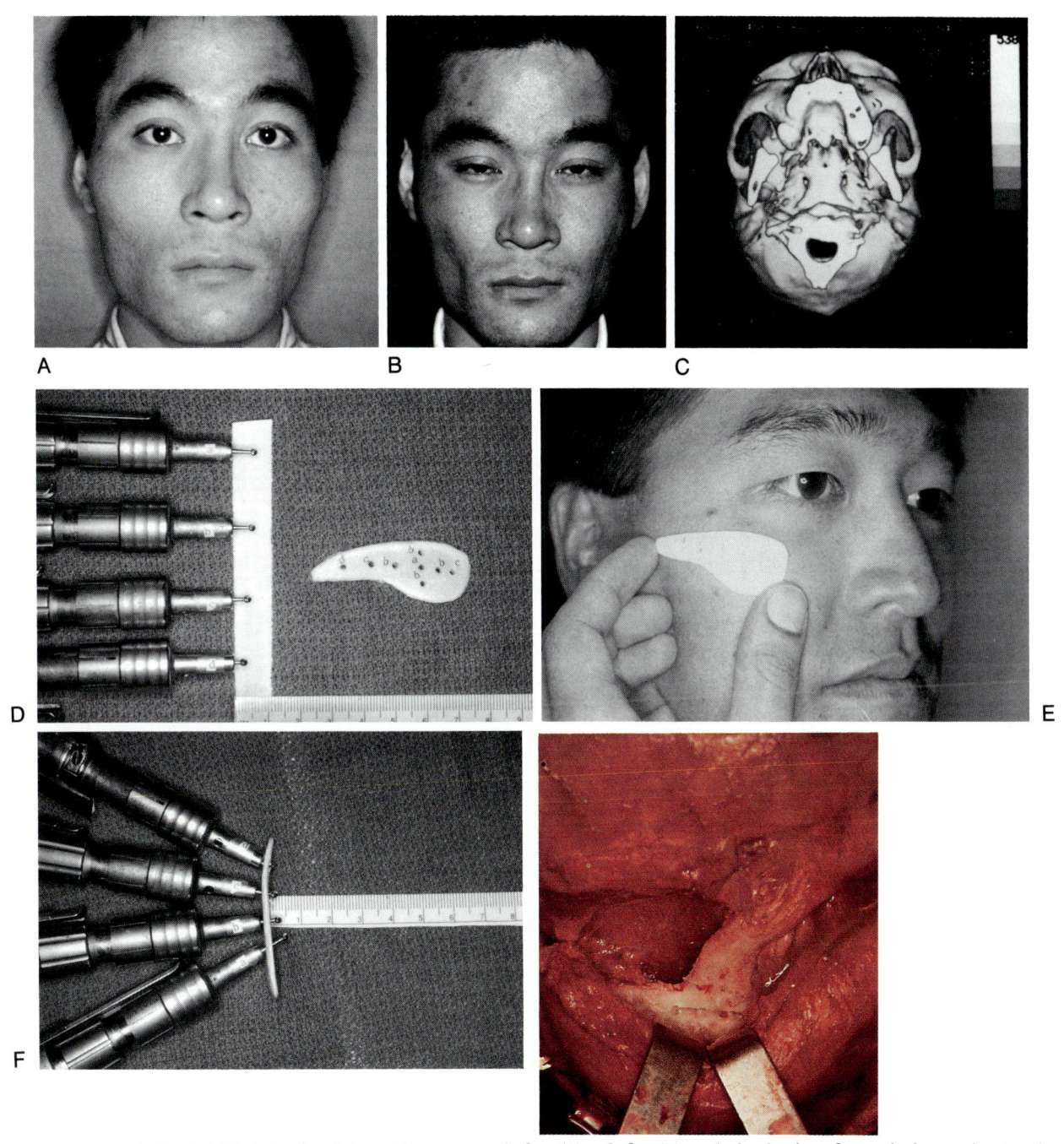

FIGURE 63–69. *A* and *B*, Facial appearance before *(A)* and after *(B)* surgical reduction of excessively prominent malar bones. *C*, Computerized tomographic (CT) scan used to analyze the amount of malar bone reduction. *D*, Template with perforations of variable length made with 4 handpieces with burs of different lengths. *E*, Template positioned over the malar bone at surgery. *F*, Four drilled holes of variable length *(left)*, which determine the depth of the reduction *(right)*.

4. MODEL SURGERY FOR FACIAL ASYMMETRY DEFORMITIES

KIM ERICKSON
DOUGLAS GOLDSMITH

Correction of complex facial asymmetry deformities is truly one of the most important and satisfying services that surgeons can offer their patients. Meticulous surgical planning is fundamental to successful treatment. Invariably, surgical treatment of patients with facial asymmetries will involve two-jaw surgery. In patients undergoing two-jaw surgery, the clinician has determined that neither the maxilla nor the mandible is acceptable. Treatment goals for these patients are exactly the same as for any patient with dentofacial deformities. The clinician strives to establish an optimal functional relationship and to position the jaws correctly, as a complex, in three planes of space, within the facial skeleton. In this section, model surgery issues related to patients with asymmetry will be highlighted. The reader is urged to review Analytical Model Surgery, Chapter 7, where model surgery procedures for two-jaw surgical treatment (Treatment Scheme III) are covered in detail.

As with all patients with dentofacial deformities, treatment planning decisions are firmly based on the presurgical data base. The primary diagnostic information will include the clinical examination, lateral and posteroanterior cephalometric radiographs, and articulator-mounted models. Important secondary components are panoramic and periapical radiographs (for interdental osteotomies) and facial and intraoral photographs.

A thorough clinical examination must be performed in a systematic fashion to accurately observe and measure (quantify) the patient's deformity. Functional problems related to the temporomandibular joints are noted and interpreted. Some asymmetry disorders are intimately associated with underlying temporomandibular joint diseases or growth disorders. Condylar hyperplasia and hemifacial microsomia are two such examples. Trauma, particularly at an early age, may also result in significant skeletal deformities that require the same thorough evaluation and careful treatment planning.

Surgical planning for the clinician is a three-step process. First, the clinician must *evaluate and quantify the deformity*. The clinician must know from where he or she is starting. Second, the surgeon must *determine appropriate clinical goals*. The surgeon must know where he or she wants to go — that is, where he or she wants the final position of the jaws to be. Last, the surgeon must *execute the plan*. He or she must be able to carry out the surgical plan by calculating the necessary net spatial changes (surgical movements) required to accomplish the clinical goals.

Experience and thoroughness are key factors in obtaining vital clinical information and in interpreting it. It may be necessary to review a patient several times before surgery in order to understand fully the complexity of the patient's deformity. The surgeon must note not only the symmetry of the jaws but also the symmetry of other important related structures, such as the eyes and ears. If these structures, particularly the orbits, are inherently asymmetric, this factor must be taken into account. From the clinical assessment, judgments will be and must be made in forming a treatment plan.

In a *frontal plane,* the clinician must make decisions related to a patient's facial midline. The surgeon must make a judgment on the acceptability of the maxillary and mandibular skeletal and dental midlines. An assessment of the position of the midline of the chin (a skeletal midline) and its relationship to the dental midline is essential. The maxillary and mandibular cant and tooth-to-lip relationships are carefully quantified and integrated into the patient's overall assessment. A small millimeter ruler, such as a Boley gauge, is very useful in making these measurements. Cant is usually measured with the patient in a supine position. The ruler is used to measure the vertical distance between the cuspids and the medial canthus bilaterally. If the orbits are inherently asymmetric, the surgeon will appropriately integrate this observation into the final treatment plan. Characteristics of the patient's smile and the effects of the muscles of facial expression are noted. When tooth-to-lip measurements are made, the patient's lips must be in repose. These are best made with the patient in a standing position. In patients with significant asymmetries, tooth-to-lip relationships will even vary between the two central incisors. Even though tooth-to-lip measurements will be correlated with the lateral cephalometric radiograph, the clinical measurements will always be superior, as the surgeon has the opportunity to ensure that the lips are in repose and can remeasure if necessary.

In the *lateral plane* (profile), the anteroposterior positions of the maxilla and mandible will be assessed as in all patients with dentofacial deformities. Upper lip support is an important feature to evaluate. An assessment of upper lip support will provide the clinician with information regarding the proper anteroposterior position of the maxilla relative to facial soft tissues. The clinician will evaluate the skin drape over the facial skeleton and make decisions related to optimal surgical positioning of the jaws in an anteroposterior plane.

Perhaps the most neglected part of a patient's clinical assessment relates to that portion of the patient's asymmetry that is present in the *horizontal plane*. Problems in *arch rotation* are often responsible for asymmetric fullness of the lips, cheeks, and mandibular angles. Ellis correctly points out that such clinical problems are occasionally noticed in patients who have undergone bimaxillary surgery for correction of symmetric deformities.[1] Asymmetries in a horizontal plane may be present even when facial midlines are correct!

To understand the nature and effect of horizontal asymmetries, it is helpful to conceptually view the patient from above. Surgeons are very familiar with viewing facial structures from this perspective. Surgeons routinely view standard CT scans (horizontal slices) of the skull and facial skeleton for various disorders. From such a perspective, the clinician can observe and judge skeletal asymmetries. Just as the clinician must make decisions related to the facial midline as viewed from a frontal plane, he or she must also make decisions related to a sagittal midline as viewed from a horizontal plane.

Prediction tracings are an important component of surgical planning. They allow the planning surgeon to estimate dental and bony changes. Prediction tracings should not be limited to lateral cephalometric views—particulary in asymmetry cases. Posteroanterior prediction tracings are performed in essentially the same manner as routine lateral tracings. "Cut outs" are repositioned on the posteroanterior cephalometric tracing. Corrections reflecting differential vertical changes and midline changes are made. As in lateral tracings, resultant bony changes can be estimated.

The concept of a *common reference plane* is important in the treatment planning for patients with facial asymmetries as well as all patients with dentofacial deformities. In Chapter 7, the importance of this is reviewed. Frankfort horizontal (FH) is the logical reference plane linking the clinical examination with the cephalometric evaluation and articulator-mounted models. A proper facebow transfer will "register" the three-dimensional relationship of the patient's maxilla and "transfer" this relationship to the articulator. When models are properly mounted on an anatomic articulator, their axis–orbital plane orientation is essentially identical to FH. It is helpful to think of the axis–orbital plane as Model Frankfort (MF). We routinely picture the articulator from its side (profile view) and understand the close relationship of the patient's FH and the articulator's axis–orbital plane. FH and MF are, in fact, "planes" and not lines. They are just as easily, and legitimately, viewed from the front (posteroanterior).

Reconstructing MF on the cephalometric radiograph is essential to ensure that the mounted models and radiograph are oriented to a common reference plane.

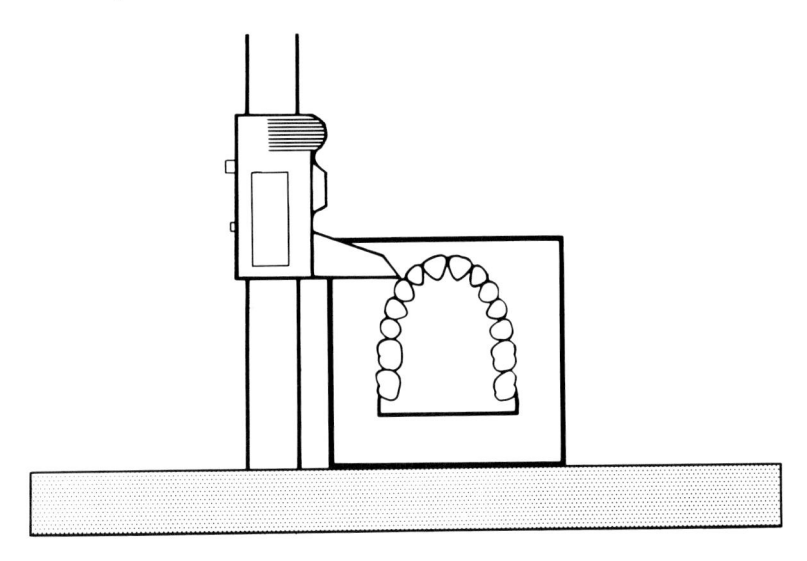

FIGURE 63-78. The Model Block is placed on end to orient the model correctly for anteroposterior measurements. A dental anteroposterior (AP) measurement of the cuspid is shown. The caliper tip is placed at a reproducible point on the mesial surface of the tooth. Both cuspids are measured and recorded. During model surgery procedures, arch rotation (symmetry in a horizontal plane) can be altered based on treatment planning decisions.

Transverse dental measurements are useful in defining the presurgical and postsurgical positions of the dental midline. *Transverse bone* reference lines (perpendicular to the reference plane of the articulator) are scribed with the caliper tip on the posterior aspect of the model bilaterally (coinciding with the tuberosities). Reference lines do not need to be recorded, as a portion of the reference line will always remain in its original position. This will allow the surgeon to judge the posterior lateral movements of the cast. This method is another way to measure desired changes or even discover unwanted changes in the horizontal plane (Fig. 63-79).

After both the maxillary and the mandibular casts have been placed in their new position, they must be carefully rechecked and interpreted by the surgeon. Changes in the position of the maxilla will lead to significant spatial changes in the position of the mandible. The postsurgical relationship between the proximal and distal segments of the mandible is particularly important to understand. After the model surgery movements are made, anticipated soft tissue changes are more easily envisioned by the surgeon. If the model surgery movements are found to be unsatisfactory, the surgical prescription must be modified and the model surgery procedures repeated. Modification of model surgery movements will require similar modifications of the lateral and posteroanterior prediction tracings. Finally, at the time of surgery, use of a reliable *vertical referent* measurement system, to double-check all surgical movements, must be part of the surgeon's technique.

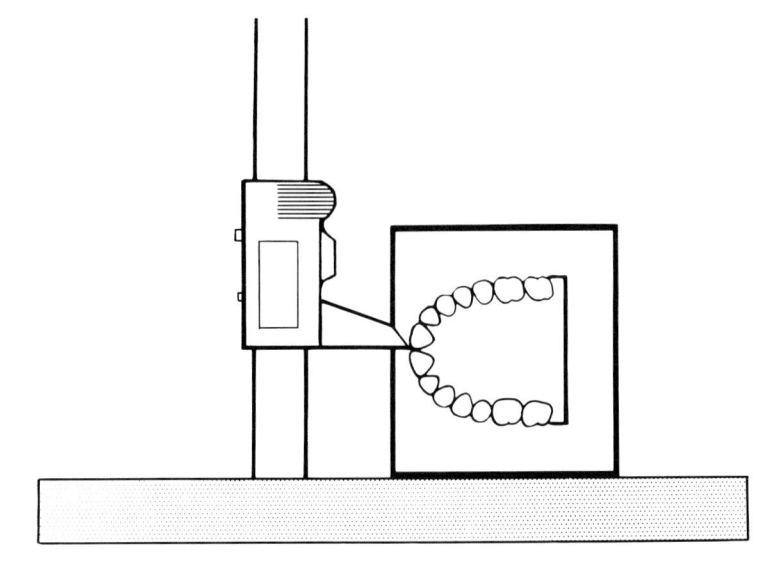

FIGURE 63-79. Transverse measurements are made with the Model Block on its side. Pre- and post-model surgery measurements must be made from the same side. For consistency, the author recommends that measurements be made from the right side. The dental midline is measured and recorded. Transverse bone reference lines are placed on the posterior aspect of the casts. From these posterior reference lines, the degree of lateral movement of the tuberosity regions can be quantified. Similar measurements can be made on mandibular models. Adjustments in arch rotation can "fine tune" the treatment of an asymmetry in a horizontal plane while the desired midline is maintained.

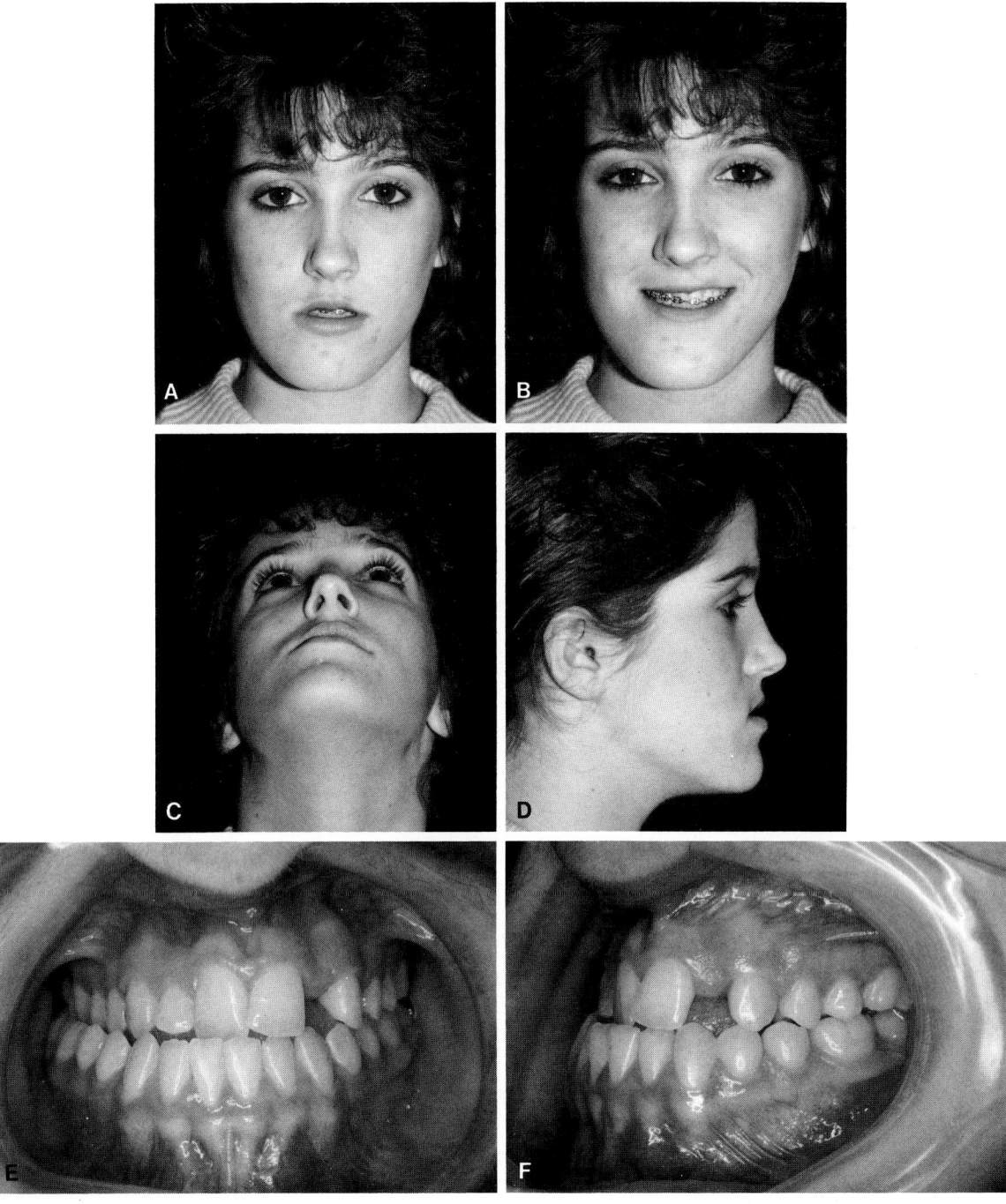

FIGURE 63–80. TWO-JAW SURGERY PERFORMED TO CORRECT A COMPLEX FACIAL ASYMMETRY. *A–D,* The patient's maxilla was long (tooth to lip) and asymmetric (abnormal cant, left side longer than right) in a frontal plane. The mandible was asymmetric with a deviation to the right. In a lateral plane, the upper jaw was deficient in an anteroposterior plane, while the mandible had undergone excessive growth. *E* and *F,* The pretreatment occlusion prior to removal of dental compensations. An arch rotation deformity was present (the maxillary left cuspid is more forward than the right cuspid). The preoperative maxillary midline was 1.0 mm left of the facial midline, while the mandible was well right of the facial midline. The maxillary left lateral incisor was congenitally missing.

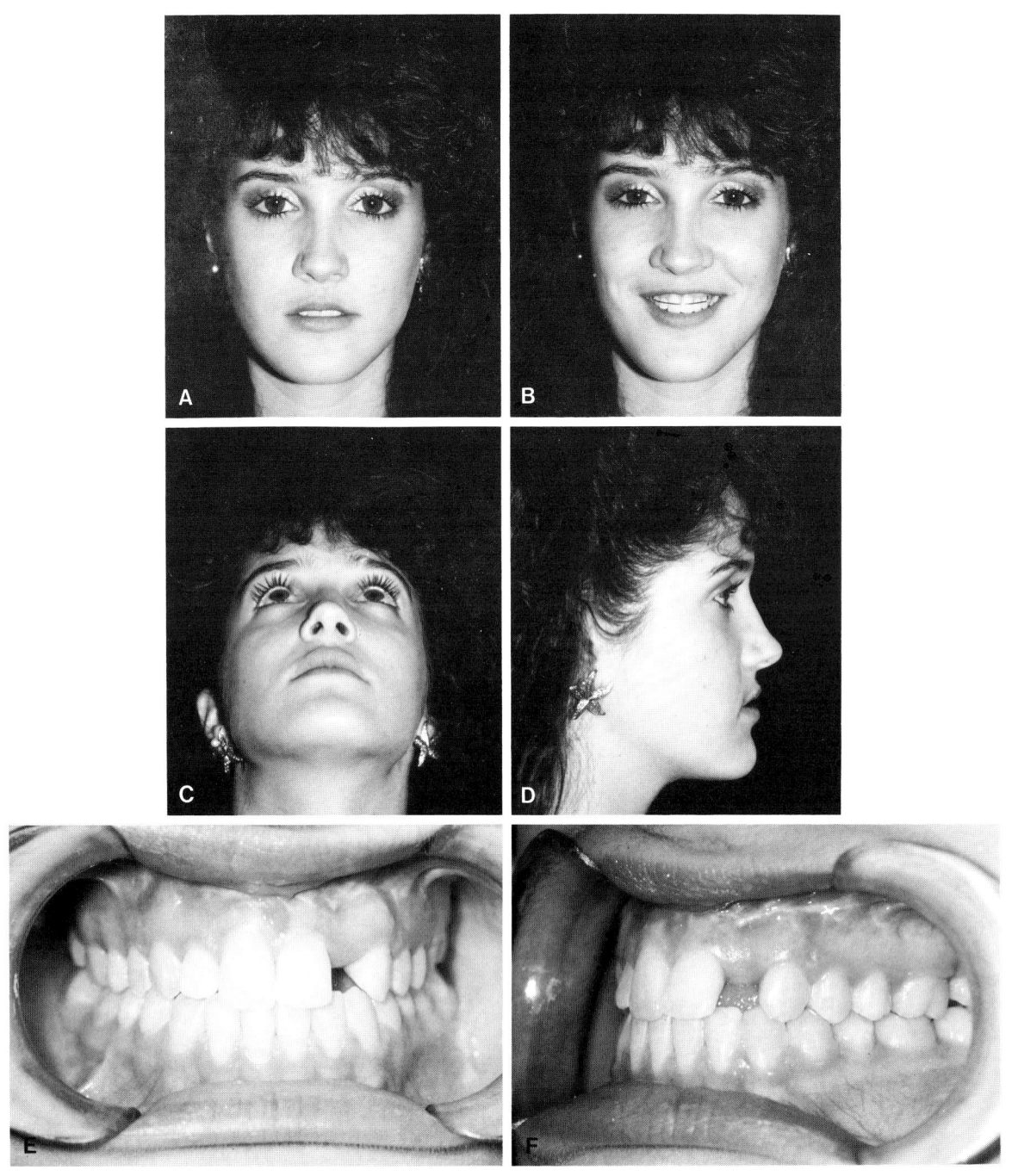

FIGURE 63–81. *A–D,* As measured from the medial canthus, there was a 3-mm vertical discrepancy between the right and left cuspids preoperatively. One half of this discrepancy was orbital in nature. The surgical prescription called for raising the left cuspid 1.5 mm relative to the right. The central incisor was raised 2.0 mm and advanced 3.0 mm. The maxillary left second molar was raised 3.5 mm. The maxillary arch was rotated to the left to correct the horizontal plane deformity. The maxillary midline was moved 1.0 mm to the right. The patient's maxillary retainer also serves as a flipper appliance to replace the maxillary left lateral incisor temporarily. *E* and *F,* The post-treatment occlusion showing the maxillary and mandibular arches in a Class I relationship. (Surgeon: Kim Erickson, Grand Rapids, MI; Orthodontist: Charles Caldwell, Grand Rapids, MI.)

REFERENCES

1. Ellis E: Accuracy of model surgery: Evaluation of an old technique and introduction of a new one. J Oral Maxillofac Surg 48:1166, 1990.

5. ORTHOPEDIC-ASSISTED MAXILLARY ADVANCEMENT IN THE CLEFT LIP AND PALATE PATIENT, USING EXTERNAL HEADFRAME TRACTION

LANCE L. LERNER
JEFFREY A. LANE

Cleft lip and palate patients are known to present with decreased horizontal maxillary growth, secondary to palatal cicatrix formation resulting from palatoplasties done when they were children.[2,7] Multiple procedures will exacerbate the amount of horizontal growth deficiency. About 25 per cent of Caucasians with unilateral cleft lip and palate develop maxillary hypoplasia that will not respond to orthodontic treatment alone.[9] This maxillary hypoplasia presents a problem, as the inelastic scar tissue can hinder large anterior advancements of the maxilla and can potentially compromise vascular flow and velopharyngeal seal during advancements of any magnitude. Our clinical experience and reported studies[3-5] have shown that it is difficult to accomplish stable, major maxillary advancements in cleft lip and palate patients. In patients with severe maxillary retrognathia, traditional Le Fort advancement and fixation techniques may not be applicable or effective. Surgical compromises may then be made to achieve some degree of occlusal harmony, while failing to attain balanced facial and skeletal morphology. To address this problem, the concept of using extraoral fixation with orthopedic traction as a tissue expansion modality was developed. The constant traction forces on the maxilla and soft palate would then utilize principles of tissue expansion.[1,6] When epidermis or mucosa is stretched, it shows an increase in the number of cells and maintains its thickness. The dermis and connective tissue, however, show significant thinning, with the collagen fibers elongated and oriented parallel to the skin. In the long term, the dermis returns to its preoperative baseline condition following expansion. Blood vessels can be rapidly expanded and show no ischemic changes or decreased flow. Rapid tissue expansion of axial blood vessels and nerves results in increases to twice the size of the original area, with no reduction in vessel wall diameter or intimal integrity and with an increase in blood flow.[10]

A technique was then developed to utilize these principles in a multistaged procedure, to attain the desired amount of maxillary advancement, and to maintain it in a stable manner.

CASE: B.M.

B.M., a 16-year-old boy with unilateral cleft lip and palate, was referred for evaluation and treatment of his dental malocclusion and severe maxillary retrognathia.

PROBLEM LIST (FIG. 63–82A to D)

1. Unilateral (left side) cleft lip and palate with a heavy palatal cicatrix.
2. Severely retrognathic maxilla with a −17-mm overjet and 4 mm of open bite.
3. Hypoplastic dorsum of nose.
4. Steep mandibular plane angle.
5. Vertically long lower one third of face.
6. Missing maxillary anterior teeth.
7. Class III occlusion.

CEPHALOMETRIC ANALYSIS (FIG. 63–82E and F)

1. SNA = 63°; SNB = 71°; ANB difference = −8°; McNamara nasion perpendicular, maxilla = −22 mm.
2. Mandibular plane angle = 49°.
3. Proportionally long lower one third of face.

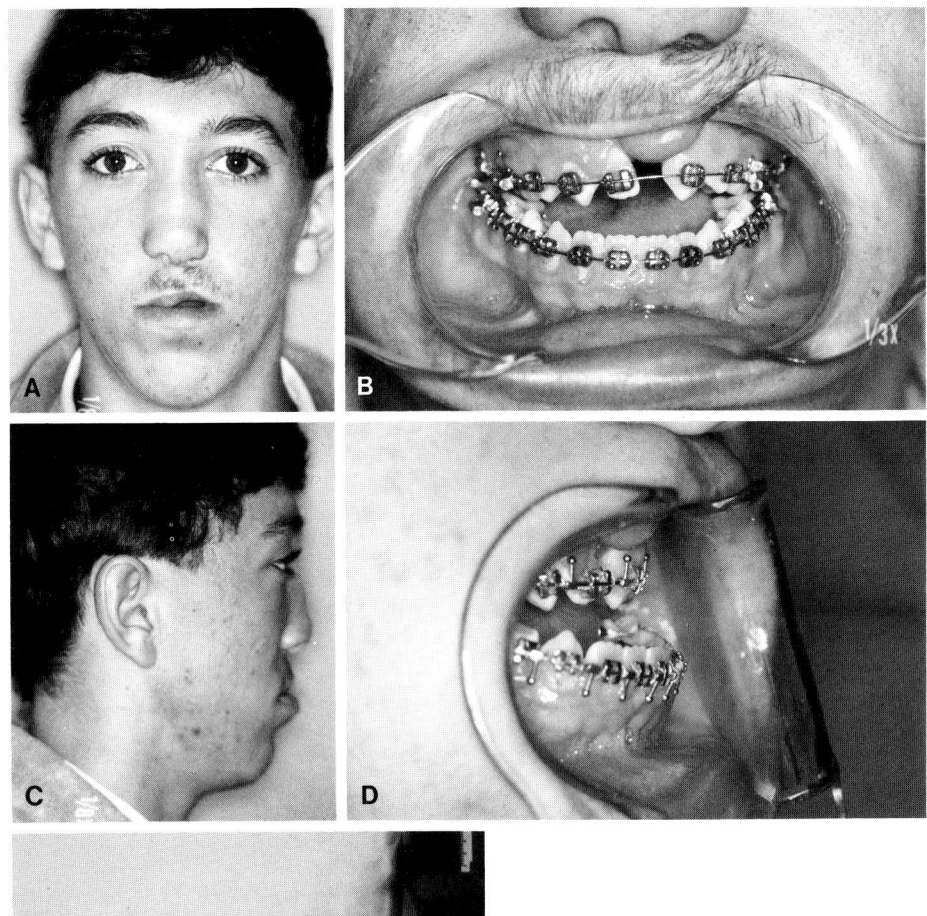

FIGURE 63-82. *A–F*, Preoperative facial and occlusal views and preoperative cephalometric studies.

Past Surgical History

1. Primary cheiloplasty at 9 weeks.
2. Ventricular septal defect repair at 3 months.
3. Palatoplasty at 18 months.
4. Four additional palatoplasties before 5 years of age to attempt to close recurrent fistulas and dehiscences.
5. Alveolar cleft closure with bone graft at 12 years.

Treatment Plan

Orthodontics

1. Presurgical—level and coordinate dental arches.
2. Postsurgical—final maximal interdigitation.

Surgical (Fig. 63-83*A* and *B*)

1. Le Fort I advancement using extraoral traction (Fig. 63-84).
2. Bone "plate" and position screw fixation.

63 — MAXILLARY AND MIDFACE DEFORMITY / **2317**

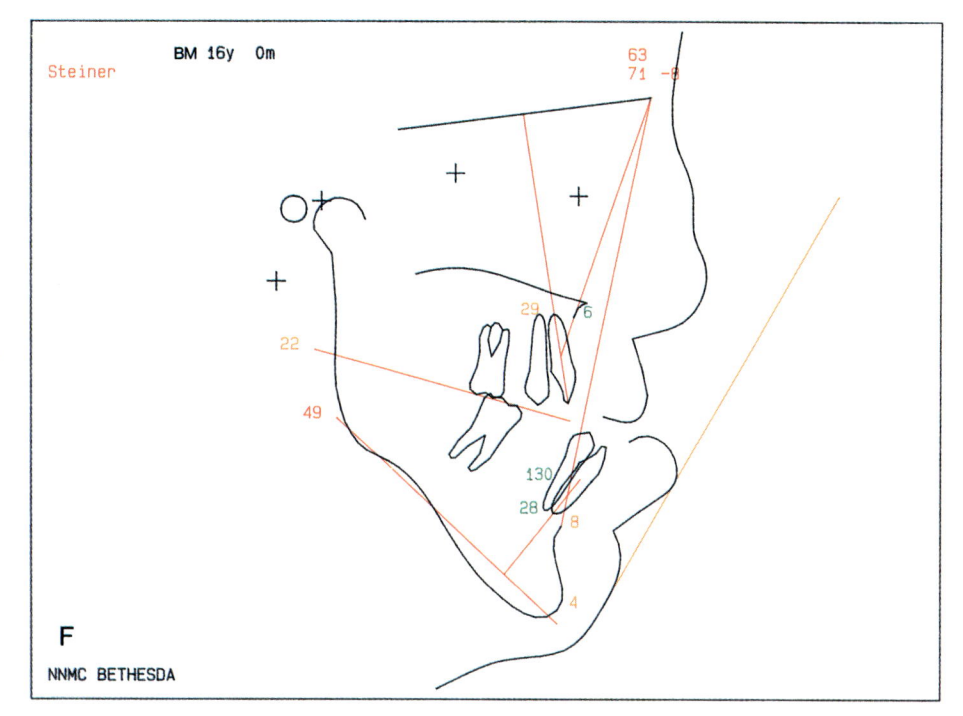

FIGURE 63–82 *Continued*

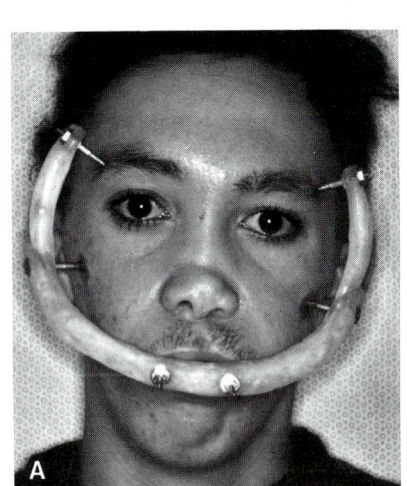

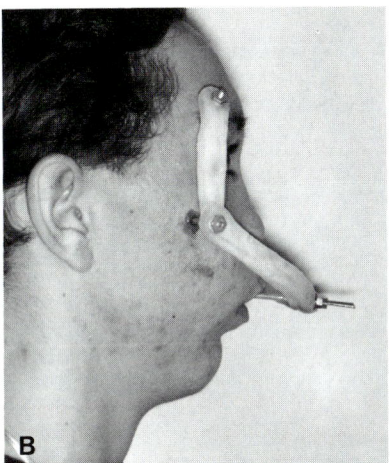

FIGURE 63–83. *A* and *B*, Headframe with traction rods.

FIGURE 63–84. Cephalogram at a maximal advancement of 23 mm.

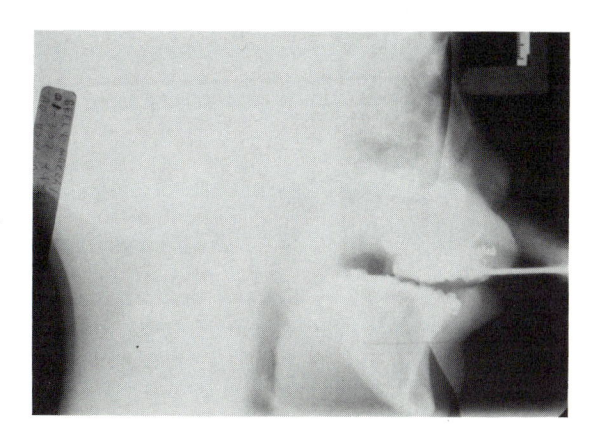

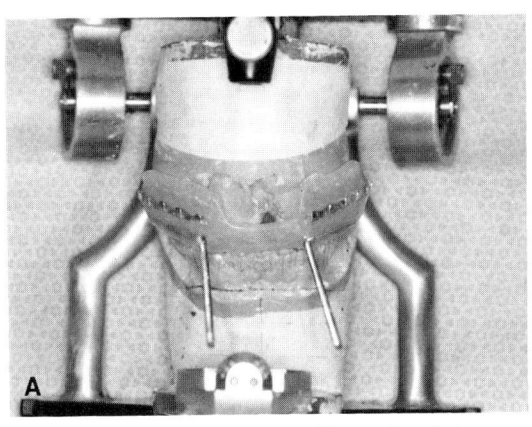

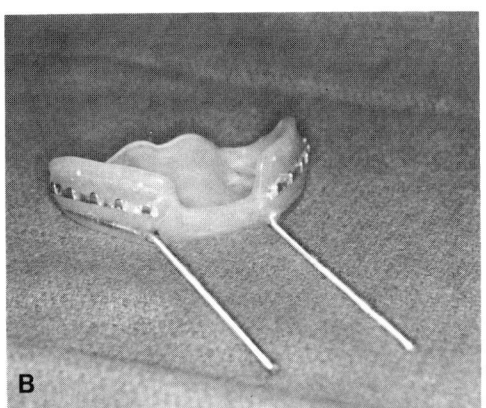

FIGURE 63-85. *A* and *B*, Maxillary splint design.

3. Postfixation stabilization with extraoral fixation.
4. Iliac crest bone harvest.
5. Genioplasty—reduction and advancement.
6. Nasal dorsum augmentation.

Prosthodontics. Postsurgical fixed restoration of maxillary anterior teeth.

TECHNIQUE

Laboratory Design

A custom maxillary tray was made that had an occlusal bite registration to act as a seating guide to orient the maxillary dentition in the tray (Fig. 63-85A and B). Undercuts were blocked out with wax during fabrication so that the splint drew. Two threaded rods were attached to the tray, parallel to the occlusal plane, and extended out of the mouth. Erich arch bars were secured to the tray. An anterior groove was placed in the tray so that the gingiva and mucosa could be observed for ischemia.

Three intermediate surgical splints were made at 4, 6, and 8 mm, to gauge the amount of surgical advancement.

Surgical Phase (Fig. 63-86)

The patient was taken to surgery, and a Le Fort I osteotomy was performed. The anterior osteotomy cuts were made 1 cm above the antral floor to facilitate future bone graft placement. The maximal amount of advancement that could be obtained intraoperatively was 6 mm. No attempt was made to fixate the maxilla, and only the mucosa was closed. The traction splint was inserted and lined with Coe Comfort as a filler. It was secured with skeletal fixation to the maxilla (dento/alveolar complex), using four Kirschner wires. Small acrylic caps were adapted to the K-wire stumps to protect the mucosa. Joe Hall Morris pins were placed in the lateral supraorbital rims and malar prominences (Fig. 63-87A and B). A custom acrylic bar was made and placed over the pins, with the threaded rods extending through metal sleeves placed in the acrylic bar and secured with hexnuts. A piece of intravenous tubing was placed on the rods extending out of mouth to protect the lips. With the use of just finger rotation, the two hexnuts were tightened intraoperatively while the maxillary gingiva was observed through the anterior splint groove for any ischemic changes. An additional 6 mm of advancement was accomplished over a period of 20 minutes.

During the next 4 weeks, the traction hexnuts were tightened, by finger pressure only, every 3 days, each time until the patient experienced an increase in pressure. At no time was any gingival ischemia or vascular compromise noted. Weekly serial cephalograms were taken to monitor progress. The maxilla was purposely overadvanced (as the amount of immediate traction release relapse was unknown), and at 4 weeks 23 mm of advancement had been obtained (see Figs. 63-84, 63-89, 63-90, and 63-91).

The patient was then taken back to surgery, the acrylic bar and traction splint were removed, and the maxilla was re-exposed. The antral membrane was removed to expose the bony antral floor and anterior wall of the maxilla. In order to fixate the

63 — MAXILLARY AND MIDFACE DEFORMITY / **2319**

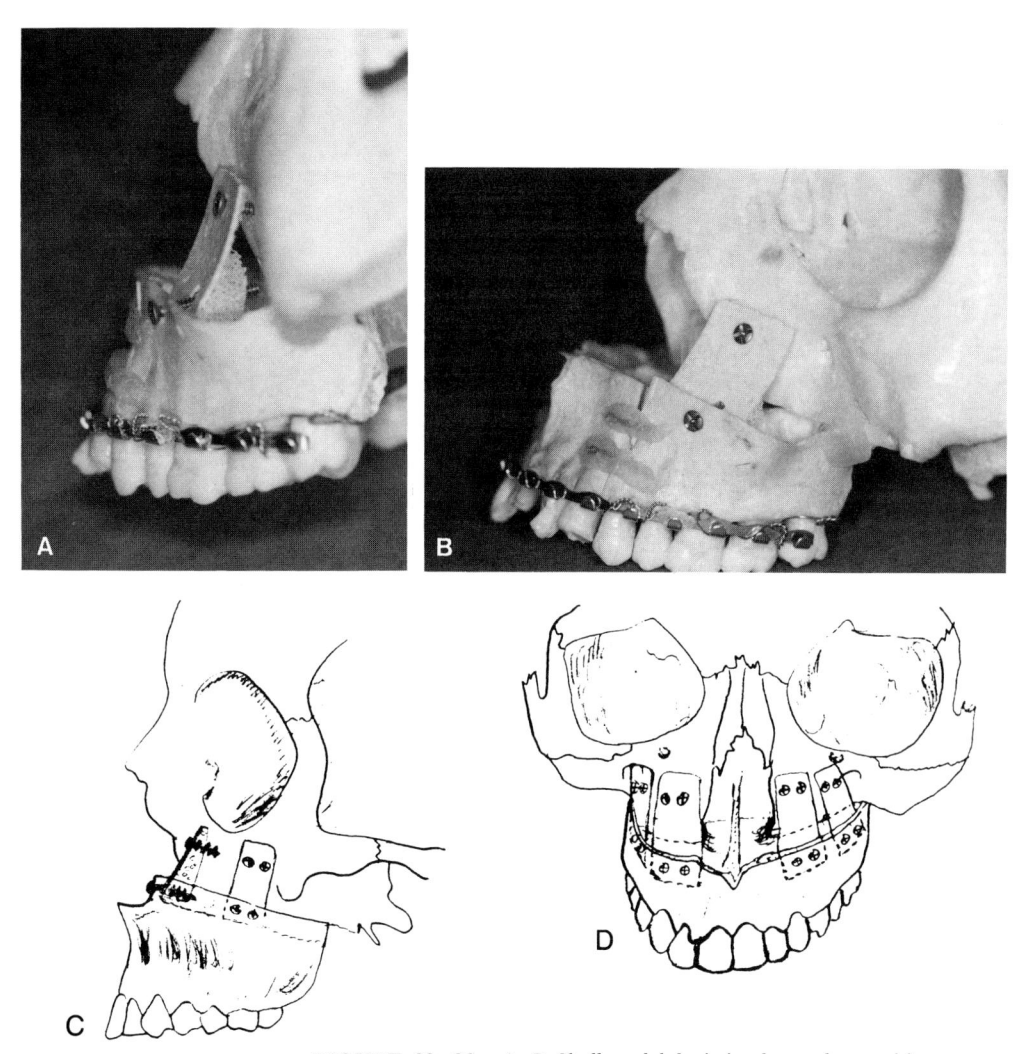

FIGURE 63–86. *A–D*, Skull model depicting bone plate position screws.

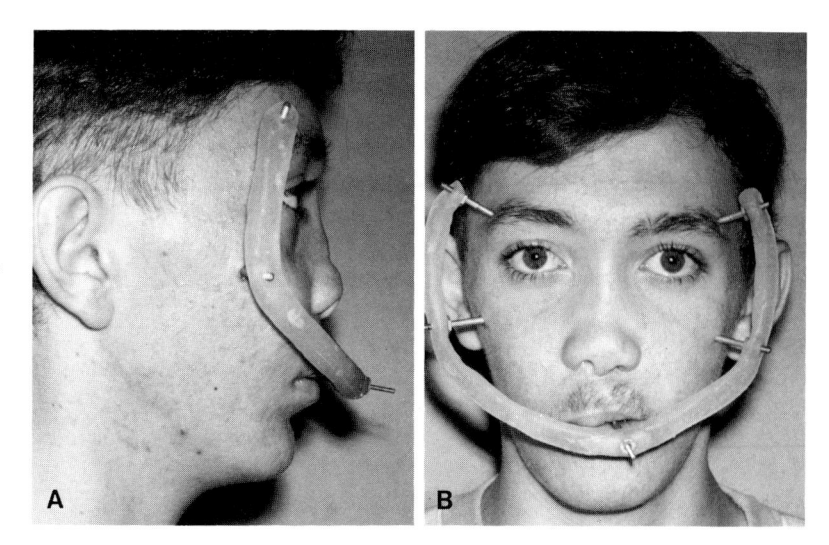

FIGURE 63–87. *A* and *B*, Stabilization (single rod) splint and headframe.

2320 / VII — ORTHOGNATHIC SURGERY

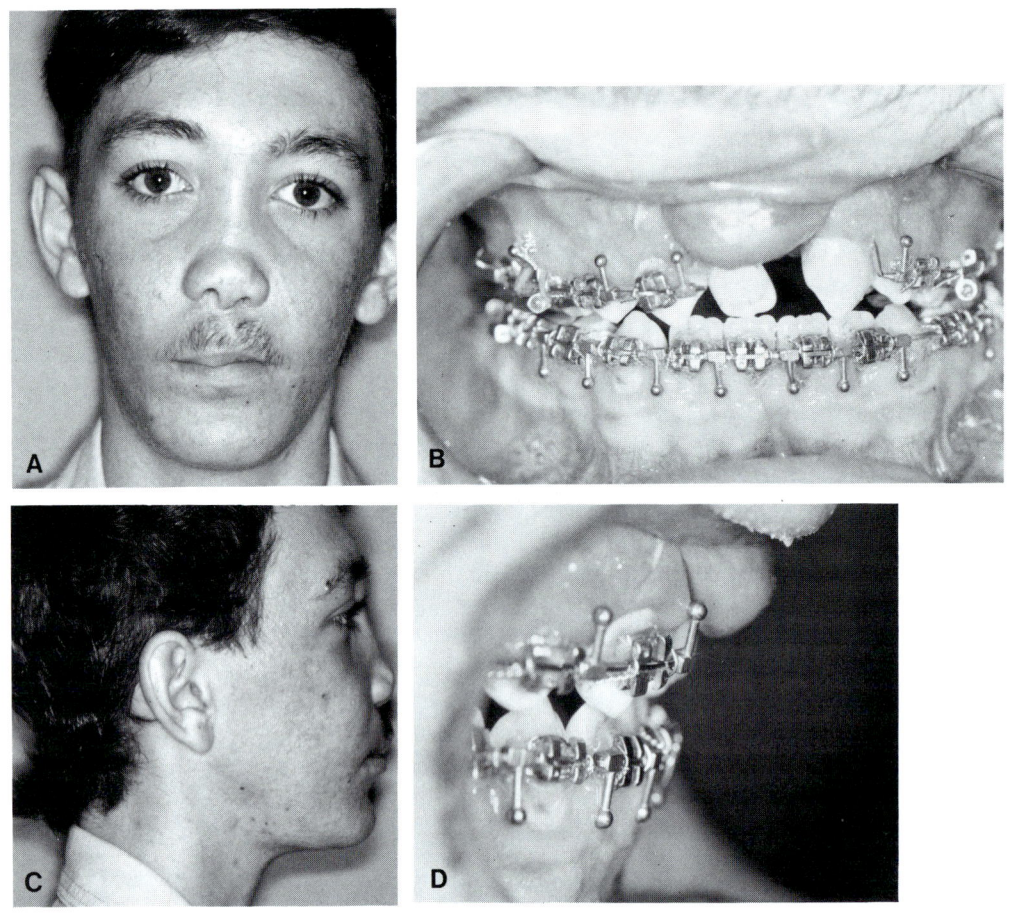

FIGURE 63-88. *A–D,* After removal of the stabilization splint and headframe.

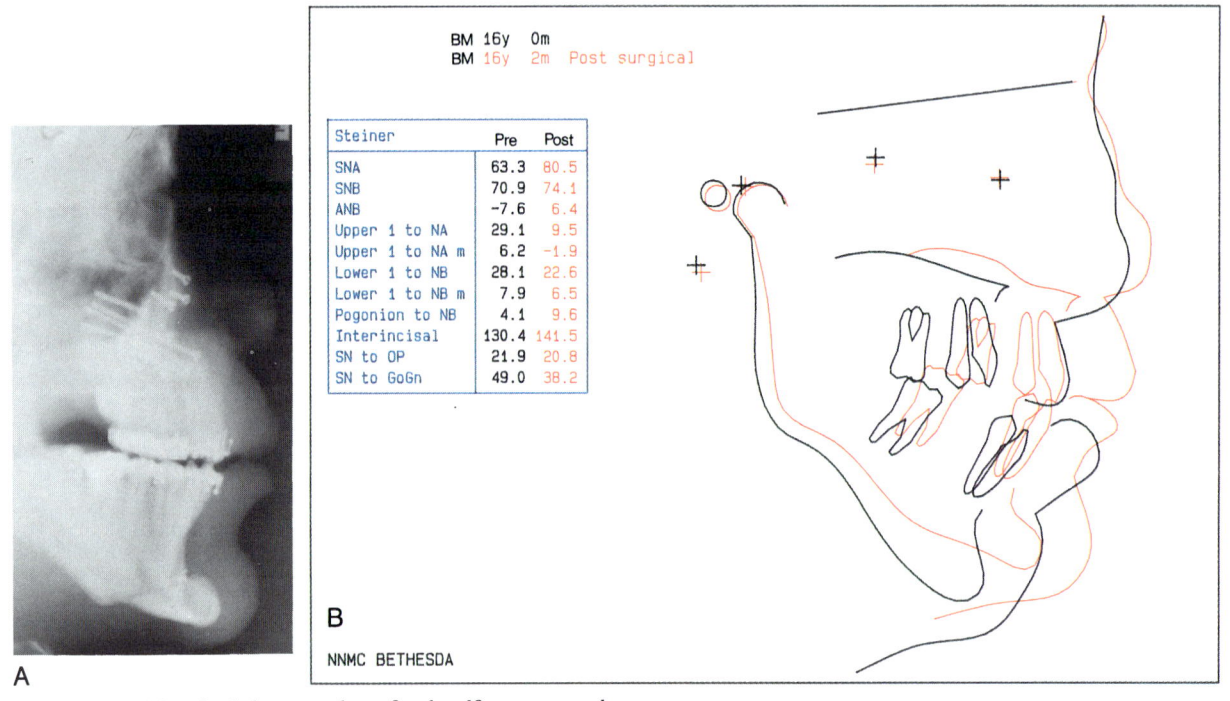

FIGURE 63-89. Cephalogram taken after headframe removal.

Steiner	Pre	Post
SNA	63.3	80.5
SNB	70.9	74.1
ANB	-7.6	6.4
Upper 1 to NA	29.1	9.5
Upper 1 to NA m	6.2	-1.9
Lower 1 to NB	28.1	22.6
Lower 1 to NB m	7.9	6.5
Pogonion to NB	4.1	9.6
Interincisal	130.4	141.5
SN to OP	21.9	20.8
SN to GoGn	49.0	38.2

BM 16y 0m
BM 16y 2m Post surgical

NNMC BETHESDA

63 — MAXILLARY AND MIDFACE DEFORMITY / **2321**

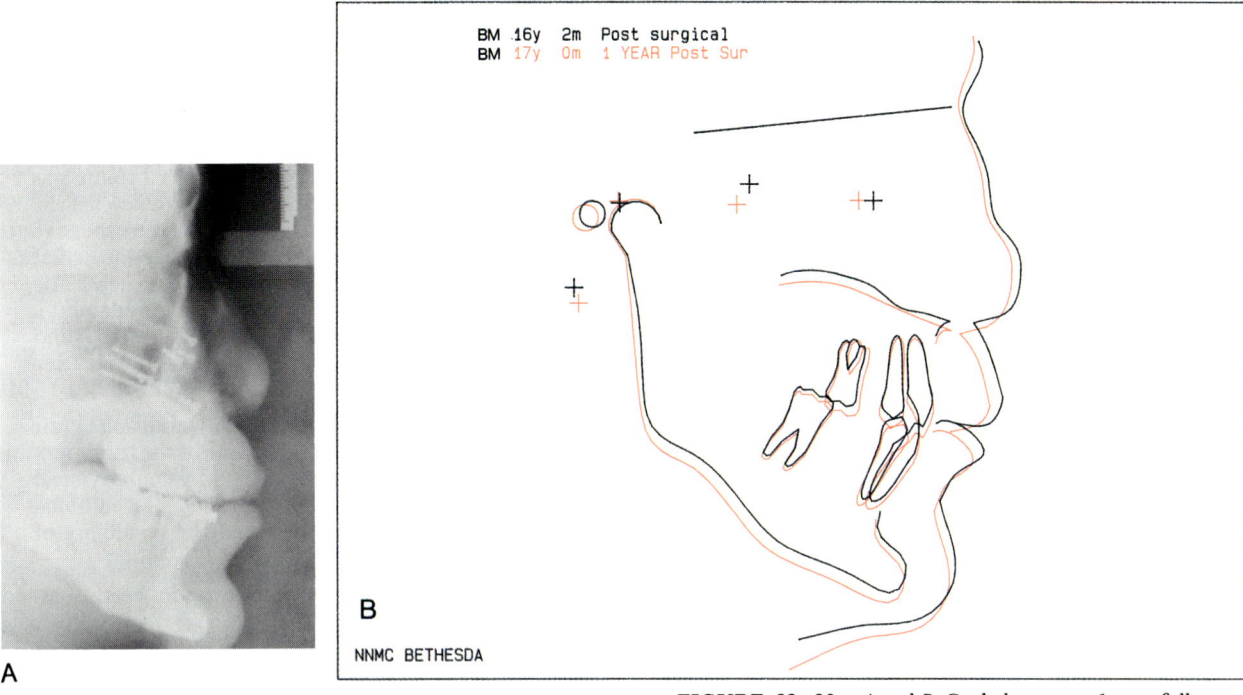

FIGURE 63-90. *A* and *B*, Cephalogram at 1-year follow-up.

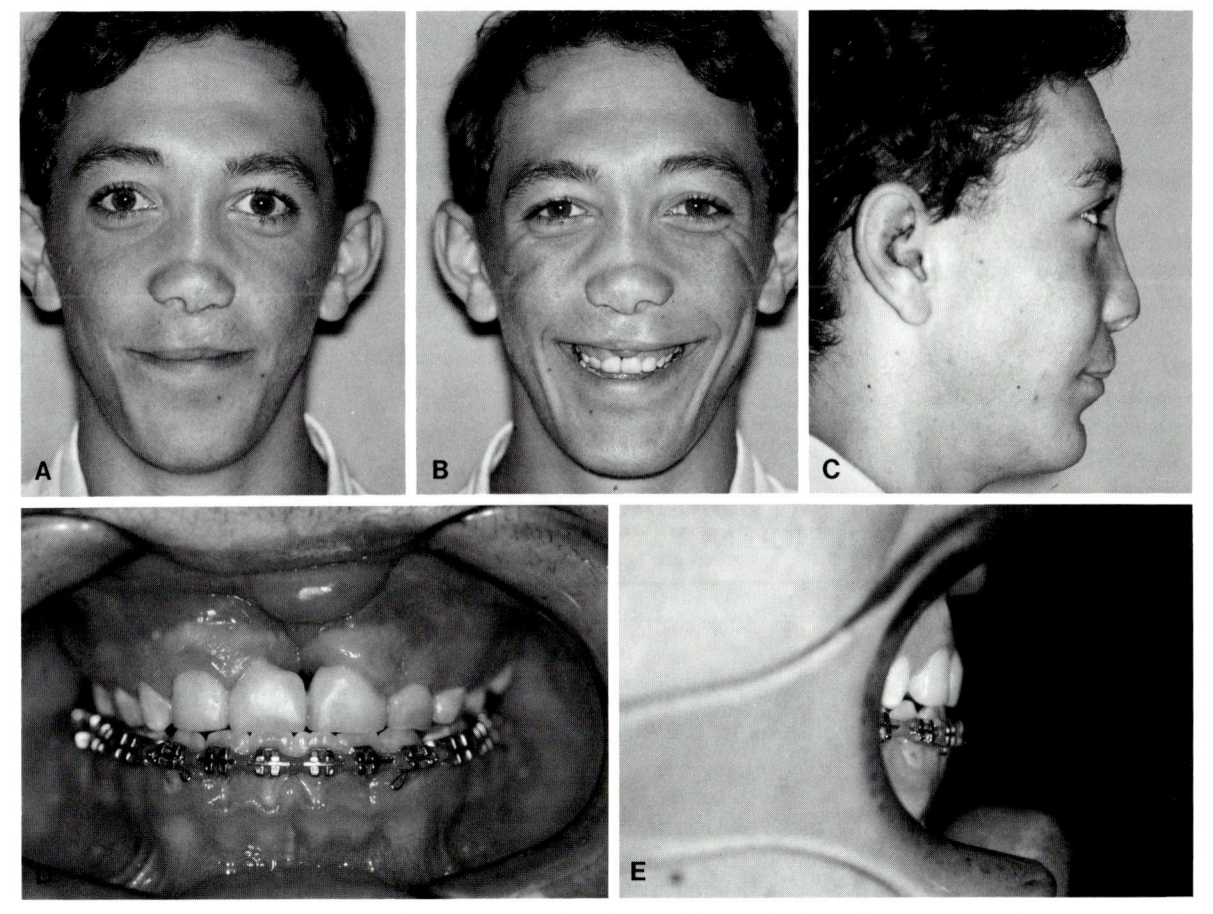

FIGURE 63-91. *A–E*, Clinical photographs at 1-year follow-up (with maxillary temporary dental restorations).

2324 / VII—ORTHOGNATHIC SURGERY

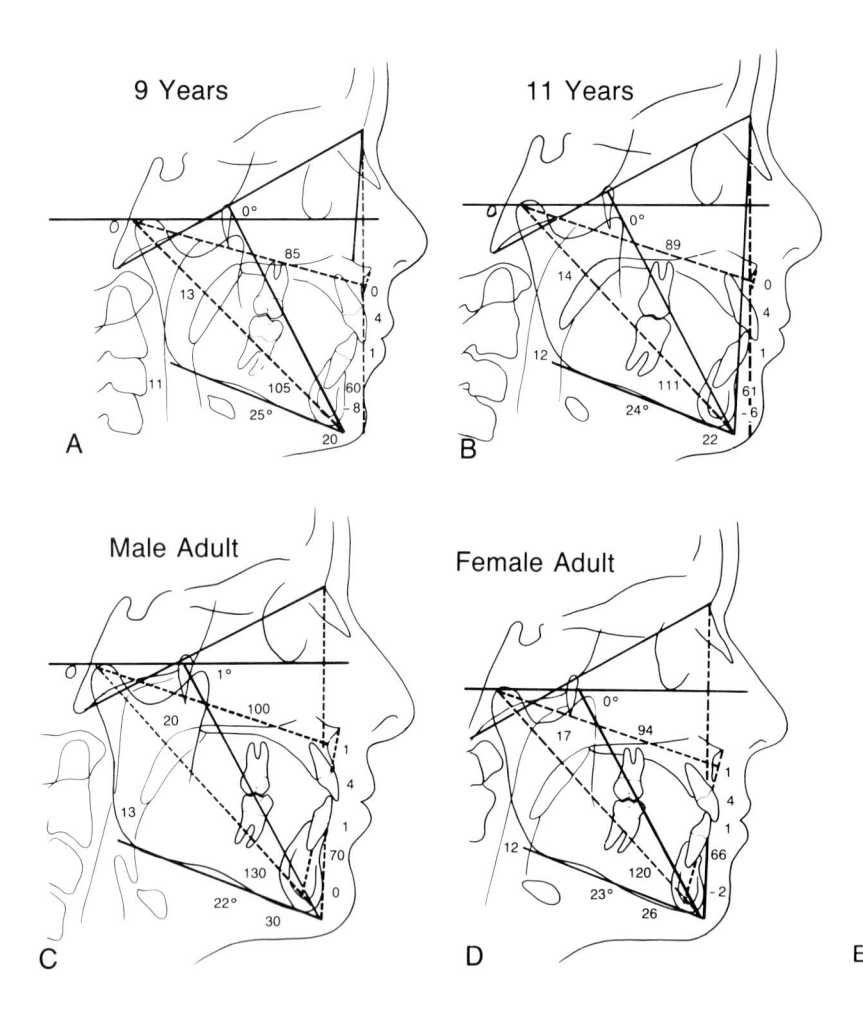

	Adult Male	Adult Female
Mandibular Length (Co·GN)	130	120
Maxillary Length (Co·pT.A)	100	94
Maxillo-Mandibular Differential	30	26
Lower Anterior Facial Height	70	66
N Perp-Point A	1	1
1̲-Point A	4	4
1̄-APo Line	1	1
N Perp-Pogonion	0	-2
Mandibular Plane Angle	22	23
Facial Axis Angle	1	0
Upper Pharynx	20	17
Lower Pharynx	13	12

CEPHALOMETRIC STANDARDS
(McNAMARA, 1983)

MAXILLARY LENGTH (MM)	MANDIBULAR LENGTH (MM)	LOWER ANTERIOR FACIAL HEIGHT (MM)
80	97 - 100	57 - 58
85	105 - 108	60 - 62
90	113 - 116	63 - 65
95	122 - 125	67 - 69
100	130 - 133	70 - 74
105	138 - 141	75 - 79

FIGURE 63–92. *A–D,* Normal dental-skeletal relationships for the cephalometric analysis of young, growing patients and of male and female adult patients. *E,* Table of cephalometric norms for adult patients. *F,* Cephalometric standards for the comparison of a skeletal part within a given patient.

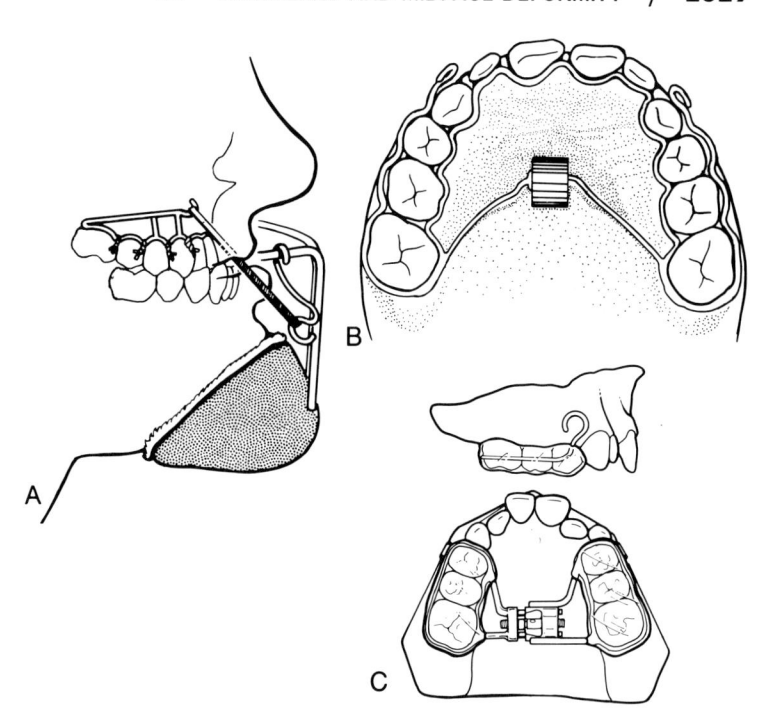

FIGURE 63-94. *A*, The face mask of Petit. *B*, A simple palatal and vestibular wire with a pearl to stimulate new tongue posturing. This appliance is worn during maxillary protraction therapy after expansion has been achieved and is most effective in treating deep bite situations, as the horizontal vector of pull will slightly open the bite. *C*, Bonded palatal expansion appliance with occlusal acrylic coverage, stainless steel framework, and protraction hooks for the attachment of elastics to the framwork of the face mask.

during protraction to transmit forces from the dentition to the maxilla. A simple palatal and vestibular wire, a removable appliance designed by Petit (Fig. 63–94*B*), can also be used during protraction therapy once palatal expansion has been achieved.

In another technique by McNamara,[7] the palatal expander is described as a framework of .045-inch stainless steel to which an expansion screw is attached (Fig. 63–94*C*). If second molars are present, an occlusal rest is extended over them to prevent overeruption of these teeth during treatment. Two hooks, to which elastics are attached, are soldered to the wire framework. These hooks usually lie adjacent to the canines or first deciduous molars. A sheet of 3-mm-thick splint Biocryl is heated and adapted to the framework and associated teeth using a Biostar thermal pressure machine. The face mask is secured to the face by stretching elastics from the hooks on the maxillary splint to the crossbar of the face mask. Heavy forces are applied bilaterally using 5/16-inch, 14-ounce elastics. The elastics vector lies in an inferomedial direction anteriorly from the hooks on the splint to the crossbar. Care must be taken that the elastics do not cause irritation to the corners of the mouth.

Hickham[5] states that 600 to 800 grams of force, per side, will effect maxillary sutural protraction. He states that the opening bite effect during the course of therapy can be avoided or reduced by placing the protraction elastics near the maxillary cuspids. Other suggestions by Hickham include (1) avoiding Class III elastics, which tend to rotate the occlusal plane quite easily but fail to advance the maxilla in its normal downward and forward direction, and (2) realizing the importance of airway obstruction as a contributor to low and forward tongue posturing. He states that even after tonsillectomy or adenoidectomy some patients may require tongue cribs on the lingual aspect of the lower incisors to correct subsequent forward posturing of the tongue.

Both McNamara[7] and Turley[11] agree that palatal expansion should begin 7 to 10 days prior to face mask delivery. The duration of expander application depends on the amount of transverse discrepancy. Optimally, once the treatment is initiated, the patient is instructed to wear the face mask on a full-time basis except during meals. Younger patients can follow this regimen especially when they understand that correction may be completed in 6 months. Older patients may not be able to adhere to this rigorous schedule, since a longer treatment time may be required.

The determination of which patients require face mask therapy can be challenging. Cephalometric values can provide important information about the relative contributions of skeletal and dental components to a malocclusion. Unfortunately, cephalometric values are often unreliable in a young child, in whom neither jaw may be identified as the obvious contributor to a Class III condition. Therefore, it is important to obtain annual cephalograms to identify the individual's dentoalveolar compensations over time as well as to evaluate disparate growth. Sue and associates[10] found that different analyses revealed different sources of skeletal discrepancies. Using SNA-SNB, these investigators found the mandible to be prognathic, but when studying Rickett's maxillary depth and facial angle, they found most cases to be maxillary retrusive. According to Turley,[11] this variability in cephalometric analysis requires the clinician to use other means to evaluate the Class III patient. Simultaneous evaluation of the patient's profile is required, since facial esthetics is a major concern with any skeletal discrepancy.

The key to successful orthopedic correction of malocclusions with face mask therapy is the patient's cooperation. Since compliance is such an important factor, it is best to treat these patients when they are young and the skeletal and soft tissues are most adaptable. Treatment success and compliance are often greatest when the child is in full deciduous or early mixed dentition. The patient must be positively reinforced to wear the appliance at all times. Turley[11] recommends a technique similar to that used for the correction of fingersucking habits. Short- and long-term goals are set, with praise and rewards given upon the attainment of each goal. At delivery of the appliance, the patient is given a card telling where the doctor can be reached during the first 24 hours, and he or she contacts the patient to check progress. Further encouragement and tangible rewards should come from the parents. A letter to the child's teacher may help eliminate any negative peer pressure felt by the child at school. Many children will decorate their appliances to make them more acceptable.

There are conflicting opinions about the stability of Class III orthopedic treatment. Delaire[2] says that "in successful cases, the facial skeleton is completely transformed. The therapeutic action has permitted, and in fact provoked, the establishment of a normal equilibrium without possibility of relapse." In contrast, Cozzani[1] cautioned that "we cannot consider a Class III malocclusion fully resolved until facial growth has ended." In addition, Jackson[6] demonstrated that the amount of relapse after treatment is directly related to the length of retention. Turley[11] anticipates relapse and recommends the overcorrection of the overjet. Well-adapted bands and a transpalatal crib can be used in lieu of the palatal expansion appliance, with use of the face mask continued at night. A removable acrylic appliance with good retention, a Class III bionator, or a Crozat or Frankel appliance can also be used. McNamara[7] corrects to a 2- to 4-mm overjet and retains with a removable stabilizing plate. In cases with profound neuromuscular imbalances, he recommends the FR-III (Frankel appliance) as an active retainer. Finally, full orthodontic therapy should follow the Phase I orthopedic therapy to provide optimal occlusion in the permanent dentition and to help control any disproportionate growth between mandible and maxilla during the prepubertal growth spurt through the judicious use of intraoral elastics.

Face mask therapy has been found to be beneficial for patients requiring maxillary protrusion. The introduction of the face mask also created new possibilities for the orthodontic treatment of cleft lip and palate patients. Friede and Lennartsson,[3] in a study with metallic implants, concluded that forward maxillary traction had a beneficial effect on the retrognathic midface of children with cleft lip and palate. In addition, Paz and associates[8] demonstrated that the face mask can be used to maintain, postsurgically, a corrected Class III malocclusion following a Le Fort I maxillary advancement.

In summary, McNamara[7] found that the treatment effects that may be seen following face mask therapy include (1) a forward and downward movement of the maxilla, (2) a forward and downward movement of the maxillary dentition, (3) a downward and backward redirection of mandibular growth, (4) a lingual tipping of the lower anterior teeth, and (5) an inhibition of mandibular growth. Accepting these effects, one can expect that treatment with a combination of face mask and bonded rapid maxillary palatal expander will be effective for those Class III patients with maxillary retrusion and will provide them with a more esthetic, functional, and stable occlusion, along with a pleasing facial profile.

REFERENCES

1. Cozzani G: Extraoral traction and Class III treatment. Am J Orthod 80:638–650, 1981.
2. Delaire J: Confection du masque orthopédique. Rev Stomatol Paris 72:579–584, 1971.
3. Friede H, Lennartsson B: Forward traction of the maxilla in cleft lip and palate patients. Eur J Orthod 3:21–39, 1981.
4. Guyer, EC, Ellis EE, McNamara JA, Behrents RG: Components of Class III malocclusion in juveniles and adolescents. Angle Orthod 56:7–30, 1986.
5. Hickham JH: Maxillary protraction therapy: Diagnosis and treatment. J Clin Orthod 25:102–113, 1991.
6. Jackson GW, Kokich VG, Shapiro PA: Experimental response to anteriorly directed extraoral force in young *Macaca nemestrina*. Am J Orthod 75:249–277, 1977.
7. McNamara JA: An orthopedic approach to the treatment of Class III malocclusion in young patients. J Clin Orthod 21:598–608, 1987.
8. Paz ME, Subtelny JD, Iranpour B: A combined face mask–orthognathic surgical approach in the treatment of skeletal open bite and maxillary deficiency. Am J Orthod. 95(1):1–11, 1989.
9. Petit H: Adaptations following accelerated facial mask therapy. *In* McNamara JA, Ribbens KA, Howe RP (eds): Clinical Alteration of the Growing Face. Monograph 14, Craniofacial Growth Series. Ann Arbor, MI, Center for Human Growth and Development, University of Michigan, 1983.
10. Sue G, Chaconas SJ, Turley PK, Itoh J: Indicators of skeletal Class III growth. J Dent Res 66:348, 1987.
11. Turley PK: Orthopedic correction of Class III malocclusion with palatal expansion and custom protraction headgear. J Clin Orthod 22:314–325, 1988.

7. THE LIP LIFT

THOMAS S. JETER
JOSEPH VAN SICKELS
GARY J. NISHIOKA

There has been a relatively recent interest in applying esthetic soft tissue procedures of the face to enhance the final results of orthognathic surgical procedures, to serve as alternative procedures, or, in some cases, to correct unfavorable surgical results. One such procedure is the lip lift, which is currently employed as a cosmetic procedure to reverse the effects of aging on the upper lip. With aging, the upper lip progressively increases in vertical height (ptosis); the philtrum flattens, losing its concave profile; and the vermilion becomes thinner, giving an unesthetic appearance associated with old age.[1,3-6,9] This procedure is commonly employed with other esthetic surgical procedures for rejuvenation of the aging face.

This procedure may potentially be used in oral and maxillofacial surgery (1) in older patients who are planning to undergo orthognathic surgery or preprosthetic surgery and whose upper lip shows undesirable effects of aging (with regard to orthognathic surgery patients, the lip lift should be seriously considered to permit unmasking of the true degree of their maxillary excess prior to final skeletal treatment planning; (2) in patients with idiopathic vertical maxillary deficiency with an acceptable anteroposterior and mediolateral position of the maxilla (this applies regardless of whether a mandibular deformity exists or not); (3) to correct

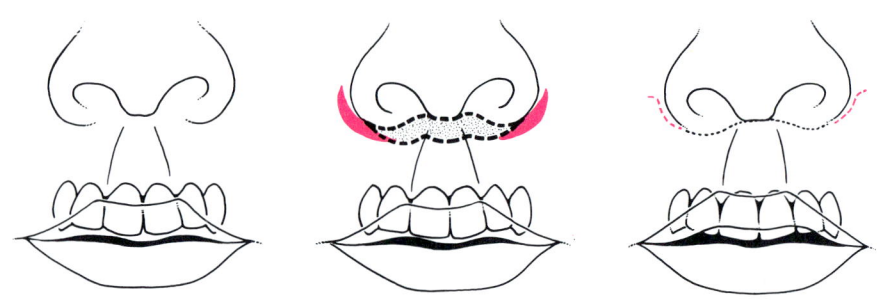

FIGURE 63-95. DIAGRAM OF THE LIP LIFT PROCEDURE. *Left,* Preoperative view. No maxillary incisors are exposed at repose. *Middle,* Elliptical excision of the skin at the time of surgery. The excision of soft tissue may be extended around the base of the nasal ala bilaterally (depicted in red) if broader shortening of the upper lip is desired. It may also be used in this manner on one side to correct asymmetric conditions. *Right,* Postoperative view showing esthetic exposure of the maxillary incisors, with the scar placed at the base of the nose. (Adapted from Jeter TS, Nishika GJ: The lip lift: An alternative corrective procedure for iatrogenic vertical maxillary deficiency: Report of a case. J Oral Maxillofac Surg 46:323–325, 1988; with permission.)

the unfavorable results of an iatrogenic vertical maxillary deficiency after a Le Fort I osteotomy, as an alternative to skeletal reoperation.

The only criterion that must be met prior to utilizing this procedure is satisfactory upper lip length. The average length of the upper lip is approximately 20 mm.[2] This procedure is not recommended if the upper lip would appear too short after decreasing the desired amount, predicted preoperatively, for esthetic exposure of the maxillary incisors.

Technique

The technique has been previously described in the literature.[7] After local anesthesia is obtained and the surgical site is prepared and draped, a wavy ellipse is marked on the skin of the upper lip, following the contours of the base of the nose (Fig. 63-95). This practice places the scar at the base of the nose, which tends to conceal it. The width of the initial ellipse is determined by pushing the lip upward with the fingers to expose the desired amount of maxillary incisor. An incision is then made with the bevel slightly backward. The skin and the orbicularis oris muscle are excised to shorten the lip. If the lip is flat and lacks pout, however, then additional skin can be excised to restore a more youthful, pouty contour. The exact amount of maxillary incisor exposed is determined at the time of surgery by placing a few temporary sutures; should more tooth exposure be needed, more skin or muscle is excised. Consequently, the initial excision should err on the conservative side. In addition, if flattening of the cupid's bow is present, more skin can be excised along the base of the nose overlying the height of contour of the cupid's bow to provide further definition. The muscular layer is coapted with 4-0 PDS or Vicryl sutures. The subcutaneous layer is closed using 5-0 PDS or nylon interrupted sutures with the knots inverted. The cutaneous surface is closed using a running 5-0 Prolene subcuticular suture or a 6-0 Prolene or nylon running suture.

REFERENCES

1. Austin HW: The lip lift. Plast Reconstr Surg 77:990, 1986.
2. Bell WH, Proffit WR, White RP: Surgical Correction of Dentofacial Deformities. Vol 1. Philadelphia, WB Saunders Company, 1980, p 118.

3. Cardoso AD, Sperli AE: Rhytidoplasty of the upper lip. *In* Transactions of the Fifth International Congress of Plastic and Reconstructive Surgery. Melbourne, Butterworth's, 1971, pp 1127–1129.
4. Fanous N: Correction of thin lips: Lip lift. Plast Reconstr Surg 74:33, 1984.
5. Gonzalez-Ulloa M: The aging upper lip. *In* Transactions of the Sixth International Congress of Plastic and Reconstructive Surgery. Paris, Masson, 1975.
6. Greenwald AE: The lip lift: Cheilopexy for cheiloptosis. Am J Cosmetic Surg 2:16, 1985.
7. Jeter TS, Nishioka GJ: The lip lift: An alternative corrective procedure for iatrogenic vertical maxillary deficiency: Report of a case. J Oral Maxillofac Surg 46:323–325, 1988.
8. Pitanguy I, Muller P, Piccolo N, et al: Esthetic surgery of the aging lip. Compend Cont Ed Dent 8:460, 1987.
9. Rozner L, Isaacs GW: Lip lifting. Br J Plast Surg 34:481, 1981.

64 MANDIBULAR DEFICIENCY

What lies behind us and what lies before us are tiny matters compared to what lies within us.
—Oliver Wendell Holmes

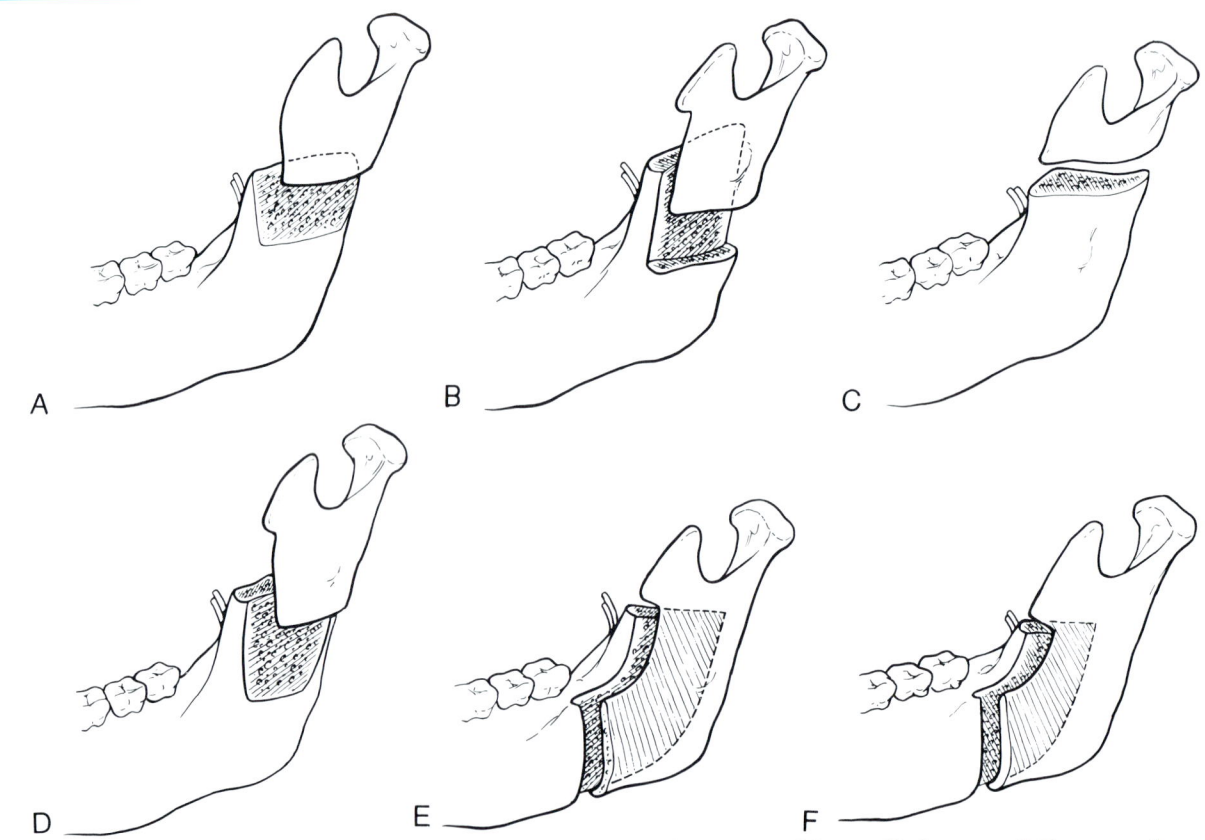

A, Perthes (1924) is credited as the first surgeon to perform a sagittal osteotomy of the mandibular ramus. *B*, Trauner and Obwegeser (1957) described "sagittal splitting" of the mandibular ramus, utilizing a transoral approach. The ascending ramus was split from the anterior to the posterior crest. *C*, By beveling the horizontal osteotomy, performed through an external approach, Kazanjian and Converse (1959) attempted to achieve better bone contact. *D*, Schuchardt's osteotomy design (1961), performed through an intraoral approach, showed an even greater step and overlap of the repositioned segments. *E*, Dal Pont (1961) changed the lateral cortical osteotomy from horizontal to vertical in the region adjacent to the third molar, thus increasing the area of bone contact even more and allowing the masseter and medial pterygoid muscles to remain in their preoperative position. *F*, Hunsuck (1968) terminated the medial cortical osteotomy just posterior to the mandibular foramen, instead of extending it to the posterior border.

64

REVIEW OF SURGICAL TECHNIQUES

ORTHODONTIC SEQUENCING, DECISIONS, AND TECHNIQUES
   Treatment Sequencing
   Arch Length Analysis
   Leveling
   Arch Width
   Anteroposterior Tooth Position
   Fixation Considerations

ANATOMIC CONSIDERATIONS IN MANDIBULAR RAMUS OSTEOTOMIES
   Position of the Mandibular Canal
   Position of Cortical Fusion in the Upper Mandibular Ramus as It Relates to the Medial Osteotomy of the SSRO
   Anatomic Study of the Position of Cortical Fusion in the Upper Ramus
   Cortical Plate Thickness in the Retromolar Area: Relationship to Rigid Fixation of the SSRO
   Anatomic Study of Cortical Thickness in the Mandibular Retromolar Area

CORRECTION OF MANDIBULAR DEFICIENCY BY SAGITTAL SPLIT RAMUS OSTEOTOMY (SSRO)

STABILITY OF MANDIBULAR ADVANCEMENT SURGERY: A REVIEW

TRANSVERSE (HORIZONTAL) MANDIBULAR DEFICIENCY
   Mandibular Expansion: Surgical Technique
   Rapid Mandibular Expansion: Orthodontic Considerations
   Classification
   Total Mandibular Augmentation
   Alteration of Mandibular Width by Symphyseal Osteotomy
   Mandibular Expansion: Age of Treatment
   Repositioning the Chin by Combined Horizontal and Oblique Anterior Mandibular Osteotomy: A New Technique

SPECIAL ADJUNCTIVE CONSIDERATIONS
   Transverse (Horizontal) Maxillary Deficiency
   The Vertical Dimension and the Deep-Bite Deformity
   Genioplasty Strategies
   Cheiloplasty
   Mandibular Angle Deficiency
   Anterior Mandibular Subapical Osteotomy
   Total Mandibular Subapical Osteotomy
   Combining Sagittal Split Osteotomy with Reduction Genioplasty
   Mandibular Deficiency Secondary to Juvenile Rheumatoid Arthritis
   Lateral Facial Reconstruction
   Mandibular Advancement in Children: Special Considerations

---

Review of Surgical Techniques

DAVID J. DARAB

Surgical treatment of mandibular retrognathia was first reported in the American literature by Blair.[2] By performing horizontal osteotomies of the mandibular ramus, the surgeon could correct both Class II and Class III malocclusions. The operative technique was carried out by passing a Gigli saw percutaneously, posterior to the condylar neck and medial to the mandibular ramus, in order to perform a horizontal osteotomy. This procedure was associated with significant problems. The pull of the lateral pterygoid and temporalis muscles on the condylar segment led to displacement with malunion and resultant anterior open bite following release of maxillomandibular fixation. Limberg[11] reviewed the surgical alternatives for correction of retrognathia. He emphasized the need for coordination of orthodontic and surgical treatment and presented alternative procedures. In these procedures, the site of operation was moved from the condylar neck, as reported by Blair, to the ramus or body of the mandible, where Limberg performed oblique osteotomies.

In 1957, Marsh Robinson reported the surgical correction of micrognathia.[12] He used an extraoral approach to perform a vertical osteotomy of the ascending ramus. A corticocancellous block of iliac crest was then interposed in the resulting osteotomy defect. This technique was modified by Robinson and Lytle,[13] who performed direct intraosseous wiring of the proximal fragment without placing a bone graft in the osseous defect. Caldwell and Amaral[3] reported the use of a vertical oblique osteotomy of the ramus with an iliac crest bone graft for the defect. In addition, they introduced decortication of the mandibular ramus to provide a greater area of contact with cancellous bone.

Hawkinson[8] first reported the "arcing" osteotomy of the ascending ramus and body. The arcing design improved bone contact for mandibular advancement procedures. This osteotomy was recommended for procedures in which rotations of the mandible were necessary, in contrast to straight or linear advancements.

Caldwell, Hayward, and Lister[4] presented a "vertical-L" osteotomy, which was modified to conform to a "C osteotomy." This was the introduction of the C osteotomy in the oral and maxillofacial surgical literature. In this article, the authors reviewed several variations in the application of the C osteotomy, which accommodated the course of the inferior alveolar nerve in the ascending horizontal ramus. Hayes introduced the "modified C-type osteotomy" by splitting the horizontal portion of the proximal segment in the sagittal plane. This procedure increased the area of bone contact following advancement.

Damage to important anatomic structures, insufficient union of skeletal fragments, postoperative relapse, and a lack of versatility of the above procedures led to the development of alternative techniques. Utilizing special instrumentation that he had developed, Ernst[7] performed the first transoral horizontal osteotomy of the ramus. Although this was a milestone in mandibular surgery, it would not be until years later that the transoral approach would become widely accepted. Kazanjian and Converse,[10] through an external approach, beveled the horizontal osteotomy to provide better adaptation of the fragments. Schuchardt[14] initiated the concept of a "step" osteotomy through the mandibular ramus that was done utilizing a transoral approach. In his technique, two parallel cuts were made: one through the medial cortex above the lingula and the second through the lateral cortex 1 cm below. With this design, the cortical plates could be separated, providing a broad area of bone contact.

In 1957, Trauner and Obwegeser[15] introduced the sagittal split osteotomy for correction of both the prognathic and the retrognathic mandible. The initial report described sagittal splitting performed in the vertical portion of the ramus. Their paper also emphasized the need for transosseous or circumferential wire fixation to provide better adaptation of the cortical surfaces and prevent postoperative movement of the proximal segment. Throughout the years, numerous authors have modified the original osteotomy design of Obwegeser in an effort to increase the area of bone contact, reduce the amount of soft tissue dissection, and enhance stability.

Dal Pont, a coworker of Obwegeser, moved the position of the lateral cut from the ramus to a position farther forward in the body.[5] This method produced a greater area of bone contact to hasten healing. Dal Pont also emphasized the importance of reducing muscular displacement. With the technique of Obwegeser, both the masseter and the medial pterygoid muscles are displaced anteriorly when the distal segment is advanced. This displacement requires prolonged fixation in order for muscular adaptation to occur, while at the same time increasing the potential for relapse and the development of an open bite. By performing an "oblique retromolar" osteotomy, described by Dal Pont, the split occurs below the inferior alveolar canal, leaving the pterygomasseteric sling attached to the condylar segment. The dento-osseous segment can now be repositioned in all dimensions without muscular displacement.

Hunsuck[9] decreased the extent of the medial osteotomy. In his technique, the medial osteotomy was carried just posterior to the mandibular foramen, thereby eliminating the need for an extension of the osteotomy to the posterior border of the ramus. Consequently, a smaller mucoperiosteal reflection is required, reducing trauma to the soft tissues and neurovascular bundle.

Epker emphasized that the "blind" stripping of the pterygomasseteric sling from the ramus is unnecessary.[6] By decreasing the extent of soft tissue dissection, intraoperative bleeding, postoperative swelling, and the risk of inferior alveolar nerve injury can be reduced.

In all of the above modifications, the sagittal split does not occur along the inferior border; rather, the inferior border remains intact on the proximal segment. Because of the thickness of the inferior border cortex, the split often occurs in an unpredictable manner along the lingual aspect of the mandible, between the inferior border and inferior alveolar canal. In 1989, Wolford and Davis[16] initiated the idea of performing an osteotomy along the inferior border to increase the predictability and decrease the difficulties and complications associated with the sagittal split technique. To accomplish this type of osteotomy, a reciprocating saw blade was specially designed. This blade allows a cut to be made through the inferior border of the mandible, extending from the buccal vertical osteotomy to the gonial notch. The main advantages of an osteotomy along the inferior border include (1) a more predictable and controlled splitting of the inferior border, (2) a greater bony interface, and (3) cortical bone sufficient to place bone screws along the inferior border.

The sagittal split technique has gained widespread acceptance for the following reasons: It is easily adaptable to correct a wide variety of mandibular anomalies; the transoral approach simplified the surgical technique while eliminating the external scar and risk to the facial nerve; and finally, sagittal splitting produced a large area of bone contact to enhance healing,[1] reducing the need for bone grafting. The surgical technique described in this chapter reflects the collective knowledge of the authors, which has been gained from surgical experience.

REFERENCES

1. Bell WH, Schendel SA: Biologic basis for modification of the sagittal split ramus osteotomy. J Oral Surg 35:362, 1977.
1a. Blair V: Operations in the jaw bone and face. Surg Gynecol Obstet 4:67, 1907.
2. Blair V: Underdeveloped jaw with limited excursion. JAMA 17:178, 1909.
3. Caldwell JB, Amaral WJ: Mandibular micrognathia corrected by vertical osteotomy in the rami and iliac bone graft. J Oral Surg 18:3, 1960.
4. Caldwell JB, Hayward JR, Lister RL: Correction of mandibular retrognathia by vertical-L osteotomy: A new technique. J Oral Surg 26:259, 1968.
5. Dal Pont G: Retromolar osteotomy for the correction of prognathism. J Oral Surg 19:42, 1961.
6. Epker BN: Modifications in the sagittal osteotomy of the mandible. J Oral Surg 35:157, 1977.
7. Ernst F: Uber die chirurgische Beseitigung der Prognathie des Unterkiefers. Zentralbl Chir 65:179, 1938.
8. Hawkinson RT: Retrognathia correction by means of an arcing osteotomy in the ascending ramus. J Prosthet Dent 20:77, 1968.
9. Hunsuck EE: A modified intraoral sagittal splitting technic for correction of mandibular prognathism. J Oral Surg 26:249, 1968.
10. Kazanjian V, Converse J: The Surgical Treatment of Facial Injuries. 2nd ed. Baltimore, The Williams & Wilkins Company, 1959.
11. Limberg AA: A new method of plastic lengthening of the mandible in unilateral microgenia and asymmetry of the face. J Am Dent Assoc 15:851, 1928.
12. Robinson M: Micrognathism corrected by vertical osteotomy of ascending ramus and iliac bone graft: A new technique. Oral Surg Oral Med Oral Pathol 10:1125, 1957.
13. Robinson M, Lytle JJ: Micrognathism corrected by vertical osteotomies of the rami without bone grafts. Oral Surg Oral Med Oral Pathol 15:641, 1962.
14. Schuchardt J: Experience with the surgical treatment of some deformities of the jaws: Prognathia, microgenia and open bite. In Wallace AB (ed): Transactions of the International Society of Plastic Surgeons, Second Congress. Baltimore, The Williams & Wilkins Company, 1961, pp 73–78.
15. Trauner R, Obwegeser H: The surgical correction of mandibular prognathism and retrognathia with consideration of genioplasty. I. Oral Surg Oral Med Oral Pathol 10:677, 1957.
16. Wolford LM, Davis WM: The mandibular inferior border split: A modification in the sagittal split osteotomy. J Oral Maxillofac Surg 48:92, 1990.

I. ORTHODONTIC SEQUENCING, DECISIONS, AND TECHNIQUES

HARRY L. LEGAN

Patients with Class II malocclusions and mandibular deficiency possess a wide range of skeletal, soft tissue, and occlusal characteristics. Optimal results are best obtained by means of a combined surgical and orthodontic approach. An analytical evaluation of the patient is necessary to decide the most appropriate treatment plan. To achieve the goals of good function, esthetics, and stability for these patients, the orthodontist and oral maxillofacial surgeon must formulate this optimal plan at the onset of treatment. Attempts to treat these patients by conventional orthodontics first, and then, if orthodontics is unsuccessful, by referring them to the surgeon will most likely produce serious compromise of the treatment and final result.

Deficient mandibular growth is not uncommon in the American population. In growing patients with mandibular deficiency, an attempt to correct the Class II 1 or 2 discrepancy with a functional appliance, such as a Monobloc or Frankel appliance is often indicated.[1] Approximately 1 per cent of the total United States adult population, however, has mandibular deficiency to the degree that surgical mandibular advancement would be required to correct it satisfactorily.

Many factors potentially contribute to the process of developing mandibular deficiency. Some factors operate at a distance from the occlusion.[2] A large middle cranial fossa, for example, may result in a posteriorly located glenoid fossa and consequently a more posteriorly positioned mandible. More often, mandibular deficiency is merely due to an inherited tendency toward a small mandible. Trauma to the mandibular condyles at a young age, with resulting functional limitations, will typically result in severe restriction of mandibular growth. Respiratory difficulties, resulting in a downward and backward posturing of the mandible, are also found in some patients with mandibular deficiency.

The orthodontic decision-making process regarding the patient with mandibular deficiency initially requires a systematic analysis of facial integumental and skeletal features in three dimensions and a decision about what procedures are necessary to produce optimal soft and hard tissue results with acceptable stability. Subsequent to the skeletal change, the direction, magnitude, and sequencing of orthodontic tooth movement are planned to accomplish the most satisfactory occlusion in the most expedient manner.

An assessment of the patient's face from the front may reveal the lower third facial height to be normal, deficient (low mandibular plane angle), or long (high mandibular plane angle). Discrepant vertical facial dimensions may necessitate additional maxillary procedures. The consistent characteristic of the patient with mandibular deficiency is obviously the retruded position of the chin, best appreciated in the profile view.[3] Chin position, however, must be related to the lips, teeth, mandibular basal bone, and neck. In many patients with mandibular deficiency, the lower anterior teeth are flared forward on the mandible in partial compensation. In these cases, the chin is deficient relative not only to the rest of the face and the neck but also to the protrusive lower lip. Either orthodontic retraction of the lower incisors (usually the better choice) or augmentation genioplasty will be necessary for good lip-chin harmony. In patients with high mandibular plane angles, the chin button may be adequate, but because of the relative downward and backward rotation of the mandible, there may not be adequate anterior projection of the chin. If two-jaw surgery with counterclockwise mandibular rotation is planned, the chin will assume a more anterior (versus inferior) projection. If mandibular advancement surgery alone is planned, a horizontal augmentation genioplasty will probably be required.

In assessing the dental relationships of patients with mandibular deficiency, crowding and protrusion of lower anterior teeth are commonly found. Maxillary incisors are generally flared in Class II, Division 1, malocclusions and are tipped lingually and hypererupted in Class II, Division 2, situations.

When considering the transverse dimension, it is necessary to ascertain whether a problem is skeletal or dental. In addition, the lower model must be advanced into a Class I relationship for accurate diagnosis of the transverse relationship. Many patients with Class II malocclusions will not demonstrate transverse problems in their pretreatment centric relationship. When the models are hand articulated into a Class I apical base relation, however, there may be an absolute transverse maxillary deficiency that needs to be corrected.

Some of the orthodontic decisions and resultant techniques used in the treatment of patients with mandibular deficiency will now be discussed.

TREATMENT SEQUENCING

Before starting surgical and orthodontic procedures, any necessary periodontal or restorative treatment should be performed. Early periodontal therapy should include reduction of inflammation, institution of good oral hygiene, and establishment of a sufficient band of attached gingiva. Caries control must be established prior to any orthodontic treatment, and permanent or temporary restorations must be placed.

Whether surgery should occur during the early or late stages of treatment is dependent upon the unique factors of each case. There are two general approaches: (1) doing most of the orthodontic tooth movement before surgery or (2) doing most of the tooth movement after surgery.

Achieving nearly all tooth movement before surgery is advocated by those who feel that (1) surgical movement of the jaws is done more accurately when the occlusion is more finished; (2) there is a reduced risk of not being able to meet treatment goals because of postsurgical orthodontic problems; (3) some orthodontic movement has to be done presurgically anyway; and (4) patients who see early facial improvement may not want to take the time to complete all necessary postsurgical orthodontic tooth movement.

The other approach is to do only that tooth movement that is absolutely necessary and indicated prior to surgery and to do the remainder after skeletal correction. There are several reasons: (1) Tooth movement requirements are more easily recognized and appreciated, and thus more precise, when the jaws are in a Class I relationship; (2) postsurgical tooth movement is probably more rapid owing to increased metabolic activity after surgery; (3) the patient's facial esthetics is improved earlier in treatment; (4) since surgery is not as precise as orthodontics, some orthodontic finishing will always be necessary postsurgically; therefore, trying to do all the orthodontic tooth movement prior to surgery will only increase the patient's total treatment time; and (5) stability is probably improved when the positions of the jaws and teeth can be guided with various orthodontic mechanisms for a longer period postsurgically.

Identifying the patient's developmental age, not chronologic age, is important for a number of reasons when planning treatment. For example, a patient with mandibular deficiency and a Class II malocclusion may be slated for either surgical or nonsurgical orthodontic correction, depending on how much growth the patient has remaining. When appropriate intervention will be most effective also is dependent on an appreciation of the patient's growth status.

Although surgery on growing patients is controversial, some practitioners have reported that surgical and orthodontic correction of mandibular deficiency in growing children has been successful.[4] Typically, though, these studies are not statistically significant. Moreover, the age at which the surgery was performed is reported as chronologic age; the more meaningful developmental age is either unknown or unreported. In addition, length of follow-up is usually not sufficient. However, assuming that reported cases of mandibular advancement surgery are mostly done on growing patients after the permanent teeth are erupted at 13 or 14 years of age, most facial growth has been completed in the majority of these patients. Consequently, postsurgical growth increments should have little effect on the occlusion achieved at surgery. However, it must be stressed that analyzing developmental age is critical and that there is really no need to take the added risk of performing surgery prior to pubertal peak velocity of growth, except when the child is experiencing extreme psychological or socialization problems because of facial appearance or when a severe functional problem is present.

ARCH LENGTH ANALYSIS

The variance between tooth mass and available arch length in the maxilla and mandible is determined by such orthodontic decisions as anteroposterior position of incisors, arch width, and treatment midline. Such discrepancies can be calculated using the occlusogram concept.[5] Extraction decisions, anchorage requirements, and mechanotherapy will depend on the existence and magnitude of arch length redundancy or inadequacy.

Arch length redundancy can be the result of overall small teeth, one small tooth (e.g., peg lateral), a missing tooth, or a disproportionately large basal bone. Possible plans for correcting these problems include (1) closing spaces orthodontically or surgically, (2) bonding or crowning small teeth, (3) inserting bridges or implants, and (4) leaving small spaces in less noticeable areas.

Arch length inadequacies can be approached in numerous ways, depending on the magnitude. Minor inadequacies of a few millimeters can be corrected by distal movement of the molars, using devices such as headgear, tipback springs, compressed coil springs, sliding jigs and elastics, removable appliances with finger springs, repelling magnets, and lip bumpers. Minimal arch length inadequacy can also be resolved, when indicated, by interproximal enamel reduction. Modifying the original treatment plan may also be an acceptable option for resolving a minor arch length inadequacy. A slight amount of arch width increase, incisor flaring, or shift of the treatment midline may eliminate an arch length inadequacy.

Large arch length inadequacies are, in some cases, best treated by extraction of teeth. The selection of which teeth to extract is influenced by many factors, including (1) arch length requirements of each quadrant; (2) the periodontal, restorative, and endodontic status of teeth in the quadrant; and (3) tooth size.

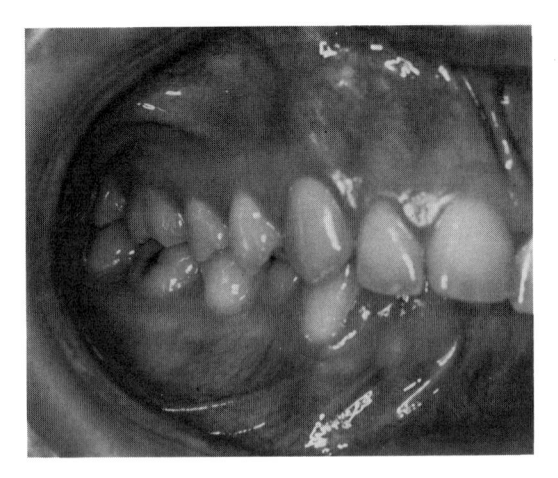

FIGURE 64–1. A 100 per cent overbite and exaggerated mandibular curve of Spee with palatal impingement by the lower incisors in a patient with Class II malocclusion and mandibular deficiency.

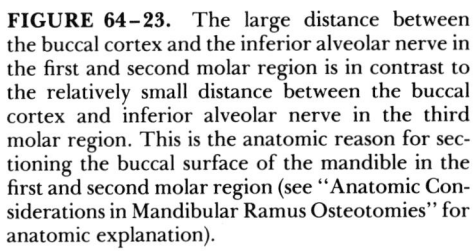

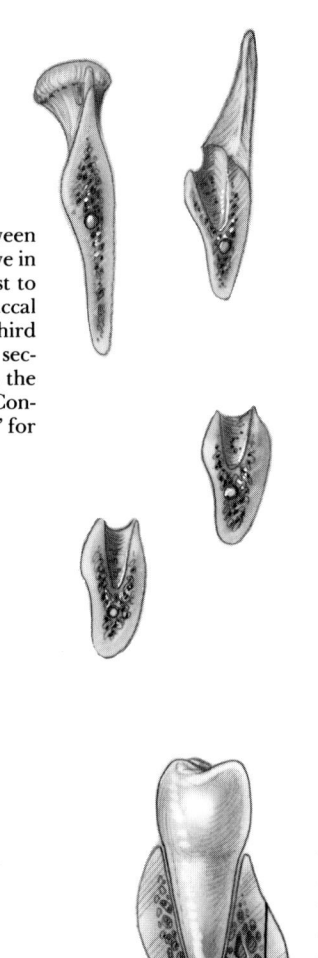

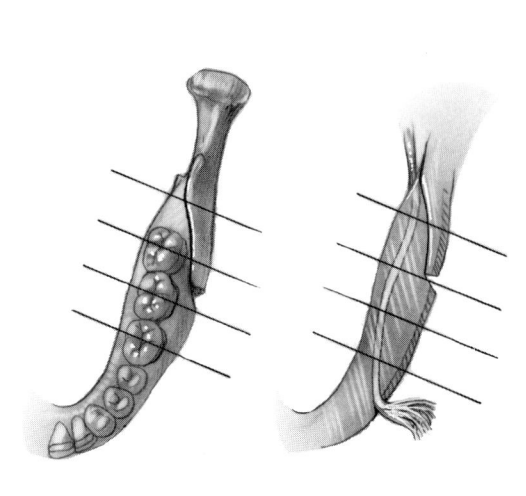

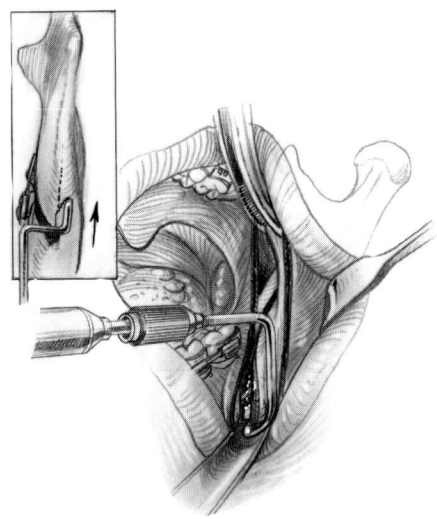

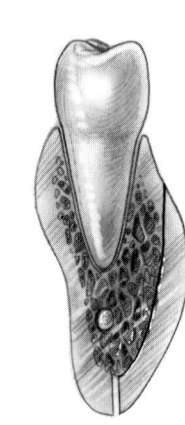

FIGURE 64-23. The large distance between the buccal cortex and the inferior alveolar nerve in the first and second molar region is in contrast to the relatively small distance between the buccal cortex and inferior alveolar nerve in the third molar region. This is the anatomic reason for sectioning the buccal surface of the mandible in the first and second molar region (see "Anatomic Considerations in Mandibular Ramus Osteotomies" for anatomic explanation).

FIGURE 64-24. The inferior border of the mandible is split utilizing blades that are offset to the left or right side to provide access for cutting on either side of the mandible. The cut is commenced anteriorly, adjacent to the vertical buccal osteotomy. The blade is oriented so that the cutting edge is parallel to the inferior border of the mandible as it bisects the buccal-lingual thickness of the cortex. The 5-mm height of the blade allows it to penetrate the inferior border cortex without damaging the neurovascular bundle. The reciprocating action of the blade is started at low speed and sunk to the approximate depth before increasing the speed. The blade is then directed posteriorly, to the distal aspect of the antegonial notch area. It is then directed immediately in a lingual direction so that it will exit through the lingual cortex anterior to the angle of the mandible at the gonial notch area. The reciprocating saw handpiece and blade should be oriented so that the blade will cut maximally up into the bone. The blade is oriented parallel to the inferior border of the mandible and should bisect the buccal-lingual thickness of the inferior border cortex. Once the saw blade has been engaged, the handpiece is rotated superiorly so that the triangular blade can cut most efficiently. The rounded shaft of the inferior aspect of the blade limits the blade from excessive vertical sectioning into the osteotomy area. The inferior border of the mandible cut is started adjacent to the vertical buccal osteotomy.

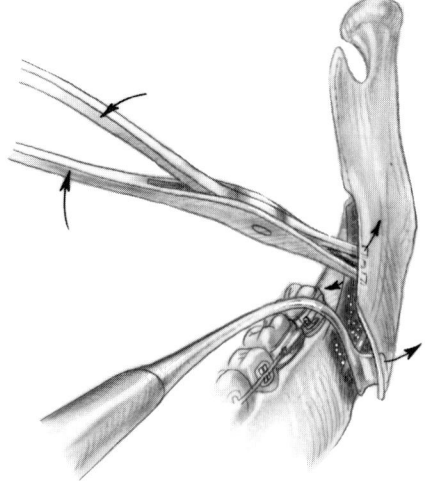

FIGURE 64-25. The Smith superior ramus separator and Smith sagittal split separator complete the split and separation.

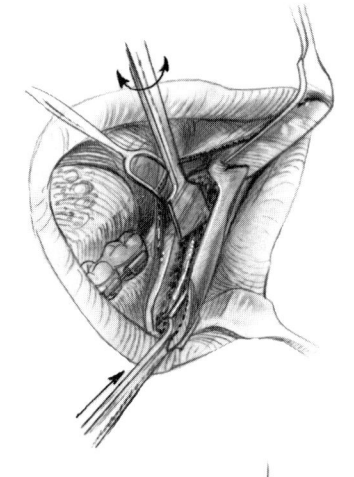

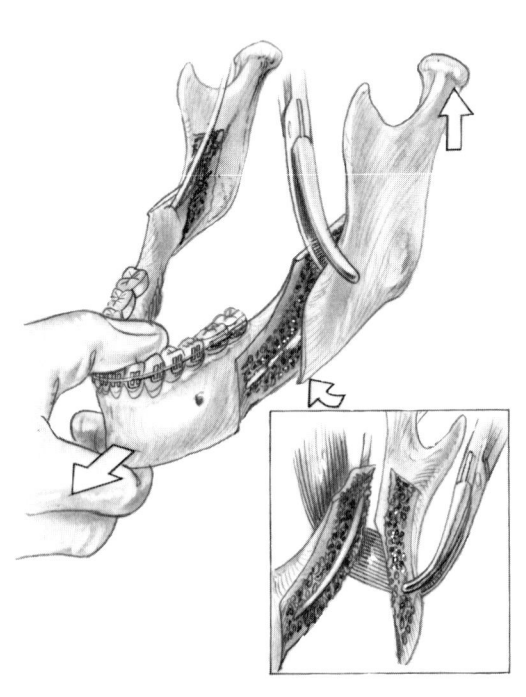

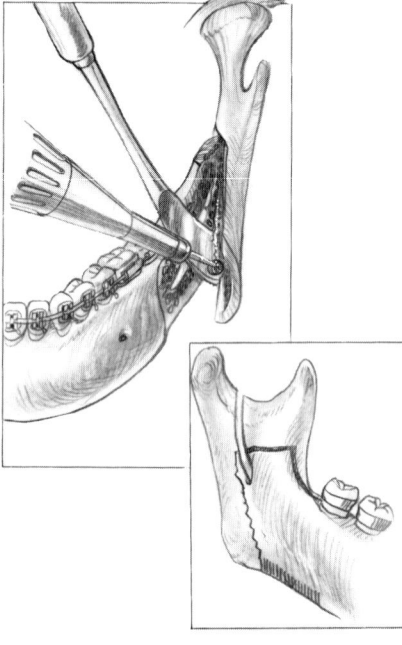

FIGURE 64-26. Spatula osteotomes are malleted to partially section the body of the mandible. Care is taken to keep the spatula osteotomes directed just subjacent to the cortical plate to prevent damage to the neurovascular bundle. If the mandible splits, the course of the neurovascular bundle must be visualized to make sure that portions of the nerve are not contained in the proximal condylar segment. A curved osteotome is used to partially split the lateromedial aspect of the ramus. An osteotome is levered against the distal segment to apply force against the inner surface of the proximal segment. An orthopedic osteotome is inserted in the split and twisted to separate the ramus segments. A bibeveled osteotome is utilized to pry the mandibular segments apart. Bone anterior to the vertical cut should be used as the principal fulcrum.

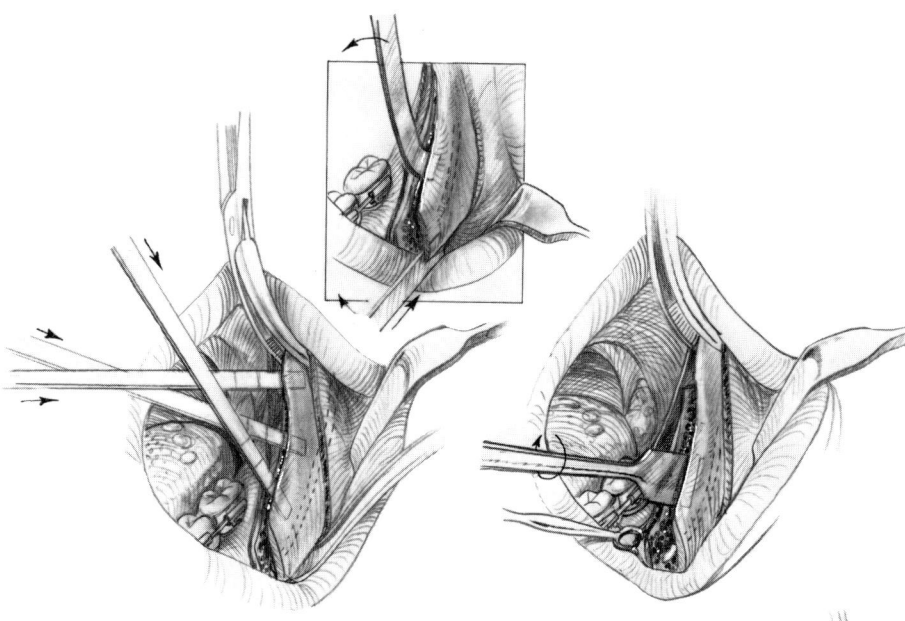

FIGURE 64-27. If separation is not complete, a splitting chisel completes the cut at the inferior border of the mandible. If the neurovascular bundle remains attached to the proximal segment, the covering bone is carefully removed with a fine osteotome, and the nerve is freed with a curette or periosteal elevator. The inset shows a fine osteotome separating the inferior alveolar nerve from the proximal segment.

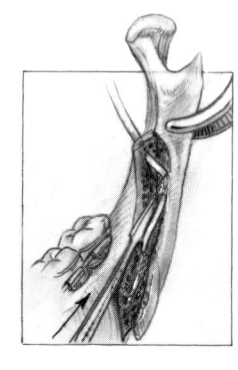

FIGURE 64-28. Completeness of separation is verified by grasping the proximal and distal segments, moving them apart in an anteroposterior direction (*arrows*), and inspecting for full separation (*inset*). Other insets show removal of protruding bone that could damage the nerve when the segments are approximated, and osteotomy lines on the medial aspect of the mandible.

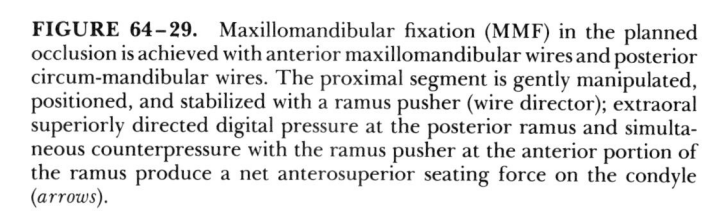

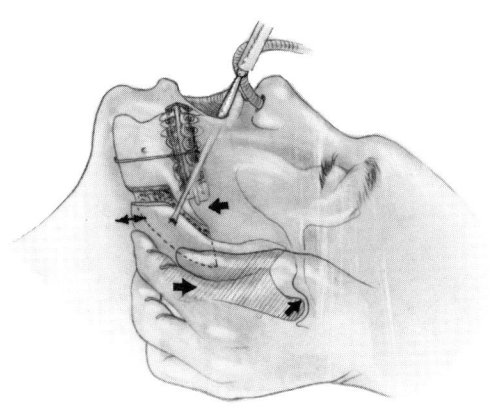

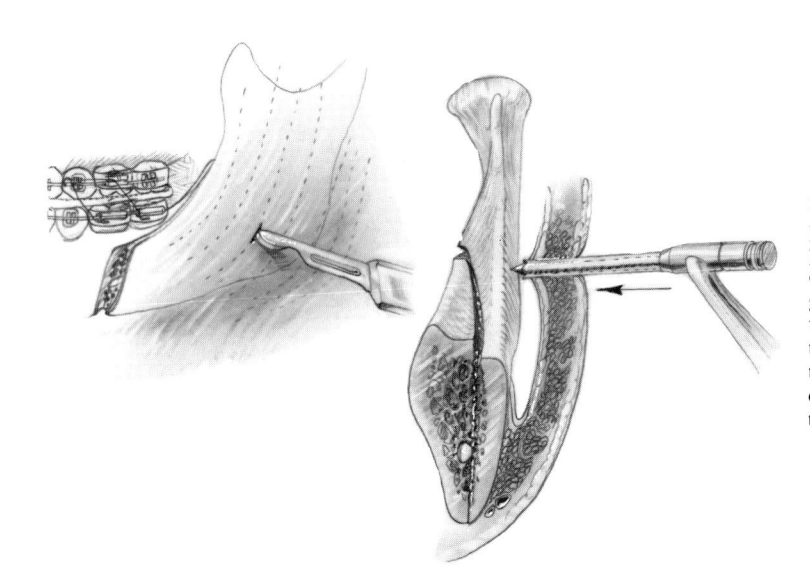

FIGURE 64-29. Maxillomandibular fixation (MMF) in the planned occlusion is achieved with anterior maxillomandibular wires and posterior circum-mandibular wires. The proximal segment is gently manipulated, positioned, and stabilized with a ramus pusher (wire director); extraoral superiorly directed digital pressure at the posterior ramus and simultaneous counterpressure with the ramus pusher at the anterior portion of the ramus produce a net anterosuperior seating force on the condyle (*arrows*).

FIGURE 64-30. When the transcutaneous approach is used, access to the osteotomy site for screw placement is gained through a stab skin incision 1 to 2 cm above the inferior border of the mandible in the gonial notch area. Following infiltration of the cheek with local anesthetic, a 4- to 5-mm incision is made through the skin only. A pointed trocar is introduced through the lumen of the drill guide and is bluntly dissected through the underlying muscle and periosteum to the lateral surface of the ramus.

FIGURE 64-31. Once the end of the drill guide is exposed intraorally, a self-retaining retractor holds the cheek tissues on the inner side away from the end of the drill guide and stabilizes the guide in place, allowing improved visualization. The necessary bone holes can be drilled, and screws placed, through one properly placed skin incision. *Top,* The tissue protector clamp is used to stabilize the tissue protector and maintain cheek retraction. A neutral drill guide insert is used in concert with the tissue protector (*arrow*). Drill holes through the proximal and distal segments are made with a slowly rotating 1.5-mm drill and a mini pin driver. A continuous flow of saline is maintained at the drill-bone interface. *Bottom,* After removing the neutral guide insert (*curved arrow*), a screw depth gauge is utilized to determine the millimetric depth of the screw hole. Position screws maintain passive separation of the proximal and distal bony segments. The screws should perforate the lingual cortex and extend 1 mm deeper than the depth of the drill hole to ensure bicortical engagement.

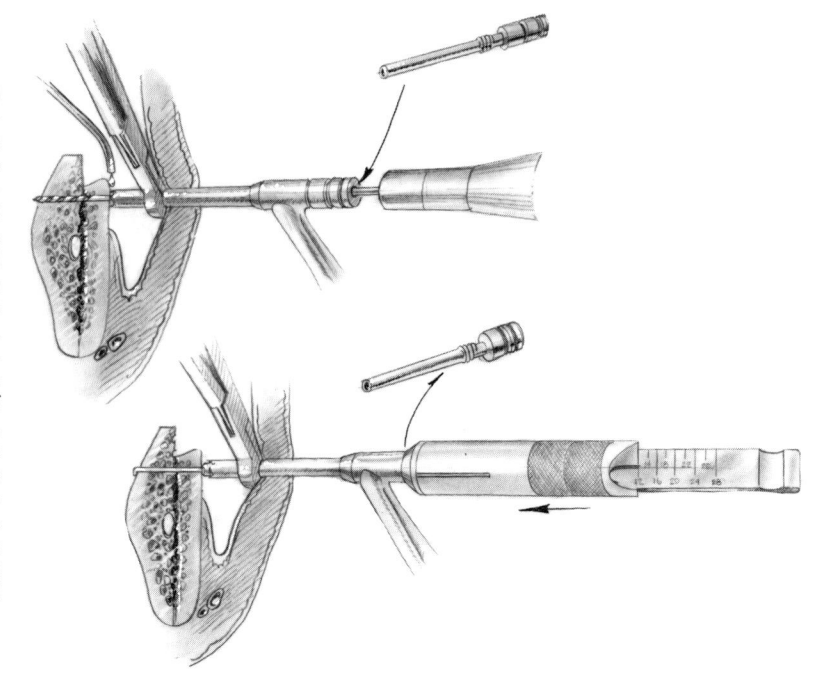

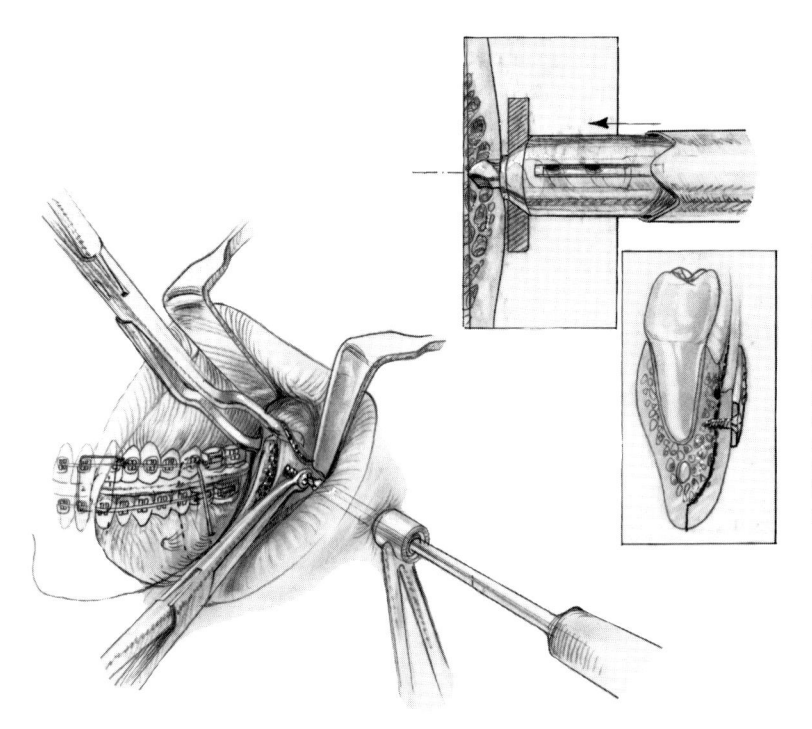

FIGURE 64-32. The inferior border of the mandible is digitally palpated to simulate the alignment of the inferior border of the mandible, consistent with the cephalometric prediction studies. The proximal and distal segments are stabilized passively in the desired position with a modified bone clamp placed initially at the area of maximal bone contact. After the drill hole is made, a 2-mm diameter screw of the required length is seated in the previously drilled screw hole on a screw-holding instrument. A Phillips-type screwdriver is inserted through the trocar to tighten the screw firmly.

FIGURE 64-33. The pattern of placement for positional screws depends on the osteotomy design and the availability of bone. A transcutaneous approach is utilized to drill holes and place three or four screws 2 mm in diameter through the superior border of the proximal and distal segments and one or two screws through the inferior border of the proximal and distal segments.

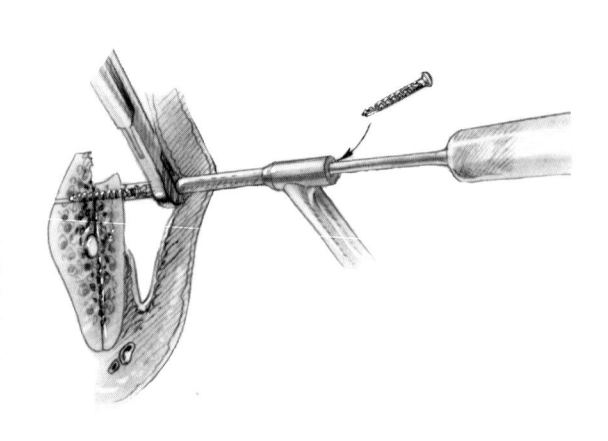

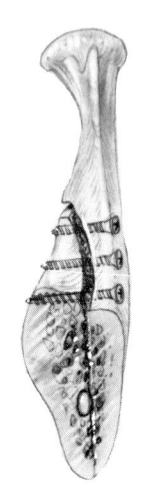

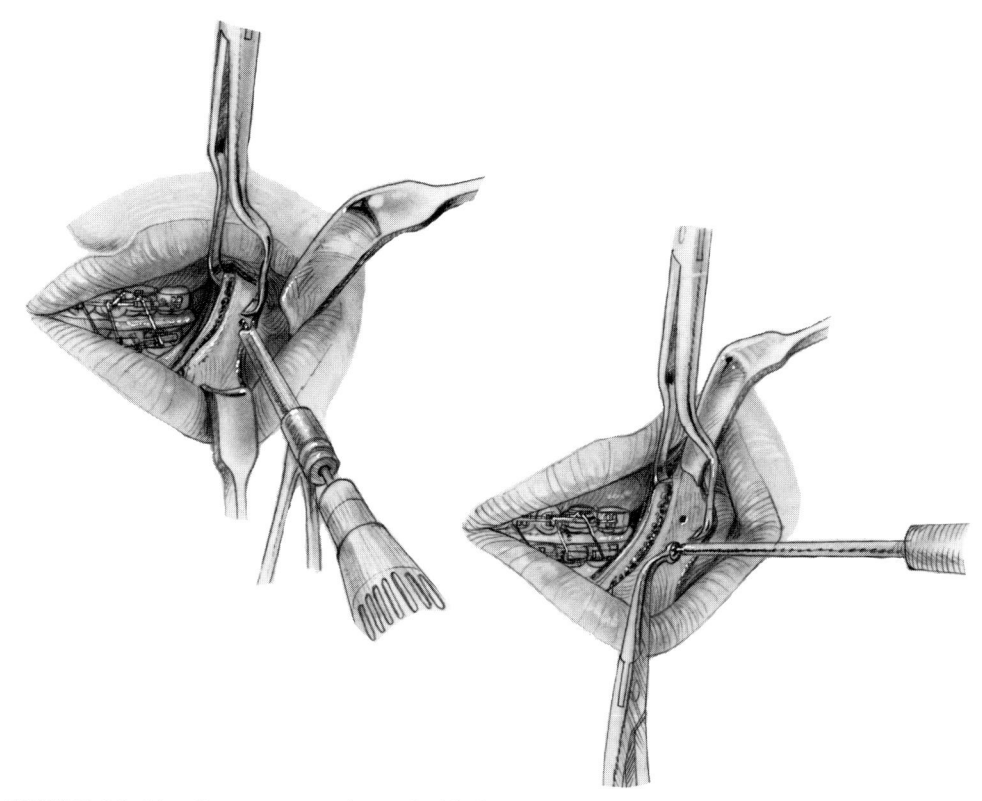

FIGURE 64-34. Great care must be used with the transoral approach to place the self-tapping screws perpendicular to the proximal segment. With teeth in MMF and segments passively stabilized with modified bone-holding forceps, a position screw is firmly tightened. In the left view, the illustrator has purposely avoided positioning the drill perpendicular to the ramus to facilitate visualization of the drill and adjunctive equipment.

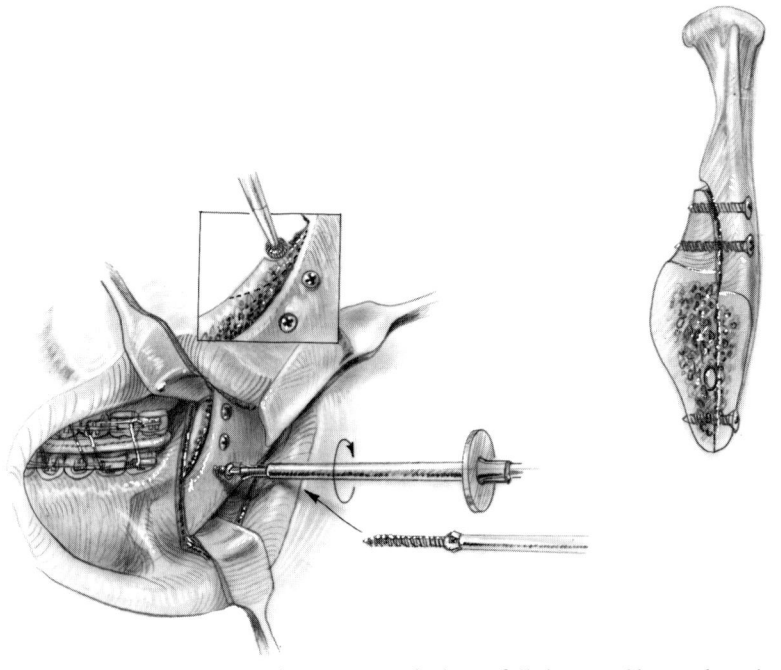

FIGURE 64-35. Three position screws may be placed anterior and superior to the inferior alveolar nerve distal to the second molar (*left*). Most frequently, one or two 2-mm screws are placed at the inferior aspect of the ramus. Two bicortical screws 2 mm in diameter are placed at the superior border, and one or two are placed at the inferior border of the mandible, avoiding the neurovascular canal. This screw placement pattern is usually feasible when the inferior border of the mandible is successfully split. Ideally, the screw at the inferior border of the mandible will transect the cortical portion of the proximal and distal segments. Screw fixation can be accomplished when there is adequate accessibility and visibility. If there has been a "bad split," it may be advisable to use the extraoral route. Position screws 2 mm in diameter will usually provide excellent fixation. To place position screws 2 mm in diameter, a 1.5-mm bone bur in a mini pin driver is used to make an initial screw hole in the proximal segment. All holes are drilled under copious irrigation. Position screws provide adequate fixation of the proximal and distal segments. These segments must, however, be aligned and held together passively as the screw engages the cortical bone of both the distal and the proximal segments. After placement of the position screws, the osteotomy site is carefully inspected by gently prying against the segments with a periosteal elevator. The medial aspect of the ramus is palpated to be sure that screws do not significantly protrude through the lingual cortex. After the screws have been placed on both sides, the MMF is released and the occlusion is checked. Clinical judgment is used at this point and is based on the stability of the postoperative occlusion. If there is an excellent Class I canine relationship with good overbite and overjet, the splint may be removed and the patient allowed to function. Finally, after removal of the drill guide, one or two mattress skin sutures are utilized to close the skin stab wound.

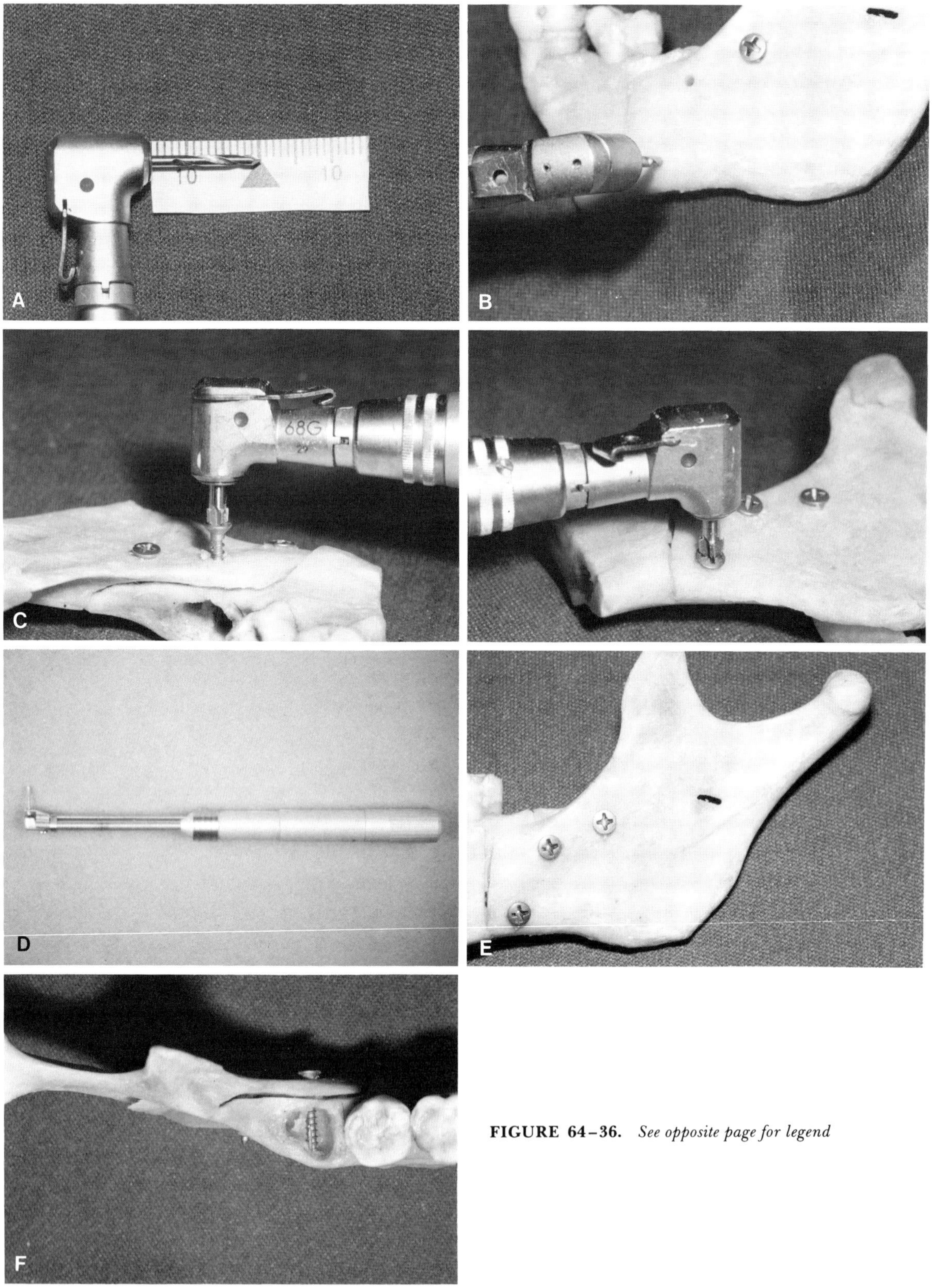

2368 / VII — ORTHOGNATHIC SURGERY

FIGURE 64-36. *See opposite page for legend*

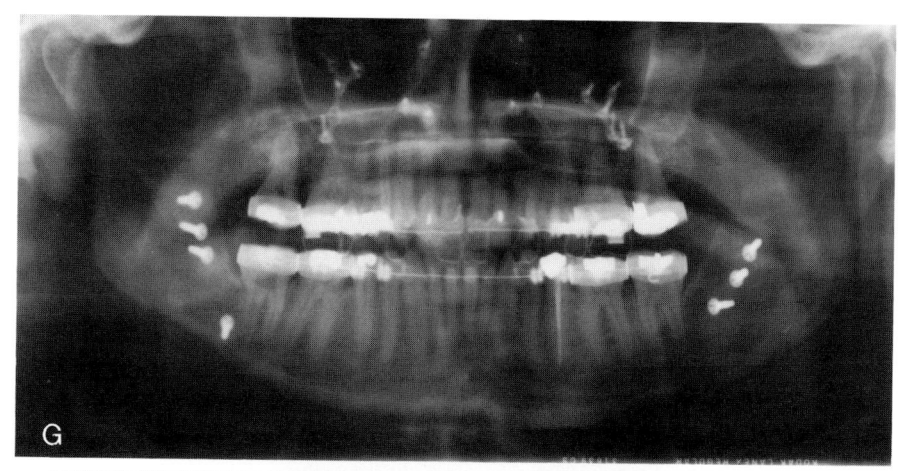

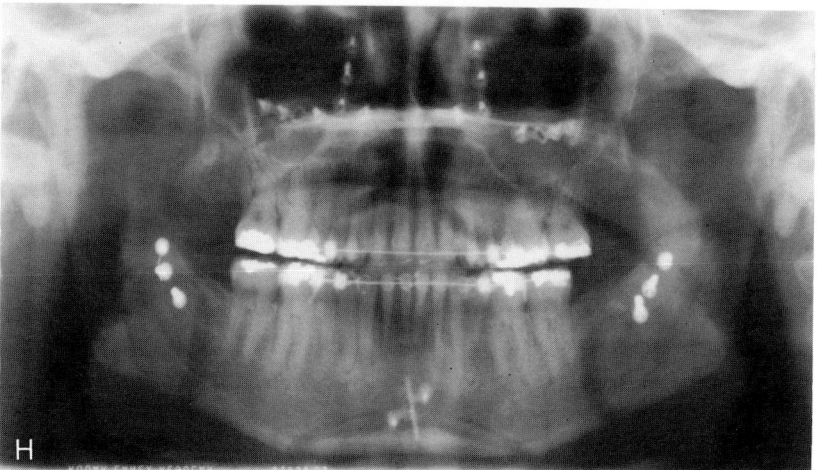

FIGURE 64–36. CONTRA-ANGLE TECHNIQUES OF RIGID INTERNAL SCREW FIXATION OF THE SAGITTAL RAMUS OSTEOTOMY, *by Anthony Farole.* We have employed a technique of contra-angle drilling and screw placement using a slow-speed contra-angle handpiece in approximately 40 sagittal ramus osteotomies (SROs) over the past 2 years. Our experiences have been most gratifying. The technique is used whenever rigid internal screw fixation is indicated or desired. There are no contraindications except when rigid internal fixation itself is contraindicated. The contra-angle technique offers the following important advantages:

1. Transoral placement of screws.
2. Perpendicular placement of screws in the direction of the sagittal split or proximal segment bone surface.
3. Very rapid and accurate placement of screws, with equal torque exerted on each screw if desired.
4. Ability to place screws in virtually any geometric pattern desired, e.g., inverted L.

Technique: After the routine SRO is completed and intermaxillary fixation is established, a single high or low wire is placed between the proximal and distal bone segments. Special attention is given to placing the proximal segment condylar position as accurately as possible with a free-hand technique similar to that discussed by Arnett. A Stryker Electric Command System with a contra-angle handpiece (or equivalent) is used with a 1.5-mm latch-type twist drill. The twist drill length is 15 mm (*A*). With the assistance of a two toe-out retractor, the first hole is drilled at the area of maximal bone contact between segments (*B*). Irrigation and high-speed selection of the control unit is used. The twist drill is then replaced with the latch Phillips-type head, and the proper screw is placed at lower speed (*C*). If additional tightening is desired, which is seldom the case, the special hand contra-angle screwdriver (Luhr) can be used (*D*). Generally, three screws are placed in an inverted-L pattern (*E*). It is virtually always possible to place one or more inferior border screws because of the versatility of the contra-angle head. The same sequence is performed on the contralateral side, making sure at all times that no bone movement of the proximal or distal segments occurs during screw placement. Intermaxillary fixation is released, and the occlusion is checked. Short-term wire, elastics, or no guided fixation is used, depending on the requirements of the particular case.

Since we began using this technique, we have not used transoral oblique placement of screws or percutaneous placement, since we feel this technique is superior. According to Foley, Frost, and colleagues (J Oral Maxillofac Surg 47:720,1989), an inverted-L pattern of screw placement offers superior transverse strength (rigidity), at least in an in vitro mechanical experimental system. Our clinical observations support this contention. First, the contra-angle system allows access to the surface of the mandible for this screw pattern placement, or others as desired (*F–H*). Second, although we are not aware of any studies proving that a perpendicular placement of screws is superior to an oblique pattern of placement, we feel that accuracy in the approximation of proximal and distal bone segments is improved (*F–H*). This accuracy has been observed by other surgeons. Third, by standardizing the setting of the percentage power of the control unit, equal torque can be placed on all screws. This factor may be important in helping to prevent proximal segment condylar torquing that may be detrimental. It is suggested that clinical competence be gained in the use of screw and plate systems in general. This increased competence, together with continuing education hands-on courses, will provide consistent predictability for this technique.

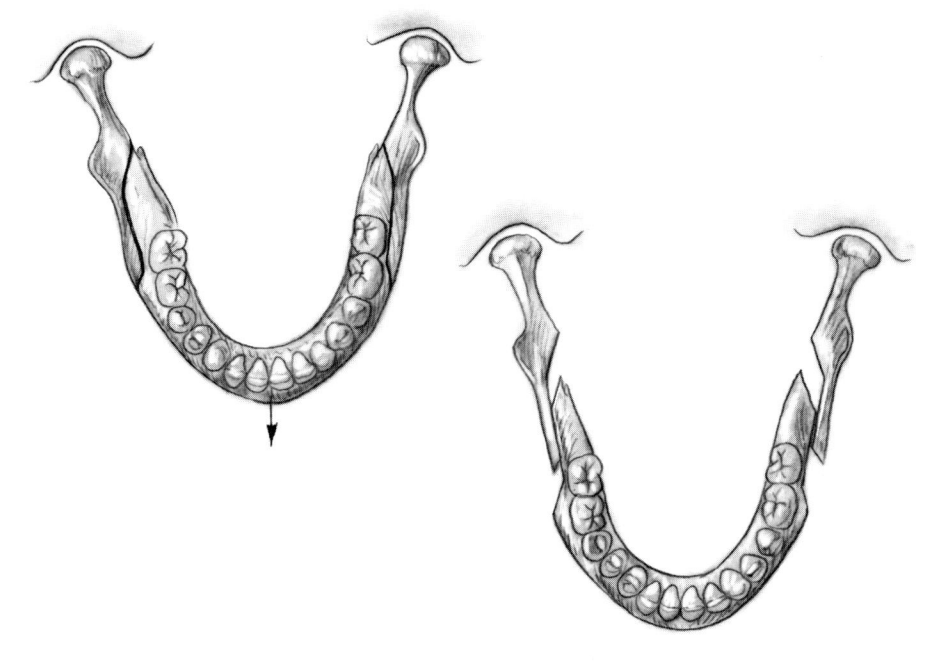

FIGURE 64-37. Ideal approximation of the proximal and distal segments has been achieved along their entire lengths. Gross interferences between the proximal and distal segments have been removed to facilitate improved apposition of the segments.

FIGURE 64-38. Whenever feasible, erupted or impacted third molar teeth are extracted 9 to 12 months before surgery. Subsequent healing of the extraction sites minimizes the possibility of a "bad sagittal split" because of the improved contact of the segments and a larger area in which to place at least two or three screws. Gross interferences between the proximal and distal segments have been removed to facilitate improved apposition of the segments. Lateral displacement of the proximal and distal segments associated with mandibular advancement, asymmetric mandibular movements, and isolated areas of poor contact between the proximal and distal segments may be improved by judicious contouring of the segments. Ideal apposition of the segments is infrequent.

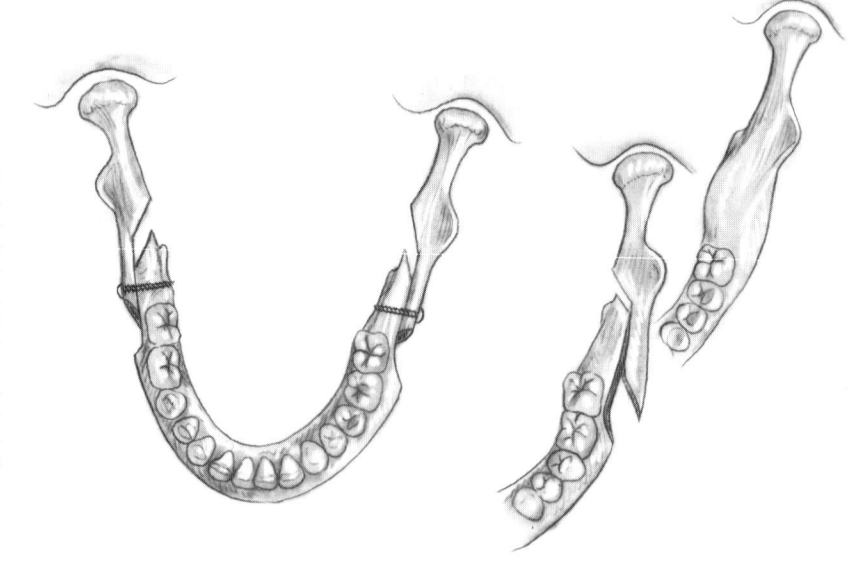

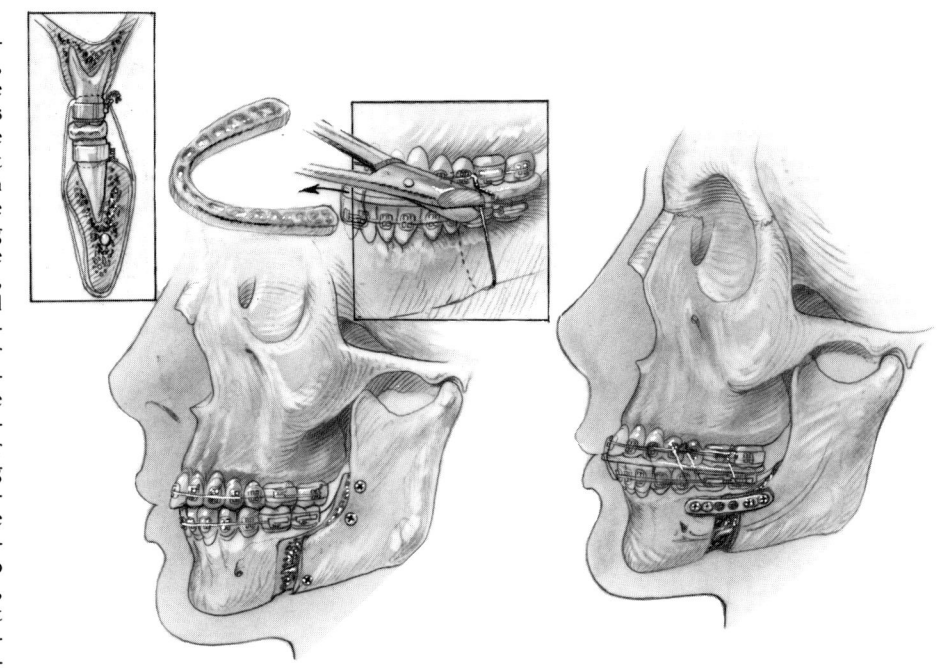

FIGURE 64-39 *Left,* When rigid fixation methods are utilized, the surgeon must release the MMF after surgery to assess whether the mandible will rotate into the planned position without distraction of the condyle from the fossa. To rotate the mandible into the splint without distracting the condyle, pressure should be applied only beneath the angles, with careful noting of the initial occlusal contact. If there is positional shifting of the mandibular teeth to achieve a maximal occlusion, the rigid fixation hardware must be removed, MMF established, and the proximal condylar fragment repositioned. Following this step, the rigid fixation hardware can be reapplied utilizing the above techniques. It should be possible to rotate the mandible into the planned position repeatedly, with minimal effort and without displacement. If an excellent occlusion results and the repositioned segments are stabilized well with screws or plates or both, consideration can be given to removing the splint and allowing the patient to progress naturally into a normal Class I occlusion. This decision is based largely on clinical judgment. *Right,* Bicortical screws provide good osseous stability, but in selected cases, it may not always be possible to place such screws without damaging the underlying teeth. In such cases, unicortical screws used in concert with mini plates usually provide sufficient stabilization of the segments. The plates must be very precisely adapted to the underlying bone to prevent condyle displacement when the screws are tightened. A neutral drill guide is used in concert with a tissue protector to facilitate symmetric drilling of a hole through the outer cortex. An example of such a need is when impacted third molar teeth are removed simultaneously with the sagittal split ramus osteotomy. In selected cases, it may be necessary to utilize two plates or a larger reconstruction plate to achieve the desired stabilization.

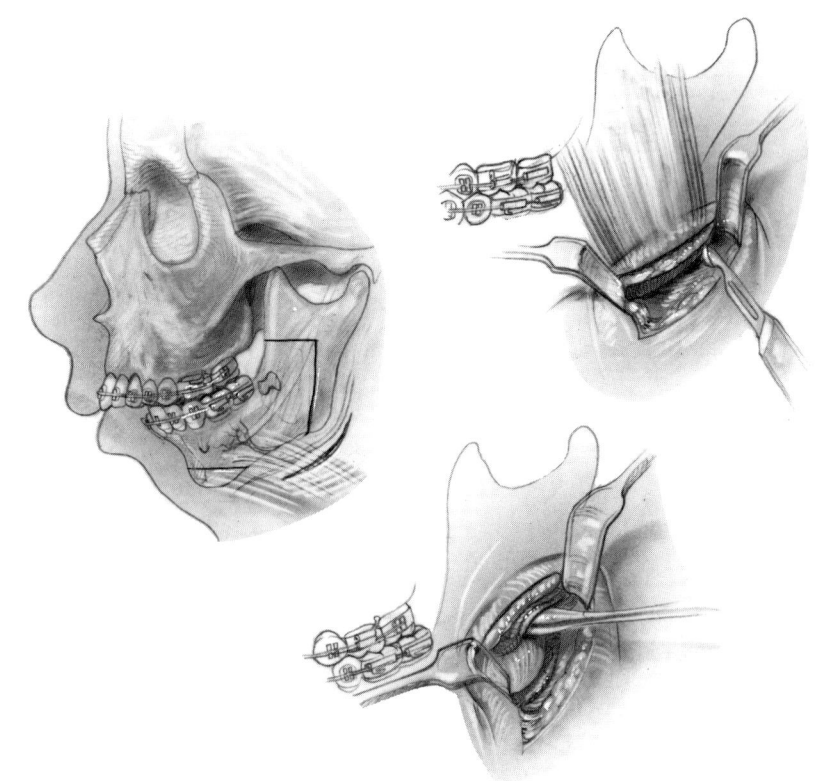

FIGURE 64-40. Limited accessibility of the oral cavity (as with microsomia), limited jaw opening, aberrant anatomy (such as excessively small mandibular rami wherein the mandibular canal is positioned very close to the inferior border of the mandible), and problematic impacted third molar teeth are relative indications for extraoral ramus surgery. Extraoral surgery requiring exposure of the mandibular ascending ramus and body of the mandible is accomplished through a retromandibular approach. When locating the incision, consideration must be given to a deeper anatomic structure that might be exposed during the dissection. The patient is placed on the operating room table in a supine position with moderate elevation of the ipsilateral shoulder and with the head rotated and extended in the opposite direction.

PLAN OF TREATMENT

Stage I (Orthodontic Treatment)

1. Mandibular arch: alignment and partial leveling without extractions.
2. Maxillary arch: lateral maxillary osteotomies and rapid palatal expansion and subsequent alignment of teeth without extractions. This plan of treatment obviated additional maxillary surgery at the time of definitive mandibular advancement surgery. Surgical removal of impacted mandibular third molar teeth by a sectioning technique minimized the removal of bone in preparation for subsequent SSROs and rigid internal fixation (approximately 1 year later).

Success with the treatment plan was contingent upon achieving rigid skeletal fixation of the repositioned mandible so that maxillomandibular fixation would be unnecessary and rhinoplasty could be accomplished simultaneously with definitive mandibular advancement surgery and submental suction lipectomy.

Stage II

1. An 8-mm mandibular advancement by bilateral SSROs and rigid internal fixation to achieve maxillomandibular harmony.
2. External rhinoplasty to reduce nasal width, increase nasal tip projection, and increase the amount of columellar exposure.
3. Removal of submental lipodystrophy by suction lipectomy.

FOLLOW-UP

After preliminary orthodontic treatment, the first stage of the surgery was accomplished. Twelve months later, after bone healing in the mandibular extraction sites was far advanced and the dental arches were coordinated, the definitive Stage II surgical procedures were achieved simultaneously. Successful use of rigid internal fixation to stabilize the surgically repositioned mandible without maxillomandibular fixation was the key to successful simultaneous nasal surgery. After this procedure was accomplished, the maxillomandibular fixation was released, and the endotracheal tube was switched from a nasal placement to an oral placement. The combined mandibular advancement, rhinoplasty, and suction lipectomy, in concert with orthodontic treatment, achieved the planned anteroposterior and vertical facial proportions, improved submental cervical esthetics, and attained the functional objectives of treatment (Fig. 64–42C, I, J, and K). Skeletal and dental stability and esthetic facial proportions have been maintained 24 months postoperatively.

Orthodontic Treatment—Stephen Chu, D.D.S., Dallas, TX
Orthognathic Surgery—William H. Bell, D.D.S., Dallas, TX
Nasal Surgery—Rod J. Rohrich, M.D., Dallas, TX

CASE 2 (Fig. 64–43)

J.R., a 26-year-old woman, was referred for treatment of her Class II, Division 2, deep bite malocclusion.

PROBLEM LIST

Esthetics (Fig. 64–43A to C)

The patient exhibited a symmetric, square face with adequate tooth exposure when in repose and when smiling (Fig. 64–43A to C).

CEPHALOMETRIC ANALYSIS. Analysis revealed an absolute skeletal mandibular deficiency with deep bite, parallel facial planes, and the mandible rotated closed (Fig. 64–43G).

OCCLUSAL ANALYSIS. A Class II, Division 2, malocclusion with excessive overjet and overbite (10 mm) was present (Fig. 64–43I to K). With the mandible positioned into a simulated Class I occlusal relationship, horizontal maxillary deficiency and esthetic vertical and sagittal facial proportions were demonstrated. There was a moderate reverse curve in the maxillary arch and a moderate curve of Spee in the mandibular arch. Mild crowding was seen in the anterior maxillary and mandibular arches.

PLAN OF TREATMENT

Orthodontic Treatment. Mandibular arch: alignment and partial leveling without extractions.

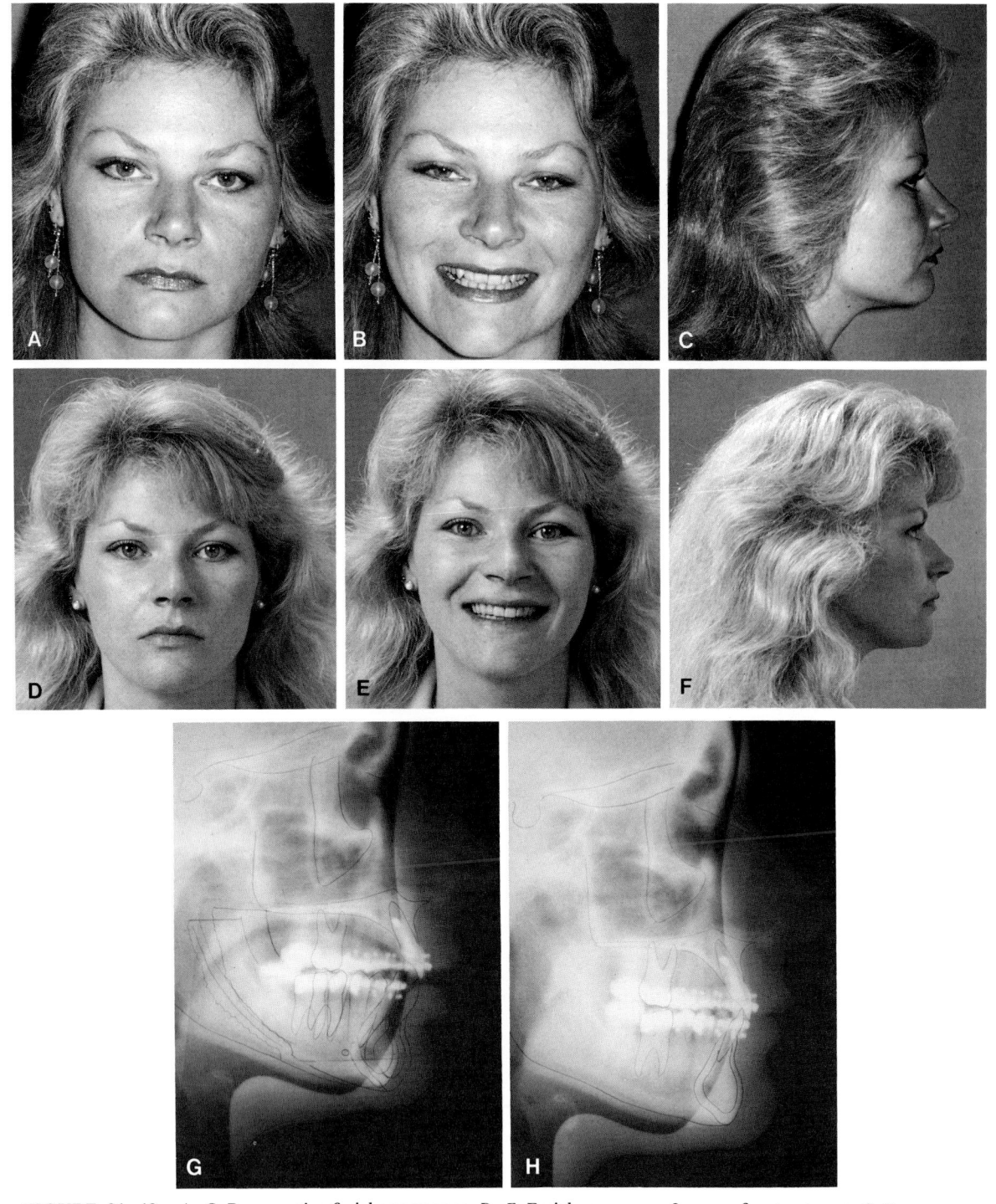

FIGURE 64-43. *A-C*, Preoperative facial appearance. *D-F*, Facial appearance 3 years after treatment. *G*, Pretreatment cephalometric radiograph. *H*, Cephalometric radiograph 3 years after treatment.

Illustration continued on following page

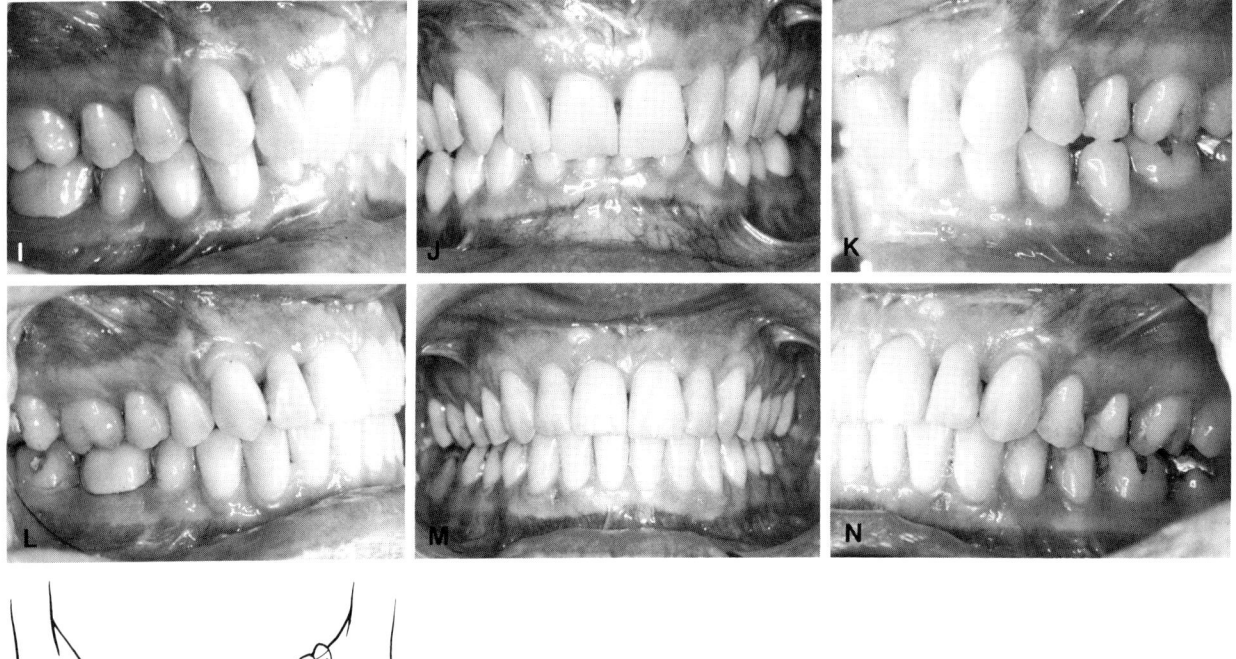

FIGURE 64–43 *Continued.* *I–K*, Pretreatment Class II deep bite malocclusion. *L–N*, Post-treatment occlusion. *O*, Reconstruction plate fixation of symphyseal osteotomy.

Surgical Treatment

1. Mandibular advancement by bilateral SSROs and rigid internal fixation to achieve maxillomandibular harmony.
2. Symphyseal osteotomy to narrow the mandible to achieve transverse harmony.

FOLLOW-UP

The surgical procedures were performed simultaneously. The combined mandibular advancement, rhinoplasty, and suction lipectomy, in concert with orthodontic treatment, achieved the planned anteroposterior and vertical facial proportions, as well as the functional objectives of treatment (Fig. 64–43*D, E, F, H, L, M,* and *N*). Skeletal and dental stability and esthetic facial proportions have been maintained 5 years postoperatively.

Orthodontist—Stephen Chu, D.D.S., Dallas, TX
Orthognathic Surgery—William H. Bell, D.D.S., Dallas, TX

IV. Stability of Mandibular Advancement Surgery: A Review

DAVID J. DARAB

The introduction of the sagittal split ramus osteotomy (SSRO) by Trauner and Obwegeser[45] more than 30 years ago significantly advanced the ability of the oral and maxillofacial surgeon to correct mandibular deformities. This technique gained widespread acceptance, for it could be easily adapted to correct a wide variety of mandibular anomalies. The transoral approach simplified the surgical technique while at the same time eliminating the external scar and minimizing risk to the facial nerve. Finally, sagittal splitting produced a large area of bony contact, which enhanced healing and reduced the need for bone grafting.[9] In spite of these many advantages, clinicians continued to be plagued with complications, including (1) injury to the neurovascular bundle, (2) inadvertent fracture, and (3) instability of the surgical result. Numerous authors have modified the original osteotomy design of Obwegeser in an effort to increase the area of bony contact, reduce the amount of soft tissue dissection, prevent proximal segment rotation,[6,11,17,19,52] and discover the ideal condyle position. Although these modifications, combined with advances in instrumentation, have simplified the surgical procedure, reducing the incidence of permanent nerve injury and inadvertent fracture, postoperative stability continues to be unpredictable.

Numerous investigators have reported postoperative relapse following mandibular advancement surgery, with an incidence ranging from 23 to 76 per cent.[21,24,25,28,33,36,37,39,44,50] Although the causes of this relapse continue to be multifactorial, investigators have stressed the importance of proximal segment control, maintaining ideal condyle position, osteotomy stabilization, and reducing muscular influences as a means of improving stability. Much in the same way that the osteotomy design and surgical techniques of the sagittal split underwent numerous modifications, fixation techniques have evolved in an effort to reduce postoperative relapse.

Initial attempts at stabilizing the repositioned skeletal fragments involved maxillomandibular fixation (MMF). This modality was derived from experience in treating maxillofacial injuries in which MMF alone was sufficient to stabilize the fractured segments. Poulton and Ware[33] demonstrated early that considerable adjustment of the teeth within the alveolar process can occur during MMF. Through intrusion of posterior teeth and extrusion of anterior teeth, the mandible can relapse without changes in the occlusal relationship. Other investigators reported similar findings after mandibular advancement surgery using MMF alone.[21,25,28,36,39,51] In addition, they noted that the majority of skeletal relapse occurred early, during the period of MMF, with little relapse occurring after this interval. Results from these and other investigations suggested that four factors contributed to relapse: (1) condyle position, (2) lack of proximal segment control at the time of surgery, (3) lack of stability of the proximal segment during healing, and (4) paramandibular connective tissue tension.[12,28,37] Of these three factors, condyle position and lack of proximal segment control have been singled out as being the most important factors in relapse following mandibular advancement.[2,12,37]

Throughout the years, an enormous volume of literature has been devoted to the topic of proximal segment control. It is important to distinguish between two aspects of proximal segment control: (1) condylar position and (2) proximal segment rotation. The importance of accurate condylar seating at the time of surgery

Improved stability in mandibular advancement surgery following screw osteosynthesis has been reported by numerous investigators.[7,8,23,44,47,48] Van Sickels and coworkers[47,48] have reported good clinical stability following mandibular advancement with percutaneous screw osteosynthesis. For small advancements, they noted anterior movement at pogonion. However, for advancements greater than 6 to 7 mm, relapse occurred, increasing with the magnitude of the advancement. In addition, they noted that screw osteosynthesis provided accurate proximal segment control. Kirkpatrick and colleagues[23] reported a 7.3 per cent mean postoperative relapse following screw osteosynthesis. No relationship was observed between magnitude of advancement and relapse. A direct comparison of combined dental and skeletal MMF and screw osteosynthesis by Darab and coworkers[7] demonstrated excellent stability in both groups. Slight anterior movement at B-point was noted in each group. Although no relationship between magnitude of mandibular advancement and posterior relapse of the mandible was identified statistically, those individuals with the greatest advancements demonstrated posterior movement. Thomas and associates[44] reported a similar net advancement in B-point during the postoperative period following lag screw osteosynthesis. They also noted greater anterior dental compensation in the wire group. The enhanced stability of screw osteosynthesis described here may result from a number of factors, including (1) the ability to assess condyle-fossa positioning and occlusal relationships at the time of surgery, (2) better proximal segment positioning, and (3) stronger osteotomy site with primary bone healing. Additional research is necessary before definitive conclusions can be reached.

Although it is not the aim of this section to describe the various techniques of screw osteosynthesis, it is important to realize that techniques differ greatly. The number of screws, placement pattern, diameter of screws, type of drill, compression versus bicortical, tapping versus self-tapping, and intraoral versus transcutaneous approach are all variables that preclude considering this a single technique. It has not been until recently that investigators have begun to evaluate these parameters. Comparison of screw placement patterns and techniques by Foley and associates[15] demonstrated that osteotomies fixated with screws placed in an inverted-L pattern were significantly more rigid than those fixated with screws placed in a linear fashion. No difference was observed between compression and bicortical positional screws placed in identical patterns. Similar investigations comparing the uniaxial pull-out strength of five commonly used screws and Kirschner pins concluded that the pull-out strength of the Kirschner pins was significantly less than that of the screws. The five-screw techniques did not differ significantly.[16] These studies stress the complexities of the many variables inherent in internal screw fixation. To categorize all screw techniques simply as "rigid fixation" is inaccurate. Until the differences between the many techniques can be evaluated, one must exercise caution when comparing results.

Reitzik advocates extraoral inverted-L osteotomies, bone grafting, and application of mesh plates to enhance stability of the surgically lengthened mandible.[34] In evaluating the treatment response of these patients, Reitzik and associates[2,34,35] report no significant changes in gonial angle, proximal segment position, or mandibular plane angle. Although they reported no mean postoperative relapse in any time interval, individual response varied greatly, and a strong positive correlation was observed between posterior relapse and the magnitude of mandibular advancement.

In conclusion, the oral and maxillofacial surgeon now has at his or her disposal numerous methods of fixating the advanced mandible after sagittal split osteotomies. All of these techniques can be categorized as either (1) skeletal fixation or (2) screw and/or plate osteosynthesis. When compared with dental MMF alone, these techniques provide superior stability for the advanced mandible. It should be emphasized that regardless of the fixation method used, there is a point at which advancement exceeds the capacity of the fixation technique, resulting in relapse.

Although relapse can be documented on lateral cephalograms, the clinical significance of this at the level of the occlusion may be negligible in the individual case. It has been suggested that relapse in large mandibular advancements (>10 mm) may be prevented by a combination of larger screws and plates, suprahyoid myotomies, and skeletal fixation.[12,47] Until quantitative data are available on large mandibular advancements, the type of fixation will continue to be chosen on the basis of the surgeon's clinical judgment.

REFERENCES

1. Arnett GW, Tamborello JA, Rathbone JA: Temporomandibular joint ramifications of orthognathic surgery. *In* Bell WH (ed): Modern Practice in Orthognathic and Reconstructive Surgery. Vol 1. Philadelphia, WB Saunders Company, 1992.
2. Barer PG, Wallen TR, McNeill RW, Reitzik M: Stability of mandibular advancement osteotomy using rigid internal fixation. Am J Orthod Dentofacial Orthop 92:403, throughout 1987.
3. Booth DF: Control of the proximal segment by lower border wiring in the sagittal split osteotomy. J Oral Maxillofac Surg 9:126, 1981.
4. Brusati R, Fiamminghi L, Sesenna E, Gazzotti A: Functional disturbances of the inferior alveolar nerve after sagittal osteotomy of the mandibular ramus: Operating technique for prevention. J Maxillofac Surg 9:123, 1981.
5. Carlson DS, Ellis E, Dechow PC: Adaptation of the suprahyoid muscle complex to mandibular advancement surgery. Am J Orthod Dentofacial Orthop 92:134, 1987.
6. Dal Pont G: Retromolar osteotomy for the correction of prognathism. J Oral Surg 19:42, 1961.
7. Darab DJ, Sinn DP, Boyd SP: Comparative stability of skeletal stabilization and screw osteosynthesis in mandibular advancement surgery.
8. Ellis E, Gallo WJ: Relapse following mandibular advancement with dental plus skeletal maxillomandibular fixation. J Oral Maxillofac Surg 44:509, 1986.
9. Ellis E, Carlson DS: Stability two years after mandibular advancement with and without suprahyoid myotomy: An experimental study. J Oral Maxillofac Surg 41:426, 1983.
10. Ellis E, Reynolds S, Carlson DS: Stability of the mandible following advancement: A comparison of three postsurgical fixation techniques. Am J Orthod Dentofacial Orthop 94:38, 1988.
11. Epker BN: Modifications in the sagittal osteotomy of the mandible. J Oral Surg 35:157, 1977.
12. Epker BN, Wessberg BA: Mechanisms of early skeletal relapse following surgical advancement of the mandible. Br J Oral Surg 20:175, 1982.
13. Epker BN, Wylie A: Control of the condylar–proximal mandibular segments after sagittal split osteotomies to advance the mandible. Oral Surg 62:613, 1986.
14. Finn RA, Throckmorton GS, Bell WH: Biomechanical considerations in the surgical correction of mandibular deficiency. J Oral Surg 38:257, 1980.
15. Foley WL, Frost DE, Paulin WB, Tucker MR: Internal screw fixation: Comparison of placement pattern and rigidity. J Oral Maxillofac Surg 47:720, 1989.
16. Foley WL, Frost DE, Paulin WB, Tucker MR: Uniaxial pullout evaluation of internal screw fixation. J Oral Maxillofac Surg 47:277, 1989.
17. Gallo WJ, Moss M, Gaul JV, Shapiro S: Modification of the sagittal ramus split osteotomy for retrognathia. J Oral Surg 34:178, 1976.
18. Guernsey LH: Stability of treatment results in Class II malocclusion corrected by full mandibular advancement surgery. Oral Surg 37:668, 1974.
19. Hunsuck EE: A modified intraoral sagittal splitting technique for correction of mandibular prognathism. J Oral Surg 26:249, 1968.
20. Isaacson RJ, Kopytow OS, Bevis RR, et al: Movement of the proximal and distal segments after mandibular ramus osteotomies. J Oral Surg 36:263, 1978.
21. Ive J, McNeill RW, West RA: Mandibular advancement: Skeletal and dental changes during fixation. J Oral Surg 35:881, 1977.
22. Jeter RS, Van Sickels JE, Dolwick MF: Modified techniques for internal fixation of sagittal ramus osteotomies. J Oral Maxillofac Surg 42:270, 1984.
23. Kirkpatrick TB, Woods MG, Swift JQ, Markowitz NR: Skeletal stability following mandibular advancement and rigid fixation. J Oral Maxillofac Surg 45:572, 1987.
24. Kohn MW: Analysis of relapse after mandibular advancement surgery. J Oral Surg 36:676, 1978.
25. Lake SL, McNeill RW, Little RM, et al: Surgical mandibular advancement: A cephalometric analysis of treatment response. Am J Orthod 80:376, 1981.
26. Leonard MS, Ziman P, Bevis R, et al: The sagittal split osteotomy of the mandible. Oral Surg 60:459, 1985.
27. Luhr HG: Skelettverlängernde Operationen zur Harmoniesierrung des Gesichtsprofils—probleme der stabilen Fixation von Osteotomiesegmenten. *In* Die Ästhetick von Form und Funktion in der Plastischen und Wiederherstellungschirurgie. Berlin, Springer-Verlag, 1985, pp 87–92.
28. MacIntosh RB: Experience with the sagittal osteotomy of the mandibular ramus: A 13 year review. J Maxillofac Surg 9:151, 1981.

29. Mayo KH, Ellis E: Stability of the mandible after advancement and use of dental plus skeletal maxillomandibular fixation: An experimental investigation in *Macaca mulatta*. J Oral Maxillofac Surg 45:243, 1987.
30. McNeill RW, Hooley JR, Sundberg RJ: Skeletal relapse during intermaxillary fixation. J Oral Surg 31:212, 1973.
31. Obwegeser H: The indications for surgical correction of mandibular deformity by the sagittal splitting technique. Br J Oral Surg 1:157, 1964.
32. Poulton DR, Ware WH: Surgical-orthodontic treatment of severe mandibular retrusion. Am J Orthod 59:244, 1971.
33. Poulton DR, Ware WH: Surgical-orthodontic treatment of severe mandibular retrusion. Am J Orthod 63:237, 1973.
34. Reitzik M: Mandibular advancement surgery: Stability following a modified fixation technique. J Oral Surg 38:893, 1980.
35. Reitzik M, Lowe A, Schmidt E: Stability following mandibular advancement using rigid internal fixation. Int J Oral Surg 10:276, 1981.
36. Sandor GK, Stoelinga PJ, Tideman H, Leenen RJ: The role of the intraosseous osteosynthesis wire in sagittal split osteotomies for mandibular advancement. J Oral Maxillofac Surg 42:231, 1984.
37. Schendel SA, Epker BN: Results after mandibular advancement surgery: An analysis of 87 cases. J Oral Surg 38:265, 1980.
38. Singer RS, Bays RA: A comparison between superior and inferior border wiring techniques in sagittal split ramus osteotomy. J Oral Maxillofac Surg 43:444, 1985.
39. Smith GC, Maloney FB, West RA: Mandibular advancement surgery: A study of the lower border wiring technique for osteosynthesis. Oral Surg 60:467, 1985.
40. Souyris F: Sagittal splitting and bicortical screw fixation of the ascending ramus. J Maxillofac Surg 6:198, 1978.
41. Spiessl B: Rigid internal fixation after sagittal osteotomy of the ascending ramus. *In* Spiessl B (ed): New Concepts in Maxillofacial Bone Surgery. 1st ed. New York, Springer-Verlag, 1976, pp 115–162.
42. Spiessl B: The sagittal splitting osteotomy for correction of mandibular prognathism. Clin Plast Surg 9:491, 1982.
43. Steinhauser EW: Advancement of the mandible by sagittal ramus split and suprahyoid myotomy. J Oral Surg 31:516, 1973.
44. Thomas PM, Tucker MR, Prewitt JR, Proffit WR: Early skeletal and dental changes following mandibular advancement and rigid internal fixation. Int J Adult Orthod Orthognath Surg 3:171, 1986.
45. Trauner R, Obwegeser H: The surgical correction of mandibular prognathism and retrognathia with consideration of genioplasty. Oral Surg 10:677, 1957.
46. Tulasne JF, Schendel SA: Transoral placement of rigid fixation following sagittal split ramus osteotomy. J Oral Maxillofac Surg 47:651, 1989.
47. Van Sickels JE, Larsen AJ, Thrash WJ: Relapse after rigid fixation of mandibular advancement. J Oral Maxillofac Surg 44:698, 1986.
48. Van Sickels JE, Flanary CM: Stability associated with mandibular advancement treated by rigid osseous fixation. J Oral Maxillofac Surg 43:698, 1986.
49. Wessberg GA, Schendel SA, Epker BN: The role of the suprahyoid myotomy in surgical advancement of the mandible via sagittal split ramus osteotomies. J Oral Maxillofac Surg 40:273, 1982.
50. Will LA, Joondeph DR, Hohl TH, West RA: Condylar position following mandibular advancement: Its relationship to relapse. J Oral Maxillofac Surg 42:578, 1984.
51. Will LA, West RA: Factors influencing the stability of sagittal split osteotomy for mandibular advancement. J Oral Maxillofac Surg 47:813, 1989.
52. Wolford LM, Bennett MA, Rafferty CG: Modification of the mandibular ramus sagittal split osteotomy. Oral Surg 64:146, 1987.

V. Transverse (Horizontal) Mandibular Deficiency

CESAR GUERRERO
GISELA CONTASTI

Transverse mandibular deficiency is frequently manifested in patients with dentofacial deformity. It is commonly managed by extractions, interproximal reduction of tooth mass, and dental compensations, which may be unstable owing to tipping of the teeth and bending of the alveolar bone. By utilizing the techniques discussed in this section and in "Transverse (Horizontal) Maxillary Deficiency," which follows, the efficiency and flexibility of treatment greatly increase and frequently preclude the need for extraction of the teeth. Surgery is often required to correct the basal bone problem. This is especially true in the narrowed and tapered arch form associated with crowded and tipped teeth, in complete telescopic bite (Brody's syndrome, Figs. 64–44 and 64–45), in certain congenital problems (whistling face syndrome, Fig. 64–46; Pierre Robin syndrome, Fig. 64–47), in maxillomandibular transverse deficiency (crocodile bite, Fig. 64–48), and in patients with mandibular transverse deficiency in whom crowded teeth have previously been treated by extraction orthodontic therapy. Some of these individuals may benefit from a surgically assisted rapid mandibular expansion and orthodontic treatment.

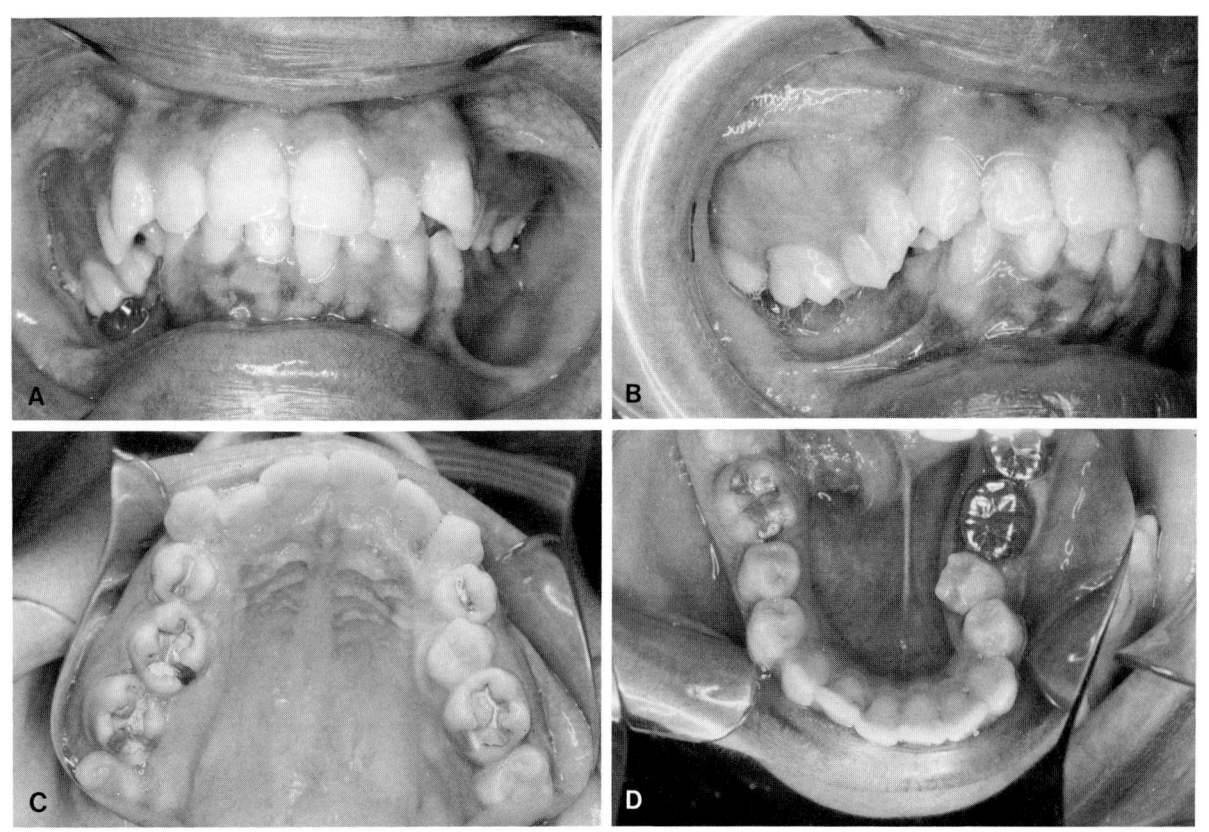

FIGURE 64–44. *A–D*, Unilateral Brody's syndrome.

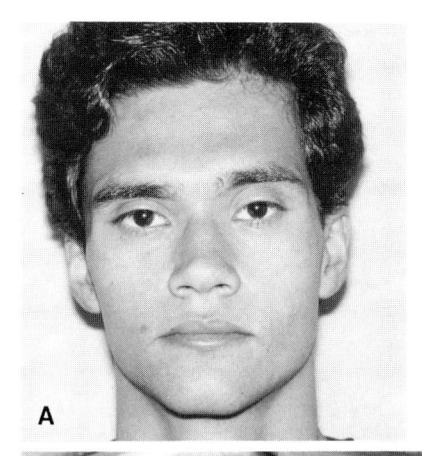

FIGURE 64-45. *A–E*, Bilateral Brody's syndrome.

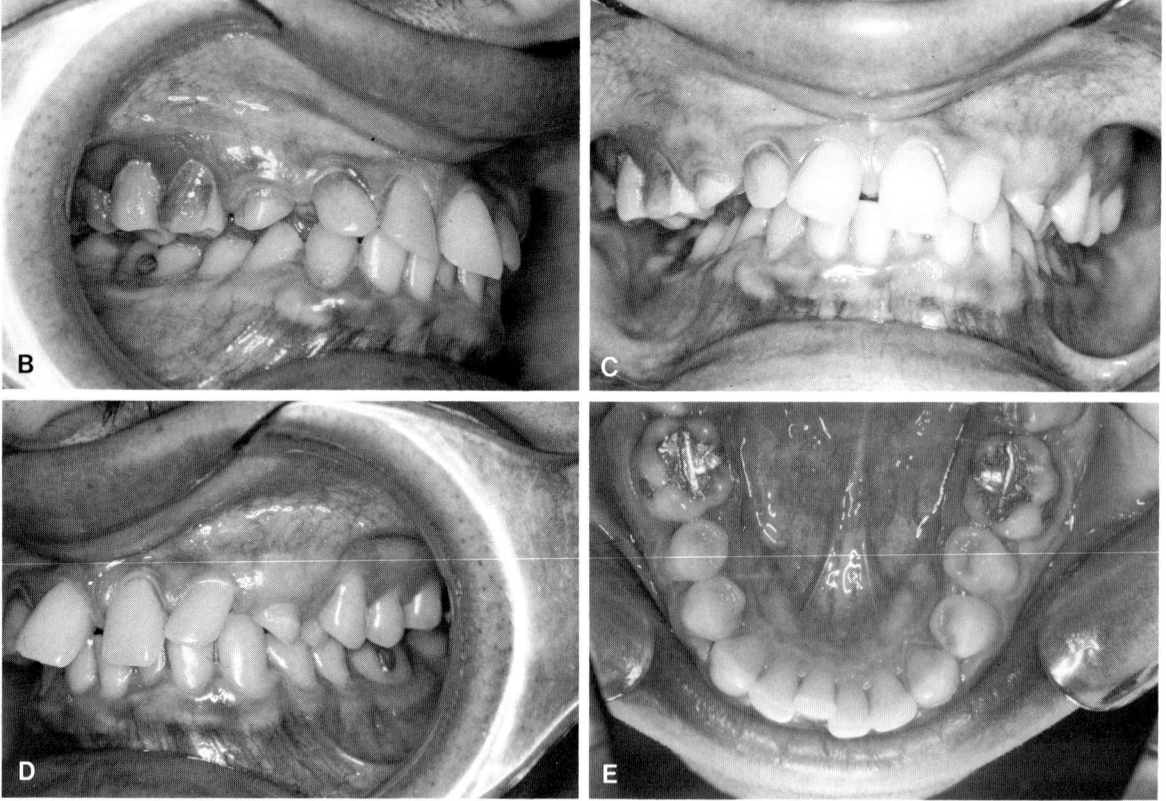

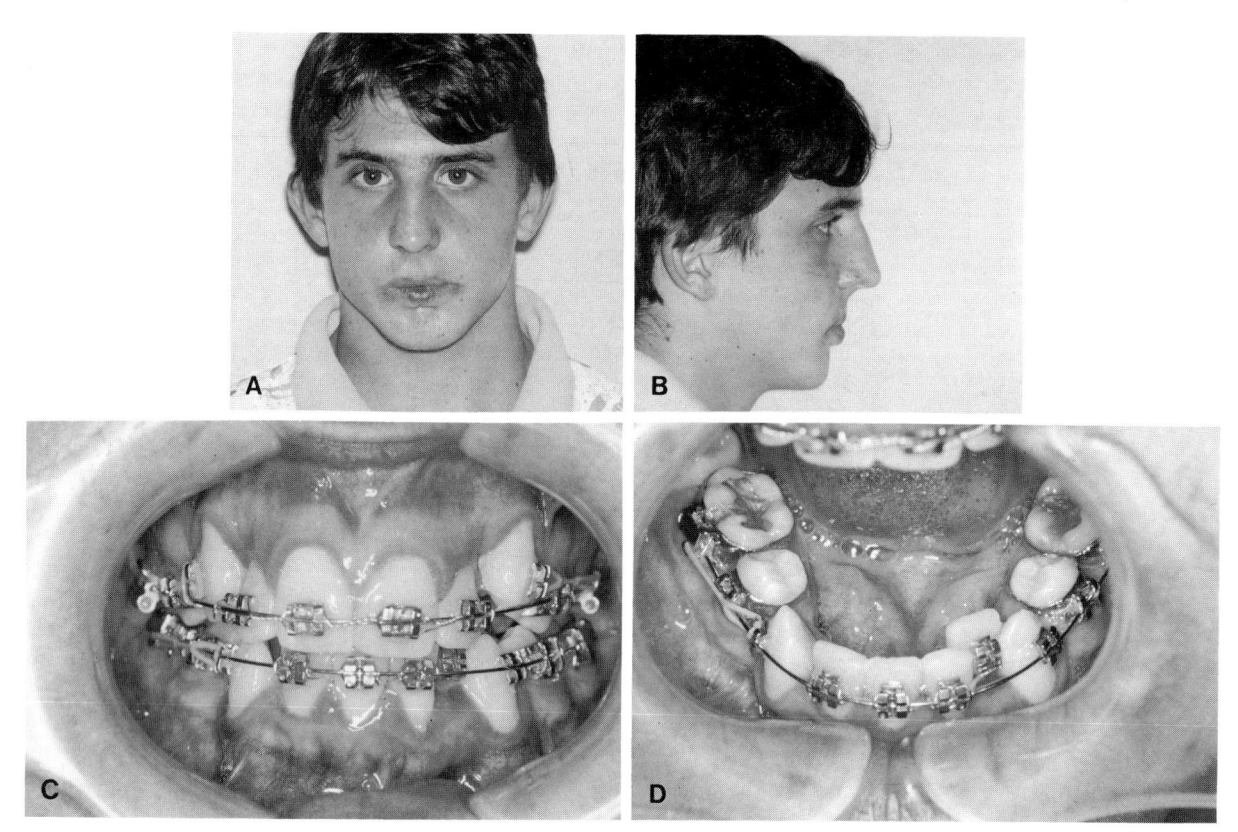

FIGURE 64–46. *A–D*, Whistling face syndrome.

Many patients manifest dental relapse in the form of crowded mandibular anterior teeth when only compensating orthodontic therapy has been performed to the exclusion of evaluating and treating the primary basal bone problem. Re-evaluation of the patient for possible retreatment leaves the clinician with few options to achieve good function, esthetics, and stability.

In addition, the clinician may encounter clinical situations in which he or she would prefer to surgically create a U-shaped arch instead of a V-shaped arch to achieve interarch compatibility. Furthermore, he or she readily appreciates the need for mandibular expansion to compensate for arch length inadequacy, proclined incisors, and an absolute basal bone deficiency.

MANDIBULAR EXPANSION: SURGICAL TECHNIQUE

Mandibular transverse deficiency can be treated by means of surgical rapid mandibular expansion facilitated by a vertical osteotomy in the symphyseal area and the use of a Haas expansion appliance. The expansion is achieved with the appliance, which is subsequently used to maintain the space while healing occurs. The *all-metal* Haas appliance is usually placed on the first molars and first bicuspids. The bars are located as anteriorly as possible to minimize interference with tongue function. The orthodontist places the expansion appliance a few days before surgery.

Rapid mandibular expansion surgery can be performed on an ambulatory basis, with the patient under either general nasoendotracheal anesthesia or intravenous

2386 / VII — ORTHOGNATHIC SURGERY

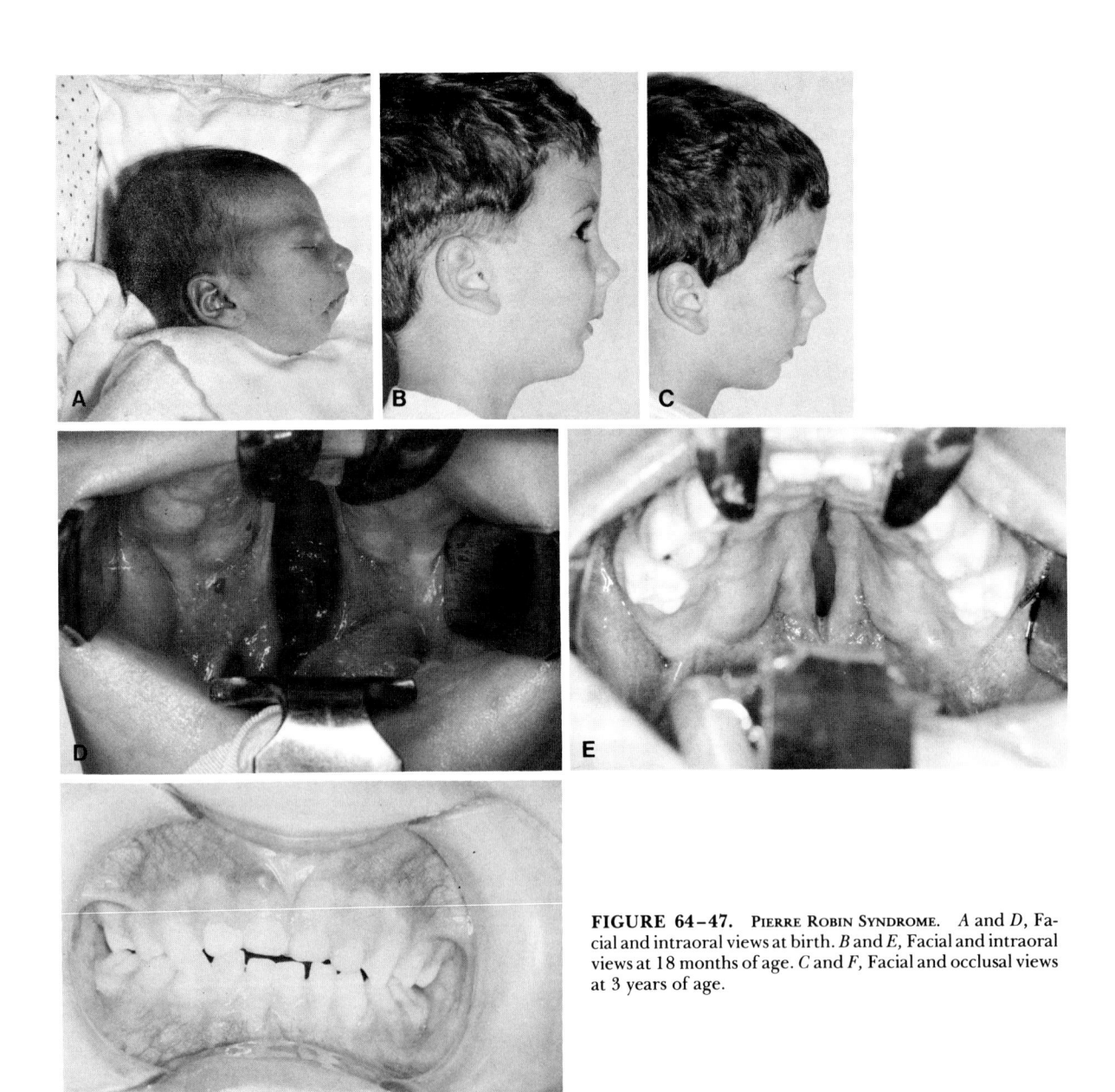

FIGURE 64-47. PIERRE ROBIN SYNDROME. *A* and *D*, Facial and intraoral views at birth. *B* and *E*, Facial and intraoral views at 18 months of age. *C* and *F*, Facial and occlusal views at 3 years of age.

FIGURE 64-48. *A* to *C*, Crocodile bite.

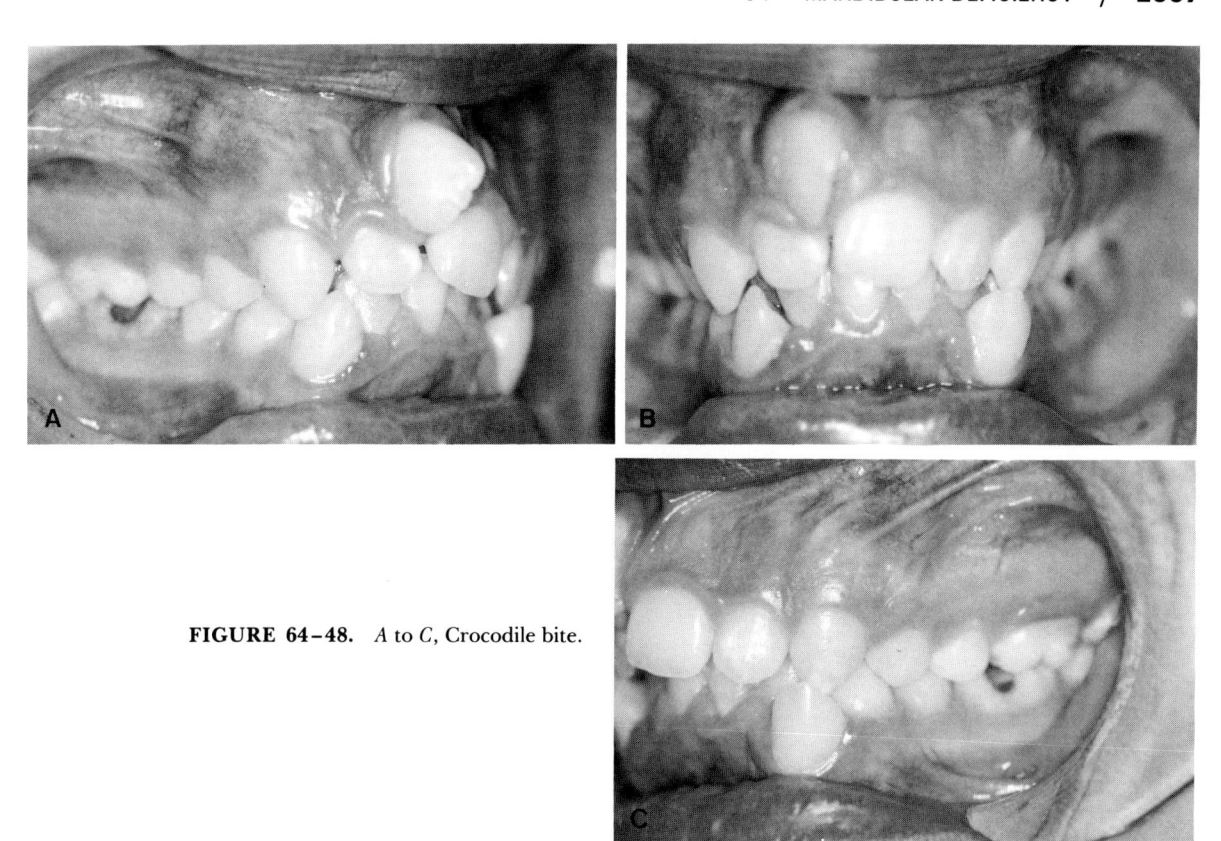

sedation. With an electrocutting knife, the incision is made 4 to 6 mm from the depth of the vestibule in the posterior aspect of the lower lip. The tissues are reflected inferiorly to the lower border of the mandible, where a channel retractor is placed. The tissues are reflected superiorly to the alveolar crest, care being taken to avoid tearing the gingival tissue. A skin hook is used to reflect the flap superiorly.

Generally, once the flaps are reflected, the roots can be seen or palpated. The inferior portion of the mental symphysis, below the level of the incisors, is *completely* sectioned with an oscillating saw blade. With the superior margin of soft tissue flap retracted, the labial cortical plate and alveolar bone immediately below the level of the incisor apices are sectioned with a No. 701 fissure bur. The symphysis is sectioned into two halves by malleting a spatula osteotome into the *partially* sectioned interdental osteotomy site. The forefinger is used at all times to avoid any tearing of the lingual flap.

Sometimes it is not possible to see or palpate the roots of the teeth. In these cases, the interdental cut is completed with a spatula osteotome oriented vertically between the two teeth and extending from the alveolar crest to the apex after minimal detachment of the gingiva between the two teeth.

The osteotomy must be meticulously performed. No vertical pressure is exerted on the mandible because it might displace the Haas appliance. Once the osteotomy is completed, the guide pin is inserted into the expansion appliance and activated. Expansion is continued judiciously. The gingival tissue, however, should not remain blanched. To expand excessively might exceed the extensibility of the gingival cuff. Care must be taken to avoid tearing the tissue because this might cause a permanent periodontal problem. The patient is seen every 48 hours until the expansion is completed. At this time, acrylic is applied over the Haas screw to stabilize and maintain the expansion.

RAPID MANDIBULAR EXPANSION: ORTHODONTIC CONSIDERATIONS

The orthodontist should base the diagnosis on the patient's records (photographs, models, and radiographs) and should design an individual treatment plan in conjunction with the surgeon. A few points should be considered:

1. *Teeth in the line of the osteotomy:* A careful analysis with periapical radiographs is made to determine the approximation of the dental roots. In addition, root length, form, and position, as well as periodontal integrity, are studied. The orthodontist should achieve satisfactory dental alignment and root divergence at the planned osteotomy sites prior to surgery and ensure that sufficient alveolar bone remains intact on both sides of the expansion. This objective can be obtained either by positioning brackets to exaggerate the inclination required or by bending the arch wire. In the former case, after the expansion therapy is complete, the brackets are rebanded in the usual position.

2. *Presurgical orthodontics:* Minimal orthodontic movements are made prior to surgery to align or level, tip or rotate, the other teeth. However, a very rotated or tipped molar should be uprighted prior to inserting the Haas appliance. Ideally, four bands are fixed on the appliance, and first premolars and first molars are typically used. The expansion screw of the appliance should be positioned as far anteriorly as possible to avoid tongue interference. We recommend that no dental compensations be made at the orthodontic appointment prior to surgery unless the appliance is constructed immediately prior to surgery by the orthodontist. Even then, as was seen in one of our cases, when the appliance was tried in the patient some 24 hours after fabrication, it did not fit because 4 to 6 mm of relapse had already occurred.

3. *Amount of expansion:* Additional research is required to determine the physiologic limits of soft tissue expansion, the effect of expansion on the temporomandibular joints, and the role of some postfixation side effects, such as torquing of the mandibular rami and alteration of intercondylar distances, as well as, for example, the effect of age differences. In our sample, there have been no temporomandibular joint complications to date. The patients were an average of 16.5 years old (ranging from 14 to 22 years old). The average follow-up was 12 months (ranging between 10 and 48 months). The amount of expansion ranged between 4 and 6.5 mm. The expansion appliance was typically activated 12 turns at the time of surgery (3 mm) until there was slight blanching of the gingival tissue. To avoid periodontal problems, the interdental soft tissue must not be torn. The patient is seen in the office every 48 hours until the desired expansion is completed (one turn per day). At that time, acrylic is applied to seal the expansion screw for the stabilization period, during which the surgical movement is maintained by the appliance.

4. *What to do with the interdental gap:* An acrylic tooth similar in color and shape to the adjacent teeth is selected. A bracket is fixed to the denture tooth and then wired to the arch wire with a wire ligature. Orthodontic tooth movement to close the space between the two teeth is not undertaken for 3 months, to ensure that new bone formation has occurred in the osseous gap.

5. *Postsurgical orthodontics:* After 3 months, light forces are applied to the teeth to close the space. The width of the acrylic tooth is reduced as the teeth are approximated. Normally, it takes approximately 6 months to complete the closing movement. The teeth are then aligned and leveled in the usual manner. Coordination of the arches and finishing orthodontics are accomplished through routine orthodontic treatment. When inadequate space still remains a problem, one of the following methods can be considered: interproximal reduction of mandibular tooth mass; or compensation of incisor inclination by labial proclination to increase arch length.

In major mandibular transverse deficiencies, a secondary mandibular expansion between the canines and laterals on either the right or the left side can be considered 6 months later.

CLASSIFICATION

Unilateral Mandibular Deficiency

The clinical presentation of this problem is usually a combination of mandibular unilateral horizontal deficiency and maxillary unilateral vertical excess on the same side because of a lack of opposing teeth. This situation allows the maxillary posterior teeth to supraerupt. The treatment plan should be designed to correct the horizontal problem by unilateral mandibular expansion, followed by maxillary surgery to reposition the supraerupted maxillary teeth superiorly.

Brody's Syndrome

CASE: M.H. (Fig. 64–49)

An 18-year-old woman was referred for treatment of her malocclusion, which was associated with Brody's syndrome (unilateral total buccal deep bite) and chin deficiency. Clinical and radiographic examination showed right vertical posterior maxillary excess, absolute unilateral mandibular transverse deficiency, and anteroposterior chin deficiency.

PROBLEM LIST

Esthetics (Fig. 64–49A to C)

FRONTAL. The nasal tip was symmetric, well balanced, and rounded; mild lip incompetence and excessive exposure of the lower lip vermilion were present.

PROFILE. Excessive exposure of the lower lip vermilion and chin deficiency were present.

Cephalometric Analysis. Anteroposterior chin deficiency was present (Fig. 64–49G).

Occlusal Analysis (Fig. 64–49I to K)

DENTAL ARCH FORM. The maxillary arch was U shaped and asymmetric; the mandibular arch was V shaped, asymmetric, and transversely deficient.

DENTAL OCCLUSION. The patient had a Class I malocclusion, a right total buccal deep bite, and a missing left maxillary second premolar.

DENTAL ALIGNMENT. There was mild crowding in the maxillary and mandibular arches.

TREATMENT PLAN

Presurgical Orthodontic Treatment

The maxillary and mandibular arches were leveled and aligned without extractions. However, braces were not placed prior to surgery in the area of the deep telescopic bite, and no attempt was made to close the space between the left maxillary first premolar and first molar teeth, as this would be closed surgically by an osteotomy and anterior repositioning of the left posterior maxillary segment (Fig. 64–49L and M).

Surgical Plan (Fig. 64–49Q)

1. Right posterior maxillary osteotomy to reposition the right posterior maxilla superiorly 7 mm by sectioning between the right maxillary canine and lateral incisor teeth.

2. Left posterior maxillary ostectomy to close the premolar space without vertical change.

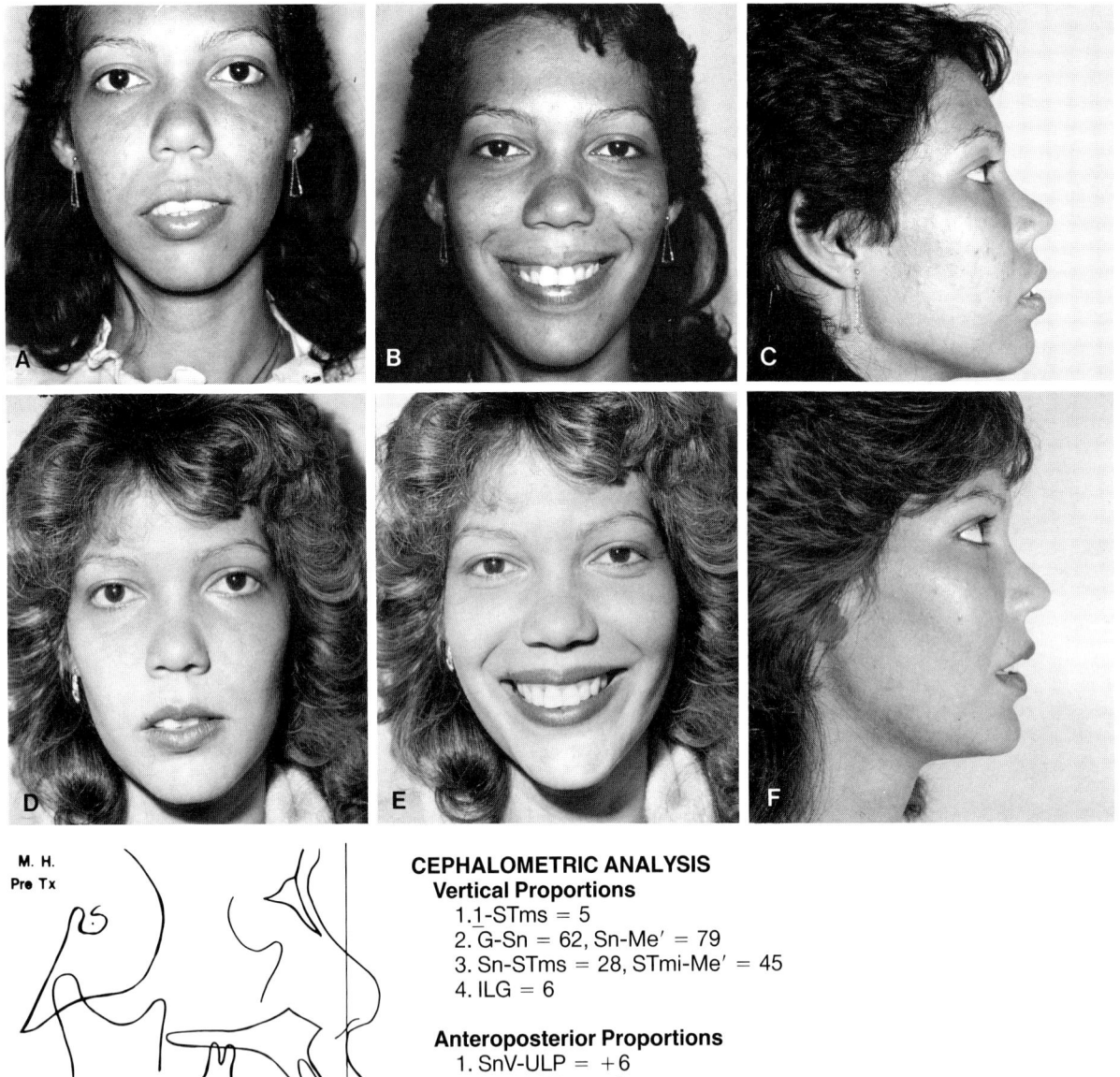

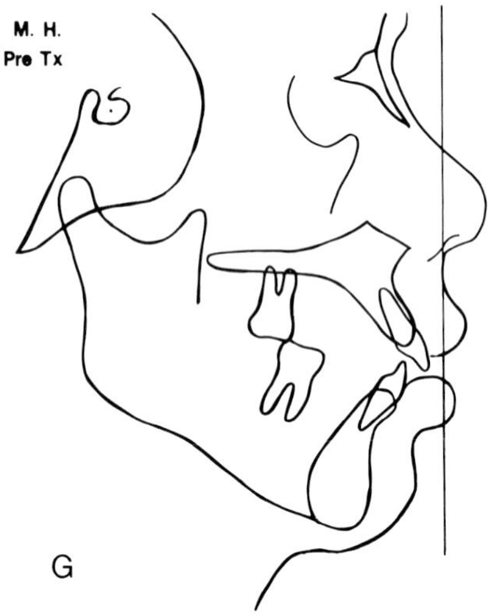

2390 / VII — ORTHOGNATHIC SURGERY

CEPHALOMETRIC ANALYSIS

Vertical Proportions
1. 1-STms = 5
2. G-Sn = 62, Sn-Me' = 79
3. Sn-STms = 28, STmi-Me' = 45
4. ILG = 6

Anteroposterior Proportions
1. SnV-ULP = +6
2. SnV-LLP = +3
3. SnV-Po' = −7
4. NLA = 93°
5. ULD = 110°

Incisor Position
1. 1-HP = 122°
2. 1-PP = 118°
3. 1-GoMe = 94°

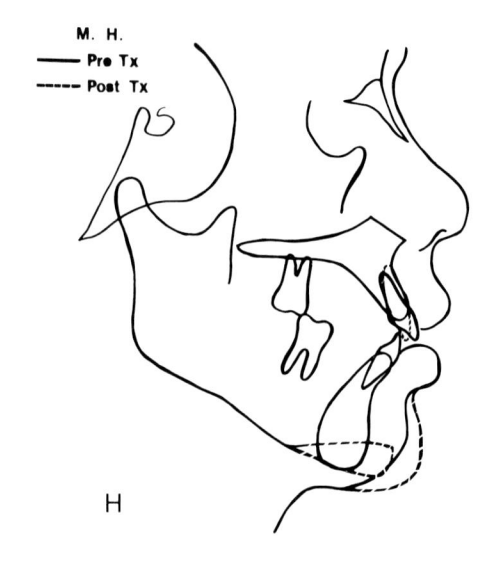

FIGURE 64-49. *A–C*, Facial appearance before treatment. *D–F*, Facial appearance after treatment. *G*, Preoperative cephalometric tracing. *H*, Composite cephalometric tracings before and after surgical and orthodontic treatment.

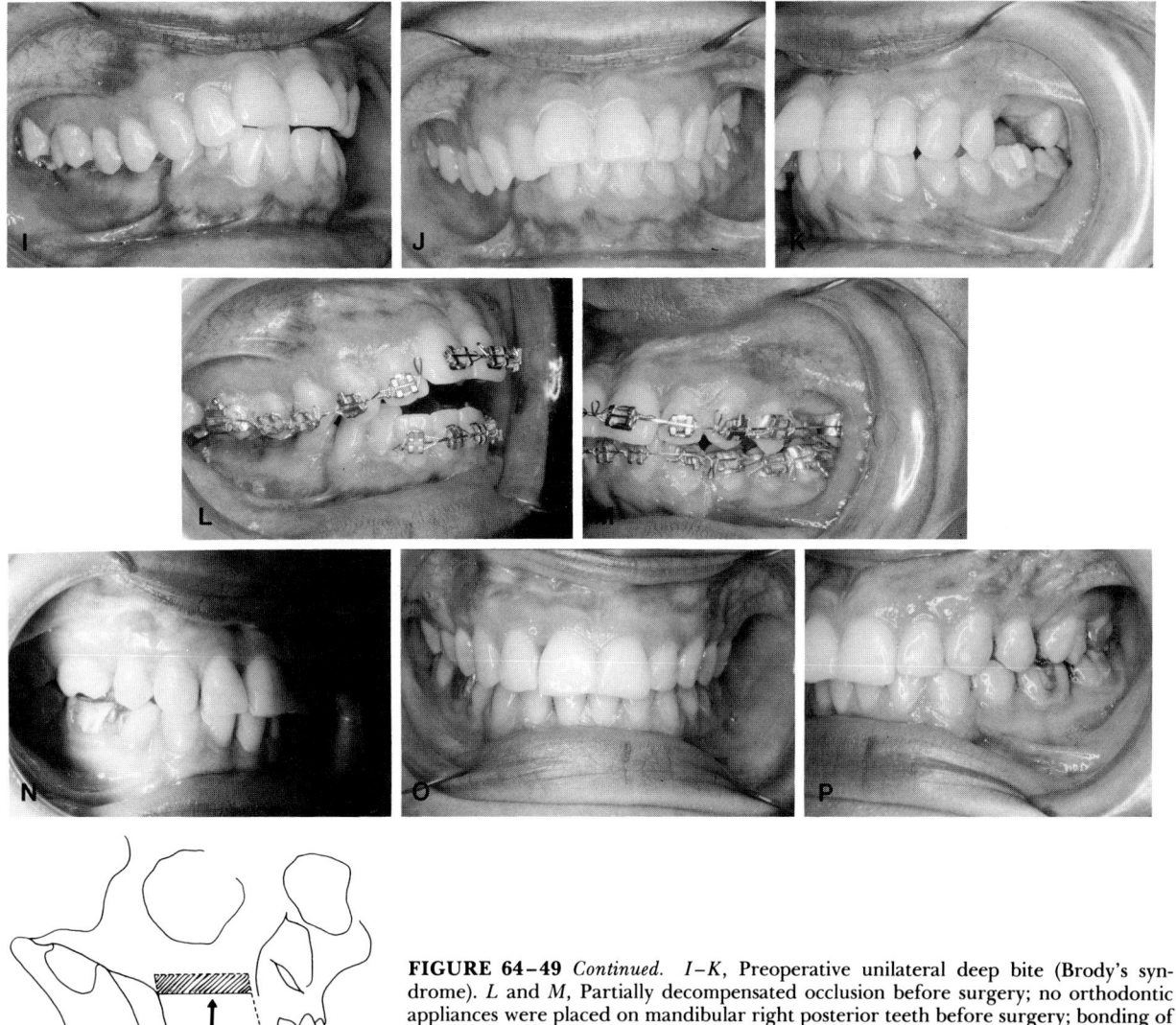

FIGURE 64-49 *Continued.* *I-K*, Preoperative unilateral deep bite (Brody's syndrome). *L* and *M*, Partially decompensated occlusion before surgery; no orthodontic appliances were placed on mandibular right posterior teeth before surgery; bonding of these teeth was accomplished after surgery. *N-P*, Postoperative occlusion. *Q*, Plan of surgery: Superior repositioning of the right posterior maxilla by posterior maxillary ostectomy; body ostectomy and advancement genioplasty.

3. A right vertical mandibular parasymphyseal osteotomy between the canine and lateral incisor teeth. The mandible would be expanded with a Haas appliance.
4. Advancement genioplasty by osteotomy of the inferior border of the mandible.

Postsurgical Orthodontic Treatment

1. Banding and bracket placement on the lower right mandibular teeth.
2. Final detailing and finishing of the occlusion.
3. Upper and lower Hawley-type removable retainers.

COMMENTS

Correcting the anatomic deformity and repositioning the segments to their normal position facilitated leveling of the occlusal plane and achievement of harmony between the dental midlines. The combined orthodontic and surgical treatment was accomplished in 14 months. The patient is 4 years out of treatment and maintains good function, esthetics, and stability (Fig. 64-49*D, E, F, H, N, O,* and *P*).

Surgeon—Cesar Guerrero, D.D.S., Caracas, Venezuela
Orthodontist—Gisela Contasti, D.D.S., Caracas, Venezuela

Bilateral Transverse Mandibular Deficiency (Crocodile Bite)

This particular dentofacial problem is relatively uncommon but represents a major challenge to the surgeon and the orthodontist when it occurs. The absolute mandibular deficiency is associated with a complete buccal overbite, a V-shaped arch, crowding, and an unesthetic, exaggerated curve of Spee. Moreover, these patients often have a triangle-shaped face with a pointed chin. Frequently, the problem is associated with maxillary transverse deficiency in which there is typically a V-shaped arch that is long in the anteroposterior dimension. The very narrow arches in these patients appear similar to those seen in some reptiles—hence the term "crocodile bite." In such cases, the orthodontist may desire to increase the horizontal dimension to create space for correction of the crowding and for achievement of harmony between the arches. Consequently, a more esthetic and symmetric smile is obtained when the unesthetic dark shadows in the buccal corridors are filled with teeth. Function is improved, as space for the tongue and for food is increased.

CASE: C.C. (Fig. 64–50)

A 17-year-old girl presented with severe maxillomandibular transverse deficiency, Class I occlusion, marked crowding, bilateral crossbite, lingual molar tipping, and maxillary and mandibular V-shaped arches.

TREATMENT PLAN

1. Surgical rapid maxillary expansion with lateral maxillary osteotomies.
2. Simultaneous rapid mandibular expansion with midline symphyseal vertical osteotomy.

PRESURGICAL ORTHODONTIC TREATMENT

1. Insertion of maxillary Haas appliance on the first premolars and first molars.
2. No active orthodontics prior to surgery.

On the day of surgery, 5 mm of maxillary expansion and 3 mm of mandibular expansion were obtained. Again, expansion in the lower arch was discontinued when blanching and stretching of the soft tissue were noted. The patient was then followed on an outpatient basis by the surgeon, who continued to activate the expansion appliance until the maxilla was expanded 9 mm and the mandible, 6 mm. At that point, acrylic was applied to the Haas device to stabilize and maintain the expansion. The orthodontist fabricated cosmetic acrylic teeth with orthodontic brackets attached and ligated these prosthetic dental units to the maxillary and mandibular arch wires. The patient was placed on a liquid diet for 2 weeks and a soft diet for the following 2 weeks; a regular diet was resumed within 6 weeks after surgery. Active orthodontic movement of the teeth with light progressive forces commenced 3 months after the surgical expansions. This treatment plan permitted correction of the following problems, without extractions:

1. V-shaped arches.
2. Maxillary and mandibular crowding.
3. Lingual inclination of molars.
4. Basal bone discrepancy.

Surgeon—Cesar Guerrero, D.D.S., Caracas, Venezuela
Orthodontist—Perla Bentolila, D.D.S., Caracas, Venezuela

TOTAL MANDIBULAR AUGMENTATION

Surgical rapid mandibular expansion can be combined with various osteotomies to correct individual growth problems and subsequent dentofacial deformities in all three dimensions of space. Horizontal, vertical, and anteroposterior growth aberrancies can be corrected simultaneously. Special attention must be paid to

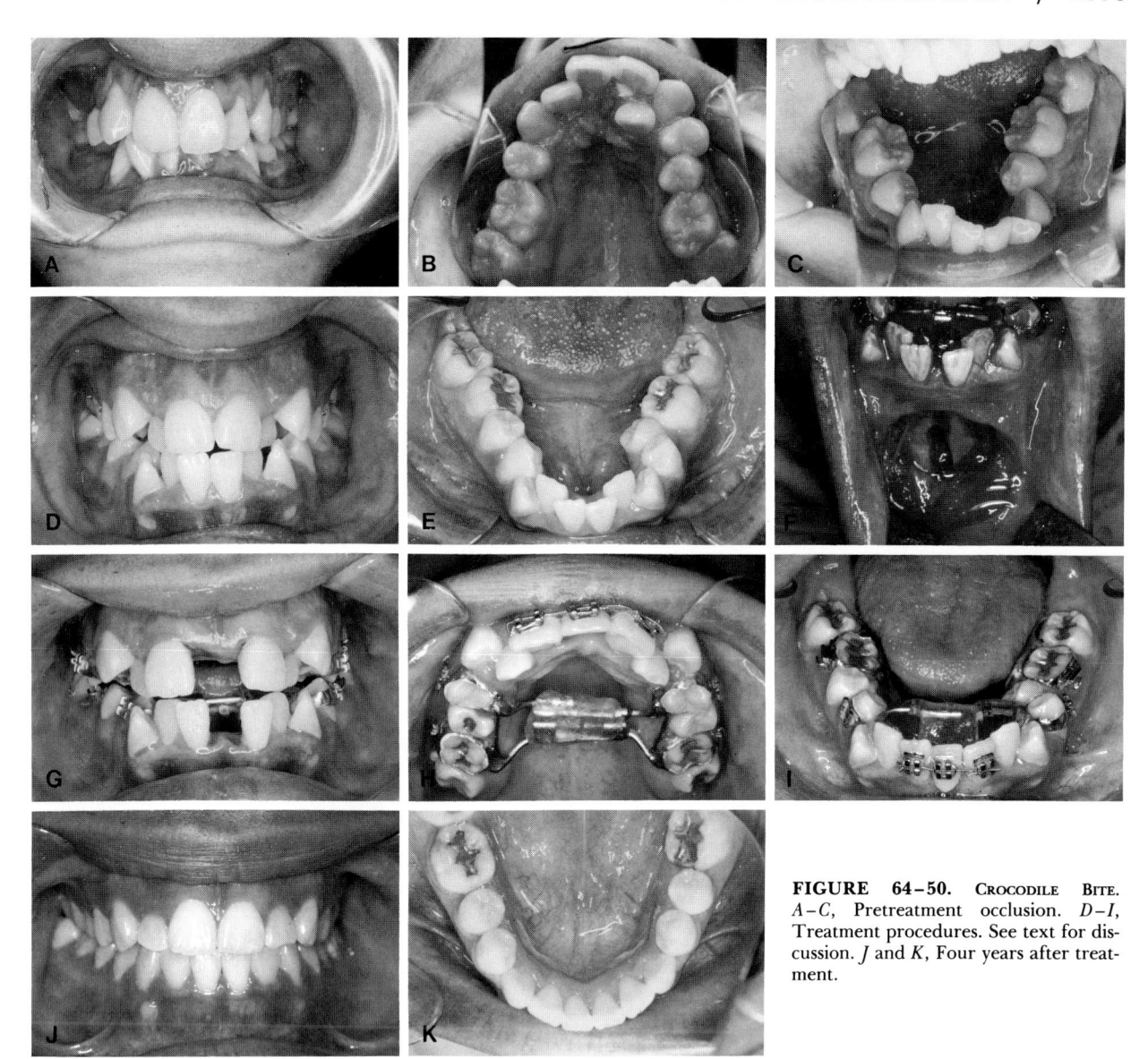

FIGURE 64–50. CROCODILE BITE. *A–C*, Pretreatment occlusion. *D–I*, Treatment procedures. See text for discussion. *J* and *K*, Four years after treatment.

proper sequencing when the surgery is performed. If there is absolute three-dimensional mandibular deficiency, the mandible must be repositioned in all three dimensions. Possible treatment options are as follows:

1. Anteroposterior mandibular advancement by sagittal split ramus osteotomies (SSROs) fixed with position screws.
2. Horizontal mandibular expansion by surgical rapid mandibular expansion with a Haas appliance.
3. Osteotomy of the inferior border of the mandible with interpositional bone graft or inferior sliding technique using bone plate and screw fixation.

Sequencing the Total Mandibular Augmentation

The chin is initially operated on by inscribing reference lines into the bone. After the osteotomy is completed, the segments are not fixed. The reference lines facilitate proper orientation at any subsequent time. The surgical assistant holds the

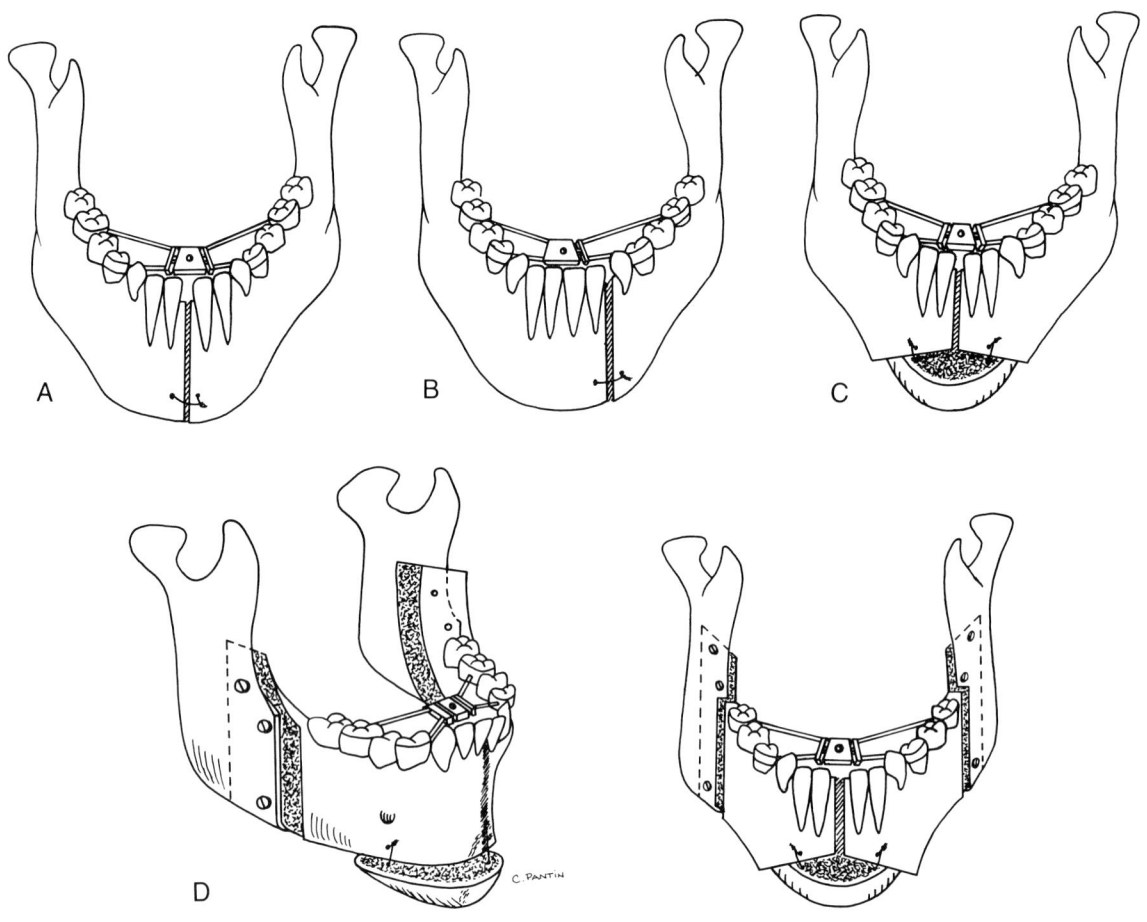

FIGURE 64–51. *A*, Midline rapid mandibular expansion. *B*, Lateral rapid mandibular expansion. *C*, Rapid mandibular expansion and genioplasty. *D*, Rapid mandibular expansion: total mandibular augmentation.

mouth closed and the mandible forward while using the reciprocating saw to protect the temporomandibular joints. A moistened 2-inch × 2-inch sponge is placed between the margins of the two bone segments.

Attention is next given to the SSRO. The procedure is completed up to the point of placing the bicortical position screws. The incisions remain open to facilitate continual monitoring of the osteotomies and fixation of the proximal and distal segments. If the vertical symphyseal osteotomy has already been performed, the surgical trauma associated with malleting and chiseling, plus the assistant's forward pressure to the symphysis region, may displace the Haas appliance and complicate the entire procedure.

Attention is now focused on the symphysis region, where the midline or lateral vertical symphyseal osteotomy is carefully completed. The expansion appliance is activated up to the point of blanching of the tissue between the incisors. Then the genial segment is fixed with bone plates or screws. When the reciprocating saw is used to complete the genioplasty, great care must be used to minimize the force transmitted to the temporomandibular joints and stabilized ramus segments. The genial segment is stabilized after the expansion is completed. A few additional millimeters of expansion may be obtained in the days after surgery by activating the expansion appliance. Finally, the soft tissue incisions are closed by routine techniques.

MANDIBULAR EXPANSION: AGE OF TREATMENT (Figs. 64–52 and 64–53)

Treatment of dentofacial deformities is based on careful coordination of orthopedics, orthodontics, and surgery. Early treatment may prevent functional and psychological problems, limit the deformity, shorten treatment time, improve results, and obtain stability. We have treated severe anteroposterior mandibular deficiencies by SSROs in patients as young as 8 to 10 years of age (except in very special situations) and have observed proportionate facial growth patterns.

The chin can be repositioned in any direction of space once the canines have erupted away from the osteotomy site. Clinical mandibular horizontal deficiency should be treated as soon as a Haas expansion appliance can be placed, by putting two metal crowns on the first deciduous molars and two bands on the first molars and fixing the expansion screw to them with 0.045-inch stainless steel wire. This procedure is possible when the child is approximately 6 years of age. Four bands are placed on the first premolars and first molars at age 8 to 10. The treatment should be done in the mixed dentition stage, when the mandible has a strong bone-healing capacity, allowing for large expansions. A second expansion in more severe cases is yet another treatment option.

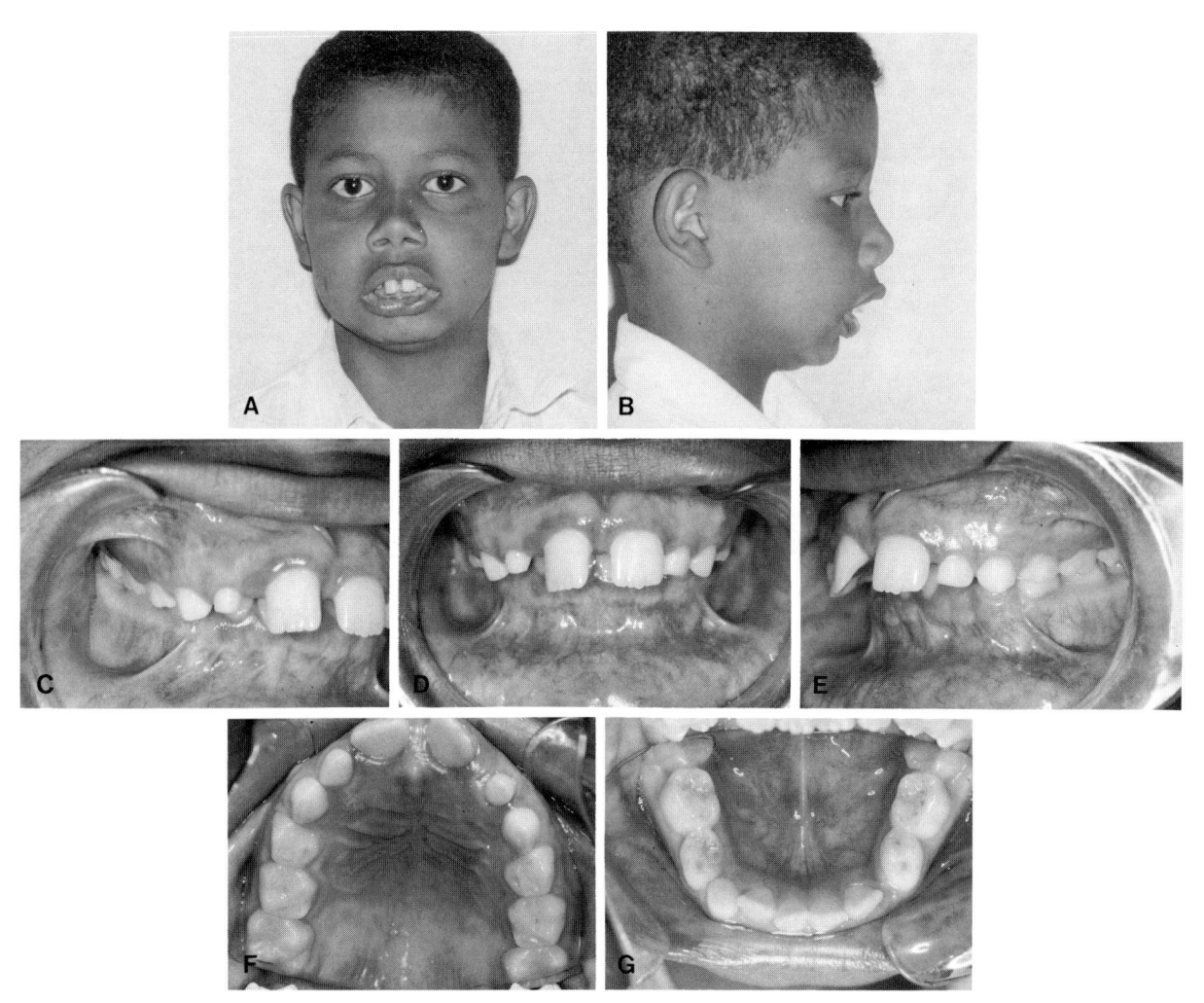

FIGURE 64–52. NINE-YEAR-OLD PATIENT WITH A BRODY ANTEROPOSTERIOR MANDIBULAR DEFICIENCY. *A* and *B*, Pretreatment facial views. *C–E*, Pretreatment occlusal views. *F* and *G*, Pretreatment intraoral views. This patient is a candidate for early rapid mandibular expansion.

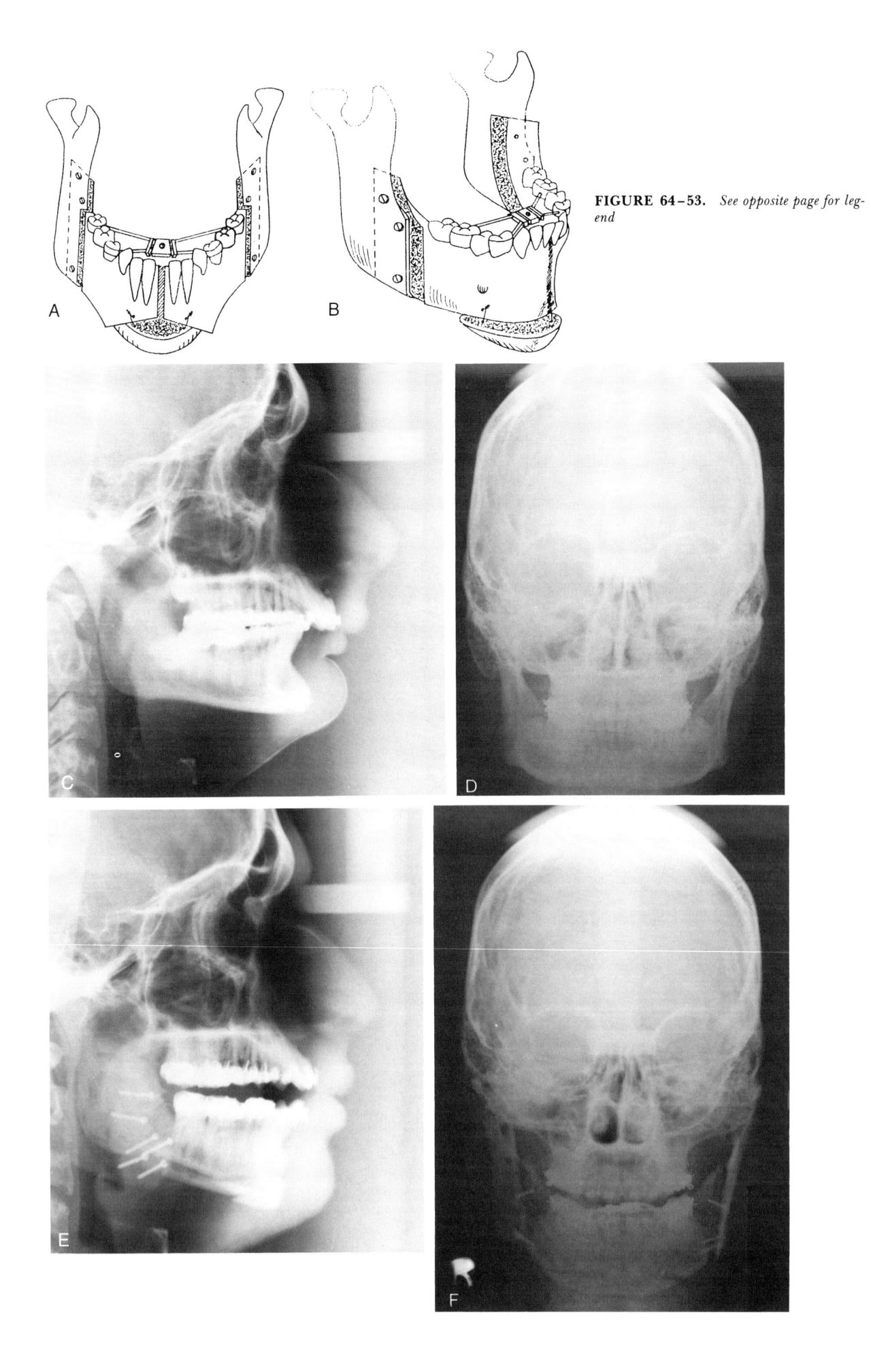

FIGURE 64-53. *See opposite page for legend*

64 — MANDIBULAR DEFICIENCY / **2397**

FIGURE 64–53. *A* and *B*, Sequence of osteotomies for total mandibular augmentation: (1) genioplasty by osteotomy of the inferior border of the mandible; (2) sagittal split ramus osteotomies; (3) midline symphyseal vertical osteotomy; (4) activation of rapid mandibular expansion appliance; (5) stabilization of repositioned genial segment. *C* and *D*, Preoperative radiographs of a patient with mandibular deficiency, deep bite, and absolute transverse mandibular deficiency. *E* and *F*, Postoperative radiographs after total mandibular augmentation by sagittal split ramus osteotomies, symphyseal osteotomy, and genioplasty by osteotomy of the inferior border of the mandible. These surgical procedures were designed to widen the mandible anteriorly and posteriorly, increase the anterior mandibular height, and lengthen the mandible in the sagittal plane of space. The surgical approach facilitated treatment of the malocclusion without the need for orthodontic extractions. *G* and *H*, Preoperative facial appearance. *I* and *J*, Postoperative facial appearance. *K* and *L*, Preoperative occlusion. *M* and *N*, Postoperative occlusion.

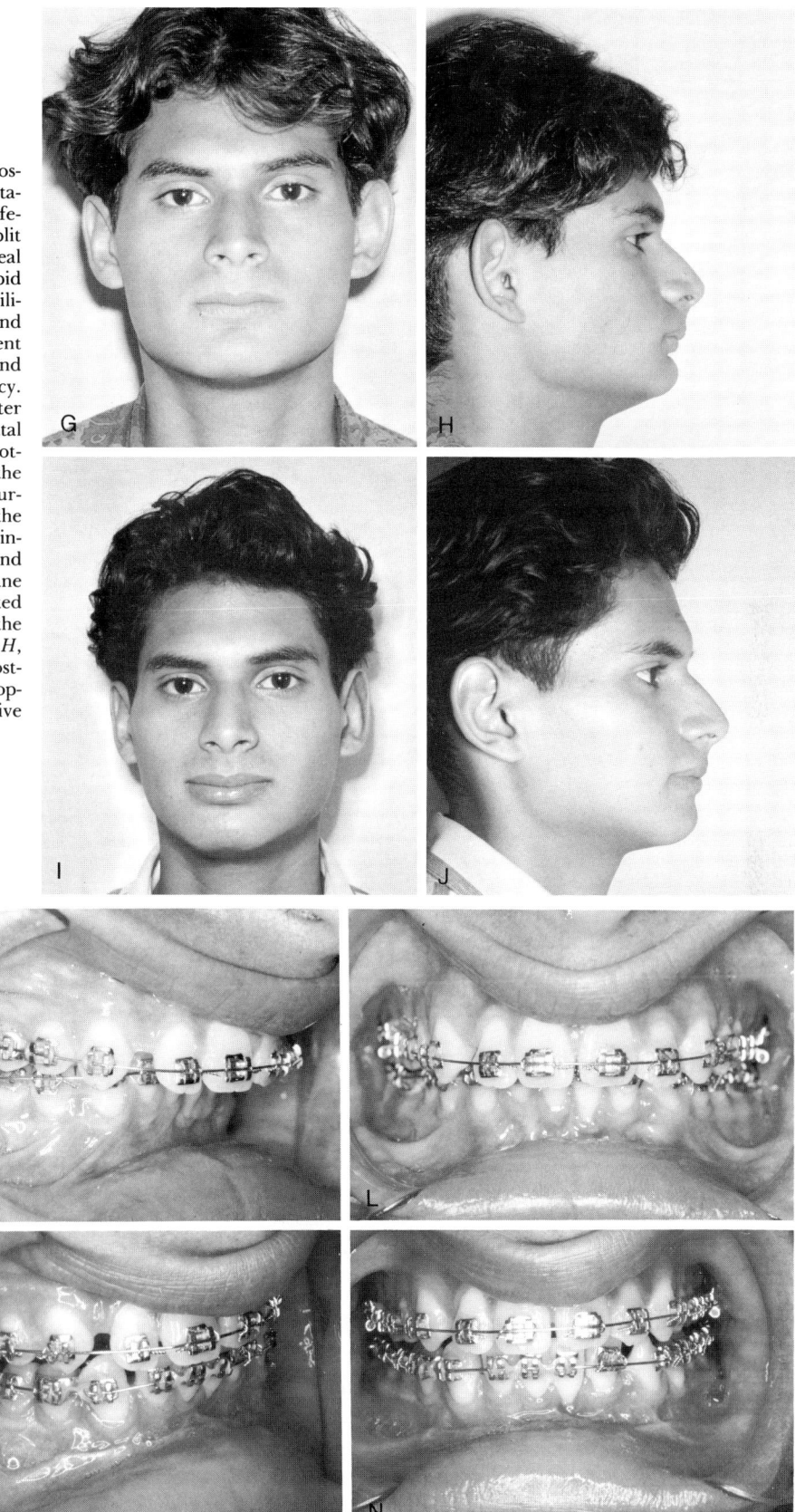

ALTERATION OF MANDIBULAR WIDTH BY SYMPHYSEAL OSTEOTOMY

WILLIAM H. BELL

Symphyseal osteotomy/ostectomy is a highly versatile surgical technique for modification of the transverse dimensions of the mandible. This procedure should be considered in the preoperative planning phases to correct absolute horizontal disharmony between the maxilla and mandible. Small-to-moderate maxillomandibular transverse deficiencies can be easily and predictably corrected by the midline mandibular osteotomy or ostectomy. Such osteotomies are usually feasible, technically easy, and predictable procedures.

Narrowing the Mandible by Symphyseal Osteotomy

A mandibular symphyseal osteotomy should be considered when Class II or Class III skeletal disharmony is corrected in the mandible only, where a small transverse discrepancy exists between the maxillary and mandibular arches after dental models are repositioned into a simulated Class I canine and molar relationship. A mandibular symphyseal osteotomy combined with ramus osteotomies produces two hemimandibles that are freely movable. By repositioning the segments and adapting them to the maxilla, the sagittal and transverse discrepancies are simultaneously corrected (Fig. 64–54A to D).

Midline mandibular osteotomy in concert with ramus osteotomies not only may correct the intermolar excess width but also may positively affect the facial esthetics by decreasing the posterior width of the mandible. The merits of this procedure must be compared with those obtained through maxillary expansion alone. A transverse discrepancy may be the result of a mild transverse deficiency of the maxilla often present in patients with Class II and III skeletal disharmonies. Midline osteotomy combined with genioplasty may be indicated in both of these deformities when a 4- to 5-mm absolute transverse discrepancy exists and maxillary surgery is not indicated to alter the sagittal or vertical position of the maxilla.

Midline mandibular ostectomy may be indicated occasionally in the presence of transverse maxillary excess. Such indications are relatively rare and must be confirmed with an orthodontic setup. When this procedure is indicated, however, the mandibular transverse and tooth size discrepancy can be corrected simultaneously by symphyseal osteotomy in concert with bilateral ramus osteotomies. A midline symphyseal osteotomy, with or without extractions, may be used to alter the transverse dimension of the mandible without ramus osteotomies in selected cases by rotation of the hemimandibles around the vertical axes of the condyles. Soft tissue constraints are not problematic with surgical procedures designed to narrow the mandible by symphyseal osteotomy/ostectomy combined with ramus osteotomies or body osteotomies.

Expansion of the Mandible by Symphyseal Osteotomy

Mandibular width changes are more complex and somewhat more limited than maxillary width changes. Although mandibular widening or narrowing is limited by the soft tissue envelope and temporomandibular joints, it is nevertheless possible to widen the mandible. Symphyseal osteotomy and mandibular orthopedic expansion facilitate mandibular transverse changes in a more controlled and predictable manner.

With meticulous attention to the details of surgical technique and the knowledge of the limitations imposed by the relative lack of gingival and mucosal extensibility,

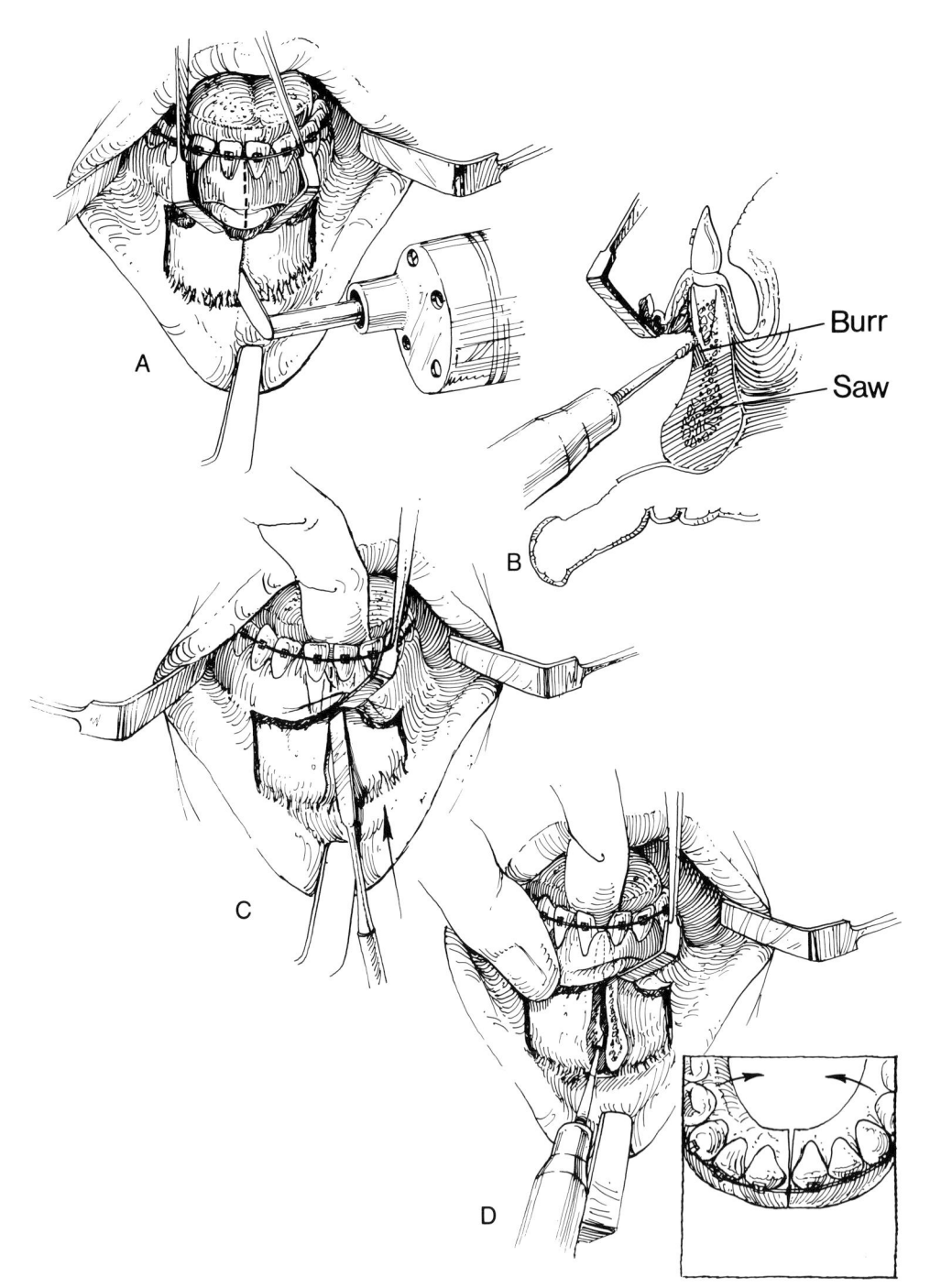

FIGURE 64–54. SYMPHYSEAL OSTEOTOMY. *A–D,* Adjunctive interdental osteotomy combined with vertical ramus osteotomies to correct crossbite. Plan of surgery: interdental osteotomy in the midsymphysis region combined with intraoral vertical ramus osteotomies. *A* and *B,* Inferior portion of the mental symphysis, below the level of the incisors, is completely sectioned with an oscillating saw blade (horizontal cross-hatched lines in *B* indicate where bone is sectioned by the oscillating saw blade); with the superior margin of the soft tissue flap retracted, the labial cortical plate and alveolar bone immediately below the the level of the incisor apices are sectioned with a No. 701 fissure bur (vertically oriented cross-hatched lines in *B* indicate where bone is sectioned with the fissure bur). *C,* The symphysis is sectioned into two halves by malleting a spatula osteotome into the partially sectioned interdental osteotomy site. *D,* The lingual aspect of the margins of the sectioned bone are ostectomized to facilitate narrowing the mandible and apposition of the two segments, which are indexed into the planned relationship with an interocclusal splint and stabilized with an arch wire. Unless there is an alteration of the vertical dimension of the two segments, it may be unnecessary to cut the arch wire in the planned osteotomy site. After the maxillomandibular fixation is in place, the sectioned repositioned mandible is stabilized with a reconstruction bone plate.

Illustration continued on following page

2400 / VII—ORTHOGNATHIC SURGERY

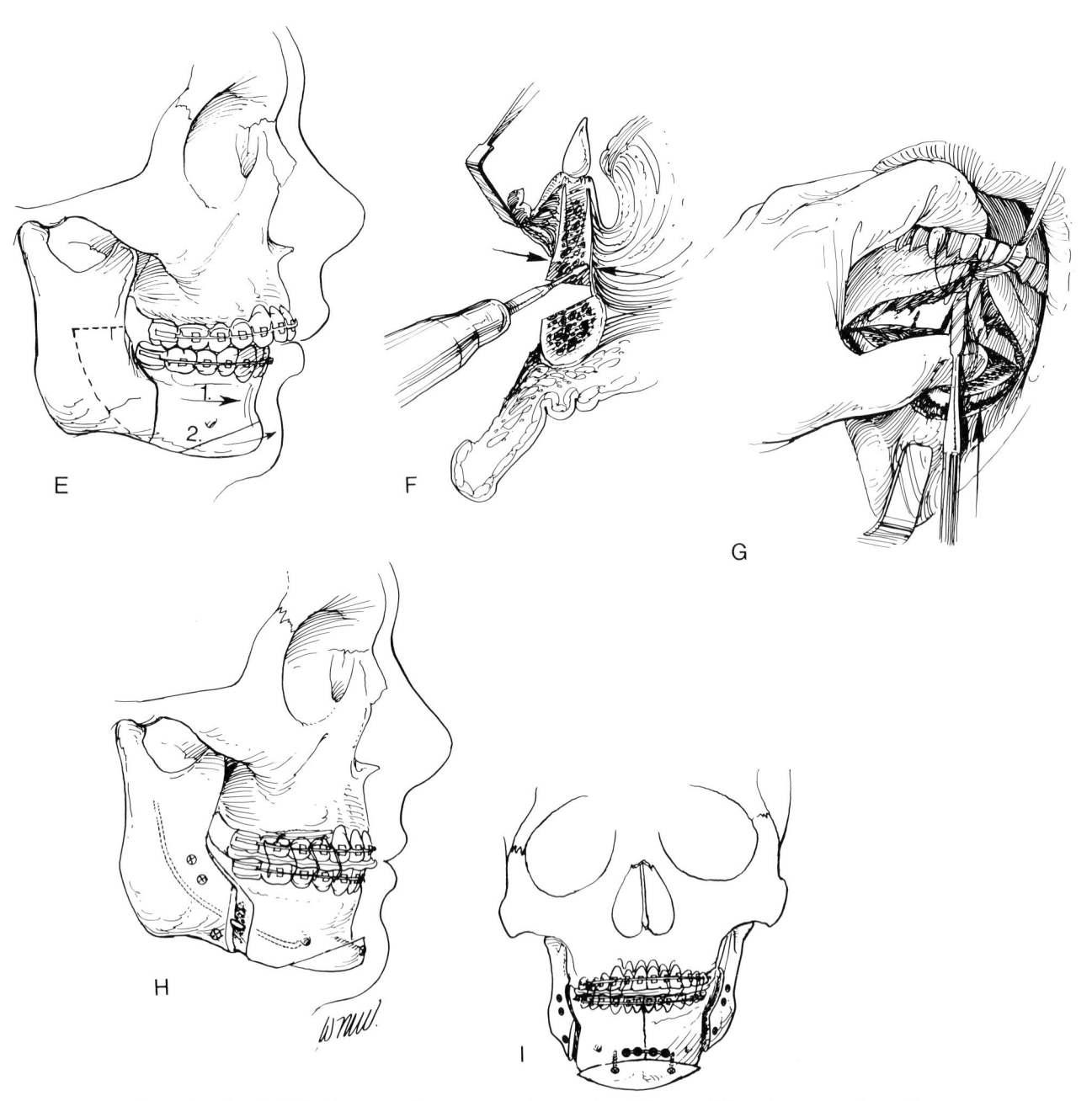

FIGURE 64–54 *Continued.* *E–I,* Simultaneous advancement and narrowing of the mandible and augmentation of the chin. *E,* Plan of surgery: sagittal split ramus osteotomies to advance mandible (1), genioplasty to augment contour-deficient chin (2), and interincisal osteotomy to facilitate narrowing of the mandible. *F,* Genioplasty is accomplished after exposure of the mental symphysis. With the mental symphysis positioned inferiorly and the superior margin of the soft tissue flap retracted, the labial cortical plate and alveolar bone immediately below the level of the incisor apices are sectioned with a No. 701 fissure bur (vertically oriented cross-hatched lines indicate where bone is sectioned; arrows indicate level of interdental osteotomy). *G,* The symphysis is halved by malleting a spatula osteotome into the partially sectioned interdental osteotomy site. *H* and *I,* After mandibular advancement, advancement genioplasty, and alteration of the transverse dimension of the mandible, the repositioned mandible is immobilized with intermaxillary wire ligatures while the mandible and chin are fixed with bone plates and screws.

J   K

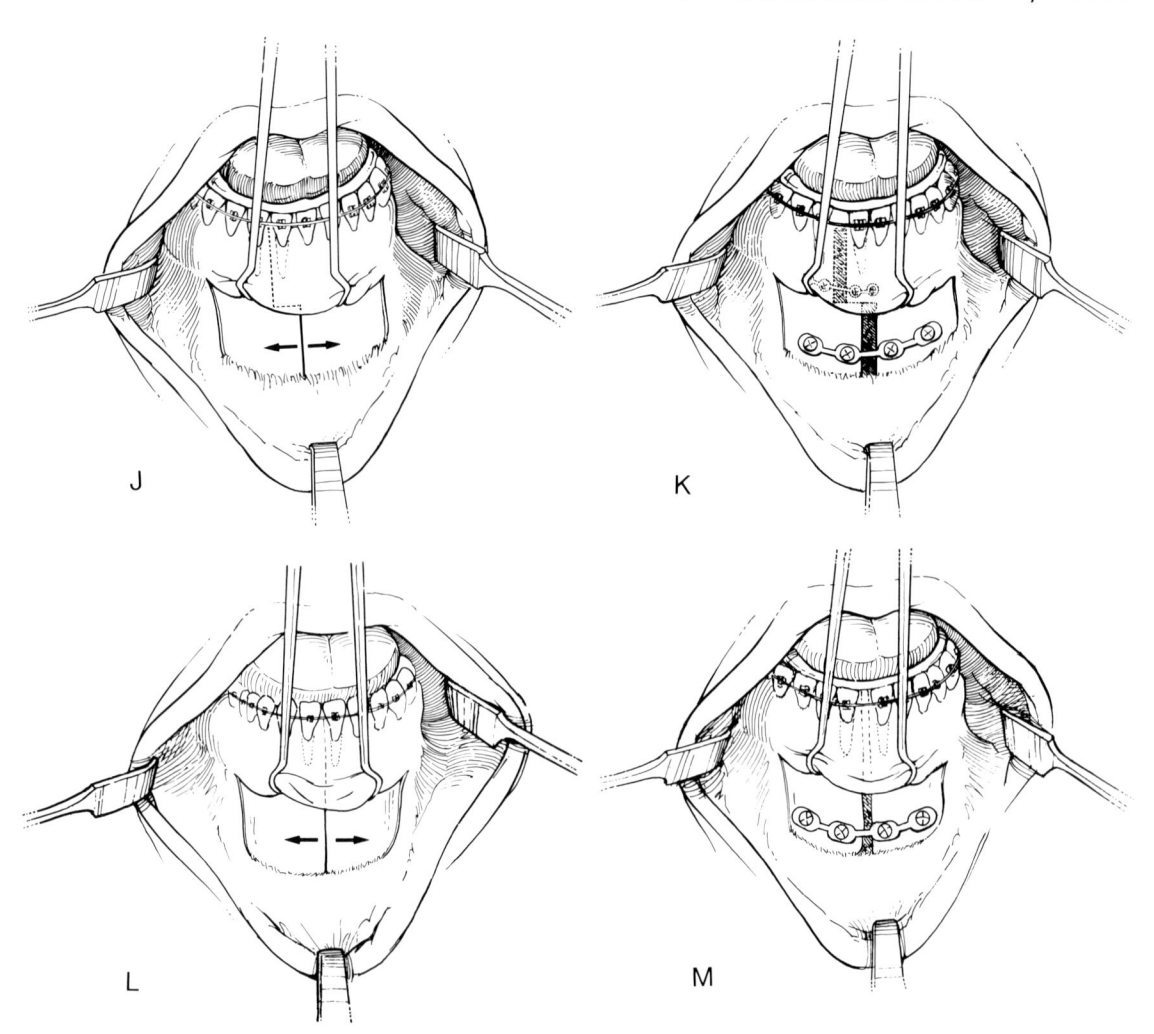

L   M

FIGURE 64-54 *Continued.* *J* and *K*, Symphyseal step osteotomy to widen the mandible. By facilitating apposition of the margins for the horizontal cuts, this procedure enhances stability of the repositioned segments of the mandible. The mandible is then stabilized with reconstruction bone plates and positional screws. Arrows indicate planned direction of movement. *L* and *M*, Vertical symphyseal osteotomy for surgical expansion of the transverse dimension of the mandible. The mandible is stabilized with a reconstruction plate and positional screws. Arrows indicate planned direction of movement. (*A–D* and *E–I* modified from Bell WH, Proffit WR, White RP Jr: Surgical Correction of Dentofacial Deformities. Vol II. Philadelphia, WB Saunders Company, 1980, pp 886, 1223, 1224; with permission.)

the anterior mandible can be surgically expanded a limited amount (Fig. 64-54*E* to *H*). Such movements are contingent upon maintaining the condylar width by rotation of condyles on their vertical axes. Additional flexibility is gained when expansion of the symphysis is combined with ramus osteotomies.

The principal indication for widening the mandible is absolute transverse mandibular deficiency (i.e., crocodile bite). An excessively tapered arch, dental crowding, and congenitally missing incisor teeth are additional reasons for use of this technique, which basically attempts to normalize basal bone position and facilitate nonextraction orthodontic treatment.

The key to immediate surgical expansion of the mandibular symphysis is proper soft tissue flap design and meticulous management of the soft tissue integument. By careful undermining of the gingiva and mucosa contiguous to the symphysis, the mandible can be immediately widened a limited amount. Success is contingent upon excellent condition of the periodontium in the planned symphyseal osteotomy site.

The lingual mucosa subjacent to the planned symphyseal osteotomy is reflected from the necks of the teeth, and the lingual tissue is protected with a periosteal elevator down to the attachment of the genioglossus muscles.

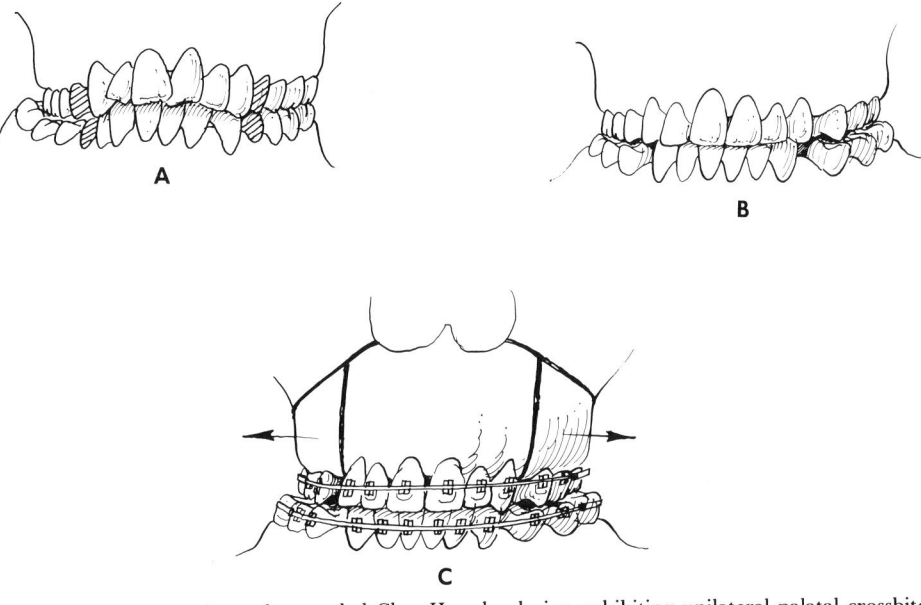

FIGURE 64–61. *A*, Severely crowded Class II malocclusion exhibiting unilateral palatal crossbite clinically with apparent necessity for extraction of four first bicuspids to alleviate arch length discrepancy. *B*, Simulated correction of Class II malocclusion to Class I cuspid relationship, with resultant worsening of palatal crossbite due to bilateral absolute transverse maxillary deficiency. Four first bicuspids have been removed to facilitate orthodontic correction of malaligned anterior teeth. *C*, Schematic depiction of three-piece segmental maxillary surgery with osteotomies through extraction sites to correct transverse deficiency following orthodontic alignment of anteriors into space created through extraction of bicuspids. (From Bell WH, Proffit WR, White RP Jr: Surgical Correction of Dentofacial Deformities. Vol I. Philadelphia, WB Saunders Company, 1980, p 525; with permission.)

ent in this type of therapy. The accentuated curve of Spee in the maxillary arch should not be leveled prior to surgery. Segmental orthodontics should be carried out in nonextraction cases, and coplanar therapy with a stepped-up anterior segment should be utilized in extraction cases to maintain the existing vertical relationships prior to ultimate surgical repositioning (Fig. 64–62).

The magnitude of the horizontal deficiency is still another consideration in planning the surgical and orthodontic treatment of transverse maxillary deficiency. If, for example, a horizontal deficiency of 10 mm is present in the intermolar area, the physiologic corrective capability of the Le Fort I downfracture technique may be exceeded. In such cases, the possibility of vascular impairment can be obviated by RPE combined with lateral maxillary osteotomies and subsequent orthodontic work, or by another surgical technique that provides dual access to the palatal and labiobuccal aspects of the maxilla.

Yet another alternative is a two-piece maxillary procedure with a midline osteotomy. The resultant diastema between the maxillary central incisors can be closed postsurgically by orthodontic movement. This treatment plan would eliminate the increased horizontal overjet that obviously would otherwise be created, but such an approach is less than ideal for several reasons. Prediction of ultimate soft tissue changes is more difficult. The maxillary incisors may move posteriorly during closure of the diastema, inducing a posterior sagittal repositioning of the upper lip that may not be esthetically tolerable to the patient being treated. In addition, extraoral traction might be required to prevent forward movement of the posterior maxillary teeth during diastema closure, or Class II elastic therapy might be required to concomitantly move the mandibular arch forward to maintain a Class I occlusion. Either occurrence greatly enhances the possibility of compromising both dental and skeletal stability, especially if both the maxilla and the mandible have been surgically repositioned.

A means of correcting mild absolute bilateral maxillary deficiency through

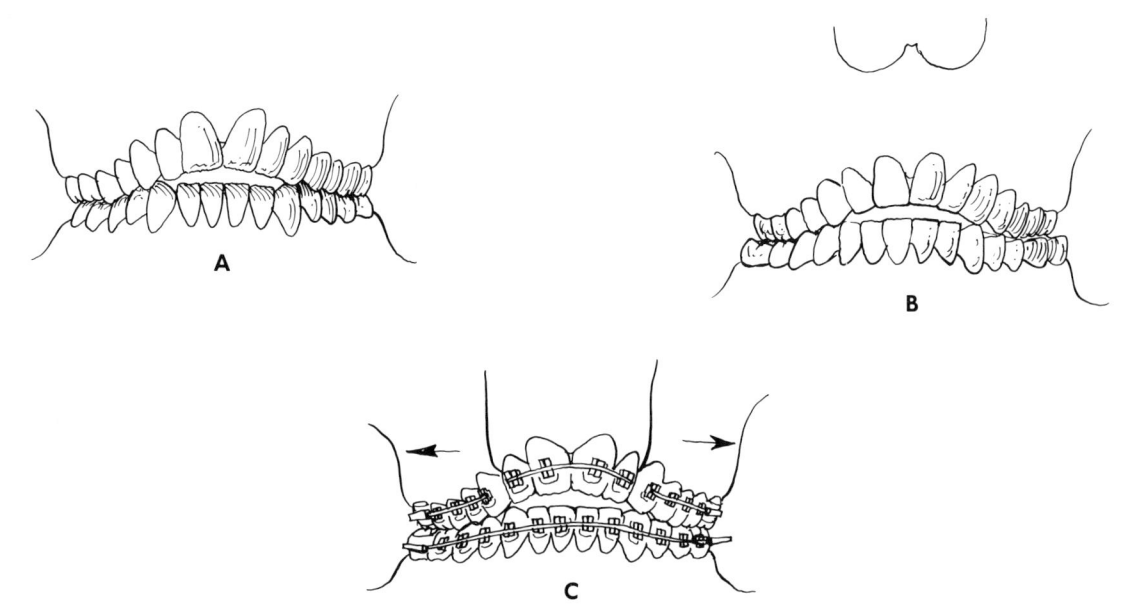

FIGURE 64-62. *A*, Class II anterior open bite malocclusion with mild bilateral palatal constriction. *B*, Simulated correction of Class II malocclusion to Class I cuspid relationship with bilateral palatal crossbite resulting from bilateral absolute transverse maxillary deficiency. *C*, Maxillary three-piece segmental surgery to correct transverse discrepancy. Segmentalized presurgical orthodontic treatment was done to align segments and prevent extrusion of anterior teeth prior to surgical correction of anterior open bite to lessen relapse potential. (From Bell WH, Proffit WR, White RP Jr: Surgical Correction of Dentofacial Deformities. Vol I. Philadelphia, WB Saunders Company, 1980, p 526; with permission.)

mandibular surgery has evolved as a viable treatment alternative.[10] The mandible is sectioned at and through the midline of the symphysis and constricted or widened as necessary, and ramus surgery is employed to facilitate advancement or reduction. Such an approach averts the need for a secondary maxillary procedure for patients who do not require maxillary surgery to correct deformity in the vertical or sagittal dimension. (See "Alteration of Mandibular Width by Symphyseal Osteotomy," p. 2398).

Absolute unilateral (true) transverse maxillary deficiencies, while rare, are encountered and should be treated by maxillary segmental surgery, with the osteotomy mesial to the most anterior tooth in palatal crossbite. The plan for orthodontic management of such patients will depend on whether extractions are necessary for the sake of aligning crowded anterior teeth. In mild arch length deficiencies, nonextraction orthodontic treatment may be facilitated by the anterior diastema that will result from such surgery (Fig. 64-63). If extractions are necessary in cases of severe crowding, routine orthodontic therapy generally should also be completed postsurgically to finish alignment and space closure.

It must be emphasized that it is extremely important to diagnose unilateral discrepancies from the existing or anticipated centric relationship and/or the maxillary and mandibular midline relationship. The evaluation must clearly determine whether the discrepancy is truly unilateral in nature or the result of a mild bilateral deficiency that elicits a functional shift from centric relation to centric occlusion with a significant lateral component as a result of interfering cusps. The treatment of such functional unilateral deficiencies should consist of one of the alternatives indicated for absolute bilateral transverse maxillary deficiency.

Finally, in some cases, the apparent maxillary deficiency may be due to the ectopic eruption of one or two posterior teeth in one quadrant, and thus be purely dental in nature. Such patients may be treated with orthodontic therapy alone or in conjunction with one-tooth or two-tooth maxillary segmental surgery to facilitate immediate repositioning and to minimize orthodontic treatment time.

A permanent increase in the width of the maxilla is attained routinely in most children by means of orthodontic mechanical expansion appliances and retention.

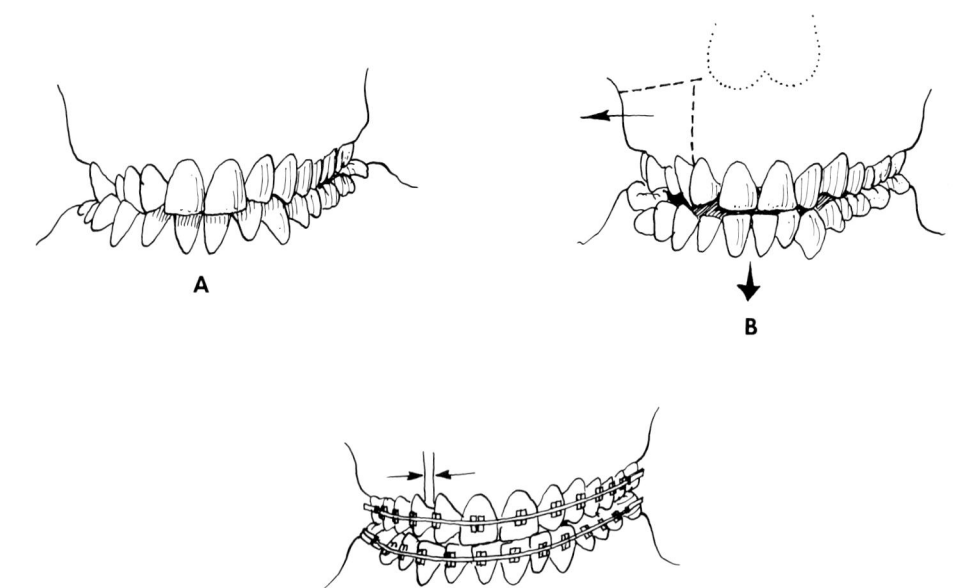

FIGURE 64-63. *A*, Absolute (true) unilateral transverse maxillary deficiency with palatal crossbite exhibited from the cuspid posteriorly. *B*, Correction of transverse deficiency through unilateral segmental maxillary surgery with osteotomy mesial to the most anterior tooth in crossbite. *C*, Utilization of diastema created by surgery to orthodontically align minimally to moderately crowded anteriors postsurgically. (From Bell WH, Proffit WR, White RP Jr: Surgical Correction of Dentofacial Deformities. Vol I. Philadelphia, WB Saunders Company, 1980, p 527; with permission.)

In adults, attempts at orthopedic RPE are frequently associated with significant problems. Inability to activate the appliance and expand the maxilla is not uncommon. In other instances, the teeth are merely pushed laterally through the bone, without midpalatal opening. Tipping of the teeth and bending of the alveolar bone are common consequences of such therapy.[15,16] Overcorrection to compensate for these undesirable changes is frequently frustrated by unpredictable and uncontrolled relapse after the palatal expansion appliance is removed.[8,14] In addition, treatment of true unilateral posterior crossbite (i.e., that secondary to true skeletal asymmetry and not just to tipping of the teeth) by means of conventional palatal expansion techniques is not feasible because a physiologic centric occlusion cannot be maintained.[4]

Most clinical failures with RPE have occurred in adults. A study by Belli and colleagues of long-term skeletal changes following rapid maxillary expansion in adults indicated that there was no significant sagittal maxillary skeletal changes throughout treatment. They concluded that there were no long-term skeletal changes following rapid maxillary expansion in adults.[7a] Various types of maxillary osteotomies have been empirically proposed to facilitate lateral movement of the maxilla by palatal expansion appliances in adults. Histologic studies have implied that the fusion of the midpalatine suture is the primary problematic area in cases resistant to mechanical expansion.[17] On the basis of this theory, midpalatal osteotomies have been performed to aid in maxillary expansion. Timms[17,18] and others[1a,12,12a,13,14a] have postulated that the midpalatal suture and the zygomaticomaxillary buttress are both problem areas. Accordingly, they have used a combination of lateral maxillary and palatal osteotomies. Still others have sectioned virtually all the maxillary bone articulations.[1,19]

By proper planning and execution, selected maxillary osteotomies can be used together with RPE appliances to achieve correction of unilateral and bilateral horizontal maxillary deficiency and the accompanying crossbites.[4]

By increasing the length of the maxillary arch, correction of crowding and malalignment of teeth and righting of anterior teeth can be accomplished without extractions. When this type of treatment is done in concert with RME, the mandibular transverse deficiency may also be treated without extraction in selected cases (see "Transverse (Horizontal) Mandibular Deficiency," by Guerrero and Contasti).

Experimental and Clinical Rationale for Surgical Widening of the Maxilla

WILLIAM H. BELL
With the assistance of JOE KENNEDY

Animal studies indicate that the effects of RPE are not limited to the dentoalveolar unit alone. As the palate is expanded, many sutures of the skull are opened and distorted when intracranial bony structures are displaced. The investigations lend support to the conclusions of Isaacson and Ingram,[9] whose study showed that force values did not change significantly prior to, during, or after the actual opening of the midpalatal sutures. Moreover, the force values recorded represented and indicated the resistance of the facial skeleton to expansion and revealed that the facial skeleton increases its resistance to expansion significantly with increasing maturity and age. These studies indicated that the point of major resistance to RPE

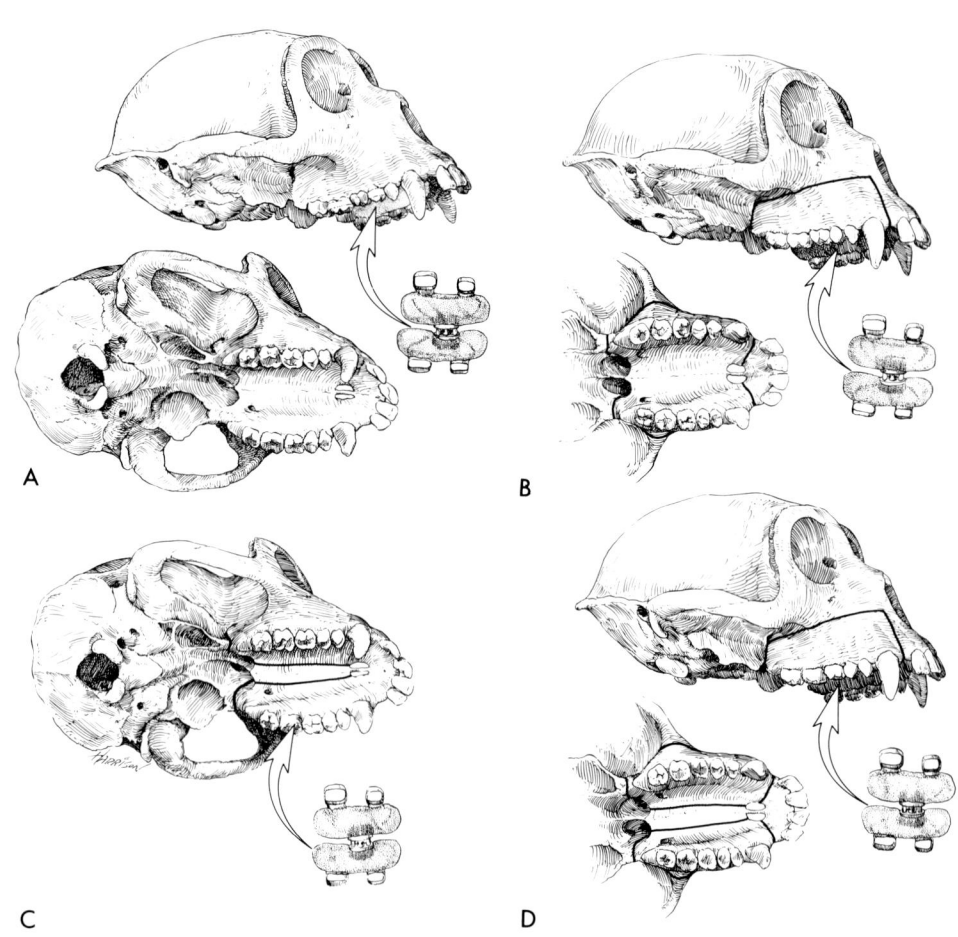

FIGURE 64-64. DIAGRAMMATIC PLANS OF TECHNIQUES UNDER STUDY. *A*, Group I contained three control monkeys. The palatal expansion appliance was activated without surgery. *B*, Group II had five animals. Horizontal subapical osteotomy of the lateral maxilla was done from the canine–lateral incisor interspace posteriorly to the pterygomaxillary suture; a posterior vertical bone incision separated the maxillary tuberosity from the pterygoid plate, and an anterior vertical bone incision was carried from the labiobuccal horizontal bone incision through the lateral incisor–canine interspace to the incisive foramen. *C*, Group III was composed of three monkeys. A parasagittal palatal osteotomy was done extending from the incisive foramen posteriorly to the horizontal process of the palatine bone; a posterior vertical bone incision separated the maxillary tuberosity from the pterygoid plate. *D*, Group IV had five monkeys. Parasagittal palatal osteotomies combined with lateral maxillary osteotomies were done. (From Bell WH, Proffit WR, White RP Jr: Surgical Correction of Dentofacial Deformities. Vol I. Philadelphia, WB Saunders Company, 1980, p 529; with permission.)

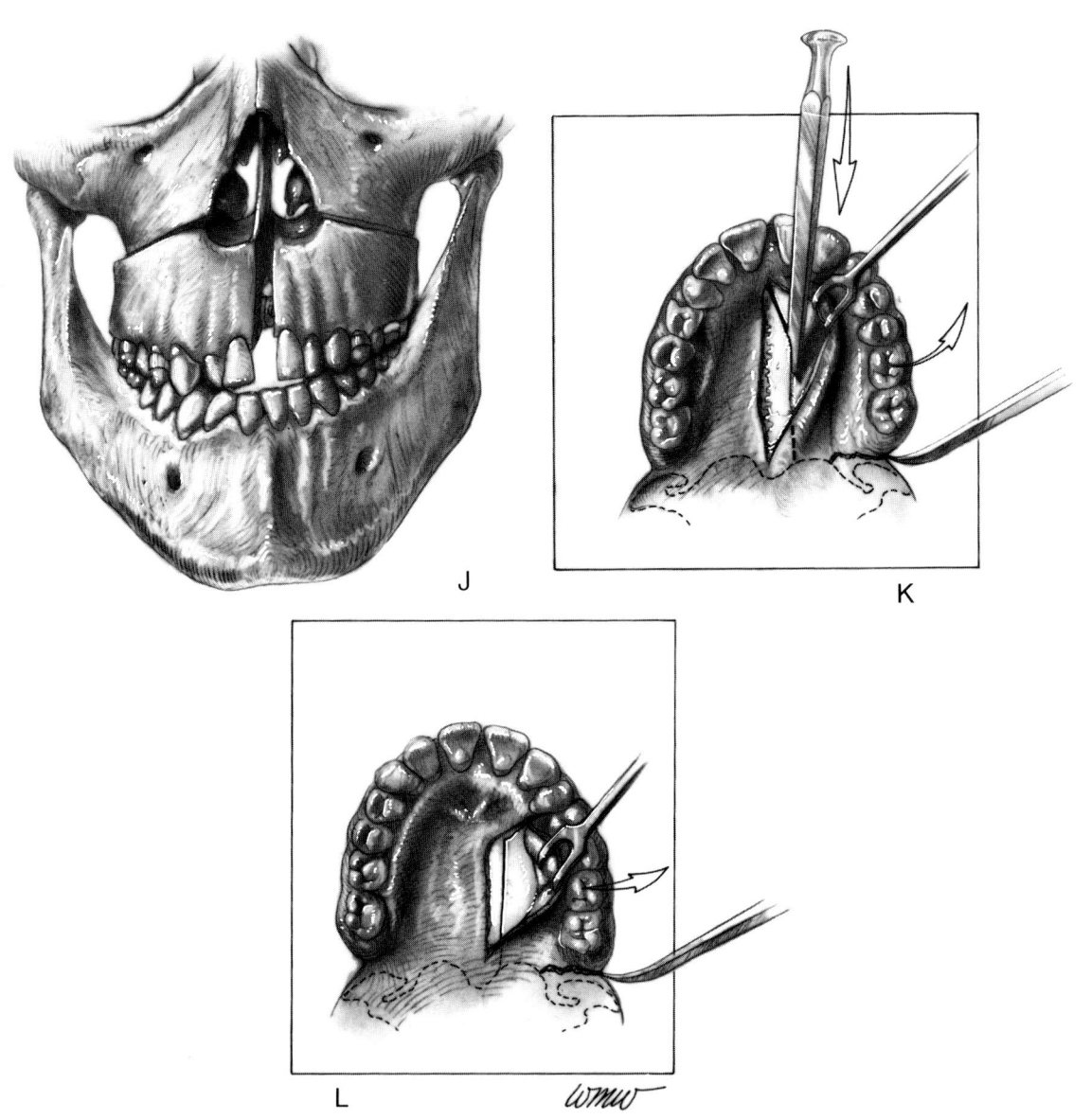

FIGURE 64–68 *Continued.* *J*, The maxillae are overcorrected 1 to 2 mm so that the lingual cusps of the maxillary buccal segments ride up on the buccal cusps of the mandibular buccal segments. *K*, Palatal bone incision for correction of complete unilateral horizontal maxillary deficiency: A midpalatal sagittal incision is made from the incisive papilla posteriorly to the termination of the hard palate. After the wound margins have been retracted bilaterally 3 to 4 mm, the parasagittal palatal cortical bone is osteotomized with a fissure bur. The bone is then completely sectioned by malleting an osteotome along the line of the osteotomy. *L*, Palatal bone incisions for unilateral expansion of the posterior portion of the maxilla: The margin of an inverted hockey stick–shaped palatal incision is raised and retracted to facilitate parasagittal and transverse palatal bone incisions. Then palatal osteotomies are combined with interproximal, lateral maxillary, and pterygomaxillary osteotomies. (From Bell WH, Proffit WR, White RP Jr: Surgical Correction of Dentofacial Deformities. Vol I. Philadelphia, WB Saunders Company, 1980, pp 534–537; with permission.)

osteotomies are feasible office procedures, and both can be accomplished with local anesthesia and sedation, with relatively little postoperative morbidity. Antibiotics are routinely used preoperatively and postoperatively to protect against infection; steroids are used similarly to reduce soft tissue swelling.

Local anesthetic with a vasoconstrictor is infiltrated into the labiobuccal vestibule for hemostasis. A horizontal incision is made through the mucoperiosteum above the mucogingival junction in the depth of the buccal vestibule, extending from the canine region to the second molar (Fig. 64–68*B*). A horizontal low-level osteotomy is made through the lateral wall of the maxilla 4 to 5 mm superior to the apices of the anterior and posterior teeth, on the same level as the occlusal plane extending from the inferolateral aspect of the piriform rim posteriorly to the inferior aspect of the junction of the maxillary tuberosity and pterygoid plate. (See Chapter 63 for individualization of Le Fort I osteotomy and anatomic considerations. This is particularly important if and when a secondary definitive low-level Le Fort I osteotomy is planned.) If the incision is properly planned and executed in this manner, sectioning of the pterygomaxillary suture is usually unnecessary. By not definitively sectioning the pterygomaxillary junction, the morbidity and blood loss are reduced to a minimum. Simultaneous extraction of lower impacted third molar teeth is frequently indicated to prepare the patient for subsequent mandibular advancement and skeletal fixation in the residual healed extraction sites.

In individuals who manifest vertical maxillary excess, the lateral maxillary osteotomies will frequently be positioned more than 5 mm above the apices of the teeth, depending on the distance between the root apices and the nasal floor. The thickened anterior portion of the lateral nasal wall is also sectioned to facilitate separation of the relatively dense nasal sutures. If indicated, a small, curved osteotome may be used to separate the tuberosity from the pterygoid plate. The opposite side is treated similarly to achieve equal mobility of the right and left sides of the maxilla (Fig. 64–68C). Selective reduction of the bone margins of the lateral maxillary osteotomy in the zygomaticomaxillary area ($\simeq$ 2 to 3 mm) may facilitate expansion of the maxillae and obviate a tendency for opening of the bite. Immediate expansion of the RPE appliance and careful clinical assessment will indicate when and if this is indicated.

A vertical incision is made through the attached gingiva and mucosa opposite the planned interincisal osteotomy site. Immediate expansion of the anterior portions of the maxilla is usually accomplished by carefully malleting a thin, sharp osteotome between the central incisors, as illustrated in Figure 64–68D. The surgeon's forefinger is positioned on the incisive papilla to feel the osteotome as it transects the palatal bone, and the osteotome is then malleted posteriorly. If the maxilla does not separate spontaneously, a spatula osteotome is malleted between the central incisors to fracture the interseptal bone. Finally, an osteotome is positioned in the interradicular space and carefully manipulated until movement of the right and left portions of the maxilla is seen (Fig. 64–68E). This simple procedure is usually done despite the fact that expansion is usually achieved with lateral maxillary osteotomies only. Preoperative assessment (with a periapical radiograph) of the planned interdental osteotomy site is always indicated to determine the feasibility of sectioning between the incisor root apices. Usually this is a feasible and safe surgical procedure.

After the bone incisions have been completed, the soft tissue wounds are closed with continuous resorbable sutures. The palatal expansion appliance is immediately activated four quarter-turns (1.0 mm). Spacing between the central incisors and midpalatal separation is noted immediately after the appliance is activated. Normally, the expansion mechanism is activated two to four quarter-turns twice a day (0.5 to 1.0 mm) until the desired amount of expansion is achieved.

The transverse changes in the maxilla are monitored every 2 or 3 days. With such an expansion regimen, midpalatal separation is achieved with virtually no pain or sensation of pressure at the maxillary articular sites. The maxillary arch width is maintained by stabilizing the appliance either by passing a piece of wire through the hole in the expansion screw and looping it around the anterior guide rod or by adding self-curing acrylic resin to the central portion of the expansion appliance. The repositioned segments are retained for 2 to 3 months with the maxillary expansion device. After this device is removed, a heavy transpalatal wire or a removable appliance is employed to maintain the maxillary arch width for an additional 9 to 10 months. Other orthodontic procedures can be initiated after the appliance is stabilized. The rapidity with which such skeletal movements are elicited prevents the stretching of the periodontal ligament fibers and intra-alveolar fibers to close the resultant midline diastema concurrently, as in conventional maxillary expansion techniques. As a result, active orthodontic force will probably be necessary to move the central incisors into juxtaposition.

If there is clinical evidence of a palatal exostosis, parasagittal osteotomies, in addition to lateral osteotomies and sectioning of the midpalatal suture, may be indicated (Fig. 64–68*F* and *G*). If extraction of impacted or partially erupted maxillary third molar teeth is indicated, they can be concomitantly removed in the same operation by slightly modifying the design of the horizontal mucosal incision: The mucosal wound margins are detached and retracted inferiorly to facilitate removal of bone and extraction of the impacted or unerupted third molar teeth. Combining extraction of four impacted third molar teeth and selected maxillary osteotomies to facilitate expansion of the maxilla is practical, timely, and useful in treating selected adolescents and adults undergoing orthodontic therapy. Additionally, it prepares the mandible for subsequent sagittal split ramus osteotomies and the use of skeletal fixation in the healed extraction sites.

CASE: G.W. (Fig. 64–69)

G.W., a 24-year-old woman, sought treatment for pain in her jaw muscles and left temporomandibular (TMJ) joint. She habitually postured her mandible forward to compensate for her Class II minimal open bite deformity. The results of the clinical assessment implicated the jaw disharmony as an etiologic factor in her TMJ dysfunction. After evaluation of her clinical records, the following problem list was developed.

PROBLEM LIST

Esthetics

FRONTAL. The patient had a symmetric, ovoid face with good balance in the upper and middle thirds; a small amount of gingiva was exposed with smiling.

PROFILE. The upper and middle thirds of the face were in good proportion; the lower lip was rolled beneath the maxillary and mandibular incisal edges and slightly everted; the chin was retropositioned.

Cephalometric Analysis

1. Good tooth-to-bone relationship, $\underline{1}$-NA 27°, 4 mm; $\underline{1}$-NB 22°, 3 mm.
2. Mandibular plane angle, GoGn-SN, 36°.
3. Retropositioned mandible (absolute mandibular deficiency).

Occlusal Analysis

DENTAL ARCH FORM. The maxilla and mandible were symmetric with mild anterior tapering.

DENTAL ALIGNMENT. There was minimal crowding in the maxillary and mandibular arches.

DENTAL OCCLUSION. Class II, Division 1, malocclusion, with a 5-mm overjet and 1-mm anterior open bite, was present. With the mandible in centric relation, there was unilateral palatal crossbite; with the mandible in a simulated corrected Class I occlusal relationship, there was transverse maxillary deficiency — 3 mm in the canine region and 5 mm in the molar region. Bolton's discrepancy of approximately 2 mm existed in the anterior 6 region, with the deficiency existing in the maxillary anterior tooth mass.

TREATMENT PLAN

Orthodontics

PRESURGICAL

1. RPE following lateral maxillary osteotomies to increase the intermolar width 5 mm and the intercanine width 3 mm and to facilitate alignment of maxillary anterior teeth without extractions.
2. Application of full banded edgewise appliances to level, align, and coordinate arches for surgical advancement of the mandible.
3. Correction of rotated maxillary and mandibular teeth.

POSTSURGICAL. Complete interdigitation of teeth and correction of residual rotations were planned.

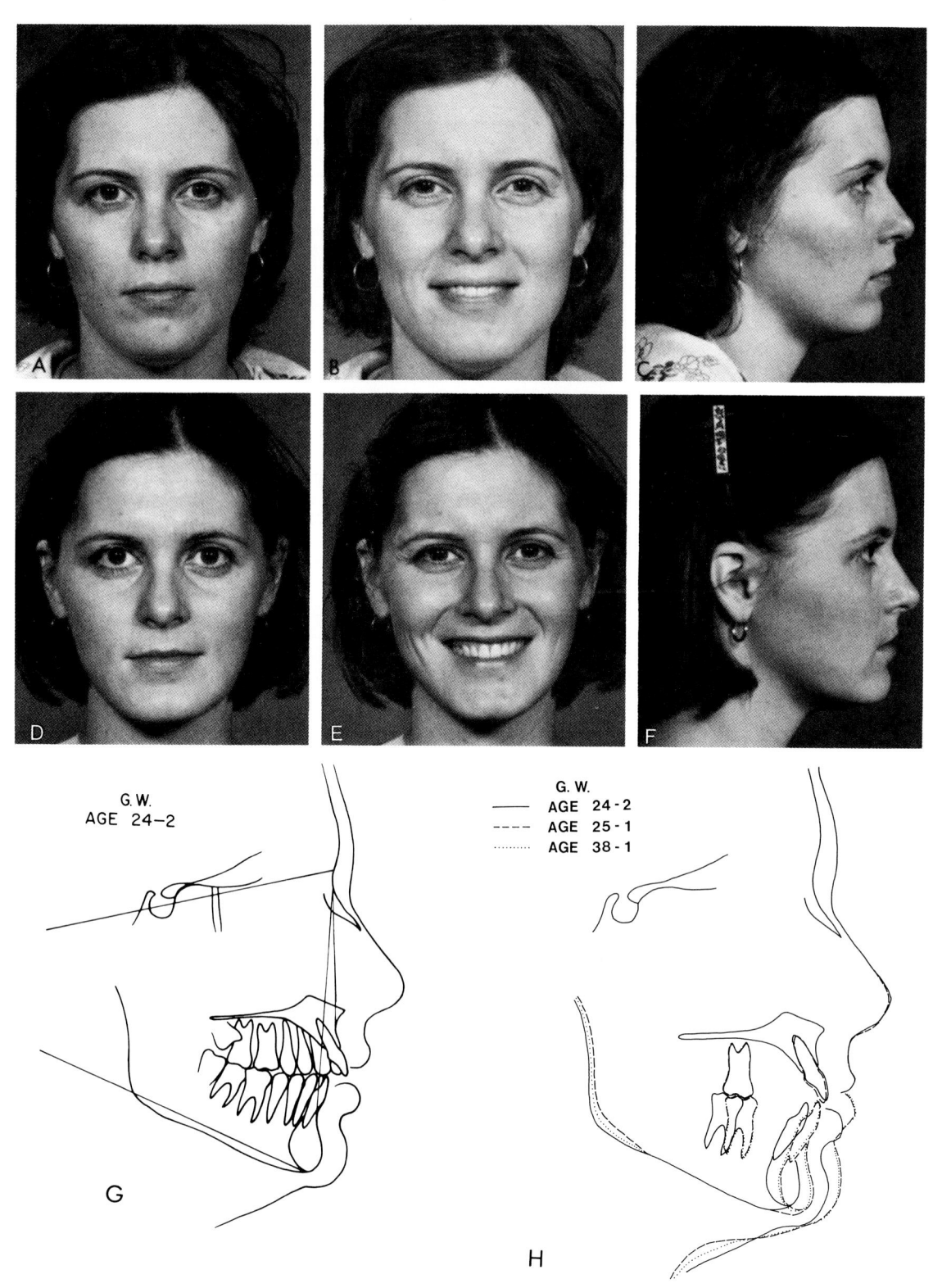

FIGURE 64–69. *A–F*, Facial appearance of 24-year-old woman before (*A–C*) and after (*D–F*) treatment. *G*, Cephalometric tracing before treatment. *H*, Composite cephalometric tracing before and after treatment.

Illustration continued on following page

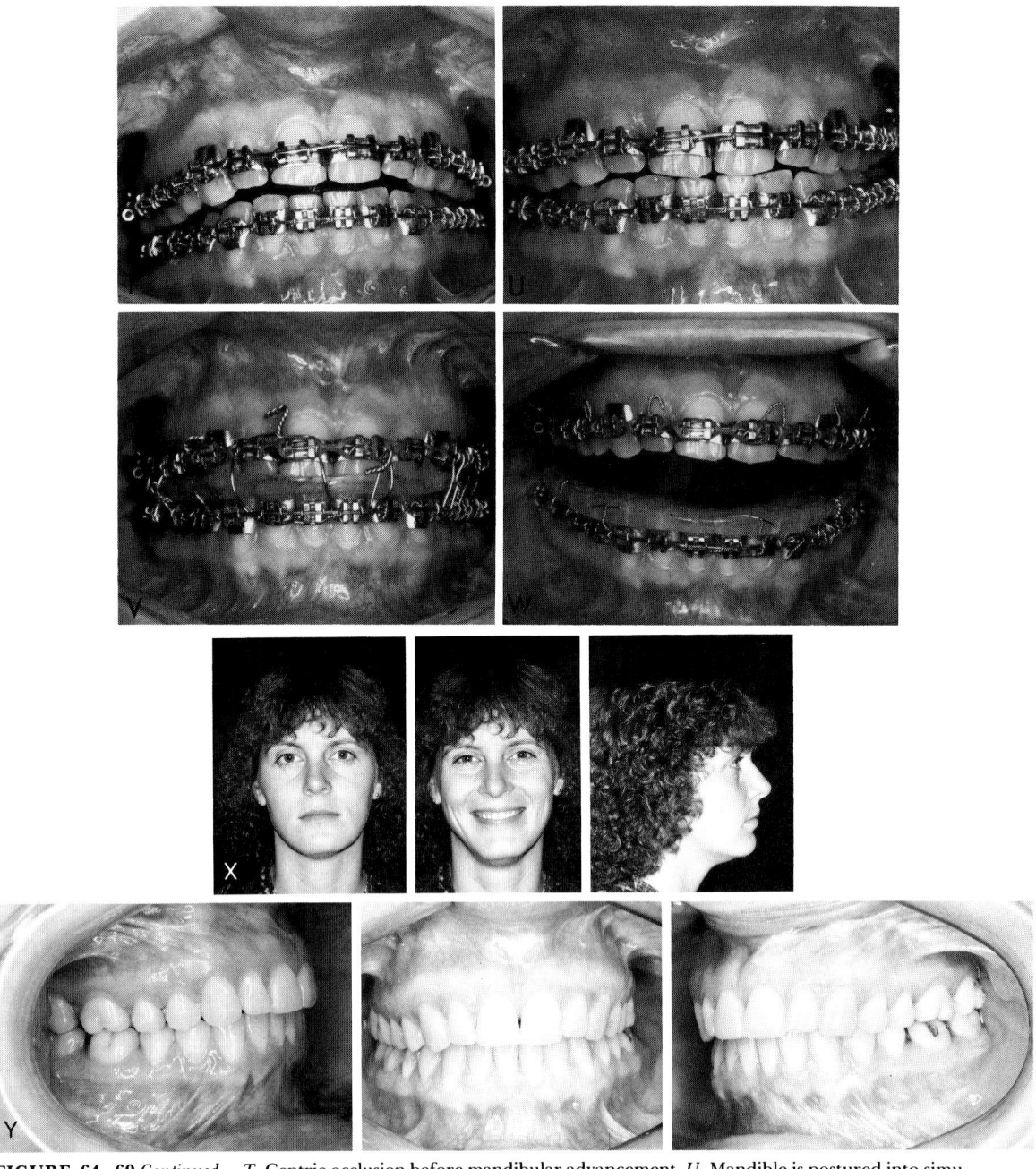

FIGURE 64–69 *Continued.* *T*, Centric occlusion before mandibular advancement. *U*, Mandible is postured into simulated corrected Class I occlusion to demonstrate that arches are adequately coordinated. *V*, Postsurgical intermaxillary fixation. *W*, Functional splint fixed to mandibular arch wire after release from intermaxillary fixation. *X* and *Y*, Skeletal and dental stability and esthetic facial proportions have been maintained 15 months postoperatively. (*A–G, L, P–W* from Bell WH, Proffit WR, White RP Jr: Surgical Correction of Dentofacial Deformities. Vol I. Philadelphia, WB Saunders Company, 1980, pp 803–806; with permission.)

Maxillary Expansion Following Modified Lateral Maxillary Osteotomy—Its Efficacy and Long-Term Stability

As pointed out by Kuo and Will, traditional maxillary expansion with a jack screw appliance is effective in widening both the dental arch and the basal bone in those patients whose circum-maxillary and palatal sutures have not yet fused. However, the fused facial sutures in the skeletally mature individual offer significant resistance to expansion forces, which often results in dentoalveolar tipping. Osteotomies of the lateral maxillary wall and palate have been used to expand the maxilla in the adult patient. In 1984, Glassman described a modified "corticotomy" involving only lateral maxillary cuts, allowing the midpalatal suture to open without palatal osteotomy.

Maxillary expansion without osteotomy typically results in an amount of basal bone expansion approximately half that of dental expansion. In other words, approximately half of the arch expansion is due to dentoalveolar tipping. As a result, significant overexpansion is recommended to achieve sufficient, stable expansion. Very little information has been reported in the literature regarding the efficacy and stability of surgical correction of transverse maxillary deficiency.

A study by Kuo and Will[12b] measured the pre-expansion and postexpansion maxillary and molar width to determine the extent of maxillary expansion achieved with dental arch expansion following modified maxillary osteotomy. Thirty patients received modified bilateral maxillary osteotomies in which bone cuts were made (with the patient under conscious sedation) through the lateral wall of the maxilla, from the piriform rim extending posteriorly to the tuberosity. The bone cut was then tapered inferiorly to terminate anterior to the pterygoid plate. No midline or palatal cuts were made. Patients began expansion on the second postoperative day using a traditional jack screw appliance, which was activated at a rate of 0.5 mm per day. Maxillary expansion ranging from 3 to 15 mm was then achieved, and expansion appliances were maintained in the mouth for 3 months after expansion was completed.

Posteroanterior head films were taken preoperatively, within 1 week of cessation of expansion, 6 months after expansion, and at debanding, wherever possible. Maxillary widths were measured between the points of greatest concavity on basal bone and between the buccal cusps of the first molars. The ratio of initial maxillary to molar expansion was 85 per cent, with nine patients showing 100 per cent. A mean of 22 months later, 98 per cent of the initial maxillary expansion remained. Eighty-four per cent of the initial molar expansion was maintained in the long term as maxillary expansion, making the modified lateral maxillary osteotomy a stable and effective procedure that is feasible on an outpatient basis, with the patient under local anesthesia and intravenous sedation. Similar stability studies have been reported by Bays[1b] and Racey,[16a] who routinely section both the palatal bone and the lateral maxilla, as we have done for some 20 years. We continue to do this because on a few occasions we have observed that the maxilla will not expand as planned with lateral maxillary osteotomies only. Sectioning the maxilla in two adds very little to the technical aspects of the procedure and is easily done with the patient under local or general anesthesia.

Posterior Bilateral Horizontal Maxillary Deficiency with Crossbite

Bilateral expansion of the posterior portions of the maxilla is accomplished by modifying the design of the bone and soft tissue incisions. A midsagittal palatal incision extending from the distal aspect of the incisive papilla to an area opposite the juncture of the hard and soft palates provides surgical access for the necessary palatal bone incisions, which are combined with vertical interdental, lateral maxillary, and pterygomaxillary osteotomies accomplished through the retracted wound margins of a vertical incision through the mucoperiosteum opposite the first premolar tooth (Fig. 64–68 B, C, and H). The thin medial wall of the maxillary sinus is not sectioned, for it offers virtually no resistance to lateral movement of the maxilla. The palatal incision averts stretching the relatively inelastic palatal mucosa and thereby facilitates widening the posterior portions of the maxilla. Immediately following surgery, the expansion appliance is inserted and activated four quarter-turns daily until the desired amount of expansion is achieved.

Unilateral Horizontal Maxillary Deficiency with Crossbite

When the crossbite is unilateral and complete (central incisor to second molar), a parasagittal palatal bone incision is combined with unilateral lateral maxillary and pterygomaxillary osteotomies before the palatal expansion appliance is placed (Fig. 64–68A to D, I, and K). The anterior maxilla is divided by malleting an osteotome between the maxillary central incisors (Fig. 64–68D). The side of the maxillary dentition that is in proper occlusal relationship acts as a buttress against which the side in crossbite is repositioned (Fig. 64–68K).

Unilateral Posterior Horizontal Maxillary Deficiency with Crossbite

When only the posterior portion of the maxilla requires expansion (canine to molar, premolar to molar, or molars only), the posterior maxillary dentoalveolar segment can be separated from the anterior portion of the maxilla through a "hockey-stick" incision that provides surgical access for the necessary palatal bone incision and interdental osteotomy wherever the crossbite begins (Fig. 64–68L). When the surgical adjustments have been completed, the expansion appliance is inserted and activated four quarter-turns a day until the desired amount of expansion is achieved. Whenever unilateral horizontal maxillary deficiency is treated by surgical and orthodontic techniques, maximum mobility of the dentoalveolar segment to be moved is desirable.

Surgical Widening of the Maxilla

With proper planning and execution, the narrow and constricted maxilla can be surgically expanded into a stable relationship with the mandible.[7] Horizontal maxillary deficiency, manifested as either bilateral or unilateral palatal crossbite, is commonly associated with vertical maxillary excess, open bite deformity, mandibular prognathism, or mandibular deficiency. Occasionally, the problem manifests independently as unilateral or bilateral crossbite in either the anterior or the posterior portion of the maxilla. In such cases, anterior or posterior maxillary osteotomies are used to correct the dysplasia. More frequently, however, when treatment priorities involve correction of the deformity and malocclusion in the horizontal, vertical, and anteroposterior planes of space, the occlusal problems defy treatment by an isolated segmental procedure. An operation to treat the individual's three-dimensional skeletal and occlusal problems is designed on the basis of the esthetic priorities established after careful clinical analysis. To accomplish this objective, the entire maxilla is mobilized and repositioned by Le Fort I osteotomy.

The design of the operation depends on whether or not teeth are extracted, the anatomy of the palatal vault, the need for leveling the maxillary occlusal plane, the magnitude of lateral movement, and the anatomic site where any transverse deficiency is located. After model surgery, a careful measurement of the transverse dimensional changes is made to determine the feasibility of surgery, the need for bone grafting, and the appropriate technique. When the amount of maxillary expansion necessary is 6 to 10 mm or less, the segments are usually moved laterally into the desired occlusal relationship by two-, three-, or four-piece Le Fort I maxillary osteotomy (Fig. 64–70). Horizontal maxillary deficiency associated with the great majority of dentofacial deformities can be managed by various modifications of the basic Le Fort I osteotomy technique. When required correction of horizontal maxillary deficiency is expected to exceed the physiologic limits of Le Fort I osteotomy and jeopardize circulation to and viability of the mobilized segments, surgery may be accomplished by combined anterior and posterior maxillary osteotomies executed through soft tissue incisions that provide simultaneous access using this technique. Cleft palate patients requiring simultaneous bilateral expansion repair of their oronasal fistulas and alveolar cleft grafting may be candidates for this procedure. Lateral maxillary osteotomies in concert with RPE and subsequent Le Fort I osteotomy constitute another option for managing transverse horizontal maxillary deficiency.

Two-Piece Le Fort I Osteotomy (Fig. 64–70)

With the maxilla in the "downfractured" position, the parasagittal palatal bone can be osteotomized from the planned anterior interdental space posteriorly to and through the horizontal plate of the palatine bone (Fig. 64–70A). The thick part of the anterior maxilla is sectioned with a fissure bur and spatula osteotome. The line of the planned osteotomy is angled laterally to an area midway between the midpalatal suture and the juncture between the horizontal and vertical parts of the maxilla (Fig. 64–70A and B). The bone in this area is very thin and is easily sectioned without tearing the attached thick palatal mucosa opposite the osteotomy site (Fig. 64–70C, E, and F). The thin posterior part of the maxilla is easily fractured by light manipulation of a periosteal elevator or similar instrument between the margins of the incompletely sectioned bone.

The index finger of the hand opposite to that used to hold the drill or saw may be positioned on the palatal bone (Fig. 64–70C and D). The bone is then completely sectioned by manipulating a periosteal elevator in the osteotomy site or malleting an osteotome along the intended line of osteotomy (Fig. 64–70D). Next, the anterior maxilla is divided by malleting a spatula osteotome between the central incisors (Fig. 64–70F). The forefinger is positioned on the incisive papilla to feel the redirected osteotome as it transects the deeper portion of the midpalatal suture and splits the interseptal bone.

When the maxilla has been divided into two segments by a sagittal osteotomy through the midpalatal suture, the cut must be made through relatively dense bone that is covered by thin mucosa (Fig. 64–70G). Therefore, when the maxilla is widened in this manner, the palatal mucosa underlying the osteotomy site is easily torn (Fig. 64–70G). For this reason, the maxilla is usually sectioned parasagittally in the area midway between the midpalatal suture and the juncture of the horizontal and vertical parts of the maxilla. Widening the maxilla by means of parasagittal osteotomies has the advantage of cutting through very thin bone that is covered by thick mucosa (Fig. 64–70E). By carefully undermining the margins of the incised palatal mucosa, lateral maxillary movement is facilitated without tearing the palatal soft tissue pedicle. (See Chapter 63 for additional details of surgical techniques.)

Three-Piece or Four-Piece Le Fort I Osteotomy (Fig. 64–70)

Maxillary expansion is frequently accomplished by means of a three-piece or four-piece Le Fort I osteotomy with or without extraction of premolar teeth.[2,6] This versatile procedure allows simultaneous three-dimensional movement of the

2428 / VII — ORTHOGNATHIC SURGERY

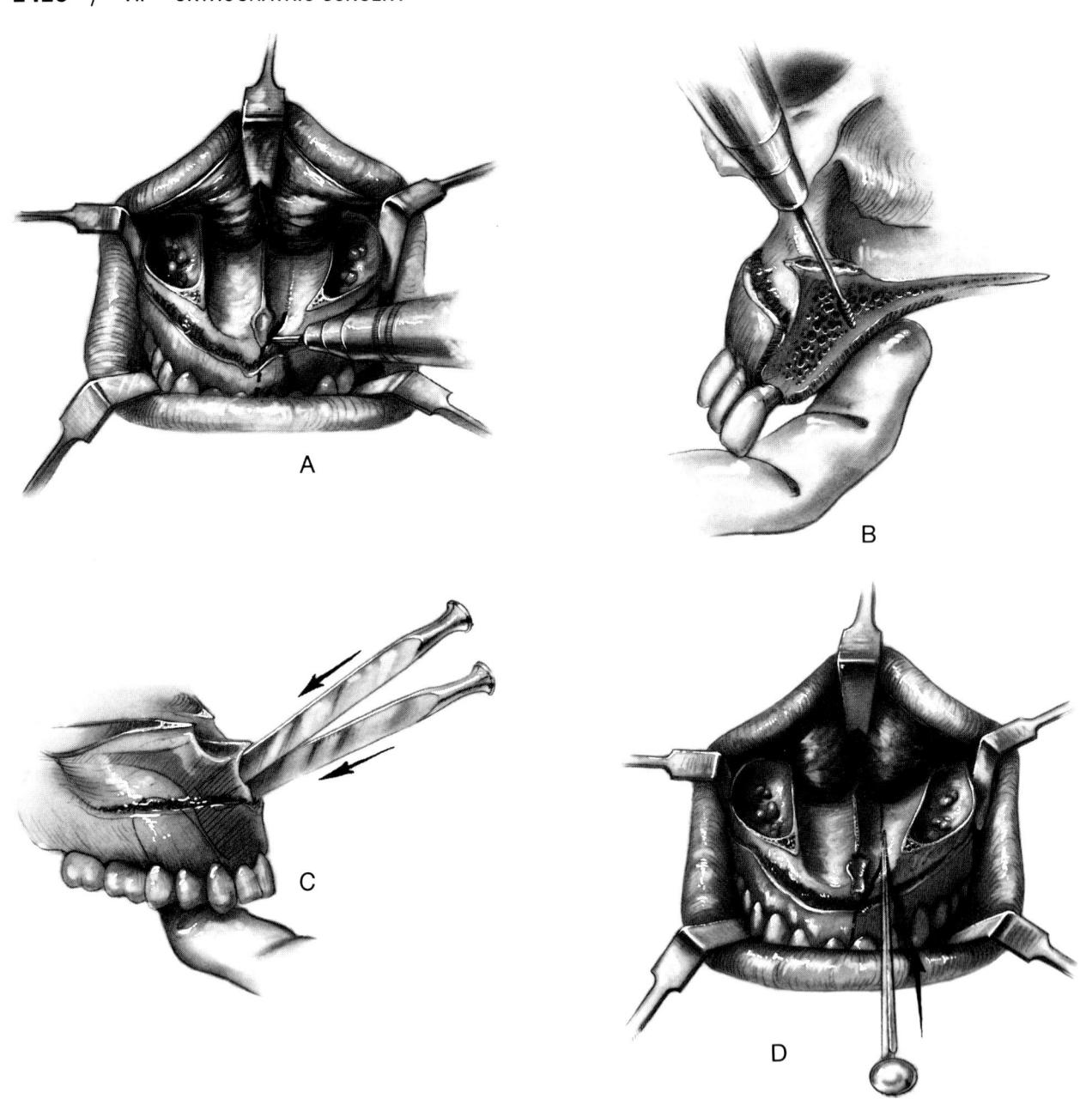

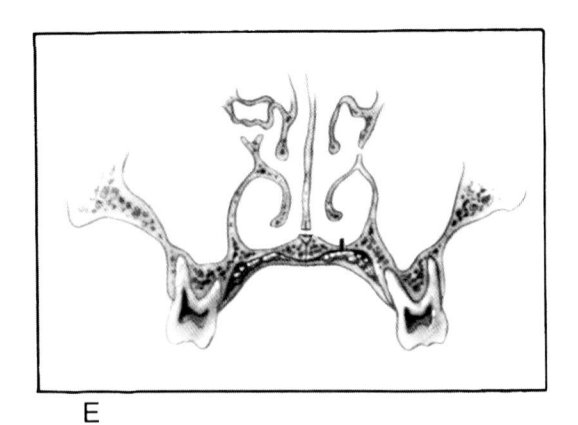

FIGURE 64-70. TWO-PIECE, THREE-PIECE, OR FOUR-PIECE LE FORT I OSTEOTOMY TO WIDEN MAXILLA. *A*, Schematic view of downfractured maxilla showing planned parasagittal palatal osteotomy. The thick portion of the anterior maxilla is sectioned with a fissure bur in a straight handpiece. *B*, Finger may be positioned on the palatal mucosa to feel the rotating bur as it partially transects the palatal cortical bone. *C*, Thick part of the anterior maxilla is partially sectioned by malleting a spatula osteotome between the central incisors; the forefinger is positioned on the palatal mucosa to feel the redirected osteotome as it transects the deeper portion of the midpalatal suture. *D*, The parasagittal palatal bone is sectioned by lightly malleting a spatula osteotome along the intended line of osteotomy. The thinner posterior palatal bone can usually be separated by manipulation of a periosteal elevator positioned between the margins of the incompletely sectioned bone. *E*, Cross-section of the maxillary molar region showing the intended line of osteotomy through thin palatal bone that is covered by thick palatal mucosa.

Illustration continued on following page

64 — MANDIBULAR DEFICIENCY / **2429**

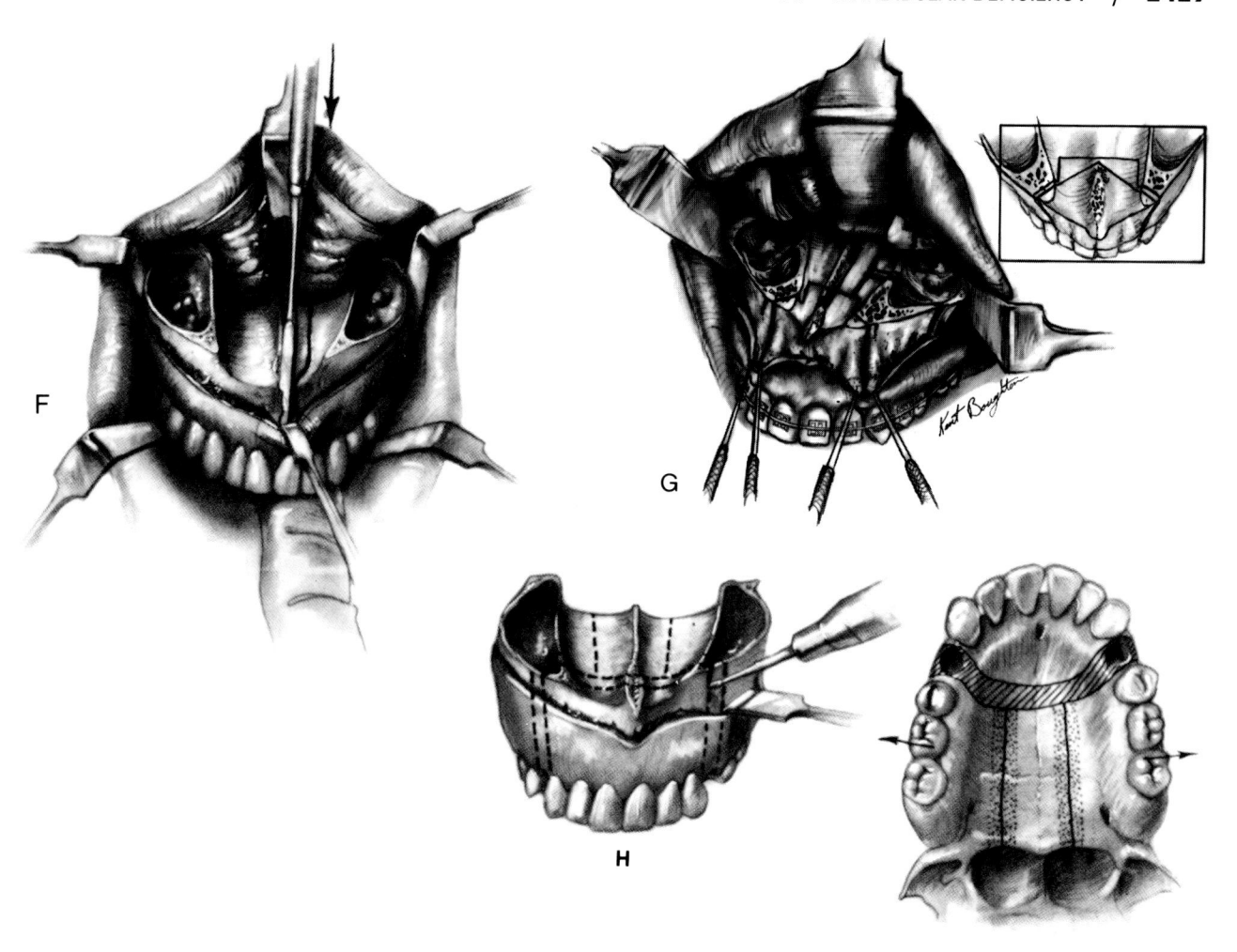

FIGURE 64–70 *Continued.* *F,* Anterior maxillae are separated by malleting a spatula osteotome between the central incisors. Finger is positioned on the incisive papilla to feel the osteotome when it transects the deeper portion of the maxilla and splits the interseptal bone. A larger osteotome is positioned in the planned incisor interradicular space and manipulated to achieve mobilization and separation of the anterior maxillae. When vertical change is not required and lateral movement is minimal, it may be unnecessary to cut the orthodontic arch wire in the planned interdental osteotomy site. If the arch wire is sectioned in several places, an interocclusal splint is usually used to index and fix the dentoalveolar segments into the planned occlusion. By careful undermining of the margins of the incisal palatal mucosa, lateral movement of the maxillae is facilitated without tearing the palatal tissue. Simultaneous lateral and forward movement of the maxillae and indexing of teeth into the splint is facilitated by lateral traction to 25-gauge wire ligatures passed around the arch bar or wire in the first molar areas. *G,* Sectioning the maxilla into three segments by Le Fort I osteotomy. In the canine–lateral incisor region, there is usually a wider and thicker zone of keratinized gingiva than is normally found in the canine-premolar region, where there is frequently a high frenum attachment and a narrower and thinner band of keratinized gingiva. Consequently, healing of a vertical incision made in this area is usually uncomplicated, and dehiscence of the wound margins is rare. Vertical interdental osteotomies in the lateral incisor–canine interspaces are connected by a transverse horseshoe-shaped palatal osteotomy distal to the incisive canal. The maxilla is sectioned tranversely to facilitate leveling of the occlusal plane and parasagittally to increase the intermolar width and improve the interdigitation of the teeth. Planned osteotomies are inscribed into the maxilla with a bur. The attached palatal soft tissue pedicle to this four-tooth incisor dento-osseous segment has been enlarged by increasing the size of the palatal bony segment. The principle may be applied to Le Fort I osteotomy techniques for repositioning one-, two-, three-, or four-tooth anterior segments. *Inset,* The conventional triangular design for comparison with the modified design that creates a larger anterior maxillary dento-osseous segment and attached soft tissue pedicle. This osteotomy design is most frequently used in nonextraction cases. See Chapter 63 for the design of the Le Fort I osteotomy. *H,* Three-piece Le Fort I osteotomy for widening the posterior maxillary dentoalveolar segment and leveling the maxillary occlusal plane by combined transverse palatal and vertical alveolar ostectomies; the palatal portion of the maxilla is sectioned by horseshoe-shaped circumpalatal osteotomy. This osteotomy design is frequently used in residual bicuspid extraction sites after segmental orthodontic alignment of the arch. *I,* Margins of horseshoe-shaped palatal bone incisions are undermined to facilitate lateral and superior movements and to prevent excessive detachment of the palatal mucoperiosteum, which is possible with large movements. Broken lines *(H)* indicate intended lines of bone sectioning; cross-hatched areas indicate intended transverse palatal ostectomy; stippled areas indicate where mucoperiosteum has been detached from the bony margins. (*A–F, H,* and *I* from Bell WH, Proffit WR, White RP Jr: Surgical Correction of Dentofacial Deformities. Vol I. Philadelphia, WB Saunders Company, 1980, pp 539–541; *G* from Bell WH: Surgical Correction of Dentofacial Deformities: New Concepts. Vol III. Philadelphia, WB Saunders Company, 1985, p 24; with permission.)

Advancement of the mandible prior to leveling of the mandibular accentuated curve of Spee will result in an occlusion in which, following fixation and splint removal, the anterior teeth and the second molars bilaterally form a tripod (Fig. 64–71B). Typically, a substantial open bite will exist distal to the canines in the cuspid-premolar-molar region, but it is easily closed with the aforementioned elastic therapy. Such sequencing of treatment may also inherently increase stability of the mandibular advancement by increasing clockwise rotation associated with forward movement of the incisors.

Although the mandibular arch should be leveled postsurgically, *the maxillary arch should be leveled prior to surgery* for several reasons. The maxillary arch typically is much easier to level and requires a minimal amount of treatment time. In addition, proper torque of the maxillary incisors must be accomplished prior to surgery to ensure that a Class I sagittal canine relationship is attained at the time of surgical mandibular advancement. If the maxillary arch is not level prior to surgery, the maxillary incisors will be too upright in most instances to facilitate a Class I canine relationship without the necessity of an anterior crossbite (or overcorrection), which is not advisable. It is also ideal for the maxillary arch, equipped with a rigid full bracket-width rectangular stainless steel arch wire, to act as a stabilizer against which a resilient mandibular arch wire and elastics may be pitted to facilitate mandibular arch leveling with little reciprocating movement of the maxillary dentition. The mandibular surgical wire will, in most cases, act also as the leveling arch after fixation and splint removal. Therefore, a light round stainless steel wire or a large, yet resilient, braided rectangular wire or nitinol should be placed immediately prior to surgery.

Surgical Options

Careful attention to the many details of esthetic, functional, and cephalometric planning studies will usually evolve a plan of treatment that will allow simultaneous correction of both the occlusal and the esthetic disharmony associated with Class II deep-bite deformity. The clinical manifestations of such patients may defy treatment without Le Fort I and interpositional bone grafting, interpositional genioplasty, and mandibular advancement surgery to achieve anteroposterior, vertical, and transverse facial proportionality (Fig. 64–72).

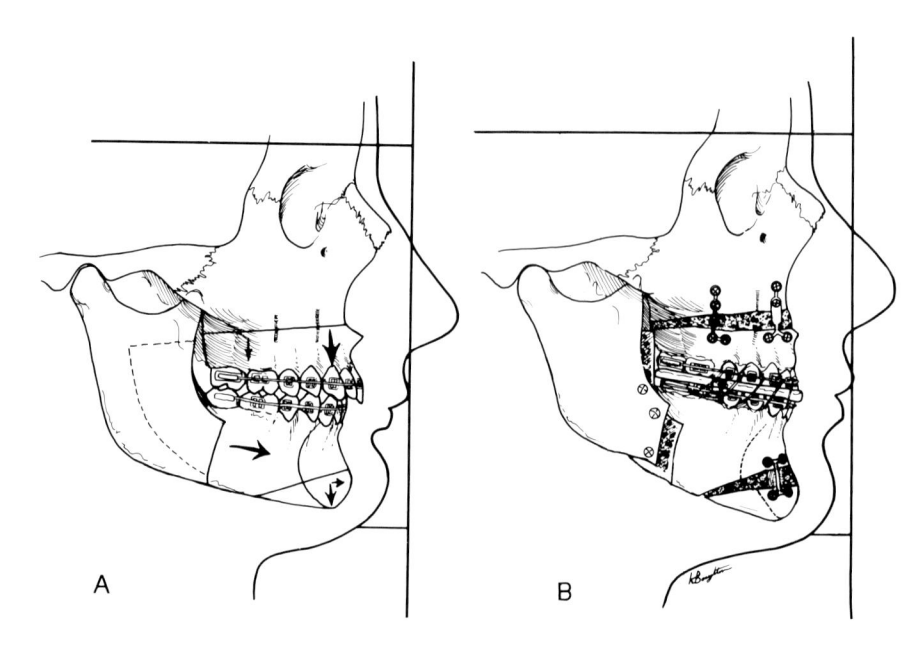

FIGURE 64–72. SURGICAL TECHNIQUES FOR CORRECTION OF CLASS II DEEP-BITE MALOCCLUSION ASSOCIATED WITH VERTICAL MAXILLARY DEFICIENCY, DECREASED CHIN HEIGHT, AND ABSOLUTE MANDIBULAR DEFICIENCY. A, Surgical plan: Le Fort I osteotomy to increase vertical dimension of maxilla, sagittal split ramus osteotomies to advance mandible and correct deep bite, and interpositional genioplasty to increase chin height. B, Postoperative result; increased facial height and Class I occlusion; interpositional bone grafts in place; maxilla stabilized by bone plates and screws. (Modified from Bell WH: Surgical Correction of Dentofacial Deformities: New Concepts. Vol III. Philadelphia, WB Saunders Company, 1985, p 173; with permission.)

Correction of the Anteroposterior Dimension

The common denominator of successful treatment of absolute mandibular deficiency involves surgical advancement of the mandible into a stable relationship with the repositioned maxilla (Figs. 64–71 and 64–72). With careful treatment planning, meticulous execution of surgical techniques, good preoperative and postoperative care, and coordination of surgery with efficient postsurgical orthodontic therapy and rehabilitation, the mandible can be advanced and the maxilla repositioned surgically with relatively few sequelae and complications.

Limited accessibility of the oral cavity, restricted jaw opening, and excessively small mandibular rami may be indications for extraoral ramus surgery. The extraoral inverted-L osteotomy is a dependable procedure for treating severe mandibular hypoplasia, typically seen in patients with juvenile rheumatoid arthritis, mandibular ankylosis, and certain syndromes (Fig. 64–73). Such persons have mandibular deficiency in the vertical and anteroposterior planes of space in addition to posterior vertical maxillary deficiency. See Chapter 57 for detailed descriptions of this technique.

Correction of the Vertical Dimension

Although the mandibular deficiency deep-bite deformity generally involves the anteroposterior dimension, the vertical and transverse dimensions are also frequently abnormal. Vertical abnormalities may be seen in the mandible, the maxilla, or both. Insufficient lower anterior facial height may be corrected by Le Fort I osteotomy and interpositional bone grafting, genioplasty with interpositional bone grafting, or total mandibular subapical osteotomy with interpositional bone grafting. These procedures are all designed to increase facial height, the amount of tooth exposure, or both. Correction of the deep bite by mandibular advancement to achieve a satisfactory overbite and overjet relationship also increases the lower anterior facial height.

Class II mandibular deficiency deep bite with vertical maxillary deficiency requires analysis and correction in all three planes of space. Multiple maxillary, mandibular, and chin surgical procedures are performed during a single operation. There may be a vertical abnormality consisting of deep bite, decreased lower anterior facial height, vertical maxillary deficiency manifested as a lack of tooth exposure when smiling, and lack of chin and mandibular body height.

CASE: M.H. (Fig. 64–74)

A 24-year-old man was referred for treatment of a severe malocclusion and a retrusive mandible (Fig. 64–74A to C). Clinical examination disclosed facial symmetry with good balance in the upper and middle thirds. The patient's symmetric, esthetic smile revealed normal exposure of gingiva (Fig. 64–74C). The upper and middle facial thirds were in good proportion, with 3 mm of upper incisor exposure when the patient was in repose. The nasolabial angle was slightly obtuse; the lower lip was rolled beneath the maxillary and mandibular incisal edges and everted. The patient's retropositioned chin and mandible contributed to the convex profile and unesthetic submental-cervical region (Fig. 64–74G and H). There was minimal crowding and malalignment of the mandibular teeth. Spaces were present between the maxillary incisors, which were slightly inclined to the labial.

The deciduous molar was extracted, and the arches were then banded and bonded with a "segmented arch" edgewise appliance. Since the patient's vertical facial proportions were within normal limits and since he desired rapid completion of treatment, early surgical intervention was proposed. The leveling would be accomplished much more efficiently by extrusion of posterior teeth after surgical treatment, since a posterior open bite would be created and there would be no occlusal forces hindering eruption of the teeth. Surgical alleviation of the transverse discrepancy was planned.

2434 / VII—ORTHOGNATHIC SURGERY

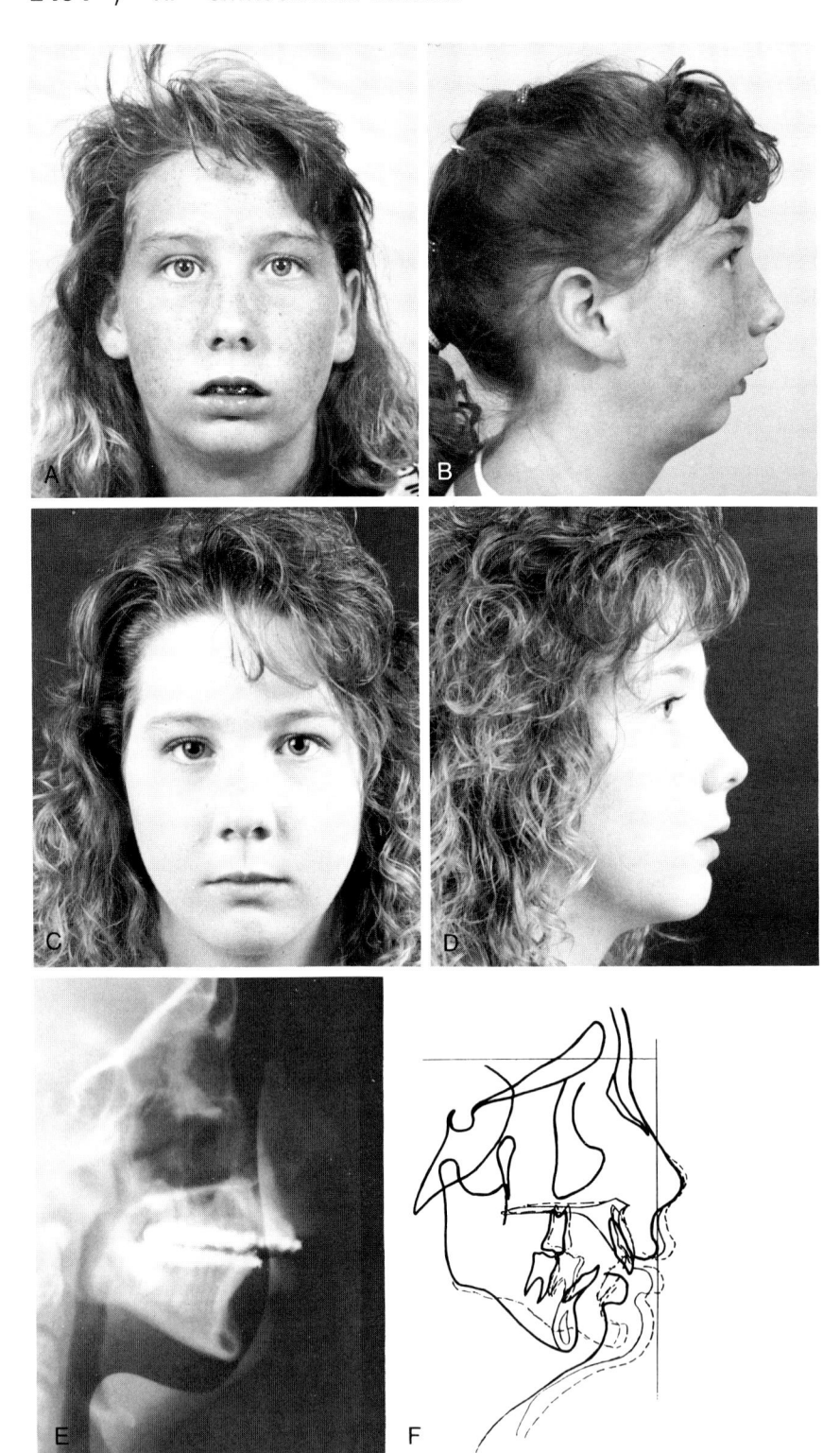

FIGURE 64–73. CORRECTION OF COMPLETE CLASS II MALOCCLUSION ASSOCIATED WITH SEVERE MANDIBULAR DEFICIENCY AND POSTERIOR VERTICAL MAXILLARY HYPOPLASIA IN 13-YEAR-OLD GIRL. *A* and *B*, Facial appearance before simultaneous mandibular advancement, superior repositioning of the maxilla, and advancement genioplasty. *C* and *D*, Postoperative facial appearance. *E*, Lateral cephalogram before surgery, showing severe mandibular deficiency and mild vertical maxillary hyperplasia. *F*, Composite cephalometric tracings before surgery (Le Fort I osteotomy, mandibular advancement, and advancement genioplasty), 3 weeks after surgery, and 1 year after surgery (solid line, before surgery; broken lines, after surgery). The initial follow-up period shows the relapse that occurred during maxillomandibular fixation. *G*, Panoramic radiograph showing impacted third molar teeth in severely retrognathic mandible. *H*, Panoramic radiograph showing various types of bone plates and screws, skeletal fixation (circum-mandibular wires), and maxillomandibular fixation that were used to stabilize the repositioned maxilla and mandible. *I*, Preoperative Class II malocclusion with 13-mm overjet. *J*, Postoperative Class I occlusion 14 months after surgery. *K*, Postoperative occlusion. *L*, Postoperative symmetric and esthetic smile. In this case involving a large mandibular advancement, a "belt and suspenders" approach to stabilization of the mandible was used—this involved *skeletal stabilization* (suspension and circum-mandibular wires) and *skeletal fixation* with bone plates and screws. Despite the use of both methods, there was some relapse during the period of maxillomandibular fixation. *M*, Alternate technique designed to achieve large advancement of the mandible. Inverted-L osteotomy with large reconstruction bone plate stabilized with 2.7-mm-diameter bone screws in the angle of the mandible, interpositional bone graft, and advancement genioplasty; the genial segment is stabilized with 18-mm-long position screw.

64 — MANDIBULAR DEFICIENCY / **2435**

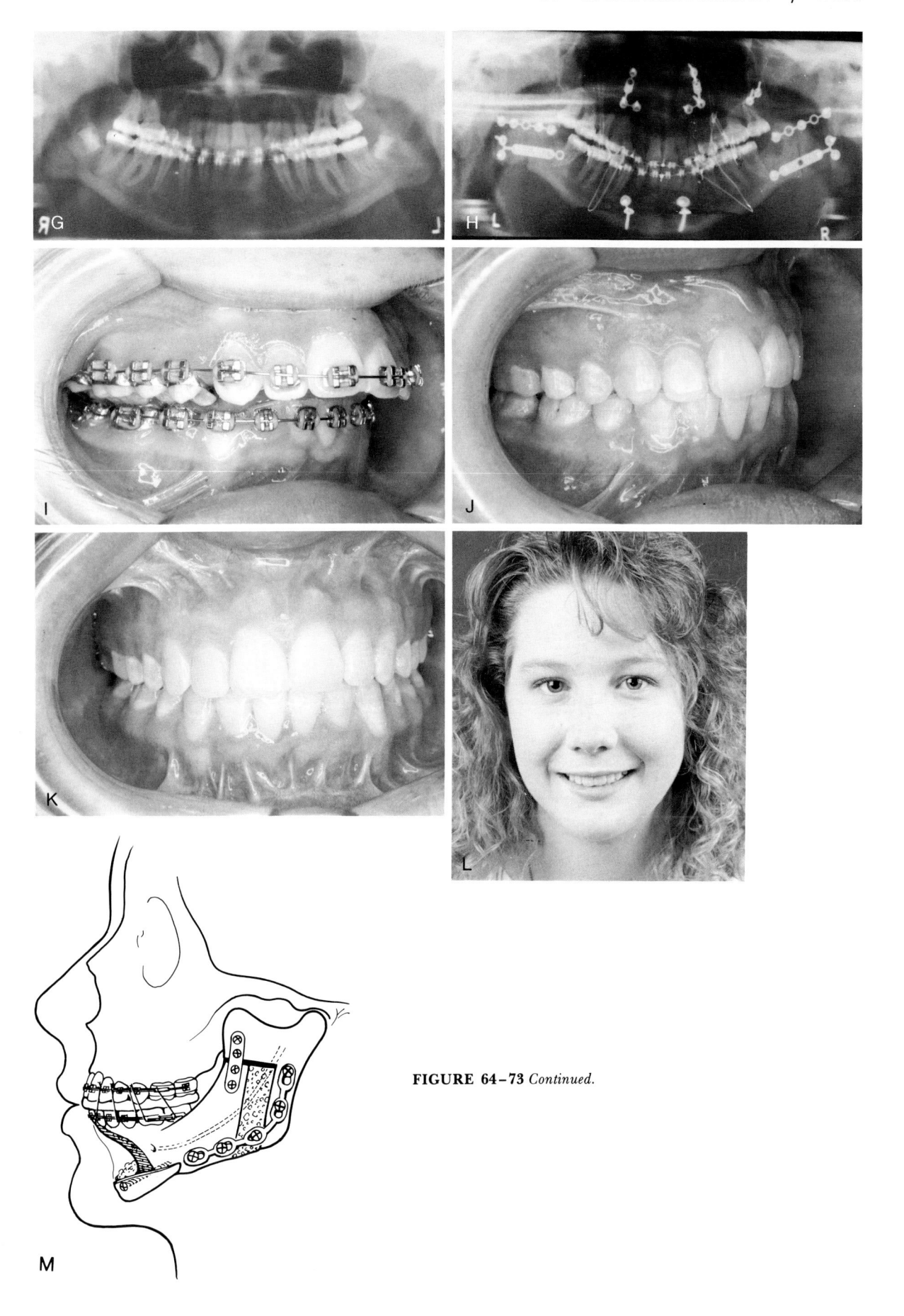

FIGURE 64-73 *Continued.*

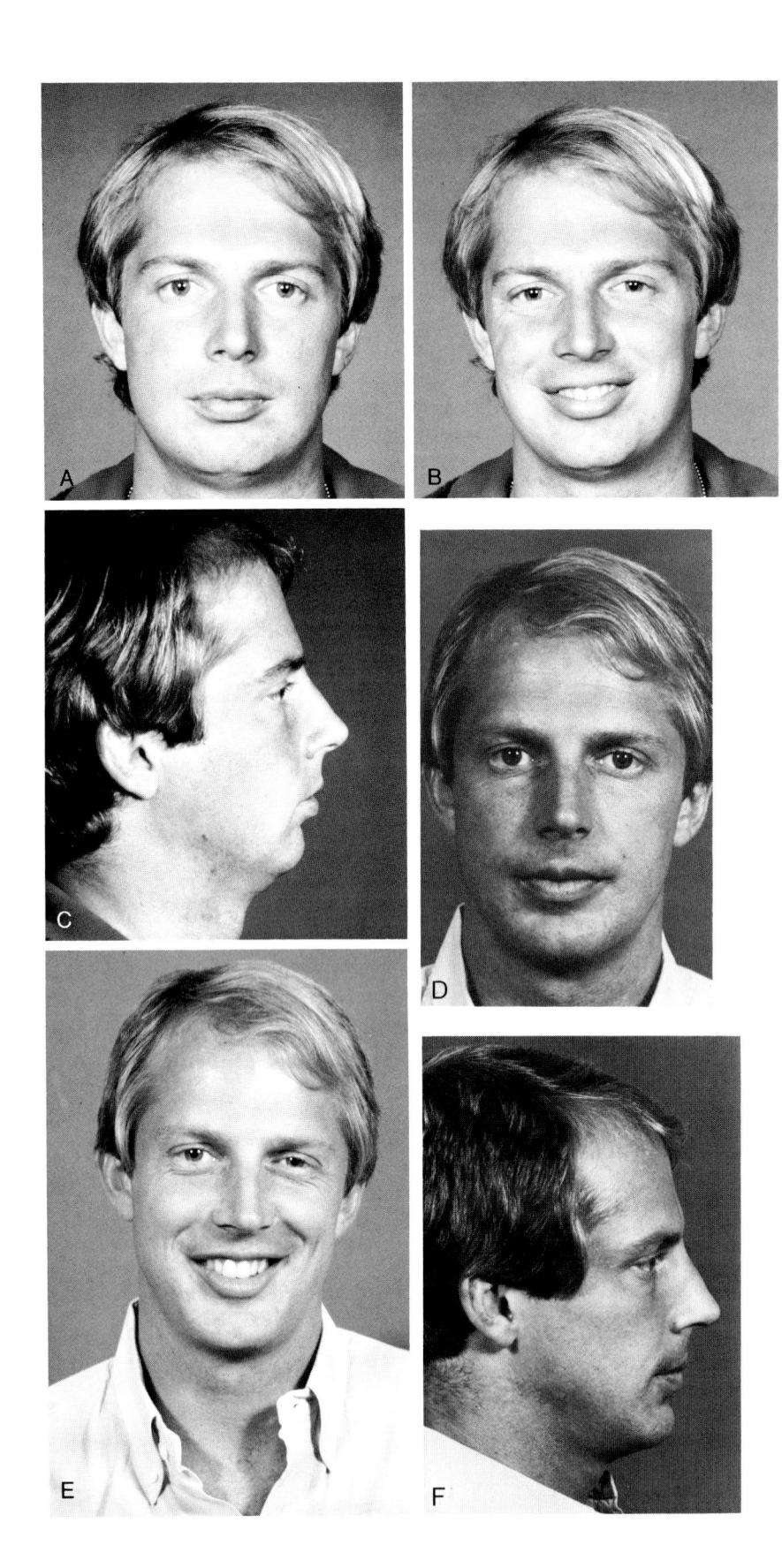

FIGURE 64–74. *A–C*, Facial appearance of 24-year-old man before treatment. *D–F*, Facial appearance after treatment.
Illustration continued on following page

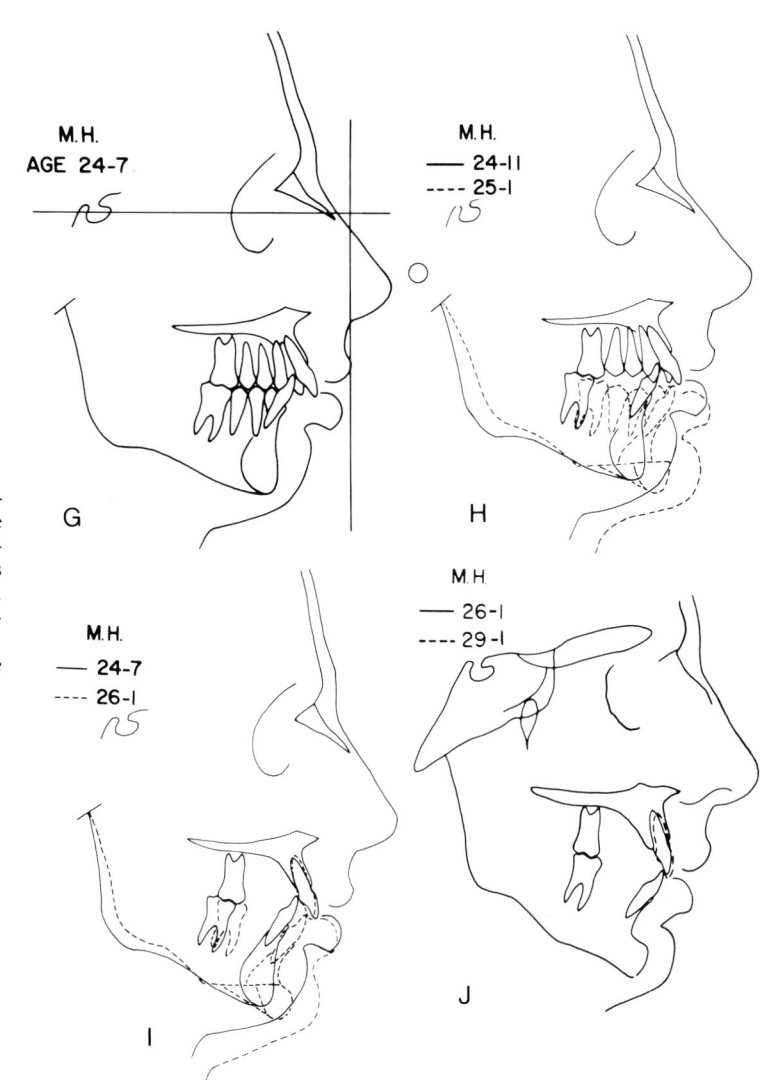

FIGURE 64–74 *Continued. G,* Cephalometric tracing before treatment (age 24 years). *H,* Composite cephalometric tracings before *(solid line)* and after *(broken line)* surgery. *I,* Composite cephalometric tracings before *(solid line)* and after *(broken line)* treatment. *J,* Composite cephalometric tracings showing skeletal stability during postoperative follow-up period.

Illustration continued on following page

Minimal alignment and leveling with rapid progression to a rectangular arch wire of sufficient dimension were the prime objectives of the presurgical orthodontic phase of treatment.

Bilateral sagittal split osteotomies of the vertical rami were performed to reposition the mandible downward and forward into a Class I canine-and-molar relationship. A genioplasty was performed concomitantly to advance the chin 8 mm in order to increase the chin prominence and improve the submental-cervical esthetics. An interdental osteotomy was made in the mandibular left central incisor–lateral incisor interspace to facilitate narrowing in the intercanine and intermolar areas. This surgery was designed to compensate for horizontal deficiency in the maxillary arch. The postoperative occlusion, which was associated with an open bite in the premolar–first molar region, was stabilized with an interocclusal wafer splint and maxillomandibular ligatures fixed to orthodontic stabilizing arch wires.

After release of maxillomandibular fixation, the interocclusal splint was removed and ligated to the lower arch wire. For 2 subsequent weeks, it was used as a functional splint to maintain the planned anteroposterior relationship. Night-time vertical elastics were worn simultaneously in the canine regions.

Upon removal of the occlusal splint, active orthodontic mechanics were resumed to readily close the posterior open bite (Fig. 64–74*M*). Initially, a light 0.016-inch lower arch wire was inserted, maintaining the 0.018-inch × 0.025-inch rectangular maxillary arch wire in place. In addition, a high-pull headgear with the outer bow anterior to the maxillary center of resistance and activated to 450 gm was worn 14 hours per day. This practice allowed for more eruption of mandibular posterior teeth than of

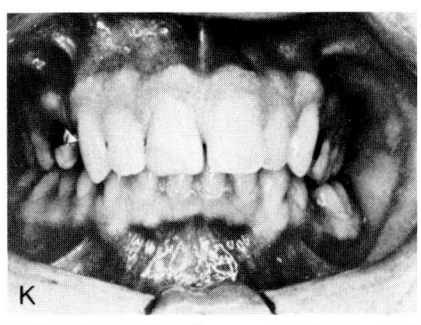

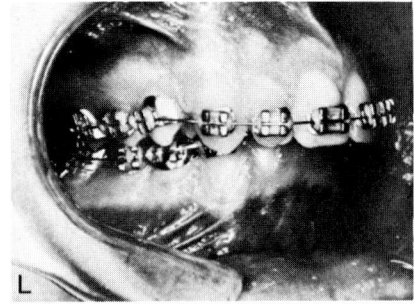

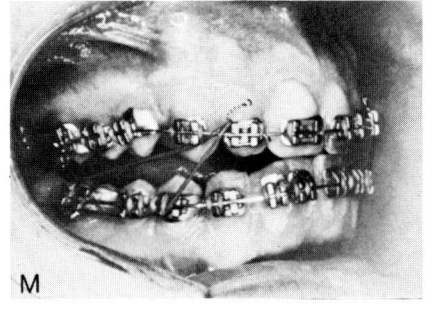

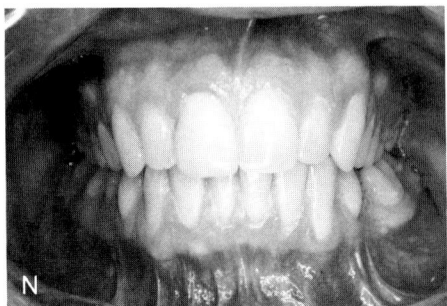

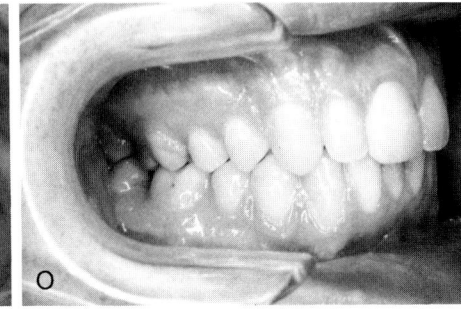

FIGURE 64-74 *Continued.* K and L, Class II, Division 1, deep-bite malocclusion before treatment. M, Occlusion after surgery at time of release from maxillomandibular fixation. N and O, Occlusion after treatment. (From Bell WH, Jacobs JD, Legan H: Treatment of Class II deep bite by orthodontic and surgical means. Am J Orthod 85:1–20, 1984; with permission.)

maxillary teeth, as was needed. In addition, a mandibular intrusive base arch was inserted at this time. When activated to heavier-than-normal forces, the base arch is an efficient means of extruding posterior teeth while maintaining sufficient intrusive force on the anterior teeth to obviate deepening of the overbite. Light Class II trapezoidal elastics were used at night.

The patient was seen by his orthodontist at 2-week intervals, and within 3 months the teeth were intercuspating well. Bands were then removed, and the patient was instructed to wear a positioner 4 hours per day and all night. After 3 months of positioner wear, an upper Hawley retainer and a lower spring retainer were placed.

To reiterate, the mandible was advanced surgically 8 mm and maintained in its new position during the postsurgical orthodontic treatment phase (Fig. 64-74H and I). At debanding, approximately 8 months after the commencement of therapy, the patient was deemed to have an excellent functional and esthetic treatment result (Fig. 64-74D, E, F, N, and O). When assessed both statically and functionally, the occlusion was considered to be very good. The anteroposterior mandibular position and Class I occlusion have remained stable over a 6-year follow-up period (Fig. 64-74J, N, and O).

Surgeon — William H. Bell, D.D.S., Dallas, TX
Orthodontist — Harry L. Legan, D.D.S., Nashville, TN

3. GENIOPLASTY STRATEGIES

WILLIAM H. BELL
KEVIN McBRIDE

Intellectual humility—prerequisite for creativity.

—Bigelow

The chin, which is one of the most obvious facial structures, has long been the object of curiosity, the basis for judging "human character," and a challenge to the surgeon interested in facial esthetics. The important role that the chin plays in facial appearance has been recognized since antiquity—ivory, bovine bone, and alloplastics are but a few of the materials that have been used clinically with variable success to augment the contour of the chin.[1] Only within the past quarter-century have surgical techniques been perfected to alter the chin contour in a reliable manner.[2-6,8] During the period when modern techniques of chin surgery were being developed, modalities for soft tissue analysis evolved concurrently.[4] Today, by prudent application of artistic sense, knowledge of the principles of facial esthetics, and proper execution of contemporary techniques of genioplasty, the maxillofacial surgeon can achieve almost any variation of three-dimensional changes in chin contour and proportions. Evaluation of submental-cervical esthetics is vital for treatment planning for chin surgery. Genioplasty and submental soft tissue surgery are readily done simultaneously and are usually complementary.

The characteristics that are considered esthetically pleasing vary according to culture, ethnic type, and even historical period. There is evidence, however, that the general characteristics associated with a beautiful face have changed very little throughout the history of Western European culture. This is also true of many other cultures—what was considered a beautiful face 2000 years ago is still regarded as esthetically pleasing today.

Western society associates certain facial features with an individual's personality. A person with a "weak" or deficient chin may subconsciously be expected to have a timid, nonathletic, unaggressive, or indecisive personality, whereas an individual with a "strong" or prognathic chin may be expected to be bold, athletic, aggressive, and decisive. The fact that our culture uses the words "weak" and "strong" to describe the chin implies subconscious association with "character" or personality trait. The hallmark of a "normal" or "balanced" face is a slightly protruding chin associated with a nose and submental-cervical morphology of normal proportions.

In general, a "weak" or retruded chin is associated with femininity and a strong or prominent chin, with masculinity. Because undesirable characteristics are associated with a weak chin, society seems to prefer facial forms with at least *some* chin prominence—more in men than in women. Even though the general public appreciates the fact that some people have more esthetically pleasing chins than others, many people do not yet realize that chin contour can be altered by surgery.

Historically, attention given to chin contour has emphasized the lateral aspect, because the retrusive chin was the most obvious and common deformity. As a consequence, results of genioplasties were evaluated on the basis of profile only. Unfortunately, the esthetic change, when viewed from the way the patient actually sees himself or herself (frontally), was sometimes compromised. Patients with the most conspicuous microgenia received the most impressive profile change, but frontal appearance was compromised unless particular attention was directed to augmenting the lateral contour during advancement.

Systematic Description of the Deformity

In evaluating facial form from an esthetic viewpoint, the absolute measurements of facial structures are not as important as the relative size and proportion of each

Since the way human beings normally posture their heads is remarkably constant, natural head position is used as a point of orientation.

All cephalometric radiographs are taken in the natural head position to orient the head to natural horizontal and vertical planes. A natural vertical is any vertical line constructed perpendicular to the normal horizontal visual axis of the patient. With the cephalometric radiographs taken in the natural head position, the natural vertical is parallel to the lateral edges of the film. By constructing a natural vertical line through subnasale, the relative prominence of the nose, lips, and chin may be assessed. Ideally, the chin should lie 1 to 2 mm behind this line and the lips slightly anterior to it. The proposed position and contour of the chin may be drawn tangential to the natural vertical reference line.

There is obviously considerable variation in individual profiles, and all patients cannot be made to fit a specific stereotype. A vertical reference line on a cephalometric radiograph provides a convenient, reproducible mechanism for determining the relationship of the chin to the remainder of the facial profile. Analysis of facial esthetics, however, is more complex than simply using a single profile reference line. A multitude of complex interrelationships among other facial structures must be considered when altering the position of any part of the face. Consequently, the final decision on where to position the chin must be made by evaluating the patient in a clinical setting. The nasolabial angle, thickness of the upper and lower lips, cheek prominence, total length of the face, submental-cervical morphology, and even general body build will affect the final decision regarding what chin contour and prominence complement an individual's face. For example, the face of a woman with fine facial features, a small nose, thick lips, and flat midfacial structures will be better balanced with a relatively retrusive chin. The 6-foot man, on the other hand, prefers a relatively prominent chin.

Anteroposterior Deficiency

Clinical and cephalometric analyses with the patient in the natural head position are used to determine the amount of soft tissue advancement needed to establish a balanced facial profile. A natural vertical reference line through subnasale is constructed on the cephalometric tracing. Subnasale, the most posterosuperior point on the curve formed by the nose and upper lip, is arbitrarily selected as the point of reference in Caucasians because it is a relatively stable landmark that moves relatively little when maxillary surgical procedures such as the Le Fort I osteotomy are performed. The facial profile is usually balanced when subnasale and chin fall on the same line or near it and the lips are slightly anterior to it (Fig. 64–76). If the nose and lips are particularly prominent, the vertical reference line is moved anterior to subnasale to establish appropriate balance with the chin. This step is usually necessary for African-Americans and Asians, who frequently manifest variable degrees of bimaxillary protrusion and lip prominence (Fig. 64–76). In such patients, the vertical reference line should lie about halfway between subnasale and the anterior prominence of the upper lip. When the chin is constructed on this line, the lips will appear less prominent, and better facial balance will be achieved. When the vertical line lies anterior to the more prominent lip, it may be desirable to move the line posteriorly to a point tangential with the more prominent lip, which then becomes the reference point for the anteroposterior position of the chin. The line is moved a few millimeters posteriorly for women, in whom a "softer" profile is preferred.

By tracing the present or proposed profile for the middle third of the face and utilizing the landmarks and criteria suggested for establishing balanced facial esthetics, the proposed profile of the lower lip and chin is drawn. The horizontal difference between the preoperative soft tissue chin position and the planned position as sketched on the profile tracing represents the amount of soft tissue augmentation required. These measurements serve as the basis for selection of the

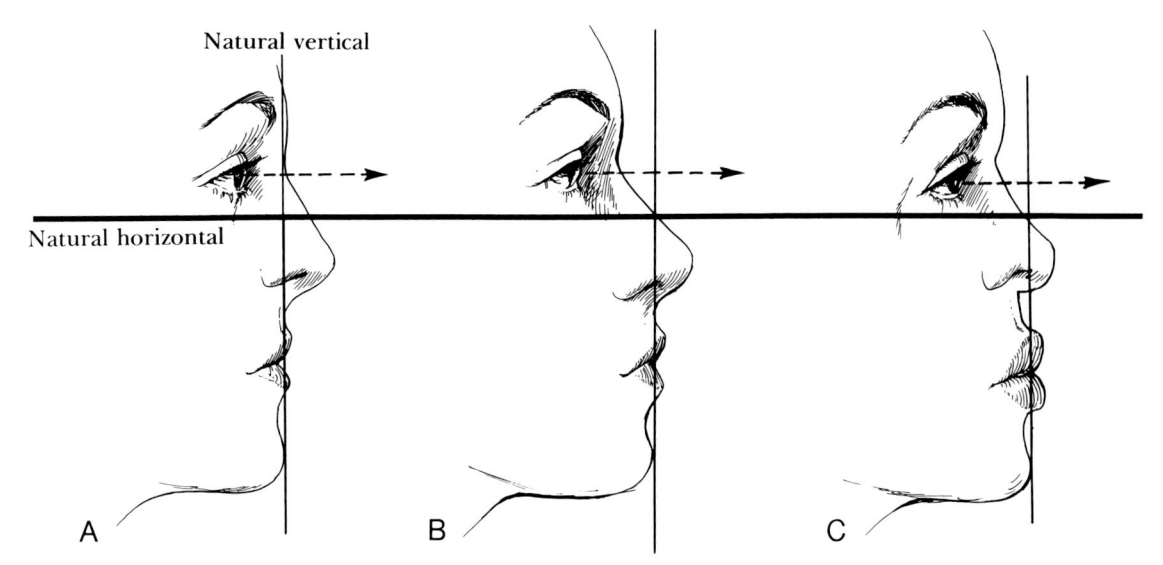

FIGURE 64–76. NATURAL VERTICAL REFERENCE LINE FOR EVALUATION OF PROFILE ESTHETICS. *A,* A natural vertical reference line is constructed to pass through the esthetic. In the balanced, relatively straight face, this line passes through soft tissue nasion and several millimeters posterior to soft tissue pogonion. The upper and lower lips are slightly anterior to this line. *B,* In more protrusive caucasoid profiles, the natural vertical through esthetic is tangent to soft tissue pogonion but passes anterior to soft tissue nasion. *C,* For African-American profiles, the vertical line is moved anteriorly to a point midway between the esthetic and the anterior prominence of the upper lip. Soft tissue pogonion should be close to this line. The lower lip should be slightly behind the upper lip. (From Bell WH, Proffit WR, White RP Jr: Surgical Correction of Dentofacial Deformities. Vol II. Philadelphia, WB Saunders Company, 1980, p 1215; with permission.)

appropriate surgical procedure to effect the desired change. The final "result" is approved or disapproved by the surgeon, who relies on his or her artistic sense of what a balanced facial profile should look like. Using this artistic sense, the surgeon may choose to simulate additional facial contour changes.

A proportioning device consisting of a clear plastic grid with horizontal and vertical reference lines can be an aid in evaluating frontal and profile facial esthetics (Fig. 64–77). Such clinical studies are made with the patient's head in a natural position.

Advancement Genioplasty

A variety of surgical techniques are available to augment a contour-deficient chin. These techniques include several variations of horizontal sliding osteotomy, free autogenous onlay bone grafts, implantation of an alloplastic material, and combinations of these methods. The horizontal sliding osteotomy of the mandibular symphysis with advancement of the mobilized segment is the technique of choice for correction of anteroposterior deficiency because the results are predictable and stable. In studying the results attained with horizontal sliding osteotomy, Bell and Dann[4] found a consistent relationship between bone and soft tissue change of 1:0.6. Soft tissue advancement was approximately 60 per cent of bone advancement. These figures, however, related to genioplasties performed with more soft tissue detachment than we currently use. Our more recent results indicate that minimal soft tissue detachment allows closer correlation between bone and soft tissue movement. We now expect soft tissue advancement to be 80 per cent of bone advancement. This observation has recently been confirmed by Polido and associates. By monitoring the horizontal advancement of the soft tissue chin brought about by advancement genioplasty and subsequent change, they concluded that for the purposes of prediction, the relation between the initial surgical, horizontal advancement of the symphysis and the ultimate horizontal advancement of the soft tissue chin is 4:3.

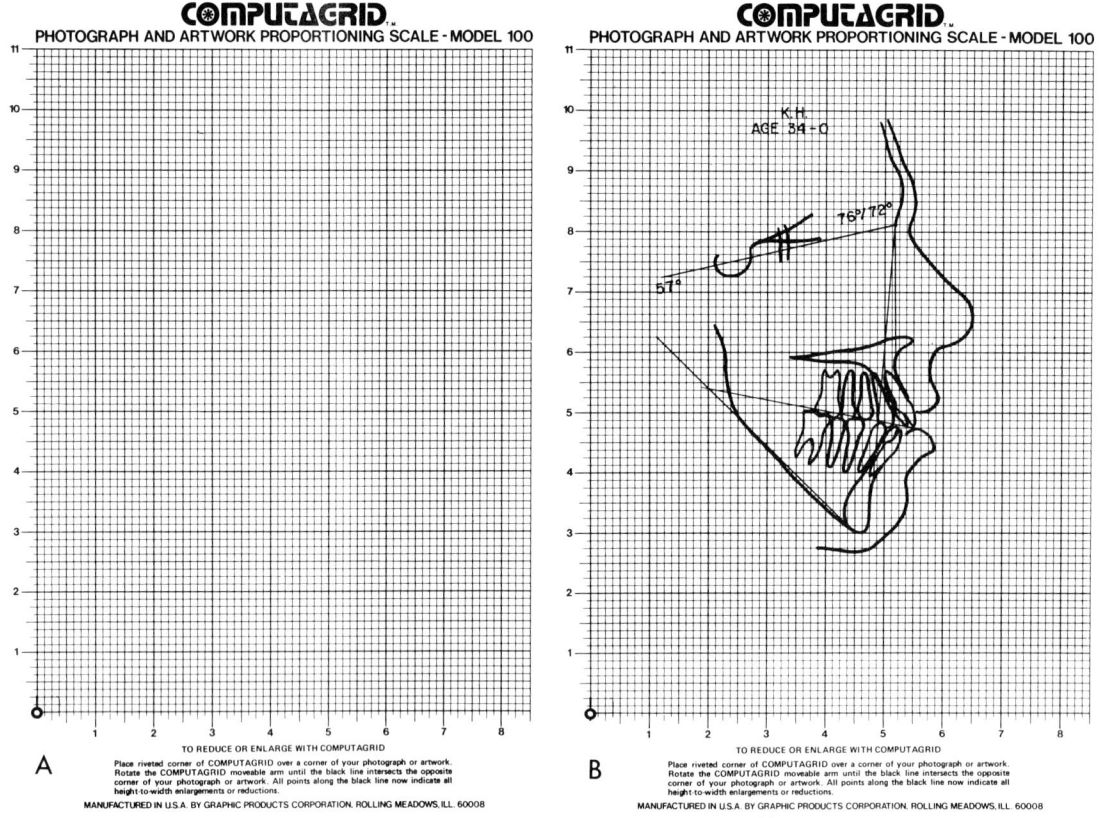

FIGURE 64-77. USE OF THE COMPUTAGRID. A, The Computagrid is a photographic and artwork proportioning device consisting of a grid of horizontal and vertical lines scribed on an 11 inch × 9 inch clear plastic sheet. It provides a series of coordinated lines to aid in evaluating frontal and profile facial esthetics. It is manufactured by Graphic Products Corporation, Rolling Meadows, IL 60008, and is sold in many art and photographic supply houses. B, Analysis of profile esthetics is facilitated by orienting a clear acetate grid over the cephalometric tracing so that grid lines parallel the natural horizontal and vertical reference lines. By following a line that passes through esthetic, the relative prominence of the lips and chin may be measured.

Sliding Horizontal Osteotomy

After the proposed chin contour is sketched on the cephalometric tracing, a template of the chin segment to be advanced is traced on an additional piece of acetate tracing paper. The soft tissue anterior and inferior to the mobilized segment and a natural horizontal line passing about 4 mm below the mental foramen are added to this template. Finally, submental surgery (rhytidectomy, suction lipectomy, or submental lipectomy) is simulated and incorporated into the planning studies.

The position of the horizontal osteotomy is controlled by the level of the mental foramen and inferior alveolar canal. The fact that the inferior alveolar canal curves superiorly as it approaches the mental foramen makes it mandatory to position the horizontal osteotomy 4 to 5 mm below the inferior edge of the mental foramen to prevent injury to the neurovascular bundle. The inferior alveolar canal can usually be identified on the cephalometric radiograph so that the distance that the canal extends below the foramen can be measured. This measurement is recorded for use at surgery and determines the posterior height of the osteotomy. The anterior height of the osteotomy is dictated by the direction in which the segment must move to produce the desired chin contour and prominence. If only horizontal augmentation is desired, the osteotomy should be made parallel to the natural horizontal. Horizontal and vertical augmentation may be accomplished by directing the anterior part of the osteotomy below the natural horizontal. Shortening is produced by directing the anterior bone incision above the natural horizontal.

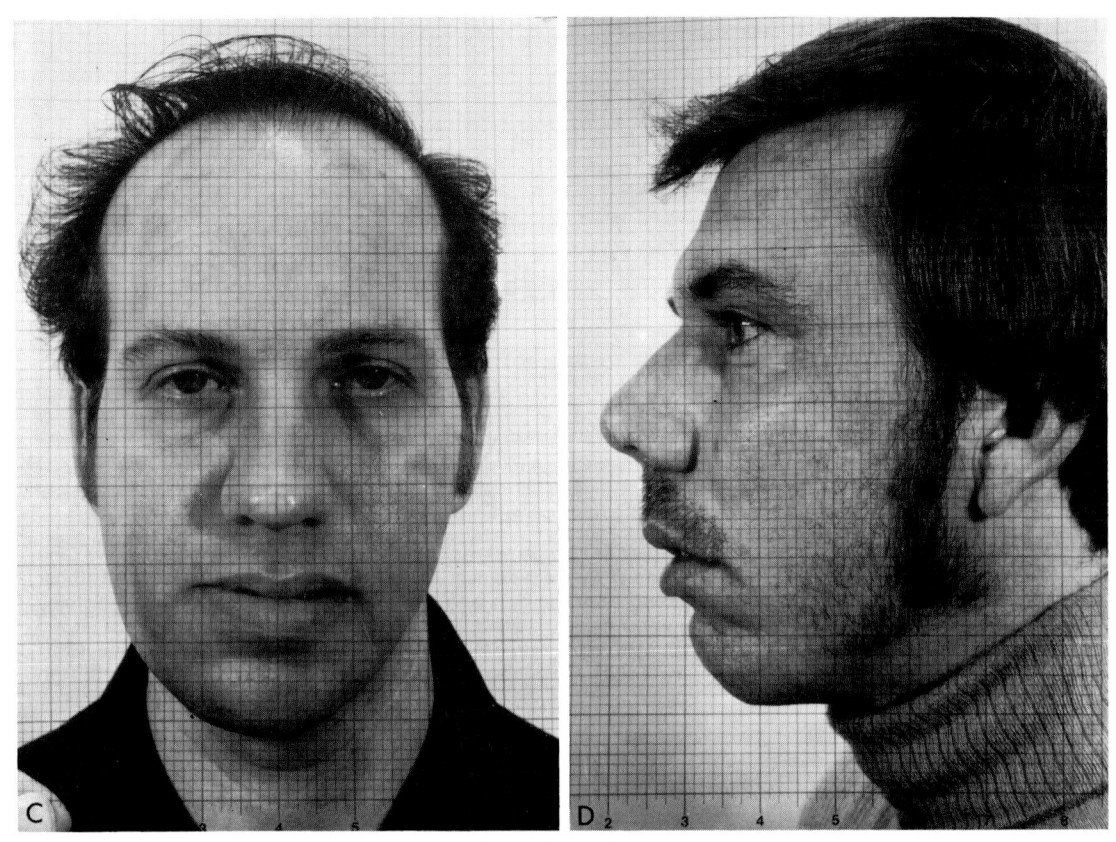

FIGURE 64-77 *Continued.* *C,* Clear plastic grid held in front of patient: A horizontal line on the grid is oriented to the natural horizontal passing through orbital rims. Balance and symmetry of facial structures are evaluated in relation to vertical lines, and vertical relationships are evaluated in relation to horizontal lines. *D,* Clear plastic grid held up to the lateral aspect of patient, whose head is held in a natural position: A horizontal line is oriented to the natural horizontal through the infraorbital rims, and the anteroposterior balance of the nose, lips, and chin is evaluated in relation to vertical lines. (From Bell WH, Proffit WR, White RP Jr: Surgical Correction of Dentofacial Deformities. Vol II. Philadelphia, WB Saunders Company, 1980, pp 1216–1217; with permission.)

The exact angle of the osteotomy is determined by advancing the chin template to coincide with the outline of the proposed chin. The template must be advanced beyond the proposed outline to compensate for the fact that the soft tissue advances only 80 to 90 per cent of the bone advancement. A line is constructed between the point where the natural horizontal line intersects the labial cortical bone on the repositioned template and a point 3 to 4 mm below the mental foramen. This line represents the position of the osteotomy needed to achieve the proposed result.

Chin augmentation by horizontal sliding osteotomy is limited by the thickness of the symphysis, angulation of the osteotomy, and anterior soft tissue attachments. Because the amount of advancement that can be achieved with sliding horizontal osteotomy is limited by the thickness of the mental symphysis at the level of the proposed cut, this dimension is measured on the preoperative cephalogram. If movement greater than the thickness of the symphysis is carried out, there will be no bone contact in the midline, and the possibility of instability of the repositioned segment, delayed healing, and relapse will be greater.

The height of the advanced segment will range between 10 and 15 mm at the anterior aspect of the symphysis. If the segment is too short, a pointed, unesthetic soft tissue chin may result; if the vertical dimension of the segment is too long, a large, knobby chin and elevation of the labiomental fold result. The specific thickness should balance with the overall height of the chin from lip margin to soft tissue

2452 / VII—ORTHOGNATHIC SURGERY

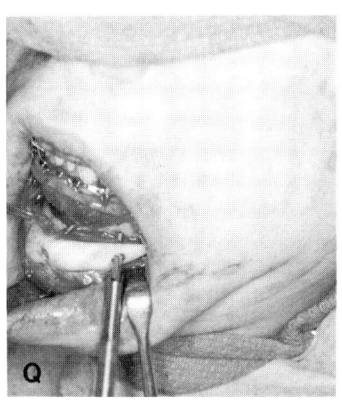

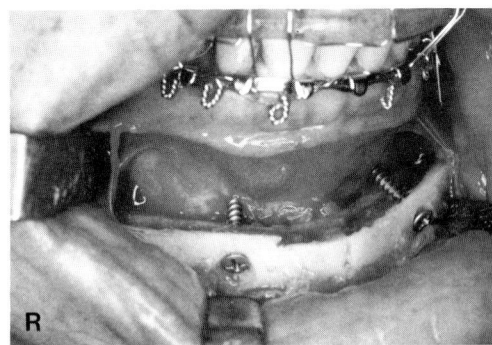

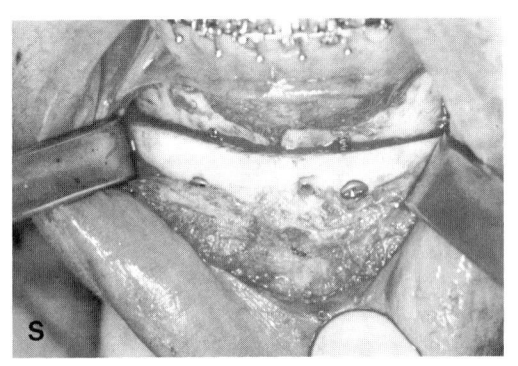

FIGURE 64–80 *Continued.* *Q*, A Phillips screw driver is used to place a 16-mm self-tapping bicortical screw to stabilize the genial segment in the desired position. Note the angulation necessary for bicortical engagement. *R*, Twelve-millimeter advancement genioplasty stabilized with two 2-mm × 16-mm bicortical screws. *S*, Five-millimeter advancement genioplasty stabilized with two 2-mm × 12-mm bicortical screws. *T* and *U*, Reduction of chin height (about 7 mm) and lateral repositioning of the chin; stabilization achieved with mini bone plates. *V* and *W*, Increasing chin height and inferior repositioning of the chin by osteotomy of the inferior border of the mandible and use of interpositional hydroxyapatite; chin stabilized with mini bone plates. *X–BB*, Use of fragmentation plate to stabilize the repositioned chin. *X*, Mini fragmentation plate is cut to the desired length with a plate-cutting instrument. *Y*, Special instrument is designed to bend the plate to the desired configuration (usually at a right angle). *Z*, Intraoperative view of the repositioned chin stabilized with two two-hole fragmentation plates; the segment is stabilized with a 2.7-mm orthopedic tap. *AA*, the genial segment is stabilized to the proximal segment with bicortical position screws, which ideally transect the labial and lingual cortical plates. In small movements, however, the genial segment may be adequately stabilized with well-positioned 2-mm unicortical self-tapping screws. *BB*, Radiograph showing stabilization of the repositioned genial segment by bicortical fragmentation plate. *CC* and *DD*, Paulus titanium bone plating systems provide a simple and effective means of stabilizing the repositioned genial segment. Millimeter gradations imprinted on the fixation device (2 to 14 mm in length) provide a means of clinically replicating the desired positional change of the genial segment. The genial segment or segments are stabilized with 5- to 6-mm-long self-tapping unicortical position screws 2 mm in diameter. A disadvantage of this bone plating system has to do with its strength when large advancement genioplasties are planned (> 10 mm). The pull of the attached musculoperiosteal pedicle and the genial segment may cause bending of the plate or instability. *CC*, Augmentation of a severely contour-deficient chin by double-step osteotomy of the inferior border of the mandible. Segments are maintained in the preplanned advanced position with three Paulus bone plates. Each of the 8-mm-thick genial segments was stabilized with 6-mm-long unicortical position screws. *DD*, Postoperative cephalometric radiograph showing the magnitude of chin advancement (18 mm). Each segment was advanced the full thickness of the symphysis (approximately 10 mm). *EE*, Pressure dressing of Elastoplast and/or tape is secured to the face with tincture of benzoin. (*E* from Bell WH, Proffit WR, White RP Jr: Surgical Correction of Dentofacial Deformities. Vol II. Philadelphia, WB Saunders Company, 1980, p 1222; with permission.) *FF*, Special versatile facial bandage may be used to stabilize the submental and submandibular soft tissue following genioplasty and/or submental lipectomy or suction lipectomy.

of the mandible with positional bone screws and bone plates (Fig. 64–80*E* to *L*). Interosseous wires, of course, may be used for interosseous fixation if bone plates or screws are unavailable.

STABILIZATION WITH POSITIONAL SCREW FIXATION

The technique of positional screw fixation offers great simplicity, versatility, and stability when repositioning the chin by osteotomy of the inferior border of the mandible (Fig. 64–80*I* to *L*). A sharp 1.5-mm twist drill, 20 mm in length, in a straight handpiece is used for intraoral drill hole placement. Because the initial penetration is usually made at an oblique angle to the dense labial cortical bone, it is useful to start the procedure by drilling a shallow pilot hole perpendicular to the bone surface with a No. 703 fissure bur. Positional screws are usually placed

64 — MANDIBULAR DEFICIENCY / **2453**

FIGURE 64–80 *Continued.*

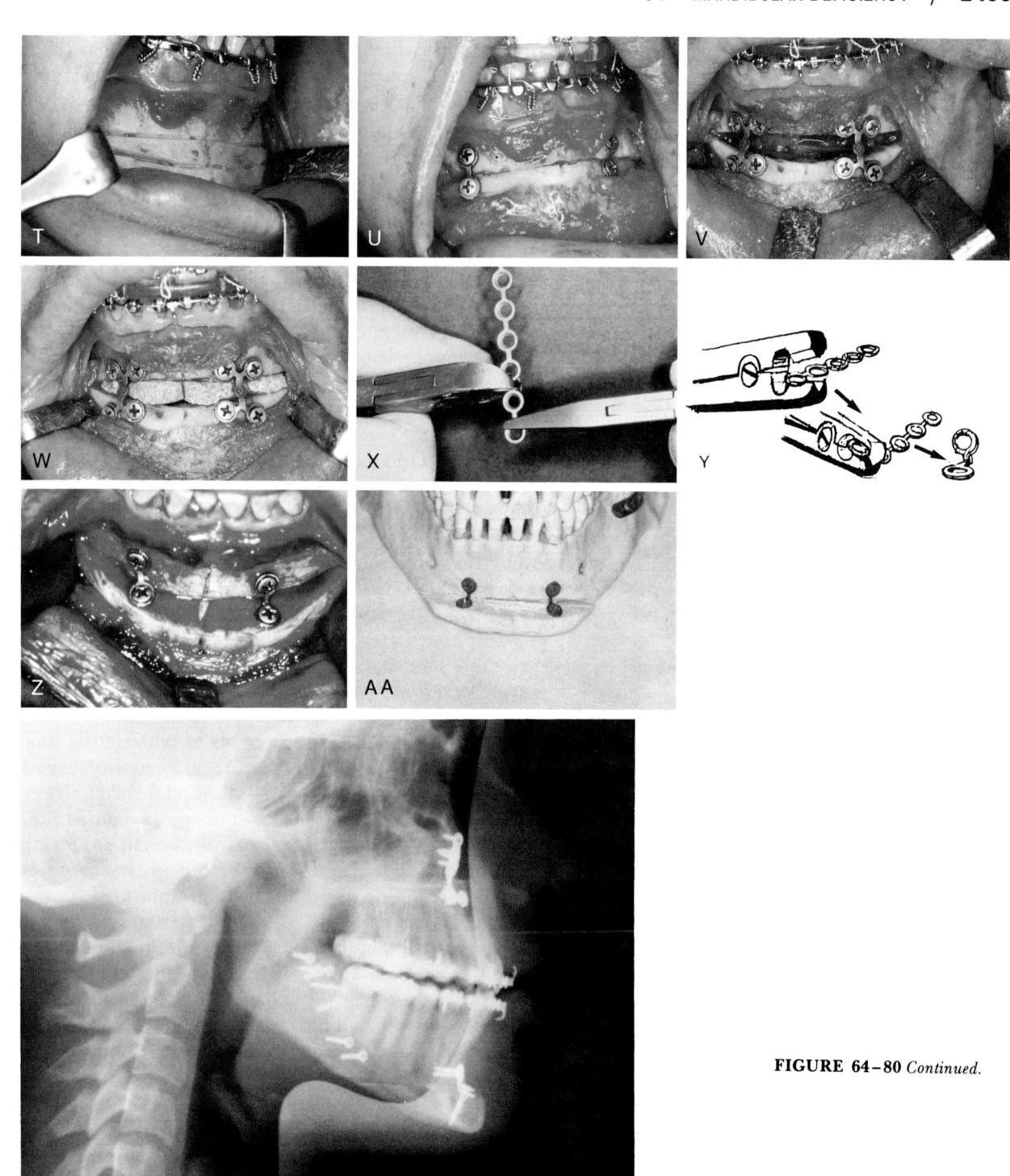

Illustration continued on following page

2458 / VII — ORTHOGNATHIC SURGERY

FIGURE 64–82 *Continued.*

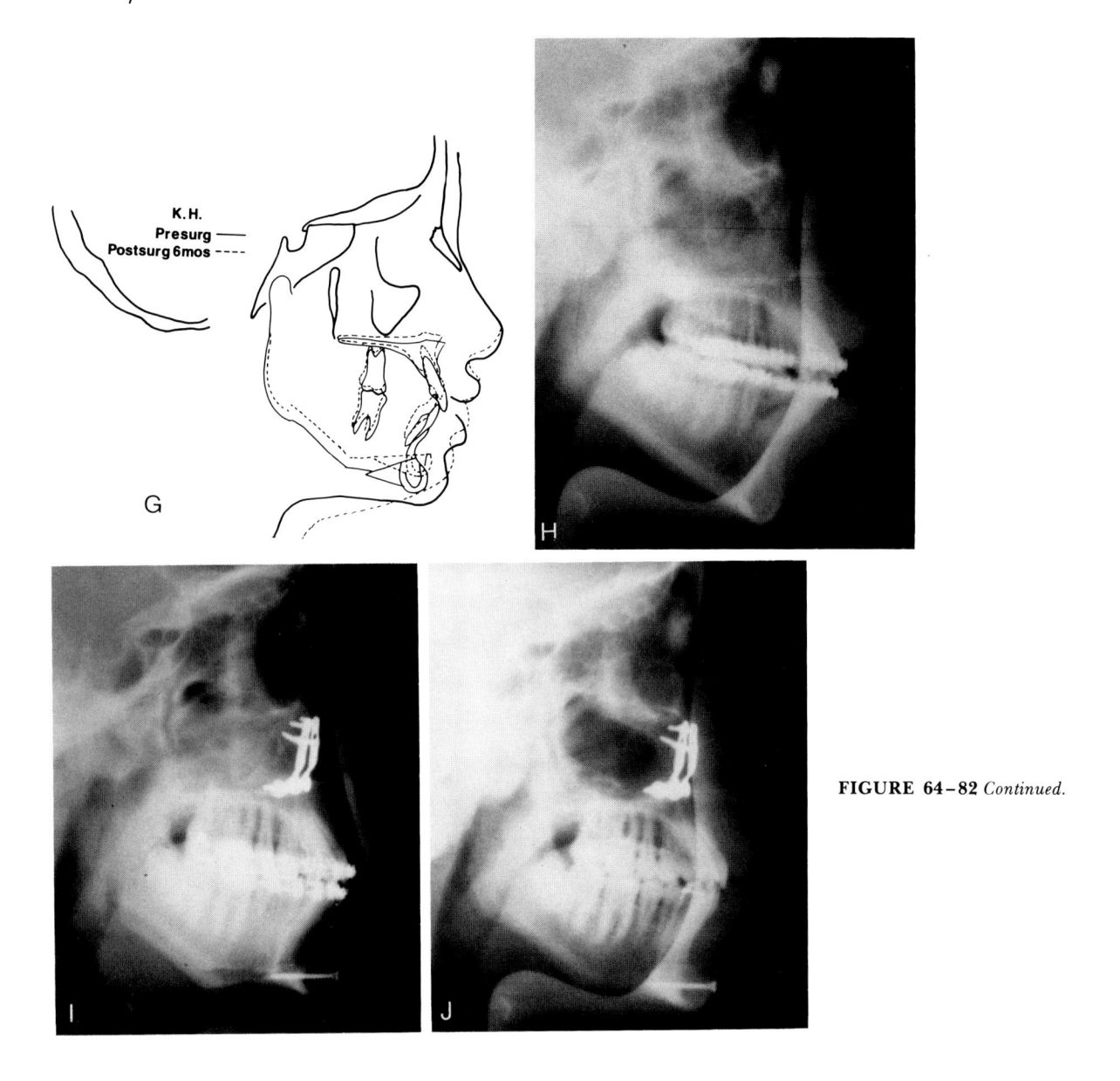

FIGURE 64–83. *A* and *B*, ANTERIOR SUBAPICAL OSTECTOMY IN THE FIRST PREMOLAR REGIONS TO RETRACT THE ANTERIOR MAXILLARY AND MANDIBULAR DENTOALVEOLAR SEGMENTS. Concomitant advancement genioplasty by horizontal osteotomy of the inferior border of the mandible positioned 5 mm below the level of the mandibular subapical osteotomy. *A*, Planned osteotomies and ostectomies are indicated by cross-hatched areas; arrows indicate direction of planned movements of the anterior parts of the maxilla, mandible, and chin. *B*, Postoperative relationships. The mandibular dentoalveolar subapical segment is stabilized with microplates and screws; the genial segment is stabilized with positional screws.

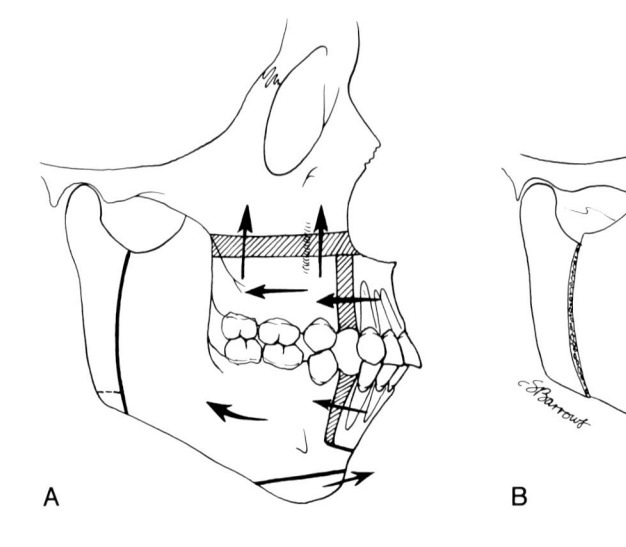

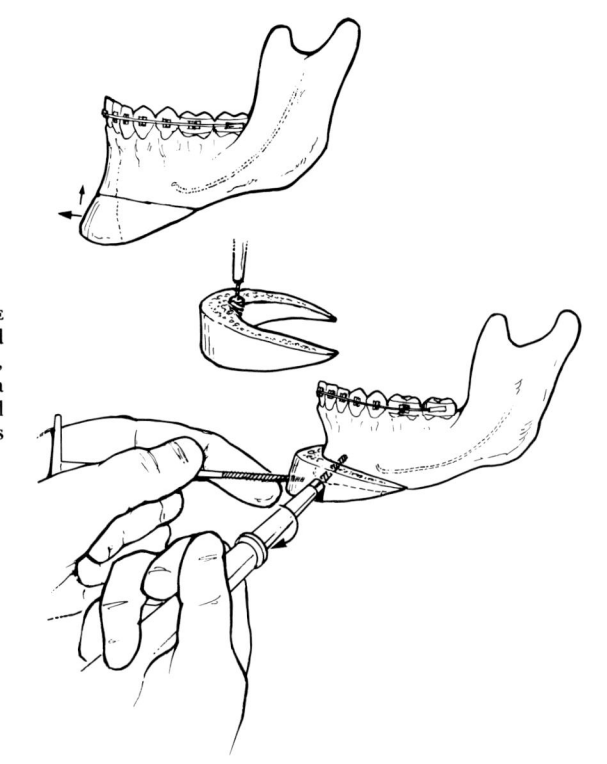

FIGURE 64–84. OVERLAPPING GENIOPLASTY MAY BE USED WHEN EXCESSIVE CHIN HEIGHT IS ASSOCIATED WITH LACK OF CHIN PROMINENCE. *Top,* A pedicled genial segment is advanced anterior to the mandibular labial cortex. *Middle,* The lingual surface of the repositioned genial segment is contoured with a large bur to control the amount of chin advancement and facilitate optimal bone-to-bone contact. *Bottom,* The genial segment is stabilized with screws positioned in the canine–lateral incisor region.

anterior mandibular cortex. By sculpting the contour of the concave surface of the genial segment with a large pineapple-shaped bur, the proximal and distal segments are brought into juxtaposition with each other and stabilized with two lag screws. In addition, the amount of chin advancement is controlled.

In cases in which the mental symphysis is thin and small, maximal chin advancement is achieved by positioning the chin on or near the inferolabial cortex of the body of the mandible. Autogenous allogeneic particulate bone marrow graft may be placed at the junction of the advanced inferior segment and anterior aspect of the proximal segment to allow additional advancement of the chin, consolidation of the repositioned segment, and augmentation of the labiomental region. Because of the additional tension on the attached soft tissues, special attention must be given to stabilizing the advanced segment. Maximal advancement and the desired vertical, sagittal, and transverse stability can be maintained with bone screw fixation to the buccal cortex of the mandible. The same technique can also be used to advance and concomitantly reposition the genial segment inferiorly. The proximal ends of the genial segment are apposed to the buccal aspect of the body of the mandible and secured in the planned position by self-tapping 2-mm bone screws, which are passed through the buccal and lingual cortices and the inferolabial aspect of the superior segment.

Large Advancement Genioplasty by Double Horizontal Sliding Osteotomy

A double horizontal osteotomy technique may be considered when the amount of advancement desired is large and exceeds the thickness of the symphysis. In such cases, the vertical chin height must be sufficient to create two separate bone segments, each of which is at least 7 to 8 mm thick. Each segment may be advanced the full thickness of the symphysis, so that almost twice as much bony advancement may be achieved compared with what is possible with a single slide (Figs. 64–85 to 64–87). Both segments remain pedicled to lingual periosteum and muscle. Because the anterior bellies of the digastric muscles are stretched farther than they

2460 / VII — ORTHOGNATHIC SURGERY

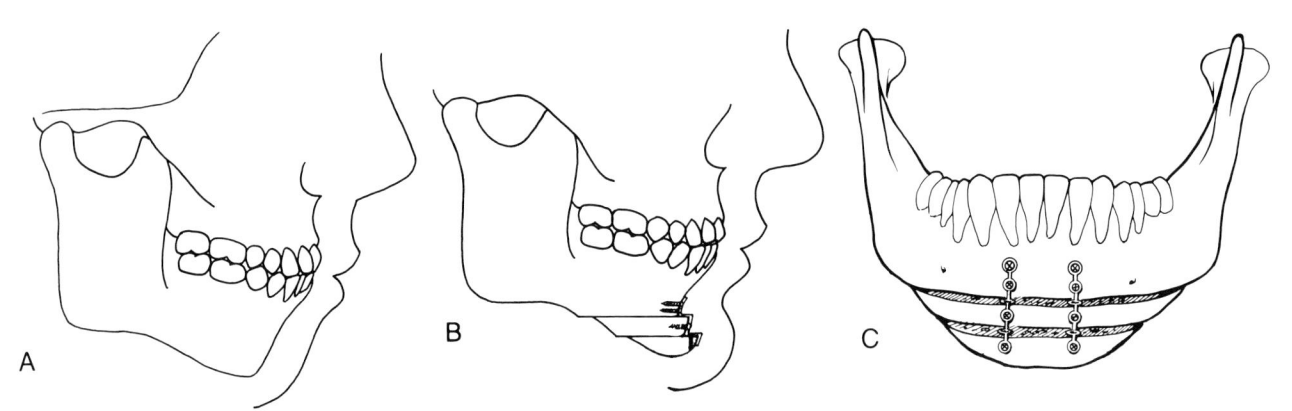

FIGURE 64–85. *A–C*, DOUBLE-STEP GENIOPLASTY. Advancement of the inferior segment is by a two-step parallel osteotomy. Stabilization and fixation of segments are accomplished with micro or mini bone plates. Particulate bone may be added to facilitate bone healing. The chin may be advanced in excess of 20 ml without creating an excessive bony step and labiomental fold. This technique has been made technically much easier with the use of bone plate and screw stabilization. Ideally, the segments should be 10 mm in height. With care, however, it is feasible to accomplish the procedure with even smaller segments (6 to 9 mm).

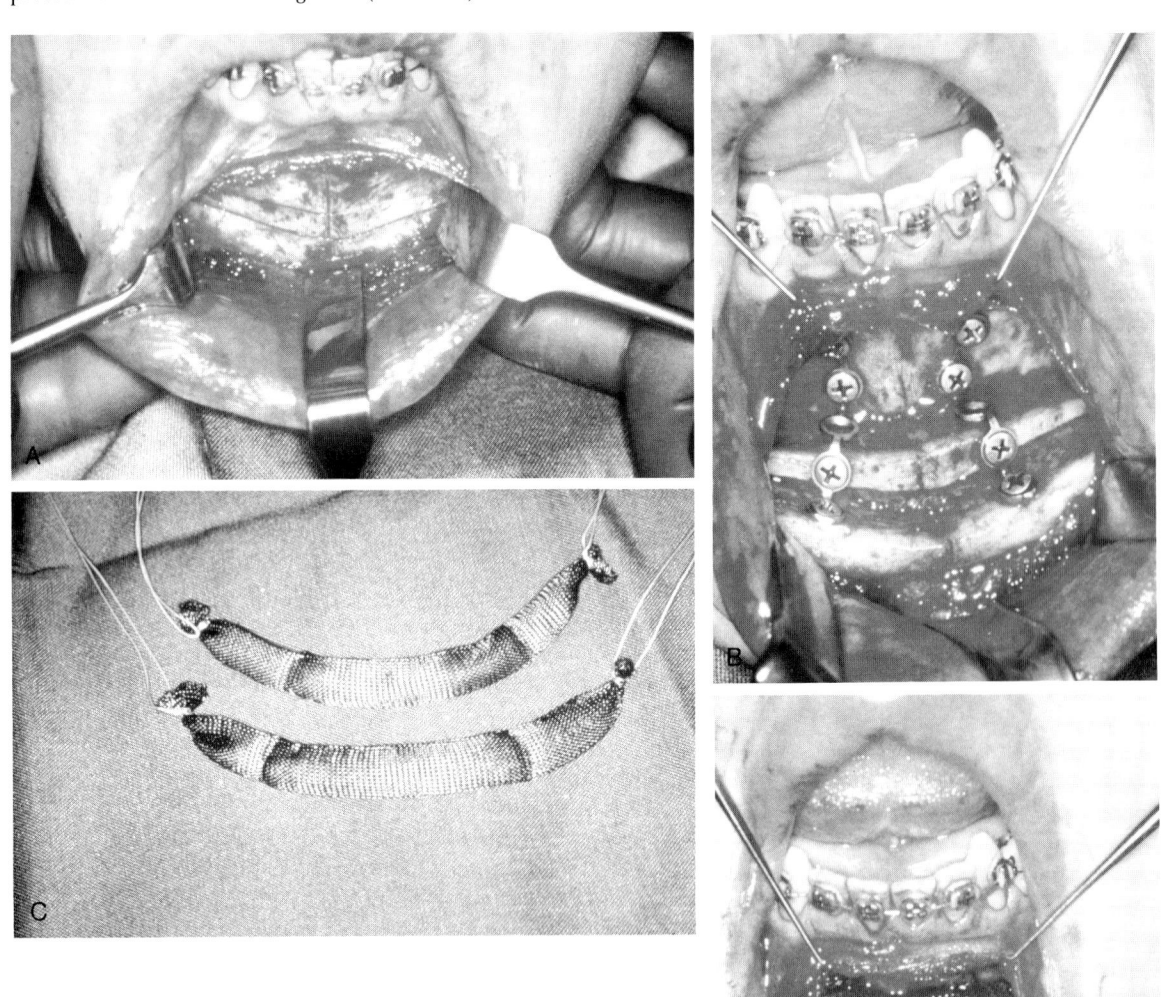

FIGURE 64–86. CASE REPORT (HANS LUHR, M.D., D.D.S.): TWO-STEP GENIOPLASTY WITH ADVANCEMENT OF 20 MM. RIGID FIXATION BY TWO MINI PLATES. *A*, Two parallel osteotomies are performed. *B*, Each of the two genioplasty segments is advanced 10 mm and rigidly fixed with two contoured steplike miniplates. *C*, Two sacks of Vicryl mesh (Ethicon, commonly used for ridge augmentation) are filled with hydroxyapatite granules. *D*, The Vicryl-hydroxyapatite implants are laid into the steps to augment the labiomental fold area.

64 — MANDIBULAR DEFICIENCY / 2461

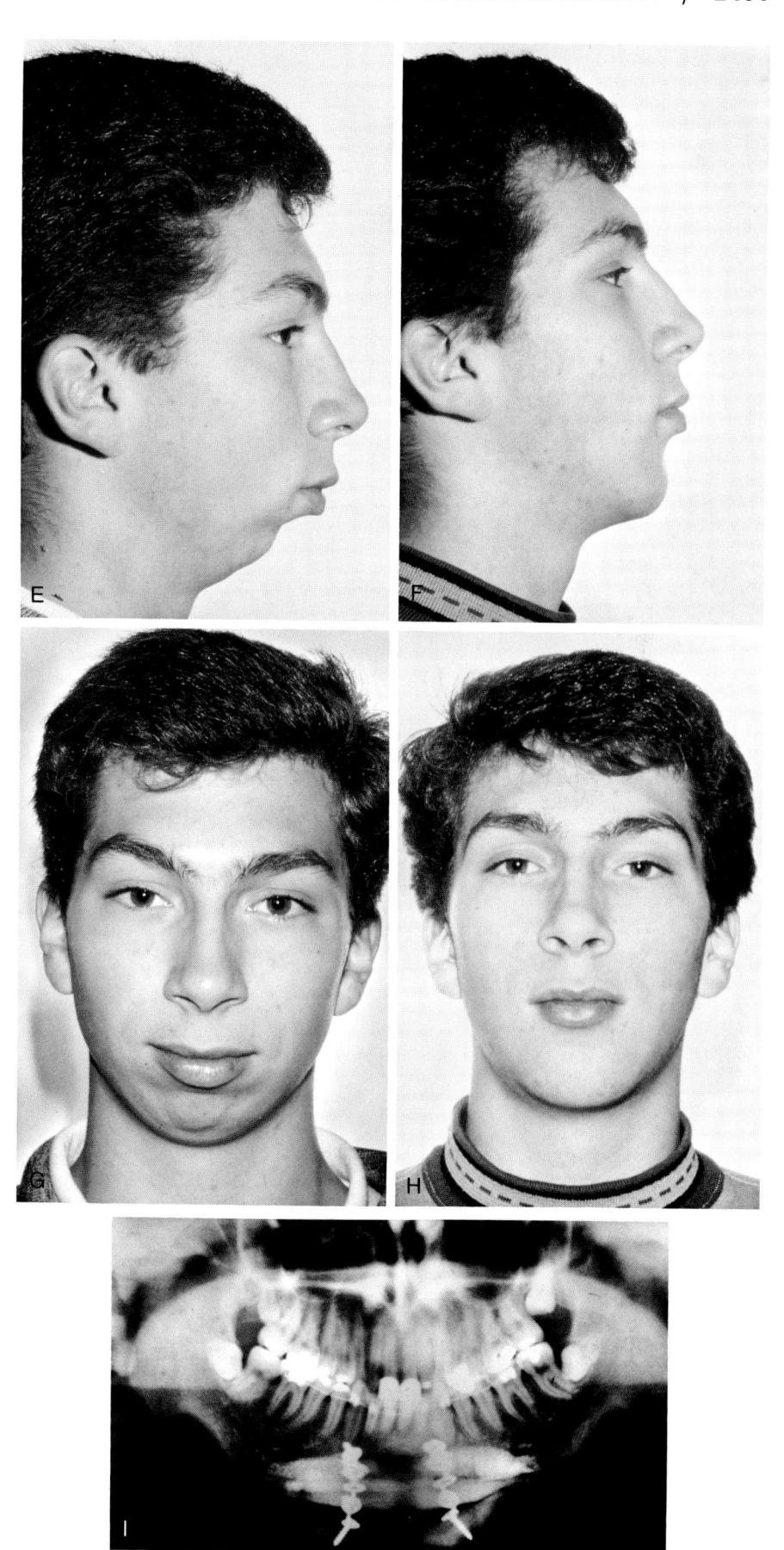

FIGURE 64–86 *Continued.* *E*, Preoperative profile of the patient showing severe chin deficiency. *F*, Postoperative results after 20-mm two-step advancement genioplasty. *G*, Preoperative frontal appearance. *H*, Postoperative frontal appearance showing well-contoured chin area (which is difficult to achieve with any onlay technique). *I*, Postoperative panoramic radiograph.

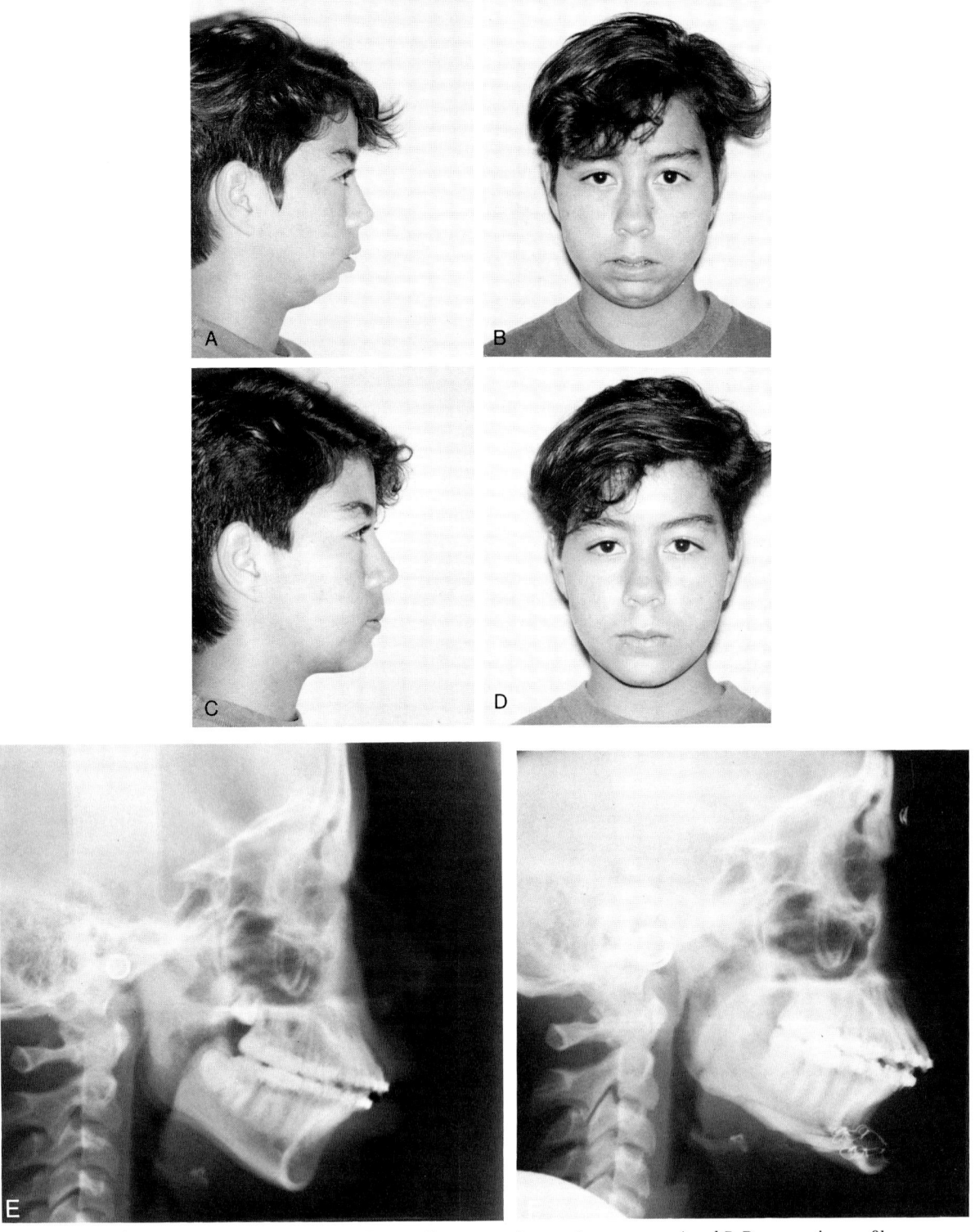

FIGURE 64–87. LARGE CHIN ADVANCEMENT BY DOUBLE HORIZONTAL SLIDING OSTEOTOMY. *A* and *B*, Preoperative profile and frontal facial views. *C* and *D*, Postoperative profile and frontal facial views. *E*, Preoperative lateral cephalometric radiograph. *F*, Postoperative lateral cephalometric radiograph.

are with a single slide, considerable care must be exercised when fixing the segments to ensure adequate stabilization. This fixation is predictably accomplished with metal plates and screws. Additional particulate marrow grafts may be placed along the lines of osteotomy on the newly created labial "steps" and between the segments to promote better healing and consolidation of the repositioned segments and augmentation of the labiomental region. Genioplasty may be combined with the insertion of alloplastic implants for larger chin advancements, as in the following case study.

CASE: M.M. (Fig. 64–88)

A 19-year-old woman with Pierre Robin syndrome (cleft palate, micrognathia, glossoptosis) was referred by her orthodontist for treatment of severe chin deficiency. The patient had received prior orthodontics; despite this treatment, which achieved a functional occlusion, there was severe anteroposterior chin deficiency. A 10-mm chin Silastic prosthesis was positioned supraperiosteally. One year later when the soft tissue was supple and more prominent, a large chin advancement was accomplished by osteotomy of the inferior border of the mandible. Fourteen months after the initial surgery, the chin and the previously placed Silastic implant were advanced 9 mm and fixed with two positional screws. A total chin advancement of 19 mm was achieved.

Surgeon—Cesar A. Guerrero, D.D.S., Caracas, Venezuela
Orthodontist—Gisela Contasti, D.D.S., Caracas, Venezuela

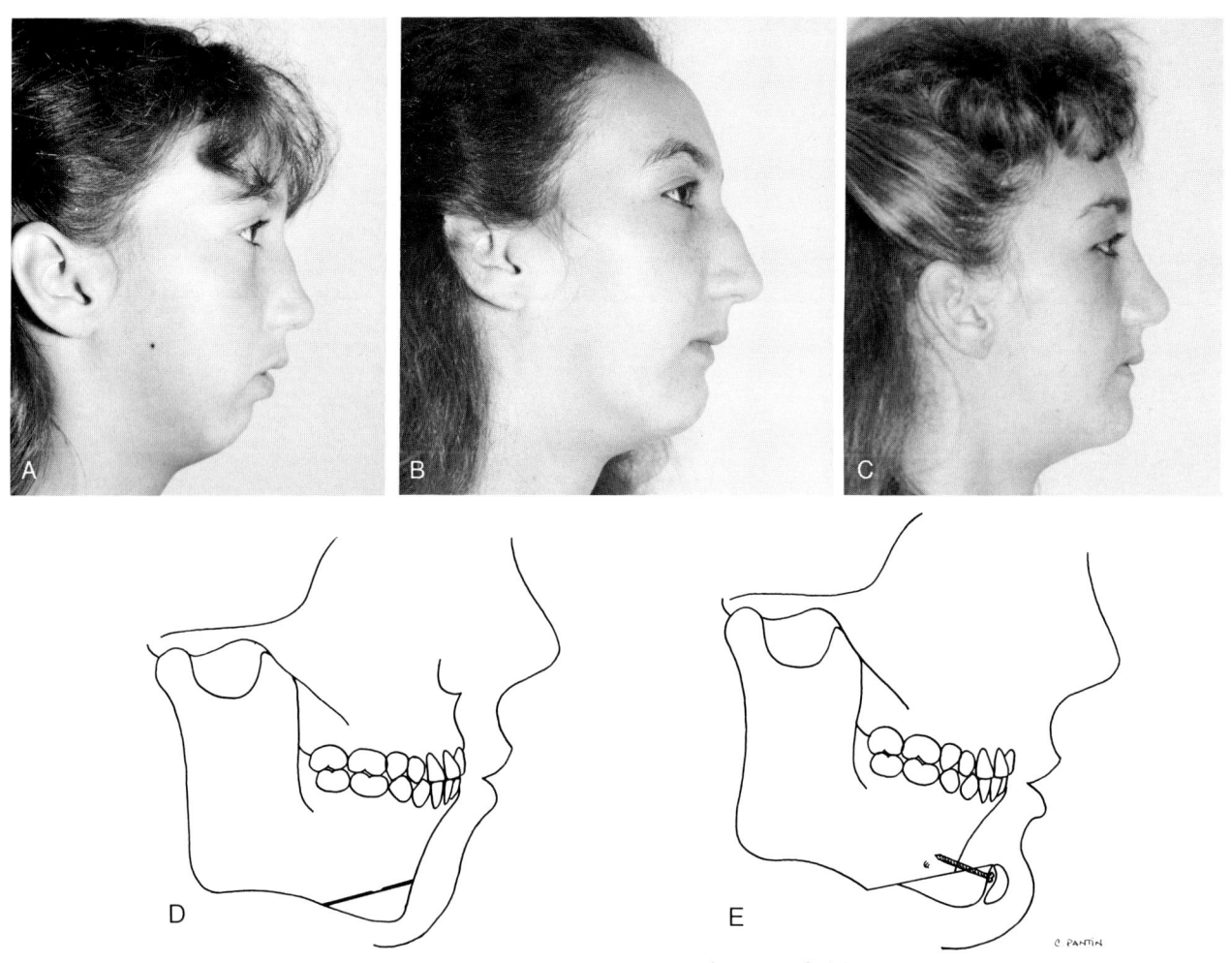

FIGURE 64–88. LARGE CHIN ADVANCEMENT. *A*, Preoperative severe facial convexity after orthodontic treatment. *B*, Postoperative facial appearance after placement of 10-mm preformed Silastic implant onto mental symphysis. *C*, Facial appearance after secondary 9-mm advancement genioplasty that included the previously placed Silastic implant. *D* and *E*, Plan of surgery to correct severe chin deficiency by two-stage genioplasty. First stage: placement of preformed Silastic implant on labial aspect of chin. Second stage: advancement genioplasty by osteotomy of the inferior border of the mandible; the genial segment is stabilized with a position screw, and the net chin advancement is 19 mm.

Soft Tissue Changes and Bone Stability Following Large Chin Advancements

Predictable soft tissue changes have been observed with most positional changes of the broad soft tissue pedicle genioplasty.[9,17] Moderately large advancement genioplasty combined with mandibular setback consistently achieves a near 1:1 ratio of soft tissue change to advancement of the osseous chin. An osseous to soft tissue proportional change of 1:0.85 has been obtained by advancement genioplasty that maintains a broad soft tissue pedicle in combination with bone plates and screws.

Careful treatment planning, meticulous surgical technique, use of a broad pedicle, and the surgeon's artistic sense constitute the sine qua non of successful and predictable chin surgery. Soft tissue changes and stabilization of the genial segment following horizontal osteotomy of the inferior border of the mandible depend on the magnitude and direction of the positional change of the genial segment, the design of the mucosal and osseous incisions, and other concomitant jaw movements. Incorrect planning, vestibular scarring, excessive detachment of soft tissue from the chin, myotomy, improper closure of the soft tissue incision, hematoma formation, genial remodeling, lack of attention to the submental-cervical esthetics, and excessive bone resorption and osseous instability all may compromise the results of chin surgery.

Advancement genioplasty by horizontal osteotomy of the inferior border of the mandible with preservation of a musculoperiosteal pedicle to the advanced genial segment is associated with relatively little bone resorption (17 per cent) and excellent osseous stability. After a mean follow-up period of 26 months, 83 per cent of the initial advancement was preserved, representing 17 per cent osseous resorption.[15] The enveloping soft tissues of the chin followed the bony movement in a ratio of 1:0.88. The broadest possible musculoperiosteal pedicle that is clinically feasible should remain attached to the advanced genial segment to minimize osseous resorption and achieve more predictable soft tissue changes (Fig. 64–89).

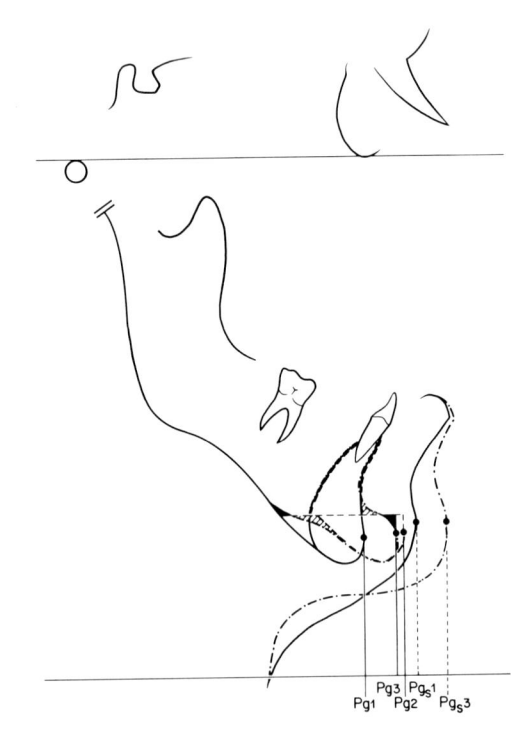

FIGURE 64–89. BONE STABILITY AND SOFT TISSUE CHANGES AFTER LARGE CHIN ADVANCEMENTS. Cross-hatched area = Bone apposition; Pg1 = preoperative position of hard tissue pogonion; Pg2 = immediate postoperative position of hard tissue pogonion; Pg3 = long-term follow-up position of hard tissue pogonion; Pg3 = long-term follow-up position of hard tissue pogonion; Pg$_s$1 = preoperative position of soft tissue pogonion; Pg$_s$3 = long-term follow-up position of soft tissue pogonion; solid area = bone resorption.

Reduction of Chin Prominence (Anteroposterior Excess)

The natural vertical reference line is used to plan surgery to reduce chin prominence in the same manner described for anteroposterior deficiency. By following the present or proposed profile for the middle third of the face and utilizing the landmarks and criteria suggested for establishing good facial esthetics, the proposed profile of the lower lip and chin is traced. The horizontal difference between the preoperative soft tissue chin position and the planned soft tissue position as sketched on the profile tracing represents the needed soft tissue change. Horizontal sliding osteotomy is the technique of choice for reducing chin prominence.

SURGICAL TECHNIQUE OF HORIZONTAL SLIDING OSTEOTOMY FOR ANTEROPOSTERIOR REDUCTION
(Figs. 64–90 and 64–91)

A reduction of chin prominence and soft tissue redraping are accomplished by horizontal osteotomy of the inferior border of the mandible when the attachment of the soft tissue to the inferior and anteroinferior portions of the repositioned segment is maintained.

By varying the angulation of the ostectomy, the chin height can be concomitantly shortened or lengthened somewhat. The magnitude of movement and the angulation of the horizontal osteotomy are determined by trial repositioning of a template of the bony and soft tissue chin. At surgery, the amount of posterior

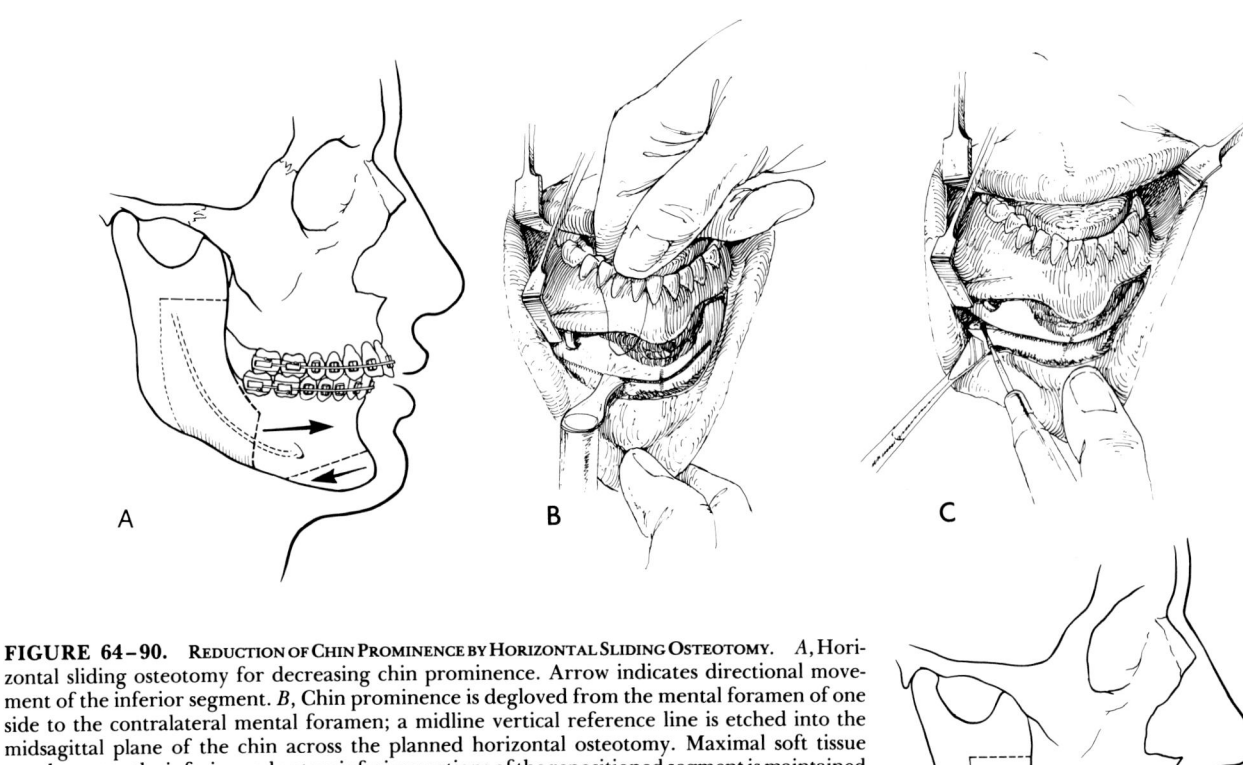

FIGURE 64–90. REDUCTION OF CHIN PROMINENCE BY HORIZONTAL SLIDING OSTEOTOMY. *A*, Horizontal sliding osteotomy for decreasing chin prominence. Arrow indicates directional movement of the inferior segment. *B*, Chin prominence is degloved from the mental foramen of one side to the contralateral mental foramen; a midline vertical reference line is etched into the midsagittal plane of the chin across the planned horizontal osteotomy. Maximal soft tissue attachment to the inferior and anteroinferior portions of the repositioned segment is maintained to optimize the result. *C*, Posterior position of the inferior segment is shortened to maintain the normal contour of the skin at the inferior border of the mandible. *D*, The inferior segment is retracted and fixed into the planned position with bone plates and screws. Maximal movement of the soft tissue to movement of the underlying osseous segment is achieved by preserving the largest possible soft tissue pedicle to the inferior and anteroinferior aspects of the repositioned segment. (*B* and *C* from Bell WH, Proffit WR, White RP Jr: Surgical Correction of Dentofacial Deformities. Vol II. Philadelphia, WB Saunders Company, 1980, p 1234; with permission.)

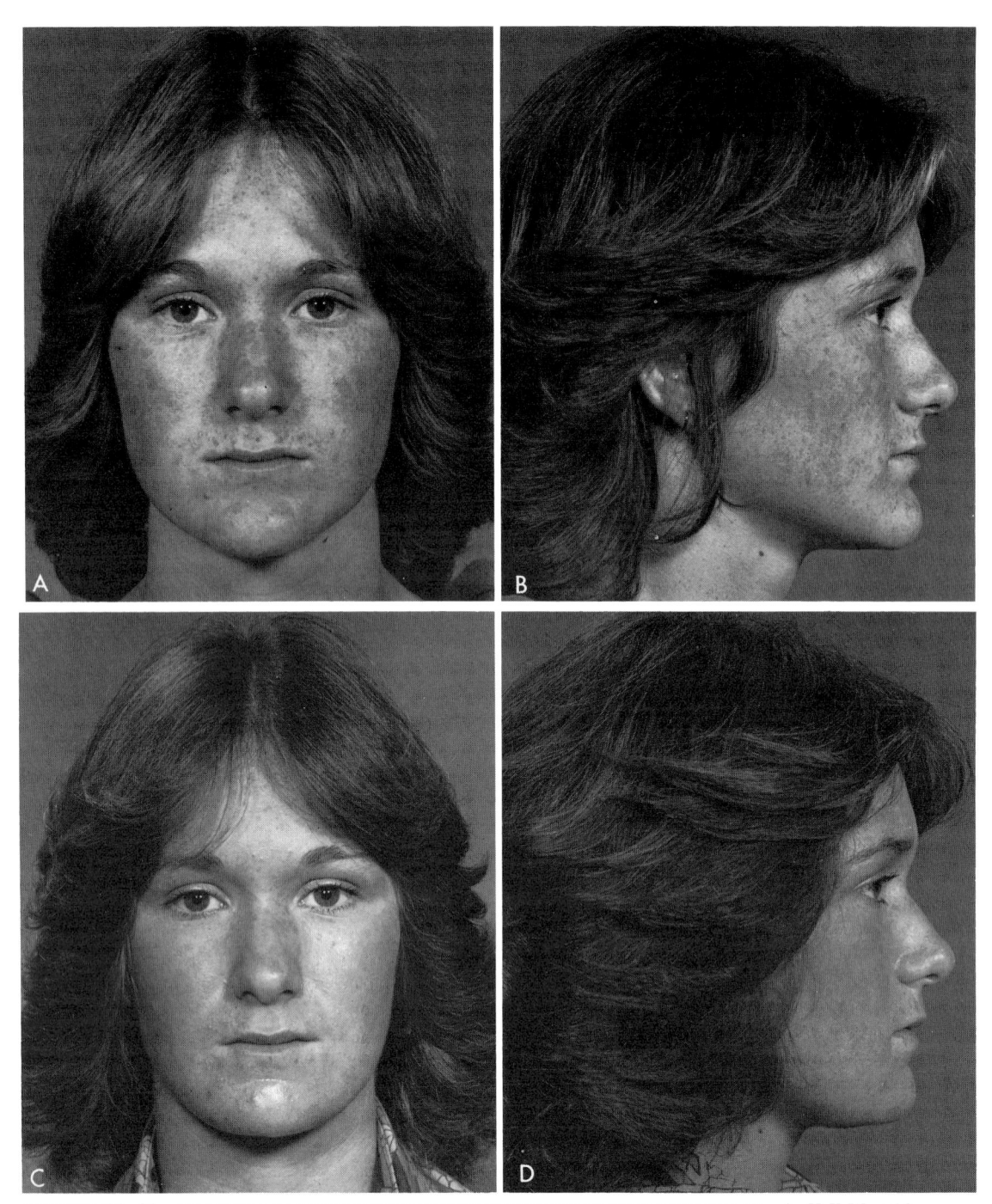

FIGURE 64–91. CORRECTION OF CHIN PROMINENCE BY REVERSE HORIZONTAL SLIDING OSTEOTOMY. *A–H,* K.W., a 16-year-old girl, was evaluated for treatment to correct her malaligned teeth and prominent chin.

Problem List

Esthetics
  1. Good midfacial contour and symmetry.
  2. Prominent chin in the anteroposterior plane of space.

Cephalometric Analysis
  1. Class I malocclusion associated with prominent chin in the anteroposterior plane of space.
  2. 1 to NB, 3 mm; NB to Po, 8 mm.

Occlusal Analysis: Class I malocclusion with moderate crowding and malalignment of maxillary and mandibular teeth.

Treatment Plan

Orthodontic Treatment: nonextraction orthodontic treatment with edgewise orthodontic appliances.

Surgical Treatment: horizontal sliding osteotomy of inferior border of mandible with posterior repositioning of segment to reduce chin prominence.

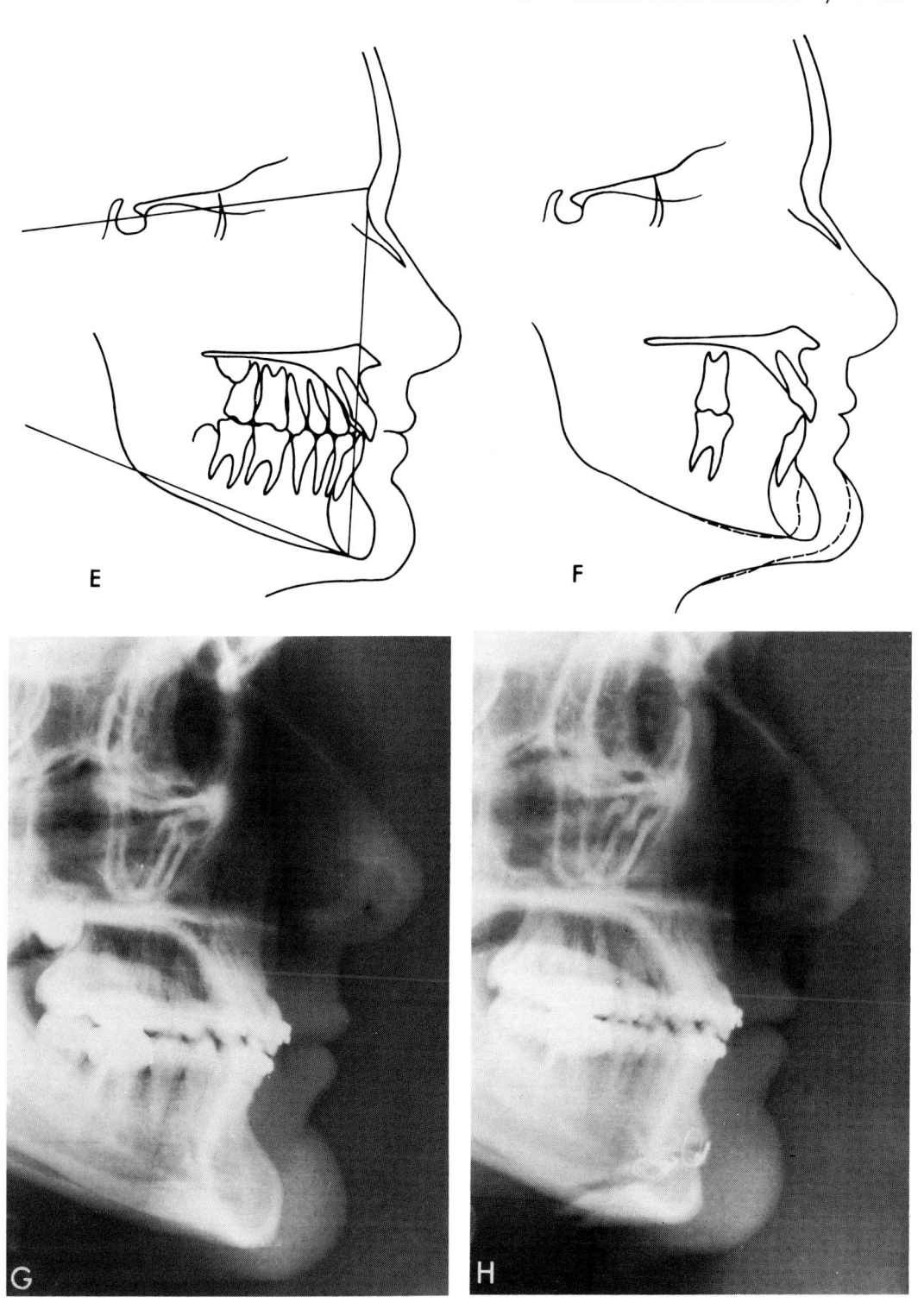

FIGURE 64–91 *Continued.*

Active Treatment

Good alignment and interdigitation of the teeth were accomplished within 12 months by orthodontic treatment. A 6-mm reduction of chin prominence was achieved by a pedicled horizontal sliding osteotomy of the inferior border of the mandible. The amount of chin reduction was consistent with the preoperative plan (the hard tissue chin was retracted 6 mm; the soft tissue chin was retracted 3.5 mm). Over a postoperative follow-up period of approximately 6 years, there has been no discernible change in the patient's profile.

A and *B*, Preoperative appearance of 16-year-old girl. *C* and *D*, Postoperative appearance after reducing chin prominence by reduction genioplasty (horizontal sliding osteotomy). *E*, Cephalometric tracing before surgery (15 years, 10 months). *F*, Composite cephalometric tracings before (*solid line*, age 15 years) and after (*broken line*, age 16 years, 1 month) surgery. *G*, Lateral head radiograph before surgery. *H*, Lateral head radiograph 18 months after surgery. (From Bell WH, Proffit WR, White RP Jr: Surgical Correction of Dentofacial Deformities. Vol II. Philadelphia, WB Saunders Company, 1980, pp 1269–1271; with permission.)

movement of the most prominent portion of the chin is not necessarily reflected by the step produced by retraction of the mobilized segment. This step, however, should be similar to the one produced on the cephalometric prediction study.

After the anterior portion of the chin is exposed as previously described, the midline of the chin and the planned horizontal osteotomy are inscribed into the chin (Fig. 64–90A and B). Vertical reference lines may also be inscribed into the lateral aspect of the mandible to indicate when the planned amount of posterior movement of the inferior segment has been achieved. The distance between vertical reference lines on the proximal and distal segments before and after the inferior segment is moved posteriorly serves as a guide to the amount of posterior movement. When the amount of retraction is in excess of 3 to 4 mm, the posterior portions of the mobilized segments are usually shortened to maintain the desired contour of the skin at the inferior border of the mandible (Fig. 64–90C). Small posterior movements have minimal effect on the contour of the inferior border of the mandible. Gradual remodeling of the repositioned segment restores the contour of the inferior border of the mandible to normal.

The repositioned inferior segment is fixed to the body of the mandible by bone plates or screws (Fig. 64–90D), The labiomental fold may be maximized by removing bone from the superior edge of the step after retraction of the symphysis. By sticking with a "game plan" based on the results of preoperative cephalometric reduction studies, bony changes are programmed to achieve rapid, predictable, and stable changes in the soft tissue drape. Submental-cervical esthetics may be compromised by reduction genioplasty, which tends to reduce the submental length and compromise the submental-cervical angle. Suction lipectomy or submental lipectomy is frequently indicated in such patients and may offset undesirable submental-cervical esthetic changes (see Fig. 64–111).

Care is exercised to avoid excessive removal of bone or retraction of the inferior border of the mandible, which will tend to obliterate the labiomental fold that is so essential for good esthetic balance in the lower third of the face. A disparate thickness of the soft tissue and bony chin can also produce unpredictable results. Successful genioplasty achieves *soft tissue* proportionality (see Fig. 64–93C to F).

The Transverse Plane

Evaluation of Transverse Deformities

Evaluation of transverse chin esthetics is best accomplished with the patient in the clinical setting, where the complex curvatures of the nose, lips, chin, malar bones, and cheeks may be studied in three dimensions while the patient is smiling and in repose. Well-oriented photographs may be used as reminders when the patient is not available, but photographs cannot be relied on for final surgical planning. Posteroanterior cephalometric radiographs are particularly useful in evaluating the bony architecture of patients with facial asymmetry.

Transverse Deficiency and Excess

A few guidelines aid the examiner in evaluating the width of the chin. The examiner must use artistic sense and analyze the transverse dimension and contour for balance with other facial structures. The width of the chin should be proportionate to the bizygomatic width — this should be a dynamic analysis based on the net effect that all of the planned positional changes of the jaws and chin have on the soft tissue drape. In the frontal view, the periphery of the face may be described as round, oval, square, tapering, or any combination of these shapes. The outline form of each third of the face should be recorded, along with the surgical changes that are needed to bring the lower third into harmony with the middle and upper thirds. Transverse reduction of the corners of a square chin to establish harmony with oval upper and middle facial thirds or broadening of a narrow, tapered chin to establish balance with a square midface is an example of a typical treatment plan. The amount of reduction or expansion is estimated preoperatively.

Widening the Chin (Transverse Deficiency) (Figs. 64–92A and 64–93)

The chin may be widened by midline sectioning following horizontal osteotomy of the inferior border of the mandible. This procedure is generally unnecessary when the horizontal osteotomy is extended posteriorly to the molar region. The lateral protuberance of the posterior ends provides important contour to the lateral aspect of the face.

Advancement of a pointed chin may not produce the desired amount of lateral or anteroposterior augmentation. In such cases, onlay bone grafts or hydroxyapatite blocks are carefully sculpted and used in concert with the sliding advancement genioplasty as interpositional grafts or implants between the bony margins created by midline sectioning of the genial segment.

Narrowing the Chin (Transverse Excess) (Fig. 64–92B)

The chin may be made more tapered by midline sectioning and excision of a triangular section of bone from the lingual aspect of the mobilized segment following horizontal osteotomy of the inferior border of the mandible. If the advanced segment is narrowed, the apposition of the proximal and distal segments is improved, the inferior segment can be advanced farther, and tension on the mental nerves is decreased. A very broad chin can be narrowed by excising a rectangular segment of bone from the midsymphyseal region. To maximize the effect on the soft tissue, the surgery is usually accomplished by maintaining as much soft tissue attachment as possible to the lateral and inferior aspects of the repositioned segments. In clinical practice, however, it is undesirable to narrow the posterior ends of the segments, which provide a symmetric, subtle increase in contour to the lateral aspect of the face as the inferior segment is advanced. The lateral protuberance of the posterior ends may *appear* too prominent at the time of surgery and may indeed stretch the mental nerves. The surgeon, however, should resist the temptation to remove these lateral protuberances, for the increased prominence is usually desirable and is an important reason for extending the horizontal osteotomy posteriorly to an area below the molar teeth.

Asymmetry of the Chin

Chin asymmetry is rarely an isolated entity; more frequently, the entire mandible is involved. Indeed, there may be compensatory changes in the midface. A facial midline is established by marking several points on the soft tissue. The middle of the forehead, the midpoint of the interpupillary distance, and the middle of the columella may be used if the midface is symmetric. Points on the lower third of the face that should intersect with this line include the middle of the philtral column, the middle of the upper and lower lips, the midpoint of the chin, and the maxillary and mandibular dental midlines. The structures on either side of the midsagittal plane should be equal in size, form, and proportion. By comparing

2470 / VII—ORTHOGNATHIC SURGERY

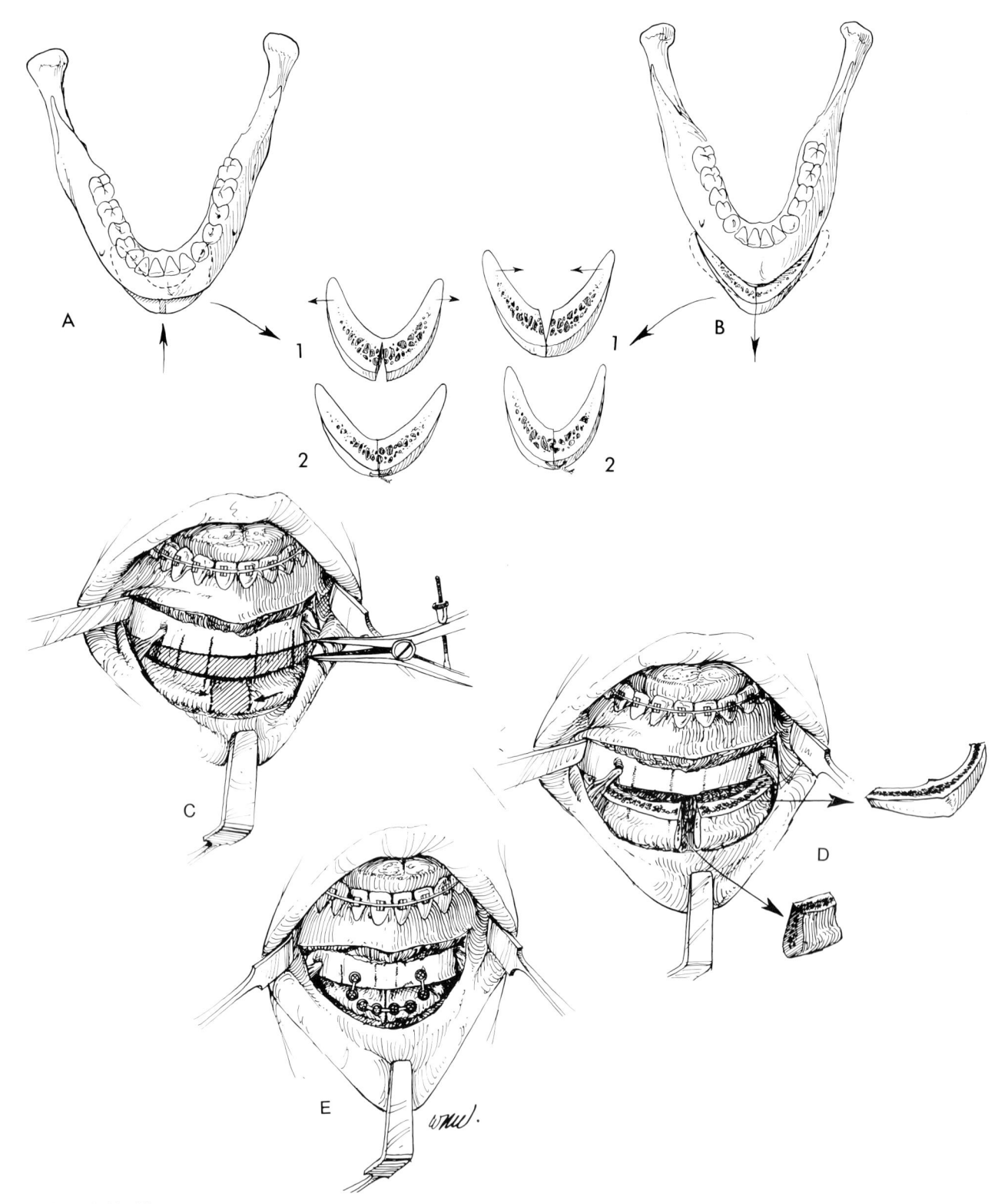

FIGURE 64-92. ALTERING THE HORIZONTAL DIMENSION OF THE CHIN BY HORIZONTAL OSTEOTOMY OF THE INFERIOR BORDER OF THE MANDIBLE. *A*, Widening the chin by midline sectioning of the chin after reduction genioplasty. *B*, Narrowing the chin by excising a triangle-shaped segment of bone from the mobilized segment after horizontal osteotomy of the inferior border of the mandible. *C*, Excessively wide chin associated with flaring of the inferior border and excessive vertical dimension of the chin. Plan of surgery: Reduction of excessive chin height by excising bone between reference marks inscribed into bone; cross-hatched areas indicate planned ostectomy sites. *D*, Horizontal and vertical segments of bone are excised from the chin. *E*, Repositioned segments are stabilized with bone plate and screws; positional changes of vertical reference lines indicate the amount of narrowing achieved. (Modified from Bell WH, Proffit WR, White RP Jr: Surgical Correction of Dentofacial Deformities. Vol II. Philadelphia, WB Saunders Company, 1980, pp 1242–1243; with permission.)

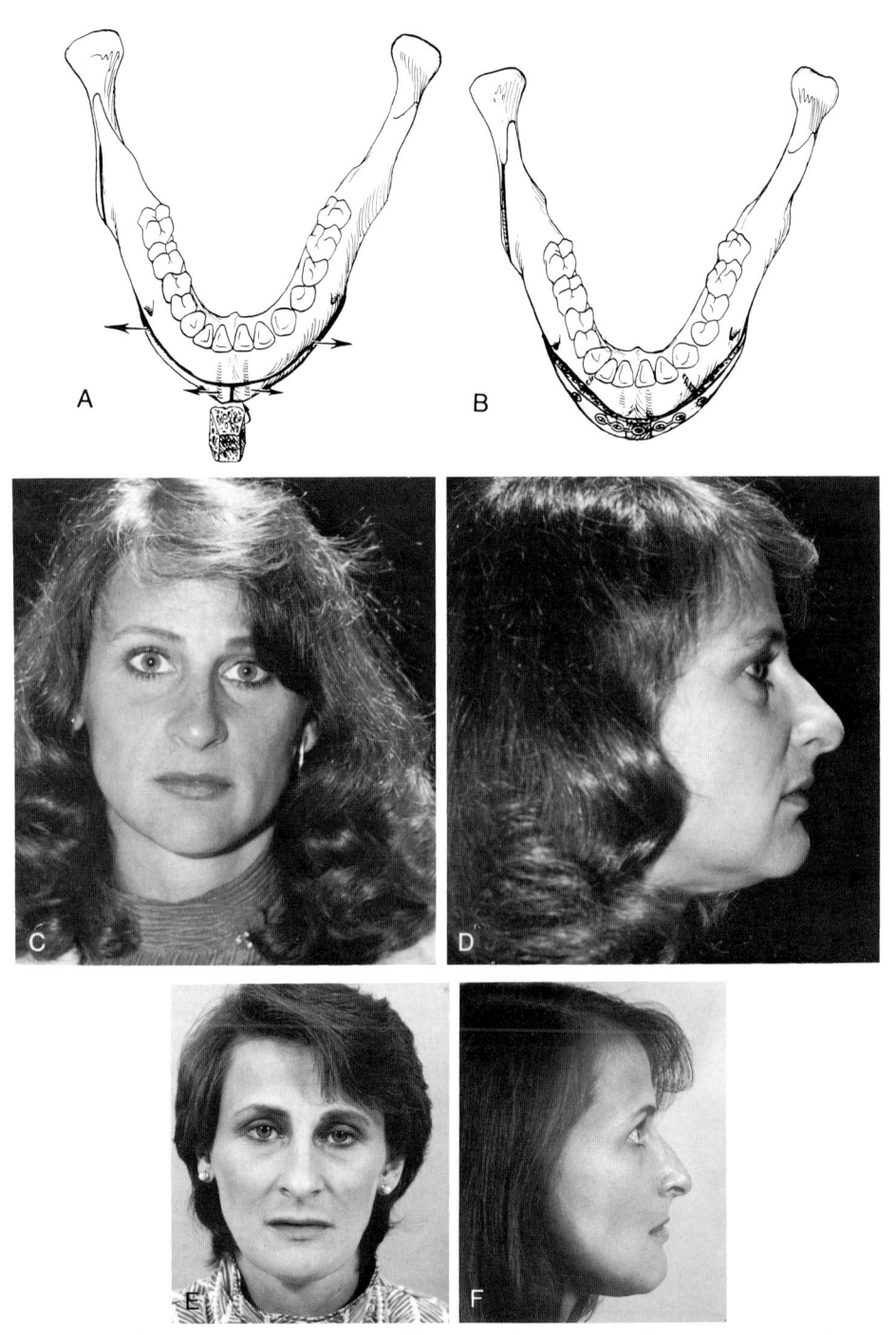

FIGURE 64–93. TECHNIQUE OF ALTERING THE HORIZONTAL DIMENSION OF A NARROW AND POINTED CHIN BY HORIZONTAL OSTEOTOMY OF THE INFERIOR BORDER OF THE MANDIBLE. *A*, Widening of the chin and mandibular body by midline sectioning of the chin and insertion of a rhomboid interpositional bone graft. Lateral dimensions of the chin and mandibular body can be differentially changed by altering the shape and dimensions of the interpositional graft or parasymphyseal osteotomies (for large lateral movements). Vertical reference lines are inscribed into bone; planned osteotomies are indicated by bold lines; arrows indicate direction of movements. *B*, Repositioned segments stabilized with bone plates and screws; positional changes of vertical reference lines indicate the amount of widening achieved. *C–F*, This patient had mandibular deficiency associated with a prominent, pointed chin and submental lipodystrophy. Surgical plan: mandibular advancement, reduction genioplasty, sectioning of the chin in two with placement of bone grafts to widen the chin, and suction lipectomy of the submental region to increase submental length and decrease the submental-cervical angle. *C* and *D* are preoperative frontal and profile views. *E* and *F* are postoperative frontal and profile views.

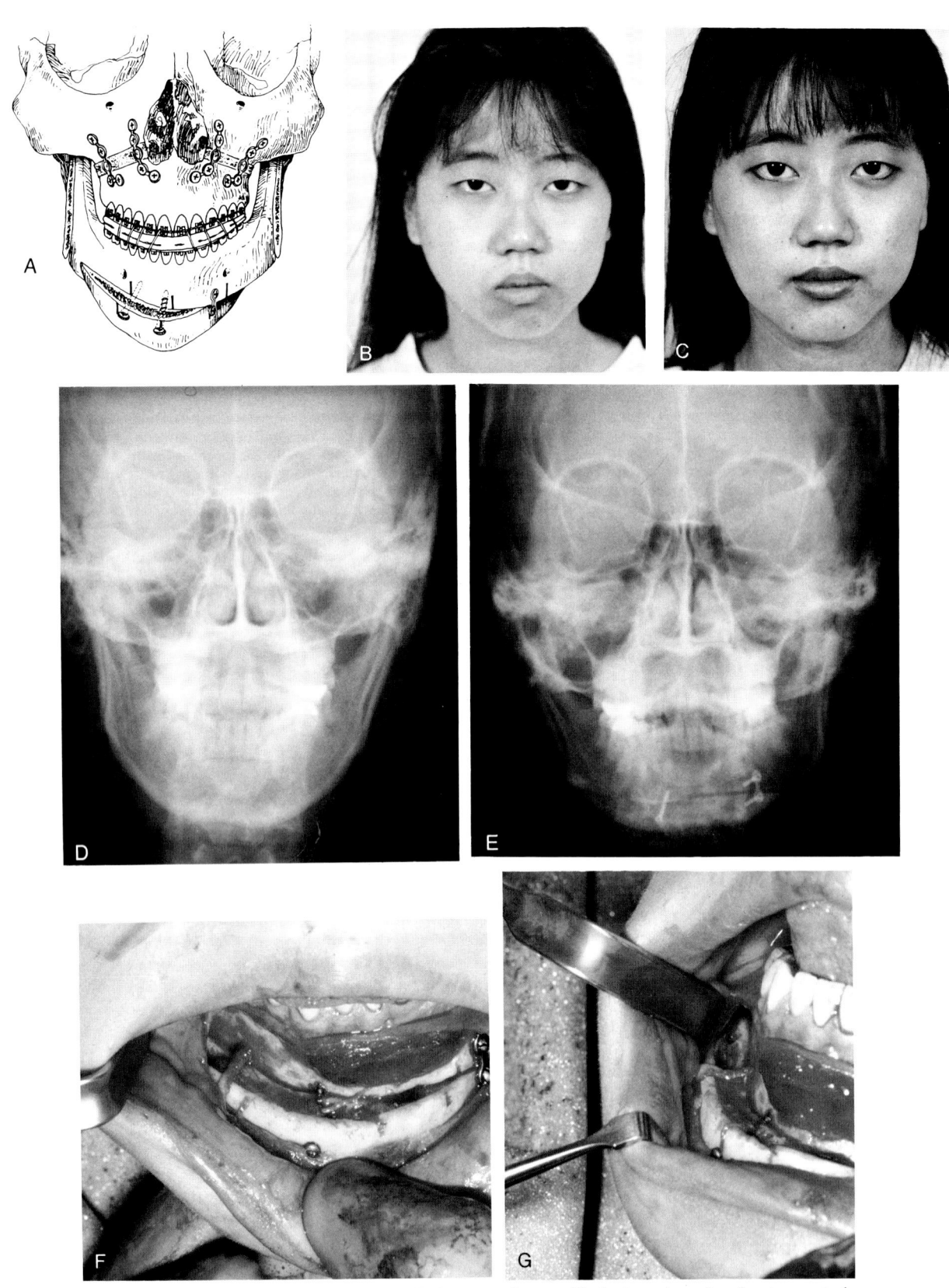

FIGURE 64-98. *A*, Correction of asymmetric mandibular excess by mandibuloplasty: lateral and anteroposterior augmentation and differential vertical height reduction of the long, flat side were achieved by stabilizing the genial segment lateral to the labial cortex of the superior segment and advancing the right side of the genial segment more than the contralateral side. *B*, Preoperative facial asymmetry. *C*, Postoperative facial appearance after mandibuloplasty. *D*, Preoperative frontal cephalogram showing facial asymmetry. *E*, Postoperative cephalogram showing improved symmetry of face. *F* and *G*, Intraoperative views of repositioned genial segment stabilized with bone plate and lag screw.

Increasing Chin Height

When it is necessary to increase the vertical dimension of the chin, a corticocancellous iliac crest bone graft, an allogeneic bank bone, or hydroxyapatite may be used in concert with horizontal osteotomy of the inferior border of the mandible (Figs. 64–99 and 64–100). Individuals who manifest a Class II deep-bite mandibular deficiency are the most logical and common candidates for such surgery. After the mobilized chin segment is fixed to the body of the mandible in the preplanned vertical and anteroposterior position by bone plates and screws, the bone graft or bone substitute is interposed between the proximal and distal segments.

An alternative method of increasing chin height without grafting involves repositioning of the genial segment by a combination of oblique and horizontal cuts to lengthen or shorten the vertical dimension of the chin (Figs. 64–101 and 64–102). To maximize the vertical change of the soft tissues, the surgery is accomplished by maintaining as much soft tissue pedicle as possible to the inferior and inferoanterior portions of the mobilized segment. The bone segment with a broadly based vascularized pedicle is easily stabilized with two screws. The osteotomy design is planned and predicted from lateral and posteroanterior cephalometric radiographs. Eight patients with anteroposterior chin prominence and vertical deficiency have been treated with superoinferior sliding and bilateral horizontal osteotomies. In addition, seven patients with anteroposterior chin deficiency and vertical deficiency have been successfully treated with inferosuperior sliding and bilateral horizontal osteotomies. This osteotomy design corrects the combined vertical deficiency and anteroposterior growth discrepancy. The patients have been followed for more than 12 months (range, 12 to 45 months; mean, 18 months). The relationship between soft tissue and osseous movement was found to be 1:0.9 in moderate discrepancies (4 to 8 mm).

Decreasing Chin Height

The individual with an excessively long chin frequently has a flat labiomental fold, mentalis muscle hyperfunction, and excessive bone height between the apices of the mandibular incisors and the inferior border of the mandible. The soft tissue of the lower lip and chin may be deficient, normal, or excessive in height. The total height of these soft tissues appears to shorten as the bony symphysis is reduced in height; consequently, it is difficult to raise the margin of the lower lip by raising the inferior border of the mandible. Shortening of the excess soft tissue with vertical reduction genioplasty, however, permits establishment of facial balance and an improved relationship between the lower incisor and the lower lip stomion.

Text continued on page 2484

FIGURE 64–99. HORIZONTAL SLIDING OSTEOTOMY COMBINED WITH INTERPOSITIONAL BONE GRAFT TO INCREASE CHIN HEIGHT AND DECREASE LABIOMENTAL FOLD. *A*, Preoperative short face syndrome deformity. Solid line indicates planned horizontal osteotomy. *B*, Postoperative view. (*A* modified from Bell WH, Proffit WR, White RP Jr: Surgical Correction of Dentofacial Deformities. Vol II. Philadelphia, WB Saunders Company, 1980, p 1237; with permission.)

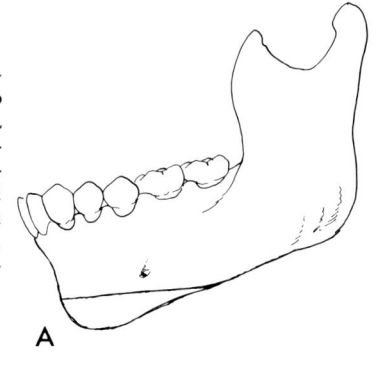

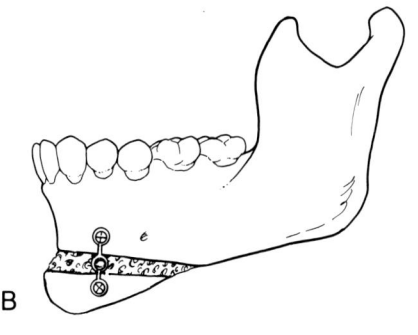

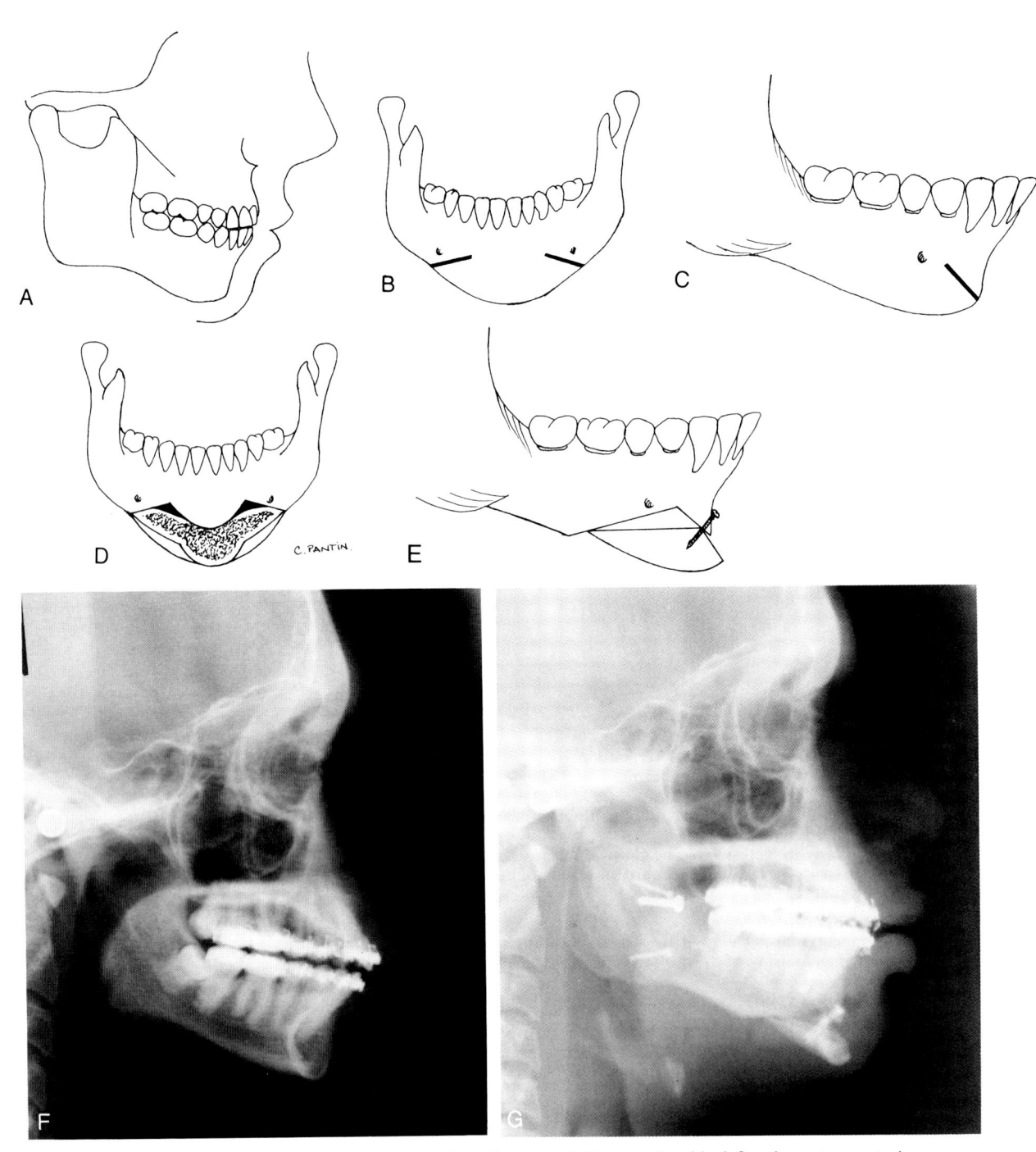

FIGURE 64–101. SURGICAL TECHNIQUE FOR INCREASING CHIN HEIGHT. *A*, Preoperative chin deformity: anteroposterior and vertical chin deficiency. *B*, Horizontal osteotomy. *C* and *D*; Oblique inferosuperior osteotomy. *E*, Anteriorly and inferiorly repositioned genial segment stabilized by position screws. *F*, Preoperative cephalogram showing mandibular deficiency associated with anteroposterior and vertical chin deficiency. *G*, Postoperative cephalogram after mandibular advancement by sagittal split ramus osteotomies and genioplasty to inferiorly and anteriorly reposition chin; genial segment stabilized by bicortical position screws.

Surgeon — Cesar Guerrero, D.D.S., Caracas, Venezuela
Orthodontist — Gisella Contasti, D.D.S., Caracas, Venezuela

64 — MANDIBULAR DEFICIENCY / **2481**

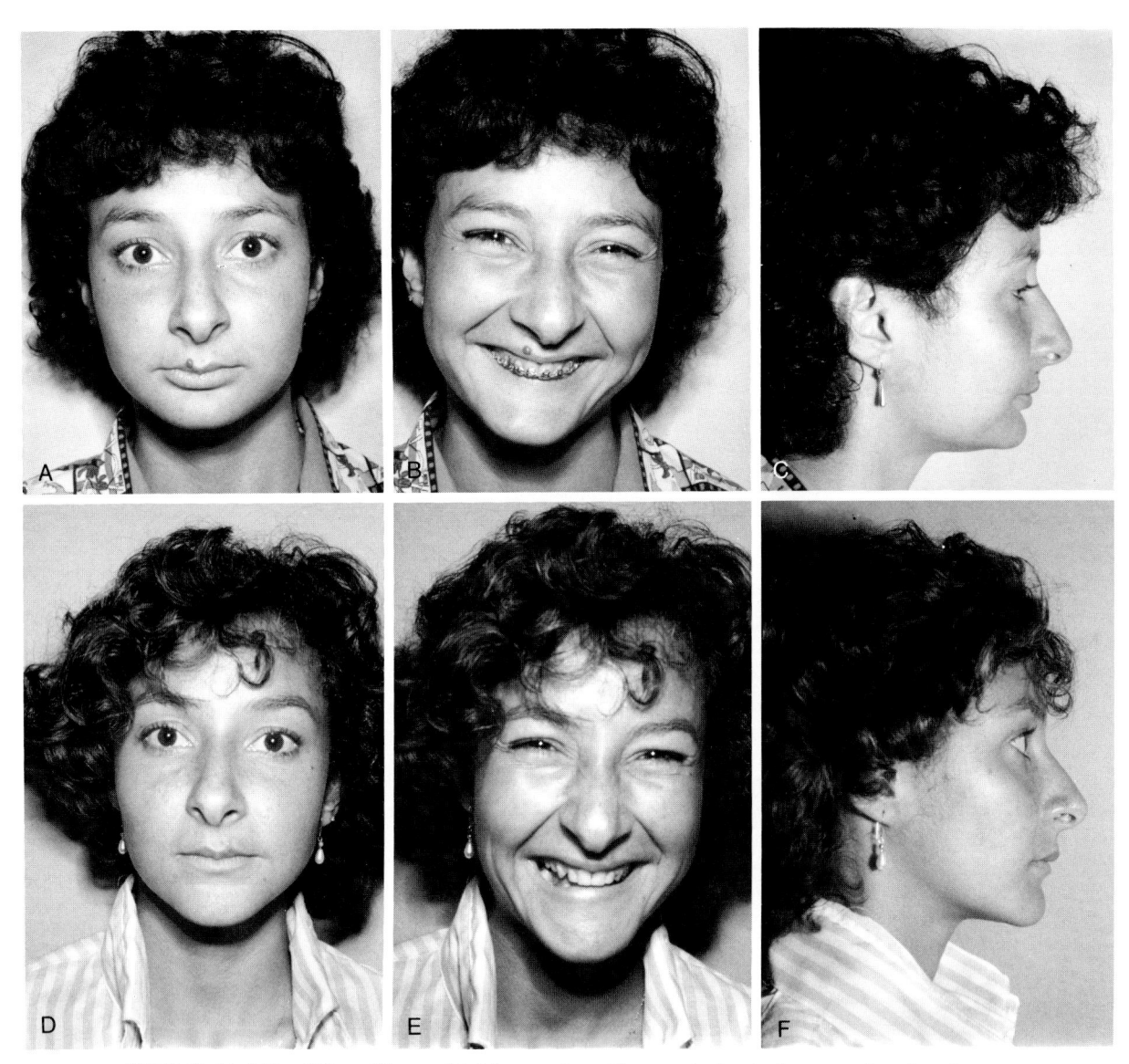

FIGURE 64–102. C.B., a 17-year-old girl, was referred by an orthodontist for correction of moderate anteroposterior mandibular deficiency associated with vertical mandibular deficiency and excessive chin prominence. She had a full Class II Division 1, malocclusion with multiple congenitally missing teeth in the mandible. The orthodontist aligned, leveled, and closed diastemas with minimal anchorage because of congenitally missing teeth.

Problem List

Esthetics
Frontal: Symmetric and proportionate upper and midfacial esthetics, vertical mandibular deficiency, pointed chin, and nevus in the upper mucocutaneous line.
Profile: Vertical mandibular deficiency, short submental length, and submental lipodystrophy.

Cephalometric Analysis
1. Vertical mandibular deficiency.
2. Deep labiomental sulcus.
3. Anteroposterior mandibular deficiency.

Vertical Proportions
1. $\underline{1}$-STm_s = 1
2. $\overline{G}$-Sn = 70/Sn = Me′ = 55
3. Sn-STm_s = 20/STm_i − Me′ = 35
4. ILG = 0

Anteroposterior Proportions
1. SnV-ULP = +12
2. SnV-LLP = −2.5
3. SnV-Po′ = 7
4. NLA = 109°
5. ULD = 109°

Illustration continued on following page

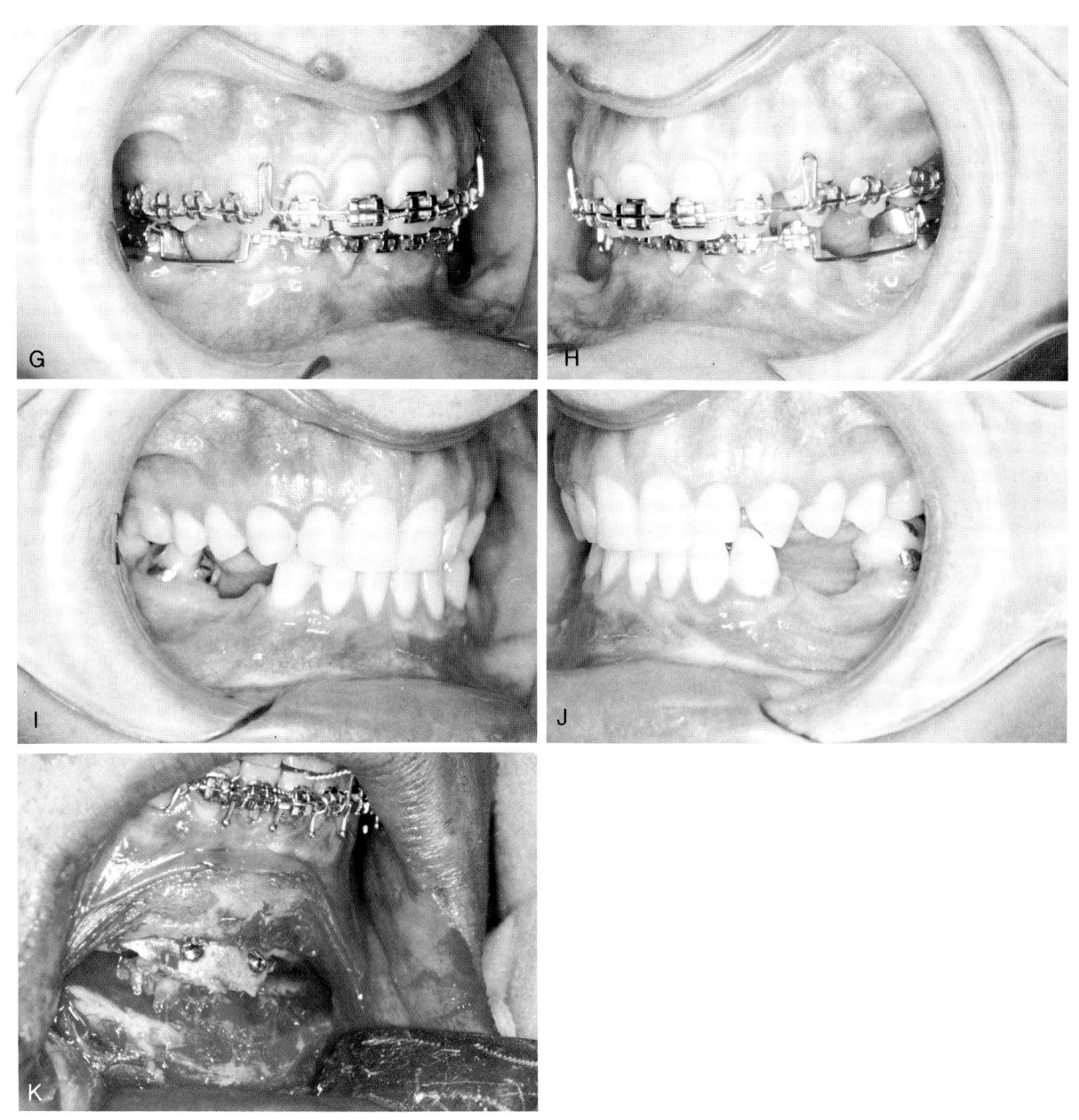

FIGURE 64-102 *Continued.*

Incisor Position
1. $\underline{1}$-HP = 101°
2. $\overline{1}$-PP = 102°
3. $\overline{\overline{1}}$-GoMe = 104°

Occlusal Analysis
Dental arch form: maxillary and mandibular arches symmetric and U shaped.
Dental occlusion: Class II, Division 1, malocclusion; multiple congenitally missing mandibular molar teeth.
Dental alignment: Mild maxillary and mandibular crowding; retroclined maxillary and mandibular incisors.

Treatment Plan

Presurgical Orthodontic Treatment: Align and level the maxillary and mandibular arches, close the diastemas, and improve the incisor inclination.

Plan of Surgery
1. Mandibular advancement by sagittal split ramus osteotomies.
2. Posteroinferior repositioning of the chin by osteotomy of the inferior border of the mandible.

Post-surgical Orthodontic Treatment
1. Final leveling and detailing of the occlusion.
2. Retention.
3. Fabrication of a temporary removable prosthesis by prosthodontist while dental implants were integrating.

64 — MANDIBULAR DEFICIENCY / **2483**

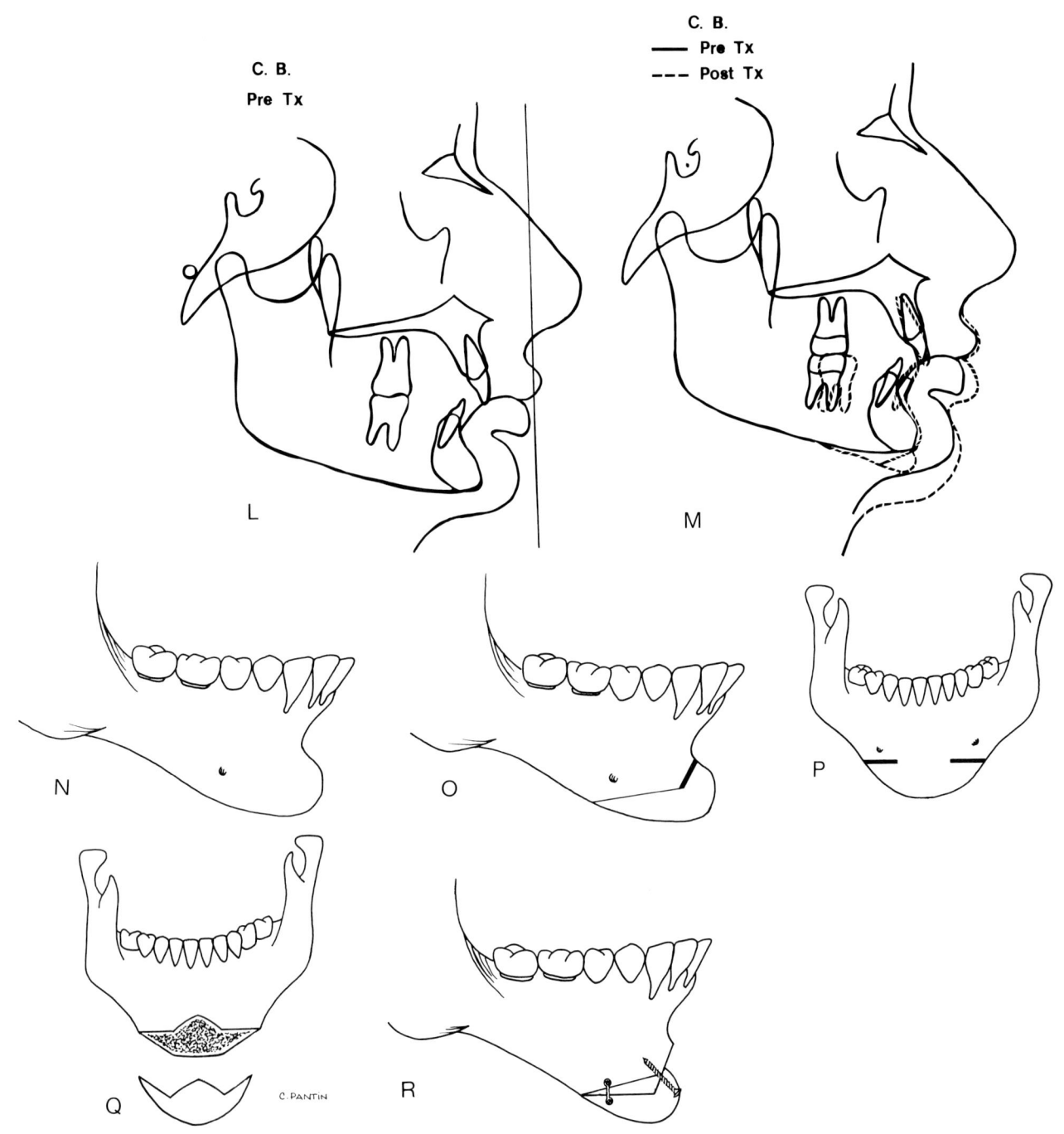

FIGURE 64–102 *Continued.*

Comments
Osteotomy design allowed correction of the vertical mandibular deficiency without the need for a bone graft. A broad soft tissue pedicle was maintained to ensure the vascularity of the repositioned genial segment and a more predictable soft tissue change. A 1:09 ratio of the soft tissue to hard tissue movement was achieved. Such genioplasties can be selectively performed as an office procedure with the patient under intravenous sedation.

Surgeon — Cesar Guerrero, D.D.S., Caracas, Venezuela
Orthodontist — Aura Marina Rodriguez, D.D.S., Caracas, Venezuela

A–C, Preoperative facial appearance. *D–F*, Postoperative facial appearance; improved submental cervical esthetics and increased lower anterior facial height. *G* and *H*, Preoperative decompensated Class II malocclusion. *I* and *J*, Postoperative occlusion. *K*, Genioplasty to increase chin height; repositioned chin stabilized by two 12-mm self-tapping positional screws. *L*, Preoperative cephalometric tracing showing mandibular deficiency with decreased lower anterior facial height. *M*, Pretreatment *(solid line)* and post-treatment *(dashed line)* cephalometric tracing showing increase in lower anterior facial height. *N–R*, Surgical technique. *N*, Vertical and anteroposterior chin deficiency. *O*, Oblique osteotomy. *P*, Horizontal osteotomy. *Q*, Plan of osteotomy. *R*, Fixation of chin with anterior and posterior position screws.

2486 / VII — ORTHOGNATHIC SURGERY

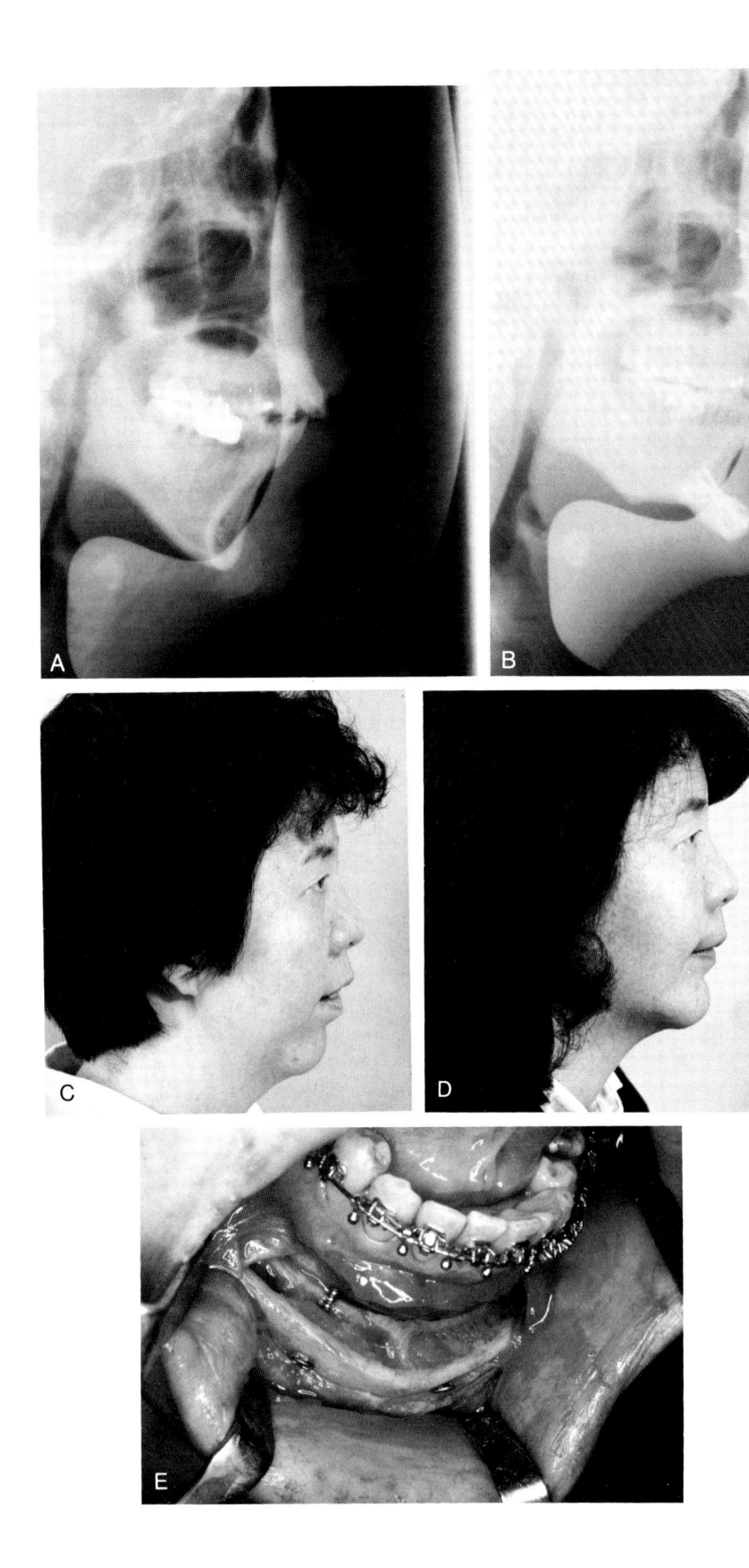

FIGURE 64-104. *A,* Lateral cephalogram of a 40-year-old woman with skeletal-type anterior open bite and relative mandibular deficiency. An unsuccessful attempt was made 10 years before to camouflage the vertical and sagittal facial disproportion with a preformed subperiosteal Silastic chin implant. Progressive osseous resorption beneath the implant and lateral migration were noted postoperatively. Effective treatment of this deformity included decompensating orthodontics, superior and posterior repositioning of the maxilla by Le Fort I osteotomy to normalize the maxillomandibular soft tissue and osseous relationship, and advancement genioplasty. *B,* Post-treatment lateral cephalogram after Le Fort I osteotomy to superiorly and posteriorly reposition the maxilla, removal of preformed Silastic chin implant, and simultaneous advancement genioplasty (10 mm) by osteotomy of the inferior border of the mandible and suction lipectomy of the submental and submaxillary regions. Chin surgery of this type is best done simultaneously with removal of the previously placed implant rather than as two independent surgical procedures. *C,* Preoperative facial appearance. *D,* Facial appearance after treatment. *E,* Intraoral view showing 12-mm chin advancement by overlapping genioplasty technique. Chin is stabilized with two position screws.

anatomic position opposite the osseous pogonion, can cause interlabial incompetence and excessive exposure of the mandibular teeth. The residual deformity may range from subtle to severe. Secondary correction to normalize the function and position of the lower lip is complex and unpredictable. Zide and McCarthy[19] have described the importance of the mentalis muscle in maintaining a normal lower lip and soft tissue pogonion position. When the mentalis muscle becomes transposed inferiorly by improper closure technique, excessive degloving, or improper incision, correction of the ptotic soft tissue and lip incompetence may be challenging, difficult, and unpredictable. In such cases, the mentalis muscle origin requires resuspension to the proper level. Nonabsorbable sutures are passed through drill holes in the alveolar bone and then through the mentalis muscles. Tightening the sutures transposes the soft tissue chin upward, allowing correction of the ptotic soft tissue chin and improvement of the lower vermilion-incisor relationship. Other soft tissue ancillary procedures may also be necessary to correct vestibular scarring.

In selected cases, soft tissue attachment to the symphyseal fragment is maintained to facilitate bony and associated soft tissue movement by vertical symphyseal osteotomy. This technique[16a] allows superior repositioning of the mentalis-periosteal complex to achieve a more normal chin contour, reduce chin ptosis, and gain lip competence.

Mentalis muscle fibers originate from an oval area of bone opposite the roots of the incisors on the anterior surface of the mandibular symphysis. Incorrect incision placement, excessive subperiosteal dissection, and improper wound closure may adversely affect the results of treatment. When genioplasty is accomplished, indiscriminant "degloving" is contraindicated. In contrast, meticulous planning and *minimal* soft tissue detachment consistent with the achievement of the planned osteotomy will minimize the possibility of postoperative undesirable transposition of the mentalis muscle attachment and lip support. A pressure dressing will assist in stabilizing the repositioned soft tissues. Techniques that advocate excessive detachment of the soft tissues to achieve greater exposure of the mental symphysis carry with them a greater risk of chin and lip ptosis. Consequently, meticulous attention to details of an anatomic closure of the soft tissues is mandatory.

Summary

Facial esthetics, in the patient in whom orthognathic surgery is considered, usually benefits from some type of genioplasty to alter one or all three dimensions of space. In the past, osteotomy of the inferior border of the mandible has been viewed as technically more difficult, lengthier, and potentially more problematic than alloplastic augmentation genioplasty. However, when accomplished by maintaining a broad soft tissue pedicle to the repositioned chin and meticulous soft tissue closure, the procedure compares favorably with other techniques in terms of morbidity and operating time, is more versatile, and produces a stable and predictable long-term result. With proper planning and execution, the genioplasty technique provides a means of concomitantly improving three-dimensional chin proportions and normalization of the associated orofacial musculature in the great majority of patients with dentofacial deformities.

REFERENCES

1. Aufricht G: Combined plastic surgery of the nose and chin. Am J Oral Surg 95:231–236, 1958.
2. Bell WH: Correction of mandibular prognathism by mandibular setback and advancement genioplasty. Int J Oral Surg 10:221–229, 1981.
3. Bell WH, Brammer JA, McBride KL, Finn RA: Reduction genioplasty: Surgical techniques and soft-tissue changes. Oral Surg 51:471–477, 1981

4. Bell WH, Dann JJ III: Correction of dentofacial deformities by surgery in the anterior part of the jaws. Am J Orthod 64(2):162–187, 1973.
5. Bell WH, Gallagher DM: The versatility of genioplasty using a broad pedicle. J Oral Maxillofac Surg 41:763–769, 1983.
6. Bell WH, Proffitt WR, White RP: Surgical Correction of Dentofacial Deformities. Philadelphia, WB Saunders Company, 1980, Chapter 12.
7. Burstone H: Integumental contour and extension patterns. Am J Orthod 29:93–104, 1959.
8. Converse JM, Wood-Smith D: Horizontal osteotomy of the mandible. Plast Reconstr Surg 34:464–471, 1964.
9. Gallagher DM, Bell WH, Storum KA: Soft tissue changes associated with advancement genioplasty performed concomitantly with superior repositioning of the maxilla. J Oral Maxillofac Surg 42:238–242, 1984.
10. Hinds EC, Kent JN: Genioplasty: The versatility of horizontal osteotomy. J Oral Surg 27:290–300, 1969.
11. Storum KA, Bell WH, Nagura H: Microangiographic and histologic evaluation of revascularization and healing after genioplasty by osteotomy of the inferior border of the mandible. J Oral Maxillofac Surg 48:210–216, 1988.
12. Moorrees C, Kean M: Natural head position, a basic consideration in the interpretation of cephalometric radiographs. Am J Phys Anthropol 16:213–214, 1958.
13. Neuner O: Correction of mandibular deformities. Oral Surg 36:779–789, 1973.
14. Obwegeser H: *In* Trauner R, Obwegeser H: The surgical correction of mandibular prognathism and retrognathia with consideration of genioplasty. Part I. Oral Surg 10:677, 1957.
15. Polido W, Regis LDC, Bell WH: Bone resorption, stability, and soft-tissue changes following large chin advancements. J Oral Maxillofac Surg 49:251–256, 1991.
15a. Precious DS, Armstrong JE, Morais D: Anatomic placement of fixation devices in genioplasty. Oral Surg Oral Med Oral Pathol 73:2–12, 1992.
16. Robinson M, Shuken R: Bone resorption under plastic chin implants. J Oral Surg 27:116–118, 1969.
16a. Rubins BC, West RA: Ptosis of the chin and lip incompetence: Consequences of lost mentalis muscle support. J Oral Maxillofac Surg 47:359–366, 1989.
17. Scheideman GB, Legan HL, Bell WH: Soft tissue changes with combined mandibular setback and advancement genioplasty. J Oral Surg 39:505–509, 1981.
18. Trimble LD, West RA: Steinmann pin stabilization after horizontal mandibular osteotomy. J Oral Maxillofac Surg 40:461–463, 1982.
19. Zide BM, McCarthy J: The mentalis muscle: An essential component of chin and lower lip position. Plast Reconstr Surg 83:413–420, 1989.

4. CHEILOPLASTY

WILLIAM H. BELL

Mandibular surgery to correct a larger anteroposterior discrepancy between the jaws, in concert with genioplasty, will usually improve lip function and posture. In a few instances, however, cheiloplasty (see Chapter 11) is required to manage the redundant everted lower lip that has been curled under the protruding maxillary incisors for so long that it can never harmonize with the upper lip without surgical intervention. The surgery may be performed in combination with ramus surgery or independently on an outpatient basis. Treatment must be planned carefully so that lip competence is achieved before undertaking cheiloplasty; if this factor is not taken into consideration, the interlabial gap might be increased (see Chapter 11).

5. MANDIBULAR ANGLE DEFICIENCY

CESAR GUERRERO

The mandibular angle deficiency must be evaluated in all three dimensions of space to obtain the best esthetic result. The angle deformity is often seen in cases of high mandibular plane angle. The deformity is typically found in the Class III open bite patient who has a tapered neck and mandibular angle vertical deficiency.

Similar morphology may be noted after mandibular angle fractures. Mandibular angle deficiency is not infrequently manifested in orthognathic surgery patients after ramus osteotomies. Problems that can and do occur are as follows:

1. Anterior rotation of the proximal segment after sagittal split or intraoral vertical ramus osteotomies. This is most commonly associated with mandibular advancements.
2. Mandibular ramus avascular necrosis after sagittal split osteotomy wherein the periosteum is excessively detached.
3. Large mandibular advancements.

Some possible surgical options for treatment of mandibular angle deficiency are as follows:

1. Mandibular ramus sagittal split osteotomy to rotate the proximal segment inferiorly and posteriorly; the proximal segment is fixed with positional or lag screws.
2. Alloplastic prosthesis.
3. Cranial bone graft fixed with lag screws.
4. Iliac crest bone graft fixed with a long, curved plate and positional screws.

Repositioning of the Mandibular Ramus

Following sagittal split ramus osteotomy, the proximal segment may be inadvertently rotated anteriorly or posteriorly. This can have a profound effect on the mandibular angle projection. Before the use of plate and screw osteosynthesis, interosseous wires were used to fix the proximal segment by various wire fixation techniques and modifications of the original Obwegeser technique. The ramus step osteotomy technique was also utilized to overcome anterior rotation of the proximal segment and loss of angle projection.

Today, however, with the use of rigid fixation and precise planning, the problems are much less common but still occur. The proximal segment can be repositioned by means of sagittal split osteotomy fixed in the desired position with positional screws. The periosteum, however, is not detached from the angle. Good esthetic and stable results can consistently be expected with this technique, which is indicated in cases after surgery in which the ramus was not well positioned. It can be accomplished in the immediate postoperative period with the patient under intravenous sedation or general anesthesia.

Mandibular Angle Alloplastic Implants

Through many years of follow-up, Silastic implants have shown better survival rates than those of other materials. The material is available in various forms— soft, hard, and gel—and can be prefabricated out of moulages or carved from blocks. A Silastic prosthesis is perhaps technically the easiest way to reconstruct the mandibular angle deficiency in all dimensions of space. Medicon is also available for the same purpose and is used in a similar manner. The mandibular angle prominence can be increased by onlaying preformed or sculpted alloplastic implants over the lateral mandibular angles below the masseter muscles. The procedure is usually accomplished with the patient under general anesthesia. The implants, which come in different shapes and sizes, are made by several different manufacturers. Such implants are usually wider posteriorly and inferiorly to simulate a natural tapered posterior facial appearance. The prosthesis is grooved to fit the lower and posterior borders of the mandible. This feature stabilizes the prosthesis and prevents displacement.

2490 / VII — ORTHOGNATHIC SURGERY

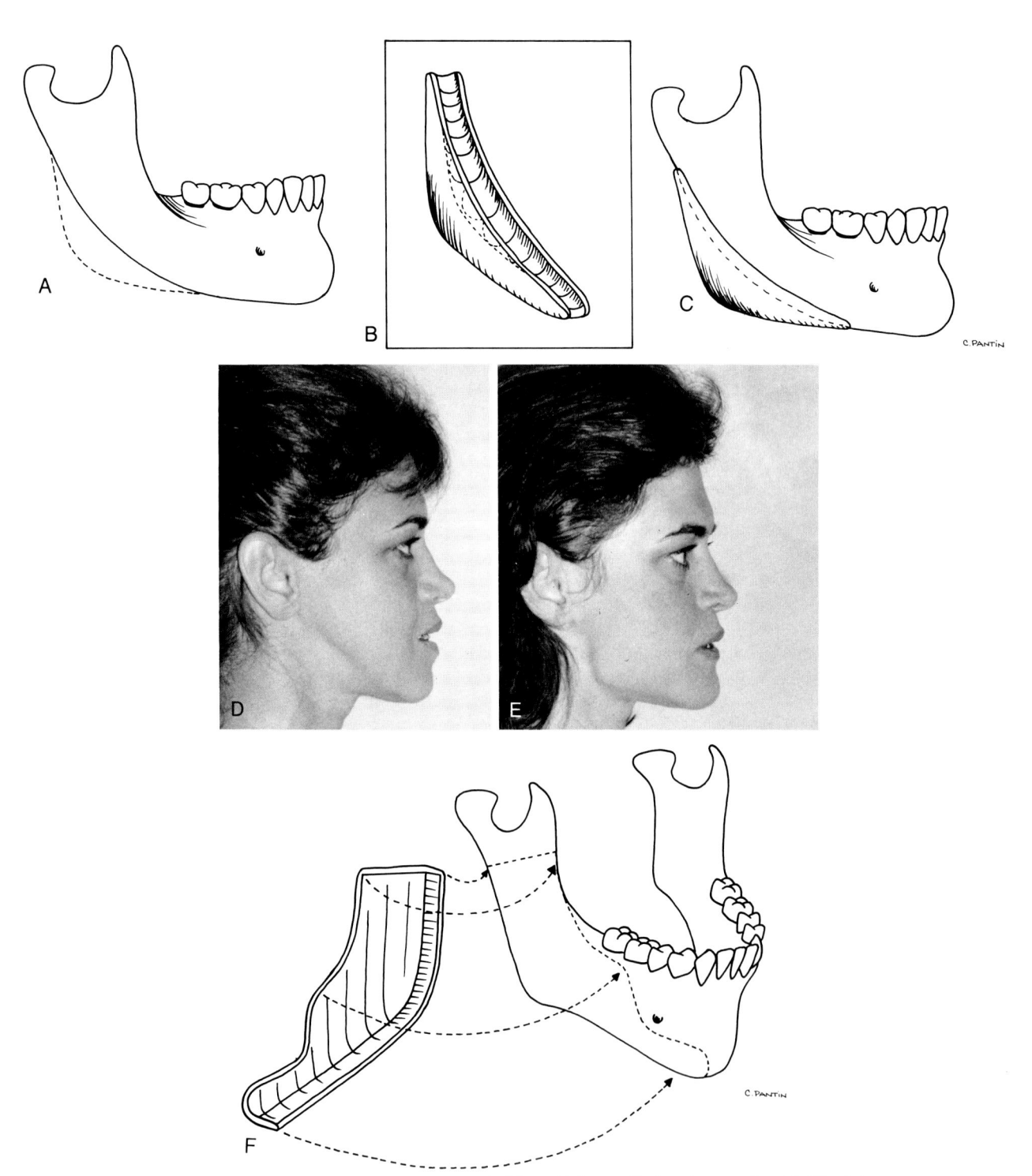

FIGURE 64–105. *A–C*, Three-dimensional augmentation of oblique high mandibular plane angle with Silastic implant. *D*, Facial appearance before surgery, showing the lack of definition of the mandibular angle. *E*, Facial appearance after application of Silastic implant to mandibular angle. *F*, Optional technique for augmentation of the mandibular angle and body with implant.

Surgical Technique

The masseter muscle is completely elevated intraorally away from the lateral and posterior aspects of the mandibular ramus. With a sharply curved J-shaped pterygomasseteric sling periosteal elevator, the muscle sling is detached from the inferior and medial aspects of the mandibular ramus and angle to facilitate passive positioning of the implant on the lateral, posterior, and inferior aspects of the mandibular ramus (Fig. 64–105A to F). Finally, the right and left angles are compared by extraoral visualization and digital palpation. Any change required is achieved by removing any excess prosthesis with a scalpel blade. After the area is well irrigated, the incision is closed in a mattress fashion, and a compression dressing is placed for 5 days. Appropriate antibiotics are used for 10 days as indicated.

Cranial Bone Graft Fixation with Lag Screws

A large amount of parietal and temporal cortical bone can be harvested without a visible scar and with only minor morbidity. In addition, cranial bone has minimal vascularization requirements and serves as a very stable onlay bone graft. The dense architecture of cranial bone is currently considered the most important reason for the lack of resorption of onlay cranial bone grafts.

Cranial bone can be used as a free or vascularized graft, maintaining the temporal muscle with or without the temporal artery. The free cranial bone graft can be used as a single layer or in two layers to reconstruct the mandibular angle in the vertical, anteroposterior, or transverse deficiency. The graft is formed from studies of the patient and his or her lateral and posteroanterior cephalometric radiographs. After the result is assessed at the time of surgery, the graft is fixed with lag screws. Cancellous bone from the inner skull table is harvested and placed around the graft. Cranial bone can be used to alter the contour of the mandibular angle, with an excellent prognosis for long-term stability.

Lack of mandibular angle definition (vertical, transverse, and sagittal deficiency) can be corrected with a free cranial bone graft fixed to the ramus with lag screws of appropriate length (Fig. 64–106).

Iliac Crest Bone Graft Fixed with Long, Curved Plates and Screws

Avascular necrosis of the proximal segment of the mandibular ramus after sagittal split osteotomy is a difficult problem that may result in pseudoarthrosis at the mandibular angle. This problem may be the result of excessive subperiosteal dissection and unnecessary prolonged surgery. The clinical consequence is a loss of the mandibular angle in the vertical, anteroposterior, and transverse planes of space. The patient typically manifests a marked depression in the lateral and posterior part of the lower face. Functionally, there may be pain and masticatory dysfunction. Radiographically, the condylar segment is rotated anterosuperiorly. There may be separation between the ramus and body segments and absence of the mandibular angle (see Fig. 64–107A to J).

An angular bone graft is harvested from the medial aspect of the anterosuperior iliac spine of the ilium for reconstruction of the angle of the mandible on the same side of the defect. A template patterned from a lateral cephalometric radiograph is prepared before exposure of the ilium to facilitate outlining and harvesting the bone graft. The three-dimensional discrepancies of the vertical ramus and body are assessed from lateral and frontal cephalometric studies. The implant is refined and sculpted to create soft tissue symmetry. The template is adapted to the lateral

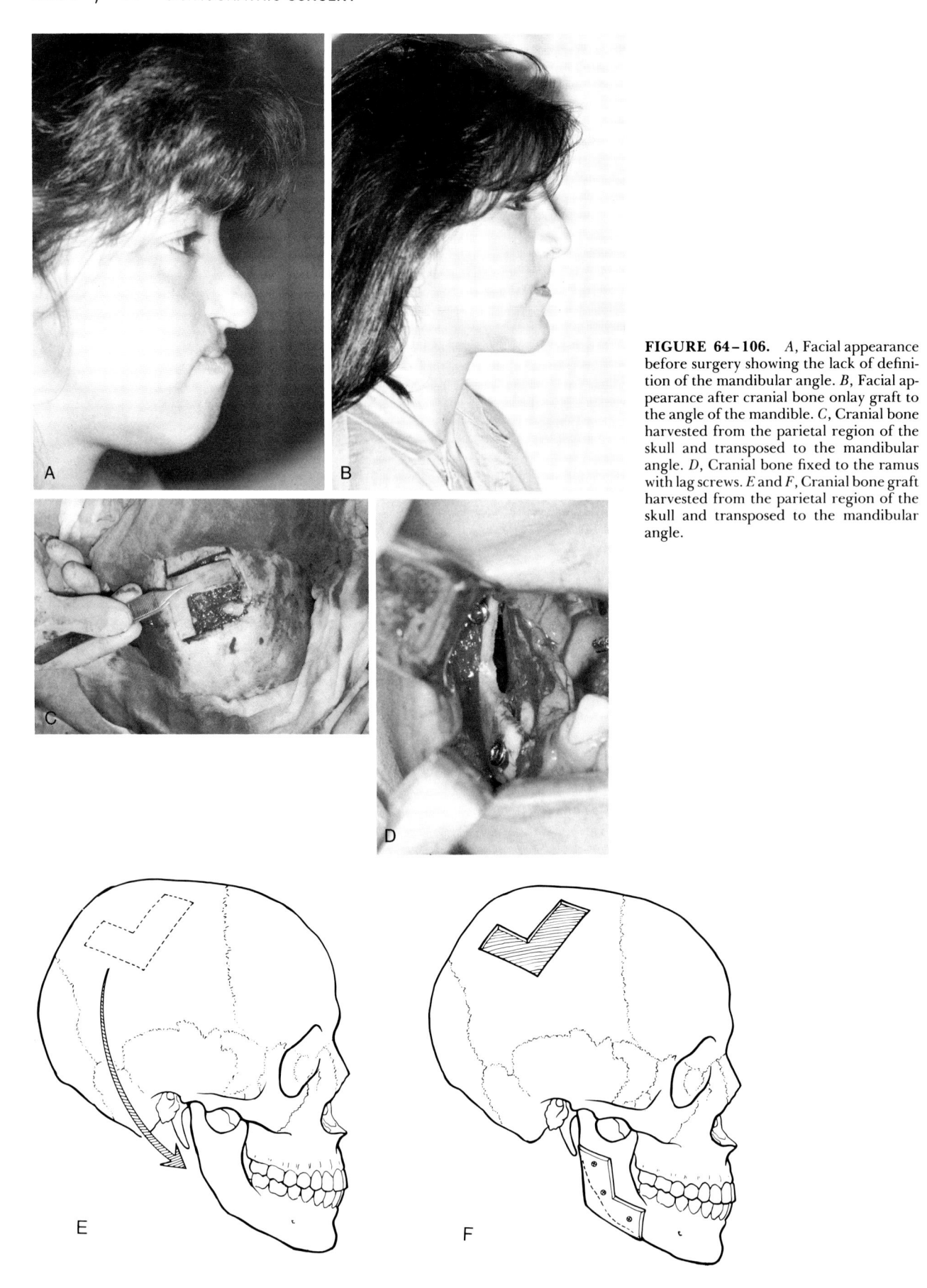

FIGURE 64–106. *A*, Facial appearance before surgery showing the lack of definition of the mandibular angle. *B*, Facial appearance after cranial bone onlay graft to the angle of the mandible. *C*, Cranial bone harvested from the parietal region of the skull and transposed to the mandibular angle. *D*, Cranial bone fixed to the ramus with lag screws. *E* and *F*, Cranial bone graft harvested from the parietal region of the skull and transposed to the mandibular angle.

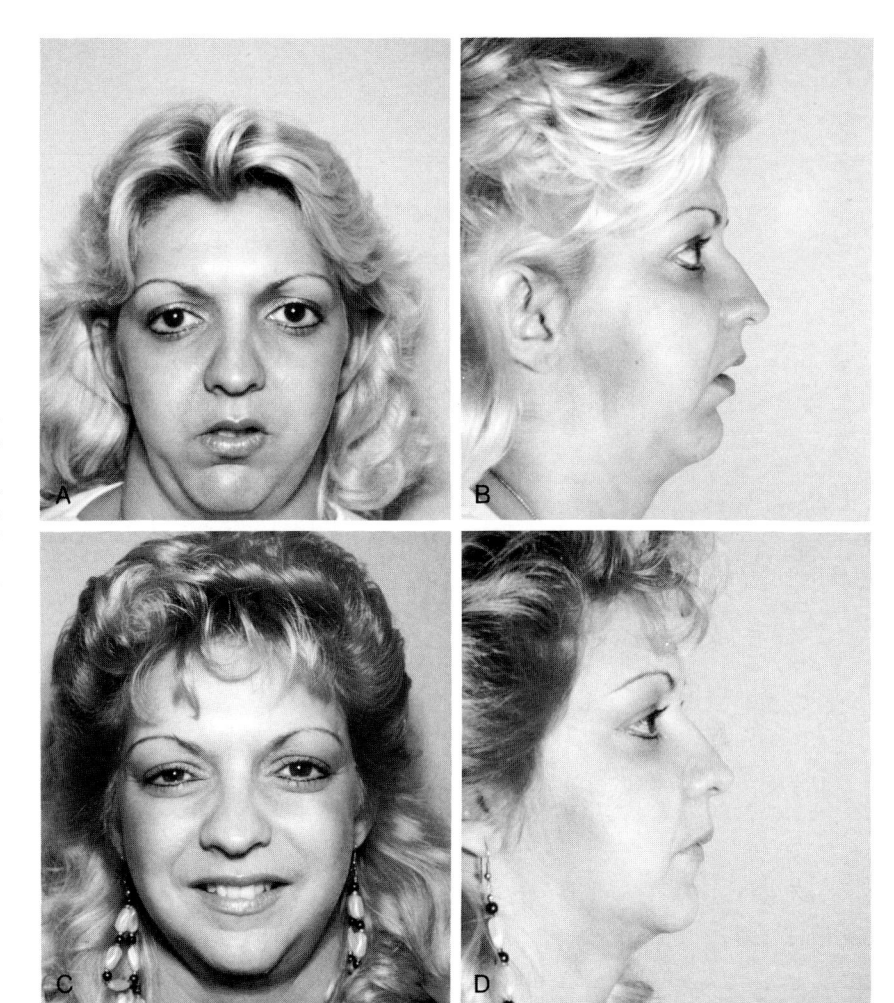

FIGURE 64-107. *A* and *B*, Facial appearance after three separate unsuccessful orthognathic surgical procedures; there was a lack of angle definition secondary to excessive anterosuperior rotation of the proximal segment following sagittal split osteotomies. *C* and *D*, Facial appearance after surgical procedures illustrated in *H*, *I*, and *J*.
Illustration continued on following page

aspect of the ilium and iliac crest, and the bone to be harvested is outlined with a pencil. The angle between the vertical and horizontal portions of the graft forms the new mandibular angle. As shown in the illustration, the implant is fashioned in such a way that it is self-stabilizing. Both Silastic and Medicon have been used for this purpose. The cancellous surface of the graft is placed against the host bone for optimal revascularization; the cortical side rests against the soft tissue to minimize resorption and promote long-term retention of the graft. Lag screws are used to stabilize the reconstructed angle.

CASE: A.P. (Fig. 64-107*A* to *J*)

A.P., a 30-year-old white woman, presented for consultation after unsuccessful orthognathic procedures to correct vertical maxillary excess, chin deficiency, and moderate Class II, Division 1, malocclusion.

FIRST SURGERY

Mandibular advancement and genioplasty were done in the first of two stages to correct the facial deformity. The patient developed avascular necrosis of the proximal segment of the right mandibular ramus.

SECOND SURGERY

Sequestrectomy was performed to remove the avascular segment. The patient manifested marked depression of the lateral mandibular angle, deviation of the chin to the right, mandibular angle pseudoarthrosis, and asymmetric Class II malocclusion.

THIRD SURGERY

A third surgery consisted of Le Fort I osteotomy to superiorly reposition the maxilla, genioplasty, and mandibular ramus osteotomy fixed with lag screws.

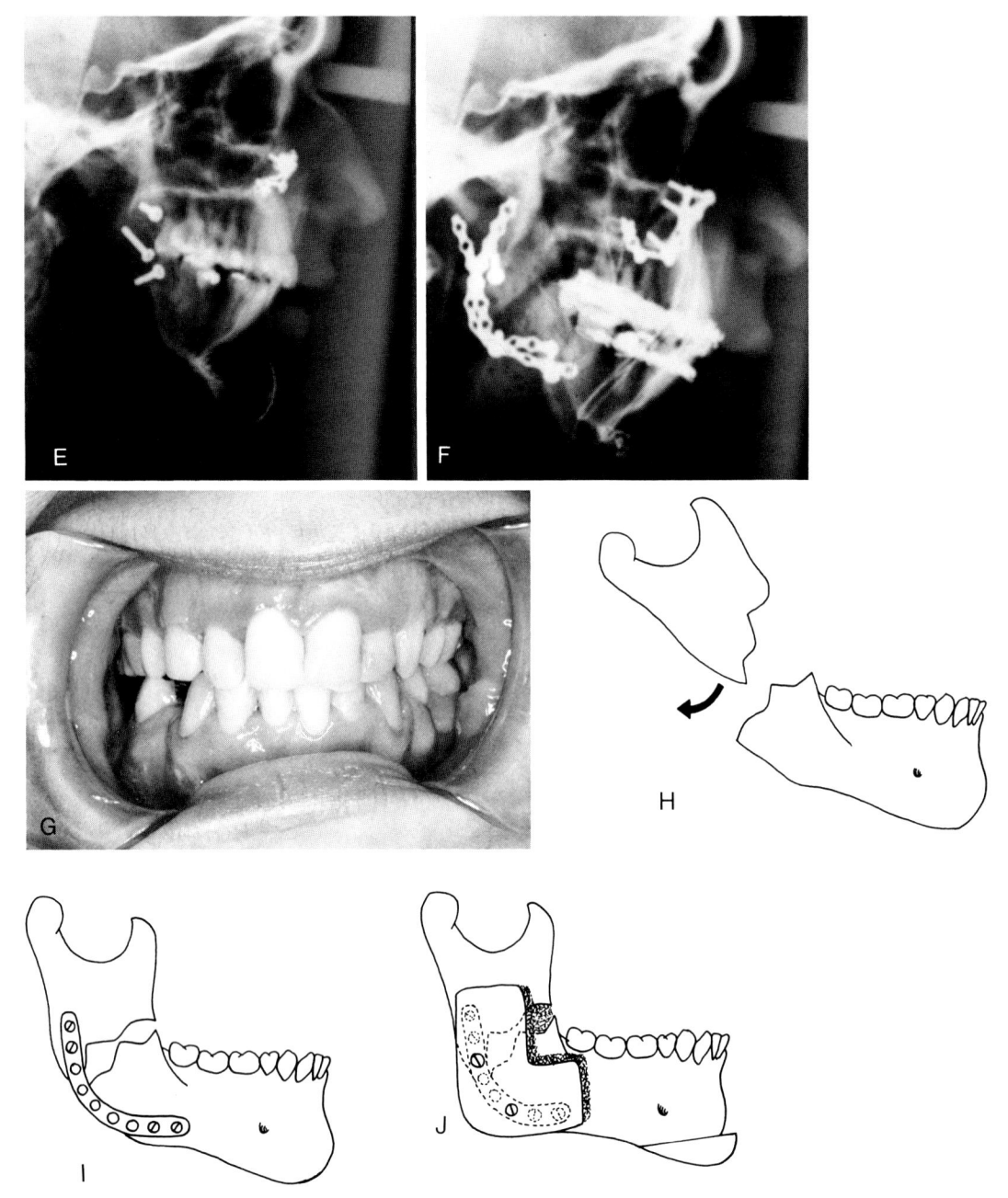

FIGURE 64-107 *Continued.* *E*, Pretreatment lateral cephalometric radiograph showing lack of angle definition. *F*, Post-treatment lateral cephalometric radiograph. *G*, Post-treatment occlusion. *H–J*, Plan of surgery: superoanterior rotation of proximal segment *(H)*; fixation of proximal and distal segments with reconstruction bone plate *(I)*; augmentation of mandibular angle contour with corticocancellous onlay bone graft stabilized with lag screws through graft and reconstruction plate *(J)*.

The patient was evaluated clinically and radiographically (Fig. 64–107A, B, and E), with the following findings:

1. Vertical maxillary deficiency (tooth to lip, −3 mm).
2. Chin deficiency and asymmetry.
3. Mandibular right angle pseudoarthrosis.
4. Loss of right mandibular angle.
5. Left mandibular angle deficiency.
6. Asymmetric Class II malocclusion.

The loss of continuity of the mandibular angle was considered the most significant problem (Fig. 64–107E). In addition, there was a need for a bone graft between the ramus and the body. An autogenous iliac crest corticocancellous bone graft was the first choice of treatment because of the multitude of previously unsuccessful surgical procedures.

SURGICAL PLAN (Fig. 64–107H to J)

1. One-segment Le Fort I osteotomy with interpositional bone graft to inferiorly reposition the maxilla, which was stabilized with mini bone plates and screws.
2. Right mandibular advancement and reconstruction of the right angle with iliac crest corticocancellous interpositional bone graft fixed with a long, curved reconstruction bone plate and screws placed through a submandibular approach.
3. Augmentation of the left mandibular angle with an iliac crest bone graft fixed with a long, curved reconstruction bone plate and screws placed through a submandibular approach.
4. Anterior and lateral horizontal sliding genioplasty.
5. Arch bars to control the occlusion.

The postoperative course was uneventful. The patient started her work 3 weeks after surgery with a very positive change in mood and personality. The bone graft became well integrated. Now, 4 years after surgery, she has maintained her facial morphology and function (Fig. 64–107C, D, F, and G).

Surgeon—Cesar Guerrero, D.D.S., Caracas, Venezuela

6. ANTERIOR MANDIBULAR SUBAPICAL OSTEOTOMY

WILLIAM H. BELL

Leveling of the mandibular occlusal plane usually is required when the mandible is advanced. Orthodontic treatment can produce leveling by extrusion of premolars, by intrusion of incisors, or by some combination of these tooth movements. It is necessary to move teeth individually in nearly all patients to obtain proper leveling of the arches. Subapical osteotomy is only occasionally a substitute for orthodontic leveling, but when significant *intrusion* of mandibular incisors is required, depressing the anterior segment surgically can facilitate treatment. This can be done at the same time as surgical advancement of the mandible or as an independent procedure.

Depressing the mandibular incisors is one way to prevent clockwise rotation of the mandible when a deep-bite mandibular deficiency problem is being corrected (Fig. 64–108A and B). The mandibular incisors should not be depressed (orthodontically or surgically) unless true supraeruption has occurred. Clockwise rotation as part of the advancement is frequently needed to correct deficient anterior facial height, and in this instance the leveling properly is done by orthodontic extrusion after surgical advancement of the mandible.

Surgical Technique of Subapical Osteotomy to Depress Incisors

The surgery is accomplished with the patient under general nasoendotracheal anesthesia. Lidocaine with a vasoconstrictor is infiltrated in the mental symphysis region for hemostasis. The incision for anterior mandibular subapical osteotomy or ostectomy is designed to maintain the circulation to the lingual and facial portions of the mobilized dental osseous segment (Fig. 64–108C). Anteriorly, the

2496 / VII — ORTHOGNATHIC SURGERY

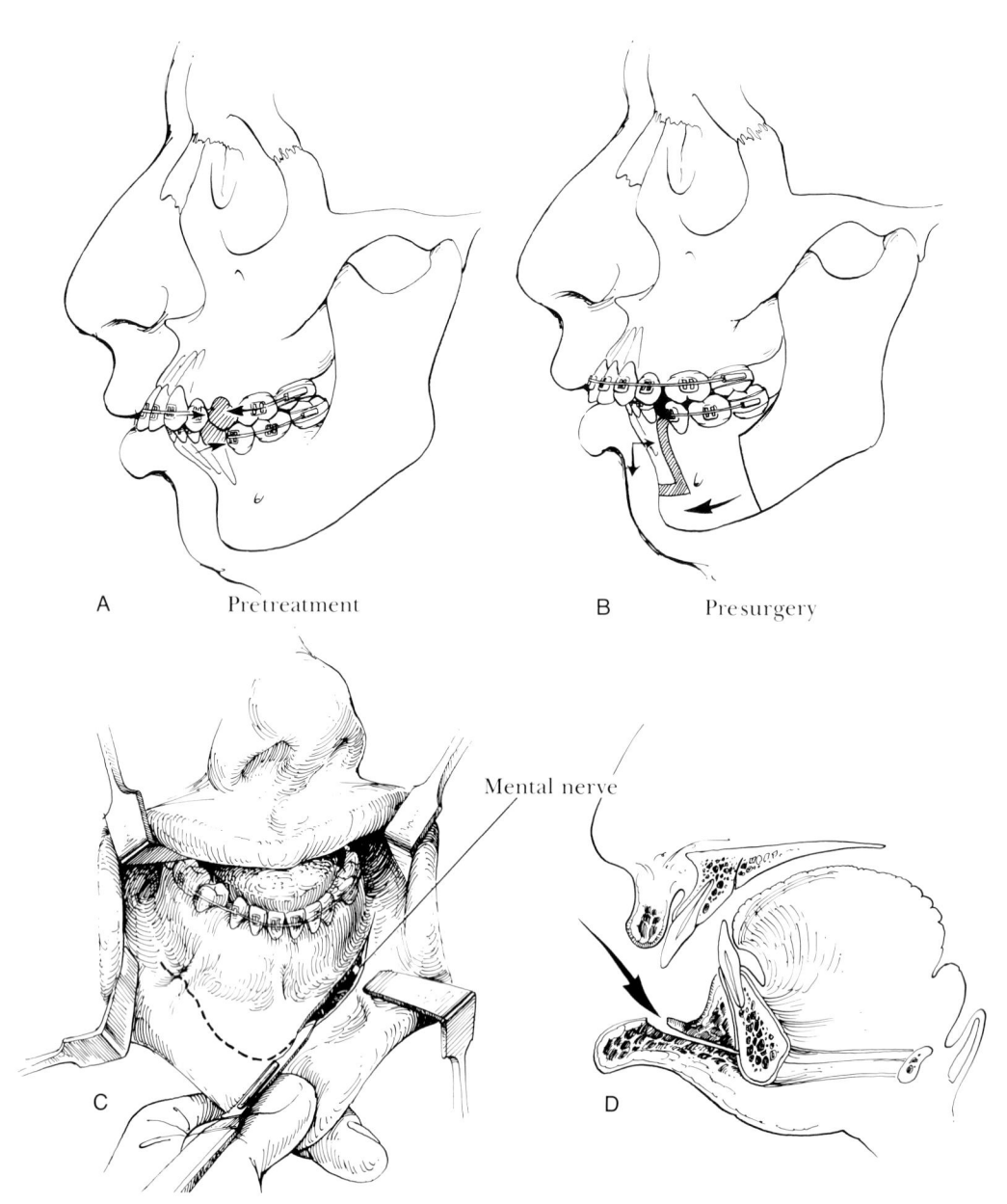

FIGURE 64–108. CORRECTION OF MANDIBULAR DEFICIENCY BY MANDIBULAR SUBAPICAL OSTEOTOMY, SAGITTAL SPLIT RAMUS OSTEOTOMIES, AND ORTHODONTIC TREATMENT. Subapical osteotomy is done to partially level the mandibular arch; the mandible is surgically advanced into a Class I occlusion by sagittal split ramus osteotomies. *A*, Typical dental, skeletal, and facial features associated with mandibular deficiency, with the mandible in centric relation and the lips relaxed. Note lip incompetence; proclination of maxillary incisors; excessive curvature of mandibular occlusal plane; deep overbite; dental compensations manifested as proclined lower anterior teeth, everted lower lip, retropositioned mandible, and Class II, Division I, malocclusion. Maxillary second premolars and mandibular first premolar teeth are extracted to allow correction of the malaligned teeth by orthodontic means. Arrows indicate the planned directional movements of teeth. The mandibular extraction space will be closed only the amount necessary to align the anterior teeth. *B*, Plan of surgery: mandibular subapical osteotomy to partially level the mandibular occlusal plane and close the residual extraction space; bilateral sagittal split ramus osteotomies to advance the mandible into a Class I canine and molar relation. Maxillary second premolar extraction space has been completely closed by orthodontic treatment with minimal retraction of the maxillary anterior teeth to preserve good esthetic balance between the upper lip and nose. *C*, Soft tissue incision for exposure of the mandible. *D*, Incision through the orbicularis oris and mentalis muscles.

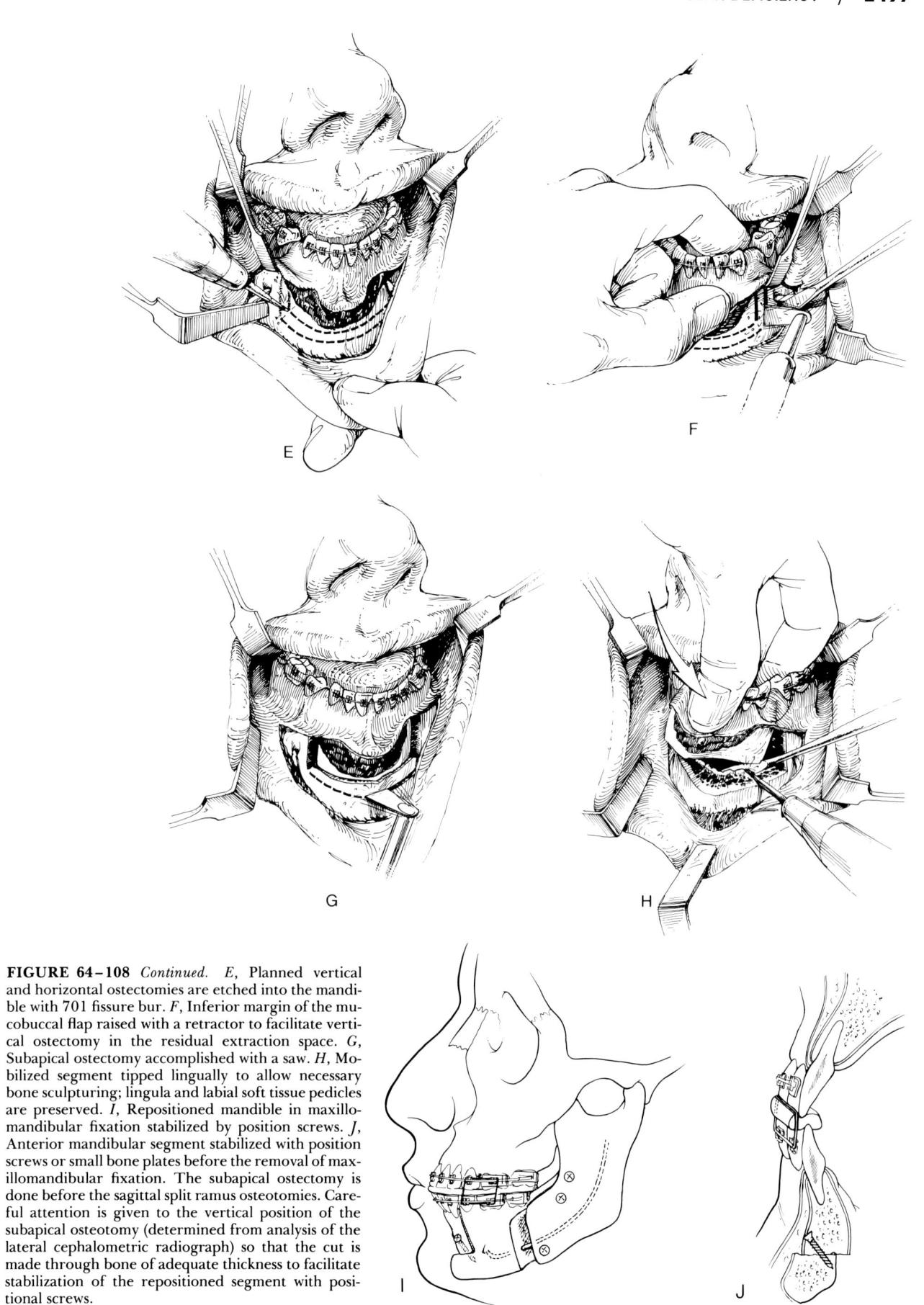

64 — MANDIBULAR DEFICIENCY / **2497**

FIGURE 64–108 *Continued.* *E*, Planned vertical and horizontal ostectomies are etched into the mandible with 701 fissure bur. *F*, Inferior margin of the mucobuccal flap raised with a retractor to facilitate vertical ostectomy in the residual extraction space. *G*, Subapical ostectomy accomplished with a saw. *H*, Mobilized segment tipped lingually to allow necessary bone sculpturing; lingula and labial soft tissue pedicles are preserved. *I*, Repositioned mandible in maxillomandibular fixation stabilized by position screws. *J*, Anterior mandibular segment stabilized with position screws or small bone plates before the removal of maxillomandibular fixation. The subapical ostectomy is done before the sagittal split ramus osteotomies. Careful attention is given to the vertical position of the subapical osteotomy (determined from analysis of the lateral cephalometric radiograph) so that the cut is made through bone of adequate thickness to facilitate stabilization of the repositioned segment with positional screws.

7. TOTAL MANDIBULAR SUBAPICAL OSTEOTOMY

MICHAEL J. BUCKLEY

The total mandibular subapical osteotomy is a surgical procedure that is available to correct a variety of dentofacial deformities (Fig. 64–109). Patients who are candidates for this procedure have mandibular dentoalveolar disharmonies and malocclusions but adequate maxillary and mandibular skeletal balance. Persons with posterior and lateral apertognathic conditions not amenable to orthodontics alone are also candidates for this procedure. In these individuals, mobilization of the entire maxillary or mandibular complex would have an unsatisfactory skeletal and esthetic change.[4,5,8]

The mandibular total subapical osteotomy was initially described by MacIntosh[9] in 1974 and has been modified several times[1,3,6,7] to decrease neurovascular damage and improve bone contact. Previous descriptions have combined the subapical osteotomy with a modified sagittal osteotomy to increase bone contact with the hope of improving stability. Previously described osteotomies have cut below the neurovascular bundle or completely removed the neurovascular bundle from the bony canal, with the hope of decreasing the potential for damage. Recent modifications by Turvey have been utilized to avoid the neurovascular bundle and simplify the osteotomy while promoting clinical stability.[2]

Surgical Procedure

Patients who have dentofacial deformities that are amenable to the total subapical osteotomy should have third molars removed several months prior to the surgical procedure. The presurgical workup includes radiographs, which help determine the position of the root apices and the neurovascular bundle. Models are mounted in the postoperative position, and a splint is constructed to stabilize the occlusal relationship.

At the time of surgery with the patient under nasoendotracheal general anesthesia, a dilute vasoconstrictor is infiltrated into the mucosa on the facial aspect of the mandible for hemostasis. A bilateral circumvestibular incision is made from the retromolar area forward. Anteriorly, the incision is carried out into the lip, and care is taken to avoid the neurovascular bundle. The mucoperiosteal flap is then elevated to expose the buccal cortical bone. At the mental foramen area, the neurovascular bundle is dissected out into the soft tissue.

The neurovascular bundle is visualized by decortication but not removed from its bony canal. The bone is scored with a small bur using rotary instrumentation, and the buccal window is removed with a small spatula osteotome. It must be remembered that the course of the mental nerve traverses superiorly and posteriorly before it exits its foramen. The cortical window therefore must be several millimeters anterior and inferior to the mental foramen. At this point, the neurovascular bundle is usually visualized in several places. Any remaining bone is then gently removed with a large diamond bur. This technique leads to less potential damage to the nerve. The neurovascular bundle must be visualized for its entire length but not removed from its canal.

In repositioning the dentoalveolar segment, it is often possible or desirable for the vertical height to change. To control this, vertical reference marks are made anteriorly and posteriorly and recorded for later use. A horizontal osteotomy is then made above the neurovascular bundle and below the apices of the teeth along the length of the mandible. This is most easily done with a micro reciprocating saw after the osteotomy line has been scored with a small bur. A finger is placed on the

64 — MANDIBULAR DEFICIENCY / **2501**

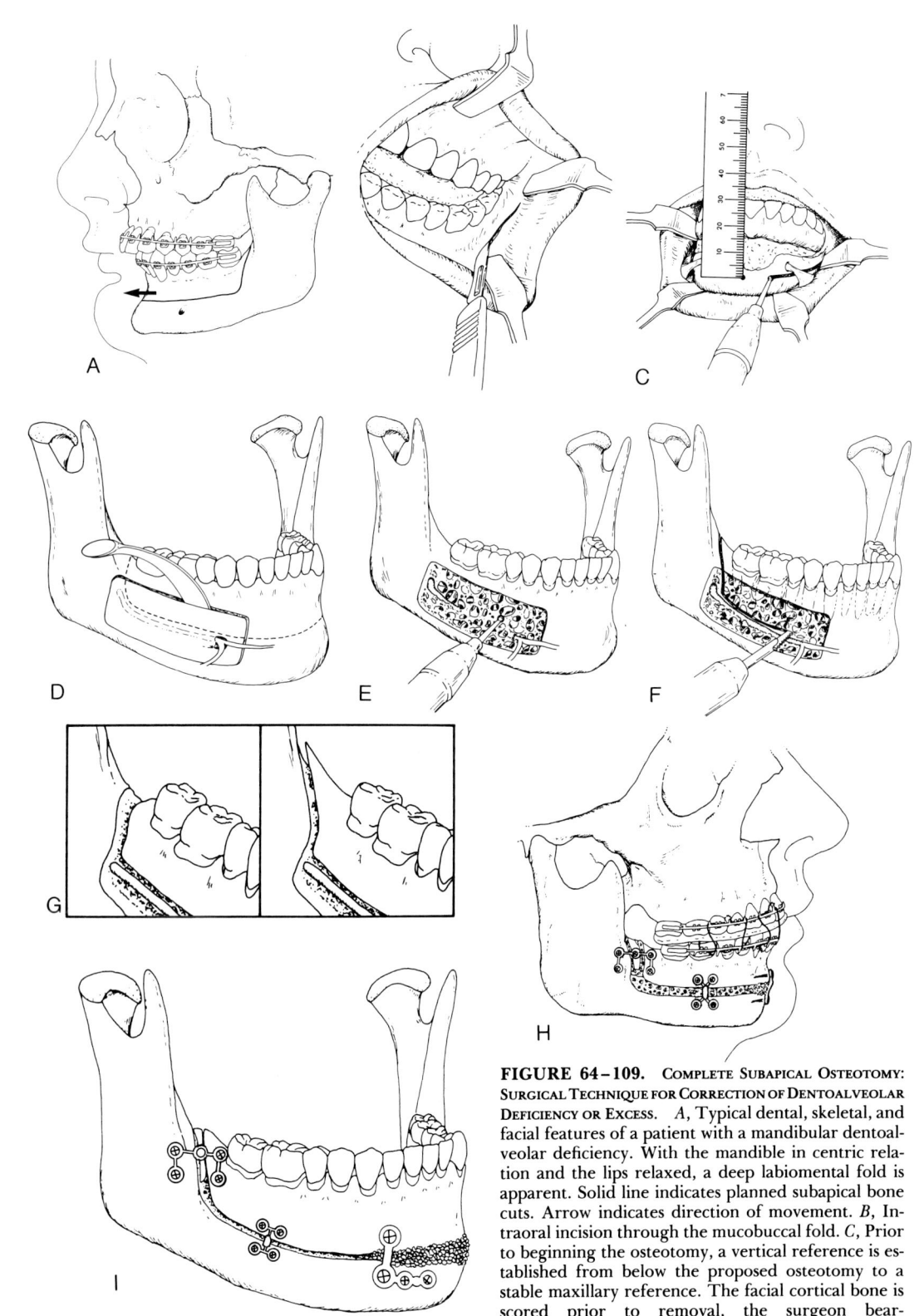

FIGURE 64–109. COMPLETE SUBAPICAL OSTEOTOMY: SURGICAL TECHNIQUE FOR CORRECTION OF DENTOALVEOLAR DEFICIENCY OR EXCESS. *A,* Typical dental, skeletal, and facial features of a patient with a mandibular dentoalveolar deficiency. With the mandible in centric relation and the lips relaxed, a deep labiomental fold is apparent. Solid line indicates planned subapical bone cuts. Arrow indicates direction of movement. *B,* Intraoral incision through the mucobuccal fold. *C,* Prior to beginning the osteotomy, a vertical reference is established from below the proposed osteotomy to a stable maxillary reference. The facial cortical bone is scored prior to removal, the surgeon bearing in mind the course of the mental nerve in the area of the mental foramen. *D,* The buccal cortical plate is undermined sufficiently and removed with an osteotome. *E,* Direct visualization of the nerve is possible in areas. A small, round diamond bur can be used to gently remove any remaining bone to ensure good visualization. *F,* The neurovascular bundle is identified but not disturbed in its position in the neurovascular canal. An osteotomy above the neurovascular canal but below the tooth apices is performed with a reciprocating saw. *G,* The two posterior vertical osteotomies are shown. For setbacks *(left),* an ostectomy is performed to allow for the setback. For advancements, an oblique osteotomy *(right)* is made to allow for bony contact and a stable area for grafting. *H,* Technique to increase lower face height and decrease the depth of the labiomental fold: Autologous bone is interposed between the separated segments. *I,* The mobilized dentoalveolar segments are stabilized by small bone plates and screws.

lingual tissue to prevent damage to the lingual vascular pedicle. The posterior osteotomy varies, depending on the movement of the dentoalveolar segment. In advancements, an oblique osteotomy is performed in the retromolar region to provide for maximal bone contact and a stable base for bone grafting. This is not a sagittal split osteotomy as previously described.[1] In retropositioning, bone is removed from a vertical osteotomy in the third molar area to accommodate the posterior movement.

The entire dentoalveolar segment is mobilized with care, utilizing small osteotomes to complete any small bone cuts and with gentle pressure from larger osteotomes. Movement of the segment in one piece is always desirable, but segmenting into two or three smaller segments is possible. This is accomplished in the traditional manner with small spatula osteotomes. The lingual vascular pedicle must be carefully protected at all times. After mobilization of the dentoalveolar segment, the new occlusal relationship is established with the acrylic splint, and maxillomandibular fixation is utilized. The condyles are seated carefully, and bone interferences are removed to acquire maximal contact between the basal bone and the mobilized dentoalveolar segment. Careful attention is then brought to the vertical dimension, where further reduction or augmentation is carried out to achieve the proper position in the three dimensions.

The cortical bone that is removed easily may be used as graft material where needed, such as at the posterior osteotomy site, or it may be morcellized and placed in gaps between the basal bone and the dentoalveolar segment. This cortical bone is usually more than adequate for grafting needs, but small quantities of additional bone can be harvested from the mandibular symphyseal area, or other suitable graft materials can be used (i.e., cranium, ilium, or allogeneic bone).

Once the dentoalveolar segment is repositioned on the basal bone, the condyles are seated, and the vertical height is adjusted, the segment is fixated in its new position. This is accomplished with bone plates utilizing monocortical screws. After copious irrigation, the anterior fibromuscular tissue is reapproximated. In large movements, this may necessitate scoring the periosteum to allow for tension-free closure. The mucosa is then closed in a water-tight manner, utilizing a horizontal mattress suture. Elastoplast or other materials are helpful in decreasing the dead space and approximating the tissue. If circum-mandibular or intraosseous fixation was utilized, maxillomandibular fixation remains for 6 weeks prior to release. This may be decreased or eliminated if rigid fixation is chosen. Light guiding elastics can be used immediately after release from fixation.

After 3 to 4 weeks, the patient is able to return to active orthodontics. The horizontal movement of the dentoalveolar segment is remarkably stable over time, with minimal movement after 1 year; however, problems with vertical instability have been shown.[2] These problems appear to have a minimal clinical effect, being easily overcome with orthodontics. With the advent of rigid fixation and more attention to bone grafting, this problem of vertical instability can be solved.

REFERENCES

1. Booth DF, Dietz VS, Gainelly AA: Correction of Class II malocclusion by combined sagittal ramus and subapical body osteotomy. J Oral Surg 34:630–634, 1976.
2. Buckley MJ, Turvey TA: Total mandibular subapical osteotomy: A report on long-term stability and surgical technique. Int J Adult Orthodont Orthognath Surg. 3:121–130, 1987.
3. Dietz VS, Gainelly AA, Booth DF: Surgical orthodontics in the treatment of a Class II Division 2 malocclusion: A case report. Am J Orthod 71:309–316, 1977.
4. Epker BN, Fish LC: The surgical-orthodontic correction of mandibular deficiency. Part I. Am J Orthod 84:408–421, 1983.
5. Epker BN, Fish LC: The surgical-orthodontic correction of mandibular deficiency. Part II. Am J Orthod 84:491–507, 1983.
6. Fitzpatrick B: Total osteotomy of the mandibular alveolus in reconstruction of the occlusion. Oral Surg Oral Med Oral Pathol 44:336–346, 1977.

7. Frost DE, Fonseca RJ, Kournik AW: Total subapical osteotomy—a modification of the surgical technique. Int J Adult Orthod Orthognath Surg 1:119–128, 1986.
8. Hohl TA, Epiker BN: Macrogenia: A study of treatment results with surgical recommendations. Oral Surg Oral Med Oral Pathol 41:545–576, 1976.
9. MacIntosh RB: Total mandibular alveolar osteotomy. J Maxillofac Surg 2:210–218, 1974.

8. COMBINING SAGITTAL SPLIT OSTEOTOMY WITH REDUCTION GENIOPLASTY

WILLIAM H. BELL

In most individuals who manifest the skeletal type of deep-bite deformity, it is technically easier to advance the mandible by bilateral sagittal split ramus osteotomies and simultaneous retraction of the chin by reduction genioplasty, accomplished by posterior horizontal sliding osteotomy of the inferior border of the mandible (Fig. 64–110). The practical result of this procedure may compare favorably with the complete subapical osteotomy, yet it is easier and less complicated to execute.

After horizontal osteotomy of the mandibular symphysis, the inferior segment is retracted to decrease the prominence of the chin. With this procedure, it is vital to first simulate the mandibular advancement and the amount of chin retraction necessary to decrease the chin prominence. The genioplasty is accomplished after minimal subperiosteal degloving of the mental protuberance. More predictable changes in the soft tissue chin are achieved by maintaining as much soft tissue attachment as possible to the repositioned symphyseal segment (see Chapter 62). The two surgical procedures are accomplished simultaneously.

The submental-cervical and labiomental regions are frequently unesthetic in patients who manifest a skeletal type of Class II deep bite and deep labiomental fold. Such patients typically have a retropositioned mandible, submental lipodystrophy, inferiorly positioned hyoid bone, parallel facial planes, and decreased lower anterior facial height. When their mandible is postured forward into a simulated Class I occlusion, they frequently manifest excessive prominence of their soft tissue pogonion and a deep labiomental fold. Because restoration of normal

FIGURE 64–110. SURGICAL AND ORTHODONTIC TREATMENTS OF SKELETAL DEEP-BITE DEFORMITY. Esthetic nasolabial proportions, repositioned mandible and chin stabilized with position screws and plates, everted lower lip, deep labiomental fold, retropositioned mandible, and Class II deep bite malocclusion. *A*, Arrows indicate planned directional movements of mandible and chin. *B*, Mandible and chin fixed in planned relationship after surgical advancement of the mandible and reduction genioplasty.

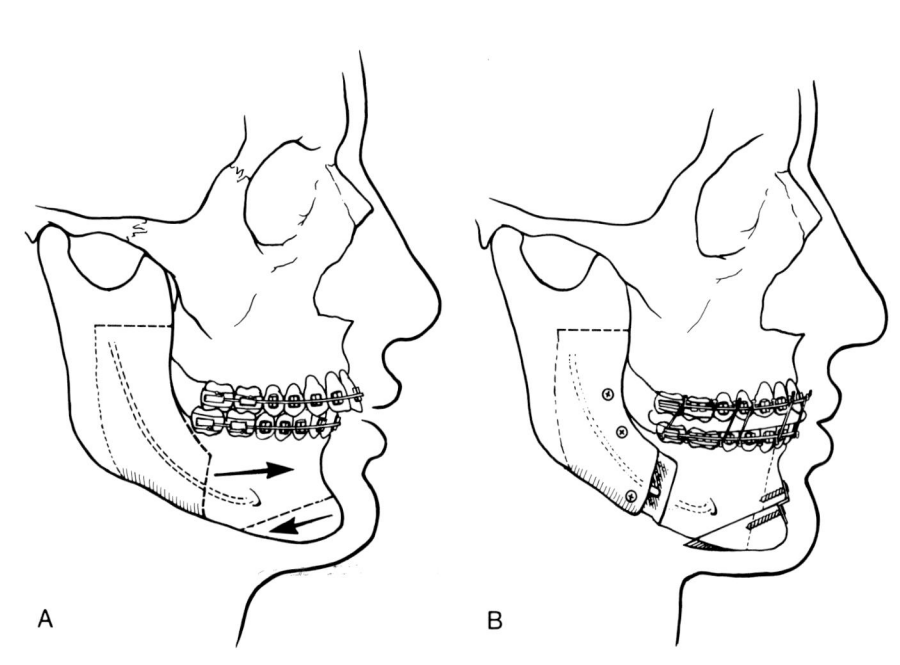

2504 / VII — ORTHOGNATHIC SURGERY

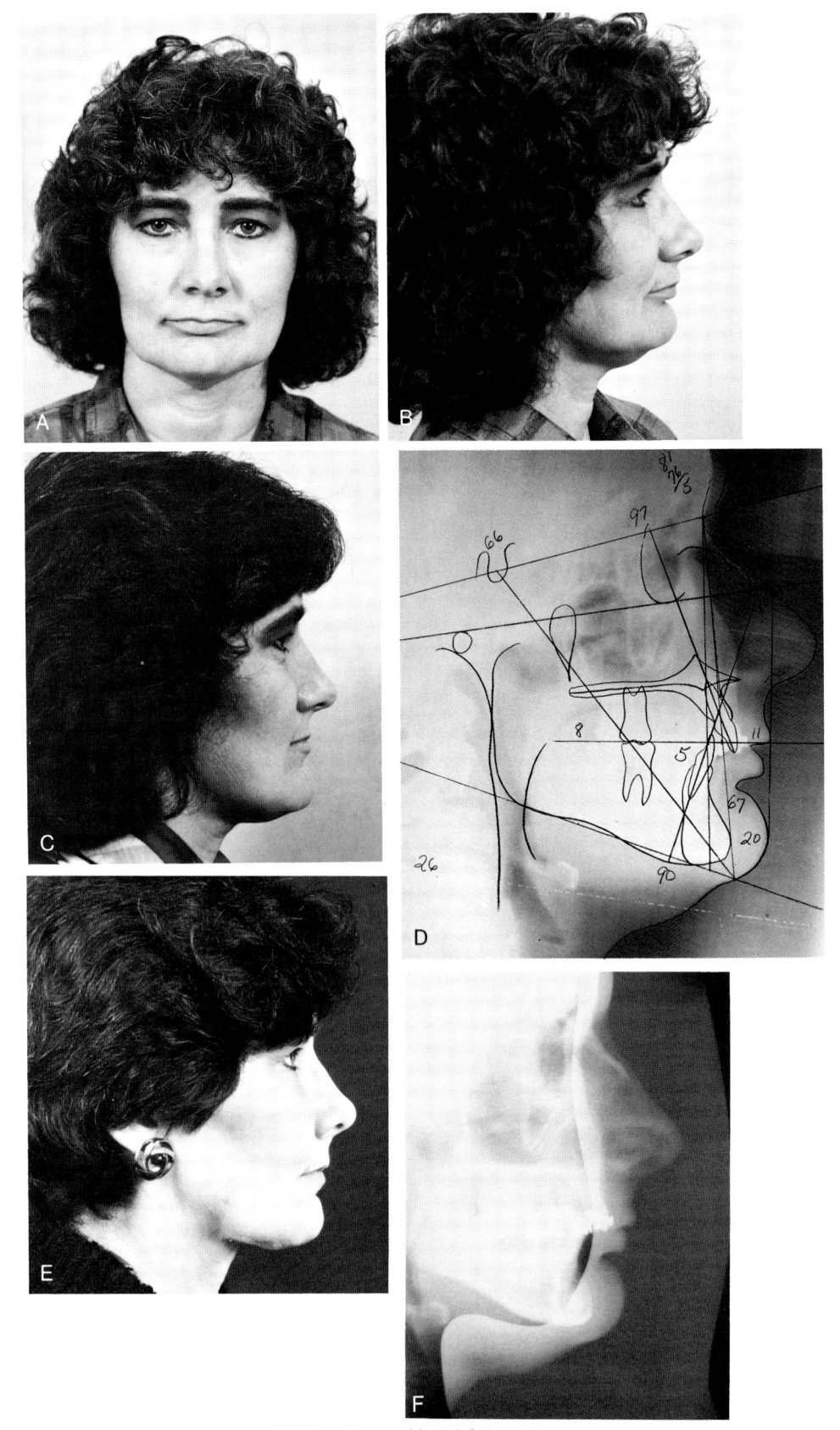

FIGURE 64–111 *See opposite page for legend*

chin–submental-cervical morphology is essential for optimal facial esthetics, mandibular advancement, reduction and/or interpositional genioplasty, submental lipectomy, and Le Fort I osteotomy with interpositional bone graft or bone substitute may all have a very positive effect on the submental-cervical and labiomental esthetics. When submental liposis is present, it can be removed by submental lipectomy or suction lipectomy at the time of mandibular advancement and genioplasty. When the submental-cervical contour deformity is caused by aging cutaneous tissue, however, rhytidectomy may be indicated.

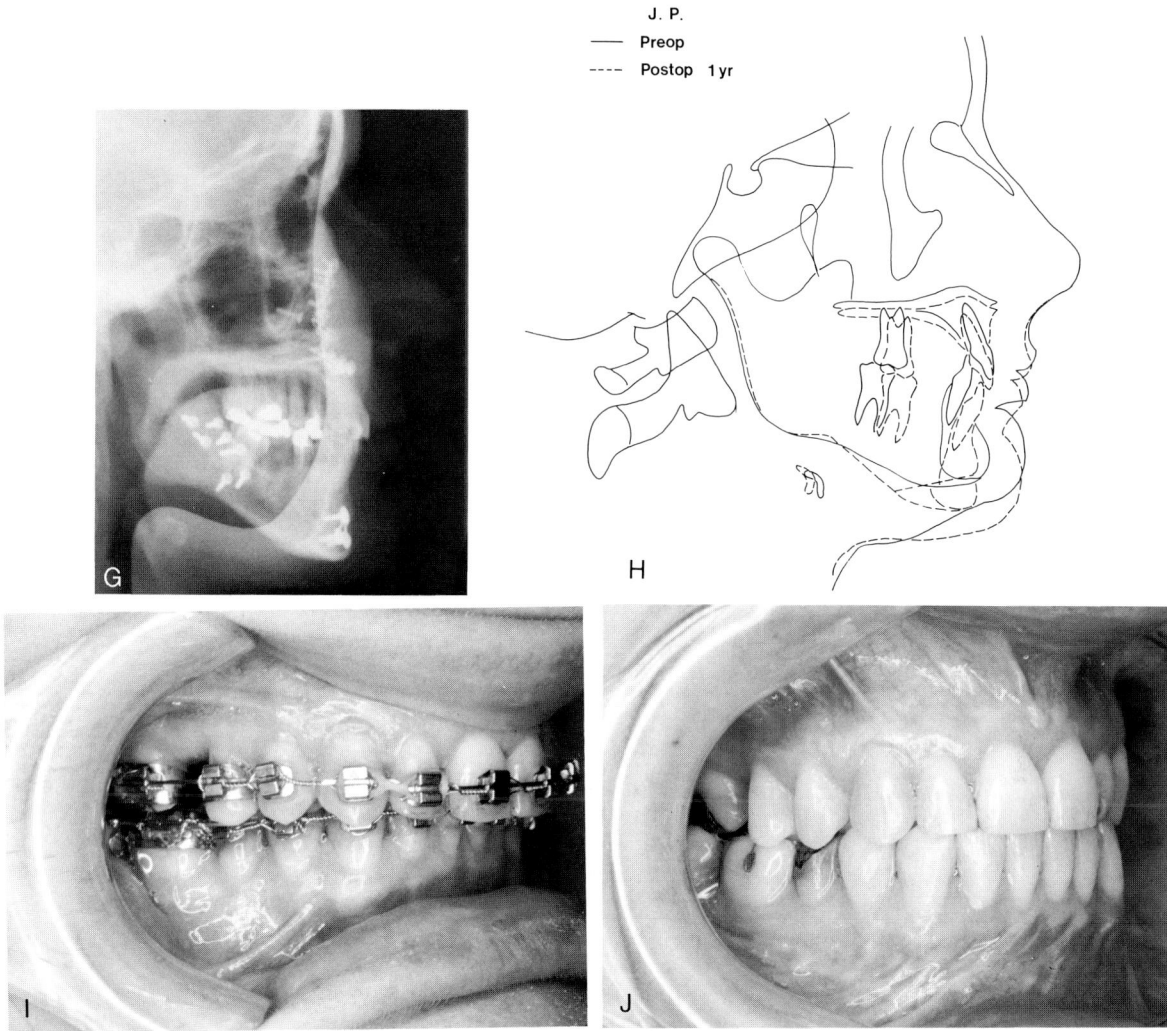

FIGURE 64–111. TREATMENT OF 35-YEAR-OLD WOMAN WITH SEVERE CLASS II DEEP-BITE MALOCCLUSION BY MAXILLARY AND MANDIBULAR OSTEOTOMIES, SUBMENTAL AND SUBMAXILLARY SUCTION LIPECTOMY, REDUCTION GENIOPLASTY, AND ORTHODONTICS. *A* and *B*, Facial appearance of 35-year-old woman with vertical maxillary deficiency, absolute mandibular deficiency, and unesthetic submental-cervical morphology before surgery. Facial appearance with simulated mandibular advancement (mandible postured forward to Class I occlusion) *(C)*; This clinical simulation, correlated with parallel cephalometric prediction studies *(D)*, indicated that the soft tissue pogonion was excessively prominent and the submental-cervical morphology was unesthetic when the mandible was advanced. These studies indicated the need for reduction genioplasty (5 mm) and suction lipectomy of the submental and submaxillary areas, which became more unesthetic when the chin prominence was reduced. *E*, Facial appearance after surgical procedures illustrated in Figure 64–106, which were combined with Le Fort I osteotomy and interpositional bone graft, as well as submental and submaxillary suction lipectomy. *F*, Cephalometric radiograph exposed with mandible in centric relation and lips in repose showing Class II deep bite, mandibular deficiency and unesthetic submental-cervical morphology. *G*, Postoperative lateral cephalogram showing balanced anteroposterior and vertical facial proportions and esthetic submental-cervical morphology. The repositioned maxilla, mandible, and chin were stabilized with bone plates and screws. *H*, Composite cephalometric tracings before *(solid line)* and after *(dashed line)* Le Fort I osteotomy and interpositional bone graft, mandibular advancement, reduction genioplasty, and submental and submaxillary suction lipectomy. *I*, Presurgical Class II deep-bite malocclusion after presurgical orthodontic treatment accomplished without extraction of teeth. *J*, Postoperative Class I occlusion after surgical and orthodontic treatment. Residual jowl appearance and lax skin will be treated in the future by rhytidectomy.

The treatment of a patient who manifests a Class II deep-bite malocclusion, decreased lower anterior facial height, and poor submental-cervical esthetics is described and illustrated in Figure 64-111. With the use of skeletal fixation, the efficiency of orthodontic treatment may be markedly increased. In such cases, postsurgical orthodontic leveling is generally started within 3 weeks after surgery.

9. MANDIBULAR DEFICIENCY SECONDARY TO JUVENILE RHEUMATOID ARTHRITIS

DOUGLAS P. SINN

Juvenile rheumatoid arthritis (JRA) is a chronic disease of childhood that affects more than 200,000 children in the United States—three times as many girls as boys. The acute febrile and polyarticular forms of the disease tend to involve the temporomandibular joints in approximately 10 per cent of patients with these types of onset. The disease is characterized by chronic synovitis at the articulation, resulting in the proliferation of epithelium, increased synovial fluid, and the presence of inflammatory infiltrate. The articular cavity becomes full and distended, periarticular inflammation is present, and blood supply to the area is increased.[2] The articular portion of the temporomandibular joint is frequently affected as a consequence of progressive damage to the cartilage and subchondral bone. Such pathologic changes in the articular surfaces frequently affect the growth and development of the mandible, alter its morphology and size, and impair dentofacial function and appearance.

The etiology of JRA is unknown at present. Infection, autoimmunity, heredity, and psychological stresses, however, have been implicated as possible contributing factors. Although the clinical course of JRA is unpredictable and varied, the prognosis is usually favorable when early diagnosis is made and proper treatment is instituted.[1]

Therapeutic exercises, prosthetic appliances, anti-inflammatory drugs, relief of myospasm by injection of local anesthetics, intra-articular injection of corticosteroids, occlusal adjustment, orthognathic surgery, and orthodontic treatment all play important roles in the treatment and rehabilitation of the child with JRA. Properly planned and executed maxillary and mandibular surgery combined with orthodontic treatment is necessary to manage mandibular deficiency and open bite deformities that children with this disorder so frequently manifest.

An example of treating mandibular deficiency in a patient with JRA is found in the following case study.

CASE: E.S. (Fig. 64-112)

E.S., a 20-year-old woman with rheumatoid arthritis, presented for evaluation of her dentofacial deformity in January 1975. Clinical, cephalometric, and radiographic studies supported the diagnosis of mandibular deficiency and vertical maxillary excess. The following problem list and treatment plan evolved.

PROBLEM LIST

Esthetics

FRONTAL. There was excessive exposure of the maxillary teeth when the patient was in repose and when she was smiling; an 8-mm interlabial gap was seen.

PROFILE. Features of the profile included mandibular deficiency and contour-deficient chin, everted lower lip, prominent nose, and a marginal nasolabial angle.

Cephalometric Analysis

1. High mandibular plane angle: GoGn-SN, 60°.
2. Maxillary and mandibular deficiency.

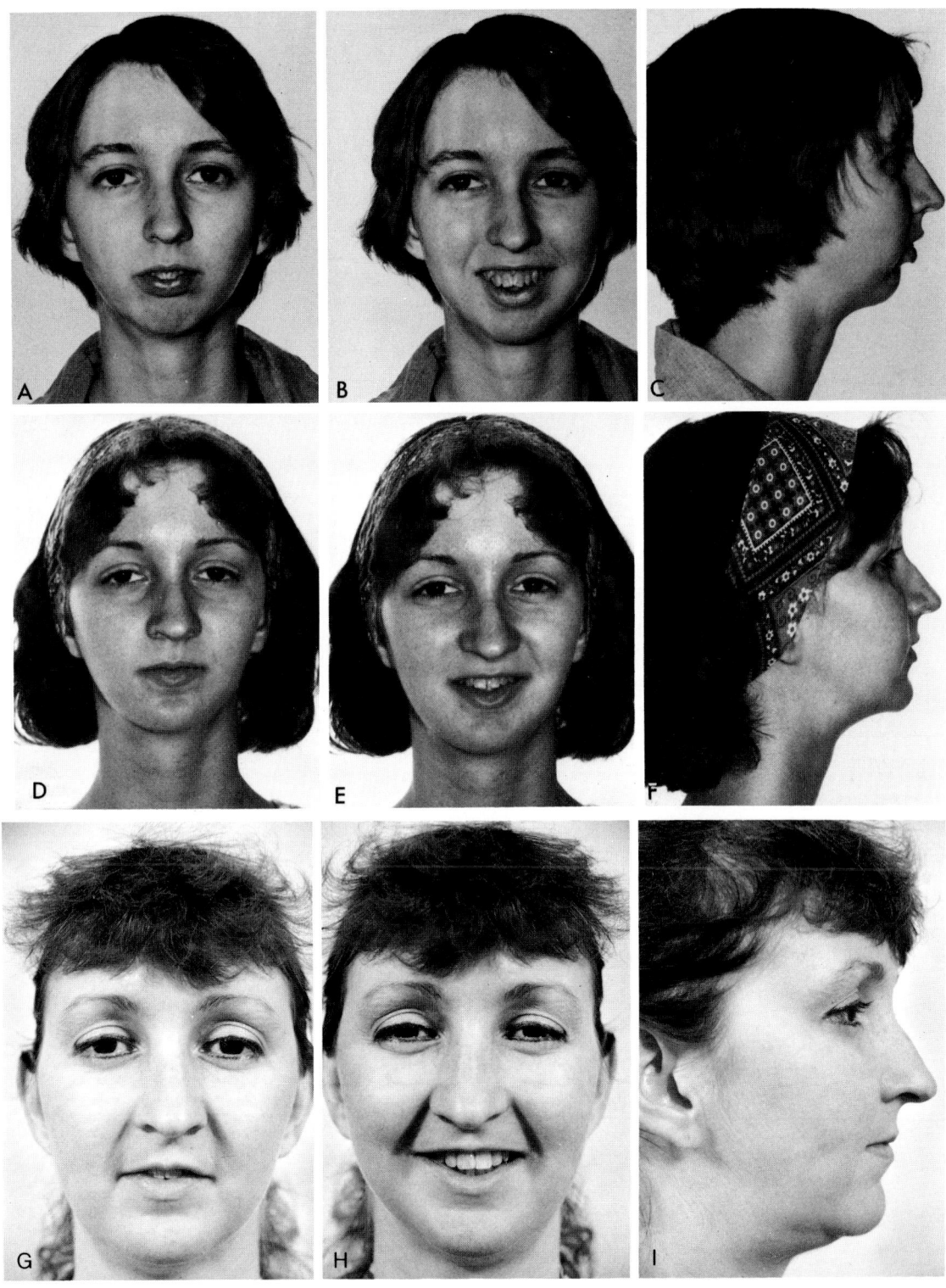

FIGURE 64–112. Facial appearance of rheumatoid arthritis patient before treatment *(A–C)* and shortly after treatment *(D–F)*. *G–I*, Facial appearance of patient 15 years after treatment.

Illustration continued on following page

2508 / VII — ORTHOGNATHIC SURGERY

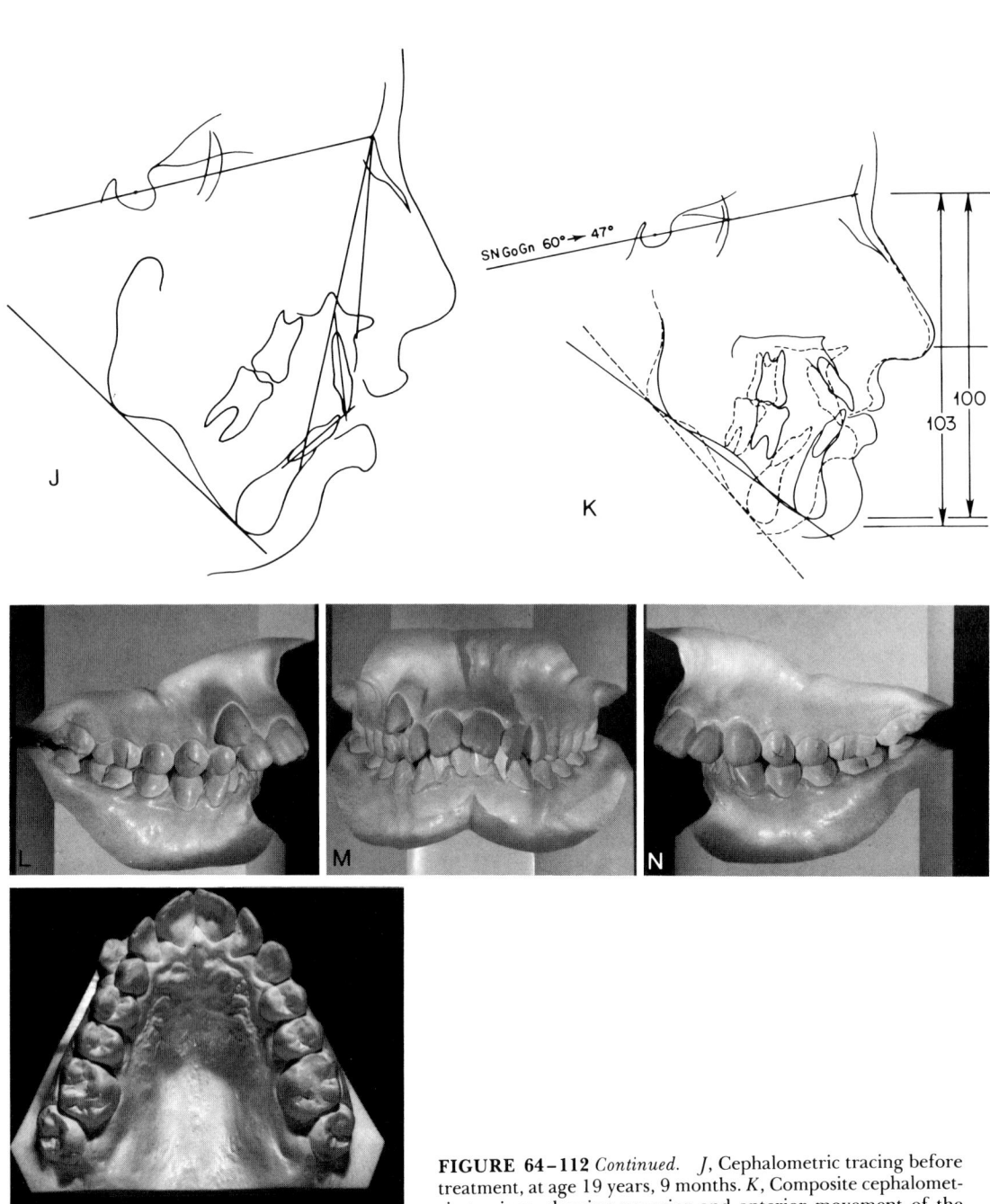

FIGURE 64–112 *Continued.* *J*, Cephalometric tracing before treatment, at age 19 years, 9 months. *K*, Composite cephalometric tracings, showing superior and anterior movement of the maxilla and mandibular advancement to a Class I occlusion. After 15 months of treatment, at age 21 years *(broken line)* and at age 21 years, 10 months *(solid line)*. *L–O*, Preoperative occlusion.

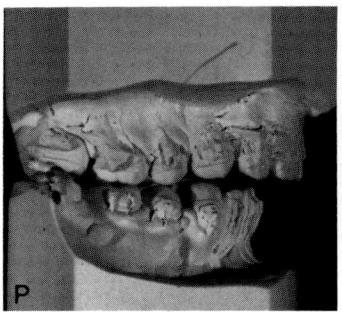

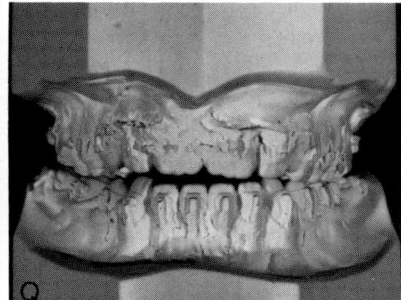

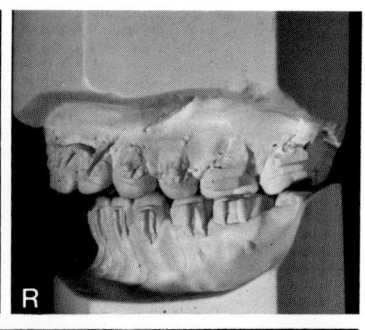

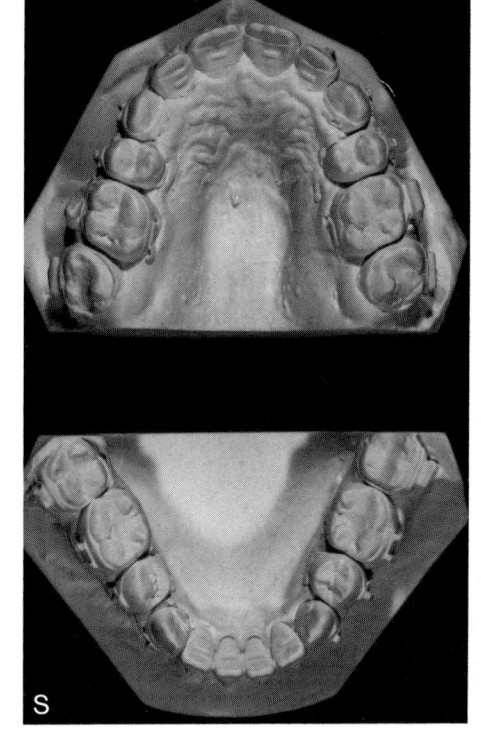

FIGURE 64–112 *Continued.* *P–S*, Presurgical occlusion after 15 months of orthodontic treatment.

Illustration continued on following page

Occlusal Analysis

DENTAL ARCH FORM. The maxillary arch was constricted and crowded.

DENTAL ALIGNMENT. Crowding of the maxillary and mandibular arches and a blocked-out maxillary right canine tooth were present.

DENTAL OCCLUSION. A Class II canine-and-molar relationship was seen.

TREATMENT PLAN

Orthodontics

PRESURGICAL

1. Extract the maxillary and mandibular first premolars to facilitate alignment of the anterior teeth.
2. Retract and align the anterior teeth by means of full edgewise orthodontic appliances.
3. Level and align the mandibular arch and relieve crowding by utilizing premolar extraction spaces.
4. Coordinate dental arches so that maxillary and mandibular arches can be harmonized by surgery.

POSTSURGICAL. The occlusion must be stabilized and detailed following release of maxillomandibular fixation.

2510 / VII — ORTHOGNATHIC SURGERY

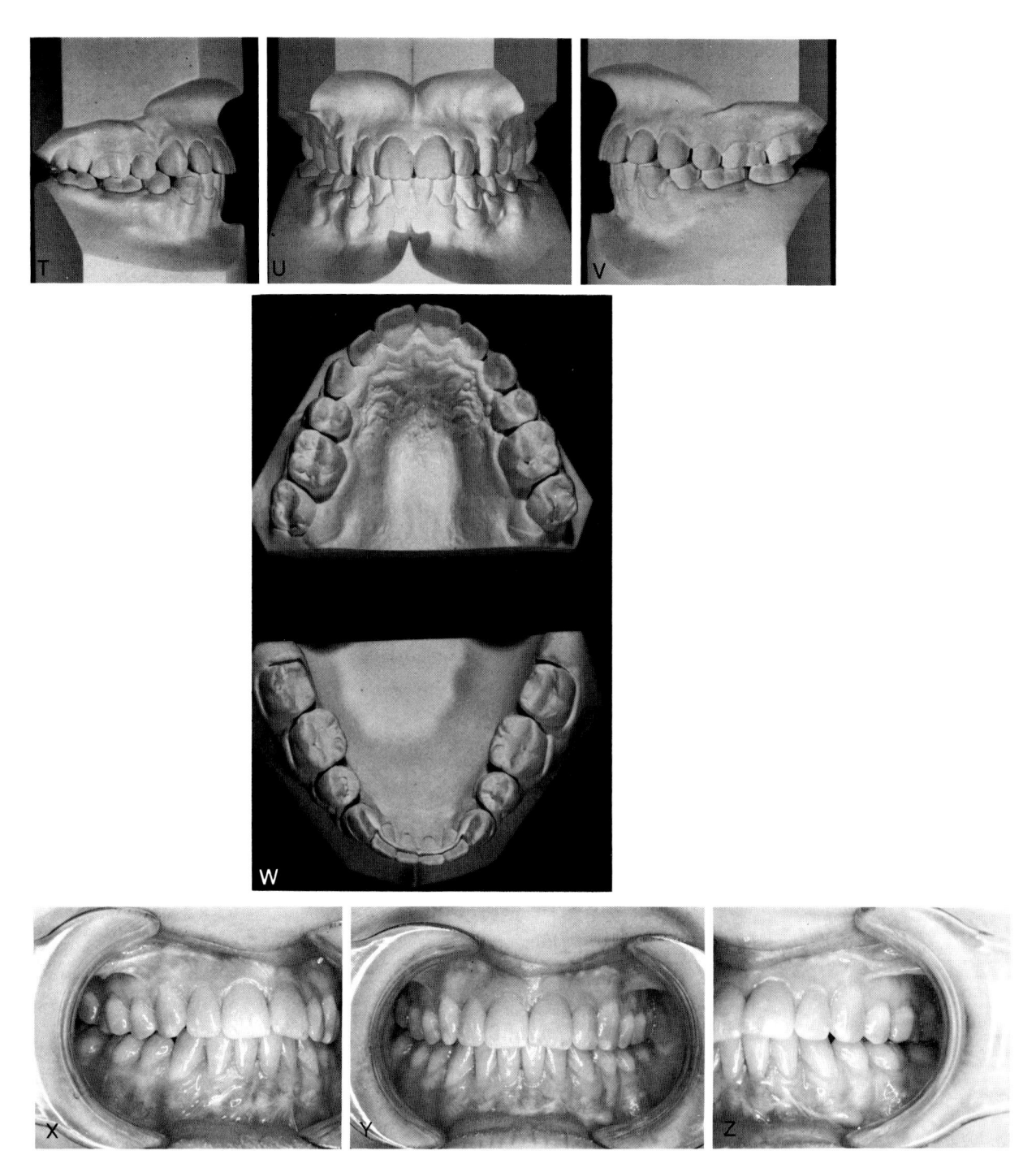

FIGURE 64–112 *Continued.* T–W, Post-treatment occlusion. X–Z, Occlusion 15 years after treatment. (A–F and J–W are from Bell WH, Proffit WR, White RP Jr: Surgical Correction of Dentofacial Deformities. Vol I. Philadelphia, WB Saunders Company, 1980, pp 834–838; with permission.)

Surgical

1. Superior and anterior repositioning of the maxilla by Le Fort I osteotomy to (a) increase the prominence of the deficient upper lip and decrease the nasolabial angle; (b) reduce the interlabial gap and improve the tooth-to-lip relationship; (c) shorten the lower anterior face; and (d) allow autorotational movement of the mandible.

2. Surgical advancement of the mandible by sagittal split ramus osteotomies to (a) reposition the mandible into a Class I molar-and-canine relationship and (b) advance the retropositioned mandible and chin.

FOLLOW-UP

Subjective

The patient had an uncomplicated course with early clinical union of the maxillary and mandibular osteotomy sites. There were no inferior alveolar paresthesias after the ramus osteotomies. Maxillomandibular fixation was maintained for 6 weeks.

Objective

The patient presented with a dentofacial deformity typically seen in patients who have JRA. Radiographic examination revealed exceedingly short mandibular rami and associated hypoplastic and deformed condyles. Aberrant growth had created a skeletal deformity similar to that seen in patients with Class II mandibular deficiency.

The presurgical orthodontic treatment was accomplished within 15 months.

The surgical plan included Le Fort I maxillary osteotomy to intrude the maxilla approximately 3 mm and advance the maxilla 6 mm. The mandible was advanced into a Class I molar-and-canine relationship by sagittal split ramus osteotomies. There were no postoperative complications, and the patient tolerated the surgery without difficulty. Ten months postoperatively, there was relatively little positional change of the mandible and virtually no movement of the maxilla. The interocclusal relationship remained stable.

There was good esthetic balance between the middle and lower thirds of the face. The anterior lower facial height was shortened 3 mm. Lip incompetence had been corrected. Esthetic facial proportions and occlusal stability have been maintained over a 15-year period of follow-up.

REFERENCES

1. Schaller J: Juvenile rheumatoid arthritis. Postgrad Med 61:177–184, 1977.
2. Turpin DL, West RA: Juvenile rheumatoid arthritis: A case report of surgical-orthodontic treatment. Am J Orthod 73:312–320, 1978.

10. LATERAL FACIAL RECONSTRUCTION

CESAR GUERRERO

Mandibular Ramus Reduction

The clinical problem of either symmetric or asymmetric transverse facial excess below the level of the zygomatic arches is a challenge in the esthetic management of some patients. This could be due to masseteric hypertrophy or unilateral masseteric hypoplasia, quadrangular mandibular shape, or mandibular exostosis. Historically, the problem has been managed by a masseter muscle partial resection, with or without the mandibular angle, through an intraoral, or extraoral approach. We have classified the problem as minor (5 mm) or major (5 to 10 mm) and have treated the minor hypertrophy by means of mandibular ramus lateral cortex removal and the major cases by an additional masseter muscle resection.

2512 / VII — ORTHOGNATHIC SURGERY

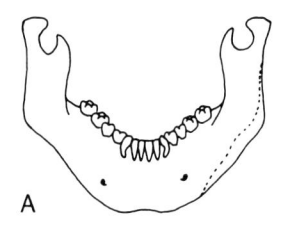

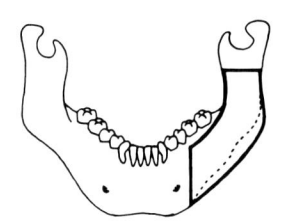

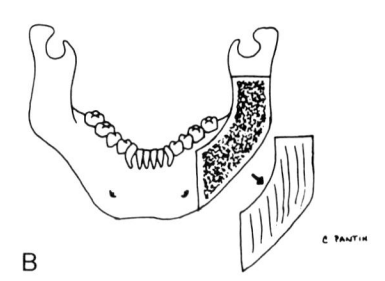

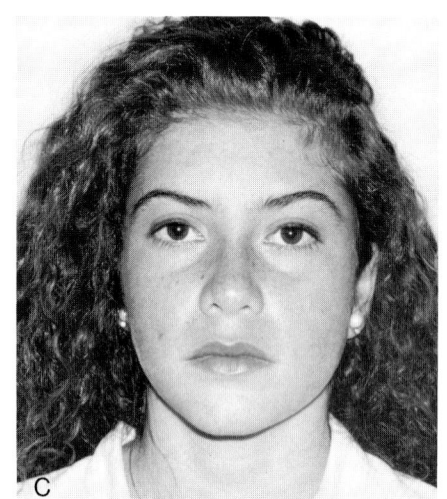

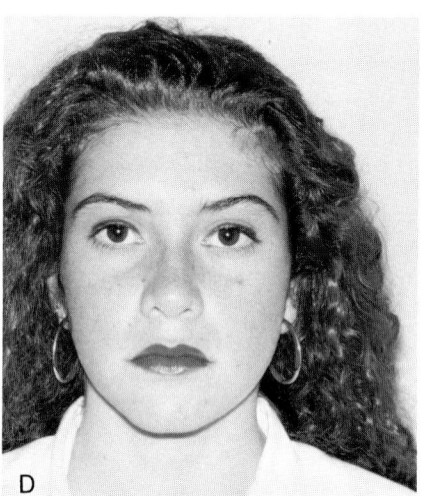

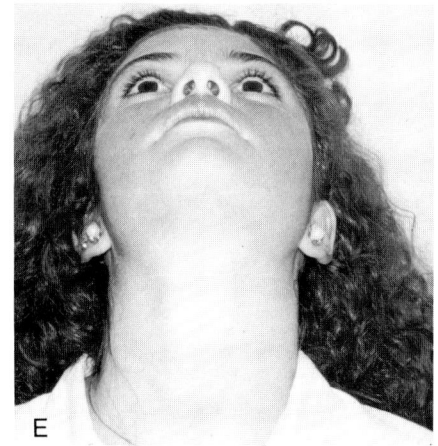

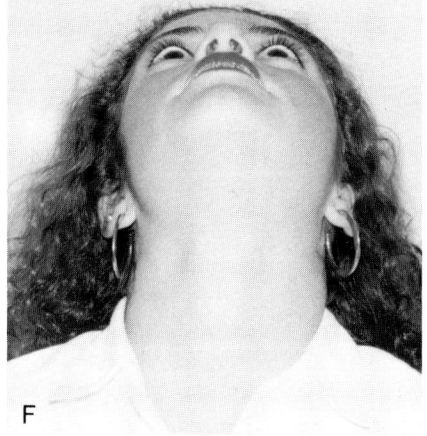

FIGURE 64–113. Narrowing the Mandibular Ramus by Sagittal Split Ramus Osteotomy and Resection of the Lateral Cortex of the Ramus. *A* and *B*, Surgical technique. *C* and *D*, Preoperative and postoperative frontal facial views. *E* and *F*, Preoperative and postoperative facial views. *G*, Preoperative frontal radiograph. *H*, Postoperative frontal radiograph showing where the lateral cortical bone was resected. *I*, Postoperative symmetric frontal cephalometric tracing.

V. Z.

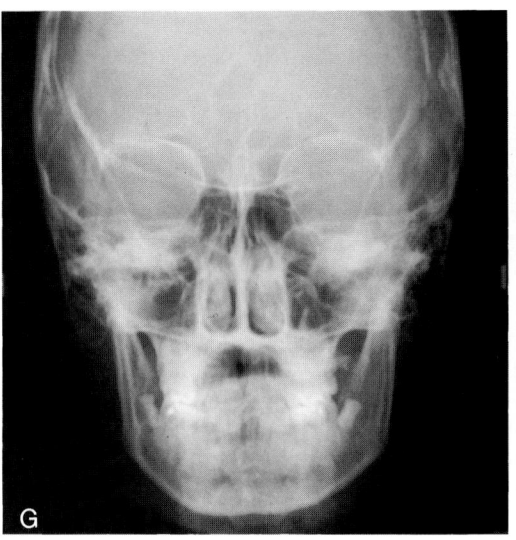

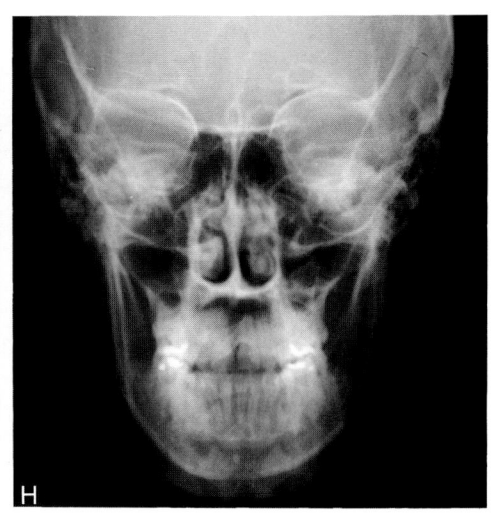

FIGURE 64–113 *Continued.*

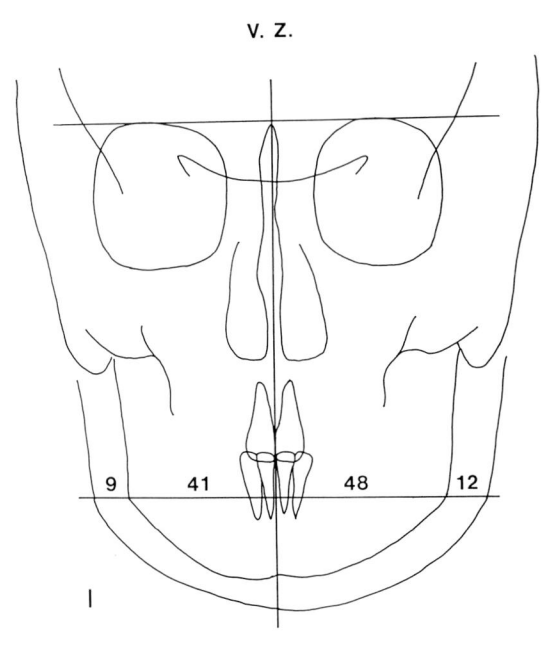

SURGICAL TECHNIQUE (Figs. 64–113 and 64–114)

A conventional sagittal split osteotomy incision is made with an electrocautery knife, the soft tissue is reflected superiorly, and a Kocher clamp is fixed to the base of the coronoid process. A subperiosteal dissection of the entire lateral aspect of the ramus is immediately performed up to the base of the condylar neck and mandibular coronoid process. A horizontal osteotomy is made with a No. 703 bur on a straight handpiece, back to the posterior border just above the antilingula. A vertical cut along the anterior border of the ramus is continued into the cortical bone, but deepened only into the cancellous bone. The vertical osteotomy in the mandibular body is individualized according to the deformity; some patients require removal of only the ramus, but others need an osteotomy forward to the premolar area. This osteotomy placement varies on the basis of the clinical findings and the posteroanterior radiograph; also, the prediction indicates the amount of bone and muscle to be removed at the time of surgery.

The osteotomy is completed at the inferior border of the mandible. Two osteotomes are positioned against the lateral cortex to avoid injury to the inferior alveolar nerve. Osteotomes are positioned to the posterior border and inferiorly to the lower border of the ramus.

Once most of the osteotomy is completed, pressure against the cortex is made laterally, and the fragment displaces laterally and is removed. A large, round bur is used to smooth the superior and anterior margins of the osteotomy. The angle can be shaped and reduced as needed. The area is well irrigated, and meticulous hemostasis is obtained before closure of the wounds.

Now attention is directed to the masseter muscle; the entire internal one half of the masseter muscle can be removed without fear of injuring the marginal mandibular branch of the facial nerve. While the lateral cortex is being resected, this removal of the muscle is done vertically and carefully to remove uniform slices to correct the transverse deformity uniformly and with as little postoperative masseteric contraction as possible to avoid permanent mandibular hypomobility and to decrease the neuromuscular rehabilitation period. Two complications may arise. One is a nerve injury (as in any sagittal split osteotomy), which can be avoided by careful inclination of the osteotomes against the lateral cortex and slow mobilization of the bone fragment laterally; if the nerve is between the two fragments, a curette is used to detach the nerve, and once it is totally free, the bone segment is excised. The second complication is a mandibular condylar neck fracture, which can occur when the osteotomy is made too high, into the cortical bone area; also, the lateral fracture must be done under direct visualization, slowly and progressively, to avoid this complication.

When the osteotomy is performed without the muscle resection, the postoperative period is very short, with minimal discomfort, the facial edema is minor, and the normal mouth opening is regained efficiently in a relatively short period of time.

Once the periosteum is transected to approach the muscle, there is resultant marked facial edema and muscle contractures; *prolonged,* aggressive mandibular neuromuscular rehabilitation is therefore mandatory (see Chapters 45 and 46).

Mandibular Ramus Augmentation (Fig. 64–115)

A common situation in facial asymmetries secondary to unilateral growth problems is the need for unilateral ramus augmentation; this problem can be approached by the use of hydroxyapatite interpositional blocks or bone grafts combined with mandibular ramus osteotomy. This technique is individualized for every patient on the basis of posteroanterior cephalometric prediction tracings; according to the goals of treatment, one or two hydroxyapatite blocks or bone grafts are used to widen the mandibular ramus cortex. Care must be taken not to

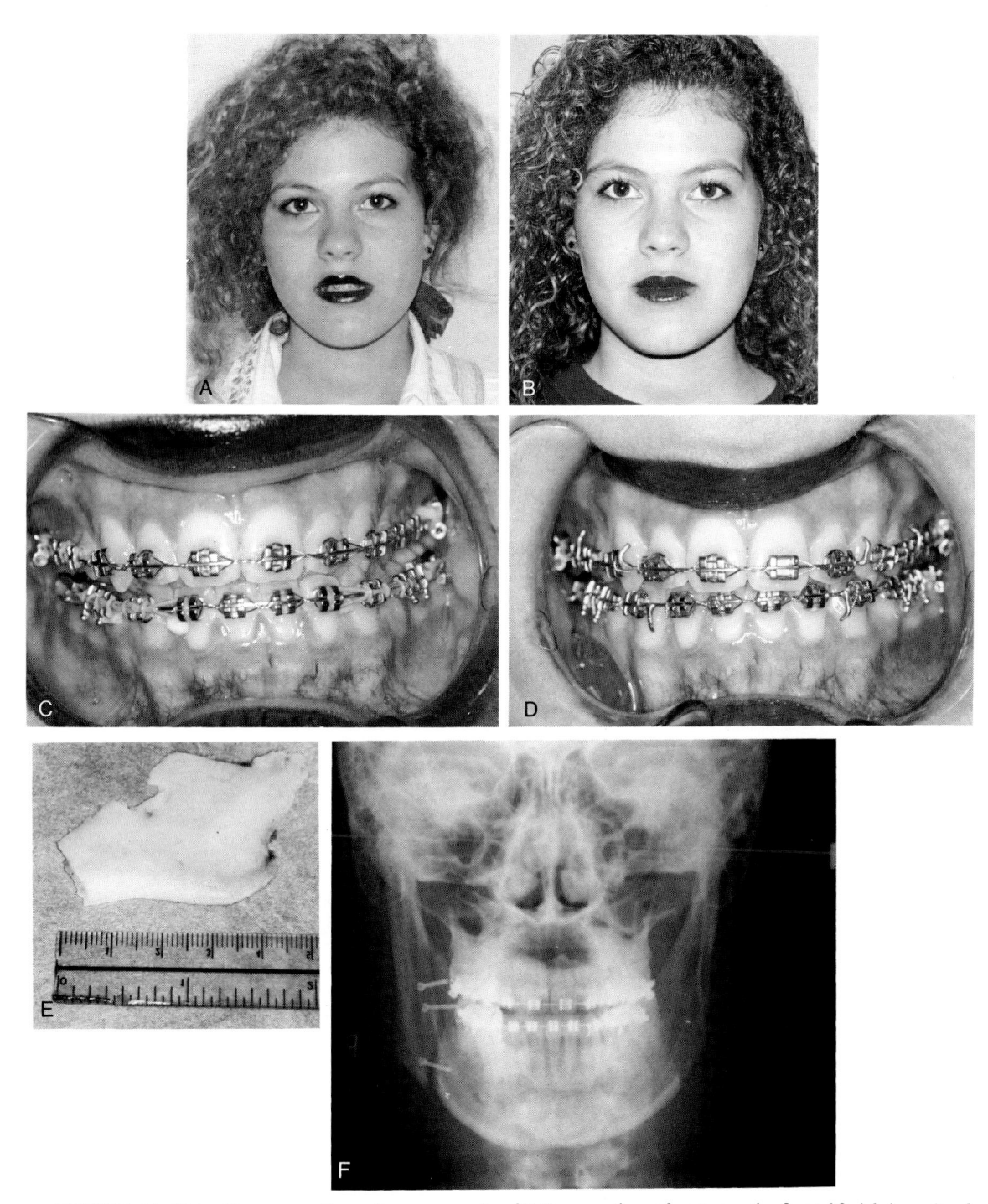

FIGURE 64–114. MANDIBULAR RAMUS REDUCTION. *A* and *B*, Preoperative and postoperative frontal facial views. *C* and *D*, Preoperative and postoperative frontal views of occlusion. *E*, Resected lateral ramus segment. *F*, Postoperative radiograph. Mandibular symmetry was achieved by unilateral sagittal split ramus osteotomy; note the contralateral ramus, where the lateral cortical plate was resected.

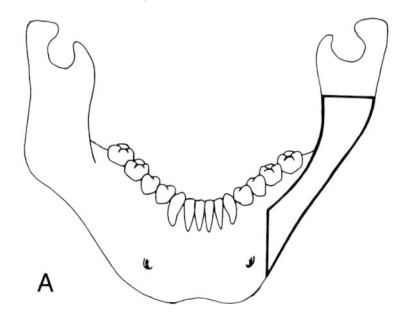

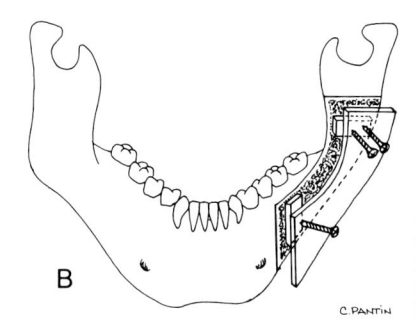

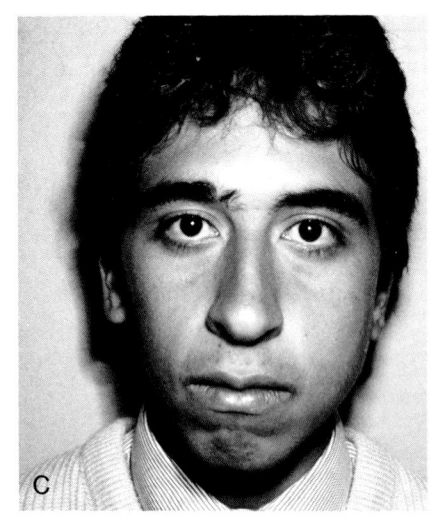

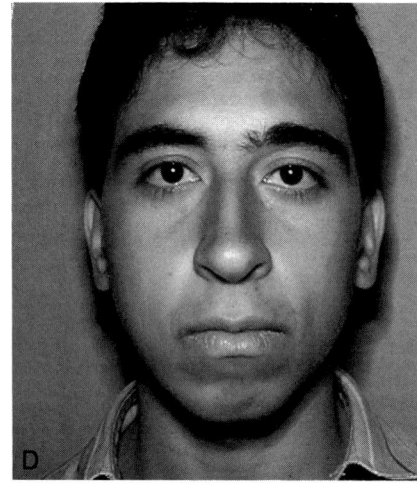

FIGURE 64–115. MANDIBULAR RAMUS AUGMENTATION BY SAGITTAL SPLIT RAMUS OSTEOTOMIES AND INTERPOSITIONAL BONE GRAFTS OR IMPLANTS. *A* and *B,* The outer cortical plate of the mandibular ramus and body is mobilized with a reciprocating saw and osteotomes. The traditional sagittal splitting technique of Obwegeser is used to section the entire *lateral* aspect of the ramus at a safe level below the sigmoid notch (5 mm). By careful subperiosteal tunneling and use of channel retractors, the lateral aspect of the ramus can be sectioned and remain vascularized by an attached muscle pedicle. The bone cut may be extended anteriorly, if necessary, to the mental foramen area. *C,* Preoperative facial photograph before sagittal split ramus osteotomies as described above. *D,* Postoperative symmetric facial appearance after increasing the ramus width by sagittal splitting procedure and interpositional hydroxyapatite.

excessively detach the musculoperiosteum from the lateral cortex. By performing the osteotomies through tunnels so that the fragment will not behave like a free bone graft but like a pedicled musculoperiosteal bone flap, avascular necrosis can be avoided, and long-term stability of the laterally positioned musculoskeletal segments is probable.

11. MANDIBULAR ADVANCEMENT IN CHILDREN: SPECIAL CONSIDERATIONS

WILLIAM H. BELL

Certain precautions must be taken when the sagittal split osteotomy technique is used in children because of their individual anatomic characteristics. Because the lingual and inferior alveolar foramina are located in a more superior and posterior position in the ramus of children than in the ramus of adult patients, the lingual horizontal osteotomy must be positioned precisely and executed carefully. The sagittal bone incision should be positioned as far laterally as possible at the junction of the lateral cortical plate and cancellous bone to obviate injury to the unerupted second molar teeth and to minimize injury to the inferior alveolar nerve (see "Anatomic Considerations in Mandibular Ramus Osteotomies," earlier in Chapter 64). Because of the propensity for "greenstick" fracturing of the inferior border of the mandible in children, it is useful to definitively section the inferior border of the mandible as described in other sections of Chapter 64. In this area, the molar teeth are located immediately subjacent to the lateral cortical plate.

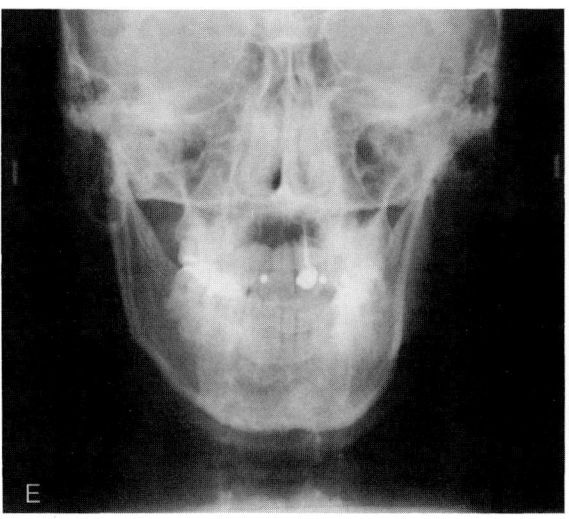

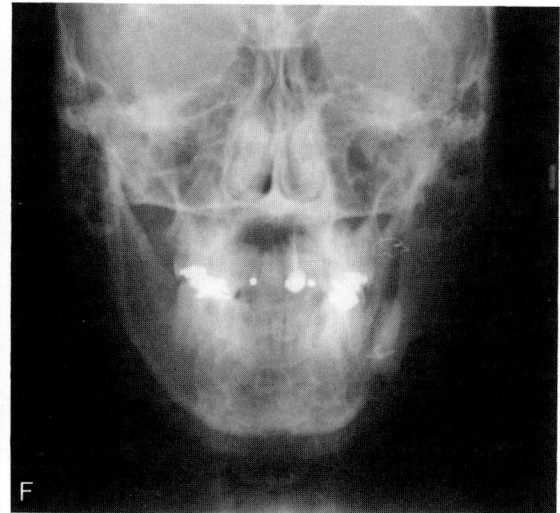

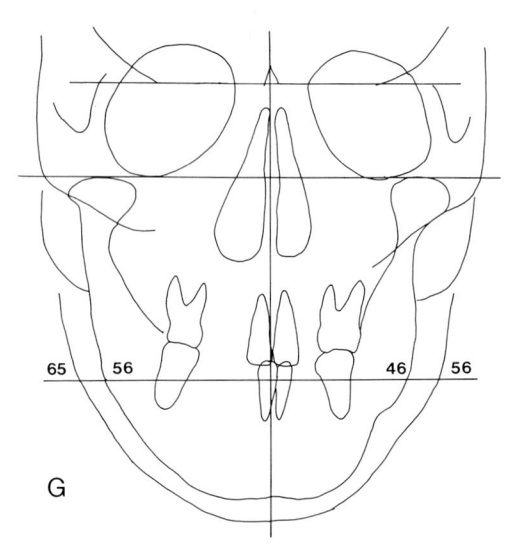

FIGURE 64–115 *Continued.* E, Preoperative frontal cephalogram showing facial asymmetry. F, Postoperative frontal cephalogram showing facial symmetry. G, Facial measurements (millimeters) of the preoperative facial asymmetry.

After the split is carefully accomplished with finely tapered spatula osteotomes, the incompletely developed third molar teeth can be curetted from the distal segment, with the proximal and distal segments separated. The reciprocating saw handpiece and blade, which is specially designed to section the inferior border of the mandible, should be oriented so that the blade will cut maximally up into the bone. The blade is oriented parallel to the inferior border of the mandible and should bisect the buccal-lingual thickness of the inferior border cortex. Sectioning the mandible in this manner facilitates splitting of the mandible and minimizes the possibility of "greenstick" fracturing of the inferior border of the mandible.

INDEX

Note: Page numbers in *italics* indicate illustrations; those followed by t indicate tables.

A alpha fibers, 1085
A beta fibers, 1085
A delta fibers, 1085–1086
A point, measurement of, 183, *183*, 188, *189*, 197, *197*
Abrasion arthroplasty, in chondromalacia, 476–477
Achondroplasia, sleep apnea and, 2037–2038
Acne, in Apert syndrome, 1896
Acquired immunodeficiency syndrome, transmission of, via allogenic graft, 1455–1456
Acrocephalosyndactyly. See *Apert syndrome*.
Adams' suspension, midfacial deformity after, *1050*, *1052*
Adenoidectomy, for speech problems, 1719
Adhesions, arthroscopic diagnosis of, 614, *614*, 651–652
  arthroscopic treatment of, 617–620, *617–620*
  orbital, 1070
  in cicatricial ectropion, 1071–1072
Adhesive capsulitis, arthroscopy of, 610–611, *611*
Adipose tissue, buccal, 379
  nasolabial fold, 380
  submental and submandibular, 377–379, *378*
  suctioning of. See *Lipectomy*.
Adolescent, growth of, biologic regulation of, 23–24, *24*
  orthognathic surgery in, craniofacial growth after, 38–44
    maxillary growth after, 1933–1954. See also *Maxillary growth, postoperative*.
  physical maturity of, indicators of, 27–38
Affricative sounds, 1689, 1689t, *1690*
Aging, attractiveness and, 1439–1442
  of baby boomers, 1440–1441
Aging face syndrome, 1427–1437
  case studies of, 1427–1430, *1428–1431*
  lip support in, 1428
  nasolabial esthetics in, 1428
  preoperative evaluation in, 1428–1429
  treatment planning for, 1428–1429
  treatment sequencing for, 1429–1430
  vertical face dimension in, 1428
Airway, nasopharyngeal, placement of, 143
  postoperative, 116, 151
Airway evaluation, preanesthetic, 130–132, *131*

Airway management, after quadrangular Le Fort II osteotomy, 1820
  in craniofacial surgery, 1841, 1891–1892, 1897
Airway obstruction, in sleep apnea, 2024–2028. See also *Sleep apnea*.
  postoperative, 115–117, 151
Ala, 287, *287*–288, *288*, 324, 2174, *2175*, *2176*
Alar base, dimension of, control of, during maxillary osteotomy, 311, 311–312, *312*
  widening of, after maxillary advancement, 297–300, *298*, *299*
Alar cartilage, *291*, 291–292, 2175, *2176*
Alar-facial junction, 288, *288*
Alar flare, 104
Alar groove, 2174, *2175*
Alar necrosis, intubation-related, 113–114
Algesimeter, 1099, *1099*
Allodynia, 1094, 1102
  evaluation of, nerve block in, 1100–1101
  pain in, 1096
Allogeneic graft, bone, 849–850, 1452–1456. See also *Bone graft*.
  cartilage, 1455
    cryopreserved, 1453, 1455–1456
    in ankylosis repair, 1522–1523, *1523*
  dura, 1454–1455
  safety of, 1455–1456
Alloplastic implant. See *Implants, alloplastic*.
Alpine anesthesia, 134
Alveolar bone height, restoration of, *1462*, 1463–1464
Alveolar crest, location of, 245, *245*
Alveolar fistula, closure of, speech and, 1722
Alveolar nerve, 1081. See also *Trigeminal nerve*.
  injury of, 997
    in Vitek-Kent prosthesis placement, 788, 789t
  microsurgical repair of, 1112–1117, *1113*–*1116*
Alveolar ridge, augmentation of. See also *Dental implants*.
  speech and, 1722, *1722*
  with bone graft, 1131–1132, 1191–1213, 1273, *1311*–*1316*, 1313, *1461*, 1463–1464. See also *Bone graft*.
  with hydroxyapatite particles, 1271, 1287–1288, *1288*, 1316, 1322, *1322*–*1324*, 1410, *1410*

Alveolar ridge *(Continued)*
  with transmandibular implant. See *Transmandibular implant*.
Ambulatory arthroscopic evaluation, 605
Ambulatory surgery, 109
  postoperative care after, 117
Amitriptyline, for post-traumatic pain, in nerve injury, 1106
Amputation neuroma, 1090, *1090*
Analgesia, definition of, 1102
  for post-traumatic neuralgia, 1106
  in interdisciplinary dentofacial treatment, 1745–1746
  postoperative, 120, 151
    after Vitek-Kent prosthesis placement, 785–786
Anatomic articulator. See *Articulator*.
Anatomic crown length, insufficient, 241, *242*, *243*
  measurement of, 239, *239*
Anatomic model. See *Model* entries.
Andy Gump deformity, *1465*
  mandibular reconstruction in, 1515–1521, *1518*–*1520*
  soft tissue graft for, 1515, *1516*
Anesthesia, 129–152
  alpine, 134
  anesthesia-surgical team positioning in, 148–149, *149*
  awakening and extubation in, 150, *151*
  condylar positioning and, *531*, 531–532, 580, 585–586
  definition of, 1102
  for arthroscopy, 605
  for lipectomy, 383–385
  for temporomandibular joint arthrography, *501*, 501–502
  for Vitek-Kent prosthesis placement, 756, 760
  head and neck evaluation for, 130–132, *131*
  hypotensive, 114–115, 135–137, *136*, *137*
  in diagnostic nerve block, 1100–1101
  in preoperative holding area, 137
  in therapeutic nerve block, 1106
  induction of, 139–140, *140*, *141*
  intraoperative management in, 135–150
  intubation in, 113–114, *114*, 141–145, *142*–*145*. See also *Intubation*.
  maintenance of, 149–150
  monitoring in, 114–115, 137–139, 149–150, 151, *152*
  patient conference for, 129–130, 130t
  patient positioning for, 137, *137*, 139, *139*, *140*

ii / INDEX

Anesthesia (Continued)
  postanesthesia care and, 151, *152*
  preoperative medication for, 132–135
  preoperative preparation for, 129–135
  preoxygenation in, 139–140
  recovery from, 115–116
  respiration rate in, 150
  risk assessment for, 130, 130t
  tube stabilization in, 145–148, *146–148*
  vascular access for, 111
Anesthesia dolorosa, 1093, 1096, 1102
Anesthesiology, endotracheal intubation in, *113*, 113–114
Angina pectoris, preoperative evaluation of, 105
Ankylosis, after Vitek-Kent prosthesis placement, 791–792, *792*
  arthroscopic diagnosis of, 651–652
  arthrotomy for, 668–673. See also *Arthrotomy.*
  condylar, costochondral graft for, 881, *890–893*
    dermal graft for, 927, *928, 943,* 943–944
  of condylar graft, 1520–1521
  postoperative, after costochondral graft, 938–945, *940–943*
    magnetic resonance imaging of, 515, *516*
    mandibular hypomobility and, 1668
    post-traumatic, 881, *890, 892–893,* 933–934
    preoperative evaluation of, 1521
    reconstructive surgery for, 1521–1524, *1522–1525*
  recurrent, prevention of, 927
  Vitek-Kent prosthesis in, 741, *742*
Anophthalmic socket, ectropion in, 1074
Anterior digastric muscles, 2180
Anterior mandibular subapical osteotomy, for arch lengthening, 2499
  for arch leveling, 2495–2499, *2496, 2497*
Anterior plagiocephaly, 1845, 1851–1855, *1852–1854*
Anteroposterior measurements, bone, 176, *176*, 188, *189*, 190, *191*
  postsurgical, 198–199, *199*
  dental, *175,* 175–176, 188, *188*, 190, *191*, 2311, *2312*
Anthropometric measurements, in malar dystopia, 1058, *1059*
Antibiotics, prophylactic, 111–112
  for hydroxyapatite implant, 857
  for transmandibular implant, 1356, 1364
  in arthroscopic surgery, 662
Apert syndrome, 1895–1899
  abnormalities in, 1849–1850
  case studies of, 1874–1876, *1876–1877*, 1897, 1898, 1913–1917, *1914–1915, 1918,* 1921, *1922–1923*
  craniosynostosis in, 1839–1842, 1846, 1849. See also *Craniosynostosis.*
  deformities in, 1896
  extremity anomalies in, 1842
  hearing loss in, 1707, 1708
  midface osteotomy for, speech after, 1728–1729
  skull development in, 2064, *2064*
  sleep apnea in, 2022, *2022*
  speech problems in, 1698, 1700, 1701, *1701*, 1702, 1720

Apert syndrome (Continued)
  surgery for, 1850, 1874–1876, *1876–1877*, 1897, 1898, 1913–1917, *1914–1915, 1918,* 1921, *1922–1923*
    craniotomy with Le Fort III osteotomy in, 2065, *2066*
    morbidity in, 1896–1897
    radical osteoclastic surgery modified after Powiertowsky in, 2064–2065, *2065*
    results of, 1896–1897
Apertognathia, post-traumatic, 989, 1000, *1003, 1010*
Appearance, aging and, 1439–1442
  physiologic function and, 1441
  psychology of, 3–10, 1439
  self-concept and, 410, 1439, 1441–1442
  speech acceptability and, 1697
Arbitrary facebow transfer, 161
Arch bar, 1658
  in Vitek-Kent prosthesis implantation, 759, *759*
  with interocclusal composite splint, 215
Arch length analysis, 2340, 2340–2341
Arch length inadequacy, treatment of, 2340, 2340–2341
Arch length redundance, treatment of, 2340
Arch leveling, orthodontic, 2341, 2341–2342, *2342*
  surgical, 62, 62, 2341, 2341–2342, *2342,* 2431, 2431–2432, 2495–2499, *2496, 2497*
Arch rotation, 169, *169*
  adjustment of, in model surgery, 194, *195*
  in facial asymmetry, 2307, *2313–2314*
Arch width analysis, 2342, 2342–2343
Arch wires. See also *Intermaxillary fixation; Orthodontic treatment; Wire fixation.*
  active, at surgery, 63
  auxiliary, 1657, *1658*
  for postoperative midline asymmetry, 80–81, *81, 82*
  in leveling of curve of Spee, 61, 61–62, *62*
  material for, 49–50, 1656, 1658
Arcing osteotomy, for mandibular advancement, 2336
Arrhythmias, sleep apnea and, 2027–2028, 2044
Arterial embolization, for postoperative hemorrhage, 121
Arterial line, for intraoperative monitoring, 138
Arteries. See specific arteries; *Vasculature.*
  of forehead, *956*, 957
  of scalp, *954*, 954–955
  of temporal region, *958*, 958–959, *959*
Arthralgia, temporomandibular joint, pain mediators in, 473, *474*, 477–480
Arthritis, arthroscopy of, 608–609, *609, 610*, 610–611, *611*
  chondromalacia and, 651. See also *Chondromalacia.*
  costochondral graft in, 894, *898*, 904, *905*
  immobilization and, 1633–1634
  juvenile rheumatoid, mandibular deficiency in, 2506–2511, *2507–2510*
  rheumatoid, costochondral graft in, 904–909, *906–912*

Arthritis (Continued)
  signs and symptoms of, 681t
  Vitek-Kent prosthesis for. See *Vitek-Kent prosthesis.*
Arthrography, 499–506, 642
  abnormal findings on, 504–506, *505, 506*
  complications of, 506
  contraindications to, 500, 500t
  development of, 499–500, 500t
  double-contrast, 499–500, 500t, 502–504, *503*
  equipment for, 501
  in disk displacement, *611,* 611–612
  increased use of, 499, 499t
  indications for, 500, 500t
  normal findings on, 504, *504*
  stepwise upgrading of, 500, 500t
  technique of, *501–503*, 501–504
  vs. arthroscopy, *611*, 611–612
  vs. magnetic resonance imaging, 507, *508*
Arthrolysis, lavage, and manipulation, arthroscopic, 617–620, 617–620, 653, 656–671, *657*, 660. See also *Arthroscopy.*
Arthroplasty, abrasion, in chondromalacia, 476–477
Arthroscope, *603*, 603–605, *604*
Arthroscopy, 595–626
  anatomic considerations in, 595–600, *596–601*
  anesthesia for, 605
  diagnostic, 608–616, 648–652
    accuracy of, 615–616, 651
    biopsy in, 652, *652*
    indications for, 608, 626
    of adhesions, 614, *614*, 651–652
    of arthritis, 608–609, *609, 610*
    of arthrosis, 610–611, *611*
    of chondromalacia, 473–476, *474–476*, 650
    of closed lock, 612–613, *613, 614*
    of disk displacement, 611–615, *612–615*
    of disk perforation, 615, *615*
    of synovial disorders, 649–650, *650, 653*
    outpatient, 605
    pathologic findings on, *601,* 601–602, *602*
  documentation in, 607, *607, 608*
  equipment for, *603*, 603–605, *604*, 655
  history of, 648
  observation and visual fields in, 606–607, *607*
  operative and surgical, 616–625, 653–659
    antibiotic coverage in, 622
    arthrolysis, lavage, and manipulation in, 617–620, *617–620*, 653, 656–657, *657*, 660
    cannulation in, 655
    complications of, 624t, 624–625, 673, 674t
    double puncture, 620–622, *621, 622*
    examination in, 655–656
    for closed lock, 617–620, *617–620*
    indications for, 626, 653, 673
    postoperative care in, 622, 657–658, 658t
    puncture technique in, *605*, 605–606, *606,* 654–655
    results of, 622–624, 623t, 653
    sclerotherapy in, 658–659, *659*

VOLUME 1—PAGES 1–828; VOLUME 2—PAGES 829–1769; VOLUME 3—PAGES 1770–2517

INDEX / iii

Arthroscopy *(Continued)*
  set-up for, 616, *617,* 653–654, *654*
  splinting in, 622
  steroids in, 622
  training for, 624t
  triangulation in, 621–622, *622,* 657
 patient preparation for, 605, 653–654, *654*
 puncture technique for, *605,* 605–606, *606,* 654–655
 staging, 643, 644t
 synovial, 649–651, *650*
 technical considerations in, 602–607
Arthrosis, arthroscopy of, 610–611, *611*
Arthrotomy, 660–670
 approaches in, 703–704
 condylar diskopexy, 660–661, *662–663*
 costochondral graft in, 671–673, *672*
 history of, 645–648
 indications for, 660, 673–674
 temporal diskopexy, 661, *664*
 temporalis myofascial flap in, 670–671, *671*
Articular artery, 954, *954*
Articular cartilage. See *Cartilage.*
Articulation. See *Speech, articulation in.*
Articulator, 179, 204, 205
 in condylar positioning planning, 629–631, *630–632*
 model mounting on, *160,* 160–163, *162*
 SAM, 202, *202*
Asthma, preoperative evaluation in, 107
Asymmetry, chin, correction of, 2469–2474, *2473–2476*
 facial, assessment of, in horizontal plane, 2307
  in lateral plane, 2307
  correction of, 241–243, *242–244*
  mandibular ramus augmentation for, 2514–2516, *2516*
 midline, postoperative, correction of, 80–81, *81, 82*
Atracurium besylate (Tracrium), in anesthesia induction, 140
Atrial natriuretic peptide, in sleep apnea, 2027
Attitude, in model measurement, 169, *169*
Audiologic tests, 1709–1716
Augmentation genioplasty, in masseter reduction, 445
 model surgery for, 181–184, 182t, *182–184*
Auricular abnormalities, hearing loss and, 1707–1708
 in hemifacial microsomia, *1536,* 1536–1537, *1537*
 correction of, 1557
 speech and, 1706–1708
Auricular artery, 959, *959*
Auricular construction, in Treacher Collins syndrome, 1609, 1610, 1614
Auriculotemporal nerve, 955, *955,* 959, *959*
Autogenous bone graft. See *Bone graft.*
Avulsion injuries, 989, 1004–1008, *1004–1008*
 of orbit, *1065,* 1065–1066, *1066*
 treatment planning for, 992
Avulsive fracture, condylar, costochondral graft in, 894–904, *895–904*
 open reduction of, 895, *899*
Axiography, 458–459, *458–460*

Axon, 1085–1086
 response of, to injury, 1089
Axonotmesis, 1087, *1087*

B point relapse, early, 588
 late, 588–591
B point stability, after bilateral sagittal split osteotomy, with rigid fixation, 558–568, 588–591
 with wire fixation, 555–557, 557t, 588–591
 after Le Fort I osteotomy, 546, 588–591
Baby boomers, aging of, 1440–1441
Baclofen, for post-traumatic neuralgia, 1106
Ball hooks, for intermaxillary fixation, 1656–1657, *1657*
Bandaging, in lipectomy, *384,* 385, 388
Basal lamina, gingival, 1339
Basilar slope, 91
Beckwith-Wiedemann syndrome, macroglossia in, 1704
Beclomethasone dipropionate (Beconase), postoperative, 151
 preoperative, 133
Beerendonk caliper, 165, 185
Bending technique, for condylar implant, 750, *752,* 777–779, 778t, *779–782*
Benign pigmented villonodular synovitis, *912,* 912–913
Benzodiazepines, preoperative, 134–135
Berkeley pump, 377, *377*
Betamethasone, for temporomandibular joint arthralgia, *479,* 479–480
 in arthroscopic lysis and lavage, 617
Beta-titanium arch wire, 1656
Bicoronal incision. See *Coronal incision.*
Bicoronal synostosis, 1846–1847, 1858, *1859–1869*
 late, 1847, 1860–1862, *1862–1863*
Bilabial sounds, 1689t, 1691, *1692*
Bimaxillary osteotomy, for open bite, *2091,* 2091–2092, *2092*
 case studies of, 2099, *2100–2103*
Binder's syndrome, 2066–2067, *2067, 2068*
 alar-facial junction in, 288, *288*
 axillary osteotomies for, 1835
 orthognathic surgery with rhinoplasty in, 277, *278–279*
Biologic width, dental, 255, 257
Biomechanics, 1957–1975
 after mandibular osteotomy, *1959,* 1959–1960, *1960*
 after maxillary osteotomy, 1961–1962
 muscular, in mandibular region, *1959,* 1959–1960, *1960*
 in midface, 1960–1962
 of bone healing, 1957–1958
 photoelastic stress analysis and, 1963–1964, *1964*
Biopsy, arthroscopic, of temporomandibular joint, 652, *652*
Bipedicled cervical flap, 1480–1481, *1481.* See also *Flap(s).*
Bird face deformity, 1997
Bird's eye, *1059*
Bite, complete telescopic (Brody's syndrome), 2383, *2383, 2384*
 in growing patient, 2395, *2395*

Bite *(Continued)*
 mandibular expansion for, 2385–2389
 case study of, 2389–2391, *2390, 2391*
 treatment of, 2383, *2383, 2384*
 crocodile, 2383, *2385*
 mandibular expansion for, 2385–2389, 2398, *2400–2401*
 case study of, 2392, *2393*
 deep. See *Deep-bite deformity.*
 open. See *Open bite.*
 unilateral deep buccal. See *Bite, complete telescopic (Brody's syndrome).*
Bite force, loss of, after muscle shortening procedures, 1631
 rehabilitation of. See *Rehabilitation.*
 surgical enhancement of, 1959–1960, *1960*
Bite registration, 162–163
 in computerized tomography, 527
 of preoperative condylar position, 527, 530
Bite splint. See *Occlusal splint.*
Bite stability, after bilateral sagittal split osteotomy, with rigid fixation, 564
 with wire fixation, 555
 after Le Fort I osteotomy, 541, 544
Biting exercises, for postoperative condylar sag, 584
Bladder catheterization, 110–111, 138, 140, *141*
Blast injuries, 989
Bleaching, dental, *225,* 225–226, *226*
Bleeding, control of. See *Hemostasis.*
 intraoperative monitoring of, 138–139
 postoperative, 121
 volume replacement for, 124–126
Blood pressure, maintenance of, in anesthesia, 137–139, 149–150
Blood transfusion, autologous, 108, 124
Blood vessels. See *Vasculature.*
Blood volume, maintenance of, 124–126
 normal values for, 138
Boley gauge, 165, 185
Bolt fixation, of condylar implant, 782–785, *783–785*
Bolton discrepancy, preoperative correction of, 56–58, *57, 58*
Bonding, composite resin, 227, *227*
Bone, assessment of, for dental implants, 1177–1178, *1181,* 1181–1182
 cancellous, 1337
 grafting of. See *Bone graft, cancellous.*
 classification of, 1232–1234, *1233, 1234*
 composite, 1233, *1234*
 cortical, 1337
 grafting of, 834, 1482–1483
 creeping replacement in, 1337
 cutting cone in, 1337
 drilling injury of, 1144, *1145*
 effects of immobilization on, 1626
 formation of, rate of, 1234
 freeze-dried, 849–850, 1453
 growth of, scintigraphic evaluation of, 1677–1684. See also *Skeletal scintigraphy.*
 guided regeneration of, 1218–1220, *1219*
 healing of, 1337–1338, 1449–1452, *1451*
 around implants, 1337–1338, 1346–1349, *1347, 1348*

VOLUME 1—PAGES 1–828;   VOLUME 2—PAGES 829–1769;   VOLUME 3—PAGES 1770–2517

Bone *(Continued)*
    implant roughness and, 1351–1353, *1352–1354*
    histology of, 1957
    muscular forces and, *1959*, 1959–1962, *1960*
    histological response of, to mechanical demands, 1957–1958
    in articular cartilage nutrition, 1635–1637, *1636*
    interfacial, 1234–1235
    irradiated, dental implants in, 1143
    lamellar, 1232, *1233*
    maturation of, 1235
    metabolic disorders of, screening for, 1231
    modeling of, 1231, *1231*, 1234–1235, *1241*
    optical chambers for, 1135–1138, *1136–1139*
    physiology of, *1231*, 1231–1232, *1232*
    radiographic assessment of, for dental implants, 1181–1182, *1182*
    regeneration of, 1449–1452, *1451*
    remodeling of, 1231, *1231*, *1233*, 1234–1235, *1235*, 1241, 1337
    with osseointegrated implants, *1162*, 1162–1163, *1232*, *1235–1240*, 1235–1241, *1256*, 1256–1258
    resorption of, with hydroxyapatite-coated implants, 1318
    shape and quality of, after tooth extraction, *1149*
    stress analysis for, 1963–1970. See also *Stress analysis.*
    stress trajectories for, 1962–1963
    supporting, 1234–1235
    thermal damage to, 1144, *1144*
    vascularization of, 1337
    woven, 1232
Bone bank, 849–850
Bone chambers, Branemark, 1135–1138, *1136–1139*
Bone conduction hearing aids, *1218*, 1218, 1721
Bone conduction implant, for hearing loss, 1721
Bone dust, cranial, 981
Bone fixation. See *Fixation.*
Bone graft, 122–123, 831–851
    allogenic, 832, 849–850, 1452–1456
    crib, 1450, 1453–1454, *1454*
    in mandibular reconstruction, 1500–1524. See also *Mandibular reconstruction.*
    hemimandibular ilium form, in mandibular reconstruction, *1501*, 1501–1502, *1502*, 1506–1507, 1510, *1510*
    indications for, 1453–1545
    rib, in mandibular reconstruction, *1505*, 1505–1514, *1506*, *1508–1512*, *1514*, *1515*
    safety of, 1455–1456
    alveolar, 1131–1132, 1191–1213, 1273, *1311–1316*, 1313, *1461*, 1463–1464
    speech and, 1722, *1722*
    alveolar height restoration by, *1461*, 1463–1464
    as matrix, 833
    autogenous, 834–849
    for midfacial augmentation, *2295*, 2295–2303, *2300–2303*
    maintenance of, 2296

Bone graft *(Continued)*
    availability of, 832
    biocompatibility of, 831–832
    block-type, 1451, *1451*
    bone continuity restoration by, 1462–1463
    bone regeneration and, 1449–1452, *1451*
    Branemark maxillary full arch, *1206*, 1207
    calvarial. See *Bone graft, cranial.*
    cancellous, 834, 1450–1451, *1451*
    vs. cortical, 834, 1482–1483
    collagen tubes for, 1221–1224, *1222*, *1223*
    cortical, vs. cancellous, 834, 1482–1483
    corticocancellous, 834
    costochondral. See *Costochondral graft.*
    failure of, Vitek-Kent prosthesis for. See *Vitek-Kent prosthesis.*
    in condylar reconstruction, 671–673, *672*
    cranial, 836–837, *837*
    anatomic basis of, 978–979
    applications of, 1483
    biologic basis of, 977–978
    bone dust, 981
    bone harvesting in, 979–984, *980–984*
    calvarial thickness and, 978–979
    complications of, 122–123, 978
    coronal approach in, *971*, 979–981, *980*
    for facial fractures, *1021*, 1021–1023, *1022*
    frontoparietal, 982, *982*, *983*
    full-thickness, 979
    harvesting of, 836–837, *837*, 975–984, 1485, *1485*, 1605, *1605*
    historical background of, 975–977
    in Apert syndrome, 1897, 1898
    in Crouzon syndrome, 1889–1890
    in Treacher Collins syndrome, 1605, *1605*
    limitations of, 978
    maxillary, for dental implants, *1206*, 1207
    methods and use of, 979–984, *980*, *982–984*
    orbital, 1066–1067
    shaving, 981
    skull chip, 981
    split-thickness, 979–981, *980*
    temporoparietal, 982, *982–984*
    vascularized, 981–984, *982–984*
    criteria for, 831–833
    endochrondral, vs. membranous graft, 1890
    failure of, 1464
    for facial prosthesis, 1525–1526, *1526*
    freeze-dried, 1453
    handling of, 1491–1492
    harvesting of, 834–849, 1482–1491, 2296–2297
    host bed vascularity for, 1452
    hydroxyapatite as substitute for, 854–871. See also *Hydroxyapatite implants.*
    ilium, 839–849, *840*, *842–844*, *846–848*
    applications of, 1483
    for maxillary sinus graft, 1282–1285, *1283–1285*

Bone graft *(Continued)*
    harvesting of, from anterior site, 839–845, *840*, *842–844*, 1486–1488, *1486–1488*
    from posterior site, 839–840, *840*, 845–847, *846–848*, 1488–1491, *1488–1491*
    nerve injury in, *1486*, 1486–1487
    morbidity and complications in, 847–849, 1486–1487, 1489
    in chin augmentation, 835
    in chin lengthening, 2477, *2477*, *2478*
    in craniofacial dysostosis, 1889–1890
    in dental prosthetics, Branemark implant, 1191–1213. See also *Dental implants, Branemark.*
    hydroxyapatite-coated implant, *1271*, 1271, *1272*, *1273*, 1288, 1316, 1324, *1324–1328*, 1407–1410, *1408–1410*. See also *Dental implants, hydroxyapatite-coated.*
    limitations of, 1131–1132
    in enophthalmos correction, 1029–1033, *1030–1034*
    in facial fractures, 1015, *1021*, 1021–1023, *1022*
    in hemifacial microsomia, for condylar process construction, 1583–1586
    revision of, 1591–1592, *1598*
    in Le Fort I osteotomy, with downsliding, 2249, *2249*
    in Le Fort I quadrangular osteotomy, 1799, 1814
    in Le Fort II quadrangular osteotomy, 1799, 1814, 1819, 1833, 1835
    in malar augmentation, *2295*, 2295–2303, *2300–2303*
    graft material for, *2295*, 2295–2302
    indications for, 2299
    technique for, *2300*, *2301*, 2989–2302
    in mandibular angle augmentation, 2491–2495, *2492–2494*
    in mandibular reconstruction, 1492–1521. See also *Mandibular reconstruction.*
    for Andy Gump deformity, 1515–1521, *1518–1520*
    for defect from angle to symphysis area, 1507–1510, *1508–1510*
    for defect from condylar neck to opposite condylar neck, 1515–1518, *1515–1518*
    for defect from condyle to opposite condylar neck, 1518–1519, *1519*
    for defect from midbody area to opposite midbody area, 1513–1514, *1514*, *1515*
    for defect from ramus across midline to opposite body area, 1510–1513, *1511–1513*
    for defect from sigmoid notch and condylar neck to ipsilateral mental foramen, 1504–1507, *1504–1508*
    for defect involving entire mandible including both condyles, *1520*, 1520–1521
    for defect of condyle to ipsilateral mental foramen, 1498–1504, *1499–1504*
    in inferior alveolar nerve repair with sural nerve graft, *1116*, 1116–1117

Bone graft *(Continued)*
  in masseter reduction, 445, 446
  in maxillary osteotomy, 71, 72
  in maxillary reconstruction, 1528–1530, *1529*
  in maxillary sinus, with simultaneous hydroxyapatite dental implants, 1277–1286, *1277–1286*, 1313–1315
  in nasal reconstruction, 305–306, *306, 307*, 835, *1024*
  in naso-orbito-ethmoid deformities, 1048
  in open bite correction, 835, *835*
  in orbital reconstruction, 1060–1067, *1061, 1063, 1064–1066*, 1605, *1605*
  in orbitozygomatic deformities, 1035–1037, *1038–1044*
  in osteotomized segment stabilization, 1027
  in post-traumatic craniofacial deformities, 1023–1025, 1027
  in ramus augmentation, in facial asymmetry, 2514–2516, *2516*
  in Treacher Collins syndrome, 1609–1610, *1610*, 1614, 1616
    for orbital construction, 1605, *1605*
    harvesting of, *1605*
    resorption of, 1604
    sources for, 1604, 1605, 1608
  infection of, 73, *73*
  mandibular, 834–835, *835*
  maxillary, Branemark, *1206*, 1207
    cranial, *1206*, 1207
  mechanical stability of, 833
  membranous, vs. endochondral graft, 977–978, 1890
  miniplate fixation of, 1016, *1024*
  nasal dorsum, 305–306, *306, 307*, 835
  onlay, 2295–2297
    fixation of, 2296
    maintenance of, 2296
  osteoconduction by, 833, 849
  osteogenesis by, 832–833, 849
  osteogenic potential of, 1482–1483
  osteoinduction by, 833, 849
  particulate bone and cancellous marrow, crib for, 1450, 1453–1454, *1454*
    in hemimandibulectomy reconstruction, 1500–1524
    for mandibular continuity defects, 1521
    in mandibulectomy reconstruction. See *Mandibular reconstruction.*
  resorption of, 1890, 2296
  retrobulbar, *1063*, 1064, *1064*, 1067
  rib, 837–839, *838, 839*. See also *Costochondral graft.*
    allogenic, 1455
      in mandibular reconstruction, *1505*, 1505–1514, *1506, 1508–1512, 1514, 1515*
      safety of, 1455–1456
    complications of, 123
    for facial fractures, *1021*, 1021–1023, *1022*
    harvesting of, 837–839, *838, 839*, 874–876, *875*, 1483–1485, *1484, 1485*
    complications of, 929
    in condylar reconstruction, 673
  selection of, 833
  storage of, 1452, 1491–1492

Bone graft *(Continued)*
  types of, 833–851
  xenogenic, 850
Bone graft chamber, Branemark, 1137, *1138*
Bone growth, as maturity indicator, 33–34, 35
  regulation of, 23, 23–24
Bone loss, with hydroxyapatite-coated dental implants, 1318
Bone marrow, condylar, magnetic resonance imaging of, 515, *515*
Bone measurements, *196*, 196–198, *197*
  anteroposterior, 175, *176*, 176, 188, *189*, 190, *191*
  in model sagittal split osteotomy, 200
  postsurgical, 198–199, *199*
  transverse, 177, 188, *189*, 192, 192, 2312, *2312*
  vertical, mandibular, *174*, 174–175, *175*, 190, *190*, 2311
    maxillary, *172*, 172–174, 186–187, *187*, 190, *191*, 2311
Bone mill, in dental implant surgery, 1166, *1166*
Bone rasp, nasal dorsum reduction, 356, *356*
Bone scan. See also *Skeletal scintigraphy.*
  of costochondral graft, 929, *930*
Bone sounding, for alveolar crest location, 245, *245*, 256, *256*
Bone spur, condylar stump, after Vitek-Kent prosthesis placement, 790–792, *792*
Bone transverse reference line, 192, *192*
Bone vertical reference line, 186–187, *187*, 196–198, *197, 198*, 2312
Bony ankylosis, after Vitek-Kent prosthesis placement, 791–792, *792*
  arthoscopic diagnosis of, 651–652
  arthrotomy for, 668–673
  postoperative, magnetic resonance imaging of, 515, *516*
  Vitek-Kent prosthesis in, 741, *742*
Brachycephaly, 1846–1847, 1858, *1859–1869*
Bracket bar, *1658*, 1658–1659
Brackets, for intermaxillary fixation, 1656–1657, *1657*
Bradykinins, release of, in chondromalacia, 473, *474*
Brain growth, in craniosynostosis, 1839–1840, 1840t
Branemark bone chambers, 1135–1138, *1137–1139*
Branemark dental implants. See *Dental implants, Branemark.*
Branemark maxillary full arch graft, *1206*, 1207
Breast development, as maturity indicator, 32, 32t
Breathing, mouth, after cleft deformity repair, 407
  after pharyngeal flap surgery, 1717, 1720
  nasal, 328–331, *329–331*
  evaluation of, 103–104, 328–329
Breathing difficulties, in sleep apnea, *2023*, 2023–2028, 2055, 2056
  in Treacher Collins syndrome, 1601, 1614
Brent's auricular construction, in Treacher Collins syndrome, 1609, 1610, 1614
Bridge, dental. See also *Dentures.*

Bridge *(Continued)*
  for transmandibular implant, 1369, *1369*
Broad soft tissue pedicle genioplasty, 2446–2456
Brody's syndrome, 2383, *2383*, 2384
  mandibular expansion in, 2385–2389
  case study of, 2389–2391, *2390, 2391*
  in growing patient, 2395, *2395*
  treatment of, 2383, *2383*, 2384
Brush directional discrimination, in neurologic examination, 1098
Bruxism, after Vitek-Kent prosthesis placement, 786, 787
  chondromalacia and, 472
  management of, 658
  masseter muscle hypertrophy and, 427
  temporomandibular joint disorders and, 472, 642
Buccal fat pad, 379
  removal of. See *Lipectomy.*
Buccal fragment, intraoperative greenstick fracture of, fixation of, *1991*, 1991–1992
Bupivacaine, for hemostasis, 112–113
Byzantine palate, 1700
Bzoch Error Pattern Diagnostic Articulation Test, 1709

C fibers, 1085–1086
C osteotomy, for mandibular advancement, 2336
Calcitite dental implants. See *Dental implants, hydroxyapatite-coated.*
Calcium triphosphate ceramic implants, 851
Caliper, Vernier, 165, *185*, 185
Caloric expenditure, in children, 125t
Calvarial bone graft. See *Bone graft, cranial.*
Calvarium, removal of, in craniosynostosis correction, 2070, *2071*
  sutures of, growth at, 2067–2070, *2069–2071*
  premature closure of. See *Craniofacial dysostosis.*
  thickness of, 978–979
Campbell's theory of condylotomy, 678, 678–679
Canalicular injuries, *1074*, 1074–1075
Cancellous bone, grafting of. See *Bone graft.*
Cancer, radiation therapy for, dental implants after, 1143
Canine(s), as lateral incisor substitute, 57, *57*
Canine eminence, 92
Cannulas, lipectomy, 376, *376*
Cant, adjustment of, in model surgery, 194, *195*
  measurement of, 156, 169, 2306
Canthal dystopia, frontal process osteotomy for, 1064–1065
  post-traumatic, 1076–1077
Canthal laxity, in Treacher Collins syndrome, 1604
Canthopexy, frontal process osteotomy with, 1065
  technique of, *1045, 1046*, 1048, 1076–1077
Canthoplasty, coronal approach in, 973, *973*

vi / INDEX

Capsular reconstruction, soft tissue patch in, 723, *724*
Capsulitis, adhesive, arthroscopy of, 610–611, *611*
Carbamazepine, for post-traumatic neuralgia, 1106
Cardiac abnormalities, in sleep apnea, 2027, 2044
Cardiovascular evaluation, preoperative, 103–105, *104*
Career opportunities, appearance and, 8
Carotid arterial flow, in hypotensive anesthesia, 136, *136*
Carpenter syndrome, 1851
  extremity anomalies in, 1842
Cartilage, articular, immobilization-induced changes in, *1633*, 1633–1634, *1635*
  nutrition of, 1635–1638, *1636*, *1637*
  repair of, 1638–1639
  temporomandibular joint, immobilization-induced changes in, 1634–1635, *1635*
  freeze-dried, 850
  nasal, *291*, 291–292, *321*, 321–322, *324*, 2175–2176, *2176*
    development of, *2066*, 2066–2067
    in Binder's syndrome, 2066–2067, *2067*, *2068*
  temporomandibular joint, composition of, 471, *471*
    degeneration of, 472–476, *472–476*. See also *Chondromalacia*.
    arthroscopy of, 601–602, *602*, 610–611, *611*, 651
Cartilage graft. See also *Costochondral graft*.
  allogenic, 1455–1456
    in ankylosis repair, 1522–1523, *1523*
  conchal, in temporomandibular joint reconstruction, 665–670, *666–669*
  cryopreserved, 1453, 1455
  in columellar augmentation, 313, *314*
  in diskectomy, 646t, 646–647, *647*, 647t, 665
  in nasal dorsum augmentation, 305–306, *306*, *307*
  in nasal tip augmentation, 308, *308*
Catheterization, urinary, 110–111, 138, 140, *141*
  venous, 111
Causalgia, 1093–1094, *1094*, 1102–1103
  evaluation of, nerve block in, 1100–1101
  pain in, 1096
Cellulosuctiontome, 374
Cementoenamel junction, in altered passive eruption evaluation, 254–255, 257
  location of, 239, *239*
Central trigeminal pathosis, 1093
Centric occlusion, 524
Centric relation, 524
Cephalometric analysis, 85–98, *89–94*, 156–157
  advantages of, 95
  after cleft deformity repair, 408–412, *409–414*
  Delaire, 89–94, *89–94*, 408–412, *409–414*, 2077–2078, *2078*
  dental, 95, *95–96*
  disadvantages of, 95–96
  for Branemark dental implants, 1178, *1179*

Cephalometric analysis *(Continued)*
  for chin deformities, in anteroposterior plane, 2441–2443, *2443–2445*
    in transverse plane, 2468–2469
    in vertical plane, 2474
  for hydroxyapatite dental implants, 1267–1268, *1268*, *1269*
  for rhinoplasty, 343
  for Vitek-Kent prosthesis, 746, *747*, *748*, 749–750
  guidelines for, 2181
  in aging face syndrome, 1428–1429
  in growing patient, 2322–2325, *2324*
  in hemifacial microsomia, *1555*, 1563, *1564*, *1565*
  in intraosseous orthodontic implant analysis, 1254–1255, *1255*
  in mandibular prognathism, 2143, 2145–2146
  in maxillary deficiency, in growing patient, 2322–2325, *2324*
  in maxillomandibular transverse discrepancies, 2403–2405, *2404*
  in open bite, 2076–2078, *2077*, *2078*
  in short mandibular ramus deformities, 1997–1998
  in sleep apnea, 2026–2027, *2031–2033*, 2031–2034, 2032t, 2033t, *2048*, 2048
  landmark identification in, 2181
  lip posture in, 2181
  Model Frankfort (MF) reconstruction in, 178–180, *181*, 2307–2309, *2308–2310*
  of post-traumatic maxillary deformities, 998–999, *1005*
  sample cases for, 96–98, *96–98*
  soft tissue esthetic, 86–88, *86–88*
  sources of error in, 2181
Cephalometric prediction tracing, 163–164
  Model Frankfort (MF) reconstruction in, 178–181, *180*, *181*, 2307–2309, *2308–2310*
Cephalometric radiography, 85, 96, 156–158
  Model Frankfort (MF) reconstruction in, 179–181, *180*, *181*, 2307–2309, *2308–2310*
  technique of, 409–412, *409–414*
Cephalosporin, prophylactic, for hydroxyapatite implant, 857
Ceramic brackets, orthodontic, stability of, 49–50, *50*
Ceramic implants, calcium triphosphate, 851
Cerebral ischemia, during hypotensive anesthesia, 114–115, 135–137
Cervical autonomic pathosis, 1093
Cervical flap, 1478–1482, *1479–1482*. See also *Flap(s)*.
  bipedicled, 1480–1481, *1481*
  skin-platysma rotation, 1478, *1479*, *1480*
  U-Y advancement, 1481–1482, *1482*
Cervicomental region, esthetic analysis of, 381, *381*
Champy plate fixation, for mandibular angle fracture, comparative stress analysis of, *1973*, 1973–1974
Champy technique, for oblique modified Le Fort III osteotomy, 1777–1779, *1777–1779*
Change Your Smile, 220, *221*, 221

Cheek bone augmentation. See *Malar augmentation*.
Cheiloplasty, in mandibular deficiency correction, 2488
  lip lift, 2331–2332, *2332*
  reduction, with maxillary osteotomy, 315–316, *316*
Cheilorhinoplasty. See also *Rhinoplasty*.
  in cleft lip repair, 394–404, *395–406*
  secondary, for bilateral deformities, 418–422, *419–421*
    for unilateral deformities, 415–418, *415–418*
  sequelae of, 404–408, *407*, *408*
  technique of, 394–404, *395–406*
  secondary functional, in cleft deformity, 408
Chemosis, subconjunctival, after quadrangular Le Fort I osteotomy, 1836
Chewing exercises, after ankylosis surgery, 1524
Children. See also *Adolescent*.
  blood volume in, 138
  caloric expenditure in, 125t
  cephalometric analysis in, 2322–2325, *2324*
  fluid and electrolyte replacement in, 125–126
  growth in. See *Growth*.
  hemifacial microsomia in, treatment of, 1542–1550, *1544–1553*. See also *Hemifacial microsomia*.
  ilial graft harvesting in, 844
  mandibular advancement in, 2516–2517
  mandibular prognathism in, 2142–2143
    surgery for, 2147–2148
  mandibular reconstruction in, costochondral graft for, 1496t, 1496–1498, *1497*, *1498*
  orthognathic surgery in, craniofacial growth after, 38–44
  Treacher Collins syndrome in. See *Treacher Collins syndrome*.
Chin, anatomy of, 2179–2180
  augmentation of. See *Genioplasty, augmentation*.
  graft harvesting from, 835, *835*
  measurement of, 175, 183, *184*
    after model surgery, 198
  prominence of, with vertical deficiency, correction of, 2402
  sagging, correction of, in transmandibular implant placement, 1358, *1359*, *1371*
  surgery of. See *Genioplasty*.
Chin asymmetry, correction of, 2469–2474, *2473–2476*
Chin augmentation. See also *Genioplasty, augmentation*.
  allogenic bone graft in, 850
  hydroxyapatite implant in, 857, 863, *863*
  nasal dorsum graft in, 835
Chin cap traction, for mandibular prognathism, 2146–2148
Chin contour, determinants of, 2440
  psychosocial aspects of, 2439
Chin deformities, anteroposterior, 2441–2468
  broad soft tissue pedicle genioplasty for, 2446–2456
  sliding horizontal osteotomy for, 2443–2446, *2446*

VOLUME 1—PAGES 1–828;   VOLUME 2—PAGES 829–1769;   VOLUME 3—PAGES 1770–2517

INDEX / vii

Chin deformities *(Continued)*
    treatment planning for, 2442–2443, *2443–2445*
    esthetic analysis for, 2439–2442, *2441, 2443*
    in Apert syndrome, 1897, 1898
    in Crouzon syndrome, 1895, 1898
    in Treacher Collins syndrome, 1606
      correction of, 1609, *1609*
    systematic descriptions of, 2439–2441
    transverse, 2468–2474
      evaluation of, 2468–2469
    vertical, 2474–2484
Chin downgraft, hydroxyapatite implant in, 862, *862*
Chin reduction. See *Genioplasty, reduction.*
Choanal atresia, in Treacher Collins syndrome, 1614
Chondrobase, cranial, development of, 2063–2067, *2063–2067*
Chondromalacia, 471–477
    arthroscopic diagnosis of, 651
    etiology of, 472
    gradations of, 472–473
    treatment of, 476, *476–477*
Chondromatosis, synovial, 650, *650*
Chronic obstructive pulmonary disease, preoperative evaluation in, 107
Cicatricial ectropion, 1071–1074, *1072, 1073*
Cicatricial entropion, 1070
Cicatricial lagophthalmos, 1070, *1070*
Circulation. See *Vasculature.*
Circummandibular wire, for two-jaw surgery, 1657, *1658*
Cleft deformities, compensatory articulation in, 1693–1694
    functional disability in, 391–392
      postoperative, 404–408, *407, 408*
    hearing loss in, 1707–1708
    hypernasal speech in, 1695–1696
    in Apert syndrome, 1841, 1842, 1896
    maxillary advancement in, with external headframe traction, 2315–2322, *2316–2321*
    maxillary collapse in, 1703, *1703*
    maxillary osteotomy in, speech after, 1723–1726, *1725–1727*
    mucocutaneous abnormalities in, *392,* 392–394, *393, 397, 397, 401*
    muscle matrix disturbances in, 2072, *2073, 2074*
    open bite correction in. See *Open bite, surgery for.*
    previously repaired, endotracheal intubation in, 113, 132
    orthognathic surgery with rhinoplasty in, 275, *276, 277*
    preoperative speech evaluation for, 104–105
    quadrangular Le Fort I osteotomy and, *1811–1813,* 1811–1815, 1816
    quadrangular Le Fort II osteotomy and, 1834
    repair of, cephalometric analysis after, 408–412, *409–414*
      cheilorhinoplasty for. See *Cheilorhinoplasty.*
      for partial bilateral labial clefts, 399, *402, 406*
      for partial unilateral labial clefts, *396,* 396, *403, 404*
      for total bilateral labiomaxillary clefts, 396–399, *397–399, 402, 403*

Cleft deformities *(Continued)*
      for total labiomaxillopalatine clefts, 394–396, *395, 400–401, 406*
      functional genioplasty after, 422, *422–424, 423*
      goals of, 392
      orofacial dysfunction after, 407–408
      secondary, for bilateral deformities, 418–422, *419–421*
        for unilateral deformities, 415–418, *415–418*
        functional, 408
      sequelae of, 404–408, *407, 408*
      techniques for, 394–404, *395–406*
      velar muscular reconstruction in, 404
    skeletal changes in, 2072, *2073, 2074*
    speech problems and, 1698–1701, *1699,* 1703, *1703*
Clicking, temporomandibular joint, 467, *467,* 489–490, 490t, 491, 643
Clonidine, preoperative, 134, 149–150
Closed lock, arthroscopic treatment of, 617–620, *617–620*
    results of, 623t, 623–624, 626
    mandibular manipulation for, 645
    temporomandibular joint, 491
      arthroscopic diagnosis of, 612–613, *613, 614*
Cluneal nerve injury, in ilial graft harvesting, 848
Coaptation, in trigeminal nerve microreconstructive surgery, 1109–1110
    maintenance of, 1110
Cochlear implant, 1721
Cold therapy, for mandibular hypomobility, 1669
Collagen, effects of immobilization on, *1642,* 1642–1643, 1644
    proteoglycans and, 1640, *1640, 1641,* 1643–1644
Collagen tubes, in bone grafting, for dental implants, 1221–1224, *1222, 1223*
Collagenases, release of, in chondromalacia, 473, *474*
Coloboma, in Treacher Collins syndrome, 1607
    correction of, 1610, *1611*
Columella, 286, 287, *287,* 288–289, 324, 2175, 2176
    surgery of, during maxillary osteotomy, 313, *313, 314*
Columella-labial angle, 267, *267*
Common reference plane, 157–159, 158t, *159,* 159t, 2307
Compensatory articulation, 1693
    speech therapy for, 1716
Complex motion tomography, of temporomandibular joint, 495, *495*
Complications, intraoperative, 65–75. See also under *Orthognathic surgery* and specific procedures.
    postoperative, 73–82, 120–126. See also *Postoperative complications* and specific procedures.
    preoperative, 49–65. See also *Preoperative preparation.*
Composite bone, 1233, *1234*
Compressed cancellous bone graft, for dental implants, 1200, *1201,* 1203, *1204*
Compression plates. See *Plate fixation.*
Computagrid, 2443, *2444–2445*
Computer imaging, in esthetic dentistry, 222–223

Computerized tomography. See *Tomography, computerized.*
Conchal cartilage graft, in temporomandibular joint reconstruction, 665–670, *666–669*
Conductive hearing loss, 1707. See also *Hearing loss.*
    treatment of, 1720–1721
Condylar ankylosis. See *Ankylosis.*
Condylar arthritis. See *Arthritis.*
Condylar deficiency, costochondral graft for, 671–673, *672*
Condylar disk. See also *Condyle.*
    anatomy of, 484–485, *485*
    disorders of, arthroscopic findings in, 602, *602*
    displacement of, 65, *65,* 77, *77.* See also *Temporomandibular joint, internal derangements of.*
      after Vitek-Kent prosthesis placement, 793
      direction of, *487,* 487–488, *488*
      with deformation, *491,* 491–493, *492*
      with reduction, *490,* 490t, 490–491
      without reduction, 491
        condylotomy for. See *Intraoral vertical ramus osteotomy.*
    movement of, 486, *486, 487,* 596
    perforation of, 493, *493*
      arthrography of, 505
      arthroscopic diagnosis of, 615, *615*
    replacement of, with costochondral graft, 918–921, 932
      with dermal graft, 926–927
    repositioning of. See also *Condyle, positioning of.*
      arthroscopic diagnosis of, *712,* 712–713, *713*
    resection of, implants in, complications of, 646t, 646–647, 647t
      temporalis fascial graft in, 713–715
      with and without autogenous interposition, 665, 714
      with temporal diskopexy, 661, *663*
Condylar disk-condyle coordination, 457
Condylar diskectomy, implants in, complications of, 646t, 646–647, 647t, 717
    interpositional materials for, 665, 714, 717, 730
    temporalis fascial graft in, 713–715
    temporalis myofascial flap in, 670–671, *671,* 717–733. See also *Temporalis myofascial flap.*
    with and without autogenous interposition, 665
    with temporal diskopexy, 661, *663*
    without replacement, results of, 665, 714, 717
Condylar diskopexy, 660–661, *662–663*
    temporal, 661, *664*
Condylar dysplasia, correction of, graft, 879–881, *880, 882–889*
    nongraft, 881, *888–889*
    timing of, 881
Condylar fracture, avulsive, costochondral graft in, 894–904, *895–904*
    open reduction of, 895, *899*
Condylar fragment, in sagittal split osteotomy, fixation of, 1990, *1991*
Condylar graft, 918–921, 932, 1493–1497
    ankylosis of, *940–943*
    costochondral, 1493–1498, *1494–1498.* See also *Costochondral graft.*

Condylar graft (Continued)
  ankylosis of, 938–945, 940–943, 1520–1521
Condylar growth, grafts and, 873–874, 932–933, 934–939
  in hemifacial microsomia, 1533, 1540–1542, 1543
Condylar implant, computerized tomography of, 498, 498–499
  development of, 737–740
  in Vitek-Kent prosthesis, 738–748, 739, 753, 753, 753. See also Vitek-Kent prosthesis.
    bending of, 773–782, 777–779
    placement of, 766, 773–779, 773–782
    securing of, 782–785, 783–785
    selection of, 773
    template for, 754, 754, 774–775, 775
  magnetic resonance imaging of, 515–516
Condylar osteomyelitis, costochondral graft in, 914, 914, 915
Condylar process, construction of, in hemifacial microsomia, 1571, 1578
Condylar reconstruction, costochondral graft in, 918–921, 932, 1493–1497, 1494–1498. See also Costochondral graft.
  in Andy Gump deformity, 1518–1521
Condylar regeneration, 895, 901
Condylar resorption, after sagittal split osteotomy, 1985
  iatrogenic, costochondral graft in, 917–922, 917–922
  dermal graft in, 926–927
Condylar sag, 65, 65, 526, 580–588
  after bilateral sagittal split osteotomy, 547–568, 580, 580–585, 581, 581t, 583
  after intraoral vertical ramus osteotomy, 690–691, 2133, 2133–2134, 2134, 2135, 2138
  after Le Fort I osteotomy, 541–547, 585, 585–588, 586t, 587
  after sagittal split osteotomy, 2134, 2138
  B-point relapse and, 588–591
  central fossa, 566–567, 567
  extracapsular, 581, 581t, 586, 586t
  intracapsular, 581, 581t, 586, 586t
  peripheral fossa, 566–567, 567
  postoperative, 77, 77
  skeletal relapse and, 534
Condylar stress patterns, 1966, 1966–1969, 1967
Condylar stump spur formation, in Vitek-Kent prosthesis placement, 789t, 790–792, 791
Condyle, as growth center, 42
  bone marrow of, magnetic resonance imaging of, 515, 515
  degenerative disease of, Vitek-Kent prosthesis in, 740–744, 741
  displacement of. See Condylar disk, displacement of.
  intraoperative, 629, 634
  fixation of, 66, 66–67, 67
  in temporomandibular joint dysfunction, 460t, 460–462, 461, 462, 484–485, 485, 486
  morphologic changes in, postoperative, 578–580, 579t, 690

Condyle (Continued)
  movement of, after bilateral sagittal split osteotomy, 547–568
    after Le Fort I osteotomy, 534–547
    after orthognathic surgery, 464–466, 465t, 466
    arthroscopic view of, 596
    in dentofacial abnormalities, 463t, 463–464, 464t
    normal, 486
    postoperative, 577–578
    recording of, 458–459, 458–460
  orientation devices for, 525–526
  position of, after condylotomy, 680, 680
    after intraoral vertical ramus osteotomy, 683, 683–684, 2133, 2133–2134, 2134, 2135, 2138
    after sagittal split osteotomy, 2134, 2138
    clinicopathologic correlates of, 529
    functional, 524
    meniscal, 524
    posterior border, 530–531
    postoperative, 690
    preoperative, wax bite recording of, 527, 530
  positioning of, 63–67, 64–67, 712, 712–713, 713
    anatomic influences on, 574–575, 575
    anesthesia and, 531, 531–532, 580, 585
    compressive loading in, 575
    determining factors in, 573–576
    gnathoretrusion studies of, 530–531
    hardware influences on, 574
    in bilateral sagittal split osteotomy, postoperative stability after, 547–568
      with rigid fixation, 558–573
      with wire fixation, 547–558
    in Le Fort I osteotomy, 534–547, 629–639
      case report of, 635–638, 635–639
      postoperative stability after, 541–547
      with firm anterosuperior pressure, 541–547
      with heavy posterior pressure, 534–541
    in mandibular advancement, 1987, 1987–1988, 1988
    intraoperative control of, 632–634, 632–635
    joint loading and, 532–534, 533t, 534
    literature review of, 524–525
    orientation devices for, 525–526
    posterior, animal studies of, 530
    postoperative adjustment of, 76–77, 77, 79
      in bilateral sagittal split osteotomy, 584–585
      in Le Fort I osteotomy, 587–588
    preoperative planning of, 63–65, 162–163, 629–631, 630–632
    radiographic assessment of, 526, 526–527
    superior-directed, 575–576, 576, 577
    surgeon influences on, 574
  posterior, developmental vs. operative, 529–530
    symptoms and, 529–530

Condyle (Continued)
  resorption of, in females, 590
  shaving of, 712
  torque of, in bilateral sagittal split osteotomy, with rigid fixation, 569–573, 570, 571
Condylectomy, for costochondral graft, 672
  for temporomandibular joint dysfunction, 645
  tissue repair after, 712–713
Condylotomy, Campbell's theory of, 678, 678–679
  closed, development of, 677–678, 678
  results of, 681t, 691
  condylar position after, 680, 680
  history of, 677–678
  intraoral, 681–700. See also Intraoral vertical ramus osteotomy.
Conformer, in anophthalmic socket, ectropion and, 1074
Conjunctival traction bands, 1070, 1071
Connective tissue, collagen in, 1640, 1640, 1641, 1642–1644
  of forehead, 955–956, 956
  of scalp, 952, 953
  of temporal region, 957–958, 958
  periarticular, immobilization effects on, 1640–1645
  proteoglycans in, 1640, 1640, 1641, 1643
Consent, for rhinoplasty, 344
Consonants. See also Speech sounds.
  articulation of, problems in, 1693, 1693–1694
Continuous passive motion, after Vitek-Kent prosthesis placement, 786–787, 787
  for mandibular hypomobility, 1669, 1671
Continuous positive airway pressure, for sleep apnea, 2028–2029, 2029, 2045
Contour deficiencies, correction of, 1464–1465, 1465
  in Andy Gump deformity, 1515–1521
  in hemifacial microsomia, 1557–1559, 1558
Contouring, cosmetic dental, 223–225, 224
Contra-angle technique, for screw fixation, in sagittal split osteotomy, 2369
Contrast media, for double-contrast arthrography, 502
Contusion, orbital, ptosis in, 1068
Copper, in Implator, 1340
Coronal incision, anatomic considerations in, 951–960
  closure of, 965, 965–966
  complications of, 966, 966–967
  for maxillary osteotomy, 967, 971
  for reconstructive surgery, 972–975, 972–977
  for trauma, 967, 968–971
  indications for, 967–975, 968–977
  scarring with, 966, 967
  soft tissue laxity after, 1023
  technique of, 961–967, 962–966
Coronal synostosis, unilateral, 1845, 1851–1855, 1852–1854
Coronoid process, tumors of, coronal approach for, 975
Coronoidectomy, 672

Coronoidotomy, after temporalis myofascial flap surgery, 733
  in intraoral vertical ramus osteotomy, 2115, 2118
Corrugator supercilii muscles, 956, *956*
Cortical bone, 1337
  grafting of, 834, 1482–1483
Corticocancellous bone graft. See *Bone graft.*
Corticosteroids. See *Steroids.*
Cosmetic contouring, dental, 223–225, *224*
Cosmetic dentistry. See *Esthetic dentistry.*
Cosmetic surgery. See also specific procedures.
  after orthognathic surgery, 232–233
  demand for, 1440–1443
  during osseointegrated implant surgery, 1433, *1434*
  patient profile in, 11–13
  satisfaction with, 1440
Costochondral graft, 873–922
  absent disk in, 932
  ankylosis at site of, 938–945, *940–943*, 1520–1521
  applications of, 1483
  biologic foundation of, 873–874
  cartilage length in, 1485
  difficulties and complications with, 929–945
  donor site complications in, 929
  failure of, Vitek-Kent prosthesis for. See *Vitek-Kent prosthesis.*
  for condylar reconstruction, 671–673, *672*
  fracture of, 932, *932, 939*
  growth of, 873–874, 932–933, *934–939*
  harvesting of, *1483*, 1483–1485, *1484*
  imaging of, 929, 929–931, *930*
  in ankylosis, 881, *890–893*
  in avulsive condylar fracture, 894–904, *895–904*
  in condylar deficiency, 1493–1498, *1494–1498*
  in congenital dysplasias, 879–881, *880, 882–889*
  in facial fractures, *1021*, 1021–1023, *1022*
  in growing child, 1496t, 1496–1498, *1497, 1498*
  in hemimandibulectomy reconstruction, 1502–1504, *1503, 1504*
  in iatrogenic disorders, 916–922, *917–922*
  in infectious disease, 914, *915, 916*
  in mandibular reconstruction, for continuity defect of condyle, condylar neck, and ramus, 1493–1498, *1495–1498*, 1496t
  in neoplastic disease, 912–914, *912–914*
  in osteoarthritis, 894, *898*, 904, *905*
  in rheumatoid arthritis, 904–909, *906–912*
  in temporomandibular joint reconstruction, 671–673, *672*
  indications for, 879–922
  infection of, 931, *931*
  lateral pterygoid muscle dysfunction in, 932
  mandibular deviation in, 932, 933
  overgrowth of, 1496t, 1496–1497, *1497, 1498*

Costochondral graft *(Continued)*
  perichondrial-periosteal sleeve for, 1485
  rib harvesting for, 874–876, *875*
  complications of, 929
  technique of, 874–879, *876–878*
  undergrowth of, 1496t, 1498
  with dermal graft, 924, *926*
Cottle test, 104, *104*, 328, *329*
Coupling factor, in bone regeneration, 1450
Cranial bone graft. See *Bone graft, cranial.*
Cranial molding, external (postural), vs. craniosynostosis, 1844–1845
Cranial nerve abnormalities, in hemifacial microsomia, 1537, *1537*
Cranial osteomuscular flap, in Treacher Collins syndrome, 1608
Cranial sutures, growth at, 2067–2070, *2069–2071*
  premature closure of. See *Craniofacial dysostosis.*
Cranial vault reshaping, in Apert syndrome, 1897, 1898, 1913–1917, *1914–1915, 1918, 1921, 1922–1923*
  in craniosynostosis. See *Craniosynostosis, surgery for.*
  in Crouzon syndrome, 1894, *1900–1912*, 1901–1913, 1923, *1924–1925*
Cranialization, in superior orbital repair, 1062
Craniofacial analysis. See *Cephalometric analysis.*
Craniofacial balance line, 91–92, *92*
Craniofacial deformity(ies), acute. See also *Fracture(s), facial.*
  congenital. See *Apert syndrome; Crouzon syndrome; Hemifacial microsomia; Treacher Collins syndrome.*
  hearing loss in, 1707–1708
  post-traumatic, 1023–1054
    bone grafting for, 1023–1025, 1027
    bony deformities in, classification of, 1027
    due to body deficit vs. bony malposition, 1027
    enophthalmos as, 1027–1033, *1028–1034*
    exposure of, 1023–1025, *1024*
    fixation methods for, 1025
    mandibular, 1054
    maxillary, 1049, *1049–1054*
    naso-orbito-ethmoid, 1037–1049, 1044t, *1045–1048, 1050–1054*
    orbital, 1057–1077. See also *Orbital deformities, post-traumatic.*
    orbitozygomatic, *1035*, 1035–1037, *1036, 1038–1044*
    principles of repair of, 1025–1027, *1026*
    soft tissue laxity and, 1023, *1024*
    speech problems in. See *Speech.*
Craniofacial dysostosis. See also *Craniosynostosis.*
  airway management in, 1841
  classification of, 1848–1851
  computerized tomography of, 1891
  extremity anomalies in, 1842, 1851
  hearing loss in, 1707, 1708
  in Apert syndrome, 1895–1899, 1913–1917, *1914, 1915, 1918, 1921, 1922–1923.* See also *Apert syndrome.*

Craniofacial dysostosis *(Continued)*
  in Carpenter syndrome, 1851
  in Crouzon syndrome, 1848–1849, 1872–1873, *1873–1875*, 1881–1883, *1882*, 1892–1895, *1900–1913*. See also *Crouzon syndrome.*
  in kleeblattschädel anomaly, 1850, *1878–1880*, 1878–1881
  in Pfeiffer syndrome, 1851
  in Saethre-Chotzen syndrome, 1851
  Le Fort III osteotomy for, speech after, 1728–1729
  mechanisms of, 2072–2073, *2072–2074*
  open bite and, 2072. See also *Open bite.*
  speech problems in, 1698, 1700, 1701, *1701*, 1702, 1720
  surgery for, airway management in, 1891–1892
    bone grafting and fixation techniques in, 1889–1890
    historical perspective on, 1889
Craniofacial growth. See also *Growth.*
  after orthognathic surgery, 38–44
  animal studies of, 38–42, *39, 40*
  clinical studies of, 42–44
  skeletal growth and, 37–38
Craniofacial prostheses, implant anchorage of, 1215–1218, *1215–1218*, 1526, *1527*
Craniofacial surgery, speech and, 1728–1729
Craniomandibular line, 94, *94*
Craniomandibular relationship, in hemifacial microsomia, 1566–1567, *1567–1569*
Cranio-occlusal plane, 94
Craniopalatal relationship, evaluation of, 412, *413, 414*
Craniosynostosis, 1839–1883. See also *Craniofacial dysostosis.*
  airway management in, 1841
  bilateral coronal, 1846–1847, 1858, *1859–1869*
  brain growth in, 1839–1840, 1840t
  calvarial sutural growth and, 2070, *2070*
  case studies of, 1851–1869, *1852–1854, 1856–1869*
  classification of, 1844–1848
  functional problems in, 1839–1842
  historical perspective on, 1839
  hydrocephalus and, 1841
  in Apert syndrome, 1839, 1842, 1843, 1846, 1849, 1874–1876, *1876–1877*
  in Carpenter syndrome, 1851
  in Crouzon syndrome, 1839, 1842, 1843, 1846, 1848, 1872–1873, *1873–1875*, 1881–1883, *1882*
  in kleeblattschädel anomaly, 1839, 1842, 1843, 1850, *1878–1880*, 1878–1881
  in Pfeiffer syndrome, 1851
  in Saethre-Chotzen syndrome, 1851
  incidence of, 1839
  inheritance of, 1839
  intracranial pressure in, *1840*, 1840–1841
  late bicoronal, 1847, 1860–1862, *1862–1863*
  metopic, 1847–1848, *1864–1867*, 1865–1867
  radical osteoclastic surgery modified after Powiertowsky for, 2070, *2071*

Craniosynostosis *(Continued)*
 sagittal, 1848, *1868–1872*
 surgery for, 1843–1848
  esthetic considerations in, 1842
  frontoforehead position in, 1842
  historical perspective on, 1843
  staging of, 1843–1844
  unilateral coronal, 1845, 1851–1855, *1852–1854*
  unilateral lambdoid, 1846, 1855, *1856–1858*
  Virchow's law and, 1839
  vs. external (postural) molding, 1844–1845
Craniotomy, with Le Fort III osteotomy, for Apert syndrome, 2065, *2066*
 for Crouzon syndrome, 2065, *2066*
Creeping replacement, 1337
Creutzfeldt-Jakob disease, transmission of, via allogenic graft, 1455–1456
Crib graft, allogenic, 1450, 1453–1454, *1454*
 in mandibular reconstruction, 1500–1524. See also *Mandibular reconstruction.*
Cricostat, 151, *152*
Cricothyroidotomy, emergency, postanesthesia, 151, *152*
Crocodile bite, *2387*
 mandibular expansion for, 2385–2389, 2398, *2400–2401*
 case study of, 2392, *2393*
Crossbite. See also *Mandibular deficiency, transverse; Maxillary deficiency, transverse.*
 in mandibular prognathism, 2145
  correction of, 2150
 in transverse mandibular deficiency, analysis and treatment of, *2342*, 2342–2343
 in transverse maxillary deficiency, 2405, 2406t, *2407*
 maxillary expansion for. See *Maxillary expansion.*
 symphyseal osteotomy for, 2398, *2400–2401*
Crouzon syndrome, 1848–1849
 case studies of, 1872–1873, *1873–1875*, 1881–1883, *1882*, *1900–1913*, 1901–1913
 computerized tomography in, 1891
 craniofacial abnormalities in, 1848–1849, 1892
 craniosynostosis in, 1839–1842, 1846, 1849. See also *Craniosynostosis.*
 middle ear anomalies in, 1707
 midface osteotomy for, speech after, 1728–1729
 skull development in, 2064, *2064*
 sleep apnea in, 2022, *2022*
 speech problems in, 1701, 1702, 1720
 surgery for, 1849, 1889–1895, *1900–1912*, 1901–1913, 1923, *1924–1925*, 2064–2065, *2065*
  airway management in, 1891–1892
  bone grafting and fixation in, 1889–1890
  Class III malocclusion correction in, 1895
  craniotomy with Le Fort III osteotomy in, 2065, *2066*
  historical perspective on, 1889
  Le Fort I osteotomy, 2287, *2288*
  morbidity in, 1892–1893

Crouzon syndrome *(Continued)*
  primary cranio-orbital, in infants, 1893–1894
  radical osteoclastic, modified after Powiertowsky, 2064–2065, *2065*
  repeat craniotomy, in young children, 1894
  results of, 1892–1893
  total midface osteotomy with advancement, 1894–1895
Crown(s), cosmetic, 228–230, *229*
Crown length, insufficient, 241, *242*, *243*
 measurement of, 239, *239*
Crura, nasal, *291*, 291–292, 322, *322*
Cryopreservation, of graft material, 849–850, 1453
Cryotherapy, for mandibular hypomobility, 1669
CT point, in cephalometric analysis, 90, *90*
Curve of Spee, in mandibular deficiency, *2340*, 2341
 leveling of, orthodontic, 61, 61–62, *62*, *2342*, 2431, 2431–2432
  surgical, 2495–2499, *2496*, *2497*
Cuspid(s), measurement of. See *Dental measurements.*
Cuspid-nose vertical referent, 177–179, *178*, 188
Cutaneous complications, of rhinoplasty, 272
Cutting cone, in bone healing, 1337

Dacryocystitis, post-traumatic, *1048*, 1074, *1074*, 1075–1076
 in medial orbital deformity, 1065
Dacryocystorhinoplasty, 1076
Dal Pont sagittal split osteotomy, 2336, 2348–2349, 2350
Date and mate selection, appearance and, 7–8
Deafness. See *Hearing loss.*
Deceleration injuries, 988
Decongestants, postoperative, 117
Deep-bite deformity, 2431–2438
 anteroposterior dimension correction in, *2431*, *2432*, 2433, *2434*, *2435*
 arch leveling in, 62, *62*, 2431–2432, *2432*
 augmentation genioplasty in, 2477, *2477–2483*
 case study of, 2433–2438, *2436–2438*
 leveling of curve of Spee in, 62, *62*
 sagittal split osteotomy with reduction genioplasty for, *2503–2505*, 2504–2506
 treatment planning for, 2431, *2432*
 vertical dimension correction in, 2433
Degenerative joint disease. See also *Arthritis.*
 arthroscopy of, 608–609, *609*, *610*
 Vitek-Kent prosthesis for. See *Vitek-Kent prosthesis.*
Delaire cephalometric analysis, 89–94, *89–94*, 408–412, *409–414*, 2077–2078, *2078*
Delaire procedure, for open bite, complications and relapse with, 2080, 2080t
 technique for, 2086–2089, *2087–2089*

Demeclocycline hydrochloride, for bone labeling, in intraosseous orthodontic implant analysis, 1255
Denasal speech, 1695–1696
Dental. See also under *Tooth (teeth).*
Dental analysis, cephalometric, 95–96, *96*
 case studies of, 97, *97–98*, *98*
Dental bridge. See also *Dentures.*
 for transmandibular implant, 1369, *1369*
Dental compensation, insufficient, 52, *52–55*
 preoperative correction of, 2181
Dental examination, preoperative, 104
Dental expansion. See *Orthodontic treatment.*
Dental extractions, in mandibular prognathism, 2148, 2149, 2150
Dental hygiene, for Branemark implants, 1182–1184, *1183*
 for hydroxyapatite-coated implants, 1319
 for orthodontic implants, 1258
 postoperative, 118
Dental implants. See also *Implants, osseointegrated.*
 Branemark, abutment examination in, 1175–1176, *1176*
  abutment placement in, 1168–1171, *1168–1172*
  abutment surgery in, 1162–1171
  acrylic-metal-framework, vs. porcelain-fused-to-metal, 1178, *1189*
  alignment devices for, 1178–1181, *1179*, *1180*
  angulated 30-degree abutment for, *1186*, 1186–1187
  applications of, with available bone, 1184–1189
  biocompatibility of, 1140–1141, *1141*
  bite rim for, 1176, *1176*
  bone assessment and alignment for, 1177–1182, *1178–1181*
  bone graft for, 1191–1213
   Branemark maxillary full arch, *1206*, 1207
   collagen tubes for, 1221–1224, *1222*, *1223*
   compressed cancellous, *1199*, 1200, *1201*, 1203, *1204*
   inlay, 1192–1195, *1193*, *1194*
   interpositional, 1200–1201, *1201*
   mandibular split, 1213–1215, *1214*
   maxillary split, with anterior fixation, 1211, *1213*
    with palatal fixation, 1207–1211, *1208*, *1209*
   results of, 1191–1192
   saddle, 1195–1196, *1196*, *1197*, 1203–1204, *1205*
   sinus, 1201–1204, *1202*, *1204*, *1205*
   types of, 1191–1192
   veneer, 1197–1200, *1198*, *1199*
  bone-metallic interface in, studies of, 1131–1147
  bone remodeling with, *1162*, 1162–1163, *1232*, 1234–1241, *1235–1240*
  bone vs. soft tissue interface for, 1146, *1146*, *1147*

Dental implants (Continued)
  case studies of, 1389, *1390, 1391,*
    1391, *1393–1402,* 1393–1403,
    1413–1425, *1414, 1415, 1418–
    1420, 1423, 1424*
  cleaning of, 1182–1184, *1183*
  conical abutment for, 1185–1186,
    1186
  countersinking in, 1154–1156,
    1154–1156
  cover screw placement in, 1159–
    1160, *1160, 1161*
  cover screw removal in, 1165–1167,
    1166–1168
  drilling in, *1150–1154,* 1151–1154
  experimental background of, 1135–
    1147, *1236–1240,* 1236–1241
  exposure in, for first-stage surgery,
    1148–1150, 1148–1151
    for second-stage surgery, 1163–
      1165, *1164, 1165*
  first-stage postoperative care in,
    1161, *1161, 1162*
  fixture placement in, 1157–1159,
    1158, 1159
  follow-up for, 1183–1184
  gingival mask for, 1177, *1177*
  gold, reactivity of, 1140, *1141*
  guided bone regeneration for,
    1218–1220, *1219*
  healing cap placement in, 1170–
    1171, *1171, 1172*
  history of, *1132–1134,* 1132–1135
  holding power of, 1141–1142, *1143*
  home care maintenance of, 1182–
    1184, *1183*
  host bed for, assessment of, 1148,
    1149, 1181, 1181–1182
    electrical stimulation of, 1143–
      1144
    experimental evaluation of, 1143–
      1144, *1144*
    irradiation of, 1143
    temperature and, 1144, *1144*
  hydroxyapatite inlay for, 1192–
    1195, *1193, 1194*
    collagen tubes for, 1221–1224,
      1222, 1223
  in irradiated bone, 1143
  insertion torque and, 1144–1145
  Le Fort I downgraft for, 1211, *1213*
  loading conditions for, 1145
  loss of, 1184
  models for, 1175–1176, *1176,
    1180,* 1180–1181
  multiplanar reconstruction imaging
    for, *1181,* 1182
  one-stage vs. two-stage procedure
    for, 1145
  orthodontic anchorage on, 1260–1261
  orthodontic treatment with, 1417–
    1421, *1418–1420*
  osseointegration of, 1146, *1146, 1147*
  overdenture for, 1187–1189, *1188,
    1189*
  physiologic response to, *1232*
  pin fixture locator splint for, 1178–
    1180, *1179–1181*
  placement of, with orthognathic sur-
    gery, 1389, *1390, 1391,* 1391,
    1393–1402, 1393–1403,
    1413–1416, *1414, 1415*
  polytetrafluoroethylene membranes
    for, 1218–1220, *1219*

Dental implants (Continued)
  porcelain-fused-to-metal, 1178, *1189*
  prosthetic overload with, 1184
  prosthetic procedure in, 1175–
    1177, *1176, 1177*
  radiographic assessment for, 1178,
    1181–1182, *1182*
  rigidity of, 1175
  rubber fixture locator splint for,
    1180, 1180–1181
  self-tapping fixtures for, 1174, *1174,
    1175*
  shape of, 1141–1142, *1143*
  single tooth, 1184–1185, *1185,*
    1189, *1190*
  site preparation for, in first-stage
    surgery, 1150–1156, *1150–
    1156*
    in second-stage surgery, 1165–
      1168, *1166–1168*
  stainless steel, reactivity of, 1140,
    1141
  success of, 1146
  surface energy of, 1142
  tapping in, *1156,* 1156–1157, *1157*
  team approach in, 1177–1182
  technique for, 1148–1171
  titanium, reactivity of, 1141, *1142*
  UCLA castable abutment for, 1187,
    1187
  zirconium, reactivity of, 1140, *1141*
Calcitite. See *Dental implants, hydroxyapatite-coated.*
  hydroxyapatite-coated, bar-and-clip at-
    tachments for, 1305–1307, *1306–
    1307*
    biointegration of, *1299–1302,*
      1299–1303
    bone loss with, 1318
    case studies of, 1319–1331, 1404–
      1412, *1404–1412*
    cleaning of, 1319
    clinical trials of, 1303–1317
    dental model for, 1319, *1319–1320*
    diagnostic planning for, 1265–1266
    fixed, clinical trials of, 1307–1317,
      1317t
      vs. removable, 1268–1269
    iatrogenic complications with, 1318–
      1319
    in anterior maxilla, technique for,
      1287–1288
    in fresh extraction sites, *1289, 1290,
      1291,* 1316, 1330, *1330, 1331*
      technique for, 1288–1293, *1289–
      1293*
    in hemimaxillectomy, 1307
    in mandibulectomy, *1311–1316,*
      1313, 1407–1410, *1408–1410*
    in posterior maxilla, technique for,
      1288
    Integral, clinical trials with, 1303–
      1317
    length of, 1305, 1305t
    mandibular augmentation for, 1271,
      1271, 1272, 1288, 1316, 1324,
      1324–1328
    materials for, 1297
    maxillary augmentation for, 1287–
      1288, 1322, *1322–1324,* 1407–
      1410, *1408–1410*
    mechanical characteristics of, 1297–
      1299, *1298*
    morbidity of, 1317–1319

Dental implants (Continued)
    mucogingival problems with, 1317–
      1318
    osseointegration of, *1299–1302,*
      1299–1303
      failure of, 1318
    overdenture, 1267, 1269
      clinical trials of, 1305–1307
    placement of, with orthognathic sur-
      gery, *1403–1412,* 1404–1412
    preservation of keratinized tissue
      for, 1293–1295, *1294*
    removal of, 1317–1319
    scientific basis for, 1297–1303,
      1298–1302
    secondary grafting around, 1295–
      1296, *1295–1297,* 1329,
      1329
    subperiosteal, *1270, 1271,* 1319,
      1319–1321
    template fabrication for, 1266–1267
    tissue reactivity of, *1299–1302,*
      1299–1303, 1317–1318
    treatment planning for, for mandib-
      ular edentulous patients, 1271,
      1271, 1272
      for maxillary edentulous patients,
        1274–1276, 1274–1277
      for partially edentulous patients,
        1266–1267
      for totally edentulous patients,
        1267–1268
      with simultaneous maxillary sinus
        grafting, 1277–1286, *1277–
        1286,* 1313–1315
  in aging face syndrome, 1427–1436
  Integral. See *Dental implants, hydroxy-
    apatite-coated.*
  maxillary, 1172–1174, *1173, 1174*
  patient satisfaction with, 1443–1446
  placement of, during orthognathic
    surgery, case studies of, 1387–
    1425
  psychological aspects of, 1443–1446
  titanium, Branemark. See *Dental im-
    plants, Branemark.*
    osseointegration of, vs. hydroxyapa-
      tite-coated implants, *1299–
      1302,* 1299–1303
    supragingival connective tissue appa-
      ratus in, 1301
  tricalcium phosphate–coated, strength
    of, 1298
Dental interdigitation, postoperative
  maintenance of, 78, *78*
  preoperative correction of, 58, *58*
Dental measurements, 185–199
  anteroposterior, 175–176, 188, *188,*
    190, *191,* 2311, *2312*
  in model Le Fort I osteotomy, 201–
    202
  in model sagittal split mandibular ad-
    vancement, 200
  transverse, 176, *177,* 188, *189,* 190,
    192, 2312, *2312*
  vertical, 170–172, *171,* 186, *186, 187,*
    190, 190, 2311, *2311*
Dental model. See also *Model* entries.
  for hydroxyapatite-coated implants,
    1319, *1319–1320*
  for transmandibular implant prostho-
    dontics, 1364, *1365, 1366*
  in post-traumatic deformity evaluation,
    990, 995, *996*

Facial nerve. See also *Nerve(s)*.
  abnormalities of, in hemifacial microsomia, 1537, *1537*
  anatomy of, 428, 704–705, *704–706*
  branches of, 704–705, *704–706*
  injury of, classification of, 1086–1088, *1087*
    ectropion and, 1071, *1072*
    in arthroscopic surgery, 624
    in masseter reduction, 433, 435
    in Vitek-Kent prosthesis placement, 788–789, 789t
    preservation of, in condylar graft placement, 876, *877*
    in coronal incision, 963–964, *964*
  temporal branch of. See *Temporal nerve*.
Facial prosthesis, implant anchorage of, 1215–1218, *1215–1218*, *1308–1310*, 1526, *1527*
  maxillary, 1525–1526
Facial reference planes. See also *Model measurement; Model surgery*.
  in hemifacial microsomia, 1562–1566, *1563–1566*
Facial sutures, growth at, 2071–2072, *2072*
  disturbances of, 2072, *2073*, *2074*
  premature closure of. See *Craniofacial dysostosis*.
Facial width, excessive transverse, mandibular ramus reduction for, 2511–2514, *2512*, *2513*, *2515*
  with masseter muscle hypertrophy. See *Masseter muscle hypertrophy*.
Fascia, temporalis, 957–958, *958*
  mobilization of, coronal approach for, 973, *974*
Fascicles, *1084*, 1084–1085
  alignment of, in nerve coaptation, 1109
  mushrooming, microsurgical preparation of, 1108
Fat, subcutaneous, as maturity indicator, 32–33, 35
Fat pad, buccal, 379
  nasolabial fold, 378
  submental and submandibular, 377–379, *378*
Fat removal. See *Lipectomy*.
Femoral cutaneous nerve, injury of, in anterior ilium graft harvesting, *1486*, 1487
Fentanyl citrate, in anesthesia, 150
Fever, postoperative, 123–124
FH plane. See *Frankfort horizontal plane*.
Fiberoptic endoscopy, for velopharyngeal function assessment, *1713*, 1713–1714, *1714*
Fibrosis, temporomandibular joint, arthroscopic diagnosis of, 651–652
Fibrous ankylosis, after Vitek-Kent prosthesis placement, 791–792, *792*
  arthroscopic diagnosis of, 651–652
  arthrotomy for, 668–673. See also *Arthrotomy*.
  postoperative, magnetic resonance imaging of, 515, *516*
  mandibular hypomobility and, 1668–1669
Vitek-Kent prosthesis in, 741, *742*
Finger spelling, 1721
Fisher-Logemann Test of Articulation Competence, 1709
Fistula, alveolar, closure of, speech and, 1722

Fistula *(Continued)*
  nasolabial, closure of, speech and, 1722, 1726
  palatal, maxillary surgery and, 1722–1727, *1725–1727*
    speech problems and, 1700, *1700*, 1710
    treatment of, 726, 1719
Fixation, intermaxillary. See *Intermaxillary fixation*.
  maxillomandibular. See *Maxillomandibular fixation*.
  rehabilitation after. See *Rehabilitation*.
  rigid internal. See *Rigid internal fixation*.
  wire. See *Wire(s); Wire fixation*.
Flap(s), cervical, 1478–1482, *1479–1482*
  bipedicled, 1480–1481, *1481*
  skin-platysma rotation, 1478–1479, *1479*, *1480*
  U-Y advancement, 1481–1482, *1482*
coronal. See *Coronal incision*.
cranial osteomuscular, in Treacher Collins syndrome, 1608
for maxillary reconstruction, 1526–1528, *1528*
frontoparietal, 982, *982*, *983*
in cleft deformity repair. See *Cleft deformities*.
ischemia of, 120–121
latissimus dorsi, *1471*, 1471–1472, *1472*
microvascular groin, cutaneous, 1569
in hemifacial microsomia treatment, 1561–1599. See also under *Hemifacial microsomia, treatment of*.
osteocutaneous, 1569–1571
mucocutaneous, in total maxillopalatine cleft repair, 394, *395*
mucoperiosteal, in gummy smile correction, 246–250, *247–250*, 257–258, *258*, 259, *259*, 260
myocutaneous, 1456–1457, *1457*
  for Andy Gump deformity, 1515, *1515*
  in irradiated tissue, 1456–1457
  indications for, 1456–1457
  technique for, 1466–1482
  types of, 1466–1482
palatal, in fistula repair, 75, *75*
pectoralis major, 1466–1469, *1466–1470*
  for Andy Gump deformity, 1515, *1515*
perfusion of, fluorescein test for, 1476–1477, *1478*
pharyngeal, for inadequate velopharyngeal valve closure, 1716–1719, *1717*, 1724–1727
skin paddle for, 1465
sternocleidomastoid, 1474–1475, *1474–1476*
tempoparietal, 982, *982*, *983*
temporalis myofascial. See *Temporalis myofascial flap*.
tissue bed dissection for, *1465*, 1465–1466
trapezius, 1472–1474, *1473*
walk-up, 1476–1477, *1477*, *1478*
Floating forehead technique, for craniosynostosis, 1843
Flossing, of dental implants, 1182–1184, *1183*
Fluid loss, intraoperative monitoring of, 138–139

Fluid replacement, postoperative, 124–126
Fluorescein test, for flap perfusion, 1476–1477, *1478*
Fluphenazine, for post-traumatic pain, in nerve injury, 1106
FM point, in cephalometric analysis, 90
Foley catheterization, 110–111, 138, 140, *141*
Forceps, microsurgical, 1111–1112, *1112*
Forehead, anatomy of, 955–957, *956*
  esthetic analysis of, 1842
  lymphatic drainage of, 960, *961*
Foreign body reaction, condylar resorption in, costochondral graft in, 918–922, *918–922*
  to dental implants, 1140–1141, *1141*
  to Vitek-Kent prosthesis, 793
Fossa. See *Glenoid fossa*.
Fracture(s), avulsive condylar, costochondral graft in, 894–904, *895–904*
  open reduction of, 895, *899*
  buccal fragment, intraoperative, *1991*, 1991–1992
    in sagittal split osteotomy, fixation of, *1991*, 1991–1992
  condylar neck, intraoperative, *1991*, 1991–1992
  costochondral graft, 932, *932*, *939*
  craniofacial, coronal approach in, 967, *968–970*
  facial. See also specific facial bones.
    bone graft for, 1015, 1021–1023, *1022*
    deformities after. See *Craniofacial deformities, post-traumatic; Maxillofacial deformities, post-traumatic*.
    direct exposure of, 1015
    enophthalmos after, 1014, *1014*, 1027–1033, *1028–1034*, 1035–1037, *1036*, *1038–1044*
    fixation of, 1015, 1016–1021, *1017–1020*
    incisions and approaches for, 1015–1016
    naso-orbito-ethmoid deformities after, 1037–1049, 1044t, *1045–1049*, *1050–1054*
    reduction of, 1015
    repair of, 1015–1023
      principles of, 1015–1016
    zygomatic arch stabilization in, 1017–1019, *1018–1020*, *1035*, *1036*, *1038–1044*, 1049, *1050–1054*
  frontal sinus, coronal approach in, 967, *969*, 975, *976*
    deformities after, 1062–1063
  frontonasal, coronal approach in, 967, *969*
  healing of. See *Bone, healing of*.
  intraoperative, in sagittal split osteotomy, fixation of, *1991*, 1991–1992
    in children, 2516–2517
  Le Fort, maxillary deformity after, 1049, *1050*, *1053–1054*
  Le Fort II, coronal approach in, 967
  Le Fort III, coronal approach in, 967, *968*
  mandibular, bone graft for, 1015, 1021–1023, *1022*. See also *Bone graft*.
    case studies of, 1000–1010
    deformity after, 993–997

Fracture(s) *(Continued)*
  fixation of, 997, 1015, 1016–1021, *1017–1020*. See also *Fixation*.
  principles of repair of, 1015–1016
  mandibular angle, screw fixation of, stress analysis of, 1971–1974, *1972–1974*
  mandibular greenstick, in sagittal split osteotomy, in children, 2516–2517
  nasal, coronal approach in, 967, *969*
  nasoethmoidal, coronal approach in, 967, *969*
  orbital, coronal approach in, 967, *968, 970*
  ramus, in sagittal split osteotomy, fixation of, *1991*, 1991–1992
    intraoperative, *1991*, 1991–1992
    unanticipated, in mandibular osteotomy, 67–69, *68–71*
  zygomatic, coronal approach in, 967, *968, 970*
Frankfort horizontal plane, 87, 157, 158–159, *159*, 159t, 179–181, *180*, 2307–2309, *2308–2310*
Freeze-drying, of graft material, 849–850, 1453
Frey's syndrome, in Vitek-Kent prosthesis placement, 788–789, 789t
Fricative sounds, 1689, 1689t, *1690*
Frontal process osteotomy, in orbital reconstruction, 1064–1065
Frontal region. See also *Forehead*.
  lymphatic drainage of, 960, *961*
Frontal sinus, fracture of, coronal approach in, 967, *969*, 975, *976*
  post-traumatic deformities of, 1062–1063
Frontalis muscle, 956, *956*
  fixation of, in ptosis repair, 1068

Gait disturbance, after graft harvesting from ilium, 1486
Galea aponeurotica, *952*, 953, 955, *956*
Gastric preparation, for anesthesia, 133–134, 141–142
General anesthesia. See *Anesthesia*.
Genial fixation devices, placement of, 2455
Genioglossus muscles, 2180
Geniohyoid muscles, 2180
Genioplasty, 1513–1514, *1514, 1515*, 2439–2487. See also *Chin*.
  after cleft deformity repair, 422, 422–424, *423*
  augmentation, allogenic bone graft in, 850
    broad soft tissue pedicle, 2446–2456
      biologic foundation of, 2446, *2447*
      screw fixation in, *2450–2454*, 2452–2455
      technique for, 2446–2452, *2447–2453*
    double sliding horizontal osteotomy in, 2459–2464, *2460–2464*
    double step, 2459–2464, *2460–2464*
    fixation device placement in, 2455
    horizontal sliding osteotomy in, 2443–2446, *2446*
    hydroxyapatite implant in, 857, *863*, 863
    implants in, 2484–2487, *2486*

Genioplasty *(Continued)*
  in Apert syndrome, 1897, 1898
  in Crouzon syndrome, 1895, 1898
  in masseter reduction, *445*
  in Pierre Robin syndrome, 2463, *2463*
  in total mandibular augmentation, 2392–2394
  model surgery for, 181–184, 182t, *182–184*
  nasal dorsum graft in, 835
  overlapping, 2456–2459, *2459*
  soft tissue changes and stability after, 2464, *2464*
  soft tissue:bone advancement relationship in, 2443
  wedge osteotomy in, 2446, *2446*
  with concurrent Le Fort I osteotomy, 2455–2456, *2456–2458*
  cheiloplasty and, 2488
  combined horizontal and oblique anterior mandibular osteotomy for, 2402
  complications of, 2487–2488
  for asymmetry, 2469–2474, *2473–2476*
  for chin lengthening, 2477, *2477–2483*
  for chin shortening, 2477–2484, *2485*
  for transverse deformities, 2468–2474
  for vertical deformities, 2474–2484
  functional, after cleft deformity repair, 422, 422–424, *423*
  in Andy Gump deformity, 1516–1521, *1517–1520*
  in maxillomandibular horizontal disharmony correction, 2398, *2401*
  in open bite correction, 2089–2091, *2090, 2091*
  in short mandibular ramus deformity correction, 1999
  in Treacher Collins syndrome, 1606
  jumping, in Treacher Collins syndrome, 1609, *1609*
  mentalis muscle positioning in, 2487
  narrowing, 2469, *2470*
  reduction, anteroposterior, 2465–2467, *2465–2468*
    with sagittal split osteotomy, 2503–2505, *2503–2506*
  widening, 2469, *2470, 2471*
Geniotomy–tongue advancement, in maxillomandibular advancement, in sleep apnea, *2052*, 2052–2053, *2053*
Gingiva, attached, 1338–1339
  free, 1338
  in implant osteointegration, 1301, *1338*, 1338–1339, *1339*
  keratinized, in dental implant surgery, 1293–1295, *1294*
  marginal, 1338–1339
  structure of, 1338–1339, *1339, 1340*
Gingival display, excessive. See *Smile, gummy*.
Gingival exposure, evaluation of, 236
  excessive. See *Smile, gummy*.
  ideal, 240–241, *241*
Gingival flap surgery, for gummy smile, 246–250, *247–250*, 257–258, *258*
Gingival height, measurement of, 239–240
Gingival hyperplasia, with transmandibular implant, 1375, *1375–1377*
Gingival inflammation, with hydroxyapatite-coated dental implants, 1317–1318

Gingival inflammation *(Continued)*
  with transmandibular implants, 1375, *1375–1377*
Gingival mask, for Branemark dental implants, 1177, *1177*
Gingival rebound, 258
Gingival sulcus, 1338
Gingivectomy, for gummy smile, clinical evaluation for, 236–240, *239*
  esthetic objectives for, 240–241, *241, 242*
  technique of, 245–246, *246, 247*, 256, 256–257, *257*, 259–261, *259–261*
Glabella, 955
Glabellar angle, in soft tissue esthetic analysis, 88
Glenoid fossa, condylar position in. See *Condyle, position of; Condyle, positioning of*.
  construction of, with costochondral graft, 879–881
  erosion of, 767–768, *768, 769*
  exposure of, hemicoronal approach for, 975, *977*
  preparation of, for Vitek-Kent prosthesis placement, 767–768, *768, 769*
Glenoid fossa implant, 752–753, *753*. See also *Vitek-Kent prosthesis*.
  computerized tomography of, *498*, 498–499
  development of, 737–740
  durability of, 792, *792*
  instability of, 772t
  magnetic resonance imaging of, 515–516
  placement of, *769–772*, 769–773
Glide sounds, 1689t, 1691, *1691*
Globe, in malar dystopia, 1060
  preoperative protection of, 1067
Glycosaminoglycans, 1640, *1640, 1641*
  effects of immobilization on, 1643
Gnathoretrusion, condylar positioning and, 530–531
Gold, in Implator, 1340
Gold dental implants, reactivity of, 1140, *1141*
Gold-samarium magnets, for prosthesis anchorage, 1526, *1527*
Goldenhar hemifacial microsomia, 1535, *1535*, 2066
Gonadal development, as maturity indicator, 32, 32t
Gonadal hormone secretion, regulation of, 23–24, *24*
Gonial arc radius method, for condylar position assessment, 526, *526*
Gore-Tex Expanded Polytetrafluoroethylene Soft Tissue Patch, in capsular reconstruction, 723, *724*
Graft. See *Bone graft; Cartilage graft*.
  bone. See *Bone graft*.
  cartilage. See *Cartilage graft; Costochondral graft*.
  dermal. See *Dermal graft*.
  dura, allogenic, in ankylosis repair, 1523–1524, *1524*
  nerve. See *Nerve graft*.
  ossicle, 1218, *1218*
  palatal, for hydroxyapatite-coated dental implants, 1295
  tissue, for hydroxyapatite-coated implants, 1295–1296, *1295–1297*
Great auricular nerve, anatomy of, 1123

Great auricular nerve graft, for trigeminal nerve repair, 1111
  harvesting technique for, 1123
Great auricular nerve transfer, in inferior alveolar nerve repair, 1114–1116, *1115*
  in lingual nerve repair, 1120, *1120*
Greater occipital nerve, 955, *955*
Greenstick fracture, intraoperative mandibular, fixation of, *1991*, 1991–1992
  in children, 2516–2517
Greenstick osteotomy, *1035*, 1037, *1039*
Greulich-Pye atlas method, for skeletal age determination, 36
Groin flap, microvascular, cutaneous, 1569
  in hemifacial microsomia treatment, 1561–1599. See also under *Hemifacial microsomia, treatment of.*
  osteocutaneous, 1569–1571
Growth, biologic regulation of, 23–38
  craniofacial, animal studies of, 38–42, *39, 40*
    clinical studies of, 42–44
    postoperative, 38–44
    skeletal growth and, 37–38
  indicators of, 27–38
    chronologic, 27
    dental, 34, 35
    facial, 37–38
    height, 27–28, *28–31*, 32t, 37
    relative significance of, 34–35
    reproductive system, 32t, 32–33
    skeletal, 33–38, *36, 37*
  maxillary, movements of, 410–411, *411*
  orthognathic surgery during, 38–44
  scintigraphic evaluation of. See *Skeletal scintigraphy.*
Growth curves, 27–28, *27–31*, 37
Growth hormone secretion, regulation of, 23–24, *24*
Guide drill, for Branemark dental implants, 1151, *1151*
Guided bone regeneration, for dental implants, 1218–1220, *1219*
Gunshot wounds, 988, 1004–1006, *1004–1007*

Haas expansion appliance, 2385, 2388
  patient age for, 2395
Hand-wrist radiography, in skeletal age determination, 35–38, *36, 37*
Hard palate. See *Palate.*
Hawley retainer, 82
Head and neck, evaluation of, preoperative, 103–105, *104*
Head and neck evaluation, preanesthesia, 130–132, *131*
Headgear, for cleft deformity–associated maxillary deficiency, 2315–2322, *2316–2321*
  maxillary protraction, for mandibular prognathism, 2146
  orthodontic, for postoperative correction, 77
  reverse-pull, for mandibular prognathism, 2146–2147
Health history, preoperative, 102–103
Hearing, after maxillary osteotomy, 1726–1727
  mechanics of, 1706

Hearing aids, 1707, 1720–1721
  bone conduction, 1721
  implanted, 1218, *1218*, 1721
  in Treacher Collins syndrome, 1610
Hearing loss, after temporomandibular joint reconstruction, 932
  in Apert syndrome, 1896
  in hemifacial microsomia, 1537
  in Treacher Collins syndrome, 1609, 1610, 1614
  speech in, 1706–1708
  treatment of, 1720–1721
Heat therapy, for mandibular hypomobility, 1669
Height, as maturity indicator, 27–30, *28–31*, 32t, 34–35, 37
Hematoma, under coronal flap, *966*, 967
Hemicoronal incision. See *Coronal incision.*
Hemifacial microsomia, 1533–1599
  bone graft in, for condylar process construction, 1583–1586
    revision of, 1591–1592, *1598*
  clinical classification of, 1537–1539, 1538t, *1538–1540*, 1540–1542
  clinical findings in, 1534–1537
  condylar process construction in, 1583–1586, 1591–1592, *1598*
  correction for abnormal lip position in, 1563–1566, *1565, 1566*
  costochondral graft in, 879–881, *880, 882–887*
  cranial nerve abnormalities in, 1537, *1537*
  craniomandibular relationship in, 1566–1567, *1567–1569*
  ear abnormalities in, *1535*, 1536–1537, *1537*
  ear canal localization in, 1562–1563, *1564*
  etiology of, 1533
  facial reference planes in, 1562–1566, *1563–1566*
  frontonasal, 1535, *1535*
  Goldenhar, 1535, *1535*, 2066
  incidence of, 1533
  microphthalmic, 1535, *1535*
  orthodontic treatment in, 1543, 1571, 1578, 1579, 1584, 1587, *1590, 1591*
  osseointegrated implants for, 1435–1436, *1436, 1437*
  ramus lengthening in, 2005–2009, *2005–2010*
  skeletal defects in, *1534*, 1534–1535, *1535*, 1536–1538, *1538–1540*, 1540–1542
  sleep apnea in, 2022
  soft tissue defects in, *1536*, 1536–1539, *1537*, 1540–1542
  tongue deviation in, 1705
  treatment of, case studies of, 1571–1599
    in growing child, 1542–1550, *1544–1553*
    orthodontic, 1543
    presurgical orthopedic, 1543, *1544–1546*
    results of, 1546–1550
    surgical, 1543–1550
  in nongrowing patients, 1553–1559
    for skeletal defects, 1553–1556, *1554–1557*
    for soft tissue defects, 1557–1559, *1558*

Hemifacial microsomia *(Continued)*
  microvascular groin flap in, 1561–1599
    case studies of, 1571–1598
    cutaneous, 1569
    osteocutaneous, 1569–1571
    patient selection for, 1562
    selection of, 1569–1571
    special problems affecting, 1562–1568
  treatment planning for, 1538t
Hemimandibular crib. See also *Crib graft.*
  allogenic, in mandibular reconstruction, *1500*, 1500–1501, *1501*
Hemimandibular ilium form, allogenic, in mandibular reconstruction, *1501*, 1501–1502, *1502*, 1506–1507, *1507*, 1510, *1510*
Hemimandibulectomy, reconstructive surgery for, 1498–1504, *1498–1504*
  allogenic hemimandibular crib for, *1500*, 1500–1501, *1501*
  allogenic hemimandibular ilium form for, *1501*, 1501–1502, *1502*
  autogenous costochondral graft for, *1502*, 1502–1504, *1503*
Hemimaxillectomy, hydroxyapatite-coated dental implants in, 1307
Hemodynamic monitoring, 138
Hemostasis, 112–113, 121
  in ilium graft harvesting, 849, 1488–1489
  in intraoral vertical ramus osteotomy, 2132
  in microreconstructive surgery, 1109
  in posterior ilium graft harvesting, 1488–1489
  in rhinoplasty, 272
  in sagittal split osteotomy, 2132–2133
  in temporomandibular joint surgery, 712
  in Vitek-Kent prosthesis placement, 789, 789t
  intraoperative, 112–113
  postoperative, 121
Hepatitis, transmission of, via allogenic graft, 1455–1456
Herbst appliance, for sleep apnea, 2029–2030, *2030*
High condylectomy, for temporomandibular joint dysfunction, 645
High Le Fort I osteotomy. See *Le Fort I osteotomy, high.*
Hinge-axis facebow transfer, 160–161
Hip. See *Ilium.*
Horizontal mandibular osteotomy, 2111, *2112*, 2113
  for chin asymmetry, 2472–2474, *2473–2474*
Horizontal plane, Frankfort, 87, 157, 158–159, *159*, 159t, 179–181, *180*, 2307–2309, *2308–2310*
  natural, 157, 158
Horizontal sliding osteotomy, for chin augmentation, 2443–2446, *2446*, 2459–2464, *2460–2464*
  for chin lengthening, 2477, *2477–2483*
  for chin reduction, 2465–2468, *2466, 2467*
  for chin shortening, 2477–2484, *2485*
Hormones, gonadal, regulation of, 23–24, *24*

Horner's syndrome, ptosis in, *1069*
Human immunodeficiency virus, transmission of, via allogenic graft, 1455–1456
Hunsuck sagittal split osteotomy, 2336, 2350
Hydrocephalus, in Apert syndrome, 1894
　in craniosynostosis, 1841
　in Crouzon syndrome, 1894
Hydroxyapatite, characteristics of, 1265
　preparation of, 1297
Hydroxyapatite implants, 854–871
　case studies of, 863–871, *864–870*
　clinical applications of, 855–857
　complications of, 856–857
　composition of, *854*, 854
　contraindications to, 857
　for dental implants, 1192–1195, *1194*
　　collagen tubes for, 1221–1224, *1222, 1223*
　histology of, *855*, 855–857
　in chin augmentation, 862, *863*, 2473, 2477, *2477, 2478*
　in chin downgraft, 862, *862*
　in chin lengthening, 2477, *2477, 2478*
　in maxillary advancement, 856, 858, *858*, 863–867, *864–868*
　in maxillary downgraft, 856, 859, *859*, 866–867, *867, 868*
　in maxillary expansion, *859*, 859–860, *860*
　in maxillary segmentalization, 860
　in midface advancement, *869*, 869–871, *870*
　in midface augmentation, 861–862, *862*
　in midface osteotomy, 861, *861*
　in ramus augmentation, in facial asymmetry, 2514–2516, *2516*
　particulate, for mandibular augmentation, 1271, *1271, 1272*, 1272–1274, 1288, 1316, 1324, *1324–1328*, 1326
　　for maxillary augmentation, 1287–1288, 1322, *1322–1324*, 1410, *1410*
　results with, 855–857
Hyperalgesia, 1103
Hyperbaric oxygen, for irradiated tissue, 1458–1461, *1460, 1461*
　preoperative, for hemimandibulectomy reconstruction, 1498
Hyperesthesia, 1103
Hypernasal speech, 1694–1696
　evaluation of, 1711
　treatment of, 1717–1719
Hyperpathia, 1094, 1103
　evaluation of, nerve block in, 1100–1101
　pain in, 1096
Hypersomnia, daytime, in sleep apnea, 2021, 2043
Hypertelorism, in craniodysostosis, 1841
Hypertension, intracranial, in Apert syndrome, 1897, 1898
　in craniosynostosis, *1840*, 1840–1841
　in Crouzon syndrome, 1894
　preoperative evaluation of, 106
　rebound, in hypotensive anesthesia, 135
Hypoalgesia, 1103
Hypoesthesia, 1103
Hypoglobus, 1060

Hyponasal speech, 1695–1696
　after Le Fort III osteotomy, 1728–1729
　after pharyngeal flap surgery, 1717, 1719
　evaluation of, 1711
　treatment of, 1719–1720
Hypopharyngeal obstruction, in sleep apnea, *2022*, 2022–2023, *2023*. See also *Sleep apnea*.
Hypotensive anesthesia, 114–115, 135–137, *136, 137*. See also *Anesthesia*.
Hypoxemia, in sleep apnea, 2044

Iliohypogastric nerve injury, in anterior ilium graft harvesting, *1486*, 1486–1487
Ilium, graft harvesting from, 839–849, *840, 842–844, 846–848*
　complications of, 122
　for maxillary sinus graft, 1282–1285
　from anterior site, 839–845, *840, 842–844*, 1486–1488, *1486–1488*
　from posterior site, 839–840, *840*, 845–847, *846–848*, 1488–1491, *1488–1491*
　morbidity and complications in, 847–849
Illouz-type cannulas, 376, *376*
Immobilization. See also *Fixation*.
　articular effects of, 1632–1639
　muscular effects of, 1626–1632
　osseous effects of, 1626
　periarticular connective tissue effects of, *1640–1643*, 1640–1645
Implants, alloplastic. See also *Hydroxyapatite implants*.
　condylar resorption after, costochondral graft in, 918–922, *918–922*
　dermal graft in, 926–927
　coronal approach in, 972, *972–973*
　for ankylosis, 1522
　for chin augmentation, 2484–2487, *2486*
　for malar midfacial augmentation, 2289–2294, *2292–2295*
　for mandibular angle deficiency, 2484–2487, *2486*, 2488–2490, *2489*
　for maxillary reconstruction, 1528–1529
　for orbital reconstruction, 1066–1067
　in conchal cartilage graft, 668, *669*
　submalar, 2293–2294, *2294*
　vs. allogenic graft, 1452–1453
　bone conduction, for hearing loss, *1218*, 1218, 1721
　cochlear, 1721
　condylar. See *Condylar implant*.
　dental. See *Dental implants*.
　endosseous. See *Implants, osseointegrated*.
　glenoid fossa. See *Glenoid fossa implant*.
　hydroxyapatite. See *Hydroxyapatite implants*.
　Lyo-dura, 647, *647*
　osseointegrated, biocompatibility of, 1337
　　biomechanics of, 1335–1337, 1354–1356, *1355*

Implants *(Continued)*
　bone healing around, 1337–1338
　　implant roughness and, 1351–1353, *1352–1354*
　bone interface in, maintenance of, 1257–1258
　case studies of, 1388–1425
　construction of, 1335–1337
　experimental background of, *1236–1240*, 1236–1241
　for dental prostheses. See *Dental implants*.
　for ear prosthesis anchorage, *1308–1310*
　for facial prosthesis anchorage, 1215–1218, *1215–1218*, 1526, *1527*
　in aging face syndrome, 1427–1436
　orthodontic, *1224*, 1224, *1225*, 1231–1261
　　advantages of, 1260–1261
　　anchorage in, 1252–1253
　　case report for, 1242–1258
　　hardware development for, 1248–1250, *1249*
　　histologic analysis of, 1255–1257, *1257*
　　limitations of, 1261
　　maintenance of rigid interface for, 1257–1258
　　mechanics in, 1250–1252, *1251*
　　preoperative evaluation for, 1242–1248, *1243–1247*
　　reactivity of, 1258
　　results of, 1253–1255, *1254, 1255*
　　soft tissue inflammation with, 1258
　　surgical technique for, 1250
　　timing of, 1253
　　treatment plan for, 1248
　　vs. orthognathic surgery, 1261
　　wires for, material for, 1258
　orthopedic, 1259–1261
　osseous interface for, 1241, 1249
　perimucosal abutments of, 1338–1339, *1339, 1340*
　perimucosal seal around, 1301, *1338*, 1338–1339, *1339*
　physiologic response to, *1162*, 1162–1163, *1232*, 1234–1241, *1235–1240*, 1255–1258, *1256*
　plaque accumulation around, 1339
　root impingement with, 1241
　transmandibular. See *Transmandibular implant*.
　with orthognathic surgery, case studies of, 1387–1425
　polyactic acid, 851
　Silastic. See *Implants, alloplastic*.
　silicone. See *Implants, alloplastic*.
　temporomandibular joint. See *Temporomandibular joint, implants for*.
　transmandibular. See *Transmandibular implant*.
　types of, 850–851
Implator, biomechanical characteristics of, 1336, 1340–1353
　constituents of, 1340
　experimental results with, 1341–1353
　mechanical characteristics of, 1336
Incisal pin, in model surgery, 198, 204, 205
Incision(s), care of, 117–118
　coronal. See *Coronal incision*.

xviii / INDEX

Incision(s) *(Continued)*
　forehead, anatomic considerations in, 955–957, *956*
　in anterior ilium graft harvesting, 1487, *1488*
　in Branemark dental implant procedure, 1148–1150, *1148–1150*
　in cleft deformity repair, for partial bilateral labial cleft, 399, *402, 406*
　　for partial unilateral labial cleft, 396, *396, 403, 404*
　　for secondary cheilorhinoplasty, 416, *416, 418, 419*
　　for total bilateral labiomaxillary cleft, 397–399, *398, 399, 402, 403*
　　for total labiomaxillopalatine cleft, 394–396, *395, 400–401, 405*
　in conchal cartilage graft, 666, *666–667*
　in condylar diskopexy, 660, *662–663*
　in condylar graft placement, 876, *877*
　in facial fractures, 1015–1016
　in iliac graft harvesting, from anterior site, 841
　　from posterior site, 841, *846*
　in intraoral vertical ramus osteotomy, 684, *685*, 2115, *2116*
　in latissimus dorsi myocutaneous flap, 1471, *1471*
　in lipectomy, 385, 386
　in masseter reduction, via extraoral approach, 442, *443*
　　via intraoral approach, *433*, 433–434
　in oblique modified Le Fort osteotomy, 1772–1773
　in pectoralis major myocutaneous flap, *1466*, 1466–1468, *1467*
　in rhinoplasty, 302–303, *303*, 349–351, *350*
　　with external approach, 360–361, *361*
　in rib harvesting, 838, *838*, 1483, 1483–1484
　in simultaneous maxillary sinus graft and hydroxyapatite dental implant placement, *1277*, 1277–1278
　in sternocleidomastoid flap, *1474*, 1474–1475
　in subtotal segmental osteotomy, for open bite, *2085*
　in temporalis myofascial flap surgery, 670, *671*, 720, *721*
　in temporomandibular joint surgery, 703–704
　　with preauricular approach, 706–709, *707–709*
　in Vitek-Kent prosthesis placement, 762–763, *763*
　in Zisser segmental osteotomy, for open bite, *2082*, 2082
　maxillary, for dental implants, 1173, *1173*
　parasagittal, in hydroxyapatite implant, *860*, 860
　retromandibular, in sagittal split osteotomy, *2371*, 2372
　scalp, anatomic considerations in, 952, 952–955, *954, 955*
　Weber-Fergusson, in maxillary reconstruction, 1528–1529, *1529*
Incisor(s), cephalometric analysis of, 95–96, *96*
　insufficient compensation of, 52, *52–55*
　lateral, missing/small, preoperative correction of, 56–57, *57*

Incisor(s) *(Continued)*
　mandibular, depression of, subapical osteotomy for, 2495–2499, *2496, 2497*
　measurement of. See *Dental measurements.*
　upper, exposure of, in Le Fort I osteotomy, 2229–2232, *2231*
Infection, after quadrangular Le Fort I osteotomy, 1815
　after quadrangular Le Fort II osteotomy, 1835
　of condyle, costochondral graft in, 914, *915, 916*
　of costochondral graft, 931, *931*
　of lacrimal sac, *1048*, 1065, *1074*, 1074–1076
　postoperative, 73, *73*, 121–122
　of Vitek-Kent prosthesis, 789, 789t
Infectious arthritis, arthroscopy of, 609, *610*
Inferior alveolar nerve, 2179
　injury of, 997
　　in sagittal split osteotomy, 2113, 2121, 2131–2132
　microsurgical repair of, 1112–1117, *1113–1116*
Inflammatory reaction, to hydroxyapatite-coated dental implants, 1317–1318
Informed consent, for rhinoplasty, 344
Infraorbital augmentation, hydroxyapatite implant in, 861–862, *862*
Infraorbital nerve. See also *Trigeminal nerve.*
　anesthesia and paresthesia of, after quadrangular Le Fort osteotomy, 1836
　injury of, 1081
　microreconstructive surgery of, 1120–1122, *1121*
Innervation. See *Nerve(s).*
Integral dental implants. See *Dental implants, hydroxyapatite-coated.*
Intelligence, speech and, 1697–1698
Intercartilaginous incision, in rhinoplasty, 302–303, *303*, 349–350, *350*
Interdental measurement, 170
　in model surgery, 185–199
Interdental splint, after Le Fort I/II quadrangular osteotomy, 1796
Interdigitation, postoperative maintenance of, 78, *78*
　preoperative correction of, 58, *58*
Interincisal angle, 95, *95*
Interincisal distance, measurement of, 1662, *1663*
Interincisal opening, range-of-motion exercises for, 1664–1666, *1665*
Intermaxillary fixation, arch wires for, 1656, 1658
　ball hooks for, 1656–1657, *1657*
　brackets for, 1656–1657, *1657, 1658*, 1658–1659
　connective tissue effects of, 1644–1645
　vs. effects of rigid internal fixation, 1645, *1645*
　disuse osteoporosis and, 1626
　elastic therapy in. See *Elastic therapy.*
　in hemifacial microsomia, 1579, 1584
　in intraoral vertical ramus osteotomy, 1667
　in Le Fort I/II quadrangular osteotomy, 1795–1796, *1796*
　in Treacher Collins syndrome, 1618

Intermaxillary fixation *(Continued)*
　intra-articular effects of, 1632–1639
　lugs for, 1656–1657, *1657*
　mandibular mobility after, vs. mobility after rigid internal fixation, 1645, *1645*
　masticatory effects of, 1625–1646
　methods of, 1656–1659, *1657, 1658*
　muscle atrophy in, 1626–1632
　　prevention of, 1629–1630, *1630, 1632*
　　vs. effects of rigid internal fixation, 1629–1630, *1630*
　occlusal splint in, 1657
　　in postoperative rehabilitation, 1657, 1659–1660, *1660*
　of mandibular fractures, 997, *997*
　of maxillary fractures, 999
　rehabilitation after. See *Rehabilitation.*
　release of, occlusal control after, 1659–1662, *1659–1662*
　temporomandibular joint changes and, 1634–1635, *1635*
　vs. rigid fixation, postoperative maxillary stability and, 1936–1937, 1938–1942
　with Vitek-Kent prosthesis, 749
Internal fixation, rigid. See *Plate fixation; Rigid internal fixation; Screw fixation.*
　wire. See *Wire fixation.*
Internal maxillary artery, preservation of, in ankylosis repair, 1521
Interocclusal splint. See *Splint(s), occlusal.*
Interproximal brush, 1182, *1183*
Interpupillary line, in facial esthetics, 236, *239*, 241
Intracranial pressure, increased, in Apert syndrome, 1897, 1898
　in craniosynostosis, 1840–1841, *1849*
　in Crouzon syndrome, 1894
Intraoperative complications, 65–75
Intraoral defect, temporalis muscle flap for, coronal approach for, 973, *974–975*
Intraoral inverted-L osteotomy, for mandibular prognathism, 2121, *2122, 2123*
Intraoral surgery, historical development of, 2111–2113
Intraoral vertical ramus osteotomy, 681–700
　case studies of, 691–698, *692, 693, 695, 697, 699*
　condylar position after, *683*, 683–684, 690–691
　evolution of, 681–684
　for prognathism, 2111–2121
　　advantages of, 2136
　　biologic considerations in, 2113–2114
　　complications of, 2131–2136
　　condylar position after, *2133*, 2133–2134, *2134*, 2135, 2138
　　healing in, 2113–2114
　　indications for, 2113
　　inferior alveolar nerve injury in, 2131–2132
　　interference with retrusion in, 2115
　　intraoperative bleeding in, 2132
　　large retrusions in, 2121
　　occlusal problems after, 2136–2137

INDEX / xix

Intraoral vertical ramus osteotomy
    (Continued)
  preoperative planning for, *2114*,
    2114–2115, *2115*
  preoperative radiographic evaluation
    in, *2114*, 2114–2115, *2115*
  rehabilitation after, 2131
  relapse after, 2135–2136, 2138
  rigid fixation in, 2119–2120, *2120*
    relapse and, 2135
  technique for, 2115–2121, *2116*,
    2117
  unfavorable osteotomy in, 2132
  vs. sagittal split osteotomy, 2113,
    2136–2137
  historical development of, 2111, *2112*
  mandibular hypomobility after, 1668,
    1668t
  patient selection for, 684
  preoperative evaluation in, 684
  rehabilitation in, 688–689, *1667*,
    1667–1668
  results of, *682*, 682–684, *683*, 689–691
  technique of, 684–688, *685–688*
  unfavorable, in intraoral vertical ramus
    osteotomy, 2132
  with symphyseal osteotomy, for cross-
    bite, 2398, *2400–2401*
Intubation, canalicular, 1075, *1075*
  endotracheal, *113*, 113–114
    after cleft deformity repair, 113, 132
    airway obstruction after, 116
    evaluation for, 130–132, *131*
    in craniofacial surgery, 1891–1892
    in temporomandibular joint surgery,
      706
    in Vitek-Kent prosthesis placement,
      758, 758, *759*
    medication for, 140–142
    nasal preparation for, 133, 143
    technique of, 141–145, *142–145*
    termination of, 150, *151*
    transtracheal block in, 142, *142*
    tube removal in, 150, *151*
    tube selection and insertion in, 143,
      143, *144*
    tube stabilization in, 145–148, *146–
      148*
  in craniofacial surgery, 1891–1892
  in dacryocystorhinoplasty, 1076
  nasogastric, 111
  postoperative, 116–117
  nasotracheal, sedated-awake, 141–
    145, *142–145*
Inverted-L osteotomy, *994*, 994–995
  for mandibular prognathism, 2121,
    2122, *2123*
Iron supplementation, for autologous
  blood donors, 108
Irradiated tissue, dental implants in, 1143
  hyperbaric oxygen for, 1458–1461,
    1460, *1461*
  myocutaneous flap in, 1457
Ischemia, during hypotensive anesthesia,
  114–115, 135–136
  flap, 120–121
  intraoperative, 73–75

Jaw. See component parts of jaw.
Job opportunities, appearance and, 8
Johnichi torque gauge, for dental implant
  holding power measurement, 1141,
  1142

Joint fusion, in Apert syndrome, 1896
Joints, synovial, effects of immobilization
  on, 1632–1639
Jones tube, in dacryocystorhinoplasty,
  1076
Junctional epithelium, gingival, 1339,
  1340
Juvenile rheumatoid arthritis, mandibular deficiency in, 2506–2511, *2507–
  2510*

Keratinized tissue, preservation of, in
  dental implant surgery, 1293–1295,
  1294
Keratocyst, odontogenic, costochondral
  graft in, *913*, 913–914
Keratopathy, exposure, 1070
Kesselring cannula, 374, 376
Killian submucous resection, for septal
  deviation, 333, *333*, 334
Kirschner wires. See *Wire(s); Wire fixation*.
Kleeblattschädel anomaly, case study of,
  1878–1880, 1878–1881
  craniosynostosis in, 1839–1842, 1850.
    See also *Craniosynostosis*.
  surgery for, 1850
Knee immobilization, 1632–1634, *1633*
Köle segmental osteotomy, for anterior
  open bite closure, 835, *835*
  for open bite, 2081

Labetalol, in anesthesia, 150
Labiodental sounds, 1689t, 1691, *1692*
Laboratory tests, preoperative, 107, 132,
  132t
Laceration, of canalicula, 1074, 1074–
  1075
  of canthus, canthal dystopia and,
    1076–1077
  of eyelid, lacrimal injury and, 1074–
    1076
  preoperative evaluation of, 1071–
    1074
  sequelae of, 1071–1074
  of nerve. See specific nerves.
Lacrimal infection, post-traumatic, *1048*,
  1065, 1074, *1074*, 1075–1076
Lacrimal sac, 2260. See also *Nasolacrimal
  injuries*.
Lacrimal trauma, 1065, 1074, 1074–
  1076, *1075*
Lag screws. See *Screw fixation*.
Lagophthalmos, 1069–1071, *1070*
Lambdoid craniosynostosis, unilateral,
  1846, 1855, *1856–1858*
Lamellar bone, 1232, *1233*
Language. See also *Speech*.
  development of, 1687
Large face syndrome, with masseter mus-
  cle hypertrophy, 441–452. See also
  Masseter muscle hypertrophy.
Laryngeal abnormalities, speech and,
  1706, 1726
Late bicoronal synostosis, 1847, 1860–
  1862, *1862–1863*
Lateral canthal advancement, for cranio-
  synostosis, 1843
Lateral canthal laxity, in Treacher Col-
  lins syndrome, 1604

Lateral crus, *291*, 291–292, 2175, *2176*
Lateral entrapment neuroma, 1091, *1091*
Lateral exophytic neuroma, 1091, *1092*
Lateral facial reconstruction, 2511–
  2516, *2512*, *2513*, *2515*, *2516*
Lateral femoral cutaneous nerve, injury
  of, in anterior ilium graft harvesting,
  1486, 1487
Lateral iliohypogastric nerve, injury of,
  in anterior ilium graft harvesting,
  1486, 1486–1487
Lateral pterygoid muscle, anatomy of,
  485, *485*
  dysfunction of, in costochondral graft-
    ing, 932
  fixation of, in Vitek-Kent prosthesis
    placement, 764, *765*, 765–767,
    766
  in hemifacial microsomia, 1537
Lateral sesamoid complex, 291–292
Lateral sounds, 1689t, *1690*, 1691
Lateral subcostal nerve, injury of, in anterior ilium graft harvesting, *1486*,
  1487
Latissimus dorsi flap, *1471*, 1471–1472,
  1472. See also *Flap(s)*.
Lawn chair position, 139, *139*
Le Fort fractures, coronal approach in,
  967, *968*
  maxillary deformities after, 1049,
  1050–1054
Le Fort I downgraft, for dental implants,
  1211, *1213*
Le Fort I osteotomy, 2211–2287. See
  also *Maxillary osteotomy; Orthognathic
  surgery*.
  advantages and disadvantages of, 2238
  B point stability after, 546, 588–591
  biologic foundation of, 2212–2218,
    2213–2217
  biomechanical factors in, 1961–1962
  case studies of, 2272–2287, *2273*,
    2274, *2276–2279*, *2281*, *2282*,
    2284–2286, *2288*
  circulatory considerations in, 2212–
    2221, *2213–2217*, 2218
  condylar positioning in, 534–547. See
    also *Condyle, positioning of*.
    case study of, 635–638, *635–639*
    compressive loading in, 575
    firm anterosuperior-directed, post-
      operative joint function with,
      541–546
    heavy posterior-directed, postopera-
      tive joint function with, 534–541
    influences on, 574–575, *575*
    intraoperative control of, 632–634,
      632–635
    preoperative planning of, 629–631,
      630–632
    superior-directed, 575–576, *576*,
      577
  condylar sag after, *585*, 585–588,
    586t, *587*
  dental considerations in, 2216–2221,
    2217, *2220*, *2221*
  dental implant placement with, *1411*,
    1411–1412, *1412*
  dento-osseous segment size in, 2218–
    2221, *2219*
  design of, anatomic basis for, case stud-
    ies of, 2222–2229, *2223–2228*
  clinical application of, 2218–2221
  dental considerations in, 2219–
    2221, *2220*, *2221*

VOLUME 1—PAGES 1–828;   VOLUME 2—PAGES 829–1769;   VOLUME 3—PAGES 1770–2517

Le Fort I osteotomy (Continued)
for high osteotomy, 2235–2237, 2235–2238, 2239–2242, 2241
for step osteotomy, 2231, 2233–2235, 2234
for traditional-level (low) osteotomy, 2229–2233, 2230, 2231, 2233
stability and, 2221
vascular considerations in, 2212–2221, 2213–2217
downsliding, 2246–2250, 2249
esthetic design for, 2235–2237, 2235–2238
for post-traumatic maxillary deformities, 1049, 1050, 1053–1054
four-piece, 2262–2264, 2262–2265
for maxillary expansion, 2408, 2410, 2411, 2427, 2428–2429
high, 2235–2237, 2235–2242
design of, 2235–2237, 2235–2238, 2239–2242, 2241
in adolescent, craniofacial growth after, 39–44
in Apert syndrome, 1897, 1898
in Crouzon syndrome, 1895, 1909–1913, 1910–1912, 2287, 2288
in deep-bite deformity, 2432, 2432–2438, 2434–2436
in facial asymmetry, 243, 243, 244
in hemifacial microsomia, 1555, 1556
in juvenile rheumatoid arthritis, 2506–2511, 2507–2510
in mandibular deficiency, in juvenile rheumatoid arthritis, 2507–2510, 2511
in maxillomandibular advancement, in sleep apnea, 2051, 2051
in open bite, complications and relapse with, 2080, 2080t
in post-traumatic maxillary deformity, 1049, 1050, 1053–1054
in short mandibular ramus deformity correction, 1999
in smile line improvement, 235, 237, 238
in vertical maxillary excess, 1944–1953, 1945–1953
indications for, 2238
inferior maxillary repositioning in, 2266–2268, 2266–2268
intraoperative fixation in, 633, 633–634, 634
malar midfacial augmentation in, 2289–2297
with bone grafts, 2295, 2295–2303, 2300–2303
with silicone implants, 2289–2294, 2292–2294
mandibular hypomobility after, 1668, 1668t
maxillary growth after, 1935–1953, 1936–1953. See also Maxillary growth, postoperative.
maxillary sectioning in, 2242–2246, 2243–2248, 2262
maxillary stability after, 50, 51, 1936–1937
biomechanical factors in, 1961–1962
model surgery for, 181–184, 182t, 182–184, 201–204, 202–204, 205
nasal surgery with, sequencing of, 2280
nasolabial changes after, 293–294, 327
avoidance of, 314–316, 316
case studies of, 294–302, 302t

Le Fort I osteotomy (Continued)
nasolacrimal anatomic considerations in, 2257–2262, 2260
occlusal considerations in, 2272–2287
orthodontic treatment in, stability of, 2272
osteotomy site exposure in, technique for, 2239, 2240
parasagittal palatal, 2265, 2265
postoperative splinting in, 634, 634, 635, 638, 638
quadrangular, 1797–1816
case studies of, 1801–1815, 1801–1816
complications of, 1815, 1835–1836
development of, 1797–1798
in cleft deformities, 1811–1813, 1811–1814, 1816
indications for, 1798, 1814–1815
intermaxillary fixation in, 1815
orthodontic treatment for, 1791–1797
results of, 1815–1816
retention methods after, 1796–1797
technique for, 1798–1801, 1799
ramping effect in, 2231–2232
reduction cheiloplasty with, 315–316, 316
rehabilitation after, 1666, 1667, 2268
rhinoplasty with, 302–316. See also Rhinoplasty.
case studies of, 275–283, 362–365, 364
for alar base deformities, 311, 311–312, 312
for nasal dorsum deformities, 303–306, 304–307
for nasal septum disorders, 313, 313–315
for nasal tip deformities, 307–310, 308–310
for nasolabial angle and upper lip deformities, 314–316, 315, 316
rigid internal fixation in, 2250–2257
with microplates, 2255–2257, 2255–2259
with miniplates, 2250–2254, 2252–2254
speech and, 1722–1727, 1723, 1725
stability after, 1936–1937
stepped, 2231, 2233–2235, 2234
temporomandibular joint function after, 541–547
three-piece, 2262–2264, 2262–2265
for maxillary expansion, 2408, 2410, 2411, 2427, 2428–2429
tooth positioning in, 2219, 2220, 2221
traditional-level (low), advantages and disadvantages of, 2232–2233
design of, 2229–2232, 2230, 2231, 2233
indications for, 2232
treatment planning for, 166–167. See also Treatment planning.
two-piece, 2264–2265, 2265
for maxillary expansion, 2410, 2427, 2428–2429
upper incisor exposure in, 2229–2232
with concurrent genioplasty, 2455–2456, 2456–2458
with external headframe traction, for cleft deformity–associated maxillary hypoplasia, 2315–2322, 2316–2321

Le Fort I osteotomy (Continued)
with Vitek-Kent prosthesis, 749, 759
zygomatic fracture in, 2241–2242
zygomaticomaxillary complex reduction in, 2304–2305, 2305
Le Fort II fracture, coronal approach in, 967
Le Fort II osteotomy, anterior, 1816
coronal approach in, 967, 971
in Treacher Collins syndrome, 1606
pyramidal, 1816, 1817
quadrangular, 1816–1837
approach in, 1832–1833
bone grafting in, 1819, 1833, 1835
case studies of, 1821–1832, 1822–1832
complications of, 1835–1836
development of, 1816–1817
indications for, 1814, 1817
maxillary downfracture in, 1833, 1835
maxillary impaction in, 1834
orthodontic treatment for, 1791–1797
overcorrection in, 1834
palatine artery identification in, 1833–1834
postoperative management in, 1820–1821
results of, 1836–1837
retention methods after, 1796–1797
technique for, 1832–1834
with maxillary cleft, 1834
Le Fort III fracture, coronal approach in, 967, 968
Le Fort III osteotomy, coronal approach in, 967, 971
in Apert syndrome, 1897, 1898, 2065, 2066
in Crouzon syndrome, 1893, 1894–1895, 2065, 2066
case studies of, 1903, 1904–1906, 1909–1913, 1910–1912
in maxillomalar advancement, case study of, 1775–1776, 1775–1777
oblique modified, 1771–1787
advantages of, 1771–1772
case studies of, 1775–1786, 1775–1787
Champy technique for, 1777–1779, 1777–1779
contraindications to, 1786
inclination of, 1772
technique for, 1772–1775
total intraoral approach for, 1786
speech after, 1728–1729
with craniotomy, in Apert syndrome, 2065, 2066
in Crouzon syndrome, 2065, 2066
with sagittal split osteotomy, in Binder's syndrome, 2067, 2068
Le Fort osteotomy, history of, 1797
Le Mesurier procedure, for cleft deformity repair, 399, 400
Lesser occipital nerve, 955, 955
Leukotriene B$_4$, in temporomandibular joint arthralgia, 473, 474, 477–480, 478
Levator anguli oris muscle, 293, 293, 2178, 2179
Levator labii superioris alaeque nasi muscle, 293, 293, 2178, 2179
Levator labii superioris muscle, 2178, 2179

Levator labii superioris nasi muscle, 293, *293*
Levator muscle, in ptosis, 1068–1069
 repair of, 1068
Lidocaine, for nasal preparation, 143
Lingual nerve. See also *Trigeminal nerve.*
 injury of, 1081
 microreconstructive surgery of, 1117–1120, *1117–1120*
Lingual sounds, 1689t, 1691, *1692*
Lip(s), abnormalities of, speech and, 1698–1699, *1699*
 anatomy of, 2178, *2179*
 cleft. See *Cleft deformities.*
 in cephalometric analysis, 2181
 postopertive care of, 118
 surgery of. See *Cheiloplasty.*
 upper, changes in, after Le Fort I osteotomy, 293–294
  case studies of, 294–302, 302t
  reduction of, during maxillary osteotomy, 315–316, *316*
  support of, evaluation of, 156
Lip lift, 2331–2332, *2332*
Lip position, abnormal, in hemifacial microsomia, 1563–1566, *1565, 1566*
Lipectomy, 373–388
 air leak method for, 375
 anatomic considerations in, 377–380, *378*
 complications of, 388
 equipment for, 375–377, *376, 377*
 facial, 373–388
 history of, 373–374
 indications for, 380–383
 mandibular nerve preservation in, 379
 parotid duct preservation in, 379
 platysma muscle preservation in, 378, *378*
 pumps for, 375
 technique of, 383–386, *384, 386*
 theoretical basis of, 374–375
 tissue elasticity and, 380
 vapor pressure vacuum in, 375
 vaporization method for, 374–375
 with mandibular setback, 381
 with maxillary repositioning, 382
 with platysma muscle plication, 385–386
Lipline, high, 253, *253*. See also *Smile, gummy.*
 low, 252, *252*
 medium, 252, *252*
Lipodystrophy, lipectomy for. See *Lipectomy.*
Lipolysis, 374. See also *Lipectomy.*
Liquid diet supplements, 119
Local anesthesia. See *Anesthesia.*
Long face syndrome, asymmetry in, orthognathic surgery and rhinoplasty in, 279–281, *280*
 cephalometric analysis in, 96, 96–97
 maxillary growth and, 1935
 transverse midface deficiency in, zygomatic sagittal osteotomy with interpositional bone grafting for, 2298–2303, *2300–2303*
Loose areolar tissue, of scalp, 952, *953*
Loudness, vocal, 1688–1689
Lower incisor–mandibular plane angle, 95, *95*
Lower lip–chin complex, assessment of, 2440–2443, *2441, 2443, 2444*

Lugs, for intermaxillary fixation, 1656–1657, *1657*
Luhr plate fixation, in Le Fort I osteotomy, 2255–2257, *2255–2259*
 in mandibular angle fracture, comparative stress analysis of, 1973, *1973–1974*
Lymphatic drainage, of face and scalp, 960, *961*
Lymphedema, in sleep apnea, 2027
Lyo-dura implants, temporomandibular joint, 647, *647*
Lysis, lavage, and manipulation, arthroscopic, 617–620, *617–620*, 653, 656–671, *657*. See also *Arthroscopy.*

M point, in cephalometric analysis, 90, *90*
Macroglossia, speech and, 1704, *1704*
Macrophage-derived angiogenesis factor, in wound healing, 1458–1459
Macrophage-derived growth factor, in wound healing, 1458–1459
Macrostomia, in hemifacial microsomia, 1536
 in Treacher Collins syndrome, 1608
Magnetic resonance imaging, contraindications to, 509t
 development of, 507
 magnet type in, 507–508
 magnetic field strength in, 507–508
 of costochondral graft, 929, *930*
 of dermal graft, *930*, 931
 of temporomandibular joint, 507–515
  contraindications to, 509t
  normal findings on, 511, *511, 512*
  postoperative, 515–516, *516*
  technologic aspects of, 507–511
  vs. arthrography, 507, *508*
 preoperative, indications for, 1792
 scanning planes in, 510t, 510–511
 suface coil for, 510
 vs. computerized tomography, 508, 509t
Magnets, gold-samarium, for prosthesis anchorage, 1526, *1527*
Malar augmentation, 2289–2297
 with bone grafts, *2295*, 2295–2303, *2300–2303*
  for transverse midface deficiency, in long face syndrome, 2298–2303, *2300–2303*
  graft maintenance in, 2296
  graft material for, *2295*, 2296–2297
  indications for, 2299
  technique for, *2301*, 2989–2302, *2300*
 with silicone implants, 2289–2294, *2292–2294*
 zygomatic sagittal osteotomy for, 2298–2303, *2300–2303*
Malar bone, absence of, in Treacher Collins syndrome, 1604, *1604*
Malar dystopia, *1058*, 1058–1062, *1059, 1061*
Malar hypoplasia, buccal fat pad removal and, 383
Malar reduction, 2304–2305, *2305*
Malocclusion, after ramus osteotomy for prognathism, 2137
 Class II, correction of, with dental implant placement, 1400–1402, *1401–1403*

Malocclusion (Continued)
 orthognathic surgery with rhinoplasty in, 273–275, *274*
 with mandibular deficiency, orthodontic treatment for, 2338–2346. See also *Orthodontic treatment, with mandibular advancement.*
 Class III, face mask therapy for, 2325–2331, *2326, 2327, 2329*
  in Crouzon syndrome, 1895
  in mandibular prognathism, 2140, 2143
   chin cap traction for, 2146–2147
   evaluation of, 2144–2146
   reverse-pull headgear for, 2146–2147
   supraeruption of second molars in, 2145
   treatment of, 2146–2152
 orthognathic surgery with rhinoplasty in, 277, *278*
 with mandibular prognathism. See *Mandibular prognathism.*
 crossbite. See *Crossbite.*
 deep-bite. See *Deep-bite deformity.*
 in Vitek-Kent prosthesis placement, 789t, 790
 open-bite. See *Open bite.*
 postoperative, orthodontic treatment for, 79–81, *80–82*
 post-traumatic, evaluation of, 988, *989*
  treatment of, 992, *995, 996*
 speech and, 1702, *1702–1703*
Mandible, as bone graft donor site, 834–835, *835*. See also *Bone graft.*
 postextraction shape and quality of, 1149
Mandibular abnormalities, in hemifacial microsomia, *1534*, 1534–1535, *1535*
Mandibular advancement. See also *Mandibular deficiency.*
 connective tissue injury and repair in, 1644–1645, *1645*
 craniofacial growth after, 43–44
 in children, 2516–2517
 in condylar dysplasia, with graft placement, 879
 in juvenile rheumatoid arthritis, 2507–2510, *2511*
 in sleep apnea. See *Maxillomandibular advancement, in sleep apnea.*
 in total mandibular augmentation, 2392–2394, *2394*
 orthodontic treatment with, 2338–2346. See also *Orthodontic treatment, with mandibular advancement.*
 patient age and, 2339–2340
 sagittal split osteotomy for. See *Sagittal split osteotomy.*
Mandibular advancement splint, 2049–2050
Mandibular alveolar process, atrophic, transmandibular implant for. See *Transmandibular implant.*
Mandibular anatomy, 2179
Mandibular angle, prominent, in masseter muscle hypertrophy, 434, *434, 435*, 441, *443, 444*, 446
Mandibular angle deficiency, 2488–2495
 alloplastic implants in, 2488–2490, *2489*
 case study of, *2493*, 2493–2495, *2494*
 cranial bone graft for, 2491, *2492*

xxiv / INDEX

Maxillary advancement. See also *Maxillary deficiency*.
  face mask therapy for, 2325–2331, *2326, 2327, 2329*
  hydroxyapatite implant in, 856, 858, *858*, 863–867, *864–868*
  in oblique modified Le Fort III osteotomy, 1771–1786. See also *Le Fort III osteotomy, oblique modified*.
  in sleep apnea. See *Maxillomandibular advancement, in sleep apnea*.
  nasolabial changes after, 297–300, *298, 299*, 302t
  planning for, 173
Maxillary alveolar-palatal cleft, Le Fort I quadrangular osteotomy for, 1814
Maxillary arch leveling, in mandibular deficiency, 2432
Maxillary artery, internal, preservation of, in ankylosis repair, 1521
Maxillary asymmetry, correction of, 241–243, *242–244*
  postoperative, correction of, 80
Maxillary augmentation, hydroxyapatite particle implant for, 1287–1288, 1322, *1322–1324*, 1410, *1410*
Maxillary cant, measurement of, 156
  model measurement of, 2306–2307
Maxillary deficiency, correction of, with dental implant, *1411*, 1411–1412, *1412*
  in cleft deformity, maxillary advancement with external headframe traction for, 2315–2322, *2316–2321*
  in growing patient, cephalometric analysis for, 2322–2325, *2324*
  mandibular excess and, 2146–2147
  oblique modified Le Fort III osteotomy for, *1775*, 1775–1776, *1776*
  orthodontic treatment for, case studies of, 1801–1814, 1821–1832
  preoperative, 1791–1797
  palatal expansion for, with face mask therapy, 2328–2331, *2329*
  quadrangular Le Fort I and II osteotomies for. See *Le Fort I osteotomy, quadrangular; Le Fort II osteotomy, quadrangular*.
  speech in, 1698–1699, 1703–1704
  tooth positioner appliance in, 1796–1797
  transverse, *2386*
    diagnosis of, 55
    preoperative compensation for, 55–56, *56*
  transverse (horizontal), 2386, 2403–2430
    absolute, 2405, 2406t
    arch-length discrepancy in, 2408, *2409*
    arch morphology in, 2408, *2409*
    bilateral, 2405, 2406t
    cephalometric analysis of, 2403–2405, *2404*
    diagnosis of, 2405–2408, 2406t
    palatal crossbite in, 2405, *2407*
    relative, 2405, 2406t
    treatment of. See *Maxillary expansion*.
    unilateral, 2405, 2406t
  vertical, in deep-bite deformity, 2433. See also *Deep-bite deformity*.
Maxillary deformities, after inadequate cleft repair, 408

Maxillary deformities *(Continued)*
  in Treacher Collins syndrome, 1601, 1606
  post-traumatic. See *Maxillofacial deformities, post-traumatic*.
  speech and, *1703*, 1703–1704
Maxillary dental implants, 1172–1174, *1173, 1174*. See also *Dental implants*.
Maxillary downfracture, Le Fort I. See *Le Fort I osteotomy*.
Maxillary downgraft, hydroxyapatite implant in, 856, 859, *859*, 863–867, *864–868*
Maxillary downgrowth, in hemifacial microsomia, 1541
Maxillary excess. See *Maxillary hyperplasia*.
  vertical. See *Smile, gummy*.
Maxillary expansion, hydroxyapatite implant in, *859*, 859–860, *860*
  inadequate preoperative compensation for, 55–56, *56*
  midpalatal osteotomy for, 2412
  planning for, 2405–2412, *2409–2412*
  rapid palatal expansion device for. See *Rapid palatal expansion device*.
  surgical, 2426–2430
  three- or four-piece Le Fort I osteotomy for, 2408, *2410, 2411*, 2427–2430, *2428–2429*
  two-piece Le Fort osteotomy for, 2410, 2427, *2428–2429*
Maxillary expansion plate. See *Rapid palatal expansion device*.
Maxillary full arch graft, Branemark, *1206*, 1207
Maxillary graft. See also *Bone graft*.
  Branemark full arch, *1206*, 1207
  with anterior fixation, for dental implants, 1211, *1213*
  with palatal fixation, for dental implants, 1207–1211, *1208, 1209*
Maxillary growth. See also *Growth*.
  abnormal, 1935–1936
  cessation of, age at, 1933
  control of, 1934
  direction of, 1935
  in long face syndrome, 1935
  movements of, *410*, 410–411, *411*
  open bite and, 1935
  postoperative, 38–44, *39, 40*
    case studies of, 1944–1953, *1945–1953*
    in vertical maxillary excess, 1933–1954
    studies of, 1937–1942, 1939t, *1939–1942*, 1941t
    animal, 1935, 1936
    rates of, 1935
    scintigraphic evaluation of, 1677–1684. See also *Skeletal scintigraphy*.
  surgical timing and, 1933–1934
Maxillary hyperplasia, cephalometric analysis in, 98, *98*
  speech in, 1703–1704
  vertical. See *Smile, gummy*.
Maxillary hypoplasia. See *Maxillary deficiency*.
Maxillary implant. See *Implants*.
Maxillary measurement. See *Bone measurements*.
Maxillary model, measurement of. See *Model measurement*.
  mounting of, 161–162, *162*
  surgery of. See *Model surgery*.

Maxillary orientation, assessment of, 411, *411*
Maxillary orthopedics, osseointegrated implants for, 1259
Maxillary osteoporosis, disuse, 1626
Maxillary osteotomy. See also *Le Fort I osteotomy; Le Fort II osteotomy; Le Fort III osteotomy; Orthognathic surgery*.
  biomechanics of, 1957–1975. See also *Biomechanics*.
  bone graft stabilization in, 1027
  complications of, intraoperative, 71–75, *72–75*
  coronal approach in, 967, *970*
  dual-arch, composite splint for, 206–215
  eustachian tube dysfunction after, 1726–1727
  for open bite. See *Open bite, surgery for*.
  for simultaneous maxillary sinus graft and hydroxyapatite-coated dental implants, *1278*, 1278–1279
  for transverse maxillary deficiency, planning of, 2408–2412, *2410, 2411*
  four-piece, for transverse maxillary deficiency, 2408, 2427–2430, *2428–2429*
  hydroxyapatite implant in, 856, 858–860, *858–860*
    case studies of, 863–871, *864–870*
    technique of, 858–860, *858–860*
  in functional genioplasty, after cleft deformity repair, 422, 422–424, *423*
  in malar dystopia correction, 1061
  in Treacher Collins syndrome, 1606
  in two-jaw surgery, rigid internal fixation for, *1992*, 1992–1994, *1993*
  incision closure in, to avoid upper lip thinning, 315, *316*
  inferior, nasolabial changes after, 300–302, *301*, 302t
  laryngeal granuloma after, 1726
  lateral wall cuts in, planning of, 173–174, *174*
  lipectomy with, 382
  mandibular hypomobility after, 1668, 1668t
  maxillary growth after, 1933–1954. See also *Maxillary growth, postoperative*.
  maxillary stability after, 1936–1937
    biomechanical factors in, 1961–1962
  modified lateral, with rapid palatal expansion device, case study of, 2420–2423, *2421–2424*
    results of, 2425
    technique for, 2415–2420, *2416–2418*
  monobloc. See *Monobloc osteotomy*.
  nasolabial changes after, 293–300, *294, 295, 298, 299*, 327
    avoidance of, 314–316, *316*
    case studies of, 294–302, 302t
  posterior, with dental implants, 1413–1416, *1414, 1415*
  postoperative complications of, 73–82
  preoperative considerations in, 49–65
  ramp inclination in, 173
  reduction cheiloplasty during, 315–316, *316*
  rehabilitation after, 1666, *1667*
  rhinoplasty with, 302–316. See also *Rhinoplasty*.
    case studies of, 273–283, 362–365, *364*

VOLUME 1—PAGES 1–828; VOLUME 2—PAGES 829–1769; VOLUME 3—PAGES 1770–2517

Open bite *(Continued)*
  orthodontic treatment for, 2079–2080
  premature facial suture closure and, 2072
  relapse of, 2181
  severity of, 2076
  skull development and, *2063*, 2063–2073
  soft tissue analysis in, 2078–2079, *2079*
  speech and, 1702–1703
  surgery for, 2074–2092
    bimaxillary, *2091*, 2091–2092, *2092*
    choice of procedure in, 2075, 2080–2081
    complications of, 2080t
    genioplasty, 2089–2091, *2090*, *2091*
    history of, 2074–2075
    Le Fort I osteotomy, 2086
    planning of, 2075–2079
    relapse after, 2080t
    sagittal split osteotomy, 2080, 2080t, 2086–2089, *2087–2089*
      relapse after, 2135–2136, 2138
    segmental osteotomy, 2081–2086
      Köle, 2081
      subtotal, 2083–2086, *2084–2086*
      Zisser, 2081–2083, *2082–2084*
    techniques in, 2081–2092
  surgically created, in hemifacial microsomia, 1546, *1548*, *1550*, *1552*
Ophthalmologic examination, preoperative, 103
Optical bone chambers, 1135-1138, *1136-1139*
Oral examination, preoperative, 104
Oral hygiene, postoperative, 117–118
Oral implants. See *Implants.*
Orbicularis oris muscle, 293, *293*, 2178, 2179
  hypofunction of, 2440
Orbital adhesions, 1070
  in cicatricial ectropion, 1071–1072
Orbital adnexal prosthesis, implant anchorage of, 1215, *1216*, 1526
Orbital augmentation, coronal approach in, *972*, 973
Orbital complications, of quadrangular Le Fort osteotomy, 1836
Orbital contusion, ptosis in, *1068*
Orbital deformities, in craniosynostosis, 1841
  in hemifacial microsomia, 1535, *1535*
  in Treacher Collins syndrome, 1601, *1602*, *1603*, 1604, 1606–1607
    correction of, 1609–1610, *1610*, 1616
  post-traumatic, 1044t, 1057–1077
    avulsive, 1065–1066, *1066*
    delayed reconstruction of, 1057–1077
    grafts and biomaterials for, 1062, 1066–1067
    naso-orbito-ethmoid, 1037–1049, 1044t, *1045–1048*, *1050–1054*
    of medial orbit, *1063*, 1063–1065, *1064*
    of superior orbit, 1062–1063
    orbitozygomatic, *1035*, 1035–1037, *1036*, *1038–1044*
    osseous, 1057–1067
      malar dystopia and, *1058*, 1058–1062, *1059*, *1061*
    reconstructive goals in, 1057
    soft tissue, 1067–1077

Orbital dystopia, post-traumatic, 1014, *1014*
Orbital fracture. See also *Fracture(s), facial.*
  bone graft for, 1015, 1021–1023, *1022*
  coronal approach in, 967, *968*, *970*
  deformity after. See *Orbital deformities, post-traumatic.*
  enophthalmos after, 1027–1033, *1028–1034*
  fixation of, 1015, 1016–1021, *1017–1020*
  principles of repair of, 1015–1016
Orbital growth, scintigraphic evaluation of, 1677–1684. See also *Skeletal scintigraphy.*
Orbital-nasal line, 325, *325*
Orbital reconstruction, bone grafting in, 1029–1033, *1030–1034*, 1525–1526, *1526*
  in Apert syndrome, 1897, *1898*, 1913–1917, *1914–1915*, *1918*, 1921, *1922–1923*
  in craniosynostosis, 1843–1844, *1854*, 1854–1855, 1860, 1861–1862, *1862*, 1867–1868
  in Crouzon syndrome, 1893–1894, *1900–1912*, 1901–1913
Orbital surround, reconstruction of, 1057–1058
Orbito-naso-ethmoid deformities, post-traumatic, 1037–1049, 1044t, *1045–1048*, *1050–1054*
Orbitozygomatic deformities, in Treacher Collins syndrome, 1601, *1602*, *1603*, 1603, 1604, 1606–1607
  post-traumatic, *1035*, 1035–1037, *1036*, *1038–1044*
Oro-facial-digital syndrome, lobate tongue in, 1704, *1704*
Oronasal fistula, iatrogenic, 75, *75*
Oropharyngeal obstruction, in sleep apnea, 2022, 2022–2023, *2023*. See also *Sleep apnea.*
Orotracheal intubation. See *Intubation, endotracheal.*
Orthodontic appliance(s), construction of, 1794, *1795*
  for sleep apnea, 2029–2030, *2030*
  operative management of, 49–50, *50*
  preoperative selection of, 49–50, *50*, *51*
Orthodontic headgear, for postoperative correction, 77
Orthodontic therapy, elastic therapy in. See *Elastic therapy.*
Orthodontic treatment. See also *Intermaxillary fixation.*
  after Vitek-Kent prosthesis placement, 788
  for deep-bite deformity, *2431*, 2431–2432
  for leveling of curve of Spee, 61, 61–62, *62*
  for mandibular prognathism, 2146–2152
    as sole treatment, 2148–2149
    case studies of, 2153–2169, *2154–2156*, *2158–2160*, *2162–2164*, *2166–2168*
    postoperative, 2152
    preoperative, 2149–2151
    pretreatment evaluation for, 2144–2146
    surgical considerations in, 2151–2152

Orthodontic treatment *(Continued)*
  for maxillary deficiency, 1791–1797
    case studies of, 1801–1814, 1821–1832
    diagnostic considerations in, 1792–1793
    intraoperative considerations in, 1795–1796, *1796*
    planning for, 1793, 1794t
    postoperative considerations in, 1796
    pretreatment records and examination in, 1791–1792
  for maxillomandibular advancement, in sleep apnea, 2049
  for open bite, *61*, 61–62, *62*, 2079–2080
    case studies of, 2092–2107
  for postoperative occlusal control, 1659–1662, *1659–1662*
  for postoperative occlusal shift, 1986, *1986*
  for post-traumatic maxillofacial deformities, 999–1000
  for root divergence at osteotomy site, 59–60, *60*, 1794–1795, *1795*
  for temporomandibular joint dysfunction, timing of, 467t, 467–468
  for tooth size discrepancy, 56–58, *57*, *58*
  for transverse maxillary deficiency, 55–56, *56*
  for vertical maxillary excess, 1944–1953, *1945–1953*
  in hemifacial microsomia, 1543, 1571, 1578, 1579, 1584, 1587, *1590*, *1591*
    in growing child, 1543
  in interdisciplinary dentofacial treatment, 1754–1757, *1755–1757*, 1759–1767, *1760–1769*. See also *Dentofacial treatment, interdisciplinary.*
  inappropriate, *61*, 61–62, *62*
  postoperative, 76, *76*, 78–82, *78–82*
    for assymetry, 79–81, *81*, *82*
    for open bite, 79, *80*
  postretention stability of, occlusal contacts and, 2272
  preoperative considerations in, 49–50, *50*
  rapid palatal expansion device in. See *Rapid palatal expansion device.*
  soft tissue changes and, 2181
  tipped brackets in, at osteotomy site, 1794, *1795*
  tooth devitalization in, 1253
  with dental implants, 1417–1425, *1418–1420*, *1423*, *1424*
  with mandibular advancement, 2338–2346
    anterior tooth intrusion in, *2341*, 2341–2342, *2342*
    anteroposterior tooth position in, 2344, *2344*
    arch length analysis in, *2340*, 2340–2341
    arch leveling in, *2341*, 2341–2342, *2342*
    arch width analysis in, *2342*, 2342–2343
    case studies of, 2374
    fixation considerations in, 2344–2346, *2345*, *2346*
    patient age and, 2339–2340
    sequencing of, 2339–2340

Orthodontic treatment *(Continued)*
  with mandibular expansion, 2388–2389
    case studies of, 2389–2392, *2390, 2391*
  with osseointegrated implants. See *Implants, osseointegrated, orthodontic.*
  with quadrangular Le Fort II osteotomy, 1821–1832, *1821–1832*
Orthodontic wires. See *Wire(s); Wire fixation.*
Orthodontist, postoperative occlusal evaluation by, 79
Orthognathic surgery. See also specific procedures.
  abbreviations and terminology for, 523
  active orthodontic wires in, 63
  ambulatory, 109
    postoperative care after, 117
  anesthesia for. See *Anesthesia.*
  antibiotic prophylaxis for, 111–112
  biomechanics of, 1957–1975. See also *Biomechanics.*
  complications of, intraoperative, 65–75
    in mandibular surgery, 65–69, *65–69*
    in maxillary surgery, 71–75, *72–75*
    postoperative, 73–82, 120–126
    preoperative, 49–65
  condylar positioning in. See *Condyle, positioning of.*
  cosmetic, demand for, 1440–1441, *1442–1445*
    satisfaction with, 1440
  during growth period, 38–44. See also *Growth.*
    animal studies of, 38–42, *39, 40*
    clinical studies of, 42–44
    skeletal maturity determination for, 27–38
  edema control in, 112
  endotracheal intubation in. See *Intubation.*
  esthetic dental procedures after. See *Esthetic dentistry.*
  eye protection in, 110
  goals of, 155, 524–525
  hemostasis in, 112–113
  in aging face syndrome, 1429–1436
  in interdisciplinary dentofacial treatment, 1759–1767. See also *Dentofacial treatment, interdisciplinary.*
  in mandibular prognathism. See also *Intraoral vertical ramus osteotomy; Sagittal split osteotomy.*
    in growing patient, 2147–2148
  in orthodontics, vs. osseointegrated implants, 1261
  in sleep apnea, 2030, 2034–2038, 2047–2058
  inadequate root divergence and, 59, *59, 60*
  inadequate transverse coordination for, 55–56, *56*
  inappropriate orthodontic movements and, *61*, 61–62, *62*
  insufficient incisor decompensation for, 52, *52–55*
  maxillary growth after, 1933–1954. See also *Maxillary growth, postoperative.*
  model surgery for. See *Model surgery.*
  nasogastric intubation in, 111, 116–117

Orthognathic surgery *(Continued)*
  orthodontic appliances in, 49–50, *50, 51*
  orthodontic treatment for. See *Orthodontic treatment.*
  patient positioning in, 109–110
  patient psychologic profile in, 11–13
  plastic surgery after, 232–233
  postoperative care in, 115–120
  preoperative data base for, 156t, 156–157
  preoperative preparation for, 49–65, 101–109. See also *Preoperative preparation.*
  pretreatment records and examination in, 1791–1792
  psychologic consequences of, 11–17, 119–120, 232–233
  rehabilitation after, 1653–1673. See also *Rehabilitation.*
  retention procedures after, 82, *82*
  satisfaction with, 15–17
  soft tissue changes with. See *Soft tissue changes.*
  speech and, 1721–1728
  splint fabrication for, 63–65, *64*. See also *Splint(s).*
  temporomandibular joint function after, 464–466, 465t, *466*, 532–591
  thermal control in, 110
  timing of, 42–45, 467t, 467–468
    maxillary growth and, 1933–1934
  tooth size disparity and, 56–58, *57, 58*
  treatment planning for. See *Treatment planning.*
  urinary catheterization in, 110–111
  vascular access in, 111
  with rhinoplasty, 271. See also *Rhinoplasty.*
    case studies of, 273–283, 362–365, *364*
    sequencing of, 281
  with Vitek-Kent prosthesis, 746–750, 759
Orthopedic implants, osseointegrated, 1259–1261. See also *Implants, osseointegrated.*
Orthopedic treatment, in mandibular prognathism, 2146–2148
Orticochea pharyngoplasty, 1726
Osseointegration, of Branemark dental implants, 1146, *1146, 1147*
  of hydroxyapatite-coated dental implants, *1299–1302*, 1299–1303
  of oral implants, 1337–1338
    experimental investigation of, 1343–1353, *1343–1354*
  of transmandibular implant, 1378–1379
    interference with, by premature loading, 1379
    loss of, 1379–1382, *1380–1382*
Osseous crest, location of, 245, *245*, 256, *256*
Ossicle graft, 1218, *1218*
Osteoarthritis. See *Arthritis.*
Osteoblast, in bone healing, 1337, 1449–1450
Osteoclast, in bone healing, 1449–1450
Osteoclastic surgery, modified after Powiertowsky, in craniosynostosis, 2070, *2071*
  in Crouzon syndrome, 2064–2065, *2065*

Osteogenesis, by bone graft, 832–833, 849, 1482–1483
Osteoinduction, by bone graft, 833, 849
Osteomyelitis, chronic condylar, costochondral graft in, 914, *914, 915*
Osteon, in bone healing, 1337
  in bone remodeling, 1233
Osteoporosis, disease, 1626
Osteotomy. See specific sites and types.
Otomandibular dysostosis, costochondral graft in, 879–881, *881, 882–887*
  overgrowth of, 933, *936–937*
Otoscopy, preoperative, 103
Overdenture, for transmandibular implant, 1367–1369, *1368, 1369*
  implanted, 1187–1189, *1188, 1189*
  prosthodontic principles for, 1367
Overlapping genioplasty, 2456–2459, *2459*
Oximetry. See *Pulse oximetry.*
Oxycephaly, 1847, 1860–1862, *1862–1863*
Oxygen, hyperbaric, for irradiated tissue, 1458–1461, *1460, 1461*
  preoperative, for hemimandibulectomy reconstruction, 1498
Oxygen gradient, in wound healing, 1458–1460, *1460*
Oxygenation, in anesthesia, 139–140, 150, *151*
Oxymetazoline hydrochloride (Afrin), postoperative, 151
  preoperative, 133, 143

Packing, intranasal, in rhinoplasty, 359–360
Pain, at ilium donor site, 122
  in nerve injury, 1093–1095, *1094*, 1096
    evaluation of, 1100–1101
    management of, 1106
  in temporomandibular joint disorders, 642
  postoperative, 120
  sympathetically mediated, 1093–1094, *1094*, 1096, 1103–1105
    evaluation of, nerve block in, 1100–1101
Pain mediators, release of, in chondromalacia, 473, *474*, 477–480, *478*, 478t
Pain relief, 1102
  for post-traumatic neuralgia, 1106
  in interdisciplinary dentofacial treatment, 1745–1746
Palatal crossbite. See also *Crossbite.*
  in transverse maxillary deficiency, 2405, 2406t, *2407*
Palatal expansion, with face mask therapy, for maxillary hypoplasia, 2328–2331, *2329*
  with rapid palatal expansion device. See *Rapid palatal expansion device.*
Palatal graft, for hydroxyapatite-coated dental implants, 1295
Palatal injury, operative, 75, *75*
Palatal obstruction, in sleep apnea, 2026
Palatal osteotomy, in transverse maxillary deficiency, 2412
  parasagittal, 2265, *2265*
Palatal plane line, 93, *93*
Palate, abnormalities of, speech problems in, *1700*, 1700–1701, *1701*, 1710

Palate *(Continued)*
  maxillary surgery and, 1722–1727, *1725–1727*
  treatment of, 1719
  Byzantine, 1700
  cleft. See *Cleft deformities*.
  deviation of, in hemifacial microsomia, 1537
Papilledema, in craniosynostosis, 1841
Parallax error, 165
Paralytic ectropion, 1071, *1072*
Parasagittal palatal Le Fort I osteotomy, 2265, *2265*
Parasymphysis, mandibular, post-traumatic deformities of, 995–997, *996*
Paresthesia, definition of, 1103
  in nerve injury, 1095
  management of, 1106
  postlipectomy, 388
Parietal artery, 959, *959*
Parotid duct, anatomy of, 428
  in lipectomy, 379
  in masseter muscle hypertrophy, 431, 435
Parotid gland, disorders of, vs. masseter muscle hypertrophy, 432
Parrot beak deformity, after Le Fort I osteotomy, 300–302, *301*, 302t
  causes of, 357
  nasal tip augmentation for, during maxillary osteotomy, 308, *308*
Patient conference, preoperative, with anesthesiologist, 129–130, 130t
  with surgeon, 107–108
Patient-controlled personal exerciser, 1669, *1671*
Pectoralis major myocutaneous flap, 1466–1469, *1466–1470*. See also *Flap(s)*.
  for Andy Gump deformity, 1515, *1515*
Penicillin, prophylactic, for hydroxyapatite implant, 857
Penile growth, as maturity indicator, 32, 32t, 35
Periarticular connective tissue, immobilization effects on, 1640–1645
Pericranium, *952*, 953–954
Perimucosal seal, around implants, 1301, *1338*, 1338–1339, *1339*
Perineurium, 1084
  suturing of, 1110
Periodontal examination, in gummy smile evaluation, 239–240
Periodontal inflammation, with osseointegrated implants, 1258
Periodontal surgery, 230, *230*, *231*
  for gummy smile, flap procedures in, 246–250, *247–250*, 257–258, *258*
  gingivectomy in, 245–246, *246*, *247*, 256, 256–257, *257*
Periodontal treatment, in interdisciplinary dentofacial treatment, 1757–1758, 1759–1767, *1760–1769*. See also *Dentofacial treatment, interdisciplinary*.
Personality traits, appearance and, 4–10
  of plastic surgery patients, 11–13
  orthognathic surgery and, 11–17
  preoperative assessment of, 1792
Petit facial mask, for Class III malocclusion, 2325–2331, *2326*, *2327*, *2329*
Pfeiffer syndrome, 1851
  case study of, 1919, *1920–1921*
  extremity anomalies in, 1842, 1851

Pharyngeal abnormalities, speech and, 1705–1706
Pharyngeal flap surgery, for inadequate velopharyngeal valve closure, 1716–1719, *1717*, 1724–1727
Pharyngeal obstruction, in sleep apnea, 2022, 2022–2023, *2023*. See also *Sleep apnea*.
Pharyngoplasty, Orticochea, 1727
Phonation, problems with, 1698
Photoelastic stress analysis, 1963–1970. See also *Stress analysis*.
  for condyle, *1966*, 1966–1969, *1967*
  for mandible, 1964–1965, *1965*
  for midface, *1969*, 1969–1970, *1970*
Photography, of post-traumatic deformities, 990–991
  preoperative, 157
  for rhinoplasty, 342–343
Physical appearance. See *Appearance*.
Physical examination, preoperative, 103–107, 156–157
Physical maturity, indicators of, 27–38
Physical therapy. See also *Rehabilitation*.
  after ankylosis surgery, 1524
  after arthroscopic surgery, 657, 658t
  after Vitek-Kent prosthesis placement, 786–787, *787*
  for mandibular hypomobility, 1669, *1669*, *1671*
Pickwickian syndrome, 2021, 2043
Pierre Robin syndrome, *2386*
  advancement genioplasty in, 2463, *2463*
  mandibular expansion in, 2385–2389
  short mandibular ramus deformity in, 2013–2017, *2013–2018*
  sleep apnea in, 2022, 2037
Pilot drill, for Branemark dental implants, 1153, *1153*
Pin fixture locator splint, for dental implants, 1178–1180, *1179–1181*
Pin pressure nociception, in neurologic examination, 1099, *1099*
Piriform rim, 324
Pitch, in model measurement, 169, *169*
  vocal, 1688–1689
  abnormal, 1696
Plagiocephaly, anterior, 1845, 1851–1855, *1852–1854*
  posterior, 1855, *1856–1858*
Plaque accumulation, around implants, 1339, 1349–1351, *1350*, *1351*
Plastic surgery. See also specific procedures.
  after orthognathic surgery, 232–233
  patient profile in, 11–13
Plate fixation. See also *Rigid internal fixation*.
  in craniofacial dysostosis, 1889–1890, 1897
  in intraoral vertical ramus osteotomy, 2119–2120, *2120*
    relapse and, 2135–2136
  in Le Fort I osteotomy, 2250–2257, *2252–2256*
    with microplates, 2255–2257, *2255–2259*
    with miniplates, 2250–2257, *2252–2254*
  in maxillary osteotomy, 71, *72*
  in orbitozygomatic deformity correction, 1037, *1038–1041*
  in sagittal split ramus osteotomy, 2355–2356, *2371*

Plate fixation *(Continued)*
  for prognathism, *2128*, 2129
    relapse and, 2135–2136
  in secondary craniofacial deformity correction, 1025
  in two-jaw procedures, *1992*, 1992–1994, *1993*
  intraoperative, in Le Fort I osteotomy, *633*, 633–634, *634*, *637*, 637
  Luhr, in Le Fort I osteotomy, 2255–2257, *2255–2259*
  in mandibular angle fracture, comparative stress analysis for, *1973*, 1973–1974
  of bone graft, 1025
  of costochondral graft, in condylar reconstruction, 672
  of facial fractures, 1015, 1016–1021, *1020*, *1024*
  of intraoperative ramus fracture, *1991*, 1991–1992
  of mandibular angle fracture, 1971–1974
    comparative stress analysis for, *1973*, 1973–1974
  of mandibular fractures, 997, *997*
  of maxillary fractures, 999
  of naso-orbito-ethmoid fractures, deformity after, *1045*, *1047*
  of unanticipated mandibular fracture, 69, *69*
  removal of, in postoperative infection, 73
  resistance of, to masticatory forces, 1961
  vs. intermaxillary fixation, postoperative maxillary stability and, 1936–1942
  vs. wire fixation, 79
  with compression plates, 1017
  with microplates, in Le Fort I osteotomy, 2255–2257, *2255–2259*
  with miniplates, 1016, *1024*
    for mandibular angle fractures, comparative stress analysis for, *1973*, 1973–1974
    in Le Fort I osteotomy, 2250–2257, *2252–2254*
  with reconstruction plates, 1017
Platinum, in Implator, 1340
Platysma muscle, 2178, 2180
  anatomic variations in, 378, *378*
  plication of, with lipectomy, 385–386
Plethysmography, respiratory induced, for nasal airway function evaluation, 1715
Pleural tear, in rib graft, 123, 838
Pneumothorax, in rib graft, 123
Pogonion, calculation of, 175, 183, *184*, 190, *191*
Polyactic acid implants, 851
Polyfascicular nerve, 1085, *1085*
Polyglactin sutures, for hydroxyapatite particulate implants, 1272
Polysomnography, 2044
  in sleep apnea, 2024, *2025*
Polytetrafluoroethylene implant, condylar resorption after, costochondral graft in, 918–922, *918–922*
  dermal graft in, 926–927
Polytetrafluoroethylene membrane, in guided bone regeneration, 1218–1220, *1219*
Porcelain laminates, 228, *228*
  in gummy smile correction, 260, *261*, 261

Porous block hydroxyapatite. See *Hydroxyapatite implants*.
Posterior articular artery, 954, *954*
Posterior auricular artery, 959, *959*
Posterior occipital artery, 959, *959*
Posterior plagiocephaly, 1855, *1856–1858*
Postoperative care, 115–120
　airway maintenance in, 115–117, 151
　analgesic, 120
　in ambulatory surgery, 117
　nutritional, 118–119
　of wounds, 117–118
　psychiatric, 119–120
Postoperative complications, 73–82, 120–126. See also specific procedures.
　donor site, 122–123
　febrile, 123–124
　fluid and electrolyte, 125–126
　hemorrhagic, 121
　infectious, 73, 121–122
　metabolic, 124–125
　segmental malposition, 76–77, *77*
　soft tissue, 73–75, *74*
　vascular, 120–121
Postoperative rehabilitation. See *Rehabilitation*.
Potassium replacement, 125
Preauricular approach, in condylar graft placement, 876, *877*
　in temporomandibular joint surgery, 706–709, *707–709*
Prediction tracings, 163–164. See also *Cephalometric analysis; Model surgery*.
　Model Frankfort (MF) reconstruction on, 178–180, *181*, 2307–2309, *2308–2310*
Premaxillary sutures, premature closure of, 2072, *2073*
Premolars, second, missing, preoperative management of, 58, *58*
Preoperative complications, 49–65
Preoperative data base, 156t, 156–157
Preoperative evaluation, of mandibular function, 1655–1656
　questionnaire for, *1654*, 1654–1655, *1655*
Preoperative orders, 109
Preoperative preparation, 49–65, 101–109
　autologous blood donation for, 108
　cardiovascular examination in, 105–106
　cephalometric analysis in. See *Cephalometric analysis*.
　condylar positioning planning in, 63–65, 162–163, 629–631, *630–632*
　for anesthesia, 129–135
　head and neck examination in, 103–105, *104*
　health history in, 102–103
　incisor decompensation in, 52, *52–55*
　laboratory examination in, 107
　model surgery in. See under *Model*.
　orthodontic, 49–50, *50, 51*, 61, 61–62, *62*
　patient conference in, with anesthesiologist, 129–130
　　with surgeon, 107–108
　photography in, 157, 342–343
　physical examination in, 103–107, 156–157
　preoperative orders in, 109

Preoperative preparation *(Continued)*
　pulmonary and respiratory examination in, 106–107
　record keeping in, 101–102, *102*
　root divergence in, *59*, 59–60, *60*
　splint fabrication in, 63–65, *64*. See also *Splint(s)*.
　tooth size equalization in, 56–58, *57, 58*
　transverse coordination in, 55–56, *56*
　treatment planning in. See *Treatment planning*.
Preoxygenation, 139–140
Pressure algesimeter, 1099, *1099*
Pressure flow technique, for nasal airway function evaluation, 1715
　for velopharyngeal function assessment, 1714–1715
Pretreatment records, recommendations for, 1791–1792
Procerus muscles, 292, *293*, 956, *956*, 2178, *2178*
Profile esthetics, 2174, *2175*, 2441–2442, *2443*
Progesterone, regulation of, 23–24, *24*
Prognathism. See *Mandibular prognathism; Maxillary hyperplasia*.
　mandibular. See *Mandibular prognathism*.
Proplast implants. See *Alloplastic implants*.
Prostaglandin E₂, in temporomandibular joint arthralgia, 473, *474*, 477–480, *478*
Prosthesis, dental. See *Dental implants; Dental prosthesis*.
　development of, 737–740
　facial, implant anchorage of, 1215–1218, *1215–1218, 1308–1310*, 1526, *1527*
　maxillary, 1525–1526
　ocular, ectropion and, 1074
　　enophthalmos of, *1028*
　　implant anchorage of, 1215, *1216*, 1526
　Vitek-Kent. See *Vitek-Kent prosthesis*.
Prosthetic bridge, for transmandibular implant, 1369, *1369*
Prosthetic speech bulb, for hypernasal speech, 1718–1720, *1719*
Proteoglycans, 471, *471*, 1640, *1640, 1641*, 1643–1644
　effects of immobilization on, 1643, 1644
Psychiatric disorders, appearance and, 9–10
Psychologic aspects, of appearance, 3–10, 439, 1441–1442, 2439
　of orthognathic surgery, 11–17, 119–120, 232–233
　of temporomandibular joint dysfunction, 645
Psychologic profile, of plastic surgery patients, 11–13
Pterygoid muscle, anatomy of, 485, *485*
　detachment of, in intraoral vertical osteotomy, condylar position and, 683–684, *2133*, 2133–2134, *2134*, 2135, 2138
　in intraoral vertical ramus osteotomy, 685, *685*
　displacement of, in sagittal split osteotomy, 2336
　dysfunction of, in costochondral grafting, 932
　fixation of, in Vitek-Kent prosthesis placement, 764, *765*, 765–767, *766*

Pterygoid muscle *(Continued)*
　postoperative biomechanics and, 1959–1962
Pterygomasseteric sling, detachment of, in sagittal split osteotomy, 2336–2337
PTFE implant. See *Polytetrafluoroethylene implant*.
Ptosis, 1067–1068, *1068, 1069*
Pts point, in cephalometric skeletal analysis, 90
Puberty, body maturity at, 27–28, *27–31*, 32t, 32–33, 35
Pulmonary complications, after rib harvesting, 929
Pulmonary evaluation, preoperative, 106–107
Pulmonary monitoring, intraoperative, 138
Pulp, changes in, after Le Fort I osteotomy, 2216–2218, *2217*
Pulse oximetry, intraoperative, 138
　postoperative, 116, 151
　preoperative, 139
Pumps, vacuum, for lipectomy, 375, *377*, *377*
Pyramidal Le Fort II osteotomy, 1816, *1817*

Quadrangular Le Fort osteotomies. See *Le Fort I osteotomy, quadrangular; Le Fort II osteotomy, quadrangular*.
Quality, vocal, 1688–1689
Questionnaire, health history, 102–103
　preoperative, *1654*, 1654–1655, *1655*

Racine adapter, endotracheal tube, *144*
Radiation therapy. See *Irradiated tissue*.
Radical osteoclastic surgery, modified after Powiertowsky, in craniosynostosis, 2070, *2071*
　in Crouzon syndrome, 2064–2065, *2065*
Radiography, cephalometric, 85, 96, 156–158. See also *Cephalometric analysis*.
　Model Frankfort (MF) reconstruction on, 178–181, *180, 181*, 2307–2309, *2308–2310*
　technique of, 409–412, *409–414*
　for dental implants, 1181–1182, *1182*
　in condylar positioning assessment, *526*, 526–527
　in interdental measurement, 170
　in masseter muscle hypertrophy, *429–431*, 429–432
　in skeletal age determination, 85, 96, 157–158, 179–181, *180*, 409–412, *409–414*
　of post-traumatic deformities, 990
　of temporomandibular joint, *494*, 494–495, *495*
Radionuclide imaging, of costochondral graft, 929, *930*
　of temporomandibular joint, 516, *517*
Radix, 286, *286*, 324, 2175
Ramping effect, in Le Fort I osteotomy, 2231–2232
Ramus, intraoperative fractures of, causes and prevention of, 2349–2352, *2350*

Ramus (Continued)
  fixation of, *1991*, 1991–1992
  post-traumatic deformities of, 994–995
  short, 1997–2019
    case studies of, *2000–2018*, 2000–2019
    cephalometric analysis of, 1997–1998
    clinical deformity in, 1997–1998
    surgical treatment of, 1998–1999
      case studies of, 2000–2019
      in Treacher Collins syndrome, 1609, *1609*, *1615*, 1616–1617
      technique for, 1998–1999
  upper, cortical fusion position in, 2349–2355, *2352*, *2353*, 2355t
Ramus procedures, *944*, 944–945. See also *Intraoral vertical ramus osteotomy; Sagittal split osteotomy*.
  condylar resorption in, costochondral graft for, *917*, 917
  dermal graft for, 926–927
  for chin asymmetry correction, 2472–2474, *2473–2476*
  for excessive transverse facial width, 2511–2514, *2512*, *2514*, *2515*
  for facial asymmetry, augmentation, 2514–2516, *2516*
    reduction, 2511–2514, *2512*, *2514*, *2515*
  for mandibular angle deficiency, 2489
  for mandibular prognathism, 2111–2113, *2112*
  in hemifacial microsomia, 1546–1550, 1553, 1556
  lengthening. See *Ramus, short, surgical treatment of.*
  mandibular angle deficiency after, 2489
  mandibular hypomobility after, 1668, 1668t
  maxillomandibular fixation in, 2119–2120, *2129*, 2129–2130, *2130*
  muscle atrophy in, 1631
  rehabilitation after, 1666–1668, *1667*
  speech after, 1728
  with dental implant placement, 1422–1425, *1423*, *1424*
Range-of-motion exercises, 1664–1666, *1665*, 1668–1669, *1669*. See also *Rehabilitation*.
  mechanical aids for, 1669, *1669*, *1671*
Ranitidine (Zantac), for gastric preparation, 134
Rapid mandibular expansion device, in transverse maxillary deficiency, 2404–2405, 2408–2410
Rapid palatal expansion device, in open bite surgery, 2084, *2084*
  in transverse mandibular deficiency, 2343, *2343*
  in transverse maxillary deficiency, 2404–2405, 2408–2410, *2409*
  in adults, 2412
  insertion of, 2415
  osteotomy with, case study of, 2420–2423, *2421–2424*
    in complete unilateral deficiency with crossbite, 2426
    in posterior bilateral deficiency with crossbite, 2425–2426
    in posterior unilateral deficiency with crossbite, 2426
  results of, 2425
  technique for, 2415–2420, *2416–2418*

Rapid palatal expansion device (Continued)
  resistance to, 2412–2415, *2413–2415*
Rasp, nasal dorsum reduction, 356, *356*
Ratchet cylinder wrench, in Branemark dental implant placement, 1158, *1158*
Reankylosis, prevention of, 927
Reconstruction plates. See *Plate fixation.*
Reconstructive surgery, advances in, 1449
  art of, 1461–1465
  bone maintenance after, 1464
  coronal approach in, 972–975, *972–977*
  elimination of soft tissue deficiencies in, 1464
  restoration of alveolar bone height in, *1462*, 1463–1464
  restoration of bone continuity in, 1462, *1462*
  restoration of facial contours in, *1464*, 1464–1465
  restoration of osseous bulk in, *1462*, 1462–1463, *1463*
  scientific basis of, 1449–1461
Record keeping, preoperative, 101–102, *102*
Reference plane, common, 157–159, 158t, *159*, 159t
Rehabilitation, after ankylosis surgery, 1524
  after arthroscopic surgery, 657, 658t
  after intraoral vertical ramus osteotomy, 688–689, *1667*, 1667–1668, 2131
  after Le Fort I osteotomy, 2268
  after mandibular surgery, 1666–1668, *1667*
  after maxillary surgery, 1666
  after plate and screw fixation, 1666
  after sagittal split osteotomy, 1666–1667, *1667*, 2131
  after Vitek-Kent prosthesis placement, 786–787, *787*
  for mandibular hypomobility, 1668–1669, *1669–1672*
  individualized, 1666–1668
  intermaxillary fixation and, 1656–1659, *1657–1658*
  mandibular function assessment in, 1655–1656
  mechanical aids for, 1669, *1669*, *1671*
  neuromuscular, 1662–1664, *1663*
    mechanical aids for, 1669, *1671*
  occlusal control during, 1659–1662, *1659–1662*
  preoperative evaluation and, *1654*, 1654–1655, *1655*
  range-of-motion exercises in, 1664–1666, *1665*, 1668–1669, *1669*, *1671*
Reproductive system measures, for growth assessment, 32–33
Resonance, vocal, 1688–1689
  evaluation of, 1710–1711
  problems with, 1695–1696
Respiratory disturbance index, in sleep apnea, 2044, 2057
Respiratory evaluation, preoperative, 106–107
Respiratory induced plethysmography, for nasal airway function evaluation, 1715
Respiratory problems, in Treacher Collins syndrome, 1601, 1614
  postoperative, 115–117
Restorative dentistry. See *Esthetic dentistry.*

Retainer, Hawley, 82
  postoperative, 82, *82*
    after mandibular prognathism surgery, 2152
Retrobulbar graft, 1064, *1064*, 1067, *1603*
Retrognathism. See *Mandibular deficiency; Maxillary deficiency.*
Retromandibular incision, in sagittal split osteotomy, *2371*, 2372
Reverse-pull headgear, for mandibular prognathism, 2146–2147
Rheumatoid arthritis, arthroscopy of, 609, *610*
  costochondral graft in, 904–909, *906–912*
  juvenile, mandibular deficiency in, 2506–2511, *2507–2510*
  Vitek-Kent prosthesis for. See *Vitek-Kent prosthesis.*
Rhinion, 324
Rhinoplasty, 268–283
  anesthesia for, 344–349, *345–348*
  approach in, selection of, 320
  bone graft for, *1024*
  case studies of, 273–283, 362–370, *363*, *364*, *366–369*
  complications of, 271–272
  conservative approach to, 320
  contraindications to, 270–271
  dorsal reduction and septal shortening in, *355*, 355–357, *356*
  endonasal, indications for, 319
  external, 268–271, 269t
    indications for, 319
    technique of, 360–362, *361*
  final inspection and closure in, 359, *359*
  for alar base deformities, *311*, 311–312, *312*
  for columellar deformities, 313, *313*, *314*
  for nasal dorsum deformities, 303–306, *304–307*
    during maxillary osteotomy, 303–306, *304–307*
  for nasal septum disorders, 313, *313–315*
  for nasal tip deformities, 307–310, *308–310*
  for nasolabial angle and upper lip deformities, 314–316, *315*, *316*
  goals of, 268
  hemostatic control in, 345
  history of, 319
  ideal face for, 268
  incisions in, 302–303, *303*, 349–351, *350*
    for external approach, 360–361, *361*
  indications for, 268
  limitations of, 270
  nasal narrowing osteotomies in, *357*, 357–359, *358*
  nasal tip problems in, 272–273
  open. See *Rhinoplasty, external.*
  preoperative evaluation in, 342–344
  revision, 369–370
  septoplasty in, 357
  skeletonization in, 349–351, *350*
  steps in, 268, 349–362
  taping and splinting in, 359–360, *360*
  technical errors in, 272–273
  technique of, 269–271
  timing of, 268
  tip-plasty in, 351–355, *351–355*
  treatment planning in, 342–344

Rhinoplasty (Continued)
  unsatisfactory esthetic result in, 272
  with cheiloplasty, in cleft deformity repair, 394–404, 395–406. See also Cheilorhinoplasty.
  with Le Fort I osteotomy, sequencing of, 2280
  with orthognathic surgery, 271, 302–316
    case studies of, 273–283, 362–365, 364
    sequencing of, 281, 2280
Rib cutter, 1484, 1484
Rib graft. See Bone graft, rib.
Rickett's E line, 86
Rigid internal fixation. See also Plate fixation; Screw fixation.
  comparative evaluation of, 1970–1974, 1972–1974
  in intraoral vertical ramus osteotomy, 2119–2120, 2120
    for prognathism, relapse and, 2135–2136
  in Le Fort I osteotomy, 2250–2257, 2252–2257
  in mandibular angle fractures, 1971–1974, 1972–1974
  in sagittal split osteotomy, 1981–1994, 2355–2356, 2365–2370, 2379–2381
    cortical thickness and, 2358–2359
    for prognathism, 2128, 2129
      relapse and, 2135–2136
    in two-jaw procedures, 1992, 1992–1994, 1993
  of mandibular fractures, 997
  rehabilitation after. See Rehabilitation.
  vs. intermaxillary fixation, mandibular mobility and, 1646
    muscle atrophy and, 1629–1630, 1630
    postoperative maxillary stability and, 1936–1942
Risorius muscle, 2178, 2179
Rod lens arthroscope, 604, 604
Roll, in model measurement, 169, 169
Root divergence, at osteotomy site, 59–60, 60, 1794–1795, 1795
Rubber band therapy. See Elastic therapy.
Rubber fixture locator splint, for dental implants, 1180, 1180–1181
Ruffini ending, static light touch detection test for, 1097–1098, 1098

Saddle graft, for dental implants, 1195–1196, 1196, 1197, 1203–1204, 1205
Saethre-Chotzen syndrome, 1851
Sagittal split osteotomy, 994, 994–995
  B point stability after, with rigid fixation, 558–591
    with wire fixation, 555–557, 557t
  bilateral, condylar positioning in. See also Condyle, positioning of.
  compressive loading in, 575
  firm anterosuperior-directed, 552–554, 552–557, 557t, 558–568
  heavy posterior-directed, 547–551, 547–552, 555–557, 557t
  influences on, 574–575, 575

Sagittal split osteotomy (Continued)
  superior-directed, 575–576, 576, 577
    with rigid fixation, 558–573
    with wire fixation, 547–558, 573
  condylar sag after, 580, 580–585, 581, 581t, 583
  temporomandibular joint function after, 547–568
  with dental implants, 1422–1425, 1423, 1424
  condylar fixation in, 66, 66–67, 67
  condylar sag after, 2134, 2138
  condyle-disk-fossa positioning in, 2378. See also Condyle, positioning of.
  cortical fusion position and, 2349–2355, 2352, 2353, 2355t
  cortical thickness in retromolar area and, 2356–2359, 2357, 2357t, 2358
  Dal Pont modification of, 2336, 2348–2349, 2350
  extraoral (retromandibular) approach in, 2371, 2372
  for deep-bite deformity, 2432, 2432–2438, 2434, 2435, 2503–2505, 2503–2506
  for mandibular advancement, advantages of, 2337
    anatomic considerations in, 2347–2359
    case studies of, 2372, 2372–2377, 2373, 2375, 2376
    complications of, 2131–2136
    in children, 2516–2517
    in deep-bite deformity, 2432, 2432–2438, 2434, 2435
    in juvenile rheumatoid arthritis, 2506–2511, 2507–2510, 2511
    technique for, 2361–2372, 2361–2372
    with rapid palatal expansion device, 2393–2394, 2394
  for mandibular arch leveling, 2495–2499, 2496, 2497
  for maxillomandibular advancement, in sleep apnea, 2050
  for open bite, case studies of, 2092–2099, 2093–2098
    complications and relapse with, 2080, 2080t
    technique for, 2086–2089, 2087–2089
  for prognathism, 2112, 2121–2129
    advantages of, 2136
    complications in, 2131–2136
    historical development of, 2111–2113
    indications for, 2121–2122
    inferior alveolar nerve injury in, 2113, 2121, 2131–2132
    intraoperative bleeding in, 2132–2133
    maxillomandibular fixation in, 2119–2120, 2129, 2130
    occlusal problems after, 2136–2137
    rehabilitation after, 2131
    relapse after, 2135–2136, 2138
    rigid fixation in, 1960, 2128, 2129
      relapse and, 1989–1990, 2135
    technique for, 2124–2129, 2125–2128
    vs. intraoral vertical ramus osteotomy, 2113, 2136–2137

Sagittal split osteotomy (Continued)
  for short mandibular ramus deformity correction, 1998–1999
  for total mandibular augmentation, 2392–2394, 2394
  free condylar fragment fixation in, 1990, 1991
  historical development of, 2111, 2112
  Hunsuck modification of, 2336
  in children, 2516–2517
  lateral cortical cut position in, 2348–2349
  mandibular angle deficiency after, 2489
  mandibular canal position and, 2347–2349, 2348
  mandibular hypomobility after, 1668, 1668t
  maxillomandibular fixation in, 2119–2120, 2129, 2130
    relapse after, 2379
    technique for, 2365
  medial osteotomy placement in, 2353–2354
  model surgery for, 181–184, 182t, 182–184, 199–201, 204
  modifications of, 2336–2337, 2350
  muscle atrophy in, 1631
  neurovascular bundle injury in, 2349
  Obwegeser-Dal Pont, for open bite, 2087
    complications and relapse with, 2080, 2080t
    technique for, 2080–2081, 2081
  plate fixation, in, 2355–2356, 2371
    for prognathism, 2128, 2129
    relapse after, 2135–2136
  proximal segment control in, 2377–2378
  rehabilitation after, 1666–1668, 1667, 2131
  relapse after, causes and prevention of, 2377–2381
  screw fixation in, 1960, 1981–1994, 2355–2356, 2365–2370, 2379–2380
    cortical thickness and, 2357, 2357t, 2358, 2358–2359
    for advancement, technique for, 1981–1985, 1982, 1983
    for prognathism, 2128, 2129
      relapse after, 1989
      relapse and, 2135–2136
      technique for, 1989–1990, 1990
    relapse after, 2379–2381
    with 2-mm bicortical screws, 1981–1994
      for advancement, condylar positioning in, 1987, 1987–1988, 1988
      occlusal shifts after, 1986
      postoperative orthodontics after, 1985–1986, 1986
      relapse after, 1985–1986
      results of, 1985–1989
      technique for, 1981–1985, 1982, 1983
      temporomandibular joint dysfunction after, 1988–1989
    for setback, 1989–1990
      relapse after, 1989
      technique for, 1989–1990, 1990
    management of buccal fragments in, 1990–1992, 1991
  speech after, 1728
  stability of, 2377–2381

VOLUME 1—PAGES 1–828; VOLUME 2—PAGES 829–1769; VOLUME 3—PAGES 1770–2517

INDEX / xxxv

Sagittal split osteotomy (Continued)
  with maxillomandibular fixation, 2379
  with screw fixation, 1989, 2379–2381, 2985–2986
  suprahyoid myotomy in, 2379
  unfavorable fractures in, causes and prevention of, 2349–2352, 2350
  fixation of, 1991, 1991–1992
  in children, 2516–2517
  with Le Fort III osteotomy, in Binder's syndrome, 2067, 2068
  with reduction genioplasty, 2503–2505, 2503–2506
  with Vitek-Kent prosthesis implantation, 749, 773
  Wolford-Davis modification of, 2337, 2349, 2352
Sagittal suture synostosis, 1848, 1868–1872
Sagittal zygomatic osteotomy, with bone grafting, for malar augmentation, 2298–2303, 2300–2303
Saline, for graft storage, 1492
SAM articulator, 202, 202
SAM facebow, 161
Samarium-gold magnets, for prosthesis anchorage, 1526, 1527
Sartorius muscle, injury of, in ilial graft harvesting, 848–849
Scalp, anatomy of, 952, 952–955, 954, 955
  lymphatic drainage of, 960, 961
Scaphocephaly, 1848, 1868–1872
Scar remodeling, 1067
Scarring. See also under Cicatricial.
  mandibular hypomobility and, 1669, 1672
  of eyelid, 1070, 1070
  repair of, 1067
  with coronal incision, 966, 967
Schwann cell, 1086
  response of, to injury, 1089
Scintigraphy, skeletal. See Skeletal scintigraphy.
Scissors, microsurgical, 1111–1112, 1112
Sclerotherapy, arthroscopic, 658–659, 659
Screw fixation. See also Rigid internal fixation.
  biomechanics of, 1960
  condylar, 66, 66–67, 67
  condylar sag and, 582
  contra-angle technique of, in sagittal split ramus osteotomy, 2369
  in bilateral sagittal split osteotomy, condylar positioning in, 558–573
  in broad soft tissue pedicle genioplasty, 2450–2454, 2452–2455
  in intraoral vertical ramus osteotomy, 2119–2120, 2120
    for prognathism, relapse and, 2135–2136
  in secondary craniofacial deformity correction, 1025
  in two-jaw procedures, 1992, 1992–1994, 1993
  of bone graft, 1025
  of condylar implant, 782–785, 783–785
  of facial fractures, 1015, 1016–1021, 1020, 1024
  of glenoid fossa implant, 771–772, 772, 772t

Screw fixation (Continued)
  of intraoperative buccal fragment greenstick fracture, 1991, 1991–1992
  of intraoperative condylar neck fracture, 1990, 1991
  of intraoperative ramus fracture, 1991, 1991–1992
  of mandibular angle fracture, stress analysis of, 1971–1974, 1972–1974
  of maxillary fractures, 999
  of unanticipated mandibular fracture, 67–69, 67–69
  of Vitek-Kent prosthesis, 755, 755
  rehabilitation after, 1666
  removal of, in postoperative infection, 73
  vs. wire fixation, 79
  with hydroxyapatite implant, 856, 858
Screw tap, for Branemark dental implants, 1156, 1156–1157
  for transmandibular implant, 1357, 1358
Sedatives, preoperative, 134–135, 141–142
Self-concept, appearance and, 4–10, 1439, 1441–1442
  orthognathic surgery and, 11–17, 232–233
Sensorineural evaluation. See Neurologic evaluation.
Sensorineural hearing loss, 1707–1708. See also Hearing loss.
  treatment of, 1720–1721
Sensory end organs, response of, to injury, 1090
Sensory nerves. See Nerve(s).
Sensory re-education, in nerve injury, 1123–1124
Septal cartilage, 2175–2176, 2176
Septo-premaxillary ligament, maxillary growth and, 1934
Septoplasty, 333–338, 333–339
  craniofacial growth after, 38–39
  during maxillary osteotomy, 314, 315
  during rhinoplasty, 357
  for sleep apnea, 2045, 2045–2046
  incisions in, 334
  Killian submucous, 333, 333, 334
  morcellation in, 336–337, 337
  overresection in, 333, 333
  steps in, 334–338, 334–339
  unsuccessful, 272
Sequestra, after quadrangular Le Fort osteotomy, 1836
Sesamoid cartilage, 291, 291–292
Sex steroids, regulation of, 23–24, 24
Sexual development, body maturity and, 27–28, 27–31, 32t, 32–33, 35
Shaving, cartilage, in chondromalacia, 476–477
  condylar, for disk repositioning, 712
Shaving graft, cranial, 981
Short face syndrome, cephalometric analysis in, 97, 97–98
Short mandibular ramus deformities. See Ramus, short.
Short stature, sleep apnea and, 2021–2022
Shunt, ventriculoperitoneal, in Apert syndrome, 1898
  in Crouzon syndrome, 1894
Sign language, 1721
Silastic implants. See Alloplastic implants.

Silicone implants. See Alloplastic implants.
Silver, in Implator, 1340
Single photon emission computed tomography, 1682–1684, 1684
Sinus, frontal, fracture of, coronal approach in, 967, 969, 975, 976
  post-traumatic deformities of, 1062–1063
  maxillary, grafting of, with simultaneous hydroxyapatite dental implants, 1277–1286, 1277–1286, 1313–1315
    hydroxyapatite communication with, 855–856
Sinus graft, for dental implants, 1201–1204, 1202, 1204, 1205
Skeletal age, determination of, 33–34, 35–38
  by hand-wrist radiographs, 35–38, 36, 37
Skeletal analysis, cephalometric, 89–94, 89–94. See also Cephalometric analysis.
  case studies of, 97, 97–98, 98
  radiographic, 85, 96, 157–158, 179–181, 180, 409–412, 409–414
Skeletal growth. See also Growth.
  regulation of, 23, 23–24
  scintigraphic evaluation of, 1677–1684
Skeletal open bite. See Open bite.
Skeletal scintigraphy, 1677–1684
  clinical applications of, 1679–1680, 1680–1682
  interpretive difficulties in, 1682, 1682
  of costochondral graft, 929, 930
  technique of, 1678, 1678–1679, 1679t
Skeleton, facial. See Bone.
Skin, of forehead, 955, 956
  of scalp, 952, 953
  of temporal region, 957, 958
Skin disorders, after rhinoplasty, 272
Skin flap. See Flap(s).
Skin graft. See Dermal graft.
Skin-platysma rotation flap, 1478–1479, 1479, 1480. See also Flap(s).
Skin tags, in hemifacial microsomia, 1536, 1536
Skoog procedure, for cleft deformity repair, 399, 401, 402
Skull, bone graft from. See Bone graft, cranial.
  development of, 2063, 2063–2073
    at chondral base, 2063–2067, 2063–2067
    growth of, at calvarial sutures, 2067–2070, 2069–2071
    premature sutural closure in. See Craniofacial dysostosis.
  thickness of, 978–979
Sleep apnea, 2021–2058
  airway development and, 2021–2024
  airway obstruction in, 2023, 2023–2028, 2055, 2056
  case studies of, 2034–2037, 2034–2039
  causes of, 2023, 2023–2024, 2027–2028
  complications of, 2023, 2044
  continuous positive airway pressure for, 2028, 2029, 2045
  craniofacial abnormalities and, 2022, 2022, 2033–2034, 2047
  diagnosis of, 2024–2028, 2025, 2026, 2031–2034, 2044
  in children, 2021–2023

Sleep apnea (Continued)
  maxillomandibular advancement for, 2045–2058, 2047–2058
    preoperative evaluation for, 2047–2050, 2048, 2049
    results of, 2053t–2055t, 2053–2055, 2054, 2057–2058
    technique for, 2050–2053, 2051–2053
  orthodontic appliances for, 2029–2030, 2030
  patient evaluation in, 2024–2028, 2025, 2026, 2031–2039, 2044, 2047
  septoplasty for, 2045, 2045–2046
  tracheostomy for, 2029, 2046, 2057
  treatment of, 2026, 2026, 2028–2030, 2029, 2030, 2034–2038, 2045–2058
    medical, 2028–2030, 2029, 2030, 2045, 2056–2057
    surgical, 2045–2058
  uvulopalatopharyngoplasty for, 2026, 2026, 2028, 2046–2047, 2056, 2058
Sleep bite, 63
Sleep disorder center, 2024
Sleep study, 2024–2025, 2025
Sliding horizontal osteotomy, for chin augmentation, 2443–2446, 2446
  for chin lengthening, 2447, 2447–2448
  for chin shortening, 2447–2484, 2485
SMAS (superficial musculoaponeurotic system) of face, 953, 957
Smile, analysis of, 236, 239, 240, 240, 253, 253
  asymmetric, 241–243, 242–244
  gummy, 235–261, 255, 255, 259–261, 260
    altered passive eruption and, 241, 242, 243, 254, 254–256
    case studies of, 1944–1953, 1945–1953
    cephalometric analysis in, 96, 96–97
    clinical examination in, 236–240, 237–239
    correction of, with dental implants, 1413–1416, 1414, 1415
    esthetic objectives for, 240–241, 241, 242
    flap procedures for, 246–250, 247–250, 257–258, 258, 259, 259, 260
    gingivectomy for, 245–246, 246, 247, 256, 256–257, 257, 259–261, 259–261
    maxillary hyperplasia and, 255, 255, 259–261, 260
    nonoperative treatment of, 1943
    oblique modified Le Fort III osteotomy for, 1777–1779, 1777–1779
    orthodontic treatment for, 1943–1953, 1945
    pathophysiology of, 1935–1936
    related problems in, 241, 242
    surgery for, 244–251, 1942, 1943–1953, 1946, 1949, 1952
      maxillary growth after, 1936–1954. See also Maxillary growth, postoperative.
      maxillary stability after, 1936–1937
Socialization, appearance and, 4–10

Socket, anophthalmic, ectropion in, 1074
  tooth, healing of, 1458–1459
    hydroxyapatite-coated implant in, 1289, 1290, 1291, 1316, 1330, 1330, 1331
Sodium citrate (Bicitra), for gastric preparation, 133, 142
Sodium replacement, 125
Sodium tetradecyl sulfate, in arthroscopic sclerotherapy, 659
Soft palate. See Palate.
Soft tissue analysis, in open bite, 2078–2079, 2079
Soft tissue changes, with orthognathic surgery, anatomic considerations in, 2174–2180, 2175–2178
  cephalometric considerations in, 2181
  facial evaluation and, 2172–2174, 2173–2175
  hard tissue changes and, 2180–2181, 2181t
  historical background of, 2171–2172
  orthodontic considerations in, 2181
  studies of, 2180–2181, 2181t
Soft tissue deformities, flap repair of. See Flap(s).
  in hemifacial microsomia, 1536, 1536–1537, 1537
  periorbital, post-traumatic, 1067–1077
  post-traumatic, 987, 1004–1006, 1004–1007
  evaluation of, 988, 989, 1067
  treatment of, 992
Soft tissue dissection, for flap repair, 1465–1466, 1466
Soft tissue esthetic analysis, 86–88, 86–88. See also Cephalometric analysis.
  case studies of, 97, 97–98, 98
  radiographic, 96
Soft tissue flap. See Flap(s).
Soft tissue injury, intraoperative, 73–75, 74–75
Soft Tissue Patch, in capsular reconstruction, 723, 724
Soft tissue resuspension, 1023, 1024
Soft tissue triangle, nasal, 291, 323, 323
Sound(s), speech, 1688–1691, 1689t, 1690–1693
  assessment of, 1709–1710
  dental factors in, 1701–1703, 1702
  frequency and intensity of, 1706
Sound waves, in speech, 1689, 1706
Spark erosion, 1188
Speech. See also Voice.
  acceptability of, 1697
    evaluation of, 1715–1716
  after craniofacial surgery, 1728–1729
    data collection and outcome measures for, 1729
  after mandibular osteotomy, 1727–1728
  after maxillary osteotomy, 1721–1727
  after orthognathic surgery, 1721–1728
    data collection and outcome measures for, 1729
  after pharyngeal flap surgery, 1719, 1724–1726
  appearance of, 1697
  articulation of, after Le Fort I osteotomy, 1722–1723
  after Le Fort III osteotomy, 1728–1729
  assessment of, 1709–1710
  compensatory, 1693
    treatment of, 1716

Speech (Continued)
  errors of, 1693, 1693–1694
  place of, 1691
  problems of, 1693, 1693–1694
    treatment of, 1716
  assessment of, 1709–1716
  breathy, 1696
  denasal, 1696
  dental problems and, 1701–1703, 1702
  development of, 1687
  disorders of, diagnosis of, 1708–1716
    treatment of, 1716–1721
  ear abnormalities and, 1706–1708
  environmental factors in, 1698
  hearing loss and, 1706–1708
  hoarse, 1696
  hypernasal, 1694–1696
    evaluation of, 1711
    treatment of, 1717–1719
  hyponasal, 1695–1696
    after Le Fort III osteotomy, 1728–1729
    after pharyngeal flap surgery, 1717
    evaluation of, 1711
    treatment of, 1719–1720
  in craniofacial dysostosis, 1842
  in hearing loss, 1720–1721
  in Treacher Collins syndrome, 1601
  intelligence and, 1697–1698
  intelligibility of, 1696
    evaluation of, 1715
    problems with, 1696
  laryngeal abnormalities and, 1706, 1726
  lip abnormalities and, 1698–1699, 1699, 1703, 1703
  mandibular abnormalities and, 1704
  maxillary abnormalities and, 1703, 1703–1704
  mechanism of, 1687–1691, 1688–1693
  nasal abnormalities and, 1705, 1720
  nasal air emission in, 1694–1695
    assessment of, 1710, 1710
    treatment of, 1716–1718
  nasal airway function and, 1720
    evaluation of, 1715
  occlusal problems and, 1702, 1702–1703
  palatal abnormalities and, 104–105, 1700, 1700–1701, 1701, 1703, 1703
  pharyngeal abnormalities and, 1705–1706
  phonation problems in, 1696
  preoperative evaluation of, with previously repaired cleft palate, 104–105
  sound of, 1697
  tongue abnormalities and, 1704, 1704–1705
  tonsils and, 1705–1706, 1718, 1719
  variables affecting, 1697–1708
  velopharyngeal valve in. See Velopharyngeal valve.
  vocal resonance problems in, 1695–1696
Speech bulb, prosthetic, for hypernasal speech, 1718–1720, 1719
Speech sounds, 1688–1691, 1689t, 1690–1693
  assessment of, 1709–1710
  dental factors in, 1701–1703, 1702
  frequency and intensity of, 1706
Speech therapy, for articulation problems, 1716
  for nasal air emission, 1716–1717

INDEX / xxxvii

Spee's curve, leveling of, orthodontic, 2341, 2341–2342, 2342
  surgical, 2495–2499, 2496, 2497
  orthodontic leveling of, 61, 61–62, 62
Splint(s), composite, for dual-arch surgery, 206–215
  fabrication of, 210–215, 210–215
    with mandible as reference arch, 206–208, 206–208
    with maxilla as reference arch, 208–209
  fabrication of, 63–65, 64
  for dual-arch surgery, 210–215, 210–215
  for Vitek-Kent prosthesis, 750
  in model surgery, 198
  surgical model for, 181–182
  in arthroscopic surgery, 622
  interdental, after Le Fort I/II quadrangular osteotomy, 1796
  mandibular advancement, 2049–2050
  maxillary advancement, 2318, 2318
  nasal, postoperative, 359–360, 360
  occlusal, 1657
    after Vitek-Kent prosthesis placement, 787–788
    in condylar positioning, for intraoperative control, 632–634, 632–635
    in preoperative planning, 630–631, 631
    in postoperative rehabilitation, 1659–1660, 1660
    postoperative, in Le Fort I osteotomy, 634, 634, 635, 638, 638
  pin fixture locator, for dental implants, 1178–1180, 1179–1181
  positioning of, 63–65, 64
  rubber fixture locator, for dental implants, 1180, 1180–1181
Splint tube, wire fixation with, in maxillary osteotomy, 72, 72–73
Split grafts. See Bone graft.
Spurs, condylar stump, after Vitek-Kent prosthesis placement, 790–792, 792
Stainless steel arch wire, 1656
Stainless steel dental implants, reactivity of, 1140, 1141
Static light touch detection, in neurologic examination, 1097–1098, 1098
Stellate ganglion block, diagnostic, 1101
  therapeutic, 1106
Stellate neuroma, 1091–1092, 1092
Stensen's duct, 428
Stereotyping, appearance-based, 6–7
Sternocleidomastoid flap, 1474–1475, 1474–1476. See also Flap(s).
Steroids, for nasal preparation, 133
  for postoperative edema, 112
  for temporomandibular joint arthralgia, 479, 479–480
  gonadal, regulation of, 23–24, 24
  subcondylar, after Vitek-Kent prosthesis placement, 791
Still's disease, costochondral graft in, 904, 905, 908–909
Stop sounds, 1689, 1689t, 1690
Stress analysis, 1963–1970
  for condyle, 1966, 1966–1969, 1967
  for mandible, 1964–1965, 1965
  for midface, 1969, 1969–1970, 1970
  fringe patterns in, 1963–1964, 1964
  in temporomandibular joint dysfunction, 1968

Stress analysis (Continued)
  of mandibular angle fracture fixation, 1971–1974, 1972–1974
  photoelastic, 1963–1964, 1964
  stress freezing in, 1964
Stress trajectories, of facial skeleton, 1962–1963
  analysis of. See Stress analysis.
Stump neuroma, 1090, 1090
Subapical mandibular osteotomy, for mandibular deficiency, anterior, 2495–2499, 2496, 2497
  total, 2500–2502, 2501
  for mandibular prognathism, 2111, 2112
Subcondylar mandibular osteotomy, 2111, 2112
Subconjunctival chemosis, after quadrangular Le Fort osteotomy, 1836
Subconjunctival ecchymosis, after quadrangular Le Fort osteotomy, 1836
Subcostal nerve, injury of, in anterior ilium graft harvesting, 1486, 1487
Subcutaneous fat, deficiency of. See Contour deficiencies.
  removal of. See Lipectomy.
Subcutaneous fat development, as maturity indicator, 32–33, 35
Subgaleal layer, 952, 953
Submalar implants, 2293–2294, 2294
Submandibular approach, in condylar graft placement, 876, 877
Submandibular fat pad, 378
  removal of. See Lipectomy.
Submental fat pad, 377–379, 378
  removal of. See Lipectomy.
Subnasale, in profile analysis, 2442, 2443
Suction curettes, lipectomy, 376, 376
Suction lipectomy, 373–388. See also Lipectomy
Suctioning, postoperative, 116
Sufentanil (Sufenta), in anesthesia, 140, 149, 150
Sulcular epithelium, gingival, 1339
Superficial musculoaponeurotic system (SMAS) of face, 293, 953, 957
Superficial temporal artery, 954, 954, 958, 958, 959
Superficial temporal fascia, 957–958, 958
  mobilization of, coronal approach in, 973, 974
Superior cranial base line, 91, 91
Supraorbital artery, 954, 954, 957, 959, 959
Supraorbital foramina, 957
Supraorbital nerve, 955, 955, 957, 959, 959
Supratip break, nasal, 265, 266
Supratrochlear artery, 954, 954, 957, 959, 959
Supratrochlear nerve, 955, 955, 957, 959, 959
Supratrochlear notch, 957
Suprazygomatic SMAS, 957–958, 958
Sural nerve, anatomy of, 1122
Sural nerve graft, for trigeminal nerve repair, 1110–1111
  harvesting technique for, 1122, 1122–1123
  in inferior alveolar nerve repair, 1113–1116, 1115, 1116
  with great auricular nerve transfer, 1114–1116, 1115

Sural nerve graft (Continued)
  with mandibular bone graft, 1116, 1116–1117
  in infraorbital nerve repair, 1121, 1121–1122
  in lingual nerve repair, 1119, 1119–1120
Surgery. See Model surgery; Orthognathic surgery; Reconstructive surgery; and names and sites of specific procedures.
Sutures, cranial, growth at, 2067–2070, 2069–2070
  premature closure of. See Craniosynostosis.
  facial, growth at, 2071–2072, 2072
  premature closure of. See Craniofacial synostosis.
  midfacial, surgery of, during growth period, 38–44
Suturing, in disk repositioning, 713, 713
  in ilial graft harvesting, 843, 848
  in microreconstructive surgery, 1110
  of coronal incision, 965, 965–966
  of dermal graft, 923–924
  of temporalis myofascial flap, 721–723, 722
  polyglactin, for hydroxyapatite particulate implants, 1272
Sympathetically mediated pain, 1093–1094, 1094, 1096, 1103–1105
  evaluation of, nerve block in, 1100–1101
Symphyseal osteotomy, for mandibular expansion, 2398, 2400–2401
  for mandibular narrowing, 2398, 2399
Syndactyly, in Apert syndrome, 1896
Synethesia, 1105
Synostosis, cranial. See Craniosynostosis.
Synovial chondromatosis, 650, 650
Synovial fluid, 649
  in articular cartilage nutrition, 1635–1637, 1637
Synovial joints, effects of immobilization on, 1632–1639
Synovial membrane, 649
Synovial pouch, of temporomandibular joint, lower anterior, 600, 600, 601
  lower posterior, 599, 599–600, 600
  upper posterior, 596, 597
Synovitis, arthroscopy of, diagnostic, 601, 601–602, 602, 608, 612, 612, 649–650, 650, 652, 652, 653
  benign pigmented villonodular, 912, 912–913
  biopsy in, 652, 652
  etiology of, 473, 474
  grading of, 477, 477t
  pain mediators in, 473, 474, 477–480, 478
  pathology of, 479
  treatment of, 479, 479–480
Synovium, anatomy of, 649
  arthroscopy of, 649
  cell types in, 649
  disorders of, 649–650, 650
Syssarcosis, 379

Tanner-Whitehouse standards, for skeletal age determination, 36
Taping, in rhinoplasty, 359–360, 360

Total mandibular augmentation, 2392–2394, *2394*
  sequencing in, 2393–2394, *2396–2397*
Total mandibular subapical osteotomy, 2500–2502, *2501*
Tracheal indication whistle, *145*, 145
Tracheal intubation. See *Intubation, endotracheal.*
  in craniofacial surgery, 1891–1892
Tracheal position, preanesthetic evaluation of, 131
Tracheostomy, in sleep apnea, 2029, 2046, 2057
  in Treacher Collins syndrome, 1621
Traction, chin cap, for mandibular prognathism, 2146–2147, 2148
  external headframe, for cleft deformity–associated maxillary hypoplasia, 2315–2322, *2316–2321*
  face mask, for mandibular advancement, 2325–2331, *2326, 2327, 2329*
  headframe, for mandibular prognathism, 2146–2147
Traction bands, conjunctival, 1070
  ectropion and, 1071
Training elastics. See *Elastic therapy.*
Transcolumellar incision, in external rhinoplasty, 360–361, *361*
Transfixion incision, in rhinoplasty, 302–303, *303, 350*, 350–351
Transfusion, autologous, 108, 124
Transjaw therapy, after Vitek-Kent prosthesis placement, 786–787, *787*
Transmandibular bridge, follow-up for, 1370, *1370, 1371*
  results of, clinical studies of, 1370–1382, 1372t–1374t, *1375–1378, 1380–1382*
Transmandibular implant, 1335–1384
  bearing capacity of, 1355
  biocompatibility of, 1337
  biomechanical characteristics of, 1336, 1340–1353
  biomechanical principles of, 1354–1356, *1355*
  bone healing around, 1337–1338, 1346–1348, *1347, 1348*
    implant roughness and, 1351–1353, *1352–1354*
  bone-implant interface with, 1343–1344, *1343–1345*
  bone loss and, 1376–1378, *1377, 1378*
  bone mineral content changes with, 1383
  complications of, 1379–1382
  components of, *1357*, 1357
  construction and biomechanics of, 1335–1337
  contraindications to, 1356
  damping capacity of, 1355
  design of, 1354, *1354*
  Dolder bar for, 1364, *1364*
  dual-photon absorptiometric investigation of, 1383
  experimental results with, 1341–1353
  fixed bridge for, 1369, *1369*
  gingival hyperplasia and, 1375, *1375–1377*
  Implator for, biomechanical characteristics of, 1336, 1340–1353
    constituents of, 1340
    experimental results with, 1341–1353

Transmandibular implant *(Continued)*
  mechanical characteristics of, 1336
  indications for, 1356, 1372
  infection and, 1379
  instrumentation for, 1357, *1358*
  loading of, bone induction by, 1382–1383
    premature, 1379
  marginal bone loss with, prevention of, 1355–1356
  material for, 1340–1342, *1341*
  osseointegration of, 1337–1338, 1378–1379
    experimental invesigation of, 1343–1353, *1343–1353*
    interference with, by premature loading, 1379
    loss of, 1379–1382, *1380–1382*
  overdenture for, 1367–1369, *1368, 1369*
  perimucosal seal around, 1301, *1338*, 1338–1339, *1339*
  plaque accumulation around, 1339, 1349–1351, *1350, 1351*
  postoperative management for, 1356, *1364*, 1364
  preoperative evaluation for, 1356, *1356, 1357*
  pretension and, 1354–1355
  prognosis with, 1384
  reconstruction with, 1364–1370, *1365–1371*
  removal of, reasons for, 1374, 1374t
  requirements for, 1335
  soft tissue response to, 1374–1378, *1375–1378*
  surgical procedure for, 1358–1364, *1359–1364*
Transnasal wiring, in canthopexy, *1045, 1046*, 1048, 1076–1077
Transtracheal block, in sedated-awake intubation, *142*, 142
Transverse facial artery, 959, *959*
Transverse mandibular deficiency. See *Mandibular deficiency, transverse.*
Transverse maxillary deficiency. See *Maxillary deficiency, transverse.*
Transverse measurements, bone, 177, 188, *189, 192*, 192
  postsurgical, 198–199, *199*
  dental, 176, *177*, 188, *189*, 190, *192*, 2312, *2312*
Transverse reference line, bone, 192, *192*
Trapezius flap, 1472–1474, *1473*. See also *Flap(s).*
Trauma, coronal flap in, 967, *968–971*
Traumatic arthritis. See *Arthritis.*
Trauner procedure, for cleft deformity repair, 399, *401*
Treacher Collins syndrome, 1601–1625
  abortive form of, 1603
  anterior open bite in, recurrence of, 1606
  asymmetry in, 1604
  bone graft in, 1609–1610, *1610*, 1614, 1616
    harvesting of, *1605*
    sources of, 1604, 1605, 1608
  breathing difficulties in, 1601, 1614
  chin deformities in, 1606
    correction of, 1609, *1609*
  combined midfacial rotation and mandibular lengthening in, 1614–1621, *1615, 1617–1621*

Treacher Collins syndrome *(Continued)*
  complete form of, *1602, 1603*, 1603
  cranial graft in, 1605, *1605*
  cranial osteomuscular flaps in, 1608
  ear abnormalities in, 1609, 1610, 1614
    correction of, 1601
  eyelid abnormalities in, 1607, *1607*
  graft resorption in, 1604
  incomplete form of, 1603
  lateral canthal laxity in, 1604
  macrostomia in, 1608
  malar absence in, 1604, *1604*
  malformations in, 1601, *1602*
  mandibular overjet in, 1617, 1618
  orbital construction in, 1616
  orbital deformities in, 1606–1607
    correction of, 1604–1605
  pharyngeal abnormalities in, 1705
  postoperative course in, 1618, 1621
  sleep apnea in, 2022, *2022*, 2037
  tracheostomy in, 1621
  treatment of, complementary procedures in, 1614
    limitations of, 1621
    objectives for, 1608
    one-step vs. two-step, 1617–1618, 1621
    priorities in, 1608
    procedures for, 1608–1610, *1609–1611*
    results of, *1612, 1613*, 1617–1622
    timing of, 1610–1611, 1623
    with severe breathing problems, 1614–1621, *1615, 1617–1621*
    without severe breathing problems, 1611–1614, *1612, 1613*
  zygomatic hypoplasia in, 1601, 1604
Treatment planning. See also *Preoperative preparation.*
  cephalometric analysis in, 85–98, 156–159. See also *Cephalometric analysis.*
  clinical examination in, 156t, 156–157
  common reference plane for, 157–159, 158t, *159*, 159t
  data base for, 156–157
  dental models for, mounting of, *160*, 160–163, *162*
  facebow transfer in, 160–161
  for mandibular surgery, 166, *174*, 174–176, *175*
  for maxillary surgery, 166–167, *172*, 172–173
  for rhinoplasty, 342–344
  for two-jaw surgery, 167–168
  guidelines for, 179–181
  model measurement in. See *Model measurement.*
  model surgery in. See *Model surgery.*
  prediction tracings in, 163–164
Trephine technique, for ilial graft harvesting, 844–845
Tri-square, 1058, *1059*
Tricalcium phosphate–coated dental implants, strength of, 1298
Trigeminal nerve, 954–955, *955*. See also *Inferior alveolar nerve; Infraorbital nerve; Lingual nerve.*
  clinical examination of, 1096–1100
  fibrosis of, surgery of, 1107–1108
  in scalp innervation, 954–955, *955*
  injury of, 1081–1124
    anesthesia dolorosa and, 1093
    anesthesia in, 1095
    axonal response to, 1089

Trigeminal nerve *(Continued)*
  central trigeminal pathosis and, 1093
  cervical autonomic pathosis and, 1093
  classification of, 1086–1088, *1087*
  clinical examination of, 1096–1100
  collateral microsprouting in, 1090
  compression, 1106–1107
  degeneration and regeneration in, 1088–1095
  diagnostic evaluation of. See *Neurologic evaluation.*
  etiology of, 1081
  fifth-degree, 1087, *1087*
  first-degree, 1086, *1087*
  fourth-degree, 1087, *1087*
  history of, 1095–1096
  in ilial graft harvesting, 848
  morphofunctional characteristics of, 1081–1095
  myelination after, 1089
  nerve trunk regeneration in, 1089–1090
  neuroma formation in, *1090–1092*, 1090–1093
    prevention of, 1106
  neuropathic events after, *1090–1092*, 1090–1095, *1094*
  observed, *1004*, 1105–1106
  pain in, 1093–1095, *1094*, 1096
    evaluation of, 1100–1101
    management of, 1106
  paresthesia in, 1095
  primary repair of, 1105
  return of sensation after, 1124
  Schwann cell response to, 1089
  second-degree, 1087, *1087*
  secondary repair of, 1105
  sensory disturbance in, evaluation of. See *Neurologic evaluation.*
    onset of, 1095–1096
  sensory end organ response to, 1089–1090
  sensory re-education in, 1123–1124
  sequelae of, 1081
  stretch, 1106–1107
  third-degree, 1087, *1087*
  transection, 1106
  treatment algorithm for, *1104–1105*, 1105–1107
  unobserved, *1005*, 1106
  microreconstructive surgery of. See *Nerve injury, microreconstructive surgery for.*
  morphology of, *1082–1085*, 1083–1086
Trigeminal pathosis, central, 1093
Trigeminal sensory evoked response testing, 1101–1102, *1102*
Trigonocephaly, 1847–1848, *1864–1867*, 1865–1867
Triploscope, 1109, *1110*
Trismus, after masseter reduction, 435
Tube, endotracheal. See *Intubation, endotracheal.*
Tumors, excision of, coronal approach for, 975
  of condyle, costochondral graft for, 912–914, *912–914*
Turbinates, 327
  enlargement of, nasal obstruction and, 332
    submucous resection for, 339–341, *339–341*
Twist drill, for Branemark dental implants, 1152, *1152*, 1154, *1154*

Two-jaw surgery, for facial asymmetry, results of, *2313–2314*
  model surgery for, 181–184, 182t, *182–185*, 205
  treatment planning for, 167–168. See also *Treatment planning.*
Two-point discrimination, in neurologic examination, 1098–1099

UCLA castable abutment, 1187, *1187*
Unilateral coronal synostosis, 1845, 1851–1855, *1852–1854*
Unilateral lambdoid synostosis, 1846, 1855, *1856–1858*
Upper incisor–palatal plane angle, 95, *95*
Upper lip support, evaluation of, 156
Urinary catheterization, 110–111, 138, 140, *141*
Uvulopalatopharyngoplasty, in sleep apnea, 2026, *2026*, 2028, *2046*, 2046–2047, 2056, 2058

Vanadium, bioreactivity of, 1340
Vapor pressure vacuum, in lipectomy, 375
Vasa nervorum, 1083
Vascular access, 111
Vascular compromise, during hypotensive anesthesia, 114–115, 135–137, *136*
  intraoperative, 73–75
  postoperative, 120–121
Vascular groin flap, cutaneous, 1569
  in hemifacial microsomia, 1561–1599. See also under *Hemifacial microsomia, treatment of, microvascular groin flap in.*
  osteocutaneous, 1569–1571
Vasculature, in Le Fort I osteotomy, 2212–2221, *2213–2217*
  of bone, 1337
  of chin, 2180
  of graft host bed, 1452
  of lips, 2179
  of maxilla, 2212–2218, *2213–2217*
  of nose, 2177–2178, *2178*, *2179*
  of scalp, *954*, 954–955, *955*
  of temporal region, *958*, 958–959, *959*
Veins. See *Vasculature.*
Velocity curves, for height measurement, *27*, *29*, *31*, *37*
Velopharyngeal valve, 1688, *1688*, 1689
  functional assessment of, 1711–1713, *1712–1714*
  inadequate closure of, 1688, *1688*, 1689, 1694–1696, *1700*, 1700–1701, 1710
  after Le Fort I osteotomy, 1723–1727, *1725*
  after Le Fort III osteotomy, 1729
  compensatory articulation and, 1693–1694, 1716
  hypernasal speech and, 1694–1696
  in palatal abnormalities, *1700*, 1700–1701
  nasal air emission and, 1694–1695, 1710
  obturator for, 1718–1720, *1719*
  pharyngeal flap surgery for, 1716, *1717*, 1717–1718

Velopharyngeal valve *(Continued)*
  orifice openings for, 1714–1715
Veneer graft, for dental implants, 1197–1200, *1198*, *1199*
Venous catheterization, 111
Ventilation, postanesthesia, 151, *152*
Ventriculoperitoneal shunt, in Apert syndrome, 1898
  in Crouzon syndrome, 1894
Vernier caliper, 185, *185*
Vertical-L osteotomy, for mandibular advancement, 2336
Vertical maxillary excess. See *Smile, gummy.*
Vertical maxillary growth. See *Maxillary growth.*
Vertical measurements, bone, 172–176, *173–175*, 190, *190*
  postsurgical, 198–199, *199*
  cuspid-nose referent, 177–179, *178*, 188
  dental, 170–172, *171*, 186, *186*, *187*, *190*, 190, 2311, *2311*
Vertical ramus osteotomy, intraoral. See *Intraoral vertical ramus osteotomy.*
Vertical reference line(s), 2312
  for profile analysis, 2442, *2443*
Vessels. See *Vasculature.*
Vestibuloplasty, for dental prosthetics, limitations of, 1131–1132
Videofluoroscopy, multiview, for velopharyngeal function assessment, 1711–1712, *1712*
Videotaping, in microreconstructive surgery, 1109
Villonodular synovitis, benign pigmented, *912*, 912–913
Virchow's law, 1839
Vision problems, in craniosynostosis, 1841
Vitek-Kent prosthesis, development of, 737–740
  durability of, 745, 792, *792*
  implantation of, anesthesia for, 756, 759, 760
  arch bar in, 759, *759*
  bleeding in, 789, 789t
  case studies of, 796–828
  cephalometric analysis for, 746, *747*, *748*, 749–750
  closure in, 784–785, *785*
  complications of, 788–793, 789t, 795–796
  condylar dislocation after, 793
  condylar implant in, 738–740, *739*, *753*, 753
    bending of, 777–779, 778t, *779–782*
    computerized tomography of, *498*, 498–499
    instability of, 776–777, 777t
    magnetic resonance imaging in, 515–516
    placement of, 773–779, *773–782*
    securing of, 782–785, *783–785*
    selection of, 773
  condylar stump spur formation after, 789t, 790–792, *791*
  condylar template in, 754, *754*, 774–775, *775*
  contraindications to, 744–745
  dural perforation after, 789t, 790
  ear injury in, 793
  equipment for, 750–755, *752–755*, 756t
  foreign body reaction after, 793

xlii / INDEX

Vitek-Kent prosthesis (*Continued*)
  fossa implant in, 752–753, *753*
    computerized tomography of, *498*, 498–499
    durability of, 792, *792*
    instability of, 772t
    magnetic resonance imaging in, 515–516
    placement in, 769–772, *769–773*
  fossa preparation in, 767–769, *768, 769*
  fossa template in, 754, *754*
  infection in, 789
  instrumentation for, *754*, 754–755, *755*, 756t, 759
  intermaxillary fixation with, 749
  joint dissection in, 764, *764*
  lateral pterygoid muscle–condylar segment repositioning in, 765–767, *765–777*
  malocclusion after, 789t, 790, 796
  nerve injury in, 788–789
  occlusal evaluation in, 784
  orthognathic surgery with, 746–750, 759
  patient preparation for, 760–762, *760–762*
  postoperative care in, 785–788
  preauricular dissection in, 762–763, *763, 764*
  preoperative planning for, 746–750
  results of, 793–796, 794t, 795t
  retromandibular-submandibular dissection in, 763, *764*
  technique of, 759–785
  with sagittal split osteotomy, 773
  indications for, 740–744, *741–744*
  loading of, 745
  splint for, fabrication of, 750
    postoperative, 787
  types of, *739*, 739–740
Voice, 1688–1689. See also *Speech.*
  parameters of, 1688–1689
  pitch of, abnormal, 1696
  resonance of, evaluation of, 1710–1711
    problems with, 1695–1696
Volume loss, intraoperative monitoring of, 138–139
Volume overload, postoperative, 125
Volume replacement, postoperative, 124–126
Vomer, 290, *2176*
Vomiting, postoperative, 117
Vowels. See *Speech sounds.*
V-Y advancement flap, 1481–1482, *1482.* See also *Flap(s).*

Walk-up flap, 1476–1477, *1477, 1478.* See also *Flap(s).*
Wallerian degeneration, 1089
Water-Pik, 118
Wax bite registration, 162–163
  for preoperative condylar position, 527, 530
  in computerized tomography, 527
Weber-Fergusson incision, in maxillary reconstruction, 1528–1529, *1529*
Wedge osteotomy, for chin shortening, 2477–2484, *2485*
  in chin asymmetry correction, 2472–2474, *2474*

Wedge osteotomy (*Continued*)
  in sliding horizontal osteotomy, 2446, *2446*
Weight loss, in sleep apnea, 2029
Weinstein-Semmes filaments, in neurologic examination, 1097–1098, *1098*
Wells pump, 377
Whistle, tracheal indication, *145*, 145
Whistling face syndrome, *2385*
  mandibular expansion for, 2385–2389
Wilkes silicone implant, in conchal cartilage graft, 668, *669*
Wire(s). See also *Orthodontic treatment.*
  arch, active, at surgery, 63
    auxiliary, 1657, *1658*
    for postoperative midline asymmetry, 80–81, *81, 82*
    in leveling of curve of Spee, *61*, 61–62, *62*
    material for, 49–50, 1258
  auxiliary, adequacy of, 50, *51*
  circummandibular, for two-jaw surgery, 1657, *1658*
  in intermaxillary fixation. See *Intermaxillary fixation.*
  orthodontic. See also *Orthodontic treatment.*
    material for, 1258
    osseointegrated anchorage for. See *Implants, osseointegrated, orthodontic.*
Wire fixation. See also *Immobilization.*
  in bilateral sagittal split osteotomy, condylar positioning in, 547–558
  in canthopexy, *1045, 1046,* 1048, 1076–1077
  in Le Fort I osteotomy, condylar positioning in, 534–547
    postoperative condylar stability and, 541–547
  in maxillary osteotomy, 71–73, *72*
  intermaxillary. See *Intermaxillary fixation.*
  interosseous, Adams' suspension, midfacial deformity after, *1050, 1052*
    in secondary craniofacial deformity correction, 1025
    of costochondral graft, *878,* 878–879
    of facial fractures, 1015, *1016*
  mandibulomaxillary. See *Maxillomandibular fixation.*
  of glenoid fossa implant, 771–772, *772,* 772t
  of mandibular angle fracture, comparative stress analysis of, *1973,* 1973–1974
  vs. rigid fixation, 79
    postoperative maxillary stability after, 1936–1942
  with Vitek-Kent prosthesis, 749
Wolford-Davis sagittal split osteotomy, 2337, 2349, 2352
Worm's eye, *1059*
Wound, gunshot, 988, 1004–1006, *1004–1007*
Wound care, 117–118
Wound healing, connective tissue repair in, 1644–1645
  during immobilization, 1644–1645
  of irradiated tissue, 1458
  oxygen gradient in, 1458–1460, *1460*
Woven bone, 1232
Wrench, ratchet cylinder, for Branemark dental implant, 1158, *1158*

Wrist-hand radiographs, for skeletal age determination, 35–38, *37, 38*
Wurzburg plate fixation, for mandibular angle fracture, comparative stress analysis of, *1973,* 1973–1974

Xenogenic bone grafts, 850
Xeroradiography, in masseter muscle hypertrophy, 432

Yaw, in model measurement, 169, *169*

Zirconium dental implants, reactivity of, 1140, *1141*
Zisser segmental osteotomy, for open bite, 2081–2083, *2082–2084*
Zone of Klein, 394
Zygomatic abnormalities, in hemifacial microsomia, 1535, *1535*
Zygomatic arch, stabilization/reconstruction of, after Le Fort fractures, 1049, *1050–1054*
  importance of, 1017–1019, *1018–1020*
  in naso-orbito-ethmoid deformities, *1050–1054*
  technique of, *1035,* 1036, *1038–1044*
Zygomatic augmentation, coronal approach in, 972, *973*
Zygomatic body, segmental depression of, correction of, *1026, 1027*
Zygomatic construction, in Treacher Collins syndrome, 1610, *1610*
Zygomatic fracture. See also *Fracture(s), facial.*
  bone graft for, 1015, 1021–1023, *1022*
  coronal approach in, 967, *968,* 970
  fixation of, 1015, 1016–1021, *1017–1020,* 1961–1962
  in high Le Fort I osteotomy, 2241–2242
  orbitozygomatic deformities after, 1037–1049, 1044t, *1045–1048, 1050–1054*
  principles of repair of, 1015–1016
Zygomatic hypoplasia, in Treacher Collins syndrome, 1601, 1604
Zygomatic nerve, injury of, in Vitek-Kent prosthesis placement, 788–789, 789t
Zygomatic-orbital artery, 959, *959*
Zygomatic osteotomy, design of, *2241,* 2241–2242
  with bone grafting, for malar augmentation, 2298–2303, *2300–2303*
Zygomatic prominence, augmentation of. See *Malar augmentation.*
Zygomatic stress trajectories, *1969,* 1969–1970, *1970*
Zygomaticomaxillary complex reduction, 2304–2305, *2305*
Zygomaticomaxillary suture, growth at, 2072, *2072*
Zygomaticotemporal nerve, 955, *955, 959, 959*
Zygomaticus major muscle, *2178,* 2179